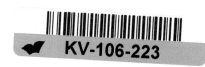

CONFERENCE CHAIRMEN

Alando J. Ballantyne, M.D.
President,
The Society of Head and Neck
  Surgeons

Paul B. Chretien, M.D.
Chairman,
Organizing Committee

Hugh F. Biller, M.D.
President,
American Society for Head and Neck
  Surgery

EXECUTIVE COUNCIL

Alando J. Ballantyne, M.D.
Hugh F. Biller, M.D.
Robert W. Cantrell, M.D.
Paul B. Chretien, M.D.
Jerome C. Goldstein, M.D.

Darrell A. Jaques, M.D.
Michael E. Johns, M.D.
Charles J. Krause, M.D.
Frank C. Marchetta, M.D.
Benjamin F. Rush, Jr., M.D.

Roy B. Sessions, M.D.
Elliot W. Strong, M.D.
Paul H. Ward, M.D.
Alvin J. Watne, M.D.
Gregory T. Wolf, M.D.

COMMITTEE CHAIRMEN

Program

Invited Speakers
Michael E. Johns, M.D.
Elliot W. Strong, M.D.

Proffered Papers
Jerome C. Goldstein, M.D.
Benjamin F. Rush, Jr., M.D.

Research Workshops
Robert W. Veltri, Ph.D.
Gregory T. Wolf, M.D.

Local Arrangements
Darrell A. Jaques, M.D.

Publication
Donald P. Shedd, M.D.
Paul H. Ward, M.D.

Promotion
John M. Loré, Jr., M.D.
Eugene N. Myers, M.D.

External Support
Helmuth Goepfert, M.D.
William A. Maddox, M.D.

Finance
Robert W. Cantrell, M.D.
Robert D. Harwick, M.D.

PROGRAM COMMITTEE

Stephen K. Carter, M.D.
Paul B. Chretien, M.D.
Jerome C. Goldstein, M.D.
Maurice J. Jurkiewicz, M.D.

Michael E. Johns, M.D.
Simon Kramer, M.D.
Gregory T. O'Conor, M.D.

Benjamin F. Rush, Jr., M.D.
Elliot W. Strong, M.D.
Robert W. Veltri, Ph.D.
Gregory T. Wolf, M.D.

TECHNICAL STAFF

PROGRAM EDITOR
Helen R. Vidockler

STEERING COMMITTEE

Stephan Ariyan, M.D.
Alando J. Ballantyne, M.D.
Hugh F. Biller, M.D.
Robert W. Cantrell, M.D.
Paul B. Chretien, M.D.
Charles W. Cummings, M.D.
Hugh O. DeFries, M.D.
Willard E. Fee, Jr., M.D.
Bimal C. Ghosh, M.D.
Helmuth Goepfert, M.D.
Jerome C. Goldstein, M.D.
Robert D. Harwick, M.D.

Arthur G. James, M.D.
Darrell A. Jaques, M.D.
Michael E. Johns, M.D.
Robert H. Johnson, M.D.
Maurice J. Jurkiewicz, M.D.
Charles J. Krause, M.D.
John M. Loré, Jr., M.D.
William A. Maddox, M.D.
Frank C. Marchetta, M.D.
Eugene N. Myers, M.D.
Arnold M. Noyek, M.D.

Benjamin F. Rush, Jr., M.D.
Donald G. Sessions, M.D.
Roy B. Sessions, M.D.
Donald P. Shedd, M.D.
Charles R. Smart, M.D.
Ronald H. Spiro, M.D.
Philip M. Sprinkle, M.D.
Elliot W. Strong, M.D.
James Yee Suen, M.D.
Paul H. Ward, M.D.
Alvin L. Watne, M.D.
Gregory T. Wolf, M.D.

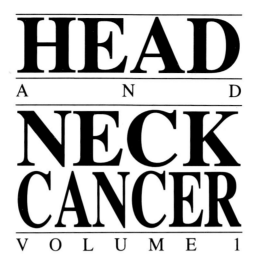

HEAD AND NECK CANCER

VOLUME 1

Proceedings of the International Conference
Baltimore, Maryland / July 22–27, 1984

PAUL B. CHRETIEN, M.D.
MICHAEL E. JOHNS, M.D.
DONALD P. SHEDD, M.D.
ELLIOTT W. STRONG, M.D.
PAUL H. WARD, M.D.

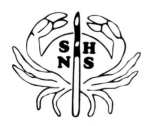

THE SOCIETY OF
HEAD AND NECK SURGEONS

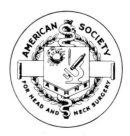

AMERICAN SOCIETY FOR
HEAD AND NECK SURGERY

1985

B.C. DECKER INC. • Philadelphia • Toronto
The C.V. MOSBY COMPANY • Saint Louis • Toronto • London

Publisher: **B.C. Decker Inc.**
               3228 South Service Road
               Burlington, Ontario   L7N 3H8

Publisher: **B.C. Decker Inc.**
               P.O. Box 30246
               Phildelphia, Pennsylvania   19103

North American and worldwide sales and distribution

               The C.V. Mosby Company
               11830 Westline Industrial Drive
               Saint Louis, Missouri   63141

In Canada: **The C.V. Mosby Company, Ltd.**
               120 Melford Drive
               Toronto, Ontario   M1B 2X5

Head and Neck Cancer, Volume 1   ISBN 0-941158-40-3

Library of Congress catalog card number: 85-070615

                    10 9 8 7 6 5 4 3 2 1

CONTRIBUTORS

AHMED ABDELAL, Ph.D.

Professor of Microbiology, Biology Department, Georgia State University, Atlanta, Georgia
Tumor-associated Antigens in Head and Neck Cancer Tissues and in Sera of Tumor-bearing Patients

ROBERT D. ACLAND, M.D.

Associate Professor of Surgery, Director, Center for Microsurgical Studies, University of Louisville School of Medicine, Louisville, Kentucky
Principles of Successful Free Tissue Transfer in the Head and Neck

MUHYI AL-SARRAF, M.D., F.R.C.P.(C), F.A.C.P.

Professor, Department of Medicine, Division of Oncology, Wayne State University; Chief, Head and Neck Service, Department of Medicine, Division of Oncology, Harper-Grace Hospitals, Detroit, Michigan
Role of Chemotherapy for Stage IV Tumors

STEPHEN ARIYAN, M.D.

Professor of Surgery and Chief of Plastic and Reconstructive Surgery, Yale University School of Medicine; Attending Physician, Yale-New Haven Hospital, New Haven, Connecticut
Osteomyocutaneous Flaps for Reconstruction of Partial Mandibulectomies

GIORGIO ARCANGELI, M.D.

Head, Division of Radiation Therapy, Instituto Medico e Di Ricerca Scientifica, Rome, Italy
Multiple Fractions Per Day in the Radiotherapy of Head and Neck Cancer: An Updated Study of the EORTC Radiotherapy Group Experience with Local Hyperthermia and Radiation

LAURE AURELIAN, Ph.D.

Professor, Department of Pharmacology and Experimental Therapeutics, University of Maryland School of Medicine, Baltimore, Maryland
HSV Antigens as Diagnostic and/or Therapeutic Markers in Squamous Cancer of the Cervix and Head and Neck

BYRON J. BAILEY, M.D., F.A.C.S.

Wiess Professor and Chairman, Department of Otolaryngology, University of Texas Medical School at Galveston, Galveston, Texas
Surgical Management of Advanced Laryngeal Cancer

VAHRAM Y. BAKAMJIAN, M.D.

Clinical Professor of Surgery (Plastic), University of Rochester School of Medicine and Dentistry, Rochester, New York and Stanford University School of Medicine, Stanford, California; Associate Chief, Department of Head and Neck Surgery and Oncology, Roswell Park Memorial Institute, Buffalo, New York
Tongue Flaps in Cancer Surgery of the Oral Cavity

DANIEL C. BAKER, M.D.

Associate Professor of Surgery (Plastic), New York University School of Medicine and The Institute of Reconstructive Plastic Surgery; Attending Surgeon, Manhattan Eye, Ear and Throat Hospital, Bellevue Hospital, New York, New York
Reanimation of the Paralyzed Face: Nerve Crossover, Cross-Face Nerve Grafting, and Muscle Transfers

HARVEY W. BAKER, M.D.

Clinical Professor of Surgery, Oregon Health Sciences University School of Medicine; Chairman, American Joint Committee on Cancer, Portland, Oregon
Staging of Head and Neck Cancer: Introduction

SHAN R. BAKER, M.D., F.A.C.S.

Associate Professor, Department of Otolaryngology, University of Michigan Medical School; Director, Division of Head and Neck Surgery, University of Michigan Hospitals, Ann Arbor, Michigan
Recent Developments in the Management of Head and Neck Cancer With Intra-Arterial Chemotherapy

ALANDO J. BALLANTYNE, M.D.

Professor of Surgery, Department of Head and Neck Surgery, The University of Texas System Cancer Center, M. D. Anderson Hospital and Tumor Institute, Houston, Texas
Selection Criteria for Modified Neck Dissection With Postoperative Irradiation for N3 Staged Cervical Metastasis

JEAN P. BATAINI, M.D.

Senior Radiotherapist, Institut Curie, Paris, France
Definitive Radiation Therapy of Cancer of the Pyriform Sinus

WILLIAM H. BEIERWALTES, M.D.

Professor, Department of Internal Medicine and Chief, Division of Nuclear Medicine, University of Michigan Medical School, Ann Arbor, Michigan
Radioiodine Therapy

ANGELA S. BELLAMY, Ph.D.

Research Fellow, Laboratory of Cellular Chemotherapy, Imperial Cancer Research Fund, Department of Neurochemistry, Institute of Neurology, London, England
Pitfalls in the Soft Agar Clonogenic Assays; Recommendations for Improving Colony-forming Efficiencies and the Potential Value of Cell Lines Derived From Head and Neck Tumors

GILEAD BERGER, M.D.

Charlie Conacher Fellow, Otolaryngology, University of Toronto Faculty of Medicine, Toronto, Ontario, Canada
Failure Analysis of T1 Glottic Carcinoma Treated With Radical Radiotherapy for Cure With Surgery in Reserve

JOSEPH R. BERTINO, M.D.

Professor of Medicine and Pharmacology and Chief, Section of Medical Oncology, Yale University School of Medicine, New Haven, Connecticut
Mechanisms of Action and Interaction of Chemotherapeutic Agents
Single Agent Versus Combination Chemotherapy in Head and Neck Cancer

HUGH F. BILLER, M.D.

Professor and Chairman of Otolaryngology, Mount Sinai School of Medicine of the City University of New York; Otolaryngologist-in-Chief, The Mount Sinai Hospital, New York, New York
Conservation Surgery of the Larynx

MELVIN A. BLOCK, M.D., Ph.D.

Clinical Professor of Surgery, University of California, San Diego, School of Medicine, San Diego, California; Chairman, Department of Surgery, Scripps Clinic and Research Foundation, La Jolla, California
Medullary Thyroid Cancer: Surgical Aspects

ERIC D. BLOM, Ph.D.

Private Practice, Head and Neck Surgery Associates, Indianapolis, Indiana
Vocal Rehabilitation After Total Laryngectomy: Current Status and Future Directions

KLAUS BOEHEIM, M.D.

Lecturer of Otolaryngology, Harvard Medical School; Dana-Farber Cancer Institute, Boston, Massachusetts
Rationale for Combination Chemotherapy as Treatment of Advanced Head and Neck Cancer

ROGER BOLES, M.D.

Chairman and Professor of Otolaryngology, Head and Neck Surgery, University of California, San Francisco, School of Medicine, San Francisco, California
Carcinoma of the Submandibular Minor Salivary Glands

BOUDEWIJN B. J. M. BRAAKHUIS, M.Sc.

Research Scientist, Department of Otolaryngology and Head and Neck Surgery, Free University Hospital, Amsterdam, The Netherlands
Nude Mice Model as a Predictive Assay in Head and Neck Cancer

JACQUES M. BRUGERE, M.D.

Head, Department of Head and Neck Surgery, Institut Curie, Paris, France
Definitive Radiation Therapy of Cancer of the Pyriform Sinus

R. NICK BRYAN, M.D.

Professor of Radiology, Baylor College of Medicine; Director of Neuroradiology, The Methodist Hospital, Houston, Texas
Intra-Arterial Cisplatin in the Treatment of Aerodigestive Squamous Carcinoma and Nasopharyngeal Carcinoma

DOUGLAS P. BRYCE, M.D., F.R.C.S.(C), F.R.C.S.(Ed.) Hon., F.A.C.S., ABOT.

Professor Emeritus, Department of Otolaryngology, University of Toronto Faculty of Medicine; Consultant in Otolaryngology, Toronto General Hospital, Toronto, Ontario, Canada
Cancer of the Larynx: Introduction
Failure Analysis of T1 Glottic Carcinoma Treated With Radical Radiotherapy for Cure With Surgery in Reserve

JOY BUCHOK, B.A.

Senior Research Assistant, Division of Oncology, Department of Medicine, University of Texas Medical School at San Antonio, San Antonio, Texas
Capillary Cloning Assay in Head and Neck Cancer

ROBERT M. BYERS, M.D.

Professor of Surgery, University of Texas Medical School at Houston; Surgeon, M. D. Anderson Hospital and Tumor Institute, Houston, Texas
Selection Criteria for Modified Neck Dissection With Postoperative Irradiation for N3 Staged Cervical Metastasis

BLAKE CADY, M.D.

Associate Clinical Professor of Surgery, Harvard Medical School; Section Chief of Surgical Oncology, New England Deaconess Hospital, Boston, Massachusetts
Cancer of the Thyroid Gland: Introduction

ROBERT W. CANTRELL, M.D.

Fitz-Hugh Professor and Chairman, Department of Otolaryngology/ Head and Neck Surgery, University of Virginia School of Medicine, Charlottesville, Virginia
Supraorbital Rim Approach to Lesions of the Craniofacial Junction
Reconstruction of the Mandible: Introduction

STEPHEN K. CARTER, M.D.

Vice-President, Anticancer Research, Pharmaceutical Research and Development Division, Bristol-Meyers Company, New York, New York
Combined Modality Chemotherapy in Head and Neck Cancer
Tumor Response to Chemotherapy and Its Measurement: Introduction

JOHN T. CHAFFEY, M.D.

Associate Professor, Department of Radiation Therapy, Harvard Medical School, Boston, Massachusetts
Combination Treatment of Head and Neck Cancer with Induction Chemotherapy

JAMES RYAN CHANDLER, M.D.

Professor and Chairman, Department of Otolaryngology, University of Miami School of Medicine, Miami, Florida
Staging of Cancer of the Larynx

DANIEL CHASSAGNE, M.D.

Chief, Department of Radiotherapy, Institute Gustave Roussy, Paris, France
Brachytherapy of Carcinoma of the Tongue (Mobile Portion) and Floor of the Mouth

PAUL B. CHRETIEN, M.D.

Professor of Surgery, University of Maryland School of Medicine, Baltimore, Maryland
Immunology and Immunotherapy: Introduction
Interrelationship of Immune Response, Circulating Proteins, and Etiologic Factors for Head and Neck Cancer

JOHN R. CLARK, M.D.

Instructor of Medicine, Dana-Farber Cancer Institute, Boston, Massachusetts
Rationale for Combination Chemotherapy as Treatment of Advanced Head and Neck Cancer
Combination Treatment of Head and Neck Cancer with Induction Chemotherapy

MICHAEL COLVIN, M.D.

Professor of Oncology and Medicine, Johns Hopkins University School of Medicine, Baltimore, Maryland
Mechanisms of Resistance to Alkylating Agents

AUSTIN COLOHAN, M.D.

Instructor, Department of Neurosurgery, University of Virginia School of Medicine, Charlottesville, Virginia
Supraorbital Rim Approach to Lesions of the Craniofacial Junction

JOHN CONLEY, M.D.

Professor Emeritus of Clinical Otolaryngology, Columbia University College of Physicians and Surgeons, New York, New York
Management of Salivary Gland Tumors: Introduction

WILLIAM C. CONSTABLE, M.B., Ch.B., D.M.R.T.

Professor and Director, Division of Therapeutic Radiology and Oncology; Professor, Department of Otolaryngology and Head and Neck Surgery, University of Virginia School of Medicine, Charlottesville, Virginia
Cancer of the Supraglottic Larynx

JAMES D. COX, M.D.

Professor and Chairman, Department of Radiation Oncology, Medical College of Wisconsin, Milwaukee, Wisconsin
Management of Clinically Occult (N0) Cervical Lymph Node Metastases by Radiation Therapy
Fractionation: Dose-Time Considerations in the Management of Carcinoma of the Upper Aerodigestive Tract

JOHN D. CRISSMAN, M.D.

Professor of Pathology, Wayne State University; Director of Anatomic Pathology, Harper Grace Hospital, Detroit, Michigan
Histopathology as a Prognostic Factor in the Treatment of Squamous Cell Cancer of the Head and Neck
Histopathologic Diagnosis of Early Cancer

ROGER L. CRUMLEY, M.D.

Clinical Professor, Department of Otolaryngology — Head and Neck Surgery, University of California, San Francisco, School of Medicine, San Francisco, California
Optimal Facial Reanimation Surgery

CHARLES W. CUMMINGS, M.D.

Professor and Chairman, Department of Otolaryngology, University of Washington School of Medicine, Seattle, Washington
Mandibular Reconstruction other than Osteomyocutaneous Homografts

HUGH O. DeFRIES, M.D., D.D.S.

Full Professor and Chief, Division of Otolaryngology, Georgetown University School of Medicine, Washington, D.C.
Mandibular Reconstruction With Homologous and Autologous Bone Grafts

LAWRENCE W. DeSANTO, M.D.

Professor of Otolaryngology/Head and Neck Oncology, Mayo Medical School and Mayo Clinic — Department of Otorhinolaryngology, Rochester, Minnesota
Treatment Options in Early Cancers of the Larynx
Curative, Palliative, and Adjunctive Uses of Cryosurgery in the Head and Neck

WILLIAM D. DeWYS, M.D.

Associate Director, Prevention Program, Division of Cancer Prevention and Control, National Cancer Institute, National Institutes of Health, Bethesda, Maryland
Interventional Approaches to Prevention: Introduction
Prevention of Head and Neck Cancer: Leads from Laboratory Research
Guidelines for Prevention: Clinical Trials

THOMAS J. DOUGHERTY, Ph.D.

Director of Graduate Research, Radiation Biology (Experimental Pathology), State University of New York at Buffalo; Head, Division of Radiation Biology, Department of Radiation Medicine, Roswell Park Memorial Institute, Buffalo, New York
Photodynamic Therapy of Solid Tumors

WILLIAM DUNCAN, F.R.C.S.E., F.R.C.P.E., F.R.C.R., F.A.C.R.

Professor of Radiotherapy, University of Edinburgh; Director, Department of Clinical Oncology, Western General Hospital and Royal Infirmary, Edinburgh
Fast-Neutron Therapy

BAHMAN N. EMAMI, M.D.

Associate Professor of Radiology and Associate Radiation Oncologist, Mallinckrodt Institute of Radiology, Washington University School of Medicine, St. Louis, Missouri
Potential Efficacy of Hyperthermia in Treatment of Head and Neck Tumors

JOHN ENSLEY, M.D.

Assistant Professor of Medicine, Wayne State University; Director of Medical Education, Harper Grace Hospital, Detroit, Michigan
Histopathology as a Prognostic Factor in the Treatment of Squamous Cell Cancer of the Head and Neck

THOMAS J. ERVIN, M.D.

Assistant Professor of Medicine, Harvard Medical School; Clinical Associate of Medicine, Dana-Farber Cancer Institute, Boston, Massachusetts
Radiobiologic Factors Influencing Fractionation in Head and Neck Cancer Therapy
Rationale for Combination Chemotherapy as Treatment of Advanced Head and Neck Cancer
Combination Treatment of Head and Neck Cancer with Induction Chemotherapy

FRANÇOIS ESCHWEGE, M.D.

Assistant Professor, Paris Sud Medical School; Department Director and Chief of Radiotherapy, Institute Gustave Roussy, Paris, France
Brachytherapy of Carcinoma of the Tongue (Mobile Portion) and Floor of the Mouth

RICHARD L. FABIAN, M.D.

Associate Surgeon in Otolaryngology, Massachusetts Eye and Ear Infirmary, Boston, Massachusetts
Combination Treatment of Head and Neck Cancer with Induction Chemotherapy

ROBERT E. FECHNER, M.D.

W. S. Royster Professor and Director, Division of Surgical Pathology, University of Virginia School of Medicine, Charlottesville, Virginia
New and Innovative Aspects of Pathology
Diagnosis of Salivary Gland Neoplasms

WILLARD E. FEE, Jr., M.D.

Associate Professor of Surgery, Stanford University School of Medicine; Chief, Division of Otolaryngology — Head and Neck Surgery, Stanford University Medical Center, Stanford, California
Treatment of Early Lesions of the Head and Neck
Management of Patients with N3 Cervical Lymphadenopathy and/or Carotid Artery Involvement

PHILIP S. FELDMAN, M.D.

Associate Professor of Pathology, University of Virginia School of Medicine; Director of Cytology, University of Virginia Medical Center, Charlottesville, Virginia
Pathologic and Cytologic Diagnosis of a Lump in the Neck

UGO P. FISCH, M.D.

Professor of ENT, University of Zurich; Head of the ENT Department, University Hospital, Zurich, Switzerland
Skull Base Surgery: Introduction
Lateral (Infratemporal Fossa) Approach to the Skull Base

THOMAS J. FITZGERALD, M.D.

Instructor of Radiation Therapy, Harvard Medical School, Boston, Massachusetts
Combination Treatment of Head and Neck Cancer with Induction Chemotherapy

PETER J. FITZPATRICK, M.B., B.S., F.R.C.P.(C), F.R.C.R.

Associate Professor of Radiology, University of Toronto Faculty of Medicine; Princess Margaret Hospital, Toronto, Ontario, Canada
Cervical Lymph Node Metastases From an Unknown Primary Tumor: The Place of Radiotherapy

SUSAN FLEMING, Ph.D.

Chief, Head and Neck Dysphagia Program, Veterans Administration Medical Center, Allen Park, Michigan
Swallowing Rehabilitation

ARLENE A. FORASTIERE, M.D.

Assistant Professor, Department of Internal Medicine, Division of Hematology/Oncology, University of Michigan Hospitals, Ann Arbor, Michigan
Recent Developments in the Management of Head and Neck Cancer with Intra-Arterial Chemotherapy

WILLIAM J. FRABLE, M.D.

Professor of Pathology, Virginia Commonwealth University Medical College of Virginia School of Medicine; Director of Surgical and Cytopathology, Medical College of Virginia Hospitals, Richmond, Virginia
Aspiration Biopsy of the Thyroid

EMIL FREI III, M.D.

Richard and Susan Smith Professor of Medicine, Harvard Medical School; Director and Physician-in-Chief, Dana-Farber Cancer Institute, Boston, Massachusetts
The Cancer Cell: Developing Knowledge and Implications for Therapy
Mechanisms of Cancer Cell Resistance: Introduction

MICHAEL FRIEDMAN, M.D.

Clinical Assistant Professor, Department of Otolaryngology — Head and Neck Surgery, University of Illinois College of Medicine, Chicago, Illinois
Computerized Tomography in the Diagnosis of Head and Neck Diseases: A Clinical Approach

PETER GARRETT, M.D.

Radiation Oncology Department, Methodist Hospital of Indiana, Indianapolis, Indiana
Management of the N3 Neck: Intraoperative Radiation

GEORGE A. GATES, M.D.

Professor and Head, Division of Otorhinolaryngology, University of Texas Medical School at San Antonio, San Antonio, Texas
Current Status of Laryngectomee Rehabilitation

ALAIN GERBAULET, M.D.

Chief, Department of Brachyradiotherapy, Institute Gustave Roussy, Paris, France
Brachytherapy of Carcinoma of the Tongue (Mobile Portion) and Floor of the Mouth

JACK L. GLUCKMAN, M.D., F.C.S.(S.A.), F.A.C.S.

Associate Professor, Department of Otolaryngology, and Director, Division of Head and Neck Surgery and Maxillofacial Surgery, University of Cincinnati College of Medicine, Cincinnati, Ohio
Total Glossectomy: Reconstruction Using Myocutaneous Flaps

HELMUTH GOEPFERT, M.D.

Professor and Chairman, Department of Head and Neck Surgery, University of Texas Medical School at Houston; Surgeon, The University of Texas System Cancer Center, M. D. Anderson Hospital and Tumor Institute, Houston, Texas
Cancer of the Larynx and Pyriform Sinus: The Surgeon's Viewpoint

DON R. GOFFINET, M.D.

Associate Professor of Radiology, Division of Radiation Therapy, Stanford University School of Medicine, Stanford, California
Treatment of Early Lesions of the Head and Neck
Management of Patients with N3 Cervical Lymphadenopathy and/or Carotid Artery Involvement
Head and Neck Brachytherapy Emphasizing Afterloading Removable Oropharyngeal Implants

JAMES H. GOLDIE, M.D., F.R.C.P.(C)

Clinical Professor of Medicine, University of British Columbia Faculty of Medicine; Head, Division of Medical Oncology, Cancer Control Agency of British Columbia, Vancouver, British Columbia
Influence of Tumor Growth Rate and Mutations on Drug Resistance

JEROME C. GOLDSTEIN, M.D., F.A.C.S.

Professor of Surgery (Otolaryngology), Albany Medical College of Union University, Albany, New York; Executive Vice-President, The American Academy of Otolaryngology — Head and Neck Surgery, Washington, D.C.
Vocal Rehabilitation After Laryngectomy: Introduction

DIONISIO GONZALES, M.D.

Head, Radiotherapy Department, Academisch Medisch Centrum, Amsterdam, The Netherlands
Multiple Fractions Per Day in the Radiotherapy of Head and Neck Cancer: An Updated Study of the EORTC Radiotherapy Group

N. DAVID GREYSON, B.Sc., M.D., F.R.C.P.(C)

Associate Professor of Radiology, University of Toronto Faculty of Medicine; Director, Division of Nuclear Medicine, St. Michael's Hospital, Toronto, Ontario, Canada
Radionuclide Imaging

VYTENIS T. GRYBAUSKAS, M.D.

Instructor, Department of Otolaryngology — Head and Neck Surgery, University of Illinois College of Medicine, Chicago, Illinois
Computerized Tomography in the Diagnosis of Head and Neck Diseases: A Clinical Approach

ANTONIO GUERRA, Ph.D.

Instituto Medico e Diricerca Scientifica, Rome, Italy
Multiple Fractions Per Day in the Radiotherapy of Head and Neck Cancer: An Updated Study of the EORTC Radiotherapy Group

OSCAR M. GUILLAMONDEGUI, M.D.

Professor of Surgery and Deputy Chairman, Department of Head and Neck Surgery, University of Texas Medical School at Houston; Surgeon, University of Texas System Cancer Center, M. D. Anderson Hospital and Tumor Institute, Houston, Texas
Treatment of Advanced Thyroid Cancer

GEORGE M. HAHN, Ph.D.

Professor, Department of Radiology, Stanford University School of Medicine, Stanford, California
Biologic Responses of Cells, Normal Tissues, and Tumors to Heat

CHRISTINE HAIE, M.D.

Assistant, Department of Radiotherapy, Institute Gustave Roussy, Paris, France
Brachytherapy of Carcinoma of the Tongue (Mobile Portion) and Floor of the Mouth

RONALD C. HAMAKER, M.D., F.A.C.S.

Private Practice, Head and Neck Surgery Associates, Indianapolis, Indiana
Management of the N3 Neck: Intraoperative Radiation
Vocal Rehabilitation After Total Laryngectomy: Current Status and Future Directions

WILLIAM N. HANAFEE, M.D.

Professor of Radiology, University of California, Los Angeles, UCLA School of Medicine, Los Angeles, California
Diagnostic Imaging: Introduction

DONALD F. N. HARRISON, M.D., M.S., Ph.D., F.R.C.S., F.R.A.C.S. (Hon.), F.R.C.S.E. (Hon.)

Professor of Laryngology and Otology and Director, Professor Unit, Royal National ENT Hospital, London, England
Head and Neck Surgery in the 1980s: The Role of More or Less

ANDREW R. HARWOOD, M.B., Ch.B., F.R.C.P.(C)

Associate Professor of Radiology and Otolaryngology, University of Toronto Faculty of Medicine; Staff Radiation Oncologist, The Princess Margaret Hospital, Toronto, Ontario, Canada
Failure Analysis of T1 Glottic Carcinoma Treated with Radical Radiotherapy for Cure with Surgery in Reserve
Definitive Radiotherapy for Glottic Carcinoma

BRIDGET T. HILL, Ph.D., F.I.Biol., F.R.S.C.

Scientific Consultant, The Head and Neck Unit, Royal Marsden Hospital; Head of the Cellular Chemotherapy Laboratory, Imperial Cancer Research Fund, London, England
Pitfalls in the Soft Agar Clonogenic Assays; Recommendations for Improving Colony-forming Efficiencies and the Potential Value of Cell Lines Derived from Head and Neck Tumors

JAN CLAUDE HORIOT, M.D.

Head, Radiotherapy Department, Centre G. F. LeClerc, Dijon, France
Multiple Fractions Per Day in the Radiotherapy of Head and Neck Cancer: An Updated Study of the EORTC Radiotherapy Group

BARRY L. HOROWITZ, M.D.

Professor of Radiology, Baylor College of Medicine, Houston, Texas
Intra-arterial Cisplatin in the Treatment of Aerodigestive Squamous Carcinoma and Nasopharyngeal Carcinoma

ADLY N. IBRAHIM, D.V.M., Sc.D.

Professor of Microbiology, Biology Department, Georgia State University, Atlanta, Georgia
Tumor-associated Antigens in Head and Neck Cancer Tissues and in Sera of Tumor-bearing Patients

IAN T. JACKSON, M.D., F.R.C.S., F.A.C.S.

Professor, Mayo Medical School; Head, Section of Plastic and Reconstructive Surgery, Mayo Clinic, Rochester, New York
Craniofacial Surgery for Congenital Deformities: Its Contribution to Surgery of the Skull

JOHN A. JANE, M.D.

Professor and Chairman, Department of Neurosurgery, University of Virginia School of Medicine, Charlottesville, Virginia
Supraorbital Rim Approach to Lesions of the Craniofacial Junction

DARRELL A. JAQUES, M.D., F.A.C.S.

Associate Professor of Surgery, Johns Hopkins University School of Medicine; Chief, Head and Neck Surgery, Greater Baltimore Medical Center, Baltimore, Maryland
Management of the Unknown Primary Tumor: Introduction

MICHAEL E. JOHNS, M.D.

Andelot Professor and Chairman, Department of Otolaryngology — Head and Neck Surgery, Johns Hopkins University School of Medicine, Baltimore, Maryland
Staging of Salivary Gland Cancers
Supraorbital Rim Approach to Lesions of the Craniofacial Junction
Chemosensitivity Assays: Introduction

MAURICE J. JURKIEWICZ, M.D., F.A.C.S.

Professor of Surgery, Emory University School of Medicine; Chief of Plastic Surgery, Emory University Affiliated Hospitals, Atlanta, Georgia
Microsurgical Reconstruction: Introduction

MICHAEL KAPLAN, M.D.

Assistant Professor, Department of Otolaryngology — Head and Neck Surgery, University of California, San Francisco, School of Medicine, San Francisco, California
Supraorbital Rim Approach to Lesions of the Craniofacial Junction

THOMAS J. KEANE, M.B., M.R.C.P.I., F.R.C.P.(C)

Assistant Professor of Radiology, University of Toronto Faculty of Medicine; Radiation Oncologist, Department of Radiation Oncology, The Princess Margaret Hospital, Toronto, Ontario, Canada
Clinical Staging of Head and Neck Cancer
Cervical Lymph Node Metastases From an Unknown Primary Tumor: The Place of Radiotherapy

JOHN A. KIRCHNER, M.D.

Professor of Surgery/Otolaryngology, Yale University School of Medicine; Attending Surgeon, Yale-New Haven Hospital, New Haven, Connecticut
Treatment of Laryngeal Cancer

JOEL C. KIRSH, M.D., F.R.C.P.(C)

Lecturer, Department of Radiology, University of Toronto Faculty of Medicine; Director, Division of Nuclear Medicine, and Staff Radiologist, Department of Radiological Sciences, Mount Sinai Hospital, Toronto, Ontario, Canada
Radionuclide Imaging

MORTON M. KLIGERMAN, M.D., M.Sc., M.A.

Henry K. Pancoast Professor of Research Oncology, Department of Radiation Therapy, University of Pennsylvania School of Medicine; Staff Attending, Department of Radiation Therapy, Hospital of the University of Pennsylvania, Philadelphia, Pennsylvania
Radiation Protection: Including a Report on the Phase I#II Study of Single and Multiple Doses of WR#2721

SIMON KRAMER, M.D., F.A.C.R.

Distinguished Professor, Radiation Therapy, Jefferson Medical College of Thomas Jefferson University; Attending Physician, Department of Radiation Therapy and Nuclear Medicine, Thomas Jefferson University Hospital, Philadelphia, Pennsylvania
Combined Surgery and Radiation Therapy in The Management of Locally Advanced Head and Neck Squamous Cell Carcinoma
Fractionation: Introduction
Hyperfractionation Studies of the Radiation Therapy Oncology Group in Patients with Advanced Squamous Cell Carcinoma of the Head and Neck

CHARLES J. KRAUSE, M.D.

Professor and Chairman, Department of Otorhinolaryngology, University of Michigan Medical School, Ann Arbor, Michigan
Management of the N3 Neck: Introduction

DENNIS B. LEEPER, Ph.D.

Professor and Director, Laboratory of Experimental Radiation Oncology, Department of Radiation Therapy and Nuclear Medicine, Thomas Jefferson University Hospital, Philadelphia, Pennsylvania
Adjuvant Hyperthermia in Radiation Therapy

DANIEL E. LEHANE, M.D.

Associate Professor, Pharmacology and Medicine, Baylor College of Medicine, Houston, Texas
Intra-arterial Cisplatin in the Treatment of Aerodigestive Squamous Carcinoma and Nasopharyngeal Carcinoma

BRUCE LEIPZIG, M.D.

Associate Professor, Department of Otolaryngology, University of Arkansas College of Medicine, Little Rock, Arkansas
Mandibular Reconstruction Other Than Osteomyocutaneous Homografts

VICTOR LING, Ph.D.

Professor, Department of Medical Biophysics, University of Toronto Faculty of Medicine; Senior Scientist, The Ontario Cancer Institute, Princess Margaret Hospital, Toronto, Ontario, Canada
Multidrug Resistance and Chemotherapy

RALEIGH E. LINGEMAN, M.D.

Morgan Professor and Chairman, Department of Otolaryngology – Head and Neck Surgery, Indiana University School of Medicine, Indianapolis, Indiana
Surgical Management of the N0 Neck

JOHN M. LORÉ, Jr., B.S., M.D.

Professor and Chairman, Department of Otolaryngology, State University of New York at Buffalo; University Chief of Otolaryngology, Buffalo Children's Hospital, Erie County Medical Center, Veterans Administration Medical Center, Buffalo, New York
Combination Radiation and Chemotherapy for Stage IV Tumors: Introduction

WILLIAM A. MADDOX, M.D., F.A.C.S.

Clinical Professor of Surgery, University of Alabama School of Medicine at Birmingham, Birmingham, Alabama
Multimodality Therapy for Advanced Epidermoid Carcinoma of the Head and Neck

MAHMOOD MAFEE, M.D.

Associate Professor, Department of Radiology, University of Illinois College of Medicine, Chicago, Illinois
Computerized Tomography in the Diagnosis of Head and Neck Diseases: A Clinical Approach

GÉRARD MAMELLE, M.D.

Assistant, Department of Head and Neck Surgery, Institute Gustave Roussy, Paris, France
Brachytherapy of Carcinoma of the Tongue (Mobile Portion) and Floor of the Mouth

ANTHONY A. MANCUSO, M.D.

Associate Professor of Radiology, University of Florida College of Medicine, Shands Teaching Hospital, Gainesville, Florida
Computed Tomography and Magnetic Resonance Imaging in the Detection and Staging of Head and Neck Cancer

LEE MARR, M.S.

Biology Department, Georgia State University, Atlanta, Georgia
Tumor-associated Antigens in Head and Neck Cancer Tissues and in Sera of Tumor-bearing Patients

STEPHEN J. MATHES, M.D.

Professor of Surgery, Anatomy and Cell Biology, and Head, Section of Plastic and Reconstructive Surgery, University of Michigan School of Medicine, Ann Arbor, Michigan
Role of the Regional Muscle Flap in Head and Neck Reconstruction

DOUGLAS E. MATTOX, M.D.

Associate Professor of Otolaryngology, Division of Otolaryngology, Department of Surgery, University of Texas Medical School at San Antonio, San Antonio, Texas
Capillary Cloning Assay in Head and Neck Cancer

MARK MAY, M.D., F.A.C.S.

Clinical Associate Professor, Department of ENT, University of Pittsburgh School of Medicine, Pittsburgh, Pennsylvania
Reanimation of the Paralyzed Eyelid Following Cancer Surgery

KENNETH J. McCORMICK, Ph.D.

Research Associate Professor of Otolaryngology — Head and Neck Surgery, University of Chicago School of Medicine, Chicago, Illinois; Research Scientist, Department of Otolaryngology — Head and Neck Surgery, University of Iowa College of Medicine, Iowa City, Iowa
Murine Subrenal Capsule (SRC) Assay in Head and Neck Cancer

JOHN BARRY McCRAW, M.D., F.A.C.S.

Professor of Plastic Surgery, Eastern Virginia Medical School; Chairman, Department of Plastic Surgery, Medical Center Hospitls, Norfolk, Virginia
Useful Arterialized Local Flaps for Head and Neck Reconstructions

IAN A. McGREGOR, Ch.M., F.R.C.S.

Honorary Clinical Lecturer, University of Glasgow; Director, West of Scotland Regional Plastic and Oral Surgery Unit, Canniesburn Hospital, Bearsden, Glasgow
Reconstruction: Yesterday, Today, and Tomorrow
Radial Forearm Flap
Reanimation of the Paralyzed Face: Introduction

BARBARA N. MEDVEC, R.N., B.S.N.

Department of Internal Medicine, Division of Hematology/Oncology, University of Michigan Hospitals, Ann Arbor, Michigan
Recent Developments in the Management of Head and Neck Cancer with Intra-arterial Chemotherapy

ROGER H. MERRICK, B.S.M.T.

Research Assistant II, Department of Otolaryngology — Head and Neck Surgery, University of Iowa College of Medicine, Iowa City, Iowa
Murine Subrenal Capsule (SRC) Assay in Head and Neck Cancer

DANIEL MILLER, M.D., F.A.C.S.

Clinical Professor in Otolaryngology, Emeritus, Harvard Medical School, Cambridge, Massachusetts; Otolaryngologist, New England Deaconess Hospital; Consultant Surgeon in Otolaryngology, Massachusetts Eye and Ear Infirmary; Chief, Head and Neck Oncology Clinic, Dana-Farber Cancer Institute, Boston, Massachusetts
Combination Treatment of Head and Neck Cancer with Induction Chemotherapy
New Treatment Modalities: Introduction

MARGARET MILLER, R.N., M.S.N.

Head and Neck Clinical Specialist, Illinois Masonic Medical Center, Chicago, Illinois
Computerized Tomography in the Diagnosis of Head and Neck Diseases: A Clinical Approach

RODNEY R. MILLION, M.D.

American Cancer Society Ashbel C. Williams, M.D., Memorial Professor of Clinical Oncology, and Director, Radiation Therapy, University of Florida College of Medicine, Shands Teaching Hospital, Gainesville, Florida
Definitive Radiation Therapy: Introduction

ENRICO MINI, M.D.

Departments of Pharmacology and Medicine, Yale University School of Medicine, New Haven, Connecticut
Single Agent Versus Combination Chemotherapy in Head and Neck Cancer

ROBERTO MOLINARI, M.D.

Chief, Head and Neck Surgical Oncology Department, Instituto Nazionale Tumori, Milan, Italy
Preliminary Intra-arterial Chemotherapy in Cancer of the Oral Cavity: Long-term Results of Combined Treatments with Surgery or Radiotherapy

EUGENE N. MYERS, M.D., F.A.C.S.

Professor and Chairman, Department of Otolaryngology, University of Pittsburgh School of Medicine; Chief, Department of Otolaryngology, Eye and Ear Hospital of Pittsburgh, Pittsburgh, Pennsylvania
Nonsurgical Rehabilitation: Introduction

CARLO NERVI, M.D.

Director, Istituto Medico e DiRicerca Scientifica, Rome, Italy
Multiple Fractions Per Day in the Radiotherapy of Head and Neck Cancer: An Updated Study of the EORTC Radiotherapy Group

CARL M. NORRIS, Jr., M.D.

Clinical Instructor, Harvard Medical School, Boston, Massachusetts
Combination Treatment of Head and Neck Cancer with Induction Chemotherapy

ARNOLD M. NOYEK, M.D., F.R.C.S.(C), F.A.C.S.

Professor of Otolaryngology and Radiology, University of Toronto Faculty of Medicine; Staff Otolaryngologist, Sunnybrook Medical Centre; Staff Otolaryngologist and Radiologist (Otolaryngology), Department of Radiological Sciences, Mount Sinai Hospital; Consultant, Department of Radiological Sciences, Toronto General Hospital, Toronto, Ontario, Canada
Radionuclide Imaging

WILLIAM R. PANJE, M.D., F.A.C.S.

Professor and Chairman, Otolaryngology — Head and Neck Surgery, University of Chicago Pritzker School of Medicine, Chicago, Illinois
Murine Subrenal Capsule (SRC) Assay in Head and Neck Cancer
Panje Procedure and Prosthetic Restoration of Speech After Laryngectomy

SHYAM B. PARYANI, M.D.

Radiation Therapist, Baptist Medical Center, Jacksonville, Florida
Management of Patients with N3 Cervical Lymphadenopathy and/or Carotid Artery Involvement

GARY R. PEARSON, Ph.D.

Professor and Chairman, Department of Microbiology, Georgetown University School of Medicine, Washington, D.C.
Advances Toward Diagnosis and Prevention of Epstein-Barr Virus EBV-Associated Malignant Disease

CARLOS A. PEREZ, M.D.

Professor of Radiology and Director, Division of Radiation Oncology, Mallinckrodt Institute of Radiology, Washington University School of Medicine, St. Louis, Missouri
Hyperthermia: Introduction
Potential Efficacy of Hyperthermia in Treatment of Head and Neck Tumors

LESTER J. PETERS, M.D.

Professor and Head, Divison of Radiotherapy, University of Texas Medical School at Houston, M.D. Anderson Hospital and Tumor Institute, Houston, Texas
Biology of Modern Radiotherapy for Head and Neck Cancer
New Aspects of Radiation Therapy: Introduction

THEODORE L. PHILLIPS, M.D.

Professor and Chairman, Department of Radiation Oncology, University of California, San Francisco, School of Medicine, San Francisco, California
Use of Radiation Sensitizers in the Treatment of Head and Neck Cancer

MARSHALL R. POSNER, M.D.

Assistant Professor of Medicine, Brown University Program in Medicine, Providence, Rhode Island
Combination Treatment of Head and Neck Cancer with Induction Chemotherapy

NEWELL PUGH, M.D.

Radiation Oncology Department, Methodist Hospital of Indiana, Indianapolis, Indiana
Management of the N3 Neck: Intraoperative Radiation

AJMEL A. PUTHAWALA, M.D.

Associate Clinical Professor, Department of Radiological Sciences, Division of Radiation Oncology, University of California, Irvine, California College of Medicine, Irvine, California; Associate Director, Department of Radiation Oncology and Department of Endocurietherapy, Memorial Medical Center of Long Beach, Long Beach, California
Role of the Interstitial Irradiation in the Treatment of Primary and Recurrent Tumors of Tonsillar Region and Soft Palate

IBRAHIM RAMZY, M.D.

Professor, Department of Pathology, University of Texas Medical School at San Antonio, San Antonio, Texas
Capillary Cloning Assay in Head and Neck Cancer

JEAN-MARIE RICHARD, M.D.

Chief, Department of Head and Neck Surgery, Institute Gustave Roussy, Paris, France

Brachytherapy of Carcinoma of the Tongue (Mobile Portion) and Floor of the Mouth

CHRISTOPHER M. ROSE, M.D.

Associate Director, Department of Radiation Therapy, St. Joseph's Medical Center, Burbank, California

Combination Treatment of Head and Neck Cancer with Induction Chemotherapy

MIRIAM P. ROSIN, Ph.D.

Assistant Professor of Pathology, University of British Columbia Faculty of Medicine; Environmental Carcinogenesis Unit, British Columbia Cancer Research Centre, Vancouver, British Columbia

Use of the Micronucleus Test to Trace the Progress of Intervention Studies with Carotenoids on Population Groups at High Risk for Oral Cancer

DAVID ROSS, M.D.

Radiation Oncology Department, Methodist Hospital of Indiana, Indianapolis, Indiana

Management of the N3 Neck: Intraoperative Radiation

MARCEL ROZENCWEIG, M.D.

Director, Clinical Cancer Research, Bristol-Meyers Company, Pharmaceutical Research and Development Division, Syracuse, New York

Issues in Defining Partial Response

H. THOMAS RUPNIAK, Ph.D.

Postdoctoral Fellow, Laboratory of Cellular Chemotherapy, Imperial Cancer Research Fund, London, England

Pitfalls in the Soft Agar Clonogenic Assays: Recommendations for Improving Colony-forming Efficiencies and the Potential Value of Cell Lines Derived from Head and Neck Tumors

BENJAMIN F. RUSH, Jr., M.D.

Professor and Chairman, Department of Surgery, University of Medicine and Dentistry of New Jersey, New Jersey Medical School, Newark, New Jersey

Intra-arterial Chemotherapy: Introduction

KUMAO SAKO, M.D.

Research Associate Professor of Surgery, State University of New York at Buffalo School of Medicine; Associate Chief, Department of Head and Neck Surgery and Oncology, Roswell park Memorial Institute, Buffalo, New York

Simultaneous Bilateral Neck Dissection

WILLIAM H. SAUNDERS, M.D.

Professor, Ohio State University College of Medicine, Columbus, Ohio

Shoulder Rehabilitation

H. DANIEL SCHANTZ, C.M.I.A.C.

Assistant Professor, Department of Pathology, University of Texas Medical School at San Antonio, San Antonio, Texas

Capillary Cloning Assay in Head and Neck Cancer

DAVID A SCHOENFELD, Ph.D.

Associate Professor of Biostatistics, Harvard Medical School, Dana-Farber Cancer Institute, Boston, Massachusetts

An Estimate of the Survival Benefit of Chemotherapy for Advanced Head and Neck Cancer and Its Implications to the Design of Clinical Trials

Is Partial Response of Value in the Chemotherapy of Advanced Head and Neck Cancer?

DAVID SCHOTTENFELD, M.D., M.S.

Professor of Public Health, Cornell University Medical College; Chief, Epidemiology and Preventive Medicine and Director of Cancer Control, Memorial Sloan-Kettering Cancer Center, New York, New York

Epidemiology, Etiology, and Pathogenesis of Head and Neck Cancer

VICTOR L. SCHRAMM, Jr., M.D., F.A.C.S.

Associate Professor, University of Pittsburgh School of Medicine; Chief, Division of Otolaryngology, Veterans Administration Hospitals, Eye and Ear Hospital, Pittsburgh, Pennsylvania

Anterior Craniofacial Surgery

DAVID E. SCHULLER, M.D.

Professor and Chairman, Department of Otolaryngology, Ohio State University College of Medicine; Director, Head and Neck Oncology Program, The Ohio State University Comprehensive Cancer Center, Columbus, Ohio

Management of the N0 Neck

JAMES W. SCHWEIGER, D.D.S., M.S.

Chief, Dental Service and Attending, Department of Surgery, Memorial Sloan-Kettering Cancer Center, New York, New York

Prosthetic Rehabilitation of the Mandibulectomy Patient

RONALD S. SCOTT, Ph.D., M.D.

Assistant Professor, Department of Radiation Oncology, University of Washington School of Medicine; Department of Radiation Oncology, University of Washington Hospital, Seattle, Washington

Potential Efficacy of Hyperthermia in Treatment of Head and Neck Tumors

DONALD G. SESSIONS, M.D.

Professor, Department of Otolaryngology, Washington University School of Medicine; Assistant Otolaryngologist, Barnes Hospital Group, St. Louis, Missouri

Composite Resection and Reconstruction with Skin Grafts for Oral Cavity and Oropharynx Cancer

ROY B. SESSIONS, M.D., F.A.C.S.

Professor of Otolaryngology — Head and Neck Surgery, Cornell Medical College; Associate Attending Surgeon, Memorial Sloan-Kettering Cancer Center; Attending Otolaryngologist, The New

York Hospital, New York, New York
Intra-arterial Cisplatin in the Treatment of Aerodigestive Squamous Carcinoma and Nasopharyngeal Carcinoma

JATIN P. SHAH, M.D., M.S.(Surg), F.A.C.S.

Associate Professor of Surgery, Cornell University Medical College; Associate Attending Surgeon, Head and Neck Service, Memorial Sloan-Kettering Cancer Center, New York, New York
The Unknown Primary: Evaluation of the Patient
The Unknown Primary: Surgical Treatment

BERNARD J. SHAPIRO, M.D., F.R.C.P.(C)

Professor, Department of Radiology, University of Toronto Faculty of Medicine; Staff Radiologist, Department of Biological Sciences, Mount Sinai Hospital, Toronto, Ontario, Canada
Radionuclide Imaging

DONALD P. SHEDD, M.D.

Chief, Department of Head and Neck Surgery and Oncology, Roswell Park Memorial Institute, Buffalo, New York
Diagnosis and Management of Early Cancer: Introduction

MARK I. SINGER, M.D., F.A.C.S.

Private Practice, Head and Neck Surgery Associates, Indianapolis, Indiana
Management of the N3 Neck: Intraoperative Radiation
Vocal Rehabilitation After Total Laryngectomy: Current Status and Future Directions

GEORGE A. SISSON, M.D.

Professor and Chairman, Department of Otolaryngology — Head and Neck Surgery, Northwestern University Medical School, Chicago, Illinois
Cancer of the Oral Cavity: Introduction

EMANUEL SKOLNIK, M.D.

Professor, Department of Otolaryngology — Head and Neck Surgery, University of Illinois College of Medicine, Chicago, Illinois
Computerized Tomography in the Diagnosis of Head and Neck Diseases: A Clinical Approach

GORDON B. SNOW, M.D., Ph.D.

Professor and Chairman, Department of Otolaryngology and Head and Neck Surgery, Free University Hospital, Amsterdam, The Netherlands
Nude Mice Model as a Predictive Assay in Head and Neck Cancer

PETER M. SOM, M.D.

Professor of Radiology and Otolaryngology, Department of Radiology, The Mount Sinai School of Medicine of the City University of New York; Chief, Head and Neck Radiology Section, The Mount Sinai Medical Center, New York, New York
Imaging of Salivary Gland Tumors

RONALD H. SPIRO, M.D.

Associate Professor of Clinical Surgery, Cornell University Medical College; Attending Surgeon, Head and Neck Service,

Department of Surgery, Memorial Sloan-Kettering Cancer Center, New York, New York
Tumors of the Parotid Gland

J. ROBERT STEWART, M.D.

Professor and Director, Division of Radiation Oncology, University of Utah School of Medicine, Salt Lake City, Utah
Deep Regional Hyperthermia: Overview of Methods and Potential Application in the Treatment of Head and Neck Cancers

HANS F. STICH, Ph.D.

Professor of Zoology, University of British Columbia; Head, Environmental Carcinogenesis Unit, British Columbia Cancer Research Centre, Vancouver, British Columbia
Use of the Micronucleus Test to Trace the Progress of Intervention Studies with Carotenoids on Population Groups at High Risk for Oral Cancer

CHARLES M. STIERNBERG, M.D.

Assistant Professor of Otolaryngology, University of Texas Medical School at Galveston; Clinical Staff, University of Texas Medical Branch Hospitals, Galveston, Texas
Surgical Management of Advanced Laryngeal Cancer

ELLIOT W. STRONG, M.D.

Professor of Surgery, Cornell University Medical College; Attending Surgeon and Chief, Head and Neck Service, Department of Surgery, Memorial Sloan-Kettering Cancer Center, New York, New York
Management of the N0 Neck: Introduction

M. STUART STRONG, M.D.

Professor and Chairman, Department of Otolaryngology, Boston University School of Medicine; Chief of Otolaryngology, University Hospital, Boston, Massachusetts
Evaluation of Patients with Advanced Head and Neck Cancer: Selection of Patients for Combination Therapy
Role of Lasers in Head and Neck Cancer

JAMES Y. SUEN, M.D.

Professor and Chairman, Department of Otolaryngology and Maxillofacial Surgery, University of Arkansas College of Medicine, Little Rock, Arkansas
Tumor Response to Chemotherapy and Its Measurement: Response Determination in Combined-modality Settings

VLADIMIR SVOBODA, M.D.

Consultant Radiotherapist, St. Mary's Hospital, Portsmouth, England
Multiple Fractions Per Day in the Radiotherapy of Head and Neck Cancer: An Updated Study of the EORTC Radiotherapy Group

A. M. NISAR SYED, M.D., F.R.C.S. (Lond.), F.R.C.S. (Edin.), D.M.R.T. (Eng.)

Associate Clinical Professor, Department of Radiological Sciences, Division of Radiation Oncology, University of California, Irvine, California College of Medicine, Irvine, California; Director, Department of Radiation Oncology and Department of Endocurie-therapy, Memorial Medical Center of Long Beach, Long Beach, California

Role of Interstitial Irradiation in the Treatment of Primary and Recurrent Tumors of Tonsillar Region and Soft Palate

G. IAN TAYLOR, M.B., B.S., F.R.C.S.(Lond.), F.R.A.C.S.

Hunterian Professor and Associate Plastic Surgeon, University of Melbourne; Consultant Plastic Surgeon, Royal Melbourne Hospital; Senior Consultant Plastic Surgeon, Preston and Northcote Community Hospital, Melbourne, Australia

Free Deep Inferior Epigastric Artery Musculocutaneous Flap and Its Application to Head and Neck Surgery
Mandibular Reconstruction with Free Iliac Osteocutaneous Flaps

DAVID B. THOMAS, M.D., Dr.P.H.

Professor, Department of Epidemiology, University of Washington School of Public Health and Community Medicine; Head, Program in Epidemiology, Fred Hutchinson Cancer Research Center, Seattle, Washington

Sinonasal, Nasopharyngeal, Oral, Pharyngeal, Laryngeal, and Esophageal Cancers: Epidemiology and Opportunities for Primary Prevention

HARVEY M. TUCKER, M.D., F.A.C.S.

Chairman, Department of Otolaryngology and Communicative Disorders, Cleveland Clinic Foundation, Cleveland, Ohio

Reanimation of the Paralyzed Face: The "Pyramid' Approach

RUTH ANN TUCKER, M.S.

Biology Department, Georgia State University, Atlanta, Georgia

Tumor-associated Antigens in Head and Neck Cancer Tissues and in Sera of Tumor-bearing Patients

MARSHALL M. URIST, M.D., F.A.C.S.

Associate Professor of Surgery, University of Alabama School of Medicine at Birmingham, Birmingham, Alabama

Multimodality Therapy for Advanced Epidermoid Carcinoma of the Head and Neck

WALTER VAN DEN BOGAERT, M.D.

Head, Radiotherapy Department, University Hospital, Antwerp, Belgium

Multiple Fractions Per Day in the Radiotherapy of Head and Neck Cancer: An Updated Study of the EORTC Radiotherapy Group

EMMANUEL VAN DER SCHUEREN, M.D.

Head, Radiotherapy Department, University Hospital, Leuven, Belgium

Multiple Fractions Per Day in the Radiotherapy of Head and Neck Cancer: An Updated Study of the EORTC Radiotherapy Group

A. W. PETER VAN NOSTRAND, M.D.

Professor, Pathology and Otolaryngology, University of Toronto Faculty of Medicine; Chief of Surgical Pathology, Toronto General Hospital, Toronto, Ontario, Canada

Failure Analysis of T1 Glottic Carcinoma Treated With Radical Radiotherapy for Cure With Surgery in Reserve

ROBERT W. VELTRI, Ph.D.

Adjunct Associate Professor, Department of Pathology, Hahnemann University School of Medicine, Philadelphia, Pennsylvania; President, American Biotechnology Co., Ltd., Kensington, Maryland

Immune Regulation in Carcinoma of the Head and Neck

STEVEN E. VOGL, M.D.

Associate Clinical Professor of Medicine, Albert Einstein College of Medicine of Yeshiva University, Bronx, New York; President, Cancer Treatment Research Foundation of New York, Scarsdale, New York

Is Partial Response of Value in the Chemotherapy of Advanced Head and Neck Cancer?
Is Combination Chemotherapy of Demonstrated Value for Advanced Head and Neck Cancer?

DANIEL D. VON HOFF, M.D.

Associate Professor of Medicine, Division of Oncology, Department of Medicine, University of Texas Medical School at San Antonio, San Antonio, Texas

Capillary Cloning Assay in Head and Neck Cancer

C. C. WANG, M.D.

Professor of Radiation Therapy, Harvard Medical School; Radiation Therapist and Head of Division of Clinical Services, Department of Radiation Medicine, Massachusetts General Hospital, Boston, Massachusetts

Brachytherapy in Head and Neck Cancer: Introduction
Brachytherapy for Selected Cancers of the Head and Neck

PAUL H. WARD, M.D., F.A.C.S.

Professor of Surgery and Chief, Division of Head and Neck Surgery, University of California, Los Angeles, UCLA School of Medicine, Los Angeles, California

Complications of Thyroid Surgery: Their Prevention, Recognition, and Management

ARTHUR WEAVER, M.D.

Professor of Surgery, Wayne State University School of Medicine; Chief, Head and Neck Surgery, Allen Park Veterans Administration Medical Center, Detroit, Michigan

Early Cancer of the Head and Neck: Diagnostic Considerations
Swallowing Rehabilitation

RALPH R. WEICHSELBAUM, M.D.

Professor and Chairman, Department of Radiation Oncology, Michael Reese/University of Chicago, Joint Center for Radiation Therapy; Chief, Department of Radiation Oncology, Divison of Biologic Science, University of Chicago Medical Center, Chicago, Illinois

Radiobiologic Factors Influencing Fractionation in Head and Neck Cancer Therapy
Rationale for Combination Chemotherapy as Treatment of Advanced Head and Neck Cancer
Combination Treatment of Head and Neck Cancer with Induction Chemotherapy

BERND WEINBERG, Ph.D.

Professor and Head, Department of Audiology and Speech Sciences, Purdue University, West Lafayette, Indiana
Speech Rehabilitation Following Total Laryngectomy: Some Perspectives

JOSEPH F. WEISS, Ph.D.

Chief, Physiological Chemistry Division, Armed Forces Radiobiology Research Institute, Bethesda, Maryland
Interrelationship of Immune Response, Circulating Proteins, and Etiologic Factors for Head and Neck Cancer

ALVIN P. WENGER, M.D.

Assistant Professor, Department of Otolaryngology, Johns Hopkins University School of Medicine; Chief of Otolaryngology — Head and Neck Surgery, Greater Baltimore Medical Center, Baltimore, Maryland
Nonsurgical Rehabilitation

RICHARD H. WHEELER, M.D.

Associate Professor, Department of Internal Medicine, Division of Hematology/Oncology, University of Alabama School of Medicine, Birmingham, Alabama
Recent Developments in the Management of Head and Neck Cancer with Intra-arterial Chemotherapy

RICHARD D. H. WHELAN, M.I.Biol.

Research Associate, Laboratory of Cellular Chemotherapy, Imperial Cancer Research Fund, London, England

Pitfalls in the Soft Agar Colongenic Assays; Recommendations for Improving Colony-forming Efficiencies and the Potential Value of Cell Lines Derived from Head and Neck Tumors

PIERRE WIBAULT, M.D.

Assistant, Department of Radiotherapy, Institute Gustave Roussy, Paris, France
Brachytherapy of Carcinoma of the Tongue (Mobile Portion) and Floor of the Mouth

ROBERT E. WITTES, M.D.

Associate Director, Cancer Therapy Evaluation Program, Division of Cancer Treatment, National Cancer Institute, National Institutes of Health, Bethesda, Maryland
Which Responses are Meaningful in Head and Neck Cancer?
Single Agent Versus Combination Chemotherapy: Introduction

JAMES E. M. YOUNG, B.Sc., M.D., F.R.C.S.(C), F.A.C.S.

Associate Clinical Professor of Surgery, McMaster University School of Medicine; Head, Head and Neck Service, St. Joseph's Hospital and McMaster University Medical Centre; Surgical Consultant, Ontario Cancer Treatment and Research Foundation, Hamilton, Ontario, Canada
The Unknown Primary: Operative Evaluation
The Unknown Primary: Prognosis and Follow-up

PREFACE

The subject of this volume is the current status of treatment and research in head and neck cancer. The major goals of the volume are to identify and evaluate recent progress in the many specialties involved in treatment and research in head and neck cancer, to discuss the interrelations of these advances, and to identify areas of investigation that hold promise of important contributions in the near future. It is intended for clinicians who seek to practice the highest levels of patient care and investigators who seek to initiate programs that will yield significant advances in the treatment of these cancers.

The volume arose from a perception by the members of the American Society for Head and Neck Surgery and the Society of Head and Neck Surgeons that the many recent advances in the various specialties contributing to treatment of head and neck cancer had not been presented in a comprehensive scientific forum. To address this need, the Societies invited 138 distinguished specialists to present these accomplishments at an international conference. Their critiques and reviews were then compiled in this volume. Their enthusiastic response to this request appears to reflect a consensus that the Societies were fulfilling a critical need.

The International Conference on Head and Neck Cancer was held in Baltimore, Maryland, July 22–27, 1984. Registration of more than 700 clinicians and investigators from 40 countries constituted the largest conference on head and neck cancer convened to date and provided the first broad interaction among the diverse specialties. The vital contribution of these interdisciplinary exchanges is reflected in the volume; the authors have rendered incisive documentations of the new contributions from their specialties to the treatment of head and neck cancer, and with mature vision, they have emphasized scientific areas in which progress is anticipated or could be anticipated and given appropriate commitments of resources and expertise.

The most important activities of the Societies are the promulgation of the highest levels of clinical practice and the commitment of impetus to programs that will improve patient care. In their evaluation of the Conference, the registrants overwhelmingly acclaimed that similar conferences at appropriate intervals should be an important function of the Societies. With this volume, the Societies solicit the readers' appraisal of the potential value of similar future publications as an authoritative source of progress in treatment and research in head and neck cancer.

The project required the dedicated efforts of many members of the Societies working in concert. Primary among these were the presidents of the Societies, who exerted the critical actions needed for the deadlines and the level of excellence projected by the Organizing Committee: The Presidents in 1981, Drs. Douglas P. Bryce (ASHNS) and John M. Loré (SHNS) gave the Committee an unequivocal mandate to proceed. In 1982, Drs. Jerome C. Goldstein (ASHNS) and Alvin L. Watne (SHNS) vigorously activated the preliminary plans. In 1983, Drs. Darrell A. Jaques (SHNS) and Paul H. Ward (ASHNS) committed the Societies to the final proposal. And in 1984, Drs. Alando J. Ballantyne (SHNS) and Hugh F. Biller (ASHNS) resolved major obstacles to ensure completion of the project.

Among the many who helped with various aspects of the project, we wish to mention three who generously provided technical services with the level of expertise and magnitude of effort needed for its success: Jane H. Chretien and Helen R. Vidockler supplied inexhaustible secretarial and administrative support for the extensive communications among the editors, authors, members of the Organizing Committee, Executive Councils of the Societies, and the publisher; and Mary E. Mansor, Associate Medical Editor, B.C. Decker, Inc., skillfully assisted the editors in their task of achieving a homogeneous presentation of the contributions.

Paul B. Chretien
Michael E. Johns
Donald P. Shedd
Elliott W. Strong
Paul H. Ward

CONTENTS

PART ONE
CURRENT PERSPECTIVES IN
HEAD AND NECK CANCER

PART TWO
CURRENT EVALUATION AND MANAGEMENT
OF HEAD AND NECK CANCER

Section One
Staging

Section Two
Diagnostic Imaging

Section Three
Surgical Management

Secton Four
Radiation Therapy

Section Five
Hyperthermia

Section Six
Chemotherapy

Section Seven
Reconstruction and Rehabilitation

Section Eight
New Treatment Modalities

Section Nine
Immunology and Immunotherapy

Section Ten
Intervention Approaches to Prevention

PART ONE

CURRENT PERSPECTIVES IN HEAD AND NECK CANCER

1. The Cancer Cell: Developing Knowledge and Implications for Therapy

EMIL FREI III, M.D.

We are in the throes of a revolution in molecular biology, and nowhere are progress and change more evident than in tumor biology. Thus our understanding of the fundamental nature of the neoplastic process, its cause, preneoplastic changes, monoclonal origin, the importance of oncogenes, clonal evolution, invasion, mediator production, heterogeneity, metastases, and proliferative and differentiation behavior—all of these represent concepts and developments that have occurred largely within the last few years. Many have major intervention implications in terms of prevention, early detection, and, particularly, treatment.

ONCOGENES

Perhaps the most exciting recent development relates to oncogenes. Although genes capable of mediating the neoplastic transformation have long been suspected, the conclusive demonstration that oncogenes exist and bear an important relation to the cancer problem required, as always, advances in sophisticated technology. Weinberg and Cooper independently demonstrated, in 1977, that if one took the DNA of a human tumor cell and transfected it into a non-neoplastic mouse cell by a technique known as calcium precipitation, the mouse cell was transformed into a tumor cell (Fig. 1). Evidence for this was multifactorial; perhaps the most conclusive evidence related to the fact that the transformed cell, when injected into a syngeneic mouse, produced a tumor, whereas the parent normal cell did not. The necessary controls included taking the DNA from normal human cells and injecting it into the mouse cell, under which circumstances no transformation to neoplasia occurred. Using restriction enzyme techniques, the isolated DNA was broken into progressively smaller fragments, and these were analyzed for transfection capability. By such reduction techniques, the specific oncogene could be separated from the whole DNA molecule. It was demonstrated that this oncogene was homologous, that is, the DNA of the oncogene was essentially similar to the DNA produced by known tumor retroviruses. In addition, it was demonstrated by molecular biologic techniques that the human oncogene was well preserved in evolution, being present down the evolutionary scale to the lamprey, that is, back some 200 million years. In short, they have been a part of life for a long time (see Fig. 1).

Once the DNA of the oncogene was demonstrated, it was found by homology studies that the oncogene, in contrast to what was suggested by the

transfection experiments, was indeed present in the DNA of normal human cells, probably all normal human cells. This suggested that the oncogene was ubiquitous and that cancer production must somehow relate to activation of the oncogene, so that gene products were produced. Let me anticipate what I am going to say by stating that that has proved emphatically to be the case. Obviously, a central theme in current work on the etiology of cancer has to do with exactly how oncogenes are activated (Fig. 2). The evidence is conclusive that there are a variety of ways in which activation can occur. First, the genes may be amplified, that is, increased in number, by any of a variety of mechanisms. Such gene amplification is known to occur in certain examples of methotrexate resistance. Second, gene alteration and activation may occur by virtue of mutation within an oncogene. Under such circumstances the nucleotide sequence in the oncogene should be altered, and this indeed has been found; the gene product, in one case protein 21, has been similarly slightly altered. Exactly why such a slight alteration in the quality, and perhaps quantity, of gene product should produce cancer in this instance is unknown. Third, the oncogene may be activated by the juxtaposition in the DNA chain of a lateral terminal repeat or insertional sequence which controls and activates the adjacent oncogene. This has been demonstrated for several oncogenes. Perhaps most

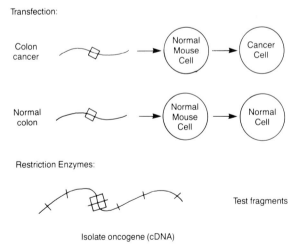

Transfection:

Oncogenic Hetroviruses: contain oncogenes that hybridize with oncogenes found by transfection.

Conserved in evolution: found in normal human cells and back to *drosophilia*.

Figure 1 Molecular biology of oncogenes: origin.

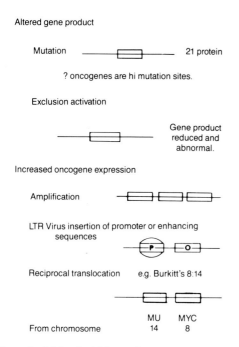

Figure 2   Molecular biology of oncogenes: activation.

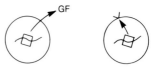

Figure 3   Molecular biology of oncogenes: products.

dramatic are the cytogenetic examples of reciprocal translocations. Thus, for many of the leukemias and lymphomas it has been demonstrated that interchanges of small bits of DNA may occur between certain chromosomes. This provides an opportunity for an activating sequence of DNA for the oncogene to be juxtaposed to the oncogene, per se, with resultant activation and gene product formation. This has been demonstrated. Tumor retroviruses in some instances may not in fact contain an oncogene, but rather a gene, which when appropriately inserted activates an oncogene (see Fig. 2).

Given an activated oncogene, how does it produce cancer (Fig. 3)? Genes, per se, are only active in that they may produce mRNA, which in turn, in the polyribosomes, produces a protein product that is the ultimate gene product and is the way our genetic material expresses itself phenotypically. Protein products of some of the oncogenes have been identified. They are enormously interesting and have major implications. They fall into at least three classes. The first are polypeptide hormones that bind to specific sites on certain DNA and thus initiate somatic cell replication. In short, they place the cell in question in a permanent proliferative state, a characteristic we know to be true for many tumors. Second, oncogenes may produce tyrosine protein kinases, enzymes that alter certain proteins. These proteins include the structural proteins of the cell which are responsible for cell shape, motility, deformability—in short, many of the characteristics of cancer cells. Enzymes require substrates, and substrates can be manipulated to inhibit the enzyme in question. Thus, already the effect of inhibition of these enzymes on cancer growth are under study, and the therapeutic implications are ap-

parent. The third class of gene products are perhaps the most interesting, and not surprinsgly they turn out to be growth factors and, in addition, growth factor receptors. Thus the oncogene may program for a growth factor capable of stimulating the host cell, as well as adjacent cells, and also produce the growth factor receptor which inserts in the membrane and allows for the growth factor produced to interact with a receptor and stimulate cell replication. Tumors grow, and it is not surprising, therefore, that they have the intrinsic mechanisms for sustaining their own growth. Minna has demonstrated that monoclonal antibodies which block growth factor receptor sites may break the cycle and thus result in tumor regression[1,2] (see Fig. 3).

PRENEOPLASIA INVASION AND METASTASIS

Oncogenes may transform cells in culture in a single step. However, we know from studies of human tumors that the neoplastic process is multistep, going from early preneoplasis through preneoplasia, and finally to neoplasia, after which there can be a continuing ascendancy of the malignant state in the form of clonal evolution. It has recently been demonstrated experimentally in vitro that at least some cells, and probably all cells, do in fact contain multiple oncogenes, and consistent with what is observed pathologically and clinically, there is a sequence of switches turning on oncogenes that leads ultimately to neoplasia. In spite of this sequence, there is evidence that tumors are monoclonal in origin, that is, at some point in the preneoplastic process, a single cell is tapped on the shoulder and told to go forth and increase and multiply (Fig. 4). Thus most tumors derive from a single cell. If this is true, how does one explain the heterogeneity of most human tumors as observed under the microscope and clinically? For example, in metastatic melanoma there may be substantial variation in pigmentation between metastases in the same patient, a situation that is seemingly not consistent with monoclonal origin. The answer is that tumor cells, in contrast to normal cells, are inherently genetically unstable and thus undergo clonal evolution. As the tu-

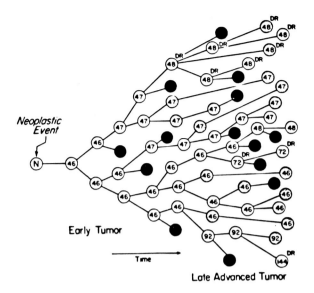

Figure 4 Clonal evolution of human neoplasia. ● = death, terminal differentiation, lethal mutant, cell loss; DR = drug-resistant mutant; 46 = Resting Cell, i.e., G_1 or G_2 Block

mor progressively increases in duration and size, there occurs progressive aneuploidy; an increasing proportion of resting cells (cytokinetic heterogeneity); an increasing proportion of daughter cells that die; and not surprisingly, therefore, an increasing risk of drug-resistant clones. Thus, tumors become increasingly heterogeneous as a result of clonal evolution. This can be demonstrated immunologically, where there is considerable variation in antigen presence among cancer cells, as evidenced by immunoperoxidase studies. The same has been demonstrated for hormone receptors, and indeed different clones from a metastatic tumor often have substantial variation in response to a given chemotherapeutic agent. It is this heterogeneity that is largely responsible for the frequent and often rapid development of drug resistance. Heterogeneity in military terms means multiple targets. If one has multiple targets, one needs multiple-target therapy, and that to the chemotherapist means combination chemotherapy. Indeed, the primary basic rationale for combination chemotherapy is tumor cell heterogeneity[5-7] (see Fig. 4).

Tumor invasion and metastases, the two established criteria for neoplasia, have moved from descriptive sciences to quantitative basic studies. It is becoming increasingly evident that tumor cells produce mediators which modify their microenvironment. Thus local invasion may be abetted by proteolytic enzymes that modify the local environmenta and decrease resistance to tumor spread. For tumors to produce metastases requires that they invade through the basement membrane of the capillary. Collagenase IV is produced by certain tumors, and Collagenase IV will disrupt capillary basement membranes, thus allowing for metastasis. Activated B-cells, and particularly myeloma cells, produce a substance known as osteoclast-activating factor. Activated osteoclasts de-

stroy bone and thus allow for myeloma cells to set up shop in this otherwise hostile environment. At least experimentally, certain breast tumor cells produce high levels of prostaglandin, some of which also activate osteoclasts, and this may be associated with the known propensity of certain types of breast cancer to produce bone metastases.

The first and seminal experimental study of metastasis was performed by Fidler almost 10 years ago. He demonstrated that B-16 melanoma cells injected into the tail vein produced very few pulmonary metastases. He postulated that the B-16 melanoma cells in these pulmonary metastases, when reinjected into the tail vein as a second-generation transplant, would produce the same number of pulmonary metastases if selection was random, but an increasing number if the cells that went to the lung were selected in some nonrandom basis. He found after 10 transfers that he had developed a B-16 melanoma line with a marked propensity to produce pulmonary metastases. Experiments demonstrating that a small proportion of cells in a primary tumor have a propensity to metastasize to specific anatomic sites have now been demonstrated experimentally in a number of circumstances. This has focused research on membrane interaction between tumor cells and the capillary endothelium of different organs as a basis for metastatic tropism. Indeed, studies of the membrane properties of cells with specific tropism indicate clear differences, and our understanding of the metastatic process at a molecular level may be forthcoming in the relatively near future.

Metastases initially grow slowly and will stop growing at about 1 mm in diameter unless they are vascularized. This is accomplished by the production of tumor angiogenesis factor, which stimulates adjacent endothelium to proliferate. The tumor is invaded with a vascular network, and subsequently the tumor may grow exponentially. However, with progressive increase in size, an increasing proportion of cells drop out of cycle, that is, the growth fraction progressively decreases. Of the several reasons for this, one relates to decreasing relative vascularity, and therefore a decreasing availability of nutrients, in particular oxygen. Thus tumors have not only a qualitatively abnormal vascular supply, but tumors of any size have relatively hypoxic centers. Since oxygen is essential for the destructive capacity of radiation and of some chemotherapeutic agents, this hypoxia represents an obstacle to therapy; hence the development of hypoxic cell sensitizers. A recent therapeutic development in this regard relates to fluorocarbons, which are colloid particles, approximately 1 percent the volume of red cells. However, they are capable of loading and unloading oxygen, as does hemoglobin, and can function as red blood cell substitutes. Moreover, because of their size, they presumably enter tumors much more readily than do the much larger red cells, particularly in hypovascular areas. Whether this is exactly what happens is uncertain, but perfluorocarbons have been demonstrated by Teicher to be capable of substantially increasing radiosensitivity of experimental hypoxic tumors.

I have discussed only several of the more exciting areas with respect to our understanding of the cancer cell. Monoclonal antibodies have allowed us to study cell differentiation with much greater precision. It develops that tumor cells represent monoclonal expansion of a given level of differentiation and thus have specific differentiation anitgens. These may be targets for monoclonal antibodies alone or, more particularly, monoclonal antibodies conjugated to chemotherapeutic agents or toxins. Finally, it has been possible experimentally to induce differentiation, as compared to proliferation, of tumor cells, and since differentiated cells are often end stage cells, such differentiation has a net therapeutic effect. There are in clinical trial today several agents which are potent differentiators in experimental tumors and are being studied with the intent of making tumor cells behave, rather than destroying them directly.

In summary, the progress achieved in cancer treatment in the past was often accomplished with relatively limited basic and bridging science information. The literally explosive nature of the development of that information during the past 5 years and into the future offer many and far more sophisticated approaches to treatment.

REFERENCES

1. Cooper GM et al. Transforming activity of DNA of chemically transformed and normal cells. Nature 1980; 284:418.
2. Krontiras TG. The emerging genetics of human cancer. N Engl J Med 1983; 309:404.
3. Busch H. Oncogenes and other new targets for cancer chemotherapy. J Cancer Res Clin Oncol 1984; 107:1.
4. Nowell P. The clonal evolution of tumor cell populations. Science 1976; 194:23.
5. Fidler IJ et al. Demonstration of multiple phenotypic diversity in the murine melanoma of recent origin. J Nat Cancer Inst 1981; 76:947.
6. Cifone MA et al. Increasing metastatic potential is associated with increasing genetic instability of clones isolated frommurine neoplasms. Proc Natl Acad Sci USA 1981; 78:6949.
7. Nicholson GL. Cell surfaces and cancer metastasis. Hosp Pract 1982; 17:75.

2. Epidemiology, Etiology, and Pathogenesis of Head and Neck Cancer

DAVID SCHOTTENFELD, M.D., M.S.

The ultimate goal of epidemiology is disease prevention. Close examination of incidence patterns and established risk factors facilitate research and intervention strategies designed to ultimately reduce cancer morbidity and mortality.

The American Cancer Society has estimated that 27,500 new cases of buccal cavity and pharyngeal cancer, and 11,100 new cases of laryngeal cancer will occur in the United States in 1984; the corresponding numbers of deaths were estimated to be 9350 and 3750, respectively.[1]

DEMOGRAPHIC PATTERNS

Buccal Cavity and Pharynx

Incidence

From 1973 to 1977, cancers of the buccal cavity and pharynx accounted for 3.4 percent of all incident malignant neoplasms in the United States, after excluding basal and squamous cell carcinomas of the skin. The most frequently diagnosed primary sites in the buccal cavity and pharynx were tongue, lip, and gum (Table 1). Among lip cancers, 84 percent were diagnosed in the lower lip and 96 percent were squamous cell carcinomas. Lip cancer was distinctive from other subsites in the buccal cavity in that it occurred significantly more commonly in white males (3.9/100,000) than in black males (0.3/100,000). Moore and Catlin described a high-risk horseshoe-shaped mucosal region which extends backward from the anterior floor of the mouth, over both lingual-alveolar

TABLE 1   Average Annual Age-Adjusted (1970 United States Standard) Incidence Rates per 100,000 Population for Buccal Cavity & Pharynx Cancer by Sex & Primary Site* (SEER Program, 1973–1977)

Primary Site	Total	Male	Female
Buccal cavity & pharynx	11.2	17.4	6.2
Tongue	2.0	3.0	1.2
Lip	1.9	3.9	0.3
Gum	1.8	2.4	1.4
Floor of mouth	1.3	2.0	0.7
Tonsil	1.1	1.6	0.7
Hypopharynx	1.0	1.7	0.4
Major Salivary Gland	0.9	1.1	0.8
Nasopharynx	0.6	0.9	0.3
Oropharynx	0.3	0.5	0.1

*Selected sulsites within buccal cavity and pharynx.

sulci and lateral margins of the anterior two-thirds of the tongue, and then finally reaches the anterior tonsillar pillar and retromolar trigone complex.[2]

More than 90 percent of oropharyngeal cancers occur in patients over 45 years of age. The average annual age-adjusted incidence per 100,000 population, based on the SEER data for 1973 to 1977, was 19.3 in black males, 16.8 in white males, 7.0 in black females, and 6.0 in white females. In patients under age 45, the incidence in men was about double that in women. With increasing age, the rate of increase accelerated more in men so that by age 70, the incidence became almost four times greater in men.

Long-term incidence patterns are not available for the United States, but may be inferred from population cancer registries. In Connecticut, over a 25-year period, buccal cavity and pharyngeal cancer incidence decreased in males from 17.9 to 16.8 per 100,000 and increased in females from 3.6 to 5.3 per 100,000 (Table 2).

Mortality

A survey of mortality in the United States from 1950 to 1969 revealed contrasting patterns for men and women.[3] Mortality among men was elevated in the Northeast, around large metropolitan areas. Morality predominated in lower socioeconomic groups. In women, the Southeastern excess of oral cancer occurred in the rural white population, in which snuff dipping was a relatively common habit.[4]

The secular trend for age-adjusted mortality in the United States from 1950 to 1979 demonstrated the predominance in nonwhite males since 1965. By 1979, buccal cavity and pharynx cancer mortality in nonwhite males was 1.7 times greater than in white males. During a period of thirty years, age-adjusted mortality decreased slightly in white males, but increased relatively by 84 percent in nonwhite males (Table 3).[5]

Data regarding patient survival have not been available on the same scale as data on mortality covering the entire United States population, or on incidence covering selected geographic areas in the United States. Mortality trends reflect both incidence and survival trends. If both incidence and mortality for a specific cancer site remain unchanged or change proportionately over a period of years, no major change

TABLE 2 Age-adjusted (1950 United States Standard) Incidence Rates per 100,000 Population for Buccal Cavity & Pharynx Cancer by Sex & Year of Diagnosis, (Connecticut, 1950–1974)

	Buccal Cavity		Pharynx	
Period	Male	Female	Male	Female
1950–54	13.3	2.8	4.6	0.8
1955–59	13.4	2.7	5.1	0.9
1960–64	14.0	3.1	5.3	1.1
1965–69	11.7	3.1	5.2	1.2
1970–74	11.8	4.0	5.0	1.3

TABLE 3 Age-Adjusted (1970 Standard Population) Mortality Rates per 100,000 Population for Buccal Cavity & Pharynx Cancer by Sex & Race (United States, 1950–1979)

	Male		Female	
Year	White	Nonwhite	White	Nonwhite
1950	6.6	4.9	1.5	2.0
1955	6.2	4.8	1.5	1.6
1960	5.9	5.2	1.6	2.0
1965	5.7	6.3	1.5	1.9
1970	5.9	7.3	1.8	2.1
1975	5.5	8.2	1.9	2.1
1979	5.2	9.0	1.9	2.4

From McKay, Hanson, & Miller[5].

in survival should be anticipated. The trend in 5-year relative survival will be influenced by the temporal trend for the percentage of cases localized at the time of diagnosis and/or by the impact of evolving methods of treatment. In general, for each of the subsites within the oral cavity and pharynx diagnosed in the 1950s and 1960s, 5-year survival was more favorable in the women (Table 4). This was partially explained by differences observed in the extent of disease at the time of initial diagnosis. For example, the striking contrast in survival for carcinoma of the tongue was reflected in the greater percentage of women (50 to 55%) than men (37 to 43%) with localized disease.[6]

International Patterns

From 1968 to 1972, incidence rates for cancer of the oral cavity showed marked geographic differences among men where alcohol and tobacco consumption were high (e.g., in France, where the age-adjusted mortality was 2.5 to 3.0 times the rate for men in the United States) or where betel quid chewing and bidi smoking were frequent (e.g., India). Among men and women in Bombay, cancer of the oral cavity and hypopharynx accounted for 50 percent of all cancers

TABLE 4 Trends in 5-Year Relative Survival* for Buccal Cavity Subsites & Pharynx Cancers in White Males (WM) & Females (WF) (1955–1959 and 1965–1969)†

	5-Year Relative Survival(%)			
	1955–59		1965–69	
Site	WM	WF	WM	WF
Lip	88	97**	84	85‡
Tongue	27	47	32	44
Floor of mouth	43	46**	42	47
Pharynx	23	29	21	30

†From end results program, National Cancer Institue (1976)

*The relative survival rate is the ratio of the observed survival rate to the expected survival rate for persons from the general population who are similar to the patient group with respect to age, race, sex, and calendar year of observation.

‡Rate has standard error between 5 and 10 percent.

TABLE 5 Age-Adjusted Incidence Rates per 100,000 Population for Oral Cavity & Pharynx Cancer in Selected Populations Throughout the World by Rank Order, Sex, and Male-to-Female Ratio (1968–1972)

Country	Male	Female	M/F Ratio
Bombay, India	33.2	12.1	2.7
Puerto Rico	25.9	6.9	3.8
Sao Paulo, Brazil	24.3	4.8	5.1
Singapore (Indian)	22.1	25.5	0.9
Quebec, Canada	15.3	3.7	4.2
Geneva, Switzerland	14.2	3.0	4.7
Connecticut	13.1	4.4	3.0
Detroit, Michigan (white)	11.3	3.8	3.0
Detroit, Michigan (black)	11.2	4.1	2.7
Hamburg, Federal Republic	9.0	3.3	2.7
Israel (all Jews)	7.4	3.4	2.2
Israel (non-Jews)	7.1	1.3	5.5
Singapore (Chinese)	6.9	1.7	4.1
Singapore (Malay)	6.0	1.6	3.8
Ibadan, Nigeria	4.2	3.2	1.3

From Waterhouse et al.[7]

(Table 5).[7] In India, especially among rural populations, tobacco was smoked, chewed and applied in a variety of ways. Carcinomas of the tongue, hypopharynx, and esophagus were attributed partially to the smoking of an uncured form of tobacco (bidi), which was dried in the sun and rolled in a dried leaf of temburni or banana. Cancer of the roof of the mouth was relatively common where reverse smoking of the lighted end of a slow-burning cheroot was practiced (e.g., Sardinia, Venezuela, Panama, and India). In Visakhapatnam, East India, almost three-quarters of the oral and pharyngeal cancers in women occurred on the hard palate.[8]

Larynx

Incidence

From 1950 to 1974, cancer of the larynx represented approximately 2 percent of all incident cancers in the United States. The incidence of laryngeal cancer increased significantly in men between the ages of 35 and 74. The disease rarely affected persons under age 35 and occurred particularly in those aged 60 to 74 years. Any apparent decline in cross-sectional incidence among males after age 75 may have represented a birth cohort rather than an age phenomenon because men born before the year 1900 did not smoke as heavily as men after 1900.[9] The incidence in women peaked between the ages of 55 and 64 years, after which there was a marked increase in the age-specific male/female incidence ratio. The male/female incidence ratio for laryngeal cancer was higher than that for lung cancer. This was true for most countries throughout the world. The decline in risk in women after age 65 years almost certainly reflected a cohort phenomenon, as the habit of smoking in women followed by at least twenty years the pattern exhibited in men.

The average annual age-adjusted incidence per 100,000 population for laryngeal cancer was 8.6 for males and 1.2 for females between 1970 and 1974. Based on the Connecticut registry, the age-adjusted incidence has not changed in males since 1960 (Table 6). In contrast to lung cancer, the incidence of laryngeal cancer was not significantly greater for blacks than for whites.

Mortality

Mortality from laryngeal cancer more than doubled in the nonwhite male during the past thirty years (1950 to 1979). Concurrently, the rate of increase in lung cancer mortality in the nonwhite male was even more significant (Table 7). Laryngeal cancer mortality in white males and females did not change materially during the same period of time, whereas lung cancer mortality increased more than threefold in white males and fourfold in white females.

The mapping of cancer mortality by county in the United States has revealed a number and variety of geographic patterns and clusters. For larynx and lung cancer during the period 1950 to 1969, mortality was increased in the urban areas of the North. Rates were higher among whites when compared with nonwhites in the rural South, and higher among nonwhites in the urban South and Northeast.

International Patterns

International variation in site-specific incidence and mortality has heightened the epidemiologic search for, and recognition of, environmental factors that are major determinants of contrasting patterns. The incidence of cancer of the larynx varies worldwide; it generally predominates in males, while the rates in females tend to persist below 1.0 per 100,000. The magnitude of larynx cancer may not vary in any constant or predictable relationship to the incidence of lung cancer in the same population. Indian men and women are at high risk for both laryngeal and oral cavity cancer, but at rather low risk for lung cancer. In the United Kingdom, incidence rates are fairly low in contrast to the high rates for lung cancer. Between 1968 and 1972, the highest laryngeal cancer incidence in males was reported from Sao Paulo in Brazil (14.1 per 100,000). The highest incidence in women was

TABLE 6 Age-adjusted (1950 United States Standard) Incidence Rates per 100,000 Population for Larynx Cancer by Sex & Year of Diagnosis* (Connecticut, 1950–1974)

Year	Male	Female
1950–54	6.1	0.3
1955–59	6.2	0.6
1960–64	8.6	0.7
1965–69	8.6	1.0
1970–74	8.6	1.2

*Includes intrinsic & extrinsic larynx & in situ cancers.

TABLE 7   Age-Adjusted (1970 Standard Population) Mortality Rates per 100,000 Population for Larynx & Lung Cancer by Sex & Race(United States, 1950–1979)

Year	White Male			Nonwhite Male			White Female			Nonwhite Female		
	Larynx	Lung	Ratio*	Larynx	Lung	Ratio*	Larynx	Lung	Ratio*	Larynx	Lung	Ratio*
1950	2.6	21.9	8.4	1.8	16.0	8.9	0.3	4.9	16.3	0.4	4.0	10.0
1955	2.7	30.4	11.3	2.3	24.1	10.5	0.2	5.1	25.5	0.4	5.1	12.8
1960	2.7	38.0	14.1	3.1	37.3	12.0	0.2	5.6	28.0	0.4	5.9	14.8
1965	2.7	47.1	17.4	3.2	45.7	14.3	0.3	7.4	24.7	0.4	7.3	18.3
1970	2.9	57.4	19.8	3.4	62.0	18.3	0.3	11.1	37.0	0.5	11.2	22.4
1975	2.7	64.1	23.7	3.9	73.7	18.9	0.4	15.3	38.3	0.6	14.3	23.8
1979	2.7	68.7	25.4	4.0	81.3	20.3	0.4	19.4	48.5	0.5	18.3	36.6

*Ratio of age-adjusted lung cancer mortality to larynx cancer mortality.
From McKay, Hanson, & Miller.[5]

reported from Bombay, India (2.6 per 100,000). In the Mediterranean countries and those lying to the east along the same latitude as India, high incidence rates of laryngeal cancer were not generally accompanied by high rates of lung cancer, but were more significantly correlated with elevated oral and esophageal cancer incidence.

The distribution and temporal trend (1955 to 1976) of laryngeal and lung cancer mortality rates varied considerably from one country to another (Table 8). In most countries, the average annual percentage increases in laryngeal cancer mortality were inconsequential over a 20-year period. Countries such as Switzerland, Finland, the United Kingdom, and Japan experienced slight decreases in laryngeal cancer mortality, whereas lung cancer mortality increased significantly. As noted by McMichael, international laryngeal cancer mortality rates correlated better with levels of population alcohol consumption than with tobacco consumption.[11]

Nasopharynx

Incidence

Nasopharyngeal cancer, a rare neoplasm in the United States, accounts for 0.2 percent of all cancers. The most common form of cancer of the nasopharynx, regardless of geography, race, or ethnicity, is nasopharyngeal carcinoma (NPC). The World Health Organization recognizes three histopathologic types of NPC: (1) squamous cell carcinoma of varying grades of differentiation, (2) nonkeratinizing carcinoma, and (3) undifferentiated carcinoma. The distinction among the three types is not often possible because of mixed patterns. The term lymphoepithelial carcinoma is used when numerous lymphocytes are found among the tumor cells. The undifferentiated or poorly differentiated forms tend to be more common in high-risk populations or in the cases occurring in children and adolescents.

From 1973 to 1977, Chinese and Filipinos were

TABLE 8   Age-Adjusted Mortality Rates per 100,000 Population for Larynx and Lung Cancer in Selected Populations Throughout the World (1955–56 and 1975–76)

Country	Larynx		Lung	
	1955–56	1975–76	1955–56	1975–76
France	8.3	11.8	16.5	36.6
Portugal	4.5	4.3	7.2	15.1
Hungary	4.0	5.8	21.1	47.8
Italy	3.7	6.5	15.3	43.2
Switzerland	3.6	3.1	26.7	47.4
Belgium	3.3	4.6	28.0	68.4
Austria	3.3	3.7	43.0	50.5
Finland	3.0	2.0	45.4	63.4
United Kingdom	2.4	1.7	52.8	72.2
USA	2.1	2.2	25.1	51.6
Canada	1.7	2.3	21.2	46.5
Japan	1.7	1.4	6.3	20.0
Australia	1.7	2.3	20.9	46.6
New Zealand	1.6	2.0	25.8	49.5
Denmark	1.0	1.7	21.9	46.0
Sweden	0.5	0.8	10.8	23.9
Norway	0.4	0.9	8.4	22.5

reported to be at extremely high risk when compared to whites or blacks (Table 9). The two- to four-fold difference between the Chinese in San Francisco and the Hawaiian Chinese appeared to be related to the origins of these populations in China. Those in San Francisco consisted mainly of immigrants from the high-risk Canton area in southern China, where it was estimated that the annual incidence was 30/100,000. The age-standardized male-to-female incidence ratio was about 2 to 3:1 for each racial group in the United States.

International Patterns

While NPC is a rare neoplasm in North America, Europe, and Japan, it is common in specific regions of China and southeast Asia. The Chinese from southern provinces of Kwangsi, Kwangtung, Fukien, and Canton are at significantly higher risk than those from the northern provinces of Peking, Tientsin, and Shanghai. Moderately high incidence rates, between 1.5 and 9.0 per 100,000 are observed among the Eskimos, Malays, Hawaiians, Tunisians, Algerians, and Sudanese. In Israel, the risks are higher in Arabs and in Jews born in Africa or Asia than in Jews born in the United States or Europe.

In the Chinese, age-specific incidence is uncommon below the age of 15 years, rises sharply until age 50, reaches a plateau until age 64, and then declines. The proportion of NPC cases occurring in children is relatively higher in populations at moderately high risk.

Nasal Cavity and Paranasal Sinuses

Incidence

Cancers of the nasal cavity and paranasal sinuses accounts for 0.2 percent of all incident invasive malignant neoplasms in the United States and less than 2 percent of all incident respiratory cancers. The average annual age-adjusted incidence for sinonasal cancers (SNC) was 0.8 per 100,000 in males and 0.5 per 100,000 in females between 1969 and 1971. Age-specific incidence in females tended to be lower than in males at every age group. Unlike lung cancer, SNC incidence did not differ significantly between blacks and whites and was relatively stable over the past 25 years in the United States.[14]

TABLE 9 Average Annual Age-Adjusted (1970 United States Standard) Incidence per 100,000 Population for Cancer of the Nasopharynx by Sex and Race (SEER Program, 1973–1977)

Race	Male	Female
Chinese (San Francisco)	15.3	8.4
Chinese (Hawaii)	6.2	2.0
Filipinos	2.3	1.1
Blacks	0.8	0.4
Whites	0.7	0.3

Mortality

Prior to 1939, sinonasal cancer deaths were not coded separately within the respiratory system. From 1950 to 1975, there were about 575 to 600 sinonasal cancer deaths reported in the United States each year. In contrast to incidence, age-adjusted mortality among black males was 1.5 times that of white males during this period of time, whereas there were no appreciable differences between white and black females. The difference between the white and black males, namely, that mortality approximated the incidence in blacks and was about half the incidence in whites, was largely due to differential survival.

International Patterns

Between 1968 and 1972, the majority of countries with cancer incidence registries reported age-adjusted rates in the range of 0.3 to 1.0 per 100,000 for males and a 2.0:1 male to female ratio. Rates between 2.0 and 3.5 per 100,000 were reported in parts of Japan, Uganda, and Zimbabwe.[7] With respect to some areas with elevated rates in Africa, Baumslag et al reported increased risk among the Bantu who used intranasal snuff.[15] African sources of snuff had higher concentrations than European sources of polycyclic aromatic hydrocarbons, nitrosamines, nickel, and chromium.

Thyroid

Incidence

Thyroid cancer accounts for approximately 1 percent of the incident cancers in the United States. In 1984, the American Cancer Society anticipated that there would be 7400 newly diagnosed cases in females and 2900 in males. The average annual age-adjusted incidence per 100,000, as determined by the United States SEER Program (1973–1977), was 5.3 in white females, 4.0 in black females, 2.4 in white males, and 1.3 in black males. The age-specific incidence in females peaked initially between 25 and 44 years of age and then again after 65 years. The age-specific incidence in males tended to fluctuate, but the overall pattern was one of gradually increasing incidence with age.[16]

An analysis by Pottern et al, of the Connecticut Tumor Registry, over the years 1935 to 1975, demonstrated a five-fold increase in age-adjusted thyroid cancer incidence with a nearly constant female:male ratio of 3:1.[17] Papillary and follicular carcinomas, which accounted for about 65 percent of the registered cell types of thyroid cancer, were responsible for the upward incidence trends in females and males aged 25 to 44, and born between 1920 and 1960. During this time period (1935 to 1975), anaplastic and medullary carcinomas, about 9 percent and 10 percent of cell types, respectively, were not increased. Carroll et al reported in New York State that thyroid cancer inci-

TABLE 10   Relative Risk* of Death from Buccal Cavity, Larynx and Lung Cancer Among Men According to Average Number of Cigarettes Smoked per Day (United States Veterans Study)

Current Cigarette Smokers (amount per day)	Relative Risk of Death		
	Lung Cancer	Larynx Cancer	Buccal Cavity Cancer
1–9	5.5	5.3	2.9
10–20	9.9	9.2	2.9
21–39	17.4	14.8	6.2
40+	23.9	32.1	12.4

*Relative to a risk of 1.0 in men who never smoked regularly.
From Kahn.[23]

dence more than doubled in persons under age 55 between 1941 and 1962, and that cohorts born between 1910 and 1950 demonstrated a doubling of age-specific incidence with each successive decade of birth.[18] These cohort patterns in Connecticut and New York State coincided with the therapeutic practice from 1920 until the late 1950s of administering ionizing radiation to children and adolescents for thymic enlargement, oropharyngeal lymphoid hyperplasia, cervical lymphadenitis, and other benign conditions of the head and neck.[19]

Mortality

Thyroid cancer mortality in the United States (1976) accounted for approximately 0.5 percent of all cancer deaths in women and 0.2 percent in men. Black females had higher mortality than white females until age 65, after which the rate declined in blacks whereas the rate in whites continued to rise steadily. Among males, the rates were similar until age 65, when the rate in blacks stabilized while the rate in whites continued to rise. During a 20-year period (1950 to 1970), mortality decreased significantly in white females and males; the female:male ratio of age-adjusted mortality was 2.0. The declining age-adjusted mortality in the face of increasing age-adjusted incidence was due to significant concurrent gains in survival, particularly in younger women and men.[20]

Prevalence at Autopsy

In autopsy studies conducted during the 1960s in the United States where the thyroid gland was examined meticulously, the observed prevalence of occult thyroid cancer varied between 1.0 and 5.7 percent, and was approximately the same in men and women.[21] Other autopsy studies revealed broad differences in prevalence ranging from 0.3 percent in Switzerland to 28 percent in Japan. The prevalence of occult thyroid cancer diagnosed at autopsy in the Hawaiian Japanese was at least four times that observed in comparable autopsy studies in Canada and the United States.[22] However, clinically apparent thyroid cancer incidence in the Hawaiian Japanese was not significantly different from that observed in whites in the United States. From these data, one may sur-

mise that the host and environmental factors that promote clinical expression of disease are distinctive from those that initiate tumorigenesis.

ETIOLOGY

Tobacco

Epidemiologic studies demonstrated that the risk of oral cavity and laryngeal (i.e., both glottis and supraglottis) cancer was increased among cigarette smokers. The degree of exposure over time, as measured by the average daily amount smoked, affected the relative risk of developing cancer in tissues of the respiratory tract and oral cavity (Table 10). When compared with nonsmokers, a prospective study of United States veterans who smoked 40 or more cigarettes per day indicated that the relative risk of dying of lung cancer was increased almost 24-fold; of laryngeal cancer, 32-fold; and of oral cavity cancer, more than 12-fold.[23]

Both laboratory and epidemiologic studies have demonstrated that exposure to cigar and pipe tobacco smoke may produce cancers, particularly of the oral cavity and larynx. Although the risk of lung cancer was less for cigar or pipe smokers than for cigarette smokers, it was significantly higher than for nonsmokers (Table 11).

Although there has been general acceptance of the tumorigenic properties of tobacco-smoke condensates, or of forms of tobacco that involve combustion,

TABLE 11   Relative Risk* of Death from Buccal Cavity, Larynx, and Lung Cancer among Men According to Cigar and Pipe Smoking (United States Veterans Study)

Smoking Type	Relative Risk of Death		
	Lung Cancer	Larynx Cancer	Buccal Cavity Cancer
Cigar only	1.7	10.3	4.1
Pipe only	2.1	—	3.1
Total pipe & cigar	1.7	7.3	4.2

*Relative to a risk of 1.0 in men who never smoked regularly.
From Kahn.[23]

the use of snuff or chewing tobacco may also cause cancers in the mouth and pharynx. Winn et al estimated a fourfold increase in the risk of oral cancer among women in North Carolina who dipped snuff.[4] The area of the mouth in contact with the tobacco powder, the gingivobuccal sulcus, was most often affected after prolonged exposure. Brinton et al observed that cigarette and pipe smoking and use of intranasal snuff were significantly associated with the risk of sinonasal cancer.[24]

Cultural differences in the use of tobacco products have led to variations in the geographic incidence and anatomic location of head and neck cancers. In countries such as India, China, Thailand, Ceylon, Afghanistan, and the Central Republic of the Soviet Union, where the use of snuff and chewing tobacco was quite common, mortality rates for oral and pharyngeal cancer were among the highest in the world.[25] Tobacco chewing by men and women in India, for example, involved mixing a paste or quid of slaked lime (calcium hydroxide), tobacco leaves, betel nuts, and catechu (an astringent powder), wrapping this in dried betel leaves, and placing this mixture in the lower posterior gingivobuccal sulcus or under the anterior two-thirds of the tongue. The physiologic effects of chewing such a mixture were curbing of the appetite and increased salivation. Pathologic consequences consisted of extensive leukoplakia and, ultimately, epidermoid carcinoma of the gingivobuccal mucosa, tongue, and extrinsic larynx.[26]

There are general principles of tobacco carcinogenesis that apply to tissues in the upper digestive tract, respiratory tract, and urinary tract. These may be summarized as follows:

1. There is a dose-response relationship, so that the level of exposure (i.e., amount smoked, chewed, or snuffed; amount of particulate phase constituents or "tar" content of the smoke; depth and mode of inhalation; duration of the habit; use of filtered versus nonfiltered cigarettes) determines ultimately the level of risk for developing a tobacco-related cancer.

2. Smoking cessation reduces the risk at a rate influenced by the amount smoked previously and the duration of the habit. Among heavy, long-term smokers, at least 10 to 15 years of abstinence from smoking may be required before the level of excess risk stabilizes and approaches the level manifested by nonsmokers of comparable age.

3. The relative risk for developing a specific type of cancer depends on the susceptibility of a tissue to various concentrations of tobacco smoke constituents and their metabolites. Within the oral cavity and extrinsic larynx, direct contact with tobacco smoke and tobacco juice is of etiologic significance. Other organs such as the pancreas and kidney are affected by systemic metabolites of tobacco after metabolic activation in the liver and target tissues.

The lighted cigarette generates about 4000 compounds which can be separated into gas and particulate phases. The major tumorigenic activity of tobacco smoke is contained in the particulate matter or "tar" fraction. The composition of the tobacco smoke is a function of the physical and chemical properties of the leaf or blends of tobacco. The carcinogenic activity of the particulate matter results from a complex mixture of interacting initiators, promoters, and cocarcinogens. The primary initiators are presumably the polynuclear aromatic hydrocarbons and volatile nitrosamines.[27]

Alcohol

The balance of epidemiologic evidence supports the view that excessive alcohol consumption increases the risk of incurring epidermoid carcinomas of the oral cavity, pharynx, larynx, and esophagus. Alcohol and tobacco act synergistically, and are the salient co-factors responsible for at least 75 percent of upper aerodigestive tract cancer deaths (Table 12). The cancer sites for which tobacco and alcohol are major determinants in the United States are reported with greater frequency in men, lower socioeconomic groups, and

TABLE 12   Estimation of Cancer Deaths Attributable to Tobacco and/or Alcohol Consumption in the United States (1983)

Type of Cancer	Estimated Deaths (1983)*		Proportion Attributable to use of Tobacco and/or Alcohol	Number of Deaths Attributable to use of Tobacco and/or Alcohol	
	Men	Women		Men	Women
Mouth & pharynx	6,300	2,850	0.75	4,725	2,138
Larynx	3,100	600	0.75	2,325	450
Esophagus	6,200	2,300	0.75	4,650	1,725
Subtotal	15,600	5,750	0.75	11,700	4,313
All cancer deaths	238,500	201,500	0.30 (men)† 0.15 (women)†	71,550†	30,225†

*From American Cancer Society (1983).
†Including lung, urinary bladder and pancreas (primarily tobacco).

with increasing age and urbanization.[28]

The clearest demonstration of the combined effects of tobacco and alcohol on the relative risk for oral and pharyngeal cancer was provided by Rothman and Keller.[29] For each level of exposure to tobacco, the risk increased with increasing level of daily alcohol exposure. However, joint exposure to tobacco and alcohol resulted in risk ratios that were 2 to $2^1/_2$ times those expected if the effects of alcohol and tobacco were only additive (Table 13). In general, the appreciable cocarcinogenic action of ethanol with tobacco occurred with levels of exposure exceeding 45 ml of ethanol per day. The subsites within the upper aerodigestive tract manifesting a higher degree of correlation with past ethanol rather than tobacco exposure are floor of mouth, supraglottis, hypopharynx, and esophagus. This has been interpreted by Kissin as suggesting a direct topical rather than systemic action for ethanol.[30]

A patient with a previous epidermoid carcinoma of the upper aerodigestive tract has an increased risk of developing a new epithelial cancer within a subsite of the oral cavity, pharynx, larynx, and esophagus. In a previously published cohort study, multiple primaries were three times more frequent in patients with cancer of the supraglottis than in those with cancer of the intrinsic larynx. In the group of patients with an antecedent carcinoma of the supraglottis, the relative risk was increased 30-fold for a subsequent cancer of the oral cavity or pharynx, 18-fold for cancer of the esophagus, and fivefold for cancer of the lung. These observations were compatible with the patterns of excessive consumption of alcohol and smoking of cigarette, cigar, and pipe tobacco that were demonstrated in these patients.[31,32]

Epidemiologic studies have stimulated interest in the biochemical mechanisms whereby alcohol consumption increases the risk of developing cancer. In animal experiments, prolonged ethanol administration may be injurious to the liver and nervous system, but has not been shown to be carcinogenic. However, human ethanol consumption may include ingestion of by-products or contaminants known to be carcinogenic and present in alcoholic beverages, concomitant exposure to tobacco, and exacerbated nutritional deficiencies.

A variety of carcinogens including nitrosamines, polycyclic hydrocarbons, fusel oils (i.e., amyl alcohol by-products of fermentation), and other mutagenic compounds have been found in different types of alcoholic drinks.[33] Nitrosodiethylamine, a carcinogen demonstrated experimentally to be organotropic for upper digestive tract tissues such as the esophagus, has been detected in apple cider distillates at concentrations of 1 to 3 parts per billion. Nitrosodimethylamine was detected in varying amounts in most beers produced all over the world. Even if one or more carcinogens were identified in specific types of alcoholic beverages, the more fundamental pathogenic relationship observed in epidemiologic studies appears to be total ethanol intake.[34]

The two most likely mechanisms whereby ethanol may act as a cocarcinogen in the initiation phase of chemical carcinogenesis involve (1) the cytotoxic effects of ethanol and its metabolites and (2) the inducing effect of chronic ethanol consumption on microsomal enzyme activity. In addition to these rather direct effects of ethanol on target tissues, a multistage process may be influenced by various nutritional deficiencies associated with excessive alcohol consumption, or by effects of ethanol on the immune system.[35]

Epstein-Barr Virus and Nasopharyngeal Carcinoma

There is mounting seroepidemiologic and experimental evidence to support the hypothesis that the Epstein-Barr virus (EBV) is an etiologic factor in NPC. The correlates of an association are: (1) patients have significantly increased antibodies (IgG and IgA) against EBV viral capsid antigen (VCA), early antigen (EA), and nuclear antigen (EBNA), and (2) the tumor cells, particularly from undifferentiated carcinomas, always contain EBV genomes. The biopsy of tumor tissue has been successfully grafted to athymic (nude) mice, and the EBV genome once again demonstrated in epithelial tumor cells. The antibody titers to VCA, EA, and EBNA increase with advancing disease. Antibodies against EA and VCA reflect active EBV infection and replication. The regular presence of EBV DNA in the epithelial elements of nasopharyngeal carcinoma and the seroepidemiologic responses prevalent in patients throughout the world support the inference that EBV is a causative agent and not a secondary passenger.[36]

The increased risk of NPC in genetically distinct subpopulations of Chinese has suggested that genetic susceptibility is necessary for tumor induction. Chinese patients with NPC demonstrate an increase in the frequency of the first-locus leukocyte antigen (HL-A2) and of the Sin-2 or BW46 locus. The A2-BW46 haplotype has been regarded both as a risk factor and as an indicator of poor survival.[37] Little evidence at present suggests that there is a common universal HLA system complex that correlates consistently with NPC,

TABLE 13 Relative Risk for Oral Cavity Cancer According to Level of Exposure to Alcohol and Smoking

Alcohol Per Day (oz)	Cigarette Equivalents Per Day			
	0	Less Than 20	20–39	40 or more
None	1.00	1.52	1.43	2.43
< 0.4	1.40	1.67	3.18	3.25
0.4–1.5	1.60	4.36	4.46	8.21
> 1.5	2.33	4.13	9.59	15.50

From Rothman and Keller.[29] Risks are expressed relative to risk of 1.00 for persons who neither smoked nor drank.

but conceivably there may be other linkages between marker HLA genes and true susceptibility genes.

Dietary Factors

A number of nutritional factors are thought to be important as modifiers of carcinogenesis. Nutritional deficiencies are commonly associated with or exacerbated by excessive alcohol ingestion. These give rise to altered mucosal integrity, enzyme and metabolic dysfunction, and morphologic abnormalities in specific target organs.

Epidemiologic studies have suggested that adequate ingestion of foods containing vitamins A and C tend to protect against epithelial tumors in the oral cavity and respiratory tract.[38],[39] After adjusting for the combined effects of smoking and drinking, individuals with low intake of vitamin A or vitamin C had twice the relative risk of oral cavity or laryngeal cancer when compared with individuals ingesting large amounts of foods containing these vitamins. Vitamin A and its provitamin, beta carotene, are needed for normal growth and differentiation of epithelial tissues. A deficiency of vitamin A leads to a loss of mucociliary epithelium in the respiratory tract and its replacement by metaplastic squamous epithelium. Vitamin A and/or its synthetic analogs have been shown to inhibit tumor induction in the respiratory tract, skin, bladder, and mammary gland model tumor systems. Possible mechanisms of action arising from vitamin A deficiency that are under investigation include (1) metabolic activation and/or DNA binding of the carcinogen during the initiation phase, (2) enhancement of metaplastic epithelial proliferation during the postinitiation phase, and (3) impairment of immune function.[40],[41] Ascorbic acid is an antioxidant that blocks the formation of carcinogenic N-nitroso compounds. The substrate for these compounds may be derived from food or cigarette smoke.[42] Whether vitamin A or vitamin C are directly protective or whether they are correlated with other dietary factors fundamentally more essential in the natural inhibition of carcinogenesis awaits explication of future research.

The Plummer-Vinson or Paterson-Kelly syndrome was noted particularly in middle-aged northern Swedish women, who frequently have poor dentition, and was characterized by iron and multiple vitamin deficiencies, achlorhydria, papillary atrophy of the tongue, glossitis, atrophy of the epithelium of the upper alimentary tract, and esophageal webs or strictures. Women with this syndrome are at increased risk of developing carcinoma of the oral cavity, hypopharynx (postcricoid), and esophagus. The epithelial changes have been attributed to complex nutritional deficiencies. Tobacco and alcohol were not major etiologic factors in carcinomas of the upper alimentary tract in the Swedish women.[28] Riboflavin deficiency causes similar epithelial lesions in animals, and McCoy has hypothesized that the common link between Plummer-Vinson disease and alcohol consumption may

be the role that iron and riboflavin play in respiratory enzyme chemistry and its relationship to rates of metabolic activation of carcinogenic precursors.[43]

The evidence available does not yet support the conclusion that EBV alone is both the necessary and sufficient cause of nasopharyngeal cancer in both high- and low-risk populations. As demonstrated in animals, chemical carcinogens may reach the nasopharynx by inhalation, ingestion, and parenteral administration. Ho proposed that Cantonese salted and dried fish, consumed traditionally from early infancy, was an important etiologic factor in NPC.[44] Because NPC was the most common cancer among southern Chinese between the ages of 15 and 34, the focus of epidemiologic attention was on risk factors prevalent during childhood. Rats fed with salted fish developed malignant nasal and paranasal tumors. Salted fish contained appreciable quantities of nitrosodimethylamine and other N-nitroso compounds. Consumption of salted fish was unusual as a dietary staple in central and northern China where NPC was less common. Thus the complex natural history of NPC may be viewed as a dynamic interaction of viral, chemical, and genetic factors.

Occupational Factors

The risk of developing laryngeal cancer in different occupations was investigated in a case-control study using the interview data of the Third National Cancer Survey.[45] The Third National Cancer Survey was a study of all incident cancers in seven cities and two states during the 3-year period from 1969 to 1971. A 10 percent probability sample of these cancer cases was interviewed to obtain more detailed epidemiologic information. The relation between laryngeal cancer and employment was studied by industry and specific job category, after controlling for smoking and drinking. Of the 17 industrial categories studied, four industries—transportation equipment, general building, lumber and wood products, and railroad—were associated with relative risks that were increased 2.0 or higher. Of 22 job categories studied, the relative risk was 4.0 or higher among sheet-metal workers, automobile mechanics, miscellaneous mechanics and repairmen, electricians, and grinding wheel operators.

Specific occupational exposure factors linked with laryngeal cancer included asbestos, diethyl sulfate, mustard gas, and isopropyl alcohol.[46] In general, duration of exposure was positively correlated with relative risk, and latency from onset of exposure extended over a period of 10 or more years. In addition, one or more studies have reported the following occupational exposures or occupations to be associated with laryngeal cancer: nickel, wood dust, grease and oil, leather, paper, textiles (textile processors and operators), and naphthalene cleaners. Workers in the textile industry may have been exposed to machine oils, acrylonitrile, or compounds of cadmium, chromium, or nickel that are either established (i.e., chromium and nickel) or presumptive respiratory tract carcinogens.[47] In many of the published reports, the number of exposed cases was small, and studies were conflicting or required confirmation and/or did not always control for smoking and drinking.

Mortality from sinonasal cancer was shown to be significantly elevated in the United States where petroleum and chemical industries were concentrated.[48,49] Brinton et al observed significantly elevated relative risks for sinonasal adenocarcinoma among males employed in industries involving exposure to wood dust (e.g., furniture manufacturing).[24] The elevated risk was noted only for sinonasal adenocarcinoma, whereas tobacco use was associated with an increased risk of squamous carcinoma.

Other occupational agents and processes linked with SNC included nickel refining (metallic nickel or nickel carbonyl, oxide, or subsulfide), chrome pigment manufacturing, mustard gas manufacturing (dichloroethyl sulfide), isopropyl alcohol manufacturing (isopropyl oil or diisopropyl sulfate), boot and shoe manufacturing (leather or wood dust constituents), textile and clothing manufacturing and tool setters and tool makers (cutting oils containing polycyclic aromatic hydrocarbons).[50,51] Formaldehyde is a ubiquitous chemical of theoretic importance in human sinonasal cancer. It is potentially an important chemical exposure in the wood products, leather, and textile manufacturing industries. Although epidemiologic data are lacking in this regard, formaldehyde inhalation experiments in rats have induced squamous carcinomas of the nasal turbinates.[52]

ETIOLOGY OF THYROID CANCER

Thyroid neoplasia develops predictably in experimental animals exposed to ionizing radiation or to any procedure that induces prolonged, excessive thyroid-stimulating hormone (TSH) secretion. Excessive TSH secretion may be produced through dietary iodine deficiency, subtotal thyroidectomy, implantation of autonomous thyrotropic hormone-secreting pituitary tumors, or by the administration of chemical goitrogens. Augmentation of neoplasia, as evidenced by shortening of the latency period or increasing tumor incidence, or both, is achieved by the prior administration of a carcinogen such as 2-acetylaminofluorene or ionizing radiation followed by experimental induction of increased TSH stimulation.

How does TSH-induced hyperplasia lead to neoplasia, and to what degree does rapid proliferation of the follicular cells independently initiate the neoplastic process? The number of cytogenetic abnormalities within the thyroid epithelium apparently increases with the duration of increased TSH stimulation. Various investigators have interpreted experimental thyroid neoplasia as being analogous to the Berenblum-Shubik two-stage hypothesis of carcinogenesis. The two-stage hypothesis presumes two consecutive processes:

(1) initiation, which is analogous to the process of genetic mutation, and (2) promotion, which is reversible and dose-dependent, often with a dose threshold requiring multiple applications after initiation. Initiators may include ionizing radiation, chemical or biologic agents, and genetic factors. The major promoting factor may reside within the hypothalamic-pituitary-thyroid axis and be triggered by an excessive secretion of TSH.[53]

Doniach suggested that experimental thyroid neoplasia resulted from the chromosomal and mutational abnormalities induced by the imposition of accelerated mitosis in a tissue in which the normal rate of cell renewal was minimal.[54] Christov has shown that irradiation of the thyroid gland in adult rats achieved the highest incidence of tumors when administered after treatment with a goitrogen and at the time of peak cellular proliferation.[55]

Iodine Deficiency

In experimental animals such as rats, mice, and Syrian hamsters, chronic iodine deficiency may eventuate into carcinoma of the thyroid after a succession of pathogenic events which include intense follicular hyperplasia, hypertrophy, and nodule and adenoma formation. The evidence in man for an etiologic association between severe iodine deficiency and thyroid cancer has consisted of increased thyroid cancer incidence and mortality, particularly of the follicular and anaplastic types, in geographic areas considered to be at high risk for adenomatous or nodular goiter.[56,57] The foci of carcinoma have usually been located in otherwise normal parenchyma rather than within hyperplastic nodules. It has even been suggested that the frequency of goiter and thyroid cancer in Switzerland diminished after the introduction of iodized table salt. Those who argued against a direct causal relationship between endemic goiter and thyroid carcinoma pointed to prior studies in geographic areas where there was no correlation (i.e., Australia, Austria, Finland, and the United States), or where the frequency of goiter was low and thyroid cancer was high (i.e., Hawaii, Iceland, and Newfoundland).[58] Other reports from Switzerland subsequent to the introduction of iodized table salt did not substantiate a continuing trend of decreasing frequency of thyroid cancer mortality, decreasing incidence of goiter, and increasing proportion of thyroid cancers that were classified as papillary.[59,60] The observation of increased thyroid cancer mortality in an endemic goiter area, i.e., where the prevalence of goiter was 10 percent or greater, may have been due to the higher proportion of anaplastic carcinomas. It has also been suggested that the highly malignant hemangioendothelioma of the thyroid occurred in geographic areas where iodine was deficient and particularly in older patients with chronic goiter. In addition, thyroid enlargement due to iodine deficiency may have obscured the existence of a cancer, and because of delay in seeking medical care, the majority of malignant tumors were diagnosed at more advanced stages. In studies conducted in the United States during 1939 to 1951, the average annual age-adjusted mortality due to thyrotoxicosis (secondary to toxic nodular goiter and the diffuse hyperplasia of Graves' disease) diminished significantly in relation to the decreasing prevalence of endemic goiter; during the same period of time, the age-adjusted mortality due to thyroid cancer increased slightly.[61] To summarize, the epidemiologic evidence that endemic iodine deficiency may have served as a cause of the follicular type of thyroid carcinoma is unconvincing, although iodine prophylaxis may have altered the histologic pattern of thyroid cancer.

Radiation

Practically all human tissues are susceptible to the tumorigenic effects of ionizing radiation. Relative risks of radiogenic thyroid tumors are enhanced when exposures occur in childhood and early adult life, in women as contrasted with men, or in relationship to the stimulated metabolic state of the organ around the time of exposure (e.g., postpubertal development, pregnancy, intercurrent endocrine dysfunction). An important factor in determining whether malignant transformation occurs in one or more cells in irradiated tissue is the quantity of radiant energy absorbed in that tissue. As ionizing radiation penetrates living tissue, it gives up its energy through random collisions and interactions with molecules in its path. This impact of photons of radiant energy gives rise to ions and reactive chemical radicals that may disrupt chemical bonds, damage DNA, and alter the number and structure of chromosomes. The capacity to cause damage is correlated with the rate and concentration of energy forces that are dissipated within a volume of tissue.[62]

Papillary thyroid cancer is the principal cell type induced by ionizing radiation. Human radiogenic thyroid cancer has been studied in populations exposed to: (1) atomic bomb explosions in Hiroshima and Nagasaki,[63] (2) fallout radiation from nuclear weapons testing,[64] (3) x-ray therapy in childhood for various benign conditions in the head and neck,[65] and (4) diagnostic or therapeutic radioactive iodine.[66]

The studies of A-bomb survivors confirmed a greater risk of radiogenic thyroid cancer among females (female:male risk ratio of 3.5) and a threefold greater risk among those exposed before age 20 when compared with survivors exposed at a later age. The published dose-response information was interpreted to be consistent with a linear, nonthreshold relationship and a minimum latency period of about 5 years postirradiation. A period of elevated risk extended beyond 30 years of follow-up.

Modan et al reported 12 thyroid cancer cases among 11,000 children given epilating doses of x-ray to the scalp for tinea capitis, where two cases would have been expected.[67] The absolute risk was esti-mated to be 6.3 excess cases per million persons per year per rad for individuals exposed to an average of 6 to 9 rads to the thyroid. The studies of children exposed to the atomic bomb (average thyroid dose of about 130 rads) or x-ray therapy for benign conditions in the head and neck (average thyroid dose varied between 120 and 790 rads) estimated that the absolute risk was around 3.4 to 3.6 excess thyroid cancer cases per million persons per year per rad.[68] Neither thyroid cancer incidence nor leukemia was noted to be increaesed following I_{131} therapy for thyrotoxicosis, possibly because of the cell destruction, rather than malignant transformation, that followed doses of approximately 7000 to 10,000 rads to the thyroid.[69]

Mouthwash and Oral Cancer

Recently, regular use of mouthwash has been suggested as a possible risk factor in the development of oral and pharyngeal cancers. In a study of 200 cases, Weaver et al reported that in a small subgroup of nonsmoking and nondrinking cases, there was a significant excess of users of mouthwash when compared with 50 control patients.[70] Blot et al, as part of a case-control study of women from North Carolina with oral and pharyngeal cancers, noted almost a twofold increase in relative risk among users of mouthwash who abstained from tobacco.[71] The estimation of increased risk in this subgroup of nonusers of tobacco was based on only 8 cases and 61 controls. There was no consistent trend in terms of frequency of daily use, or whether the mouthwash was taken in full strength or diluted form. Similarly, in the study of Wynder et al, daily mouthwash use was associated with increased risk in women who were nonsmokers and nondrinkers, but no dose-response effect was demonstrable in the women, and no effect was observed in the men.[72] In each study, the difference in chronic mouthwash use between cases and controls was not limited to the period immediately preceding diagnosis. It is possible that commercial mouthwashes, which contain various flavoring and coloring agents as well as significant amounts of ethanol, may be irritating and injurious to the oral mucosa after prolonged and regular use, but it is not possible at this time to infer any causal association.

REFERENCES

1. American Cancer Society: Cancer Facts and Figures. 1984.
2. Moore C, Catlin D. Anatomic origins and locations of oral cancer. Am J Surg 1967; 114:510–513.
3. Blot WJ, Fraumeni JF Jr. Geographic patterns of oral cancer in the United States: Etiologic implications. J Chron Dis 1977; 30:745–757.
4. Winn DM, Blot WJ, Shy CM, et al. Snuff dipping and oral cancer among women in the southern United States. N Engl J Med 1981; 304:745–749.
5. McKay FW, Hanson MR, Miller RW. Cancer mortality in the United States: 1950–1977. National Cancer Institute Monographs (No. 59) Washington, DC: US Government Printing Office, 1982.

6. Axtell LM, Asire AJ, Myers MH. Cancer patients survival. (Report No. 5) Washington, DC: US Government Printing Office, 1976.
7. Waterhouse J, Muir CS, Correa P, et al. Cancer incidence in five continents. (Vol III). Lyon: IARC Scientific Publication No. 15, 1976.
8. Reddy CR. Carcinoma of hard palate in India in relation to reverse smoking of chuttas. J Natl Cancer Inst 1974; 53:615–619.
9. Rothman KJ, Cann CI, Flanders D, et al. Epidemiology of laryngeal cancer. Epidemiol Rev 1980; 2:195–209.
10. Dunham LJ, Bailar JC. World maps of cancer mortality rates and frequency ratios. J Natl Cancer Inst 1968; 41:155–203.
11. McMichael AJ. Increases in laryngeal cancer in Britain and Australia in relation to alcohol and tobacco consumption trends. Lancet 1978; 1:1244–1247.
12. Shanmugaratnam K. Nasopharynx. In: Schottenfeld D, Fraumeni JF Jr, eds. Cancer epidemiology and prevention. Philadelphia: WB Saunders, 1982:536–553.
13. Schottenfeld D. The epidemiology of cancer: An overview. Cancer 1981; 47:1095–1108.
14. Redmond CK, Sass RE, Roush GC. Nasal cavity and paranasal sinuses. In: Schottenfeld D, Fraumeni JF Jr, eds. Cancer epidemiology and prevention. Philadelphia: WB Saunders, 1982:519–535.
15. Baumslag N, Keen P, Petering HG. Carcinoma of the maxillary antrum and its relationship to trace metal content of snuff. Arch Environ Hlth 1971; 23:1–5.
16. Schottenfeld D, Gershman S. Epidemiology of thyroid cancer. CA 1978; 28:66–86.
17. Pottern LM, Stone BJ, Day NE, et al. Thyroid cancer in Connecticut 1935–1975: An analysis by cell type. Am J Epidemiol 1980; 112:764–774.
18. Carroll RE, Haddon W Jr, Handy VH, et al. Thyroid cancer: Cohort analysis of increasing incidence in New York State, 1941–1962. J Natl Cancer Inst 1964; 33:277–283.
19. Greenspan FS. Radiation exposure and thyroid cancer. JAMA 1977; 237:2089–2091.
20. Ron E, Modan B. Thyroid. In: Schottenfeld D, Fraumeni JF Jr, eds. Cancer epidemiology and prevention. Philadelphia: WB Saunders, 1982:837–854.
21. Sampson RJ, Key CR, Buncher CR, et al. Thyroid carcinoma in Hiroshima and Nagasaki. Prevalence of thyroid carcinoma at autopsy. JAMA 1969; 209:65–70.
22. Fukunaga FH, Yatani R. Geographic pathology of occult thyroid carcinomas. Cancer 1975; 36:1095–1099.
23. Kahn HA. The Dorn study of smoking and mortality among US veterans: Report on 8½ years of observation. J Natl Cancer Inst 1966; 19:1–125.
24. Brinton LA, Blot WJ, Becker JA, et al. A case-control study of cancers of the nasal cavity and paranasal sinuses. Am J Epidemiol 1984; 119:896–906.
25. Schottenfeld D. Snuff dipper's cancer. N Engl J Med 1981; 304:778–779.
26. Schonland M, Bradshaw E. Upper alimentary tract cancer in Natal Indians with special reference to the betel chewing habit. Br J Cancer 1969; 23:670–682.
27. Wynder EL, Hoffman D. Tobacco. In: Schottenfeld D, Fraumeni JF Jr, eds. Cancer epidemiology and prevention. Philadelphia: WB Saunders, 1982:277–292.
28. Schottenfeld D. Alcohol as a co-factor in the etiology of cancer. Cancer 1979; 43:1962–1966.
29. Rothman K, Keller AZ. The effect of joint exposure to alcohol and tobacco on risk of cancer of the mouth and pharynx. J Chron Dis 1972; 25:711–716.
30. Kissin B. Epidemiologic investigation of possible biological interactions of alcohol and cancer of the head and neck. Ann NY Acad Sci 1975; 252:374–384.
31. Berg JW, Schottenfeld D, Ritter F. Incidence of multiple primary cancers. III Cancers of the respiratory and upper digestive system as multiple primary cancers. J Natl Cancer Inst 1970; 44:263–274.
32. Schottenfeld D, Gantt RC, Wynder EL. The role of alcohol and tobacco in multiple primary cancers of the upper digestive system, larynx, and lung: A prospective study. Prev Med 1974; 3:277–293.
33. Lieber CS, Garro A, Gordon GG. Alcohol as a mutagen, carcinogen, and teratogen. In: Lieber CS, ed. Medical disorders of alcoholism: pathogenesis and treatment Philadelphia: WB Saunders, 1982:526–550.
34. Tuyns AJ. Alcohol. In: Schottenfeld D, Fraumeni JF Jr, eds. Cancer epidemiology and prevention. Philadelphia: WB Saunders, 1982:293–303.
35. Schottenfeld D. Epidemiology of cancer of the esophagus. Semin Oncol 1984; 11:92–100.
36. De The G, Zeng Y. Epstein-Barr virus and nasopharyngeal carcinoma. In: Evans PHR, Robin PE, Fielding JWL, eds. Head and neck cancer. New York: Alan R Liss, 1983:43–51.
37. Simons MJ, Day NE. Histocompatibility leukocyte antigen patterns and nasopharyngeal carcinoma. Natl Cancer Inst Monogr 1977; 47:143–146.
38. Graham S, Mettlin C, Marshall J, et al. Dietary factors in the epidemiology of cancer of the larynx. Am J Epidemiol 1981; 113:675–680.
39. Marshall J, Graham S, Mettlin C, et al. Diet in the epidemiology of oral cancer. Nutr Cancer 1982; 3:145–149.
40. De Luca L, Maestri N, Bonanni F, et al. Maintenance of epithelial cell differentiation. The mode of action of vitamin A. Cancer 1972; 30:1326–1331.
41. Sporn MB. Retinoids and carcinogenesis. Nutr Rev 1977; 35:65–69.
42. Mirvish SS. Blocking the formation of N-nitroso compounds with ascorbic acid in vitro and in vivo. Ann NY Acad Sci 1975; 258:175–180.
43. McCoy GD. A biochemical approach to the etiology of alcohol-related cancers of the head and neck. Laryngoscope 1978; 88:59–62.
44. Ho JHC, Huang DP, Fong YY. Salted fish and nasopharyngeal carcinoma in Southern Chinese. Lancet 1978; 2:826.
45. Flanders WD, Rothman KJ. Occupational risk for laryngeal cancer. Am J Public Hlth 1982; 72:369–372.
46. Decoufle P. Occupation. In: Schottenfeld D, Fraumeni JF Jr, eds. Cancer epidemiology and prevention. Philadelphia: WB Saunders, 1982:318–335.
47. Flanders WD, Cann CI, Rothman KJ, et al. Work-related risk factors for laryngeal cancer. Am J Epidemiol 1984; 119:23–32.
48. Hoover R, Fraumeni JF Jr. Cancer mortality in US counties with chemical industries. Environ Res 1975; 9:196–207.
49. Blot WJ, Brinton LA, Fraumeni JF Jr, et al. Cancer mortality in US counties with petroleum industries. Science 1977; 198:51–53.
50. Roush GC. Epidemiology of cancer of the nose and paranasal sinuses: Current concepts. Head Neck Surg 1979; 2:3–11.
51. Cecchi F, Buiatti E, Kriebel D, et al. Adenocarcinoma of the nose and paranasal sinuses in shoemakers and woodworkers in the province of Florence, Italy (1963–1977). Br J Ind Med 1980; 37:222–225.
52. Pera F, Petito C. Formaldehyde: A question of cancer policy. Science 1982; 216:1285–1291.
53. Nadler NJ, Mandavia M, Goldbert M. The effect of hypophysectomy on the experimental production of rat thyroid neoplasms. Cancer Res 1970; 30:1909–1911.
54. Doniach I. The effect of radioactive iodine alone and in combination with methylthiouracil and acetylaminofluorene upon tumor production in the rat's thyroid gland. Br J Cancer 1950; 4:223–234.
55. Christov K. Thyroid cell proliferation in rats and induction of tumors by X-rays. Cancer Res 1975; 35:1256–1261.
56. Cuello C, Correa P, Eisenberg H. Geographic pathology of thyroid carcinoma. Cancer 1969; 23:230–239.
57. Wahner HW, Cuello C, Correa P, et al. Thyroid carcinoma in an endemic goiter area, Cali, Colombia. Am J Med 1966; 40:58–66.
58. Ramalingaswami V. Iodine and thyroid cancer in man. In: Hedinger CE, ed. Thyroid cancer. Berlin: Springer-Verlag, 1969:111–123.
59. Thalman A. Incidence of malignant goiter at the Berne Patho-

logical Institute during the period 1910–1960. Relation to iodine prophylaxis against endemic goiter. Schweiz Med Wschr 1954; 84:474–478.

60. Walthard B. The influence of the iodine prophylaxis of goiter on the frequency of cancer of the thyroid gland and on its structure. In: Pitt-Rivers R, ed. Advances in Thyroid Research. Oxford: Pergamon Press, 1961:350–351.

61. Riccabona C. Hyperthyroidism and thyroid cancer in an endemic goiter area. In: Dunn JT, ed. Endemic goiter and cretinism: continuing threats to world health. Washington DC: Pan American Health Organization, 1974:156–165.

62. Upton AC. The biological effects of low-level ionizing radiation. Sci Am 1982; 246:41–49.

63. Beebe GW. The atomic bomb survivors and the problem of low-dose radiation effects. Am J Epidemiol 1981; 114:761–783.

64. Conard RA. Summary of thyroid findings in Marshallese 22 years after exposure to radioactive fallout. In: DeGroot LJ, ed. Radiation-associated thyroid carcinoma. New York: Grune and Stratton, 1977:241–257.

65. Hempelmann LH, Hall WJ, Phillips M, et al. Neoplasms in persons treated with x-rays in infancy: Fourth survey in 20 years. J Natl Cancer Inst 1975; 55:519–530.

66. Dobyns BM, Sheline GE, Workman JB, et al. Malignant and benign neoplasms of the thyroid in patients treated for hyperthyroidism: A report of the cooperative thyrotoxicosis therapy follow-up study. J Clin Endocrinol Metab 1974; 38:976–998.

67. Modan B, Ron E, Werner A. Thyroid cancer following scalp irradiation. Radiology 1977; 123:741–744.

68. Shore RE, Woodward ED, Hempelmann LH. Radiation-induced thyroid cancer. In: Boice JD, Fraumeni JF Jr, eds. Radiation carcinogenesis: epidemiology and biological significance. New York: Raven, 1984:131–138.

69. Boice JD Jr, Land CE. Ionizing radiation. In: Schottenfeld D, Fraumeni JF Jr, eds. Cancer epidemiology and prevention. Philadelphia: WB Saunders, 1982:231–253.

70. Weaver A, Fleming SM, Smith DB. Mouthwash and oral cancer: Carcinogen or coincidence? J Oral Surg 1979; 37:250–253.

71. Blot WJ, Winn DM, Fraumeni JF Jr. Oral cancer and mouthwash. J Natl Cancer Inst 1983; 70:251–253.

72. Wynder EL, Kabat G, Rosenberg S, et al. Oral cancer and mouthwash use. J Natl Cancer Inst 1983; 70:255–260.

3. New and Innovative Aspects of Pathology

ROBERT E. FECHNER, M.D.

Microscopic examination of tissue continues to be the sole manner in which the unequivocal diagnosis of cancer is made. The light microscope and routine histologic techniques that have been used for more than a century remain the diagnostic mainstays. Nonetheless, additional methods have become available that go beyond what can be accomplished by examining histologic sections. Electron microscopy or immunohistochemistry may provide discriminating information that is crucial to an accurate diagnosis, especially in small- cell, undifferentiated neoplasms. As therapeutic regimens are developed that are effective against one neoplasm but not another, it is increasingly important to make pathologic diagnoses as accurate as possible.

The next step, after the diagnosis of a malignant neoplasm, is to predict its biologic behavior. This has met with only partial success. In the past, the pathologist has relied on subjective evaluations to classify tumors as "well-differentiated," "high grade," and so on. Unfortunately, the subjectivity in the interpretation of such "measurements" has limited their value. Attempts to quantitate a variety of histologic parameters, as by the Jakobsson method,[1] continue to be refined. The studies by Crissman are especially notable.[2]

A desire for more objective methods of assessing the cellular features of tumors has stimulated development of new techniques, including the use of new instruments that provide a wide variety of methods for examining cytologic detail. Many of the methods circumvent the shortcomings of subjective interpretations by precisely measuring parameters with computer-assisted techniques. These methlologic advances must be exploited to the fullest if new insights are to be gained that will lead to a better understanding of the biologic potential of neoplasms. Some of the techniques to be discussed have not been applied to head and neck cancers, whereas others have been applied in only a limited number of patients. Data obtained from the study of tumors outside the head and neck region may or may not be applicable, but if the techniques are useful in evaluating tumors from other sites, they deserve to be explored for their possible relevance to head and neck cancer.

The ensuing discussion includes a brief mention of electron microscopy and the importance of proper harvesting of neoplastic tissue. This is followed by descriptions of techniques that may become useful in the initial diagnosis of head and neck cancer and techniques that may be helpful in predicting the behavior of cancer.

HARVEST OF TISSUE

The opportunity for the best pathologic diagnosis requires forethought and clinical judgement regarding the proper harvest of tissue. For example, if the differential diagnosis includes malignant lymphoma, fresh frozen tissue should be taken for immunologic studies and cell suspensions for flow cytometry. It is no longer acceptable to take a biopsy from a patient with possible lymphoma and plunge it into formalin. In other situations, correct fixation for examination with the electron microscope is necessary. A frozen section of the tumor may be required to demonstrate the need for electron microscopy. For instance, an adult with a polypoid mass in the nose may have an undifferentiated tumor on frozen section that could be melanoma, lymphoma, esthesioneuroblastoma, or undifferentiated carcinoma. By realizing this differential problem, the pathologist can take additional pieces of fresh tumor for immediate fixation in an appropriate fixative such as glutaraldehyde.

Another technique for harvesting neoplastic tissue is fine-needle aspiration. The cellular material is smeared, stained, and microscopically examined in the same manner as routine cytologic specimens. Fine-needle aspiration has been used extensively for decades in the Scandinavian countries, and it is now becoming widely employed in the United States.[3] In essence, a suspension of tumor cells is aspirated through a needle 0.6 to 1.0 mm in external diameter (essentially 22-gauge). The procedure usually does not require a local anesthetic, and several passes can be made into different parts of the tumor. Many areas of the lesion are sampled rather than the single core obtained with a cutting needle of larger gauge. Fine-needle aspiration does not implant the tumor in the needle track, and there are virtually no complications.

Fine-needle aspiration is highly cost-effective as a definitive diagnostic procedure. It also provides cells in a suspension that is suitable for study by flow cytometry, an important technique (to be discussed). Because of the negligible morbidity, a lesion can be repeatedly aspirated over a period of time, thereby providing cells for sequential studies that may detect alterations in tumor kinetics during therapy.

ELECTRON MICROSCOPY

One technique that has been available for about 20 years is electron microscopy. This tool is of great value in visualizing cytoplasmic structures (e.g., premelanosomes or melanosomes in melanoma or striations in rhabdomyosarcoma.) Defining cell shapes beyond what can be seen by the light microscope can also be useful. Under the electron microscope, the cells of esthesioneuroblastoma have elongated cell processes that are not perceptible by light microscopy, a feature that separates the lesion from lymphoma and other small-cell tumors that may be confused with esthesioneuroblastomas. Numerous other situations could be described in detail, but space limitations preclude this.

In a preliminary study, Incze et al studied biopsies of normal mucosa from smokers, nonsmokers, and reformed smokers in an attempt to judge malignancy by ultrastructural examination.[4] Some patients had concurrent cancer or had had cancer in the past. Twenty-eight ultrastructural abnormalities were sought in the nucleus, nucleolus, cytoplasm, basement membrane, cell attachments, and stroma. Nonsmokers and reformed smokers had an average of 1.2 abnormalities per cell; smokers without cancer had 2.3 abnormalities, and smokers with cancer had 6.3 abnormalities. These observations are in keeping with a stepwise progression of structural abnormalities toward the occurrence of cancer during a clinically latent period. Of particular interest is the lack of abnormalities in the reformed smokers, including one who had had morphologic abnormalities before he quit smoking. The authors point out that this method of study provides the clinican with an objective assay of the severity of mucosal alterations induced by tobacco.

TECHNIQUES APPLICABLE TO THE DIAGNOSIS OF CARCINOMA AND CARCINOMA IN SITU

Looking at an individual cell and deciding that it is malignant is an impossible task. Many benign tumors and reactive processes contain cells with every abnormal feature that can be found in malignant cells. This means that the diagnosis of malignant squamous cells requires indubitable evidence of invasion, evidence that is often lacking in small biopsies. Furthermore, some lesions have abnormal squamous cells that are confined to the epithelium, and although they may be transformed cells (i.e., malignant cells), they cannot be separated from abnormal benign cells. Some intraepithelial lesions with abnormal cells are diagnosed as atypia or dysplasia, whereas others are diagnosed as carcinoma in situ. Despite this sharp division in words, it is nonetheless an arbitrary distinction. As Ober wisely said, carcinoma in situ is "a diagnosis of opinion, not of fact."[5] It is obvious that an invasive carcinoma must begin from cells located within the epithelium, and that there is a stage in which noninvasive malignant cells exist. Until it becomes possible to recognize malignant cells, short of invasion, the term carcinoma in situ serves little purpose. It might be replaced with a more general term such as "intraepithelial neoplasia," coupled with a modifier such as "mild" or "severe nuclear atypia." Indeed, lesions that do not fulfill the traditional definition of carcinoma in situ (full-thickness involvement by malignant-appearing cells) will be followed by invasive carcinoma as frequently as lesions called carcinoma in situ.[6]

The meticulous studies by Auerbach et al suggested that atypia and so-called carcinoma in situ are reversible in cigarette smokers who quit smoking. Their data disclosed that nearly 16 percent of 1644 cigarette smokers had carcinoma in situ at the time of autopsy, and 99 percent had atypia. By contrast, none of the ex-cigarette smokers had carcinoma in situ, and only 25 percent had mild atypia, figures similar to those who had never smoked. It is likely that the ex-smokers had a high frequency of atypia and carcinoma in situ at the time they were smoking, but it did not persist after smoking was discontinued.[7]

The cells of invasive cancer have alterations that can be measured by several techniques, and it is possible to see these same changes in the cells of non-invasive lesions. The goal is to identify carcinomas before they become life-threatening, when minimal therapy should be curative.

Two techniques have been developed in the last few years that are altering profoundly the pathologist's approach to diagnosis. One is the immunoperoxidase method that identifies antigens in ordinary paraffin-embedded tissue sections, thereby needing no special tissue harvesting. Tissue blocks obtained years ago can be recut and examined for specific antigens. A great deal of information can be obtained by staining the ''old'' tissue, and there is an instant clinical follow-up interval.

The second technique, the ability to produce highly purified antibodies by the hybridoma method, has enhanced the value of the immunoperoxidase staining process. These two methods will now be looked at in detail. Compared to other techniques (to be discussed), they probably form the most immediately applicable methods for the study of abnormal cells and extracellular structures that are important in the study of cancer.

MONOCLONAL ANTIBODIES

The production of monoclonal antibodies by the hybridoma technique takes advantage of mice myeloma cells that are not secreting any immunoglobulins and that are immortal in vitro. Therefore, they are a vehicle that can be fused with normal plasma cells that *are* producing a single antibody. These fused cells literally become an antibody factory. Not all of the antibodies can be used for immunohistochemical studies for a variety of technical reasons, and there may be problems of cross-reaction and nonspecificity that accompany any antibody. Nonetheless, this technique is yielding, almost daily, new antibodies that are of diagnostic value.

There are three major ways that monoclonal antibodies can be used: in vitro tissue analysis, serologic analysis, and in vivo radioimaging and therapy. The last-mentioned is at an experimental stage, and its use has been restricted by undesirable cross-reactivity and hypersensitivity to mouse immunoglobulin. Nonetheless, it represents a rich area for further investigation.[8]

The second major use of monoclonal antibodies is the serologic diagnosis of cancer. Its usefulness is limited to tumor antigens that are released by the cells, but luckily, many abnormal glycoproteins and glycolipids are located on the tumor cell membranes. Moreover, they are highly antigenic and often (but not invariably) shed into the blood. Whether wide-scale surveys against these antigens can serve as effective screening for cancer is still unclear. It is more likely that they will be used to monitor disease in patients already known to have cancer.[9,10]

The third use of monoclonal antibodies is on tissue in vitro (immunohistochemistry). The application of these antibodies has been enormously enhanced by the immunoperoxidase technique that will now be discussed in detail.

IMMUNOHISTOCHEMISTRY INCLUDING THE IMMUNOPEROXIDASE METHOD

Immunologic methods of studying neoplasms include the use of immunofluorescence and immunoperoxidase techniques for demonstrating cellular features including hormones, enzymes, oncofetal antigens, and other compounds. These markers sometimes allow sharp distinction between small cell tumors that otherwise lack distinguishing features by light microscopy. Immunofluorescence requires fresh tissue that is snap-frozen. Tissue sections are cut on a cryostat and stained either by the direct or the indirect method. The direct method employs a fluorochrome (fluorescein or rhodamine) conjugated to the specific antibody that is applied directly on the tissue. The indirect method requires a second step. In addition to applying the antibody to the tissue, a fluorochrome-labeled antibody directed against the globulin fraction of the first antibody is added. Regardless of the method of labeling, the antigen-antibody reaction requires activation by ultraviolet light in a dark-field microscope. The lack of permanence of the sections used for fluorescence, and the difficulty in correlating the fluorescent images with the histopathology as viewed with conventional light microscopy have limited the usefulness of this method.

Without a doubt, the development of immunoperoxidase techniques constitutes one of the most fundamental new tools for the characterization of antigens in normal and neoplastic cells as well as extracellular elements. The sensitivity is at least equal to, and usually exceeds, that of the immunofluorescent methods already mentioned. The immunoperoxidase test does not require conjugated antibodies and avoids many of the disadvantages of the conjugation procedure, such as inactivation of enzyme and denaturation of the antibody.

The immunoperoxidase technique relies on bridges of antibody that connect the antigen to peroxidase. In the final step, the tissue is incubated with hydrogen peroxide and a chromogen (usually diaminobenzidine). If the antigen is present, the chromogen is oxidized and assumes a brown color, a reaction that takes place only at the precise point where the antigen is bound to the peroxidase. Sections are then stained with hematoxylin and coverslipped with a resin that produces permanent sections. One can see the exact cells where the brown granules mark the site of the antigen-antibody reaction.

Now that we know that the methodology is available for accurate identification and localization of innumerable intra- and extracellular substances, how can this be exploited? Can it help in the diagnosis of cancer? Can it help in judging the prognosis of cancer?

Let us digress for a moment to consider some current avenues of research into the characteristics of malignant cells and their interaction with the stroma that they permeate. The study of stroma may seem an odd way to approach the diagnosis of cancer, but nonetheless, many alterations occur around malignant cells. It is possible that they could have diagnostic importance.

Epithelium is intimately associated with the basement membrane that the cell produces. By electron microscopy two layers are evident: the lamina rara and the lamina densa. Although the molecular interactions are not fully understood, there are two substances, laminin (a proteoglycan macromolecule) and type IV collagen, that are unique to the basement membrane.

Barsky et al have demonstrated that malignant tumors elaborate an enzyme that preferentially digests type IV collagen.[11] Moreover, a positive correlation between the amount of collagenolytic activity of the malignant cells and their metastatic potential has been demonstrated.[12] Antibodies to both type IV collagen and to type IV collagenase have been prepared. Thus one can show the loss of basement membrane by staining tissue sections with antibody to type IV collagen. The potential value of this has been demonstrated on intraductal, noninvasive carcinomas of the breast that are completely surrounded by intact basement membrane. Sometimes, small protrusions of epithelium are seen that raise the differential diagnosis of an irregular contour of noninvasive cancer versus a small focus of invasion. When the sections are stained for type IV collagen, the protrusions lack type IV collagen immediately beneath the cells, although it is present under the adjacent nonprotruding cells. The protruding foci presumably are the earliest manifestation that a noninvasive carcinoma is becoming invasive.[11]

The pertinence of these observations to squamous carcinoma revolves around the difficulty of assessing invasion of small, unoriented biopsies (usually from the larynx). If the biopsy comes from a lesion that is not an obvious cancer clinically, the diagnosis rests solely on the histologic findings. We have already stated that we cannot rely on cytologic abnormalities to tell whether the cells are malignant. Detached nests of epithelium may suggest invasion, but they also may be only tangential sections of hyperplastic epithelium. Even serial sections often fail to verify continuity of the nests with the overlying epithelium, thereby suggesting carcinoma. By use of the immunoperoxidase technique with antibody to type IV collagen, the absence of the basement membrane around these isolated nests might prove to be an excellent criterion of malignancy. Conversely, the presence of type IV collagen would be evidence for a benign process. The diagnostic applicability of staining the basement membrane must be carefully evaluated because malignant cells sometimes form basement membranes, although they are usually incomplete. Paradoxically, adenoid cystic carcinoma produces large quantities of basement membrane that are visible with the light microscope as the amorphous, acellular material that contributes to the distinctive pattern of this neoplasm.

In addition to the destruction of the basement membrane, there is considerable interplay between malignant cells and stroma. Carcionomas often stimulate excessive connective tissue formation, and in some carcinomas, such as breast, most of the palpable mass is the reactive connective tissue rather than the epithelium. Indeed, the matrix of human breast cancer cells has been shown to be mitogenic for fibroblasts.[13] In another organ, the endometrium, the distinction between atypical hyperplasia and carcinoma is a common problem, and a desmoplastic (fibrous tissue) response has been suggested recently as a criterion for the diagnosis of carcinoma.[14] In other words, a stromal change is sometimes more helpful than the epithelial alterations. The recognition of even a minute focus of desmoplastic response in the endometrium is easy to recognize because fibrous tissue is normally completely absent.

Desmoplasia is not so easily recognized in the mucous membranes of the upper aerodigestive system where fibrous tissue is a normal constituent. This necessitates identifying other markers of malignancy within connective tissue. One substance that is increased within the connective tissue of neoplasms is the enzyme cathepsin B. Cathepsin B may be secreted by malignant cells or the cancer may stimulate its formation by non-neoplastic stromal cells. This protease degrades collagen and stromal proteoglycans and presumably enhances the spread of malignant cells. The enzyme is localized at the advancing edge of the tumor in a rabbit model,[15] and in another animal tumor (melanoma) the elevation of cathepsin B is correlated with the metastatic potential.[16] Human breast carcinomas contain far higher concentrations of the enzyme than do benign breast tumors,[17] and increased levels have been found in human colon and lung cancers.[18]

Fibroblasts derived from human basal cell carcinomas can secrete high levels of collagenase.[19] Even though desmoplasia reflects an increase in the amount of collagen, it is possible that high levels of collagenase are a manifestation of the vigorous turnover of collagen during the connective tissue reaction. Squamous carcinomas of the oral cavity and larynx have variable levels of collagenase when extracts of tumor are analyzed in vitro, and Abramson et al showed that high collagenase activity correlated with poor survival in patients with squamous carcinoma at these sites.[20]

What can be identified in cells that may be useul markers of abnormal function, either in preneoplastic or neoplastic cells? To bridge the prior discussion regarding stromal changes, Barsky et al have demonstrated large quantities of type IV collagenase in breast carcinoma cells.[11] Obviously, this destroys the basement membrane. The enzyme would not only permit the cells to invade the stroma, but it presumably could destroy the basement membrane around lymphatic or vascular channels, thereby promoting the chance for metastasis.

There are several intracytoplasmic constituents that can be expressed abnormally in either benign or malignant squamous cells. One example is involucrin, which, unlike keratin, is a single-molecular-weight species. It is normally located near the cell membrane of squamous cells. Murphy et al used the immunoperoxidase technique to study cutaneous lesions and found that the cells of the normal epidermis had diffuse staining in the upper third.[21] On the other hand, patchy staining occurred in carcinoma in situ. The cells of invasive squamous cell carcinomas were negative for involucrin, whereas the cells of pseudoinvasive hyperplasia at the base of a benign lesion (keratoacanthoma) were focally positive. This provides the possibility for distinguishing between pseudoepitheliomatous hyperplasia and microinvasive carcinoma in other sites.

A major intracytoplasmic constituent of squamous epithelium is keratin, which corresponds with the tonofilaments seen ultrastructurally. Keratin is a family of several members with molecular weights ranging between 40 to 67 kilodaltons. The largest keratin polypeptides are produced only in the most mature squamous cells. Winter et al, using electrophoresis, found that cell cultures of murine cutaneous squamous cancers failed to synthesize the largest keratins.[22] They extended their electrophoretic studies to human cutaneous and vaginal carcinomas where they made the same observation.[23]

Thomas et al found that a large keratin (63 kilodalton) was only focally present in human cutaneous squamous cancer. They used rabbit antibodies with the immunoperoxidase technique. Paradoxically, cutaneous carcinoma in situ (Bowen's disease) showed increased staining for the 63-kilodalton keratin.[24] Loning et al examined normal, inflamed, "premalignant," and carcinomatous oral mucosa. There was variable staining of keratin in dysplastic epithelium of leukoplakic lesions. Large keratins were present in the carcinomas.[25] All of these studies are preliminary, and their use in a diagnostic or prognostic capacity is unknown.

A practical application of the immunohistochemical identification of keratin has been shown by Taxy et al, who found that all undifferentiated nasopharyngeal carcinomas contained keratin.[26] This provides a clear separation from malignant lymphoma, with which these lesions are frequently confused, especially when they occur initially as metastases in the cervical lymph nodes of young people.[27]

Molecular biology is another approach to the identification of tumor-specific markers. A few cancers have been associated with the abnormal expression of cellular oncogenes. Perhaps the best characterized example is the protein designated p21 of the *ras* oncogene in a cell line derived from human bladder cancer. The oncogene differs by only a single amino acid from the corresponding normal protein.[28] It is theoretically possible to produce monoclonal antibodies that would distinguish between these two compounds.[29] Ideally, these could be adapted to the immunoperoxidase technique and recognized in individual cells.

ALTERATION IN BLOOD GROUP ANTIGENS

The ABH blood group antigens are normal constituents on the cell surface of many cells, including squamous epithelium. The antigens are decreased or absent in about 85 percent of neoplasms, including squamous carcinoma.[30] Conversely, carcinoma in situ of the oral cavity has an increase in the type 2 chain of the H antigen.[31] The type 2 chain H antigen is an immediate precursor of the A and B antigens. A deficiency of enzymes necessary to convert H antigen to A antigen has been demonstrated using monoclonal antibodies and immunofluorescence in oral cavity lesions judged to be premalignant.[32]

The loss of A and B antigens and/or the accumulation of H antigen has been investigated in a small number of lesions in the upper aerodigestive tract. Dabelsteen et al used immunohistochemical techniques to examine epithelium from nine patients with laryngeal carcinoma who had blood type A. They found that in four out of nine squamous carcinomas were completely devoid of blood group antigen A, four had a few patches of cells with retained antigen, and only one tumor had a majority of cells with retained antigen.[33] Lin et al, using the red cell adherence method, found that antigens were absent in 15 of 24 laryngeal cancers, partially lost in eight, and completely retained in only one.[30]

The altered ABH antigenicity of most invasive carcinomas has led to its study in noninvasive, abnormal epithelium. Dabelsteen et al noted that dysplastic epithelium adjacent to two laryngeal carcinomas retained their blood group antigens.[33] Conversely, Lin et al found that there was a gradual loss of antigen corresponding to a transition from normal to dysplastic cells to overt laryngeal carcinoma.[30] Their observation that morphologically normal epithelium adjacent to cancer was devoid of antigens in 10 cases has potentially great implications. It suggests that antigen-depleted cells may have declared their malignant potential at a time when the cells are still morphologically normal. The most intriguing patients were four whose initial biopsy specimens were benign, but in which the cells had a complete loss of antigens. All four patients subsequently developed carcinoma. This kind of information might be applied prospectively on a clinical basis. A biopsy of squamous epithelium failing to show A or B antigens could serve as a stimulus to pursue the possibility that the patient had a cancer that had not yet been identified or that the patient was at a high risk to develop cancer.

CYTOGENETICS

Cytogenetics is the morphologic study of chromosomes from squashed cells arrested in metaphase. The chromosomes are photographed through a microscope, enlarged, and arranged to show their karyotype. An individual chromosome may have an increased quantity of DNA manifest by enlargement of part or all of the chromosome. Abnormal configurations include chromosomes in the shape of a ring, deleted fragments, or fragments transplanted onto other chromosomes. All of these abnormalities are called marker chromosomes and can correlate with biologic behavior. The tumors from 53 patients with well-differentiated transitional cell carcinomas of the urinary bladder were examined for marker chromosomes. Out of 33 patients with marker chromosomes, 32 had recurrent tumor. On the other hand, only 1 of 20 patients had recurrence when their neoplasms lacked marker chromosomes, even though by histologic examination the tumors from both groups were similar.[34]

There is ample evidence that there is a relation between biologic behavior and abnormal karyotypes.[35] We are unaware of karyotyping of squamous cancers of the head and neck.

FLOW CYTOMETRY

A flow cytometer examines individual cells suspended in a liquid medium and measures a variety of physical and biochemical properties. Several thousand cells can be analyzed in a matter of minutes. Many flow cytometers can segregate different subpopulations of cells, a method referred to as cell sorting. Single cell suspensions are easy to prepare from fluids such as blood or bone marrow. Solid tumors, however, pose a problem because the cells must be detached from one another, and they must also be separated from the stroma either physically or with enzymes. Such preparations often contain stromal debris, damaged cells, or fragments of cells that result in confusing measurements.[36] Refinements of techniques leading to better individual cell recovery are a specific focus of research in several laboratories.

The principle of flow cytometry is based on individual cells flowing at high speed, one by one, through a sensing area where either electrical or optical signals are generated. The signals can be derived from fluorescence, light scatter, electrical resistance of cells, or light absorbance. By means of one or another of these modalities, physical and biochemical properties, such as cell size and nucleic acid levels, can be measured. Flow cytometry should prove useful in quantitating surface antigens and receptors. Fluorescence probes bound to specific antibodies can be measured with great accuracy. The action and eventual fate of injected monoclonal antibodies used for therapeutic purposes in humans could be closely followed with this technique.

The flow cytometer is attached to a computer that stores and processes the data as computer-drawn histograms. If DNA is being measured, the DNA histogram not only tells what proportion of cells have abnormal quantities of DNA, but it can identify subpopulations of cells. Measurements of DNA content by flow cytometry are of comparable accuracy to data derived by other techniques such as microspectrophotometry or thymidine labeling. Furthermore, flow cytometry takes only a fraction of the time required by the other techniques.[36,37]

Flow cytometry can evaluate tumor kinetics. A histogram of normal cells has two major peaks. One corresponds to cells in the presynthetic (G_1) phase of the cell cycle, when the cells have a normal diploid number of chromosomes, and the other peak consists of cells with a tetraploid complement of DNA in the postsynthetic/mitotic phases (G_2 and M respectively). A minority of cells with variable quantities of DNA are located between these peaks. They are the cells synthesizing DNA (the S phase) that will reach the final tetraploid quantity prior to cell division. The proportion of cells synthesizing DNA is a measure of the proliferative activity of the overall cell population.

The application of flow cytometry to the diagnosis of solid tumors is hampered by the technical aspects already mentioned. Nonetheless, it has shown its potential in the prognostic correlation of some lymphomas,[38] and cancers of the colon.[39]

DNA analysis has also shown how heterogenous the cells of a cancer are. In a colon cancer mapped by taking fine needle aspirations from different parts of the tumor, two populations of tumor cells were more or less mixed throughout the tumor. However, there were areas in which the majority of cells had nearly the same DNA content and therefore were a single population. Thus, in part, the tumor was an anatomic mosaic.[40] Only a few squamous carcinomas have been examined, but heterogeneity of cell populations has been found.[41] The increasing awareness of the heterogeneity of tumors is important. The concept needs to be kept in mind when using therapeutic regimens that are based on cycle- or phase-specific chemotherapeutic agents.

Aneuploid tumors are usually associated with greater microscopic abnormalities, more frequent metastases, and a worse prognosis than tumors that are diploid. In some cases of colon carcinoma, patients with metastatic disease who have diploid tumors do better than those with metastatic disease of the same stage whose tumors are aneuploid.[39]

CYTOPHOTOMETRY

A simple technique for assessing the quantity of DNA in individual cells involves scraping the cords with a wooden stick during microlaryngoscopy. The cells are smeared immediately on a slide, fixed in 95 percent ethanol, and stained with a fluorescent dye that has an affinity for DNA. Accurate quantitation of DNA within the individual cell can be attained by using a microcomputerized cytophotometer. Bjelkenkrantz et al studied smears from patients who had moderate-to-severe dysplasia in the tissue biopsy.[42] Fourteen of the patients did not have hypertetraploid cells on cytophotometry. Eleven of these patients had no progression of disease and only one developed cancer. Conversely, five of the seven patients with moderate-to-severe dysplasia that had hypertetraploid cells eventually developed carcinoma, and one additional patient required frequent therapy for recurrent dysplasia. The difference in the rate of cancer between the two groups was statistically significant. The potential of this technique for selecting the patient at high risk for subsequent carcinoma is obvious.

The DNA content varies in the different cells of an individual laryngeal carcinoma. In order to easily convey this variation, mathematical expressions have been derived. Bocking et al expressed the DNA ''grade of malignancy'' on a scale of 0 to 3.[43] Patients with a DNA grade of 0 to 1 had a mean survival of 1.5 years (p<0.0001). Clinical stage and mode of therapy were not taken into consideration. Holm carried out a similar study that included clinical staging. He found that patients with carcinomas that were diploid or had lower than normal values had a longer survival, even when they were in advanced clinical stages.[44]

AUTORADIOGRAPHY WITH TRITIATED THYMIDINE

Tritiated thymidine is a radioactive marker that is incorporated into nuclear DNA if the cell is in the synthetic phase of DNA formation. Thymidine can be given intravenously, and biopsy of the neoplasm obtained a few hours later for assessment of the amount of incorporated thymidine. Alternatively, fresh tumor can be incubated in vitro with thymidine. The latter is the most widely used, and it has recently become a fairly standardized procedure so that the results from different laboratories can be meaningfully compared.

The method consists of incubating thin slices of fresh tumor under hyperbaric conditions in a balanced salt solution for approximately 2 hours. The tissue is then fixed in formalin, embedded in paraffin, sectioned, and mounted on glass slides. The slides are placed in a liquid photographic emulsion for 2 weeks, developed, and stained with hematoxylin and eosin. Using an ordinary light microscope, one sees the silver grains that have precipitated at the site of the radioactive thymidine. These are the nuclei that have incorporated the thymidine during the S phase. The percentage of labeled cells is the thymidine labeling index. Thymidine labeling permits visualization of the relationships of the labeled cells to other constituents in the tumor. One can be certain that the examined sections are representative when a tumor has variable patterns, different degrees of differentiation, or large areas of fibrosis.

Prioleau et al discuss one way in which autoradiography could have diagnostic utility.[45] They showed that the S-phase cells in a verrucous carcinoma were confined to the basal and parabasal region. This distribution contrasts with nonverrucous squamous cancers that have S-phase cells throughout all zones except in the most mature keratinized cells.

The proportion of tumor cells in S phase has been correlated with the aggressiveness of the tumor. This holds true for carcinoma of the breast, carcinoma of the urinary bladder, and lymphomas.[46]

S phase has been measured in squamous cancers of the upper aerodigestive tract by immunofluorescence. The antibody is antiguanosine directed against single-strand DNA. DNA is single strand prior to replication, and the cells are marked at that time. This leads to a labeling index comparable to that obtained with tritiated thymidine, and the data have the advantage of being obtained shortly after the biopsy.[47]

COMPUTER-ASSISTED IMAGE ANALYSIS

Computer-assisted image analysis capitalizes on the fact that most neoplasms have nuclei with abnormal shapes. Some of these abnormalities may be so subtle that the naked eye cannot perceive them. Computer-assisted image allows precise quantitation of the shapes of either nuclei or nucleoli, and it can be performed on ordinary tissue sections or smears. The nuclei of malignant cells are transmitted by a camera lucida to a digitizer platen, where the image of the cell is several inches wide. An illuminated stylus is used to manually trace the perimeter of the nucleus or nucleolus. The digitizer platen electronically senses the movements of the stylus and converts the impulses into readings that the computer can calculate regarding the shape or area of the nucleus.

Nuclear roundness is defined as the degree to which the nuclear cross-section approximates a perfect circle. A perfectly round nucleus has a roundness factor of 1.0. The factor is never less than 1.0 because the circumference of a circle is the smallest perimeter that can enclose a given area. As the nucleus becomes progressively noncircular, larger perimeters are required to enclose a given area. The technique is reproducible with less than 10 percent variation between different examiners. The drawback of the technique is the 3 to 4 hours required to examine enough nuclei for statistical adequacy (about 600 nuclei).

Initial studies on prostatic cancer vividly demonstrate the possible value of nuclear roundness. As with squamous cancer, prostatic cancer has a range of both cytologic and architectural differentiation. As expected, patients with well-differentiated tumors almost always have a good prognosis, and patients with poorly differentiated tumors have a dismal outlook. Most patients have tumors of intermediate differentiation, which is again analogous to squamous cancer, and it is impossible to predict accurately the tumor that will metastasize. A group of 27 men with carcinoma of the prostate treated only with radical prostatectomy were followed for at least 15 years or until metastases were detected. Fourteen men developed metastases, although some of these patients had tumors that were histologically identical to tumors from patients who did not develop metastasis. All of the patients with metastases had a high roundness factor.[48]

Computer-assisted image analysis has also been used to study primary melanomas of the uveal tract. Gamel et al measured 18 parameters and combinations of parameters in the nuclei and nucleoi.[49] The circumference of the nucleoli was one feature that highly correlated with survival (p=0.00001). In this particular tumor, mathematical analysis indicated that only 50 cells were sufficient to provide discriminating data. Refinements continue to be made and the time to analyze adequately this particular tumor is about 40 minutes of a technician's time.[50]

The correlation of nuclear or nucleolar roundness with metastatic potential is an empiric observation. It is, however, a logical extension from the occurrence of nuclear abnormalities in malignant cells. It is not difficult to conceive that changes in the function of the nucleus could alter its structural integrity, and that this might correspond to certain basic tumor properties including metastatic potential.

In conclusion, there are many recent technologic advances that should enhance our understanding of neoplastic diseases. We must not forget, however, that the use of the light microscope and routine tissue sections will continue to be a major source of useful information. This instrument is not new, but the pathologist who uses it can be innovative by his observations, open-mindedness, and critical thinking. During the last 10 years, thoughtful study of routine tissue has seen a separation of necrotizing sialometaplasia from malignant salivary gland tumors,[51] and the distinction of the virally induced verruca vulgaris of the larynx from verrucous carcinoma.[52] There has been the rediscovery of the juxtaoral organ of Chievitz, a normal structure near the angle of the jaw that may be confused with squamous carcinoma.[53] The understanding of the pathology of salivary gland tumors relies almost exclusively on light microscopy, and continual progress is being made in recognizing variants with their clinical implications. For example, the study of tumors that were unheard of 10 years ago (e.g., salivary duct carcinoma and polymorphic low-grade adenocarcinoma) is yielding valuable prognostic information.[54,55] The imagination with which techniques are used is more important than the novelty of the

technique itself. Old techniques that continue to yield new information are not to be shunned as long as they are productive.

REFERENCES

1. Jakobsson PA. Histologic grading of malignancy and prognosis in glottic carcinomas of the larynx. In: Alberti PW, Bryce DP (eds). *Centennial Conference on Laryngeal Cancer.* New York: Appleton-Century Crofts, 1973; 847–852.
2. Crissman JD, Liu WY, Gluckman JL, Cummings G. Prognostic value of histopathologic perimeters in squamous cell carcinoma of the oropharynx. Cancer. (In press)
3. Feldman PS, Kaplan MJ, Johns ME, Cantrell RW. Fine-needle aspiration in squamous cell carcinoma of the head and neck. Arch Otolaryngol 1983; 109:735–742.
4. Incze J, Vaughan CW Jr, Lui P, et al. Premalignant changes in normal appearing epithelium in patients with squamous cell carcinoma of the upper aerodigestive tract. Am J Surg 1982; 144:401–405.
5. Ober WB. Recent ideas in the pathology of endometrial carcinoma. In: Brush MG, King RJB, Taylor RW (eds). *Endometrial Cancer.* London: Baillere Tindall, 1977; 111–117.
6. Hellquist H, Olofsson J, Grontoft O. Carcinoma in situ and severe dysplasia of the vocal cords. A clinicopathological and photometric investigation. Acta Otolaryngol 1981; 92:543–555.
7. Auerbach O, Hammond EC, Garfinkel L. Histologic changes in the larynx in relation to smoking habits. Cancer 1970; 25:92–104.
8. Weinstein JN, Parker RJ, Keenan JM, et al. Monoclonal antibodies in the lymphatics: Towards the diagnosis and therapy of tumor metastases. Science 1982; 218:1334–1335.
9. Sears HF, Herlyn M, Del-Villano B, et al. Monoclonal antibody detection of a circulating tumor-associated antigen: II. A longitudinal evaluation of patients with colorectal carcinoma. J Clin Immunol 1982; 2:141–149.
10. Bast RC, Klug TL, St. John E, et al. A radioimmunoassay using a monoclonal antibody to monitor the course of epithelial ovarian cancer. N Engl J Med 1983; 309:883–887.
11. Barsky SH, Siegal GP, Jannotta F, Liotta L. Loss of basement membrane components by invasive tumors but not by their benign counterparts. Lab Invest 1983; 49:140–147.
12. Liotta LA, Tryggrason K, Garbisa S, et al. Metastatic potential correlates with enzymatic degradation of basement membrane collagen. Nature 1980; 284:67–68.
13. Kao RT, Hall J, Engel L, Stern R. The matrix of human breast tumor cells is mitogenic for fibroblasts. Am J Pathol 1984; 115:109–116.
14. Norris HJ, Tavassoli FA, Kurman RJ. Endometrial hyperplasia and carcinoma. Diagnostic considerations. Am J Surg Pathol 1983; 7:839–847.
15. Kramer RH, Vogel KG, Nicolson GL. Solubilization and degradation of subendothelial matrix glycoproteins and proteoglycans by metastatic tumor cells. J Biol Chem 1982; 257:2678–2686.
16. Sloane BF, Dunn JR, Honn KV. Lysosomal cathepsin B: Correlation with metastatic potential. Science 1981; 212:1151–1153.
17. Poole AR, Tiltman KJ, Recklies AD, Stoker TAM. Differences in secretion of the proteinase cathepsin B at the edges of human breast carcinomas and fibroadenomas. Nature 1978; 273:545–547.
18. Crissman JD, Sloane B, Ryan R. Correlation of cathepsin B and metastatic potential in malignant neoplasia. Lab Invest 1984; 50:13A. (Abstract)
19. Bauer EA, Uitto J, Walters RC, Eisen AZ. Enhanced collagenase production by fibroblasts derived from human basal cell carcinomas. Cancer Res 1979; 39:4594–4599.
20. Abramson M, Schilling RW, Huang CC, Salome RG. Collagenase activity in epidermoid carcinoma of the oral cavity

and larynx. Ann Otol 1975; 84:158–163.

21. Murphy GF, Flynn TC, Rice RH, Pinkus GS. Involucrin expression in normal and neoplastic human skin. A marker for keratinocyte differentiation. Lab Invest 1984; 50:42A. (Abstract)

22. Winter H, Schweizer J, Goerttler K. Keratins as markers of malignancy in mouse epidermal tumors. Carcinogenesis 1980; 1:391–398.

23. Winter H, Schweizer J, Goerttler K. Keratin polypeptide composition as a biochemical tool for the discrimination of benign and malignant epithelial lesions in man. Arch Dermatol Res 1983; 275:27–34.

24. Thomas P, Said JW, Nash G, et al. Profiles of keratin proteins in basal and squamous cell carcinomas of the skin. An immunohistochemical study. Lab Invest 1984; 50:36–41.

25. Löing T, Staquet M-J, Thivolet J, Seifert G. Keratin polypeptides distribution in normal and diseased human epidermis and oral mucosa. Immunohistochemical study on unaltered epithelium and inflammatory, premalignant and malignant lesions. Virchows Arch A Path Anat Histol 1980; 388:273–288.

26. Taxy JB, Battifora H, Hidvegi D. Nasopharyngeal carcinoma: Electron microscopy and a comparison of three antikeratin antisera. Lab Invest 1984; 50:59A. (Abstract)

27. Giffler RF, Gillespie JJ, Ayala AG, Newland JR. Lymphoepithelioma in cervical lymph nodes of children and young adults. Am J Surg Pathol 1977; 1:293–302.

28. Reddy EP, Reynolds RK, Santos E, et al. A point mutation is responsible for the acquisition of transforming properties by the T24 human bladder carcinoma oncogene. Nature 1982; 300:149–152.

29. Borowitz MJ, Stein RB. Diagnostic applications of monoclonal antibodies to human cancer. Arch Pathol Lab Med 1984; 108:101–105.

30. Lin F, Liu PI, McGregor DH. Isoantigens A, B, and H in morphologically normal mucosa and in carcinoma of the larynx. Am J Clin Path 1977; 68:372–376.

31. Dabelsteen E, Vedtofte P, Hakomori S, Young WW Jr. Accumulation of a blood group antigen precursor in oral premalignant lesions. Cancer Res 1983; 43:1451–1453.

32. Dabelsteen E, Graem N, Hakomori S, Young WW Jr. Monoclonal antibodies in the diagnosis of epithelial premalignant lesions. Bull Cancer 1983; 70:127–131.

33. Dabelsteen E, Mygind N, Henriksen B. Blood group substance A in carcinomas of the larynx. Acta Otolaryngol 1974; 77:360–367.

34. Falor WH, Ward RM. Prognosis in early carcinoma of the bladder based on chromosomal analysis. J Urol 1978; 119:44–48.

35. Wolman SR. Cytogenetics and cancer. Arch Pathol Lab Med 1984; 108:15–19.

36. Braylan RC. Flow cytometry. Arch Pathol Lab Med 1983; 107:1–6.

37. Lovette EJ III, Schnitzer B, Keren DF, et al. Application of flow cytometry to diagnostic pathology. Lab Invest 1984; 50:115–140.

38. Diamond LW, Nathwani BN, Rappaport H. Flow cytometry in the diagnosis and classification of malignant lymphoma and leukemia. Cancer 1982; 50:1122–1135.

39. Wolley RC, Schreiber K, Koss LG, et al. DNA distribution in human colon carcinomas and its relationship to clinical behavior. J Natl Cancer Inst 1982; 69:15–22.

40. Petersen SE, Bichel P, Lorentzen M. Flow-cytometric demonstration of tumor-cell subpopulations with different DNA content in human colo-rectal carcinoma. Europ J Cancer 1978; 15:383–386.

41. Nervi C, Badaracco G, Morelli M, Starace G. Cytokinetic evaluation in human head and neck cancer by autoradiography and DNA cytofluorometry. Cancer 1980; 45:452—459.

42. Bjelkenkrantz K, Lundgren J, Olofson J. Single-cell DNA measurements in hyperplastic, dysplastic and carcinomatous laryngeal epithelia, with special reference to the occurrence of hypertetraploid cell nuclei. Analyt Quant Cytol 1983; 5:184–188.

43. Bocking A, Adler C-P, Common HH, et al. Algorithm for a DNA-cytophotometric diagnosis and grading of malignancy. Analyt Quant Cytol 1984; 6:1–8.

44. Holm L-E. Cellular DNA amounts of squamous cell carcinomas of the head and neck region in relation to prognosis. Laryngoscope 1982; 92:1064–1069.

45. Prioleau PG, Santa Cruz DJ, Meyer JS, Bauer WC. Verrucous carcinoma. A light and electron microscopic, autoradiographic, and immunofluorescence study. Cancer 1980; 45:2849–2857.

46. Meyer JS. Cell kinetic measurements of human tumors. Hum Pathol 1982; 13:874–877.

47. Cinberg JA, Chang TH, Hebbard P, et al. An application of immunocytology to the analysis of the cell kinetics of upper respiratory and digestive tract squamous carcinoma. Cancer 1983; 51:1843–1846.

48. Diamond DA, Berry SJ, Jewett HJ, et al. A new method to assess metastatic potential of human prostate cancer: Relative nuclear roundness. J Urol 1982; 128:729–734.

49. Gamel JW, McLean IW. Computerized histopathologic assessment of malignant potential: A method for determining the prognosis of uveal melanomas. Hum Pathol 1982; 13:834–837.

50. Gamel JW, McLean IW. Computerized histopathologic assessment of malignant potential. III. Refinements of measurement and data analysis. Analyt Quant Cytol 1984; 6:37–44.

51. Fechner RE. Necrotizing sialometaplasia. A source of confusion with carcinoma of the palate. Am J Clin Pathol 1977; 67:315–317.

52. Fechner RE, Mills SE. Verruca vulgaris of the larynx. A distinctive lesion of probable viral origin confused with verrucous carcinoma. Am J Surg Pathol 1982; 6:357–362.

53. Tschen JA, Fechner RE. The juxtaoral organ of Chievitz. Am J Surg Pathol 1979; 3:147–150.

54. Garland TA, Innes DJ, Fechner RE. Salivary duct carcinoma: An analysis of four cases with review of literature. Am J Clin Pathol 1984; 81:436–441.

55. Evans HL and Batsakis JG. Polymorphous low-grade adenocarcinoma of minor salivary glands. A study of 14 cases of a distinctive neoplasm. Cancer 1984; 53:935–942.

4. Head and Neck Surgery in the 1980s: The Role of More or Less

DONALD F. N. HARRISON, M.D., M.S., Ph.D., F.R.C.S.,
F.R.A.C.S.(Hon.), F.R.C.S.E.(Hon.)

Those of us who practice the craft of operative surgery are by nature activists and, in our earlier years, optimists. During the past twenty years, my initial youthful enthusiasm has been replaced by a period of calm optimism, and now possibly some degree of pessimism (Fig. 1). However, the wide range of conditions that I have been privileged to treat gave me an opportunity to review the whole field of head and neck pathology (Table 1), and the judgments that I present here are based on personal experience rather than a concentrate of oncologic literature. On reflection, this is patently untrue, for no rational individual would ignore the many thoughtful contributions on this subject published by that mentor of Head and Neck Oncology, John Conley.[1-3] In many ways I feel that I am merely translating his concepts and wisdom into my own brand of English.

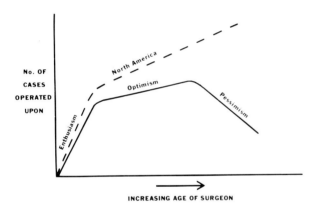

Figure 1 Schematic representation of decision to operate in relation to age of surgeon.

TABLE 1 Personal Experience with Head and Neck Cases — 1963–1983

Site of Malignancy	Number of Patients
External and middle ear	63
Nose and paranasal sinuses	297
Bony maxilla	34
Postnasal space	115
Orbit	29
Tonsil — palate	174
Tongue — floor of mouth	182
Hypopharynx	284
Salivary glands	64
Thyroid	57
Larynx	1045
Other sites (lung — neck etc)	126
	2470

In selecting a particular procedure for any individual patient, the surgeon is influenced by his personal philosophy and past experience, as well as by his own technical capability. If we are to understand the many factors that influence decision making and the variations in attitudes among oncologists, it is essential to consider briefly the training and work patterns of head and neck surgeons.

Despite the expenditure of considerable amounts of money and work, our knowledge of the genetic biochemical disorders recognized as human cancer remains minimal. Although the major cause of the four principal head and neck carcinomas—oral cavity, pharynx, larynx, and esophagus—seems likely to be tobacco, the revenue gained by all governments from this plant ensures that no effective action is ever likely to occur![4] Epidemiologic studies give little indication of meaningful reduction in absolute numbers of those affected. What has changed within the last twenty-five years has been our acceptance that a more professional approach is needed if patients who are curable are to be cured.

The combined approach to any cancer requires the availability of a wide range of expertise, none more so than when dealing with head and neck tumors. Since individuals of equal experience are not often available in most combined clinics, democratic discussion is invariably weighed toward a particular discipline. However, the desire for improvement in the overall poor long-term control rate, resistance to the crippling and mutilating effect of many orofacial resections and the pressures from medical oncologists searching for a clearly defined role, has resulted in the ostracism of the purely surgically oriented individual.

The fundamental principles of excisional surgery within the head and neck region were clearly established 30 years ago. Although enhanced by modern developments in anesthesia and antibiotics, and by an increased knowledge of surgical anatomy and pathology, these principles remain much the same. What is surely changing, and this is vitally important to my prime thesis, is the acknowledgment in many countries that the head and neck surgeon requires special training. Cancer can rarely be managed by any single individual, and the modern head and neck surgeon requires some knowledge of all facets of oncology as well as technical expertise in both excisional and reconstructive surgery. The credit for establishing this dictum lies with the American Society for Head and Neck Surgery (ASHNS), which incidentally includes both pathologists and radiotherapists.[5] Fortuitously many of the present-day experienced surgeons within this field possess a strong training in general and plastic surgery, with, in my instance, ophthalmology for good measure.

However, the mere acquisition of the necessary technical skills together with support from paramedical and other oncologically oriented colleagues is not enough. The selection of patients for elective surgery is a problem fraught with philosophic and ethnic implications. Will the advantages of successful surgery outweigh the risks and disability? Am I really able to perform the procedure at an acceptable level of competency?[6] Such queries form the basis for my evaluation of the position of major excisional surgery within the 1980s, in the hope that we may continue to ask ourselves, "What is the best treatment for *this* patient suffering from *this* particular disease?"[7] While not wishing to pursue the somewhat hazardous subject of why individuals take up the often stressful discipline of surgical oncology, it is probably of some relevance when considering the topic of decision making. A study by Wright in 1980 suggested that when compared with the general population, surgeons showed a significant need to achieve control, resist change, persist methodically and conventionally in a task, and sustain positions of influence.[8]

POSSIBLY TOO MUCH

The head and neck surgeon is possibly unique in that he is committed to treating a life-threatening disease in an exposed area of the body that has fundamental physiologic functions together with considerable aesthetic noticeability.[2] Much of his surgery, aimed at cure or long-term palliation, is associated with some degree of mutilation and interference with physiologic function. In many parts of the world, such disabilities preclude social acceptance or even survival. Even in the more developed countries, it is only recently that the significance of the social implications of sudden facial disfigurement and its importance in meaningful rehabilitation has attracted the attention of social workers and similar welfare groups.

Even the best of external prostheses are an obvious form of camouflage, and the damage to self-image may be considerable.

In the 1940s the overriding premise was to cure the cancer and save the patient's life by a heroic act of surgical extirpation. Surgical procedures are now becoming more varied, custom-designed for each patient and their disease, and generally more conservative. Frequently, elective conservative procedures are combined with other modalities in the hope of achieving success without associated disability. Such expectations are rarely achieved! Indeed conservation surgery within the head and neck requires at least twice as much experience and skill as so-called radical extirpation!

In order to justify the concept of radical excision, some thought must be given to the practicality of obtaining "clear" margins, whether macroscopically or histologically, and the effect of technical failure. A fundamental concept of oncologic surgery is that for localized cancer, complete excision must be performed with adequate surgical margins if cure is to be expected.[10] However, there are site differences; within the oral cavity positive margins for carcinoma contribute to both local recurrence and eventual treatment failure.[11] This may not be so within the larynx following conservation surgery.[12]

Theoretically, postoperative residual tumor proliferates and results in gross recurrence. However, in a study of 72 patients in whom postoperative radiotherapy was given for detectable residual tumor, provided the latter was given within 6 weeks, recurrence was reduced to 31 percent for those with microscopic disease and 50 percent for those with macroscopic tumor.[13] This supports other evidence that the combination of surgery and radiotherapy in advanced head and neck cancer results in fewer recurrences than does either modality alone. However, in a larger series, the local failure rate was 39 percent even when the margins of resection were said to be satisfactory (at least 5 mm) and 73 percent when the margins were unsatisfactory.[14] The recurrence rates were no higher with more extensive primaries, possibly because the surgical removal of gross tumor left only a microscopic burden for postoperative radiotherapy. Accepting that all patients with a high risk of postoperative recurrence should be irradiated prophylactically to therapeutic doses, microscopic cancer found at the margins of intended curative resection significantly reduces local control, particularly within the oral cavity and pharynx. Every effort must be made to accomplish microscopically "complete" surgical resection, and although such margins do not guarantee control of the primary tumor, the improved incidence of local recurrence may improve prognosis.

The patient pays a price for such a philosophy, and "cure at any cost," even if one could accurately define such an expression, is no longer acceptable. The ability to reconstruct and, to some extent, rehabilitate has enlarged our armamentarium to an astounding degree. "Because we can, we do," and some of these formidable surgical procedures require analysis from the detached viewpoint of patient benefit.

Conservation Surgery of the Larynx

Despite the fact that the larynx is the most common site of cancer within the head and neck, its natural history and pattern of spread having been clearly identified by whole organ serial sections, and more attention has been paid to laryngeal surgical techniques than those for any other organ, management of laryngeal cancer remains obscure. It is impossible to quantify the relative roles of primary laryngectomy, conservation surgery, radiotherapy, and combination therapy. I have recently investigated some of the underlying reasons for the confusion,[15] concluding that the intrinsic errors in classification and the varying means used for end-stage reporting are together responsible for an inability to compare like with like.

Obviously, tumor confined within the laryngeal framework can be successfully removed by total laryngectomy, leaving as the primary goal the restoration of functional speech. The present emphasis on a variety of surgical reconstructive techniques designed to produce effective postlaryngectomy speech relates to a failure in a selected group to achieve esophageal speech. However, assessment of all forms of laryngectomy speech has in the past been largely subjective, and there is a danger that once again surgical technique will precede objective evaluation.

Conservation procedures on the larynx have evolved through an understanding of surgical anatomy, including embryologic development and pattern of spread. Although cancer does recur locally after conservation surgery, the technique of horizontal supraglottic laryngectomy is clearly effective, provided it is appreciated that critical areas such as anterior commissure, subglottis, and paraglottic space must be precisely evaluated. In experienced hands the operation is obviously curative, although many reports make little reference to objective assessment of the postoperative voice or the problems associated with swallowing and decannulation.[16] Ignoring the errors in classification, the results of radiotherapy for many patients considered suitable for such surgery are compatible, leaving the patient with a complete larynx! Although re-evaluation of laryngectomy specimens reveals instances in which conservation surgery would have been possible,[17] such retrospective studies ignore the need for whole patient assessment, such an essential aspect of oncologic practice.

Indications for the various types of vertical frontolateral laryngectomies have been recently reviewed.[18] The criteria are more easily clarified, but again tend to relate to lesions suitable for primary radiotherapy. In radiation failure the procedure offers an alternative to total laryngectomy, but requires a maturity in preoperative evaluation and surgical skills that challenges many surgeons.

While accepting the difficulties of assessing with accuracy the true extent of all except the earliest of laryngeal cancers, the experienced oncologic team is now able to advise each patient as to the most acceptable means of obtaining long-term control with the least disability. In selected patients this may entail conservation surgery, but such techniques require judgment and experience, not necessarily available or suitable to all patients in all countries.

Neck Dissection

The control or prevention of metastasis to the cervical lymph nodes is a major unresolved problem in the management of head and neck cancer. Although the anatomic location of the cervical lymph nodes has been known for many years, there has been disagreement as to the method of classifying metastatic disease in these nodes (N). It is now believed

that the presence of a single, small, homolateral metastatic node has a distinctly better prognosis than a large node or multiple nodes. The term "fixed" is not reproducible, being defined by surgeons as "immobile" and radiotherapists as "attached to deeper structures."

Recently, representatives from the American Joint Committee (AJC) and the International Union Against Cancer (UICC) have agreed on a common N classification (Fig. 2), which appears to be more clinically realistic. Since Crile described radical neck dissection in 1906,[19] it has been known that this operation does not always control cervical metastasis. Massive and fixed nodes that extend into surrounding tissues or involve skin or skull base, as well as relatively inaccessible nodes in the superior mediastinum or lower neck, are nonresectable. Even in the clinically negative neck, there are recurrences of 7.5 to 24 percent,[20] depending on the site and control rate of the primary lesion. Removal of the spinal accessory nerve, an essential feature of the classic neck dissection, is accompanied by a varying degree of postoperative disability. In a 1979 report on 788 radical neck dissections, the major surgical complication rate was 16.2 percent, with an overall rate of 50.8 percent.[21] Of these patients, 20.4 percent had regional recurrences, and although many of these problems are predictable, it is hardly surprising that consideration should be given to the "functional neck dissection."

In 1967, a technique was described for removing the node-bearing tissues of the neck while preserving the spinal accessory nerve and other structures. Since the upper portion of this nerve runs through node-bearing tissue in the anterior superior part of the neck, patients had to be selected carefully, but the method has attracted attention, particularly in the high-risk clinically negative neck. Valid comparisons between the two techniques from the viewpoint of the patient's permanent morbidity must consider the total treatment program. Radiation therapy contributes significantly to the total disability, irrespective of which type of

---

N - REGIONAL LYMPH NODES

Nx - Minimum requirements to assess the regional node cannot be met.

N0 - No clinically positive node.

N1 - Single clinically positive homolateral node. 3 cm or less in diameter.

N2 - Single clinically positive homolateral node, more than 3 cm but not more than 6 cm in diameter, or multiple clinically positive homolateral nodes, none more than 6 cm in diameter, or clinically positive bilateral or contralateral nodes, none more than 6 cm in diameter.
(This N2 category can be broken down into N2a, N2b and N2c)

N3 - Clinically positive homolateral node(s), one more than 6 cm in diameter.

Figure 2 Classification of regional neck nodes agreed upon by American Joint Committee (AJC) and International Union Against Cancer (UICC), December 1983.

neck dissection is employed. This is particularly relevant since many conservation dissections are combined with postoperative radiotherapy.[23]

Prophylactic radiation may be given to the clinically negative neck or as an adjuvant to neck dissection in the treatment of clinically positive nodes. One of the principal problems in determining the success of these varying concepts is the well-established error in clinical staging. Analysis of 1,048 neck dissection specimens by De Santo et al[20] revealed an understaging of 30 percent in N0 disease and 40 percent in N1 disease. These errors are themselves underestimates since they ignore undetectable micrometastatic deposits.

A 2-year recurrence rate of 7.5 percent in pathologically negative necks serves as a reference point for the evaluation of other treatments, such as prophylactic radiation and functional neck dissection. However, a determinant failure rate of 4 percent has been reported for one series of 152 patients with N0 necks treated with 5000 rads of irradiation, the investigators claiming that dermal irritation and fibrosis are always temporary.[2;4] In another report, however, the local recurrence rate was only 3.5 percent for 476 functional neck dissections, the majority of patients with positive histologic findings receiving postoperative irradiation![25]

The difficulty in establishing a rational approach to the problem of controlling or avoiding cervical metastatic disease lies in the varying factors present in many authoritative publications. The clinically negative neck, with an incidence of undetected metastatic disease, in possibly 3 percent, may present varying problems dependent on the site and extent of the primary tumor. Functional neck dissection, which is technically more difficult, is not suitable for identifiable disease in the upper neck where nodes lie close to the accessory nerve. Positive nodes in the operative specimen necessitate postoperative radiotherapy which may increase postoperative disability. The classic radical neck dissection may be associated with serious complications, particularly in the irradiated neck. These may be acceptable in the presence of clinically detectable disease, but not in N0 diseae, in which prophylactic radiotherapy may be both safer and effective. The combination of radical surgery and postoperative radiation still seems the best choice for detectable metastasis. The role of functional neck dissection is as yet ill-defined.

Hypopharyngeal Cancer

Carcinoma of the hypopharynx, although uncommon, poses a surgical challenge possibly unequalled within the head and neck. Despite the limitations to effective excision posed by superior extension to relatively inaccessible regions, the postcricoid tumor offers an opportunity for wide excision. Except in the treatment of the extremely rare small carcinoma, radiotherapy has played a minimal role in the initial therapy in recent years. The best results were reported by Pearson in 1966,[26] this paper being subject to considerable criticism. Radiotherapy is frequently followed by stenosis, the very symptom most of these patients need to have relieved.

Since the minimal excision will be pharyngolaryngectomy with total thyroidectomy, it is the replacement of the pharynx which has occupied the attention of surgeons since Wookey in 1942.[28] However, the length of the cervical esophagus is variable, and in patients with extension of tumor inferiorly, adequate excision of the esophagus may be difficult if not impossible. My own evaluation of pharyngolaryngectomy specimens suggested that inadequate excision as well as an involved tracheoesophageal wall were possible reasons for a high local recurrence rate following this operation.[29] In selected patients, total esophagectomy might be indicated to ensure an adequate excision (Fig. 3). Tumors with a vertical length greater than 5 cm have a poor prognosis[30] probably because such extensive tumors frequently penetrate the muscular wall and are then in the tissue of the neck. An association with cervical and mediastinal metastasis is also likely, and the presence of palpable cervical metastasis seriously affects prognosis.

The mainstay of pharyngoesophageal replacement has always been the skin flap. By means of cervical skin techniques, this progressed to the deltopectoral and, more recently, myocutaneous flap. All carry a low operative mortality, but a high incidence of local complications and a lengthy hospital stay. The revascularized intestinal autograft has recently reappeared,[31] and although it requires a lengthy operation, it seems to be suitable for localized lesions when the inferior extension is accessible. Manubrial resection is done routinely when there is doubt regarding involvement of the tracheoesophageal wall, and it may assist in providing access to the lower limits of the cervical esophagus. The technique is uncomplicated and preferable to the "sternal split".[32]

The real challenge has come from the use of a transposed abdominal viscus for a one-stage reconstruction; colon via the anterior mediastinum and stomach through the vacant posterior mediastinum have both been used with varying degrees of success. The choice has been evaluated in a paper written in 1979,[33] but increasing experience with both techniques suggests that, in skilled hands, both are successful. Colon would appear to have a less predictable blood supply, and its use is accompanied by more complications. My experience with 104 gastric "pull-up operations" has been associated with a 15 percent hospital mortality rate, but in less experienced hands 40 percent of patients might die in the hospital from postoperative complications.[34] Gastric transposition, however, possesses the advantages of a one-stage, cosmetically acceptable procedure with adequate excision inferiorly and no abdominal anastomosis. It is doubtful whether gastric transposition is more successful than other less complex procedures in curing patients, but it does offer the patient trouble-free swallowing and

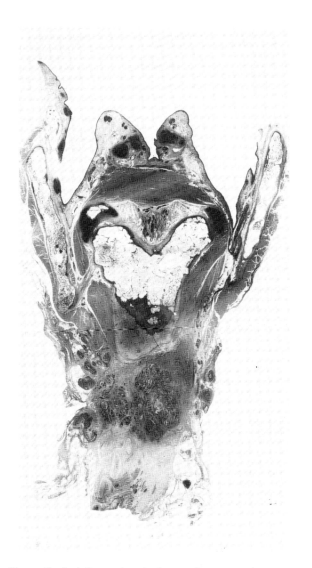

Figure 3 Serially sectioned pharyngolaryngoesophagectomy specimen showing clear margin below tumor. Note paratracheal node.

minimal long-term morbidity.[35] Because of the late stage at presentation, the poor prognosis attached to the development of cervical and mediastinal metastasis, and the restriction on adequate superior excision, it is doubtful whether 5-year survivals for postcricoid carcinoma will exceed 40 percent. However, viscus transposition in experienced hands offers a maximum opportunity for adequate excision together with excellent cosmetic and functional rehabilitation. Without such expertise, or in unsuitable patients, repair with a single-stage myocutaneous flap would appear more sensible.

External and Middle Ear

Surgical excision of the rare tumor localized in the external auditory meatus or middle ear is a formidable exercise and should be viewed in relation to expected benefit to the patient. Despite its accessible position, squamous carcinoma of the external ear canal is an aggressive disease spreading rapidly to middle ear, parotid gland, skull base, and related lymph nodes. Radical excision followed by radiotherapy offers the best prospect of control, but few localized tumors have been reported, and these lesions are usually incorporated with carcinoma arising within or involving the middle ear and mastoid.

Apart from Lewis,[36] and Goodwin and Jesse,[37] few surgeons have extensive personal experience with radical surgery for malignant tumors in this region. The major therapeutic problem with temporal bone involvement is incomplete resection of disease, for there is little chance of cure with postoperative radiotherapy if disease is left in situ. Even with the use of computerized axial tomography, it is difficult to be certain that the tumor is resectable. In the 100 cases reported by Lewis, 20 percent had disease outside the temporal bone resulting in positive margins following surgery. An additional 10 percent had unresectable tumor despite encouraging preoperative investigations. Even with a 70 percent resectability, the local recurrence rate was 40 percent. Postoperative radiotherapy still gave an overall 5-year cure rate of only 25 percent.

This surgery is formidable even in experienced hands using hypotension, high speed air drills, and careful dissection. Lewis's operative mortality is now 5 percent, with little reference to morbidity or disability figures. Such specialized surgery must be compared with the results from primary radiotherapy, usually preceded by radical mastoidectomy. Lederman's figures of 30.7 percent 5-year survival obtained in 1965 remain much the same today,[38] although now based on 250 patients. Surgery for radiotherapy failures has proved useful for palliation, but unsuccessful in producing long-term cure. It appears likely that the long-term results with skilled radiotherapy match those obtained with experienced surgery, but without the considerable morbidity attached to excisional surgery.

A similar controversy exists regarding glomus tumors of the temporal bone. The advances made in neurologic surgery have brought the radical extirpation of even the most vascular and extension lesions within the realm of feasibility. This apprach to the infratemporal fossa and skull base was pioneered by Fisch in 1978,[39] and its use in the removal of glomus tumors has been reported by Jackson et al[40] and by Jenkins and Fisch.[41] Despite the vascularity of the lesion, the need for over 4 units of blood, the 10-hour operating time, and the complexity of the surgery, mortality rates are reported as zero. Postoperative permanent cranial nerve deficiencies range from 10 to 18 percent, with a varying incidence of other surgically related disabilities. The team approach is emphasized with the need to include neurosurgeons. "These neoplasms represent monumental challenges to even the most experienced of neurotologic surgeons."[40]

It is difficult to summarize the rationale that supports the concept of early, primary, radical excision.

Certainly extirpation is possible in many glomus tumors, and as elsewhere, the smaller the better. Many patients are young and growth rate is often slow. The original concept of radioresistance arises from early experience with carotid body tumors, which usually present with a much larger mass than glomus jugulare tumors. Glover and Block[42] reported six patients treated with radiotherapy, all with several cranial nerves involved. Follow-up varied from 5 to 18 years; all except one (dying from unrelated causes) remained alive and free from further neurologic deficits. Modern radiotherapeutic techniques might enhance response even in large tumors, and even in the young patient, the risk of radiation-induced neoplasms would appear to be minimal.

Despite the formidable advances made in the surgical approach to the skull base, technical ability must not be allowed to supersede common sense. In a few specialized centers, selected cases may well require such surgery. However, it is doubtful whether a critical examination of the advantages of such surgery at present justifies its general acceptance as the treatment of choice in preference to skilled radiotherapy.

Juvenile Angiofibroma

Much of the confusion regarding the management of this often vascular benign lesion, which occurs predominantly in males, is due to inadequate classification. Although no effective means exists for determining preoperatively the relative amounts of stroma and angioma, and thus its vascularity, its extension can be determined by the use of angiography, tomography, and CT scanning.

The four types described by Fisch[43] accurately delineate those extensions that pose problems in surgical excision—the accepted method of management. When they are confined to nasopharynx, posterior nose, pterygomaxillary fossa, sphenoidal sinus, or maxillary sinus, near-total removal is possible by means of a lateral rhinotomy with, perhaps, preoperative selective embolization. Extension to the infratemporal fossa, orbit, and parasellar region necessitates an infratemporal approach, which should allow adequate removal. The residual functional loss consists of complete conductive loss as well as loss of sensation in the area of the mandibular nerve. Infiltration of the cavernous sinus, the region of the optic chiasma, or the pituitary fossa prevents complete removal. In lesions that are undergoing involution, residual tumor probably remains quiescent, although postoperative regrowth may be rapid even in older patients (Fig. 4). Radiotherapy is reserved in most instances for lesions considered inoperable or for recurrences following inadequate removal. However, many consider primary radiotherapy to be contraindicated if alternative treatment is available, because of the young age of the patients with this condition. Cummings reviewed the relative risks of both primary surgery and radiotherapy.[44] Accepting that certain assumptions were necessary relating to risks of general anesthesia, radio-

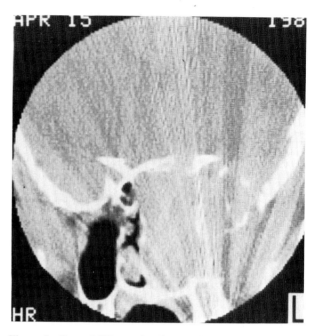

Figure 4 Coronal CT scan showing massive erosion of left pterygoid region and clinoid region from an angiofibroma occurring in a white Greek male aged 24 years following removal of a fibrous angioma 2 years previously.

graphic investigation, reduction in operative blood loss, surgery, and radiation, he concluded that the relative risks of management by primary surgery or radiotherapy were similar—fatal complications in 1 in 500 cases. Despite this imaginative analysis, most surgeons believe that this lesion should be treated by radical surgery, the approach being tailored to the anticipated extent.

In this section, I have examined some of the surgical procedures for which it is possible that, with the best intentions, we may be guilty of overenthusiasm. We live in an age of technical expertise, and it would seem unlikely that such an aggressive and dynamic specialty as head and neck surgery could be accused of doing too little. However, the subject deserves attention.

PERHAPS TOO LITTLE

Even the poorly equipped head and neck surgeon has rarely been accused of lack of enthusiasm for expanding the borders of surgical excision. Today, when most such individuals are well trained and working in an environment that permits the most radical of operative procedures, it seems unlikely that any surgeon could be accused of undue technical reticence!

No matter how the end-staging is calculated, the success rate in controlling cancer of the paranasal sinuses remains poor. This is related partly to the late stage of presentation, but also to the complex anatomy of the region, whereby most tumors of the maxillary sinus have involved the adjoining ethmoids at initial diagnosis. Combination therapy (surgery, radiotherapy, and possibly chemotherapy) is now used in a variety of ways; individual modalities have long proved to be less effective. Although no generally accepted system of classification has yet evolved, and most systems now used possess serious intrinsic defects, I have produced a plan that relates "T" grouping to the anatomic site of the tumor. This is because residual neoplasm is invariably found following radiotherapy, and success is then related to the likelihood of radical resection. Extension of primary surgery to include orbital contents, pterygoid region, or facial skin offers worthwhile palliation, but probably has not affected long-term cure rates. However, some mention must be made of the publications of Sakai et al.[46] By combining limited sinus surgery with radical radiotherapy and chemotherapy, they have reduced the incidence of total maxillectomy to 22 percent. In claiming a 5-year cumulative survival rate of 54 percent, they admit a systemic metastatic rate of 10 percent! The concept is of interest, but the classification system makes it difficult to compare their results with the more generally accepted figures of 30 percent long-term cure.

Although tumor remaining in the apex of the orbit or in the pterygoid region is virtually impossible to remove surgically, concern has long been expressed for neoplasms occurring primarily in the ethmoid labyrinth or olfactory area. The relatively slow-growing adenocarcinoma or localized olfactory neuroblastoma has previously been treated by the combination of radiotherapy and lateral rhinotomy. The latter operation provides exclent access,[47] but allows only an inadequate means of wide resection of the cribriform plate and associated dura. Recent investigation of the surgical pathology of this region illustrates the close relationship of cribriform plate to lateral ethmoidal masses[48] (Fig. 5). Since the plate, which is usually only 1 mm thick, has perforations for the passage of the olfactory nerves, there is a preformed communication between the nasal cavity and the cranial surface of the dura. In the case of olfactory tumors, all must be considered as having involved the olfactory bulbs despite the absence of radiologic evidence of bony erosion (Fig. 6).

The gradual development of the craniofacial approach to the cribriform plate area as a safe, standard procedure for the experienced head and neck surgeon, requiring no neurosurgical assistance, has resulted in an opportunity for primary radical surgery in selected tumors involving the ethmoid labyrinth and cribriform plate. Results obtained by Tony Cheesman in our Institution after 70 operations were as follows: only two patients had minor complications, zero mortality rate, and no instances of cerebrospinal leakage. However, postoperative radiotherapy may result in necrosis of the fascial graft and prolapse of the frontal lobes. Except in patients with noncurable conditions, such as chondrosarcoma, adequate local resection is usually possible.

The acceptable cosmetic appearance, low morbidity, and excellent exposure associated with this now

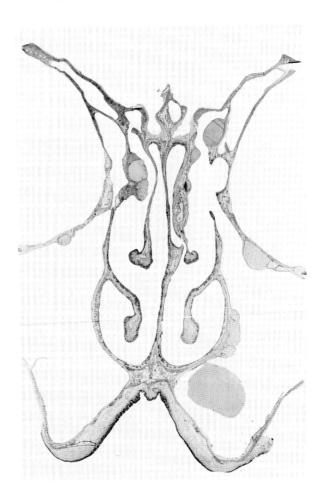

Figure 5 Serial section cut at 5 μ through normal midface to illustrate small area of cribriform plate and its close relationship to ethmoidal block.

routine operation offer an important opportunity for extending the surgical management of ethmoidal tumors. However, in the majority of antroethmoidal neoplasms, this region is only one of the areas where disease may remain. Although the apex of the orbit is accessible by the posterosuperior approach obtained from within the anterior cranial fossa, extension to the chiasma limits the margins of excision. Anything less radical for such tumors must now be considered inadequate surgery.

Surgery of the Tongue

An area in which most surgeons are reluctant to carry out the necessary radical resection is the tongue. When compared with a series of over 100 total glossectomies carried out without the benefit of endotracheal intubation or tracheostomy, reported by Whitehead in 1891,[49] the incidence of advanced tongue cancer has diminished in the Western world, although it continues to be common in Southeast Asia.

There are clear differences between the incidence, presenting symptoms, and management of tumors growing in the mobile anterior two-thirds of the

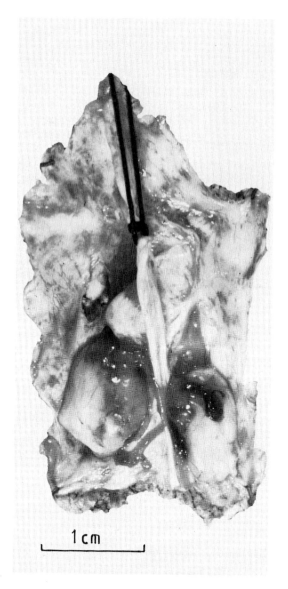

1 cm

Figure 6 Operative specimen of dura and olfactory bulbs removed via craniofacial approach. Essential surgery for olfactory neuroblastoma?

tongue (classified as oral cavity) and those in the less accessible fixed posterior one-third (oropharynx). However, such differences are related only to site for the tongue is one organ. The lingual septum exists for the attachment of the transverse muscular fibers, and there is no barrier to the spread of tumor either across the tongue or from anterior to posterior regions. Limited primary excision of small neoplasms arising within the anterior tongue is effective and not associated with marked disability. However, more radical resection is undoubtedly disabling, and since it is invariably carried out following radiation failure and with the hope of retaining some residual tongue, it is invariably inadequate. Local recurrence rates of 40 to 60 percent have been reported even when the margins of excision have been reported as clear.[50,51] Examination of total glossectomy specimens illustrates the variability of

tumor differentiation within invididual specimens and the presence of micrometastatic tumor deposits within 2 cm from the macroscopic margins of the tumor.[52] Since the greatest width of the adult tongue is 6.0 cm and a T2 oral cancer is defined as no more than 4 cm, surgical excision would have to be about 5.9 cm across the tongue base to ensure adequate margins!

It is this concept, together with the abhorrence of removing such a useful organ as the tongue, which has encouraged primary radiotherapy as the initial treatment of most tongue cancers. Parsons, Million, and Cassisi report a local control rate for a minimum of 2 years for tongue base tumors of over 60 percent for T1 to T3 lesions treated by primary irradiation.[58] The near impossibility of accurately estimating the real extent of the tumor in a painful tongue or inaccessible tongue base is exemplified by similar control rates for all except the very advanced tumors. Few failures were salvaged by subsequent surgery. Thawley et al,[54] using a combination of radiation and surgery for a greater number of patients, had a similar control rate, possibly because subsequent surgery was limited to partial glossectomy and supraglottic laryngectomy. There is little doubt that in all except the very advanced lesion most surgery will be carried out following radiotherapy. Residual or recurrent disease is usually obvious in this organ. However, limited excision is rarely effective, and the concept of early total glossectomy would surely enhance long-term control rates. Use of the pectoralis myocutaneous flap is a major contribution to the rebuilding of the floor of the oral cavity, where its bulk is of value. If the larynx is left in situ, reasonable vocal communication is possible together with adequate swallowing. However, examination of glossectomy and laryngectomy specimens suggests that in neoplasms involving the tongue base, allowing the larynx to remain in situ will jeopardize tumor control (Fig. 7). Local disease recurred in 26 percent of the cases reported by Thawley,[54] suggesting inadequate surgery, although in my own experience,[52] extension along the linguotonsillar sulcus to the lateral pharyngeal wall proved difficult to control.

It is suggested, therefore, that these factors be considered when resecting radiation failures in both anterior and posterior tongue. Early total glossectomy, possibly allowing preservation of the larynx, might then enhance long-term cure rates without producing unacceptable disability.

Adenoidcystic Carcinoma in the Head and Neck

Despite representing no more than 10 percent of all salivary neoplasms, this tumor has a unique natural history, confusing even the most experienced oncologists. The relevant factors that influence survival and must be considered when planning therapy have been demonstrated by Spiro, Huvos, and Strong.[55] Emphasizing that clinical staging, as advocated by the American Joint Committee for the parotid and submandibular glands, offers a more reliable prognostic

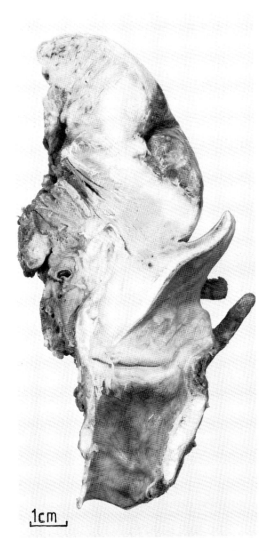

Figure 7 Total glossectomy and laryngectomy specimen showing extension of tumor to pre-epiglottic region.

1cm

guide than the histologic appearance, they reported a 5-year survival rate of 69 percent which dropped to 22 percent within 20 years.

Distant metastases were found in 43 percent of patients, one-third dying within 2 years of confirmation. However, a unique feature of this neoplasm is that 20 percent of patients survived 5 to 14 years after discovery of pulmonary metastasis, which was often solitary. The underlying problem with adenocystic carcinoma is the undetected extension, often perineurally, well outside the macroscopic extent of the tumor. Conley and Dingman had a 42 percent incidence of at least one local recurrence,[56] and although these patients may survive many years and many operations, local recurrence usually indicates incurability. When this tumor occurs within the paranasal sinuses, perineural and bone involvement is usually extensive, whatever the clinical and radiographic findings. All must be considered grade 3 and the prognosis poor. Local recurrence rate is greater with minor salivary gland tumors because of the impossibility of adequate monobloc resections within the nasal, oral, and pharyngeal cavities. Actuarial survival is significantly lower in patients with submandibular gland tumors because of a reluctance to excise digastric, mylohyoid, and hyoglossus muscles, lingual and hypoglossal nerves, the floor of the mouth, and possibly portions of the mandible. Conley has said that the "biggest operation that can be rationally developed is the best," for one can never rely entirely on clear margins with the ever-present threat of distant perineural spread.[56] This philosophy entails the removal of hard and soft palate, alveolus, pterygoid plates, and muscles, together with the contents of the nasal cavity, for even an apparently small palatal lesion. Combinations of more extensive initial surgery, postoperative radiotherapy, and possibly adjunctive chemotherapy, although this may improve the frequency of distant metastasis, may enhance local control. However, such an approach requires careful patient selection as well as favorable tumor sites. Whether the associated disabilities can be justified by a worthwhile increase in local control and possibly reduction in late-stage systemic metastasis is as yet unknown.

HOW DO WE KNOW WE ARE DOING THE RIGHT THING?

Although there is undoubtedly a sense of technical achievement in successfully performing a complex surgical operation, the prime purpose of our efforts is to cure each patient of malignant disease while producing the least possible interference with normal physiology and well-being. Since none of these praiseworthy motives can be measured objectively, and we now live in the age of computers and statisticians, it is essential for any self-respecting oncologist to be able to justify his opinions and therapy by means of figures and graphs. The rationale behind this totally erroneous concept has been superficially explored by me, utilizing a simple flow chart.[57]

INPUT—THERAPY—CURE RATE

The clinical oncologist, unlike the statistician, is aware that tumor growth is a reflection of intrinisic growth rate, histologic type, tumor-host relationships, and difficulty of diagnosis. Consequently, there must always be inherent weaknesses in any system of classification, and these vary with the anatomic site.[45] In addition, there is lack of uniformity between systems used throughout the world; there may not even be agreement on anatomic definitions. How often, one wonders, is it possible to evaluate objectively the available information with sufficient accuracy to describe the true dimensions and extent of any primary tumor or regional metastasis? If not, how important are such errors of assessment? Are such criteria sufficient to formulate an indication of prognosis and are the data recorded accurately enough to allow retrospective analysis? Such anxieties are well founded since they represent unknown, and often unsuspected, errors of input which in themselves may effectively nullify suggested improvements in treatment.

Even more disturbing is the variety of ways in which cancer survival figures are calculated and presented. Stell and Morton recently examined this problem in depth, utilizing 362 patients with carcinoma of the hypopharynx and an untreated group of 254 patients who had died from cancer.[58] Apart from illustrating the varying results from these various analyses, they found that medium survival time was a poor estimation of average survival. A similar and more expansive review can be found in Mould's book, *Cancer Statistics*, published in 1983.[59] However, it is still common to find a wide range of variance in presentation of end results of treatment within many journals and textbooks. How then can we judge the long-term effects of our therapy when both the input and output contain such potential errors? If we are to accept a plea for more radical surgery, together with greater usage of both radiotherapy and chemotherapy, then surely serious attention must be paid to the construction of meaningful, realistic systems of classification and clearly defined end-stage statistics.

CONCLUSIONS

The acceptance of the head and neck surgeon as a specialist in his own right, requiring specific experience in addition to basic training within a related surgical field, has provided an increased challenge to develop surgical oncology. I have attempted to identify several areas in which more radical, even adventurous surgery might improve local tumor control. There are also areas in which the available evidence may suggest that less radical excisions may be effective, although experience and informed judgment are paramount in making such a decision. Combined clinics, with their need for open, justified decision making, must surely be the best protection for the patient against the overenthusiastic applied anatomist. However, well-trained technically competent surgeons working with adequately equipped and staffed facilities, aided by a competent oncologic team, must surely offer each patient the best opportunity of cure. Although much progress toward this goal has been made in the 1980s, we cannot be sure whether we are doing too much or too little operating. Perhaps our salvation lies in actually asking the question!

REFERENCES

1. Conley J. Changes in head and neck surgery. Am J Surg 1983; 146:425–428.
2. Conley J. Trends in minimizing deformity in head and neck resections. J Laryngol 1983; 97:1047–1052.
3. Conley J. Ethics in head and neck surgery. Arch Otolaryngol 1981; 107:655–657.
4. Moore C. Changing concepts in head and neck surgical on-cology. Am J Surg 1980; 140:480–486.
5. Bryce DP. In pursuit of excellence. Arch Otolaryngol 1982; 108:757–758.
6. Schuknecht HF. To treat or not to treat - a difficult question. Laryngoscope 1982; 1393–1394.
7. Harrison DFN. The natural history of some cancers affecting the head and neck. J Laryngol 1972; 86:1189–1202.
8. Wright MR. Self perception of the elective surgeon and some patient perception correlates. Arch Otolaryngol 1980; 106:460–465.
9. Addison C. The social implications of sudden facial disfigurement. Social Work Today 1978; 9:18–20.
10. Looser KG, Shah JP, Strong EW. The significance of "positive" margins in surgically resected epidermoid carcinomas. Head Neck Surg 1978; 1:107–111.
11. Shah JP, Cendon RA, Farr HW. Carcinoma of the oral cavity—factors affecting treatment failure at the primary site and neck. Am J Surg 1976; 132:504–507.
12. Bauer WC, Lesinski SG, Ogura J. The significance of positive margins in hemi laryngectomy specimens. Laryngoscope 1975; 85:1–13.
13. Mantravadi RVP, Haas RE, Skolnick EM. Postoperative radiotherapy for persistent tumor at the surgical margin in head and neck cancer. Laryngoscope 1983; 93:1337–1340.
14. Vikram B, Strong EW, Shah JP, Spiro R. Failure at the primary site following multimodality treatment in advanced head and neck cancer. Head Neck Surg 1984; 6:720–723.
15. Harrison DFN. Correlation between Clinical and Histological Staging in Laryngeal Cancer. Ph.D. Thesis, University of London, 1983.
16. Bocca E, Pignatabo O, Oldini C. Supraglottic laryngectomy: 30 years experience. Ann Otol Rhinol Laryngol 1983; 92:14–18.
17. Russ JE, Sullivan C, Gallager HS, Jesse RH. Conservation surgery of the larynx: a reappraisal based on whole organ study. Am J Surg 1979; 138:588–596.
18. Mohr RM, Quenelle DJ, Shumrick DA. Verticofronto lateral laryngectomy. Arch Otolaryngol 1983; 109:384–395.
19. Crile G. Excision of cancer of the head and neck with special reference to the plan of dissection based upon 132 operations. JAMA 1906; 47:1780–1786.
20. De Santo L, Holt JJ, Beahrs OH, O'Fallon WM. Neck dissection: is it worthwhile? Laryngoscope 1982; 92:502–509.
21. McGuirt WF, McCabe BF, Krause CJ. Complications of radical neck dissection: a survey of 788 patients. Head Neck Surg 1979; 1:481–487.
22. Bocca E, Pignatarro O. A conservation technique in radical neck dissection. Ann Otol Rhinol Laryngol 1967; 76:975–979.
23. Schuller DE, Reiches NA, Hamaker RC, Lingeman RE, Weisberger EC, Suen JY, Conley J, Kelly DR, Miglets AW. Analysis of disability resulting from treatment including radical neck dissection or modified neck dissection. Head Neck Surg 1983; 6:551–558.
24. Rabuzzi DD, Chung CT, Sagerman RH. Prophylactic neck irradiation. Arch Otolaryngol 1980; 106:454–455.
25. Calearo CV, Teatini G. Functional neck dissection—anatomical grounds, surgical technique, clinical observations. Ann Otol Rhinol Laryngol 1983; 92:215–222.
26. Pearson JG. Radiotherapy of carcinoma of the oesophagus and postcricoid region in South-East Scotland. Clin Radiol 1966; 17:242–249.
27. Harrison DFN. Thyroid gland in the management of laryngopharyngeal cancer. Arch Otolaryngol 1973; 97:301–302.
28. Wookey H. Surgical treatment of carcinoma of the pharynx and upper oesophagus. Surg Gynec Obstet 1942; 75:499–506.
29. Harrison DFN. Pathology of hypopharyngeal cancer in relation to surgical management. J Laryngol 1970; 84:349–367.
30. Stell PM, Ramadan MF, Dalby JE, Hibbert J, Raab GM, Singh SD. Management of post-cricoid carcinoma. Clin Otolaryngol 1982; 7:145–152.
31. Harrison DFN. The use of colonic transplants and revascularized jejunal autografts for primary repair after pharynglaryngoesophagectomy. Proc Roy Soc Med 1964; 57:1104–1107.

32. Harrison DFN. Resection of the manubrium. Br J Surg 1977; 64:347–377.

33. Griffiths JD, Shaw HJ. Cancer of the laryngopharynx and cervical esophagus. Arch Otoloaryngol 1973; 97:340–346.

34. Stell PM, Ramadan MF, George WD. Postcricoid carcinoma: the place of visceral transposition. Clin Oncol 1982; 8:17–20.

35. Harrison DFN. Surgical management of hypopharyngeal cancer. Arch Otolaryngol 1979; 105:149–152.

36. Lewis JS. Temporal bone resection: review of 100 cases. Arch Otolaryngol 1975; 101:23–25.

37. Goodwin WJ, Jesse RH. Malignant neoplasms of the external auditory canal and temporal bone. Arch Otolaryngol 1980; 106:675–679.

38. Lederman M. Malignant tumours of the ear. J Laryngol 1965; 79:85–119.

39. Fisch U. Infratemporal fossa approach to tumors of the temporal bone and base of the skull. J Laryngol 1978; 92:949–967.

40. Jackson CG, Glasscock ME, Harris PF. Glomus tumors. Arch Otolaryngol 1982; 108:401–406.

41. Jenkins HA, Fisch U. Glomus tumors of the temporal bone. Arch Otolaryngol 1981; 107:209–214.

42. Glover, GW, Block J. Glomus jugulare tumors–radiotherapy or surgery. Br J Surg 1972; 59:947–953.

43. Fisch U. The infratemporal fossa approach for nasopharyngeal tumors. Laryngoscope. 1983; 93:36–44.

44. Cummings BJ. Relative risk factors in the treatment of juvenile nasopharyngeal angiofibroma. Head Neck Surg 1980; 3:21–26.

45. Harrison DFN. Critical look at the classification of maxillary sinus carcinomata. Ann Otol Rhinol Laryngol 1978; 87:3–9.

46. Sakai S, Homki A, Fuchimata H, Tanaka D. Multidisciplinary treatment of maxillary sinus carcinoma. Cancer 1983; 52:1360–1364.

47. Harrison DFN. Lateral rhinotomy: a neglected operation. Ann Otol Rhinol Laryngol 1977; 86:756–759.

48. Harrison DFN. Surgical pathology of olfactory neuroblastoma. Head Neck Surg 1984; 7:60–64.

49. Whitehead W. A hundred cases of entire excision of the tongue. Br Med J 1891; 1:961–965.

50. Schleuning AS, Summers CW. Carcinoma of the tongue; a review of 220 cases. Laryngoscope 1972; 82:1146–1454.

51. Skolnick EM, Saberman MN. Cancer of the tongue. Otolaryngol Clin N Am 1969; 2:603–615.

52. Harrison DFN. The questionable value of total glossectomy. Head Neck Surg 1983; 6:632–638.

53. Parsons JT, Million RR, Cassisi NJ. Carcinoma of the base of the tongue: results of radical irradiation with surgery reserved for irradiation failures. Laryngoscope 1982; 92:689–696.

54. Thawley SE, Simpson JR, Marks JE, Perez CA, Ogura J. Preoperative irradiation and surgery for carcinoma of the base of the tongue. Ann Otol Rhinol Laryngol 1983; 92:485–490.

55. Spiro RH, Huvos AG, Strong EW. Adenoidcystic carcinoma: factors influencing survival. Am J Surg 1979, 138:579–583.

56. Conley J, Dingman DL. Adenoidcystic carcinoma in the head and neck. Arch Otolaryngol 1974; 100:81–90.

57. Harrison DFN. The value of multimodal treatment and new approaches to therapy. Head Neck Cancer 1983; 18:223–247.

58. Stell PM, Morton RP. ''Average'' survival times after treatment of cancer. Clin Oncol 1982; 8:293–303.

59. Mould RF. Cancer statistics. Medical Science Series, Bristol: Adam Hilger Ltd, 1983.

5. Biology of Modern Radiotherapy for Head and Neck Cancer

LESTER J. PETERS, M.D.

In recent years our understanding of the biology of radiotherapy, as it affects the management of patients with head and neck cancer, has improved significantly. This is particularly true with regard to modified radiation dose fractionation schedules, and the increasing use of combined modality treatment strategies. Although clinical practice is certainly possible without an understanding of radiobiology, familarity with the basic concepts permits a better appreciation of the strengths and weaknesses of the various treatment strategies and offers a rational approach for future modifications of technique so as to improve the therapeutic outcome.

CELLULAR EFFECTS OF IONIZING RADIATION

Cell Death

Cellular radiation biology has its origins in the development of techniques to assay clonogenic cell survival, i.e., the ability of single cells to grow into visible clones analogous to those formed by bacteria when plated onto an appropriate culture medium. The ability to form a clone is dependent on the reproductive integrity of the cell, and thus, from the point of view of radiation biology, cell death is defined as loss of reproductive integrity or clonogenic capacity.[1] While morphologic disruption of a cell is clearly incompatible with reproductive survival, the converse is not true; in other words, a cell may appear intact morphologically, but may have lost its reproductive capability by virtue of injury to its genetic apparatus. This is the most common mode of cell death following exposure to ionizing radiation, and the bulk of experimental evidence points to DNA as being the critical target for radiation injury for the majority of cell types. Radiation injury to DNA is expressed when cells attempt mitotic division. This is not necessarily the first division after radiation exposure, and pedigree studies have shown that mitotic death may occur after several apparently successful cell divisions have been accomplished. The essence of clonogenic survival, however, is the ability to reproduce indefinitely, and even cells that retain the capability of several mitotic divisions before undergoing mitotic death are considered sterilized by irradiation.

Less frequently, cell death following radiation injury is not linked to cell division and is therefore termed "interphase death". Unlike mitotic death, interphase death occurs soon after radiation exposure, presumably as a result of damage to the plasma membrane; histologically, it creates the impression of extreme sensitivity of the cell type to ionizing radiation. Classic interphase death with cell lysis is manifested by certain classes of lymphocytes. Another more recently described mode of interphase death is apoptosis,[2] a process by which defunct cells collapse into electron-dense bodies with preservation of organelles and are subsequently phagocytosed by adjacent parenchymal cells. In the head and neck region the serous cells of the salivary glands, which have a slow turnover rate, undergo acute interphase death after modest doses of radiation.[3] The mechanism by which this occurs has not been fully elucidated.

Loss of Tissue Function

Unlike reproductive integrity, the vegetative functions of most mammalian cells are not detectably altered by doses of radiation in the range used clinically. Thus, loss of function of an organ following irradiation is not due to loss of an increment of function of individual cells, but rather to a depletion of the total number of functional cells in the tissue. Depending on the kinetic and organizational status of a particular tissue, its functional response to radiation may vary widely. In general, tissues that are rapidly turning over and have definable stem cell, maturation, and functional cell compartments manifest radiation injury soon after exposure, with a rate of onset that is not greatly dose-dependent. Examples of such tissues include most epithelia and the bone marrow. Depending on the extent of stem cell depletion, these tissues may recover essentially all of their function following irradiation. These types of tissues have been termed type H (Hierarchical) (Fig. 1).[4]

However, tissues characterized by low cell turnover rates and populations of functional parenchymal cells that retain the ability to revert to a reproductive function in the event of tissue loss manifest more delayed radiation injury. At the time of onset, such injury is dependent on radiation dose and tends to increase in severity with time due to an "avalanche" phenomenon, i.e., the drawing into the division cycle of cells harboring latent reproductive injury. These tissues are termed type F (Flexible) (Fig. 2).[4] Examples of such tissues with reference to radiotherapy in the head and neck region include bone, neuroglial, and endocrine tissues.

PATHOGENESIS OF ACUTE AND LATE REACTIONS

Acute reactions to radiation therapy are arbitrarily defined as those whose onset normally occurs dur-

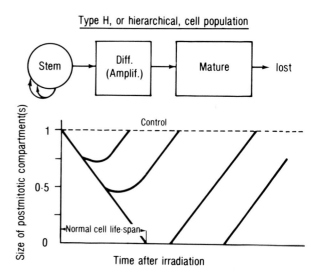

Figure 1 *Top*, A schematic representation of a type H cell population. *Bottom*, Theoretic response of a type H cell population to a range of single doses of ionizing radiation. During this period of zero input to the mature compartment of newly born mature cells, the total number of these cells declines linearly at a rate equal to that characteristic of steady-state conditions of the tissue concerned. The onset of the complete depletion occurs at a time equal to normal mature cell longevity. Recuperation sets in later the higher the dose. (From Michalowski.[4])

ing a conventional course of treatment. This allows for therapeutic modifications to be made in the event that acute reactions are excessive. Conversely, late radiation reactions have their onset months or years after radiation therapy is completed, and treatment decisions involving late reactions can only be made on a probability basis.

Acute reactions are usually associated with denudation of epithelia. In the head and neck region the most significant acute reactions involve the mucous membranes of the aerodigestive tracts, which are rapidly proliferating tissues. The skin is also an acutely reacting tissue, although the severity of skin reactions is usually less than that of the mucous membranes because of the skin-sparing effect of megavoltage radiation beams. Acute epithelial reactions result from radiation killing of stem cells in the basal layer. Death of these cells has no immediate clinical consequence, but the physiologic loss of cells in the superficial layers of the epithelium is not made good, and after a lag period of approximately 1 to 2 weeks for the mucous membranes and 2 to 3 weeks for skin, epithelial denudation occurs. This denudation triggers a regenerative response in the stem cells surviving radiation injury, and this acts to offset the depletion of stem cell compartment by irradiation. In most persons this regenerative response can keep pace with weekly doses of the order of 900 to 1000 rads in five fractions, and this is the main reason for the common use of this fractionation schedule. If more intensive dose schedules are adopted, it is often necessary to introduce a split in the treatment regimen to enable epithelial regeneration to catch up before resuming therapy. The severity of acute mucosal reactions varies inversely with the volume of tissue irradiated and also with the site. Acute reactions in the oral cavity are less well tolerated than those in the pharynx, whereas severe reactions in the larynx may be associated with acute edema, causing compromise of the airway.

A completely different pathogenesis underlies the acute response manifested by salivary tissue to irradiation. The salivary glands are not rapid turnover tissues, and according to general radiobiologic principles, they would not be expected to manifest an acute radiation response. However, the serous cells of the salivary glands are uniquely susceptible to acute interphase death following radiation exposure. This causes a rapid reduction in the volume and quality of saliva (Fig. 3).[5] Reduction in salivary flow is associated with loss of taste, increased friability of the mucous membranes, and aggravated risk of dental caries and periodontal disease. Unlike the epithelia of the mucous membranes, the surviving cells of the salivary glands do not regenerate themselves rapidly or completely, and recovery from radiation injury is therefore slow and usually incomplete.

Late reactions may occur in a variety of slowly proliferating tissues following irradiation of the head and neck region, including vascular and connective tissues, bone, endocrine glands, and the central nervous system. Since these tissues are not actively proliferative, the duration of a course of treatment does not significantly affect their tolerance to radiation

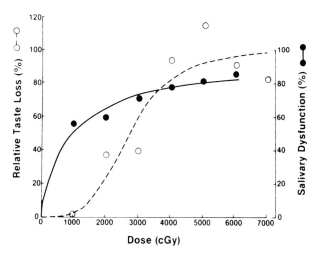

Figure 3 Dose-response curves for salivary dysfunction and taste loss in patients during radiotherapy for head and neck tumors. Abscissa is cumulative radiation dose. Closed circles and solid lines represent the dose-response curve for salivary dysfunction, defined as the percentage decrease in salivary flow rate measured at a particular radiation dose relative to the preradiotherapy flow rate. Open circles and dashed line represent the dose-response curve for taste loss. (From Mossman[5])

therapy. However, the sensitivity of these tissues is markedly dependent on the size of dose per fraction used, the tolerance being much greater for a smaller size of dose per fraction. Therefore, large incremental-dose fractions are generally discouraged, and when such fractions are used, the total doses must be judiciously set. In particular, formulations based on the NSD, TDF, or CRE systems cannot be used to determine equivalent doses when large-size doses per fraction are employed without risking severe late normal tissue injury. The differential effects of fraction size and overall treatment time on the doses necessary to produce equal acute and late radiation reactions are summarized in Figure 4.[6]

FACTORS AFFECTING RADIOSENSITIVITY

Multiple factors can modify cellular radiosensitivity and thus affect the observed response to a given dose of radiation.

Oxygen

As early as 1904, it was observed that interference with the blood supply of irradiated skin reduced the intensity of the erythema that was produced. However, it was not until the early 1950s that it was appreciated that the presence of molecular oxygen at the time of irradiation rather than the metabolic state of cells determined their radiosensitivity.[7] The presence of molecular oxygen appears to fix labile radiation injury that would otherwise be repaired within milliseconds of irradiation. Thus, although the same number of radiochemical lesions are produced by irradiation in the presence or absence of oxygen, many

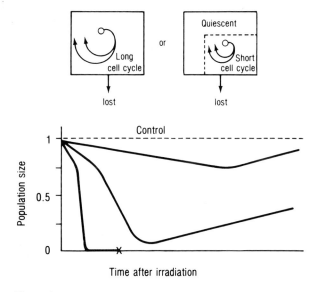

Type F, or flexible, cell population

Figure 2 *Top,* A schematic representation of a type F cell population. *Bottom,* Theoretic response of a type F cell population to a range of single doses of ionizing radiation. The first, slower phase of depopulation is followed by the "avalanche" if the dose is large enough. The overall rate of depletion is inversely related to dose, the more severe damage developing earlier. (From Michalowski[4])

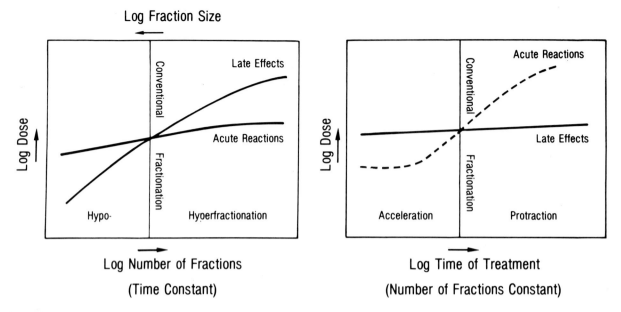

Figure 4 Effect of changes in time-dose relationships in fractionated radiotherapy on acute and late normal tissue reactions. Curves represent isoeffective doses for a given level of reactions, normalized to the point designated "conventional fractionation", i.e., 1.8 to 2.0 Gy, five fractions per week. *Left,* With overall time held constant, a change in the number (and size) of dose fractions has a relatively greater effect on the isoeffective doses for late effects than for acute reactions. In particular, it should be noted that hypofractionation carries the risk of overdosage for late effects if doses are adjusted to equalize acute reactions. *Right,* The effect of varying overall time of treatment, with the number of fractions held constant. The influence of time on the isoeffect dose for acute reactions is complex. If the treatment time is less than the turnover time of the tissues in question, registration of the radiation injury will occur after treatment is completed, and the ensuing regenerative response will not affect the isoeffect dose. When the treatment time extends into the regeneration phase, however, the isoeffect dose for a given acute reaction increases steeply, flattening off again as treatment times exceed the most active regenerative spurt. With any protraction beyond conventional treatment times, acute reactions are preferentially spared, leading to excessive late effects if doses are made isoeffective for acute reactions. Thus, both hypofractionation and protraction are hazardous strategies if based on acute normal tissue reactions. (From Peters[6])

more are repaired if oxygen in absent. The range of oxygen tensions over which the maximum change in radiosensitivity occurs is from 0 to 20 mmHg. Within this range there is considerable variability among cell types as to the effect of oxygen tension on cell survival. Oxygen is usually considered to be dose-modifying, i.e., the dose required to produce a certain level of cell survival is greater by a constant factor in the absence of oxygen than in well oxygenated conditions. This factor is known as the oxygen enhancement ratio (OER), which, for most mammalian cells, is the order of 2.5 to 3. There is some evidence that the OER may be somewhat lower for small-sized doses per fraction or low dose-rate irradiation because of the preponderance of cell killing by single-hit mechanisms.[8]

Since the range of partial pressures of oxygen over which cellular radiation sensitivity varies most markedly is well below the PO^2 of venous blood, the clinical relevance of the oxygen effect is not immediately apparent. However, in 1955, Thomlinson and Gray combined histologic observations with oxygen diffusion calculations to predict that radiobiologic hypoxia would exist in human solid tumors.[9] Although direct evidence of radiobiologic hypoxia cannot be obtained from human material, there is abundant indirect evidence that these conditions exist, and all solid ex-

perimental tumors show evidence of the presence of radioresistant hypoxic cells.

In contrast to the situation in which a subpopulation of cells is located remote from blood vessels and is therefore radiobiologically hypoxic, the situation can exist in normal tissues, and possibly in tumors as well, in which, by virtue of shunting of blood through arteriovenous anastomses, whole populations of cells can be marginally hypoxic and thus somewhat more resistant to radiation than they are under fully oxygenated conditions.[10]

Because of the magnitude of the oxygen effect and the unequivocal evidence of the presence of radiobiologic hypoxia in experimental animal tumors, many treatment strategies aimed at overcoming the resistance of such cells have been tested. These strategies include the use of hyperbaric oxygen, mixtures of oxygen and carbon dioxide (to induce vasodilatation), chemical analogs of oxygen, metabolic approaches to inhibit oxygen consumption, selective vasoconstriction in normal tissues, and tourniquet hypoxia. A fair summary of the clinical results of these strategies is that the beneficial results have been associated with the use of large fractional doses of radiation, whereas with conventionally fractionated radiation, results have been disappointing.[11] This suggests that the oxygen status of hypoxic cells surviving one dose of radiation improves during the interval between fractions, a process termed ''reoxygenation''.

Because many human tumors are cured by doses of radiation that would be inconsistent with the presence of a significant number of hypoxic tumor cells, and because strategies to improve tumor control based on the oxygen effect have been largely unsuccessful with conventionally fractionated treatment, it can be concluded that reoxygenation does, indeed, occur in those human tumors controlled by radiation therapy. The failure of reoxygenation is a possible cause of failure to control a given tumor, but it is only one of many.

Cell Age in the Division Cycle

Experiments with synchronized cell populations have demonstrated significant variations in the radiosensitivity of the same cell type as it traverses the division cycle. In virtually all cell lines the late G2 and mitotic phases are the most sensitive, the next most sensitive phases being late G1 and early S. Many cell lines show a peak of resistance in late S phase, and those with a long G1 phase also tend to show a peak of resistance in early G1. In spite of these differences, however, cell killing by radiation is not phase-specific as is the case with certain chemotherapeutic agents, and cells in all phases of the division cycle are susceptible to radiation killing. By delivering a course of radiation in multiple fractions, the chances of irradiating a given cell in a sensitive phase of the division cycle are increased, particularly with respect to cell populations that have a moderately rapid turnover rate. This applies both to acutely reacting normal tissues and to tumors. Conversely, late-reacting normal tissues with a very low turnover rate would not be sensitized to any extent by redistribution during a conventional course of therapy. This results in a net gain in the therapeutic ratio between tumor control and late normal tissue injury.

Quality of Radiation

The biologic effect of a given absorbed dose of radiation varies markedly according to the quality of the radiation. The relative biologic effect (RBE) of a given beam in relation to a reference standard is calculated as the dose of the reference standard divided by the dose of the beam in question to produce the same biologic effect. In relation to ^{60}Co gamma rays, kilovoltage x-rays are somewhat more effective, rad for rad, by a factor of 10 percent to 15 percent. Recent data suggest that high-energy electrons and protons are also more biologically effective by about the same factor.

All the beams of x-rays, gamma rays, electrons, and protons are characterized as having low linear energy transfer (LET), i.e., the density of ionization produced by such beams is sparse. On the other hand, irradiation with heavy nuclear particles, such as fast neutrons or heavy nuclei, produces tracks of dense ionization, and these beams are said to have high LET (Fig. 5).[12] High LET beams are much more damaging, rad for rad, to biologic material than are low LET beams. No constant factor is applicable for stating this difference in biologic effect, however, because the shape of the survival curves of cells irradiated with high LET radiations is different from that following low LET radiation. The most notable differences are that the shoulder of the radiation survival curve is markedly reduced or abolished and the terminal slope is steeper. In addition, there is less dependence on molecular oxygen and on cell age as determinants of radiati/n survival. Furthermore, cells show liseen simultaneously by participating physicians from each service. At that time, the patient's pretherapy examination was reviewed and all patients were staged according to the American Joint Committee for Cancer Staging System.[10]

All 114 evaluable patients received their chemotherapy as induction chemotherapy prior to definitive treatment. All patients receiving chemotherapy on this protocol were hospitalized at the Dana-Farber Cancer Institute, the Children's Hospital Medical Center, or the Beth Iw LET radiation will have the highest RBE for high LET radiation.

A

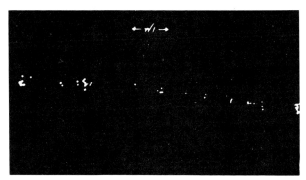

B

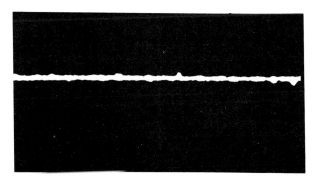

Figure 5 *A*, Cloud chamber tract of a fast electron illustrates that ionization occurs in clusters. Successive clusters are separated by approximately 1 μm. *B*, Cloud chamber tract of a proton ejected by a neutron; note the high density of ion pairs. (From Bacq ZM, Alexander P.[12])

Drugs

Many drugs are capable of modifying radiation response when given in conjunction with radiation. This may be due to independent cytotoxicity or to interactive reactions, as defined below:

1. *Independent action.* The total effect of the combination is equal to that of the agents given separately. All cytotoxic agents have an element of independent action, although some interact with radiation as well.
2. *Additivity.* Not only are independently induced lethal events cumulative, but sublethal lesions inflicted by the two agents may interact to cause increased lethality. In situations where cell killing results only from single-hit lethal lesions or where complete repair of sublethal lesions occurs in the time between administration of the two agents, additivity reduces to independent action.
3. *Supra-additivity (Synergism).* Interaction between two agents results in cell killing greater than that ascribable to additivity. An example of supra-additivity is the interaction of actinomycin-D and radiation.
4. *Sub-additivity (Antagonism).* Interaction between two agents results in cell killing less than that ascribable to additivity or independent action. Radioprotection by sulfhydryl-containing compounds is an example of sub-additivity.

Definition of the type of interaction between radiation and drugs is difficult and requires a complexity of analysis not usually possible in clinical settings. The most valid technique for studying interactions is to generate single-agent dose-response curves for each of the two agents being studied and to construct isobolograms defining a given level of effect for different doses of the two agents in combination, based on assumption of zero or maximum additivity. This results in what is known as the envelope of additivity,[14] outside of which supra- or subadditive interactions can be presumed to occur (Fig. 6).[15] In clinical practice the term synergism is frequently misused to describe any situation in which an increased reaction is observed, when, in fact, this could be due to independent action, additivity, or even subadditive interaction rather than true synergism.

Regardless of their mode of interaction, the combination of cytotoxic drugs and radiation will increase cell kill, and this usually translates into an increased tumor response. Unfortunately, however, the same applies to normal tissues, so that normal tissue reactions, both acute and late, are also exacerbated unless total radiation doses are reduced. The experience with concomitant intra-arterial 5-FU (5-fluorouracil) and radiotherapy at UT M.D.Anderson Hospital illustrates this point.[1];6 From the radiobiologic perspective, the use of interactive combined modalities invalidates many of the predictors of radiation response, for example, changes in fractionation and dose rate. Since drug exposure at the cellular level is difficult to measure and constantly changing after administration, experimental measurement of parameters of interactive combined modalities is extraordinarily complex, and clinical dose schedules must be determined empirically. On the other hand, sequential (noninteractive) combined modality therapy involves only independent toxicity, and well-established radiobiologic parameters may be applied, thus reducing the risk of substantial over- or underdosage. For this reason, sequential combined modality therapy is now usually favored, and several preliminary reports have indicated encouraging results in uncontrolled studies with combination chemotherapy given before definitive surgery or radiotherapy.[17,18] It is too soon, however, to conclude that this approach will improve the overall long-term results of therapy, and a recent randomized clinical trial resulted in poorer survival of the patients receiving adjuvant chemotherapy before and after definitive radiation therapy.[19] Experimentally, improved therapeutic outcomes have been achieved with alternating schedules of chemotherapy and radiation therapy,[20] the rationale being that modest doses of radiation given between cycles of chemotherapy will prevent the emergence of drug-resistant subpopulations of tumor cells. This approach has not been tested clinically in head and neck cancer.

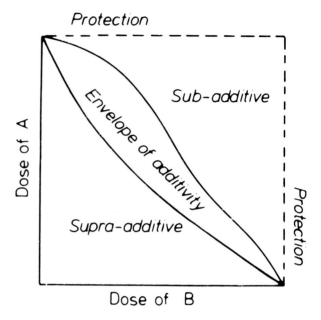

Figure 6 Recommended terminology for interactions between two agents, based on an isobologram. (From Steel GG, Peckham MJ.[15])

Heat

Hyperthermia is an investigational mode of therapy capable of modifying and complementing ionizing radiation.[21] In contrast to radiation therapy, hyperthermia is preferentially toxic to cells at low pH (usually corresponding to areas of hypoxia and aner-obic metabolism) and to cells in the S phase of the division cycle. In addition, relatively mild hyperther-mia of 42 to 43°C sensitizes cells to irradiation both by reducing the shoulder and increasing the slope of the radiation cell survival curves. Since tumors are in general less well perfused than normal tissues, it is frequently posible to induce higher temperatures within tumors than in surrounding normal tissues, thus pro-viding a therapeutic advantage. Unfortunately, the sound biologic rationale for combined hyperthermia and irradiation is not matched by the technology nec-essary to accurately heat and monitor interstitial tem-peratures. The head and neck region is particularly difficult for hyperthermia because of intolerance of the central nervous system to heating and poor patient tolerance because of pain. Although data are lacking, it is also likely that the avascular cartilages of the lar-ynx would be at increased risk of thermal injury. For these reasons, application of hyperthermia in head and neck cancer has been essentially limited to treatment of inoperable neck masses.

ALTERED FRACTIONATION SCHEDULES

Radiation dose fractionation schedules have evolved empirically over the years, with a general tendency toward protraction of treatment to prevent acute mucosal reactions from interrupting the course of radiotherapy. So-called conventional fractionation schemes vary in different parts of the world, but in the United tates the term "conventional fractiona-tion" is generally held to mean incremental doses of 180 to 200 cGy delivered 5 days per week for periods of 6 to 8 weeks. Recently, on the basis of radiobiol-ogic considerations, attempts have been made to im-prove the therapeutic ratio by using multiple dose fractions per day. There are two distinct rationales for the use of more than one daily dose fraction, and this is reflected in the following terminology:

1. *Accelerated Fractionation.* Overall treatment time is reduced by giving two or more daily dose frac-tions of close to conventional size.
2. *Hyperfractionation.* The overall time is conven-tional or slightly protracted, but an increase in to-tal dose is achieved by giving two or more small dose fractions on each treatment day.

The major difference from conventional treat-ment with accelerated fractionation is the shortening of overall treatment time, whereas with hyperfrac-tionation it is a reduction in size of dose-per-fraction with a corresponding increase in total dose. The basic concept underlying accelerated fractionation is pre-vention of treatment failure due to tumor cell regen-eration during treatment. This is more likely when clonogenic cells are characterized by a short potential doubling time. The use of accelerated fractionation protocols in the treatment of head and neck cancer is

limited by severe acute mucosal reactions, which often necessitate an interruption in treatment. Such a break defeats the main rationale for accelerated fractiona-tion. To avoid this limitation, one may use the tech-nique of concomitant boost, by which a second daily treatment is given to a reduced "field-within-a-field" on certain days during the basic course of therapy. Recent analysis of results of the concomitant boost technique as practiced at UT M.D. Anderson Hospital revealed an actuarial local-regional disease control rate at 2 years of 65 percent in a series of 53 patients with advanced nodal or primary disease.[22] Of these pa-tients, only three required an interruption in treatment because of excessive acute reactions.

In contrast, hyperfractionation has its rationale in the different ways in which acute and late radiation responses are affected by dose fractionation (see Fig. 4). Conventional fractionation schedules are limited in total dose by late normal tissue injury. The use of smaller fractions increases the tolerance of late-react-ing normal tissue and therefore allows the total dose to be increased. This increased total dose has a greater relative effect on acutely reacting tissues, and insofar as most tumors resemble kinetically acutely reacting tissues, an improvement in therapeutic ratio for tumor control in relation to late normal tissue injury may be anticipated.

The choice of strategy, i.e., whether to use ac-celerated fractionation (concomitant boost) or hyper-fractionation in a given clinical circumstance, de-pends basically on the tumor's cell kinetics: the greater the regenerative potential of the tumor, the more ac-celerated fractionation would be preferred. The re-verse, however, is not the case, i.e., hyperfraction-ation would not be the preferred strategy for extremely indolent tumors, since the rationale for hyperfraction-ation depends on tumors behaving kinetically in a fashion similar to acutely responding normal tissues. On radiobiologic grounds, very indolent tumors would be best treated with high LET radiation since cell ra-diosensitivity in different phases of the division cycle varies much less with such beams, and resistance con-ferred by failure of redistribution between dose frac-tions is minimized.

The niche for hyperfractionation would therefore be in the treatment of tumors with intermediate turn-over rates, i.e., potential doubling times of the order of a few weeks.

RATIONALE FOR INTERSTITIAL RADIOTHERAPY

The same basic considerations that apply to frac-tionated irradiation also apply to low-dose-rate con-tinuous irradiation. However, implantation techniques do offer certain advantages where they are technically feasible. Radiobiologically, interstitial therapy com-bines the benefits of both hyperfractionation and ac-celerated fractionation since low-dose-rate continuous irradiation is equivalent to a large number of very small fractions, while continuous exposure reduces the duration of treatment much more than can be achieved with an external beam technique. Furthermore, interstitial therapy permits the volume of high-dose radiation to be kept small, owing to the rapid fall-off of dose around implanted sources, allowing normal structures outside the target volume to be preferentially spared. The disadvantages associated with the interstitial technique relate mainly to the increased risk of inadequate dosage to part of the tumor or risk of normal tissue injury associated with "hot spots" adjacent to individual radioactive sources. Provided the technical skills are available, however, and patients for interstitial therapy are carefully selected, this technique is one of the most effective means of radiotherapy available.

DOSE RESPONSE CURVES FOR TUMOR CONTROL PROBABILITY

For tumor to be controlled, it must, by definition, contain no surviving clonogenic cells. When the average number of surviving clonogens per tumor is known, the probability of zero survivors in a particular tumor is obtained from Poisson statistics, e.g., $p = e^{-n}$, where n is the average number of surviving clonogenic cells per tumor. For example, if the probability of cure is 50 percent, then n = 0.693. This does not mean that there is a fraction of a cell surviving in each tumor, but rather that half the tumors contain no surviving clonogens and are cured, while the other half contain one or more and will recur. For a homogeneous population of tumors, a very marked change in tumor control probability occurs over a small dose range, e.g., (Fig. 7),[23] if the TCD_{50} of a population of tumors, each containing 10^8 clonogenic cells, was 65 Gy, tumor control would increase from a little over 5 percent at 60 Gy to a little under 85 percent at 70 Gy. In clinical practice tumor control probablity curves are never so steep because of the heterogeneity of the clinical material, and in some analyses no dose-response relationship has been demonstrated (Fig. 8). The issue of dose-response relationships for control of human tumors by radiotherapy is of great impor-

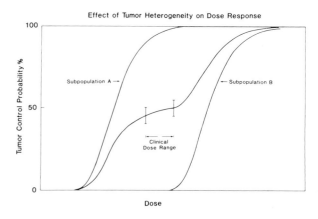

Figure 8 Effect of tumor heterogeneity on observed tumor control dose-response. This simple example is based on two equal subpopulations of tumor differing substantially in their radiocurability for any reason. If the clinical dose range were in the region indicated, even with tumor control probability rates defined accurately to within ±5 percent, no significant dose-response for tumor control could be demonstrated.

tance since it affects the philosophy of radiotherapy, with regard to both dose prescription and accuracy of treatment planning and delivery. Clearly, if tumor control is not considered to be dose-dependent, these aspects of radiotherapeutic practice become less critical. Even when no dose-response relationship can be demonstrated for various types of human cancer, it is inescapable that tumor control is dose dependent for individual cancers, unless one postulates subpopulations of tumor cells that are absolutely resistant to ionizing radiation. This has never been demonstrated, and the only circumstance in which it could be true is when a geographic miss occurs and part of the tumor is not adequately irradiated. Thus, any analysis of clinical dose-response relationships must include a critical assessment of radiotherapeutic technique and quality control.

Notwithstanding these inherent difficulties, significant dose-response relationships have been demonstrated for a variety of tumors in the head and neck region.[24]

RATIONALE FOR SHRINKING FIELDS

The concept of dose-response relationship for tumor control based on the number of clonogenic cells to be sterilized underlies the use of shrinking field techniques in radiotherapy and combinations of radiation and limited surgery. Since cell killing by radiation is essentially an exponential function of dose, it follows that the dose required for a given level of tumor control probability is directly proportional to the logarithm of the number of clonogenic cells in the tumor (Fig. 9).[25] Thus, subclinical extensions of disease can reach the same probability of tumor control as gross palpable tumor after treatment with a lower total dose. This is true even when one assumes that the radiosensitivity of cells in small and large aggre-

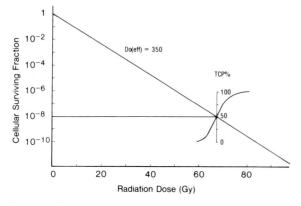

Figure 7 Diagram illustrating the relationship between D0 (eff) with fractionated irradiation and the tumor control probability (TCP). (From Fletcher GH, et al.[23])

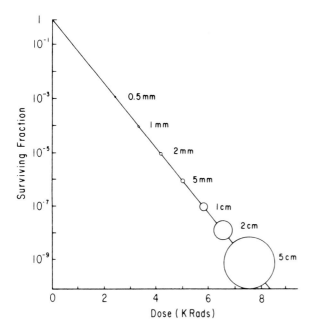

Figure 9 Representative of a fractionated survival curve for 200-rad increments based on an "effective DO" of approximately 350 rad. If a dose of 6500 rad results in a given (say 80%) probability of controlling a lesion 2 cm in diameter, the dose to produce the same level of control probability for deposits of the same tumor of different sizes can be read from the figure. To simplify, the assumption is made that the cellular radiosensitivity and clonogenic fraction of cells in lesions of different size is constant. In practice, both would tend to be higher for smaller lesions. (From Peters LJ, et al.[25])

gates is identical. In fact, since the former have a higher growth fraction, one would predict them to show increased radiosensitivity. However, the proportion of clonogenic cells in small tumors are also more likely to be higher, so that these two influences would tend to cancel out. The ideal dose distribution to be achieved in radiotherapy is one in which the physical dose is graded to provide a homogeneous tumor control probability throughout the treatment volume rather than a homogeneous dose distribution. This is normally achieved by the so-called shrinking field technique, or the use of body contours to provide built-in dose gradients to the site of maximum disease bulk.

TUMOR REGRESSION AND REGROWTH

Although, by definition, a tumor is controlled only if there are no surviving clonogenic cells remaining at the completion of radiation therapy, this does not necessarily mean that there will be no morphologically viable cells, since these cells may be reproductively dead but not yet have manifested mitotically linked death. The rate of regression of tumors following radiotherapy varies widely and is determined by many factors, including the turnover rate of the tumor, its cellularity versus stromal content and necrosis, and the efficiency of removal of dead tissue from the tumor site. In general, tumors with the most rapid

cellular turnover rate respond most rapidly to radiotherapy; those with a low cell turnover rate respond slowly and historically have been termed radioresistant.

Prognostic Significance of Tumor Regression Rates

The prognostic significance of residual tumor at the completion of a course of radiotherapy varies according to the type of tumor. Most squamous cell carcinomas of the upper aerodigestive tracts have a moderately rapid turnover rate, and the presence of gross residual tumor at the end of a course of radiotherapy is associated with a lower probability of tumor control (Table 1).[26] For this reason, additional boosts or limited surgical procedures are frequently carried out to remove residual disease following a planned definitive course of treatment. From the radiobiologic viewpoint, the most plausible explanation for the fact that residual tumor at the end of treatment carries a worse prognosis is that complete tumor regression is almost axiomatically associated with full reoxygenation of tumor cells during treatment. Conversely, when a tumor does not regress completely it is possible, but by no means certain, that reoxygenation may not have been complete.

Biopsies in the Postirradiation Period

Differences in rate of regression of tumors following radiotherapy lead to difficulty in interpretation of biopsies taken in the postirradiation period. Because radiation killing generally is not expressed until cells attempt mitosis, it is impossible to determine, on the basis of histologic examination, whether apparently intact tumor cells do, in fact, retain clonogenic ability. For this reason biopsies of residual tumor in the absence of any clinical evidence of regrowth should be discouraged. Such biopsies do not aid in diagnosis and increase the risk of radionecrosis. Patients with residual disease at the end of treatment should therefore be closely followed, and biopsy confirmation of recurrence should be sought only in the presence of clinical regrowth.

TABLE 1 Clinical Evaluation of the Status of the Primary Lesion at the End of Treatment in Squamous Cell Carcinoma of the Faucial Arch Tonsillar Fossa, and Base of the Tongue in All Stages: 1948–1970 (Analysis in January 1976)

Present*	Residual Tumor Present*	No Residual Tumor
Recurrence of primary tumor	71/117 (60 7%)	76/249 (30.5%)
No recurrence of primary tumor	46/117 (39.3%)	173/249 (69.5%)

*X^2 30.135; $p < 0.005$
From Barkley and Fletcher.[26]

COMBINATION OF IRRADIATION AND SURGERY

The same basic rationale underlies the boosting of gross disease with extra radiation doses or its removal with limited surgery. Frequently, the latter is to be preferred since the total dose of radiation can then be kept down to reduce the risk of normal tissue complications. The concept of elective treatment of subclinical disease with radiation doses causing little or no morbidity was pioneered by Fletcher,[27] and has recently been extensively reviewed.[28] When radiation precedes surgery, a dose of the order of 50 Gy in 25 fractions over 5 weeks is usually adequate to sterilize subclinical disease. However, when radiation is given postoperatively, as is more usually the case in head and neck cancer, the extent of "subclinical" residual disease varies widely owing to altered proliferation kinetics in the healing phase, and tumor cells are more likely to be in a state of radiobiologic hypoxia owing to disturbance of the tissue planes. Higher doses may therefore be necessary postoperatively, depending on an assessment of the risk of residual disease after surgical dissection.

The combination of limited surgery with radiotherapy exploits the strengths of both modalities: with surgery, gross disease can usually be extirpated but microscopic residual disease cannot be excluded, whereas with radiotherapy, microscopic disease is most easily sterilized and failures are more likely at sites of gross tumefaction. Perhaps the most successful application of this complementary aspect of the two modalities in head and neck cancer has been the abandonment in all but a few cases of radical neck dissection at UT M.D. Anderson Hospital in favor of limited "functional" neck dissections supplemented by radiotherapy or the use of limited surgical procedures to remove residual disease following a basic course of radiation therapy to the neck.[29]

The sequencing of radiation and surgery is a trade-off between the radiobiologic advantages of preoperative irradiation and the practical and logistic advantages of operating first. The advantages of preoperative irradiation can be summarized as follows: radiotherapy is more effective in a surgically undisturbed bed; tumor regression resulting from radiotherapy may facilitate surgical dissection; and the risk of implantation or dissemination of viable cells at the time of surgery is greatly reduced. On the other hand, preoperative irradiation carries the following disadvantages: accurate surgical staging is precluded; margins of surgical resection are difficult to define; and delays in wound healing occur when major resections are undertaken after preoperative irradiation. For these reasons, the majority of combined procedures in the United States use radiation postoperatively. However, the option for preoperative treatment should not be overlooked, especially when a tumor is marginally resectable and a surgical cut-through is likely, or when a tumor is rapidly growing, in which case gross recurrence may rapidly follow surgery even before postoperative irradiation can be initiated.

The essential rationale of combined radiation and surgery is that the two modalities complement each other. Thus, it is important that the use of each modality be planned accordingly. For example, if postoperative irradiation is deemed necessary on the basis of the extent of primary disease in a patient with a node-negative neck, there is no need to dissect the neck since any subclinical disease in this region will be effectively sterilized by the postoperative radiation therapy. Conversely, in a patient whose primary tumor is planned for definitive radiation therapy, but in whom a neck dissection is indicated on the basis of bulk nodal disease, efforts should be made to choose beam energies and port arrangements to avoid excessive doses to the neck that will increase the risk of surgical complications.

Surgery in a Previously Irradiated Field

Attempted surgical salvage of recurrence or surgery for complications of radiation therapy call for specialized techniques and for a thorough understanding of the pathophysiology of the irradiated tissues by the surgeon. As indicated previously, acute radiation reactions are mainly due to a depletion of stem cells in rapid turnover tissues, such as epithelia, whereas late radiation injury results from a progressive depletion of functional cells in slowly proliferating tissues. In the context of surgery months to years after previous high-dose radiation therapy, devitalization of the vasculoconnective tissues is a major deterrent to healing. Indeed, as explained in Figure 2, surgical trauma may precipitate an avalanche of cell death in previously irradiated, late-responding normal tissues, so that attempted conservative excision of a small area of osteoradionecrosis, for example, leads only to a larger volume of necrosis. Neck dissections after previous irradiation call for the avoidance of trifurcate incisions, since these frequently lead to flap necrosis and exposure of underlying vessels. With excellent surgical technique, neck dissections can usually be accomplished following previous radiotherapy without importation of new tissue. However, when major resection is necessary, the only really satisfactory way of insuring wound healing following previous high-dose radiotherapy is to import new tissue with an intact blood supply and fibroblastic vitality. This is possible through the use of pedicle flaps and/or free microvascular grafts.

THE THERAPEUTIC RATIO

For the majority of head and neck cancers, the dose-response curves defining tumor control and normal tissue injury overlap. If the curve for tumor control lies to the left of that for dose-limiting normal tissue injury (Fig. 10), the therapeutic ratio is said to be positive, whereas if it lies to the right of that for normal tissue injury, the therapeutic ratio is negative,

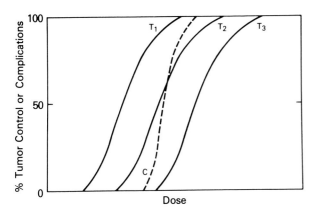

Figure 10 The therapeutic ratio relates the probability of tumor control to that of a treatment complication for a given dose of radiation. If curve C represents the dose-response relationship for an unacceptable normal tissue injury, and curves T1, T2, and T3 represent tumor control probabilities for say three increasing stages of the same tumor, the therapeutic ratio would be strongly positive for T1 with a high percentage of uncomplicated cures possible; marginally positive for T2 with a maximum of 20 to 25 percent of uncomplicated cures possible; and negative for T3, for which curative treatment by radiotherapy would be contraindicated. (From Peters LJ.[6])

and radiotherapy is generally contraindicated except for palliation. The possible outcomes of radiation therapy with respect to tumor control and normal tissue injury are: tumor control without complications, tumor control with complications, failure of tumor control without complications, and failure of tumor control with complications. The therapeutic ratio is maximized when the greatest number of patients experience the first of these outcomes. The use of radiation treatments that are too conservative will unduly increase the number of patients experiencing failure of tumor control, whereas excessive escalation of dose will increase the proportion of severe complications. The ultimate goal of all radiotherapy research is to increase the therapeutic ratio either by rendering tumors more susceptible to cure by ionizing radiation or by making normal tissues more resistant to injury.

REFERENCES

1. Puck TT, Marcus PI. Action of x-rays on mammalian cells. J Exp med 1956; 103:653.
2. Searle J, Kerr JFR, Bishop CJ. Necrosis and apoptosis: Distinct modes of cell death with fundamentally different significance. Pathol Annu 1982; 17:229.
3. Kashima HK, Kirkham WR, Andrews JR. Postirradiation sialadentis: A study of the clinical features, histopathologic changes and serum enzyme variations following irradiation of human salivary glands. Am J Roentgenol 1965; 94:271.
4. Michalowski A. Effects of radiation on normal tissues: Hypothetical mechanisms and limitations of in situ assays of clonogenicity. Radiat Environ Biophys 1981; 19:157.
5. Mossman KL. Quantitative radiation dose-response relationships for normal tissues in man. II. Response of the salivary glands during radiotherapy. Radiat Res 1983; 95:392.
6. Peters LJ. Biology of radiation therapy. In: Thawley SE and Panje WR, eds. Comprehensive management of head and neck tumors, Philadelphia: WB Saunders, 1985, in press.
7. Read J. The effect of ionizing radiation on the broad beam root. Part X. Br J Radiol 1952; 25:89 and 154.
8. Hall EJ. Radiation dose-rate: A factor of importance in radiobiology and radiotherapy. Br J Radio 1972; 45:81.
9. Thomlinson RH, Gray LH. The histological structure of some human lung cancers and possible implications for radiotherapy. Br J Cancer 1955; 9:539.
10. Hendry JH. Quantitation of the radiotherapeutic importance of naturally hypoxic normal tissues from collated experiments with rodents using single doses. Int J Radiat Oncol Biol Phys 1979; 5:971.
11. Henk JM. Does hyperbaric oxygen have a future in radiation therapy? Int J Radiat Oncol Biol PHys 1981; 7:1125.
12. Bacq ZM, Alexander P. Fundamentals of Radiobiology. 2nd Ed. New York: Pergamon Press, 1961, p 1.
13. Withers HR, Thames HD Jr, Peters LJ. Biological bases for high RBE values for late effects of neutron irradiation. Int J Radiat Oncol Biol Phys 1982; 8:2071.
14. Steel GG. Terminology in the description of drug-radiation interactions. Int J Radiat Oncol Biol Phys 1979; 5:1145.
15. Steel GG, Peckham MJ. Exploitable mechanisms in combined radiotherapy chemotherapy: The concept of additivity. Int J Radiat Oncol Biol Phys 1979; 5:85.
16. Goepfert H, Jesse RH, Lindberg RD. Arterial infusion and radiation therapy in the treatment of advanced cancer of the nasal cavity and paranasal sinuses. Am J Surg 1973; 126:464.
17. Weaver A, Fleming S, Kish J, Vandenberg H, Jacobs J, Crissman J, Al-Sarraf M. Cis-platinum and 5-fluorouracil as induction therapy for advanced head and neck cancer. Am J Surg 1982; 144:445.
18. Weichselbaum RR, Posner MR, Ervin TJ, Fabaian RL, Miller D. Toxicity of aggressive multimodality therapy including cis-platinum, bleomycin and methotrexate with radiation and/or surgery for advanced head and neck cancer. Int J Radiat Oncol Biol Phys 1982; 8:909.
19. Stell PM, Dalby JE, Strickland P, Fraser JG, Bradley PJ, Flood LM. Sequential chemotherapy and radiotherapy in advanced head and neck cancer. Clin Radiol 1983; 34:463–467.
20. Looney WB, Hopkins HA, Kovacks CJ, Moore JV, Trefil JS, Rawley R, Carter WH Jr. Single and combined "radiation-cyclophosphamide" modality therapy in experimental solid tumors. Adv Radiat Biol 1983; 10:305.
21. Manning MR, Cetas TC, Miller RC, Oleson JR, Conner WG, Gerner EW. Clinical hyperthermia: Results of a phase I trial employing hyperthermia alone or in combination with external beam or interstitial radiotherapy. Cancer 1982; 49:205.
22. Knee R, Peters LJ. Concomitant boost radiotherapy for advanced squamous cell carcinoma of the head and neck. Radiotherapy and Oncology 1985 (in press).
23. Fletcher GH, Withers HR, Peters LJ. Boost in radiotherapy: rationale and technique. In: Chu FCH, Laughlin JS, eds. Proceedings of the Symposium on Electron Beam Therapy. New York: Memorial Sloan-Kettering Cancer Center 1981:107.
24. Thames HD Jr, Peters LJ, Spanos W, Fletcher GH. Dose response of squamous cell carcinomas of the upper respiratory and digestive tract. Br J Cancer 1980; 41(Suppl IV):35.
25. Peters LJ, Withers HR, Fletcher GH. Alternatives to radical neck dissection: The M.D. Anderson approach. Aust Radiol 1980; 24:303.
26. Barkely HT Jr, Fletcher GH. The significance of residual disease after external irradiation of squamous cell carcinoma of the oropharynx. Radiology 1977; 124:493.
27. Fletcher GH. Clinical dose-response curves of human malignant epithelial tumors. Br J Radiol 1973; 46:1.
28. Fletcher GH. Lucy Wortham James Lecture: Subclinical disease. Cancer 1984; 53:1274–1284.
29. Jesse RH, Ballantyne AJ, Larson D. Radical or modified neck dissection: A therapeutic dilemma. Am J Surg 1978; 136:516.

6. Combined Surgery and Radiation Therapy in the Management of Locally Advanced Head and Neck Squamous Cell Carcinoma

SIMON KRAMER, M.D., F.A.C.R.

The combined use of surgery and radiation therapy in locally advanced squamous cell carcinoma of the head and neck has been the practice for many years and has given rise to a voluminous literature.[1-6] Most recently, Strong in the Janeway Lecture of 1983 has given an excellent overview of the subject.[7] Since the addition of chemotherapy is now being investigated intensively, and since the early results are quite favorable, it would seem important to define now just how far we have come with the surgery and radiation therapy management and whether we can reach a consensus on best current management by these two modalities so that we can establish a baseline or benchmark for comparison with the results of future studies. The number of patients with advanced but potentially curable squamous cell carcinoma of the head and neck is not large. An estimate made in 1977 shows that at the time probably only 500 patients were available to be entered into prospective controlled trials[8] (Table 1). Even if that number were to be doubled, the need to utilize these patients optimally makes clear the need to define precise questions and end points and the need to prioritize the allocations of patients to such studies.

Can we establish and adopt certain premises on the basis of what is known today? First, how valuable is combined surgery and radiation therapy in locally advanced tumors as compared with surgery alone? It is important here to define the end point we use to measure any advantage. Although survival is the ultimate aim of all our treatment, I would suggest it is a poor end point to use in these studies. The mortality of these patients is high, from new primary tumors in the air and food passages, from distant metastases, and from deaths relating to the ravages of their life style. These causes probably account for mortality in 40 percent of all patients treated. Probably none of these deaths can be prevented by any form of locoregional treatment. Therefore, it is suggested that locoregional control of the disease is a more suitable end point for treatment comparisons. Unfortunately, there are few controlled prospective trials that compare the results of surgery with those of surgery combined with radiation therapy. Most of the studies are observational and retrospective reports. Most deal with preoperative radiation and surgery compared with surgery alone. In studies in which some patients are treated by combined therapy and other patients are treated by surgery alone, it is extremely difficult to assess the validity of the results.[9,10] Few, if any, of them indicate the reason for the choice of combined therapy versus single-mode therapy. One might suspect that even on a stage-by-stage basis, patients with more advanced disease would be submitted to combined therapy, but neither this nor the contrary is made clear. Failure to improve results by combined therapy could result from such a bias, but in the absence of such information we simply have no way of knowing. On the other hand, studies in which combined therapy is compared with historic controls are subject to the criticisms of using historic controls. Yet the vast majority of these studies indicate an advantage in terms of locoregional control for combined surgery and radiation therapy.[4,5,11] Perhaps the most convincing data are those published recently by Vikram, Strong, Shah, and Spiro from the Memorial Sloan Kettering Cancer Center.[12-15] Here the results of surgery followed by postoperative radiation therapy utilized in previously untreated patients between January, 1975 and December, 1980 were compared with the results in patients treated by surgery only between 1960 and 1970. These comparisons are dramatic. When looking at failure at the primary site (Fig. 1), a very meaningful reduction is seen both where the surgical specimen showed satisfactory margins of tumor clearance and more so when there were unsatisfactory margins. Equally dramatic results are shown in the case of metastatic neck nodes in a comparison of three methods of treatment, namely, surgery alone, 2000 rads preoperatively followed by surgery, and surgery and 5000 rads postoperatively as shown in Figure 2. Particularly noticeable is the improvement in neck failure when multiple-level metastases are present in the neck. These authors also point

TABLE 1 Estimate of Patient Numbers for Clinical Trials (Head and Neck Cancer, USA 1977)

Total H & N Cancer (6% of 690,000)		41,400
Localized	36%	
Regional	44%	= 18,216
Disseminated	20%	
Uncommon or different biology		6,000
Available no. of patients		12,216
In nonparticipating institutions	60%	7,326
Potentially available		4,800
Entered into trials	10%	500
Neutron trials		?

(Ref. 8)

Supported in part by the National Cancer Institute, Division of Cancer Treatment, Grant CA 11602

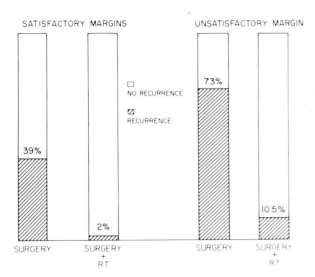

Figure 1 Historical comparison of the local recurrence rates in patients treated with surgery or with surgery and postoperative radiation therapy. (From Vikram et al.[12])

out the importance of multiple-level involvement in neck nodes with regard to distant metastases (Fig. 3) and this confirms the statement already made by others that patients with multiple positive neck nodes run the highest risk of the development of distant metastases. The authors also confirm the prominence of a second malignant neoplasm as a cause of failure in these patients which becomes particularly prominent after the second year (Fig. 4). Incidentally, the value

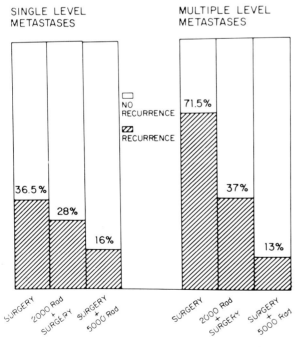

Figure 2 Comparison of the rates of recurrences in the neck among patients treated with surgery alone or surgery with 2000 rads preoperative irradiation, and patients treated with surgery and 5000 to 6000 rads postoperative irradiation. (From Vikram et al.[13])

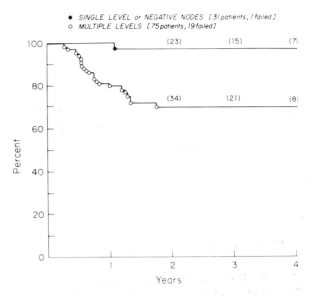

Figure 3 Comparison of the incidence of distant metastases between patients with single level or no cervical nodal metastases pathologically and patients with multiple-level metastases. (From Vikram et al[14])

of combining radiation with surgery for control of positive neck nodes, as shown initially by Strong[16] and later by Barkley et al[17] is generally accepted even by authors who fail to find any other advantage in combination therapy. This advantage remains whether radiation is given preoperatively or postoperatively. On the basis of the information available at present, I consider that the first premise has been established, namely, *that the combination of surgery and radiation therapy is advantageous for locally advanced, but still operable head and neck cancer.*

Next we must consider the best way of combining surgery and radiation therapy. Should radiation therapy be given preoperatively, postoperatively, intraoperatively, or as sandwich therapy, that is, both

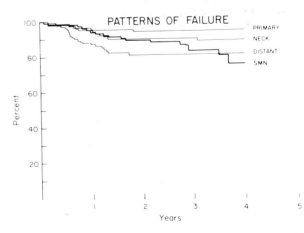

Figure 4 Comparison of the rates of relapse of the head and neck cancer at the primary site, neck, and distant sites with the rate of appearance of second malignant neoplasms (SMN). (From Vikram et al.[15])

Oral Cavity or Oropharynx

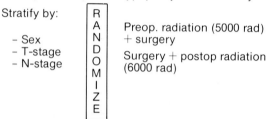

Stratify by:

- Sex
- T-Stage
- N-Stage

RANDOMIZE

Preop. radiation (5000 rad) + surgery

Surgery + postop radiation (6000 rad)

Rad. ther. (6500–7000 rad) (plus surgery for salvage)

Supraglottic larynx or hypopharynx or maxillary sinus

Stratify by:

- Sex
- T-stage
- N-stage

RANDOMIZE

Preop. radiation (5000 rad) + surgery

Surgery + postop radiation (6000 rad)

Figure 5 Schema for RTOG Study 73–03. A controlled study to determine the value of radiation therapy alone or in combination with surgery for squamous cell carcinoma of the oral cavity, pharynx and larynx.

pre- and postoperatively. Little is known about sandwich therapy in head and neck cancer; it is being intensively investigated at other sites, primarily the genitourinary tract and the gastrointestinal tract. Intraoperative therapy originally suggested by Patterson 40 years ago has its proponents, but is being used primarily when not all tumor can be removed at the time of surgery. The main discussion here centers on preoperative versus postoperative irradiation. Preoperative irradiation has been used both in relatively low doses (2000 rads in one week) and in high doses (5000 rads in 5 to 6 weeks). There seems to be rather general agreement that the higher preoperative dose is more effective, although surgery is delayed. Five thousand rads in 5 weeks, given in five daily fractions per week, is considered a maximum safe dose since surgical complications after higher preoperative doses rise precipitously. Postoperative radiation at a dose of 5000 to 6000 rads has been used and appears to be safe and tolerable. Only a few prospective randomized trials to test preoperative versus postoperative irradiation have been undertaken. Vandenbrouck et al undertook such a study,[18] but it had to be abandoned because the surgical complications after preoperative irradiation were too high. In the small number of patients reported, however, postoperative irradiation seemed to have a distinct advantage both in local control and in survival. The Radiation Therapy Oncology Group undertook a study in 1973 (RTOG 73-03), testing 5000 rads delivered preoperatively versus 6000 rads delivered postoperatively.[19] This study tested the comparative value of preoperative radiation versus postoperative radiation and definitive radiation therapy with surgery reserved for rescue in the oral cavity and oropharynx. In the hypopharynx and supraglottic larynx, only two arms were used, namely, preoperative

radiation and postoperative radiation (Fig. 5). A total of 354 patients were entered, of whom 320 were evaluable, with a median follow-up period of 60 months (Table 2). Pertinent to the current discussion, 277 evaluable patients were entered into either the preoperative or postoperative arm (Table 3). As can be seen in Table 4, about 90 percent of all patients were in stages III and IV. Results are shown in Table 5, which shows that the estimated survival rate was better in the postoperative cases, but it did not reach statistical significance, whereas loco-regional control, expressed as an estimated 4-year competing risk rate, showed a statistically significant better result for postoperative radiation (Table 6). When evaluating the status of all patients at the time this report was prepared, it can be seen (Table 7) that the difference in

TABLE 2 RTOG 73–03 Study

Patients entered	354
Cancelled	12
Ineligible	17
Maxillary sinus	5
Patients analyzed	320

TABLE 3 RTOG 73–03 Study: 320 Patients Analyzed

Region	Preop RT & Surgery	Surgery & Postop RT	Def. RT & Surg Salv	Total
Oral cavity	20	20	19	59
Oropharynx	23	23	24	70
Supraglottic larynx	58	60		118
Hypopharynx	35	38		73
Total preop and postop RT	277			

TABLE 4 RTOG 73–03 Study (Preop vs Postop Radiation Therapy): Patient Characteristics by Region

	Oral Cav.	Oropharynx	Supra. Larynx	Hypopharynx
% Stage II	8	13	12	6
% Stage III & IV	92	87	88	94
% Male	82	83	76	88

TABLE 5 RTOG 73–03 Study (Preop vs Postop RT): Estimated* 4–yr Survival Rates by Treatment and Region

Region	Preop	Postop	Total
Oral cavity	34	32	33
Oropharynx	26	38	32
Supraglottic larynx	41	47	44
Hypopharynx	18	28	25
All regions	33	38	36
p = 0.10			
Pts. compl. planned R_x	40	45	

*Est. by Kaplan-Meier Method

TABLE 6   RTOG 73–03 Study (Preop vs Postop RT): Estimated 4–yr Competing Risk Loco-regional Control Rates by Treatment & Region

Region	Preop	Postop	Total
Oral cavity	40	44	42
Oropharynx	47	61	54
Supraglottic larynx	53	77	64
Hypopharynx	50	61	55
All regions	48	65	57
p = 0.04			
Pts. compl. planned R$_x$	56	74	

TABLE 7   RTOG 73–03 Study (Preop vs Postop RT): Case Status (All Cases)

Status	Preop (136)	Postop (141)
% No disease		
Alive NED	45	56
Dead no rec.		
% Disease present		
Alive with rec.	55	44
Dead with rec.		
Site of first failure		
% Persis. or rec. loco/reg.	39	23
% Metastasis	13	16
% Both	2	5
p = 0.09		

outcome is largely due to a difference in control at the loco-regional site, whereas the incidence of distant metastases is quite similar. It can also be seen that the loco-regional control is markedly different when the cause of death is considered. Our incidence of second primary tumor is lower than that reported by Vikram et al; cervical node involvement as cause of death is practically nonexistent, and the relatively high incidence of deaths unrelated to the treated head and neck tumors is shown (Table 8). Finally, looking at

TABLE 8   RTOG 73–03 Study (Preop vs Postop RT): Cause of Death (All Cases)

	Preop (136)*	Postop (141)*
% Treated primary	29	16
% Second primary	7	8
% Cervical nodes	1	3
% Distant metastasis	15	15
% Treatment related	8	6
% Unrelated	11	11
% Unknown	3	8

*Numbers in parenthesis refer to number of patients.

TABLE 9   RTOG 73–03 Study (Preop vs Postop RT): Treatment Complications ("Severe" Complications)

	Preop RT & Surg. (135)*	Surg. & Postop RT (139)*
Surgical	18%	14%
Radiation	14%	20%

*Numbers in parenthesis refer to number of patients evaluated.

complications of the treatment (Table 9), it can be seen that there is only a minimally higher incidence of severe surgical complications in the preoperative group and a slightly higher radiation complication rate in the postoperative group. Severe surgical complications include delayed healing, fistula formation, carotid blowout, failure of graft, and death. Severe radiation complications include necrosis, esophageal and tracheal stenosis, severe fibrosis, edema with respiratory obstruction, and death. In all the parameters tested, we could find no advantage for preoperative radiation. Thus, we have good evidence to conclude as our second premise established that: *In general, postoperative radiation therapy is more useful than preoperative radiation in patients with locally advanced, but operable disease*; radiation therapy should be started as soon as possible after surgery; 5000 to 6000 rads in 5 to 6½ weeks is an effective and safe dose.

Next we need to examine the extent of surgery to be performed in conjunction with radiation therapy. There is a need to define the term "debulking procedure". A procedure that leaves behind gross tumor is not useful from a curative point of view. The term itself is misleading and should not be used. If used at all it should imply removal of all gross tumor with at worst residual microscopic tumor in the specimen. As far as the primary tumor is concerned, it appears that most surgeons feel that a classic radical resection is indicated as if no postoperative radiation will take place. The question whether less margin around the tumor is acceptable in the light of postoperative radiation remains moot. The question of an elective neck dissection in the case of a clinically negative neck is less easily defined. If the neck is negative clinically, but the primary tumor is such that there is considerable likelihood of subclinical disease in the neck, particularly when the management of the primary calls for surgical invasion of the neck, most surgeons seem to prefer concomitant radical neck dissection. Most radiation oncologists, on the other hand, feel that subclinical disease in a clinically negative neck can be controlled by adequate postoperative radiation therapy. The Radiation Therapy Oncology Group endeavored to institute a trial on classic radical neck dissection versus a modified radical neck dissection with postoperative radiation therapy, but this failed because no agreement could be reached on what constituted a modified radical neck dissection. At any rate, it seems fair to say that when the neck is negative, or only the first node station is involved and postoperative radiation therapy is planned, preservation of the spinal accessory nerve can often be achieved. Thus, premise number 3 reads: *Extent of surgery for the primary site - classic resection. Neck dissection; if neck positive–yes, if neck negative–?*.

In summary, then, it seems that these findings are established:

1. That in the management of primary operable advanced loco-regional squamous cell carcinoma of

the head and neck, combined therapy is advantageous in leading to better loco-regional control.

2. That postoperative radiation therapy is to be preferred to preoperative radiation therapy; a dose of between 5000 and 6000 rads in 5 to 6 weeks is generally acceptable and safe and should be instituted as soon as possible postoperatively, preferably within 4 to 6 weeks.

3. That the surgery to be performed is to be classic resection of the primary with or without radical neck dissection.

With this baseline of best current management established, we must recognize that we have probably reached a plateau because of technical limitations both of surgery and radiation therapy. Of course, many questions remain unanswered: Extensive research is proceeding in radiation therapy using such adjuvants as sensitizers, protectors, and local hyperthermia, changes in fractionation, particularly hyperfractionation, and particulate irradiation such as neutrons, heavy nuclei, or pi-mesons. If any of these can be shown to make a major contribution, they will obviously change the best current management. But meanwhile I would suggest that the highest priority for future studies in this group of patients now lies in determining the optimal use of adjuvant chemotherapy. Again, in combining chemotherapy, surgery, and radiation therapy, there is a universe of variables. Many pilot studies have already been reported. The combination of cisplatin with one or another agent seems most promising. In order to utilize the scarce patient material to best advantage, we should now prioritize studies tailored to the patterns of failure in specific regions and specific sites. We have been somewhat prone to lump together head and neck cancer. The head and neck contains many different structures, and each of these gives rise to tumors with different biology, different modes of spread, and different metastatic patterns. There is some commonality of problems, but it is no greater than, say, in the lower genitourinary tract. Yet no urologist would lump together tumors of the bladder, prostate, and urethra and draw general conclusions from such a composite experience. I would also suggest that the TNM grouping for stage IV in the American Joint Commitee staging is too broad. T4N0 tumors have a far better chance of loco-regional control and a lower incidence of distant metastases than T4N2 or T4N3 tumors.

Can we identify the patterns of failure in locally advanced tumors in different regions of the head and neck? Loco-regional control remains a problem and continues to be dominant in the oral cavity, oropharynx, and glottic larynx. In the nasopharynx, supraglottic larynx, and hypopharynx, particularly when there is extensive nodal disease, distant metastases cause death as frequently as local failure. Common to all regions are the problems of new primary tumors and mortality from unrelated causes, both due to the

ravages of life style. Some 30 to 40 percent of these patients die from alcoholism, inanition, and new primary tumors in the air and food passages, particularly the lung and esophagus. If this area could be addressed by appropriate psychosocial intervention, the potential gain would be enormous, but I must confess to a sense of frustration in trying to modify the life style of these patients in our present societal framework, and even if it were possible, one wonders how effective it would be at this late point in time.

In dealing with the tumor problems, ideally one should study all patients with a comprehensive combination of modalities. Induction therapy would start with several courses of chemotherapy (this would allow us to study response before proceeding to further loco-regional treatment). This would then be followed by surgery, then postoperative radiation therapy, and finally maintenance chemotherapy. In point of practice, few patients tolerate or accept such rigorous treatment. Since there are good reasons to deliver the chemotherapy early on, the next best schema might be as shown in Figure 6, that is, to induce with several courses of chemotherapy, then follow with surgery and postoperative radiation therapy, with standard therapy as control. Because of a number of considerations, the Radiation Therapy Oncology Group chose to put the surgery first, and then to randomize to the study arm versus the control arm (Fig. 7). This study is now ongoing in the RTOG for stage III tumors and has been agreed upon for stage III and IV tumors as an Intergroup Study with most large cooperative groups participating. Patient accession should be excellent and answers forthcoming within a reasonable period of time. While it is gratifying to see such a consensus developed, I would suggest that different schemata addressing more specific questions also be considered. Possibly such studies could be done consecutively, or those of us not committed to the Intergroup Study could undertake them. In patients in whom metastatic disease in the face of loco-regional control is a major factor in poor survival, as in advanced supraglottic larynx and hypopharyngeal tu-

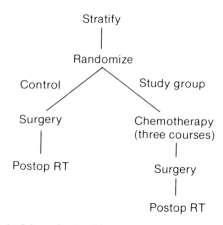

Figure 6 Schema for Combined modality therapy in advanced SCC Head & Neck (Stage III & IV).

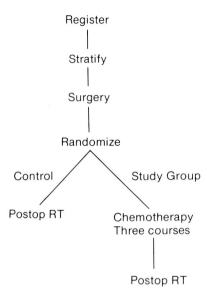

Figure 7   Schema for therapy of advanced SCC Head & Neck (Stage III & IV).

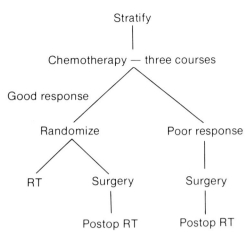

Figure 9   Proposed schema for treatment of Stage III laryngeal tumors.

mors, particularly with large nodal disease, it might be more appropriate to devise a study specifically addressing the question of controlling subclinical distant metastases. Perhaps chemotherapy might be given more appropriately here as maintenance therapy after the loco-regional disease has been dealt with. Figure 8 shows the schema for such a study. I realize one might lose something in loco-regional control by postponing chemotherapy, but by concentrating on this group of patients, an answer might be obtained more quickly and more decisively.

Next we should consider whether and how the quality of life of our patients can be improved. Reconstructive surgery has had excellent results both in function and cosmesis following resections in the oral cavity and oropharynx. But the loss of the voice following laryngectomy remains an overwhelming dis-

ability. Unfortunately, up to now radiation therapy as a single mode has had much worse results in stage III and IV laryngeal tumors than surgery and radiation therapy combined.[20,21] But now that the initial response to cisplatin-containing regimens is favorable, one should consider the possibility of omitting surgery in relatively less advanced stage III laryngeal tumors. Perhaps of less high priority but nonetheless important, I would suggest a study to test this possibility (Fig. 9). Even a modest increase in the number of patients who could retain their larynx following an initial favorable response to chemotherapy would be worthwhile.

Committing a group of patients to prospective randomized studies is always a serious, difficult, and expensive undertaking. The commitment must usually extend over several years so that meaningful patient numbers can be accumulated. If we realize that advances in oncology are stepwise, since we have no magic bullet yet, such studies are mandatory to demonstrate these advances. If we could reach a broad consensus on the group of studies I have suggested, unhampered by territorial imperatives, and pool our resources nationally, we would be able to answer a good many questions within the next 5 years, questions to which we have no answers at present.

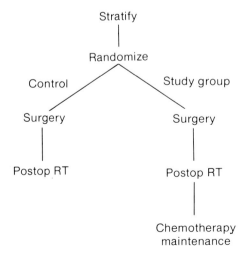

Figure 8   Protocol for patients with high risk for distant metastases (Multiple neck nodes-Stage IV-supraglottic larynx, hypopharynx).

REFERENCES

1. MacComb WS, Fletcher GH. Planned combination of surgery and radiation in treatment of advanced primary head and neck cancers. Am J Roentgenol Radium Ther Nucl Med 1957; 77:397–414.
2. Buschke F, Galante M. Radical preoperative roentgen therapy in primarily inoperable cancers of the head and neck. Radiology 1959; 73:845–848.
3. Bryce DP, Rider WD. Preoperative irradiation in the treatment of advanced laryngeal carcinoma. Laryngoscope 1971; 84:1481–1490.
4. Jesse RH, Lindberg RD. The efficacy of combining radiation therapy with a surgical procedure in patients with cervical metastases from squamous cell cancer of the oropharynx and hypopharynx. Cancer 1975; 35:1163–1166.
5. Fletcher GH, Jesse RH. The place of irradiation in the man-

agement of the primary lesion in head and neck cancers. Cancer 1977; 39:862–867.

6. Ogura JH, Biller JF. Preoperative irradiation for laryngeal and laryngopharyneal cancers. Laryngoscope 1970; 80:802–810.

7. Strong EW. Multidisciplinary management of head and neck cancer, update and prospects. Janeway Lecture, 1983 American Radium Society annual meeting.

8. Kramer S. Cancer of the head and neck: A challenge and a dilemma. Sem Oncol 1977; 4:353–355.

9. Eisbach LJ, Krause CJ. Carcinoma of the pyriform sinus. A comparison of treatment modalities. Laryngoscope 1977; 87:1904–1910.

10. Schuller DE, McGuirt WF, Krause CJ, McCabe BF, Pflug BK. Symposium: Adjuvant cancer therapy of head and neck tumors. Increased survival with surgery alone vs combined therapy. Laryngoscope 1979; 89:582–594.

11. Perez CA, Marks J, Powers WE. Preoperative irradiation in head and neck cancer. Sem Oncol 1977; 4:387–397.

12. Vikram B, Strong EW, Shah JP, Spiro R. Failure at the primary site following multimodality treatment in advanced head and neck cancer. Head Neck Surg 1984; 6:720–723.

13. Vikram B, Strong EW, Shah JP, Spiro R. Failure in the neck following multimodality treatment for advanced head and neck cancer. Head Neck Surg 1984; 6:724–729.

14. Vikram B, Strong EW, Shah JP, Spiro R. Failure at distant sites following multimodality treatment for advanced head and

neck cancer. Head Neck Surg 1984; 6:730–733.

15. Vikram B, Strong EW, Shah JP, Spiro R. Second malignant neoplasms in patients successfully treated with multimodality treatment for advanced head and neck cancer. Head Neck Surg 1984; 6:734–373.

16. Strong EW. Preoperative radiation and radical neck dissection. Surg Clin North Am 1969; 49:271–276.

17. Barkley HT Jr, Fletcher GH, Jesse RH, et al. Management of cervical lymph node metastases in squamous cell carcinomas of the tonsillar fossa, base of tongue, supraglottic larynx, and hypopharynx. Am J Surg 1972; 124:462–467.

18. Vandenbrouck C, Sancho H, LeFur R, Richard JM, Cachin Y. Results of a randomized clinical trial of preoperative irradiation versus postoperative in treatment of tumors of the hypopharynx. Cancer 1977; 39:1445–1449.

19. Kramer S, Gelber R, Snow J, Marcial V, Lowry L, Davis L. Preoperative versus postoperative radiation therapy in advanced squamous cell carcinoma of the head and neck: Final report on study 73-03 of the Radiation Therapy Oncology Group. Am J Clin Oncol (CCT) 1983; 6:150–151. (Abstract 25).

20. Lustig RA, MacLean CJ, Hanks GE, Kramer S. The patterns of care outcome studies: Results of the national practice in carcinoma of the larynx. Int J Rad Onc Biol Phys 1984; 10:12.

21. Wang CC. Supraglottic carcinoma: Selection of therapy and results. Am J Clin Oncol (CCT) 1984; 7:109. (Abstract 1)

7. Mechanisms of Action and Interaction of Chemotherapeutic Agents

JOSEPH R. BERTINO, M.D.

During the past decade, development of effective chemotherapy of head and neck cancer has progressed rapidly. Several agents have been described with single-agent activity, and combinations of these drugs have been developed that cause tumor regression in the majority of patients with advanced or recurrent disease. Several studies are now in progress that integrate chemotherapy with definitive therapy for this disease (surgery and/or irradiation).

This chapter will review the mechanism of action of these drugs, and indicate limitations as well as possibilities for improved use in combination.

CHEMOTHERAPEUTIC AGENTS WITH ACTIVITY IN PATIENTS WITH CANCER OF THE HEAD AND NECK REGION

Although many drugs have been tested for anticancer activity in head and neck cancer,[1,2] three drugs have been tested in a sufficient number of patients to establish that they have significant activity in this disease. These are methotrexate (MTX), cisplatin (DDP), and bleomycin. Although fluorouracil (FU) has not

been tested extensively as a single agent in patients with head and neck cancer, a review of its pharmacology is also included because of its activity in combination with MTX and DDP in the treatment of head and neck cancer.

Methotrexate

MTX has been studied extensively in patients with head and neck cancer over the past decade. This drug is probably the single most effective chemotherapeutic agent in this disease (30 to 50% response rates), although remissions are usually only partial, and response duration short.[1,2] In combination, MTX has been used with FU, bleomycin, and DDP.

Mechanism of Action. It is now well documented that the major action of MTX is inhibition of the enzyme dihydrofolate reductase (DHFR) (Fig. 1). Inhibition of this enzyme activity rapidly leads to depletion of intracellular levels of tetrahydrofolate coenzymes, essential for thymidylate biosynthesis and for purine synthesis.[3] Recent work has also shown that MTX is retained in cells for long periods as a consequence of an enzymatic process that adds additional glutamates (up to 5) to the molecule.[4] This may be an important determinant of MTX action since cells

Supported by NIH grants CA 08010 and CA 08341

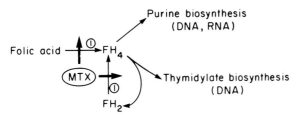

Figure 1 Inhibition of dihydrofolate reductase (1) by MTX. Inhibition of this enzyme leads to depletion of tetrahydrofolate (FH_4) and consequently decreased synthesis of thymidylate and purines. In the synthesis of thymidylate, dihydrofolate (FH_2) is produced, and tetrahydrofolate must be regenerated via dihydrofolate reductase.

capable of this conversion may be expected to be more susceptible to cell kill by this drug.[4]

Resistance to MTX. Patients with head and neck cancer may not respond to this drug if sufficiently high intracellular concentrations of the drug are not achieved (owing perhaps to limited transport or to inability to polyglutamylate the drug or to the cells' ability to rapidly resynthesize the MTX target enzyme dihydrofolate reductase.[3] On a kinetic basis, cells in G0, i.e., not "in cycle," would also be unaffected by MTX.[5,6]

Acquired resistance, i.e., resistance occurring after a response has been obtained, may be due to one of three mechanisms: impaired uptake of MTX into cells, an increase in the level of the enzyme dihydrofolate reductase, or an alteration in this enzyme, so that it binds MTX less well.[7] All of these mechanisms of resistance have been noted in experimental tumor systems, including human squamous cell carcinoma cells grown in vitro. Recent studies have led to the startling discovery that elevation of dihydrofolate reductase is due to gene amplification, i.e., an increase in the gene copy number coding for this enzyme, rather than an increase in the rate of transcription of the gene.[8] In experimental systems, both gene amplification and impaired transport appear to be more commonly observed to occur than alteration of DHFR to a form that binds MTX less well than the sensitive cell.

The mechanisms of resistance to MTX in patients with head and neck cancer have not yet been documented but recent studies in patients with leukemia[9,10] and small cell cancer[11] indicate that small increases in gene copies of DHFR (2–4) may be associated with MTX resistance.

The use of high-dose MTX with leucovorin rescue may therefore be rational from several points of view: (1) better permeability and intracellular levels of the drug in tumor cells may be produced, (2) modest levels of resistance (transport, elevated levels of DHFR) may be overcome, and (3) increased polyglutamate formation may occur, thus resulting in increased retention of the drug.[4] Unfortunately, resistance even to high doses of MTX with leucovorin occurs rapidly, owing perhaps to accumulation of reduced folates rather than development of true MTX

resistance. This point clearly is deserving of further study.

Clinical Pharmacology. Although MTX is well absorbed in low doses (up to 50 mg), larger doses should be given parenterally, since absorption is less quantitative as MTX doses are increased.[12] The drug is excreted primarily unchanged by the kidney ($t^{1}/_2$ = 2.5 hours), although with larger doses, a significant amount of the drug is inactivated by hydroxylation at the 7 position (7-OH MTX).[13] Dichloro-MTX is more rapidly metabolized to the 7-hydroxy compound and is therefore an attractive agent for intra-arterial use, in which high local concentrations of drug are desired with rapid metabolism once the drug leaves the perfused organ, so that systemic toxicity does not occur.[14]

Toxic Effects. Since MTX inhibits DNA synthesis, the two tissues of greatest importance and most susceptible to MTX side effects are the bone marrow and the gastrointestinal epithelium. The oral mucosa and the small intestinal epithelium appear to be more sensitive to the effects of this drug than the large bowel. Marrow suppression results in a circulating WBC and platelet nadir at day 9 or 10 after a single dose, and recovery by day 14 to 21. Mucositis and diarrhea may occur 4 to 7 days after MTX and usually improves by day 14.

Nausea and vomiting are relatively uncommon with MTX treatment, even when high doses of the drug are administered. Less common side effects are skin rash (about 10% of patients), conjunctivitis, serositis (pleural or peritoneal pain), and photosensitivity. Transient liver abnormalities are commonly seen (increase SGOT), but liver fibrosis and cirrhosis are uncommon, and usually seen only in patients with psoriasis treated with this drug for long periods of time.[15] CNS toxicity can also occur with intrathecal administration of MTX, or when the drug is used with whole brain irradiation.

Renal toxicity, especially with high doses of MTX, can also occur, presumably as a consequence of precipitation of MTX in the kidney tubules. This is a serious event since the renal impairment results in prolonged high blood levels of the drug, which may lead to pancytopenia.[16] Therefore, it is our practice to screen patients with a creatinine clearance and to employ hydration and alkalization in patients receiving doses larger than 250 mg/m^2.[17]

Severe toxicity may also occur in patients with pleural effusions or ascites since MTX may enter these spaces and only slowly be released, thus giving prolonged blood levels. If patients with this "third space" are to be treated, extreme care and careful plasma monitoring of MTX levels should be done. Treatment of patients with MTX at doses of 250 mg/m^2 or higher should only be carried out in institutions where serum MTX levels are available and can be obtained the same day as drawn. While serum creatinine levels are useful, and toxicity may be predicted when the 24-hour serum creatinine increases to greater than 50 percent

TABLE 1   Commonly Used Dosage Schedules of Methotrexate

Dose	Schedule	Leucovorin rescue
5-10 mg/day	Daily until toxicity	No
15-25 mg/day x 5	Every 3 - 4 weeks	No
30-60 mg/m²	Weekly	No
200-250 mg/m²	Weekly to biweekly	At 24 - 36 hrs
3-7 g/m²	Weekly to biweekly	At 24 hrs

of the pretreatment level, one-third of patients with the potential for serious toxicity are not detected with this test alone.[17]

Which Dose of MTX? There have been many doses of MTX employed for the treatment of head and neck cancer, ranging from oral use of 5 to 10 mg/day to weekly or biweekly treatments of 3 to 7 g/m² with leucovorin rescue. As a single agent, the two most convenient dosage schedules are 30 to 60 mg/m² IV weekly without rescue, and 120 to 240 mg/m² IV weekly with leucovorin rescue, started 24 hours after MTX (Table 1). We prefer the latter schedule with rescue because we believe that the toxicity of this regimen is less than with regimens not employing leucovorin. With higher doses (3 to 7 g/m²), the requirement for hydration and alkalinization and the cost may not be worth the possibly slightly higher response rates noted.[18]

Single agent MTX has largely been supplanted by combination chemotherapy, but the principles of administration and monitoring of this drug apply when this drug is used in combination therapy as well.

5-Fluorouracil

Although it has been used as a radiosensitizing agent in this disease, 5-fluorouracil has not been studied extensively in patients with head and neck cancer. Recent studies show that 5-FU has excellent activity when combined with MTX,[19] or with cisplatin.[20]

Mechanism of Action. Two sites of action of FU have been identified: inhibition of thymidylate synthase by the nucleotide of 5-FU (namely, 5-fluorodeoxyuridylate) or incorporation into RNA as 5-fluorouridylate (Fig. 2).

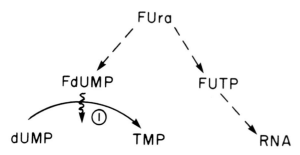

Figure 2 Mechanism of action of 5-FU. 5-FU is converted to 5-fluorodeoxyuridylate (FdUMP), an inhibitor of (1), thymidylate synthase (TS), or to fluorouracil triphosphate (FUTP), which may be incorporated into RNA. Other abbreviations used are dUMP, deoxyuridylate; TMP, thymidylate.

Toxicity. Since 5-FU inhibits cell growth in most cells by inhibition of DNA synthases, its toxicity is similar to that of MTX (on bone marrow, gastrointestinal epithelium). Unlike MTX, it causes diarrhea as a common side effect, presumably because of colorectal mucosal cell toxicity. Less common side effects of 5-FU administration are skin rash, photophobia and conjunctivitis, and cerebellar dysfunction. Also like MTX, the drug is not usually the cause of nausea or vomiting.

Resistance to 5-FU usually occurs by deletion or decreased activity of the enzyme that activates this base to the nucleotide form.[21] Since this enzyme activity utilizes phosphoribosyl pyrophosphate (PRPP) as the cofactor, compounds that deplete PRPP stores (e.g., hypoxanthine, allopurinol) lead to decreased 5-FU effects, and compounds that cause an increase in PRPP levels (e.g., MTX, 6-mercaptopurine) increase 5-FU cytotoxicity.[22]

Clinical Pharmacology. When given intravenously in the usual dose (600 mg/m²), 5-FU is rapidly cleared ($t_{1/2}$ = 15 min).[23] Since the drug is metabolized by the liver, patients with liver damage are at increased risk of toxicity. Because the drug is absorbed to a variable degree when administered by mouth, oral administration is not usually recommended. During recent years, continuous intravenous administration of the drug has been popular; in this circumstance, larger doses are tolerated (1000 mg/m²/day for five doses), and limiting toxicity is gastrointestinal rather than bone marrow. Allopurinol administration will allow larger doses of 5-FU to be safely administered, but it is not yet clear whether this provides a therapeutic benefit.

Bleomycin

Bleomycin, actually a mixture of bleomycins, is a group of antitumor antibiotics that was first discovered by Umezawa. The drug has activity primarily in patients with lymphoma, testicular cancer, and squamous cell cancers. Its role in head and neck cancer is currently limited to its use in combination regimens.

Mechanisms of Action. Bleomycin has been shown to interact with DNA and cause chain scission. This process appears to require a ferrous iron–oxygen complex.[24] Natural resistance and possibly acquired resistance may occur when inactivating enzymes are present (bleomycin hydrolase).[25]

Toxic Effects. Unlike the other agents discussed, bleomycin does not have significant toxicity to marrow stem cells; thus marrow impairment is not a serious problem with this drug. The basis for this lack of marrow toxicity is not clear, but may relate to the presence of bleomycin hydrolase in marrow cells. Thus this drug may be used in full doses in myelosuppressed patients or in combination with agents whose dose-limiting toxicity is to the bone marrow.

Mucositis and skin toxicity are commonly noted with this drug and are a function of intensity of drug administration (mucositis) and total dose (skin toxicity). These side effects are reversible when the drug is discontinued. Fever, malaise, and myalgia are common, especially with higher doses, and can be managed with administration of antihistamines and antipyretics. These effects are noted several hours after drug administration and usually do not last longer than 24 hours. In 1 percent or less of patients treated, particularly patients with lymphoma, a severe pulmonary cardiovascular collapse syndrome has been noted, and patients with lymphoma or with pulmonary or cardiac disease should receive a test dose with 1 mg before instituting standard therapeutic doses.

Pulmonary fibrosis is the most worrisome toxicity to this drug and is almost, but not always, related to total cumulative dose.[26] If this toxicity is not recognized early so that treatment can be stopped, it can progress to a fatal outcome. Therefore, the total bleomycin dosage is usually limited to 300 mg of drug, since the risk increases with increasing drug dosage. Patients who have had previous lung irradiation or are over 70 are at greater risk for this complication.

Clinical Pharmacology. Bleomycin is usually administered either IV or IM, but can be given SC or intra-arterially. The drug is rapidly excreted by the kidney, and kidney function impairment can lead to delayed clearance of the drug and an increase in toxicity.

Experimentally, continuous infusion of bleomycin leads to less host toxicity and a greater antitumor effect.[27] Clinically there is some evidence for improved therapeutic index, but conclusive studies have not yet been done.[28]

Bleomycin, when used concomitantly with other agents causing mucositis (MTX, x-ray), may lead to severe mouth ulceration and therefore should be used in decreased dosage when this toxic additive effect is possible.

Clinical Use. As mentioned, bleomycin is used primarily in combination regimens to treat patients with head and neck cancer. The optimum dosage schedule for this drug in combination for the treatment of head and neck cancer patients has not been established, but intermittent as well as continuous infusion schedules have been used.

Cisplatin

Cisplatin (cis-diamminedichloro platinum, DDP) is a platinum coordination complex that has broad-spectrum antitumor activity in man. It is effective in testicular, ovarian, and squamous cell carcinoma, and is a major new agent for the treatment of head and neck cancer.[29] As a single agent, a response rate of approximately 30 percent has been reported.[30] Originally discarded because of renal toxicity, the drug was found to be safe when administered with forced hydration.[31] Several new analogs are now in clinical trial and may eventually supplant cisplatin because of less renal toxicity. Of great importance is the ability of cisplatin, when used with several other agents, to give additive or synergistic activity. Thus, it is almost always used in combination in the clinic. Drugs that give additive or synergistic cell kill when combined with DDP are bleomycin, 5-FU, mitomycin-C, VP-16, and vinblastine. There is also evidence that DDP is a radiosensitizing agent, and this drug is being evaluated in combination with irradiation in the clinic.

Mechanism of Action. Cisplatin is a reactive molecule and has been found to be capable of cross-linking DNA.[32] In general, however, there is no cross-resistance to alkylating agents. Drug-resistant cell lines have been produced, but the mechanism(s) whereby cells become resistant remains unclear.

This drug is administered intravenously or intra-arterially. Following drug administration, the drug is rapidly protein-bound and persists in the serum for a long time. High concentrations of platinum, as measured by atomic absorption, persist in liver, intestines, and kidney, and only 20 to 40 percent is excreted into the urine within the first few days following drug administration.[33]

Toxicity. Moderate-to-severe nausea and vomiting are usually seen after administration, and many patients have prolonged anorexia, malaise, and weight loss lasting days to weeks. Nausea may be decreased by administering the drug as a continuous intravenous drip for 24 to 120 hours, with no loss in antitumor activity. Nausea and vomiting may also be controlled using high doses of droperidol.[34]

Nephrotoxicity is usually the dose-limiting toxicity of DDP, and as mentioned, this can be prevented by pretreatment and posttreatment hydration.[35] Even with hydration, transient increases in serum creatinine may occur in the second posttreatment week. Therefore it is essential to monitor renal clearance before using this drug and each time a new course is administered. Toxicity can be augmented by other drugs, such as aminoglycoside antibiotics, and if possible, these drugs should be avoided when using cisplatin. The renal toxicity produced by cisplatin may also lead to impaired excretion of other drugs, such as MTX, and when these drugs are used in combination, the potential for increased toxic effects should be kept in mind. Continued administration of cisplatin may lead to a cumulative irreversible loss of renal function and to abnormalities of electrolyte balance, particularly hypomagnesemia.[35] Of interest is recent work indicating that renal toxicity is diminished when hypertonic saline is used with this drug; presumably the increased chloride load protects the kidney from cisplatin damage. Thiosulfate has also been used to protect the kidney from cisplatin damage, presumably by inactivating the drug. Howell has used this compound intravenously together with intraperitoneal administration of cisplatin to decrease systemic toxicity of the drug.[36]

Myelosuppression is less commonly observed as a dose-limiting toxicity, but cisplatin may augment the expected myelotoxicity observed when used with other marrow-suppressing drugs (e.g., vinblastine, VP-

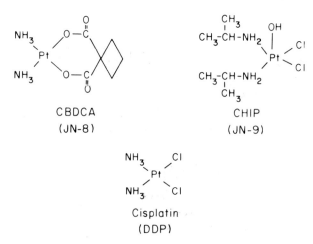

Figure 3 Analogs of DDP in clinical trial.

16). Anemia frequently occurs and may be severe, requiring blood transfusions. Other toxicities associated with cisplatin administration are hearing loss for high frequencies and peripheral sensory neuropathies. The latter are usually dose-related.

Clinical Use. Several studies have shown that cisplatin is an active agent in the treatment of head and neck cancer, although there is lack of good dose-response data. Doses of 80 to 120 mg/m^2 have been shown to be effective, and response rates of 25 to 40 percent with this drug as a single agent have been reported. The drug has also been used intra-arterially and may be more effective via this route than when used intravenously, although comparative studies have not been done.

New Platinum Analogs

Several platinum analogs have been evaluated in recent years in phase I and II trials (Fig. 3). At least two compounds have emerged as promising new agents, i.e., equal or better antitumor effects with less renal and gastrointestinal toxicity.[37,38] At present, limited studies in head and neck cancer have been carried out, but both drugs should be available for clinical use in the near future.

COMBINATION CHEMOTHERAPY

Drugs are used in combination to (1) produce additive or synergistic tumor cell kill, and (2) decrease the potential for development of drug resistance. Additive or synergistic cell kill may be obtained if the drugs employed have different limiting toxicities and different mechanisms of tumor cell kill (e.g., bleomycin and methotrexate). However, the empiric use of drug combinations, based only on toxicity considerations, can sometimes lead to drug antagonism rather than synergy. An example of this phenomen is the simultaneous use of methotrexate and asparaginase. Asparaginase can completely block the antitumor effects of methotrexate.[39] Sequencing of drugs used in combination may also be crucial; in experimental systems the sequence of methotrexate followed by fluorouracil one or more hours later leads to synergistic tumor cell kill, whereas the opposite sequence leads to less than additive tumor cell reduction.[40]

Goldie and Coleman have recently formulated a model that has been useful in devising new strategies to eliminate the possibiliy that drug-resistant mutants will emerge, thus resulting in tumor regrowth after chemotherapy.[41] Based on this model, the use of two or more different drug combinations in an alternating sequence is advocated. One test of this hypothesis that may have produced a higher rate of cures in advanced Hodgkin's disease is the use of MOPP (mechloramine, Oncovin, prednisone, procarbazine) and ABVD (Adriamycin, bleomycin, vinblastine, Dacarbazine) in alternating sequences for several cycles.[42] This hypothesis is currently being tested by several major clinical cooperative groups. It is important to emphasize that in order for this hypothesis to be adequately tested, the combinations used must be *equally* effective.

From experimental work of both murine and human cells in tissue culture, drug-resistance mutants are present in frequencies of one in 10^4 to 10^6 cells; therefore, the possibility that drug resistance to a single agent will develop following treatment in human solid tumors containing 10^9 to 10^{11} cells (1 to 100 g of tumor) is very high. Additionally, certain drugs with different mechanisms of action may share the same transport mechanism, and resistance to one may mean resistance to several drugs (e.g., vinblastine, Adriamycin, actinomycin D).[43]

Thus the argument for the use of drugs in combination is compelling, if the combinations are based on solid experimental and clinical data indicating that they produce an increase in therapeutic index.

REFERENCES

1. Bertino JR, Boston B, Capizzi R. The role of chemotherapy in the management of cancer of the head and neck: A review. Cancer 1975; 36:752–758.
2. Wolf GT, Chretien PB. The chemotherapy and immunotherapy of head and neck cancer. In: Suen JY, Myers EN, eds. Cancer of the head and neck. New York: Churchill Livingstone 1981:782.
3. Bertino JR. "Rescue" techniques in cancer chemotherapy: use of leucovorin and other rescue agents after methotrexate treatment. Semin Oncol 1977; 4:203–216.
4. Galivan J. Evidence for the cytotoxic activity of polyglutamate derivatives of methotrexate. Mol Pharmacol 1980; 17:105–110.
5. Hryniuk WM, Fischer GA, Bertino JR. S-phase cells of rapidly growing and resting populations. Differences in response to methotrexate. Mol Pharmacol 1969; 5:557–564.
6. Johnson LF, Fuhrman CL, Abelson HT. Resistance of resting 3T6 mouse fibroblasts to methotrexate cytotoxicity. Cancer Res 1978; 38:2408–2412.
7. Bertino JR, Srimatkandada S, Carman MD, Schornagel JH, Medina WD, Moroson BA, Cashmore AR, Weiner HL, Dube SK. Mechanisms of methotrexate resistance in acute leukemia. In: Golde DW, Marks PA, eds. Normal and neoplastic hemtopoiesis. New York: Alan R. Liss, Inc., 1983:465.

8. Alt FW, Kellems RE, Bertino JR, Schimke RT. Multiplication of dihydrofolate reductase genes in methotrexate-resistant variants of cultured murine cells. J Biol Chem 1978; 253:1357–1370.

9. Carmen MD, Schornagel JH, Rivest RS, Srimatkandada S, Portlock CS, Bertino JR. Clinical resistance to methotrexate due to gene amplification. J Clin Oncol 1984; 2:16–20.

10. Horns RC, Dower WJ, Schimke RT. Gene amplification in a patient treated with methotrexate. J Clin Oncol 1984; 2:2–7.

11. Curt GA, Carney DN, Cowan KH et al. Unstable methotrexate resistance in human small cell carcinoma associated with double minute chromosomes. N Engl J Med 1983; 308:199–202.

12. Chungi VS, Bourne DWA, Dittert LW. Drug absorption VIII: Kinetics of GI absorption of methotrexate. J Pharm Sci 1978; 67:560–561.

13. Lankelma J, Van der Klein E. The role of 7-hydroxymethotrexate during methotrexate anti-cancer therapy. Cancer Lett 1980; 9:133–142.

14. Cleveland JC, Johns DG, Farnham G, Bertino JR. Arterial infusion of dichloromethotrexate in cancer of the head and neck: A clinicopharmacologic study. In: Zuidema GD, Skinner DB, eds. Current topics. J Surg Res 1969; 1:113–120.

15. Nyfors A. Benefits and adverse drug experiences during long-term methotrexate treatment of 248 psoriatics. Dan Med Bull 1978; 25:208–211.

16. Bleyer WA. Methotrexate: clinical pharmacology, current status and therapeutic guidelines. Cancer Treat Rev 1971; 4:87–101.

17. Pitman SW, Frei E III. Weekly methotrexate-calcium leucovorin rescue: effect of alkalinization on nephrotoxicity; pharmacokinetics in the CNS; and use in CNS nonHodgkin's lymphoma. Cancer Treat Rep 1977; 61:695–701.

18. Pitman SW, Meller D, Weichselbaum R, Frei E III. Weekly high-dose methotrexate with leucovorin rescue as initial adjuvant therapy in advanced squamous cell carcinoma of the head and neck. A pilot study. In: Salmon SS, Jones JE, eds. Adjuvant therapy of cancer. Amsterdam: Elsevier/North Holland, 1977:467.

19. Pitman SW, Kowal CD, Bertino JR. Methotrexate and 5-fluorouracil in sequence in squamous head and neck cancer. Semin Oncol 1983; 10:15–19.

20. Kish J, Drelichman A, Weaver A, Jacobs J, Bergsman K, Al-Sarraf M. Cisplatin and 5-fluorouracil infusion in patients with recurrent and disseminated cancer of the head and neck. Proc Am Soc Clin Oncol 1982; 1:193.

21. Heidelberger C. Fluorinated pyrimidines and their nucleosides. In: Sartorelli S, Johns D, eds. Antineoplastic and immunosuppressive agents. New York: Springer-Verlag, 1975:193.

22. Cadman E, Heimer R, Davis L. Enhanced 5-fluorouracil nucleotide formation after methotrexate administration: explanation for drug synergism. Science 1979; 205:1135–1137.

23. MacMillan WE, Wolberg WH, Welling PG. Pharmacokinetics of fluorouracil in humans. Cancer Res 1978; 38:3479–3482.

24. Suzuki H, Nagai K, Akutsu E, Yamaki H, Tanaka N, Umezawa H. On the mechanism of action of bleomycin strand scission of DNA causes by bleomycin and its binding to DNA in vitro. J Antibiot 1970; 23:473–480.

25. Miller WEG, Schmidseder R, Rohde HJ, Zahn RK, Scheunemann, H. Bleomycin-sensitivity test: application for human squamous cell carcinoma. Cancer 1977; 40:2787–2791.

26. Rudders RA, Hensley GT. Bleomycin pulmonary toxicity. Chest 1973; 63:626–628.

27. Sikic BI, Collins JM, Mimnaugh EG, Gram TE. Improved therapeutic index of bleomycin when administered by continuous infusion in mice. Cancer Treat Rep 1978; 62:2011–2017.

28. Krakoff IH, Cuitkovic E, Currie V, Yeh S, Lamonte C. Clinical pharmacology and therapeutic studies of bleomycin given by continuous infusion. Cancer 1977; 40:2027–2037.

29. Rosensweig M, Van Hoff DD, Slavik M, Muggia FM. Cis-diamminedichloroplatinum, a new anti cancer drug. Ann Int Med 1977; 86:803–812.

30. Prestayko AW, D'Aoust JC, Issell BF, Crooke ST. Cisplatin (cis-diamminedichloroplatinum II). Cancer Treat Rev 1979; 6:17–39.

31. Mead GM, Jacobs C. The changing role of chemotherapy in the treatment of head and neck cancer. Am J Med 1982; 73:582–595.

32. Haynes DM, Cuitkovic E, Golbey RB, Scheiner E, Helson L, Krakoff IA. High dose cis-platinum diamminedichloride: amelioration of renal toxicity by mannital diuresis. Cancer 1977; 39:1372–1381.

33. Munchausen LL. The chemical and biological effects of cis-dichlorodiammineplatinum (II), an antitumor agent, on DNA. Proc Natl Acad Sci USA 1974; 71:4519–4522.

34. DeConti RC, Tofnress BR, Lange RL, et al. Clinical and pharmacologic studies with cis-diamminedichloroplatinum (II). Cancer Res 1973; 33:1310–1315.

35. Mason BA, Dambra J, Grossman B, Catalano RB. Effective control of cisplatin-induced nausea using high-dose steroids and droperidol. Cancer Treat Rep 1982; 66:243–245.

36. Madias NC, Harrington JT. Platinum nephrotoxicity. Am J Med 1978; 65:307–314.

37. Markman M, Howell SB, Pfeifle CE, Lucas WE, Green MR. Intraperitoneal chemotherapy with high dose cisplatin and cytarabine in patients with refracting ovarian carcinoma and other malignancies confined to the abdominal cavity. Proc Am Soc Clin Oncol 1984; 3:165.

38. Calvert AH, Harlane SJ, Newell DR, Siddik ZH, Jones A, McElwain TJ, Raja S, Wiltshaw E, Smith IE, Peckham MJ, Baker J, Harrup KR. Early clinical studies with cis-diammine-1,1-cyclobutane dicarbonylate platinum II. Proc Am Assoc Cancer Res 1982; 23:129.

39. Pendylala L, Cowens JN, Mittleman A, Creaven PJ. Clinical pharmokinetics of cis-dichloro-trans-dihydroxy-bis-isopropylamine platinum IV (CHLP). Proc Am Assoc Cancer Res 1982; 23:127.

40. Capizzi RL. Schedule-dependent synergism and antagonism between methotrexate and asparaginase. Biochem Pharmacol 1974; 23(Suppl 2):151–161.

41. Bertino JR, Sanicki WL, Linquist CA, Gupta VS. Schedule-dependent antitumor effects of methotrexate and 5-fluorouracil. Cancer Res 1977; 37:327–328.

42. Goldie JH, Coldman AJ, Gadauskas GA. Rationale for the use of alternating non-cross-resistant chemotherapy. Cancer Treat Rep 1982; 66:439.

43. Bonnadonna G. Chemotherapy strategies to improve the control of Hodgkin's disease: The Richard and Linda Rosenthal Foundation Award Lecture. Cancer Res 1982; 42:4309.

44. Brockman RW, Yagisawa Y, Ling V, et al. Modes of acquiring resistance to chemotherapeutic agents. In: Sregenthaler W, Luthy R, eds. Current chemotherapy. Proc 10th Int Congress of Chemotherapy, Washington D.C.; Amer Soc Microbiol 1978: 97–102.

8. Combined Modality Chemotherapy in Head and Neck Cancer

STEPHEN K. CARTER, M.D.

Squamous cell carcinoma of the head and neck area accounts for 5 to 6 percent of all malignant tumors diagnosed yearly in the United States. Unfortunately, at the time of diagnosis, the majority of head and neck lesions are large and not easily cured by local control modalities. Head and neck cancers include six broad sites, and the 5-year survival rates are low for all of them. This indicates a great need for additional or improved modalities of treatment.

The patterns of failure in patients treated for primary head and neck cancer are predominantly local and regional with a significant metastatic component which is clinically underestimated in comparison to autopsy findings.

Strong has studied the sites of treatment failure in 798 patients with epidermoid cancers of the oral cavity, pharynx, and supraglottic larynx treated at the Memorial Sloan-Kettering Cancer Center.[1] Surgery was the modality of treatment in 90 percent of the patients. Local-regional failure was the major failure pattern observed. Distant metastases occurred in only 11.7 percent of the patients, but were much more common with tumors of the nasopharynx (39.5%), tonsil (18.6%), base of tongue (16%), and pharynx (15.9%). As might be expected, stage was the most important prognostic variable for local-regional relapse. A multivariate statistical analysis of the incidence of distant metastases at the various anatomic sites reveals a significant difference in the likelihood of distant metastases based on stage of disease, but shows no significant impact for site.

When time to recurrence was analyzed, 54.3 percent of the 359 initial occurrences (in the group of 798 studied) occurred within the first 6 months. This includes 57 patients who were never rendered disease-free by initial treatment. A total of 74.9 percent of the recurrences were seen within 1 year, 82.7 percent within 18 months, and 89.7 percent within 2 years. Three recurrences were observed at 86 months or later.

Lindberg has studied the site of first failure in 3616 patients at the M.D. Anderson Hospital treated over a 15-year period from 1960 to 1974.[2] The sites included were oral cavity, oropharynx, nasopharynx, supraglottic larynx, glottic larynx, hypopharynx, and paranasal sinus. In the patients treated with surgery, the incidence of primary failure varied from 3.7 percent in glottic cancer to 23.4 percent in cancer of the paranasal sinus. Cervical node failure ranged from 6.4 percent in paranasal sinus legions to 24.4 percent in hypopharyngeal legions. No patient had distant metastases in glottic legions compared to 12.4 percent in hypopharyngeal legions. The sites of failure after radiotherapy were slightly higher, but similar in distribution.

Overall distant metastases were the only manifestations of disease in 7.2 percent of patients (262/3616). What is unknown is what the ultimate metastatic failure would be if total local control were achievable.

Distant metastases are not a major cause of death in patients with squamous cell lesions of the head and neck area. The major cause of demise is usually recurrent local and regional disease. When autopsies are performed, the incidence of metastatic disease is in the range of 40 to 51 percent.[3] This would indicate that if full local control could be achieved for these patients, metastatic failure would become a problem of great significance, and adjuvant systemic treatment would have to receive a higher clinical research priority.

Head and neck cancer is a disease that offers a full panoply of combined modality opportunities involving chemotherapy (Fig. 1). Nearly all the various combinations of drugs with surgery and/or radiation can be recommended in the treatment of these squamous cell tumors. As with all solid tumors, the therapeutic need is a mixture of loco-regional control and metastatic control. Many head and neck cancers are diagnosed in a locally advanced (stage III–IV) state in which loco-regional control with surgery and/or x-ray therapy is difficult to achieve. Chemotherapy (Table 1) can be used with the goal of enhancing local control with primary therapy. Chemotherapy can also be used to attack micrometastatic disease outside the surgical field or irradiation port. This latter approach is traditionally called adjuvant chemotherapy, the drugs being administered after surgery and/or x-ray therapy. The use of drugs to increase local control is increasingly being called neoadjuvant chemotherapy, the

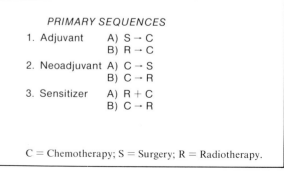

Figure 1 Chemotherapy in combined modality setting for head and neck cancer.

TABLE 1 Chemotherapy in a Combined Modality Setting
for Head and Neck Cancer

Type	Target
Adjuvant	Micrometastasis
Neoadjuvant	Local-regional disease
Sensitizer	Local-regional disease

drugs being given prior to the surgery and/or x-ray therapy. While it is important to conceptually separate adjuvant from neoadjuvant chemotherapy, there are practical overlaps which cannot be avoided which make analyses of effects tricky. It is the purpose of this paper to review the theoretic rationales, design, analysis, and interpretation of combined modality trials in this disease, with emphasis on neoadjuvant chemotherapy.

In any trial involving primary therapy of a solid tumor, three efficacy end points must be balanced against the morbidity of the therapy as well as the mortality risk:

1. Local control with no evidence of residual cancer. In head and neck cancer, this is evaluated both macroscopically and microscopically. Macroscopically, local control means all visible tumor removed by surgery or x-ray. Microscopically, local control means no tumor at the margins of the resection after surgery and/or negative biopsies after irradiation.
2. Relapse-free (or disease-free) survival (RFS), which involves therapy as the zero point and relapse as the end point. This can be measured as a median, mean, or overall survival curve, which can be actuarily projected or an absolute curve after long-term follow-up. Cure can be defined as RFS at 5 years or longer for head and neck cancer, but not for all solid tumors, some exceptions being breast cancer and malignant melanoma.
3. Overall survival (OS), which utilizes either diagnosis or first therapy as the zero point and death as the end point. This is measured in the same way as RFS. It is assumed that RFS and OS will strongly correlate but this does not necessarily have to be the case as has been demonstrated in the adjuvant chemotherapy of breast cancer.[4]

The three end points of a combined modality trial involving chemotherapy in head and neck cancer differ depending on whether the conceptual thrust is

TABLE 2 Role of Chemotherapy and the
Most Direct Efficacy Determinant

Type	Efficacy Determinant
Adjuvant	Relapse-free survival
Neoadjuvant	Regression of primary tumor and nodes
Sensitizer	Local-regional control

neoadjuvant or adjuvant (Table 2). In a neoadjuvant trial, the major goal is to first improve local control. It is also hoped that the local control, when achieved, will be long-term to the extent that "cure" can be claimed. Therefore, the efficacy evaluation of the neoadjuvant drug trial is identical to the evaluation of surgical or radiotherapeutic trial of primary disease. It must be clearly demonstrated that administering the drug prior to the local control will give superior efficacy by one or more of three end points just mentioned without an undue increased morbidity or mortality.

In an adjuvant drug trial, local control is an essential preliminary component of the therapeutic thrust and is not itself an end point of the study. The goal of adjuvant chemotherapy is to eradicate microscopic metastatic disease remaining outside the field of local control. In actuality, "adjuvant" chemotherapy could also have impact on microscopic residual disease existing at the margins of a resection or within a radiation port. Despite this, the end points in adjuvant trials are only RFS and OS and *not* the rate of local control.

The concept of neoadjuvant chemotherapy becomes complicated when irradiation is the loco-regional control modality in use. The complication arises because many of the commonly used cytotoxic drugs in head and neck cancer have been shown experimentally to function as radiation sensitizing agents. These include methotrexate, cisplatin, bleomycin, and 5-FU, which are the most commonly used drugs. These drugs may enhance the cell kill of x-ray therapy if they are given just prior to or concomitant with it. Drug sensitization is conceptually different from neoadjuvant cell kill, although the practical result may be very difficult, if not impossible, to differentiate. The efficacy end points of a "sensitization" and a "neoadjuvant" drug trial with radiation therapy would be identical.

NEOADJUVANT CHEMOTHERAPY

Neoadjuvant trials in head and neck cancer require large numbers for meaningful evaluation because the variables are numerous, and subsets, which can exist within the therapeutic flow, are also large in number. It is unfortunate that the great majority of reported neoadjuvant trials are in fact only pilot studies with small numbers. As pilot studies, they are interesting and point up the need for large-scale randomized studies. They do not validate the use of neoadjuvant drug treatment as part of everyday practice.

The variables in neoadjuvant chemotherapy can be broken down into five major categories (Table 3). In the first category, the disease itself, there exists (1) the heterogeneity of sites with their multiple natural histories of presentation, spread, response to therapeutic modalities, and patterns of relapse; (2) the stage (stage III versus stage IV) and operability; and (3) tumor differentiation.

The second category involves the drug treatment

TABLE 3 Variables in Neoadjuvant Chemotherapy

Disease
  Site
  Stage (III vs IV)
  Differentiation
Drug Treatment
  Drugs chosen
  Number of cycles
  Route (IA vs IV)
  Intensity
Patient Variables
  Age
  Nutritional status
  Co-morbidity
  Performance status
Local Control
  Surgery vs x-ray
  Surgery → x-ray vs x-ray → surgery
  Criteria for operability
  Surgical technique
  Radiation dose and port
Adjuvant Chemotherapy
  Yes vs no
  Drugs(s) chosen

itself. This begins with the drugs chosen.

The choice of drugs for neoadjuvant use had been exclusively based on drugs active against advanced recurrent disease. Since a multiplicity of active drugs exist, the possible combination regimens are numerous. Table 4 lists the single agents with some reported activity and the two-, three-, and four-drug combinations, derived from these drugs, which have actually been investigated in neoadjuvant trials. These are only a small percentage of the combinations that could be investigated.

TABLE 4 Drug Variables for Neoadjuvant Chemotherapy in Head and Neck Cancer

Single Agents
  Cisplatin
  Bleomycin (Bleo)
  Methotrexate (MTX)
  5-Fluorouracil (5-FU)
  Vincristine (VCR)
  Vinblastine (VLB)
  Mitomycin C
  Cyclophosphamide (Cytoxan)
Two-Drug Combinations
  Cisplatin + 5-FU
  Cisplatin + Bleo
  Cisplatin + MTX
  5-FU → MTX
Three-Drug Combinations
  Cisplatin + Bleo + MTX
  Cisplatin + Bleo + VCR
  Cisplatin + Bleo +5-FU
  Cisplatin + 5-FU + VLB
  Cisplatin + Bleo + VLB
  Cisplatin + Bleo + MMC
  MTX + Bleo + 5-FU
Four-Drug Combinations
  Bleo + 5-FU + MTX + VCR (+ Hydrocortisone)
  Bleo + Cytoxan + MTX + 5-FU
  Cisplatin + MTX + Bleo + VCR

The most commonly used drug has been cisplatin; bleomycin, methotrexate, and 5-FU also are commonly used. Cisplatin and methotrexate, generally considered to be the most active drugs against advanced head and neck cancer, have response rates of 30 to 50 percent, depending on such variables as disease extent, prior treatment, site, performance status, and nutritional status.[5] Bleomycin has been attractive as a component of combination regimens because it does not cause myelosuppression. Continuous infusion of 5-FU has recently gained in popularity because it is not myelosuppressive on this schedule and synergism with cisplatin appears to exist.

Hong et al performed a study designed to compare the relative effectiveness and toxicity of weekly intravenous methotrexate (MTX) and intermittent low-dose cisplatin in the treatment of recurrent head and neck cancer, the goal being palliation with minimal toxicity.[6] The patients had recurrent disease, either regional or distant, after prior treatment with surgery and/or radiation therapy. The MTX dose was 40 mg/m^2 weekly and the cisplatin dose 50 mg/m^2 days 1 and 8 by 6-hour infusion repeated at 4-week intervals.

A total of 44 patients were entered into the study between 1979 and 1981. Thirty-eight patients were considered evaluable for tumor response. With MTX, there were four partial responses in 17 evaluable patients, for a response rate of 23.5 percent. After cisplatin, there was one complete and five partial responses in 21 evaluable patients, for a response rate of 28.6 percent. The median survivals were 6.1 months (MTX) and 6.3 months (cisplatin). This study has demonstrated that cisplatin and MTX are comparable in this patient population at the dose levels utilized.

After the choice of drugs had been made, the next question involves the number of cycles to be administered. The number of cycles has ranged from one to three in the studies reported to date, and it has become obvious that with more cycles the initial response of the primary tumor is greater. Whether this enhanced response, with increasing cycles, actually improves local control and survival remains to be determined. It is now generally believed, however, that only one cycle is probably inadequate to test the neoadjuvant hypothesis.

The next consideration in Table 3 is the dilemma of route, schedule, and intensity. There is a long history of intra-arterial drug treatment of head and neck cancer, particularly with methotrexate.[7] In recent years, intra-arterial cisplatin has gained in popularity, but to date no prospectively randomized trial exists to support the use of intra-arterial chemotherapy over standard systemic routes in head and neck cancer.

The variables of schedule are important, particularly with methotrexate, bleomycin, and 5-fluorouracil. Methotrexate has been utilized on a plethora of schedules with and without calcium leucovorin. When the extensive data base on methotrexate is analyzed, there is no schedule that stands out clearly as the one of choice. In addition, several prospectively randomized trials have failed to demonstrate any advantage for high-dose methotrexate with calcium leucovorin over lower doses without rescue. The important schedule questions with bleomycin and 5-FU revolve around whether continuous infusions are beneficial in comparison to IV push. With bleomycin, some groups believe that efficacy is improved on continuous infusion, although a randomized trial to support this hypothesis has not been published. With 5-FU, there is a toxicity difference with infusion since myelosuppression is no longer dose-limiting on this schedule. What this does to the efficacy is essentially unknown at this time.

Intensity of drug treatment is another unanswerable question. Should the drugs be given at their "MTD" as if recurrent disease were being attacked, or should doses be attenuated somewhat since severe toxicity might impair the potential to delivery prompt and appropriate local control. With cisplatin, the dilemma concerns high- vs low-dose schedules.

Veronesi et al have compared high-dose cisplatin (120 mg/m^2) with a low-dose regimen in 61 patients (59 evaluable) with stage III + IV measurable disease, some of whom had failed on prior radiotherapy. With high-dose cisplatin, responses were seen in 5/31 (16%) as against 5/28 (17.8%) after the low-dose regimen. This would indicate that, in the population studied, there was not a meaningful dose-response effect for cisplatin as a single agent.

The Wayne State Group has randomly compared cisplatin + 5-FU 96-hour infusion with cisplatin + 5-FU 600 mg/m^2 Day 1 and 8 by bolus IV injection.[9] A total of 43 patients were randomized and 37 are deemed evaluable. With infusion 5-FU, the response rate is 76 percent (13/17). With bolus 5-FU, the response rate is only 20 percent (4/20). This difference is statistically significant with the P 0.01. The bolus group had more severe leukopenia while the incidence of stomatitis in those receiving continuous infusion was 35 percent. It thus appears that the 96-hour infusion of 5-FU is superior in combination with cisplatin.

The third category of variables in neoadjuvant chemotherapy are prognostic indicators of response to drug treatment, local control therapy, and survival; these variables are age, nutritional status, co-morbidity, and performance status. In any trial of neoadjuvant therapy, data related to these variables must be analyzed for purposes of comparison.

The fourth category involves the methods of, and adequate delivery of, local control therapy. These methods are surgery alone, irradiation alone, or surgery combined with preoperative vs postoperative x-ray therapy. The operative procedure utilized should be appropriate for the site and stage in question. Irradiation has the variables of the port outlined, the dose and fractionation chosen, and adequacy of administration. If the local control is not standardized in a neoadjuvant trial, the data must be analyzed within the subsets of the different local control approaches.

The fifth and final category relates to whether adjuvant chemotherapy is used after local control treatment. If so, it will complicate the interpretation of RFS and OS data.

Analysis of Results

The analysis of results, particularly survival, in neoadjuvant trials must reckon with tremendous heterogeneity of zero points, or denominators which can be picked as the therapeutic flow develops. Figure 2 demonstrates that flow in a hypothetical situation starting with 100 patients. As can be seen, between 10 and 20 denominators exist within the therapeutic flow. In studying the existing trials, reported to date in the literature, it is impossible to develop a meaningful breakdown along the lines of Figure 2. There are only bits and fragments available in the papers, and sometimes it is impossible to fully understand what denominators have been chosen for survival analysis.

An example of the complexity in interpreting trials, particularly with small numbers, is shown in a trial recently reported by the Walter Reed Army Medical Center.[10] They treated 18 patients with newly diagnosed stage III–IV lesions deemed unresectable. The first treatment was neoadjuvant chemotherapy with sequential 5-FU (600 mg/m^2) and methotrexate (125 mg/m^2) weekly for six courses. The second treatment was full-course radiotherapy. Those who achieved local control of the primary, but had residual neck disease, underwent radical neck dissection. Those who were free of disease after local treatment received four cycles of adjuvant chemotherapy with vinblastine, bleomycin, and cisplatin. Of the 18 treated, four had CR and 10 PR after neoadjuvant chemotherapy. After x-ray therapy, 6/18 achieved local control and 9/18 after surgery. Five patients received the three-drug adjuvant regimen. Relapses have occurred in two of these five and in five of nine overall with a median follow-up time of 12 months. The actuarial disease-free survival is 23 percent at 6 months. The toxicity was significant with one drug-related death. Thus it appears that this has not improved survival, but the complexities are so great that individual effects are hard to dissect.

Neoadjuvant Regimens

The most commonly used neoadjuvant regimen is cisplatin plus bleomycin. to date, six different single-arm series have been reported (Table 5). The numbers tend to be small, with 65 being the largest and four of the series involving less than 40 evaluable patients. Three of the series involve one cycle, and the other three, two cycles. Complete response rates range from 0 to 25 percent with no apparent correlation with the number of cycles administered. The overall response rates range from 48 to 88 percent with five of six falling in the 71 to 88 percent range, indicating reasonable comparability, given the great heterogeneity discussed previously. In none of these six papers is there enough data on long-term survival

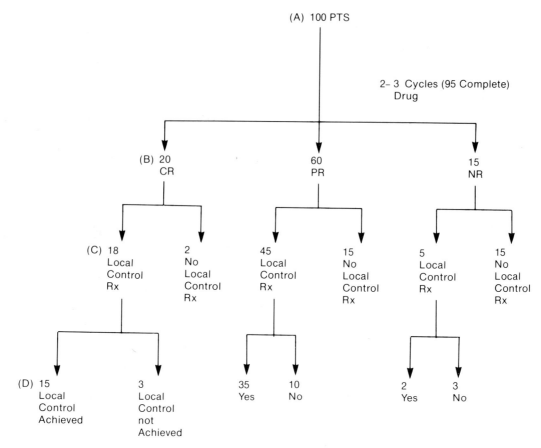

Figure 2 The Christmas tree-shaped flow in neoadjuvant chemotherapy and the heterogeneity in zero points and denominators for analyzing relapse-free survival (RFS) and overall survival (OS).

Zero point and denominator for measuring RFS and OS

1. A 100
2. B 95
   B 80 CR + PR
   B 20 CR
3. C 68 undergoing local control Rx
4. D 52 achieving local control

TABLE 5   Cisplatin plus Bleomycin Neoadjuvant Therapy

Investigation	Dose Cisplatin mg/m²	Dose Bleomycin µ/m²	No. of Cycles	Local Control Therapy	No. of Evaluable Patients	No. of CR	% CR	No. of PR	% PR	% Overall Response
Randolph et al[11]	120 D1	10 D3–10	2	RT	21	4	19	11	52	71
Hong et al[12]	120 D1	15 D3–10	1	Surg + RT or RT	39	8	21	22	56	77
Glick et al[13]	80–100 D1 24-hr infusion	15 D3	2	RT	29	0	0	14	48	48
Elias et al[14]	100 D1	15 D5–9 + MTX	1	Surg and RT	22	4	18	12	55	73
Spauling et al[15]	80 D1	VCR 1D3 6 hrs later 15 D3–7 infusion	2	Surg	50	11	22	33	66	88
Peppard et al[16]	100 D1	30 D2–5 + VCR D2	1	Surg + RT or RT	65	16	25	36	55	80

to judge whether this type of treatment is having an impact on this parameter.

The most interesting combination regimen at this time is cisplatin plus 5-FU by 96-hour or 120-hour infusion. The logic of the continuous infusion of 5-FU is that myelosuppression is minimal on this schedule, and therefore both drugs theoretically could be administered at nearly full therapeutic dose levels. This approach has been pioneered by the group at Wayne State University. In their initial evaluation, they studied 26 patients with inoperable stage IV disease.[17] Inoperability, based on the surgical evaluation, meant that the primary legion and/or the regional nodes could not be removed with cancer-free margins. The dose of cisplatin was 100 mg/m^2, given by 4-hour infusion (with hydration and mannitol) and followed by 1000 mg/m^2 per day of 5-FU continuously infused for 4 days. The course was repeated after 3 weeks.

In this initial study, all 26 patients completed two courses. After the second course, they observed 5 complete (19.2%) and 18 partial (69.3%) responses for a total response rate of 88.5 percent. After these two courses, six patients had radical resection, six had radiotherapy followed by resection, and 12 had radiotherapy only. Two patients had negative histology for tumors at the time of surgical resection after drug.

The follow-up time was too short, and the numbers too small, to speak meaningfully about the survival in this group. However, the 88.5 percent response rate was impressive and clearly indicated that this regimen needed further study in a combined modality setting.

In a follow-up study, the Wayne State Group decided to give full-dose 5-FU, 1000 mg/m^2 per day by 120-hour infusion, with cisplatin at a dose of 100 mg/m^2 for three courses every 3 weeks.[18] The patients treated had either stage III or IV measurable local disease without distant metastases. Thirty-five patients were treated and 32 completed three courses. After one course of drugs, two patients had achieved complete response (CR) and 25 partial response (PR). After two courses, there were 13 CR and 19 PR. At the completion of the final course, there were 21 CR (66%) and 9 PR for a 94 percent overall response rate.

After achievement of CR, 8/22 went on to have radical surgery with six showing no histologic evidence of cancer in the specimen. Seven of these eight patients received postoperative radiotherapy. Eight of the 22 CRs were subsequently given curative intent irradiation. All subjected to biopsy prior to their x-ray therapy and four (50%) were negative for tumor. Of the 11 PRs, five received radical surgery and four radiation therapy. The follow-up time is too short to speak meaningfully about survival.

Weaver et al have published the largest experience on neoadjuvant cisplatin + 5-FU infusion from the Wayne State Group.[19] The patients had stage III and IV squamous lesions with measurable disease and without distant metastases. Patients with a serum creatinine above 1.5 mg/100 m^2 or a blood urea nitrogen

above 20 mg/100 m^2 were excluded. The dose of cisplatin was 100 mg/m^2 with hydration and mannitol dieuresis. The 5-FU dose was 1000 mg/m^2 for 5 days by continuous 24-hour infusion. Three cycles were administered at 3-week intervals.

A total of 61 patients were entered into the study, and 58 completed three cycles of drug as planned. One patient died from aspiration pneumonia after the second course, and two patients who were receiving simultaneous radiation for esophageal cancer developed severe leukopenia. Complete responses were observed in 33 (54%) patients, and 24 (39%) achieved partial response status. Thirteen of the 33 with CR underwent surgery, and nine had no histologic evidence of tumor, either in the primary site or in the radical neck specimen. Biopsies of 8 additional patients prior to irradiation were also negative. An additional 15 patients who had less than total clinical response also underwent resection after drug treatment. Twenty-two had postoperative x-ray therapy, and another 23 had only irradiation for local control.

The toxicity was generally quite acceptable, according to the authors. Hematologic toxicity was severe in four patients and life-threatening in one.

An attempt to develop the tree-shaped analysis is limited by the incompleteness of the data reporting (Fig. 3). Until we get these data in a more complete

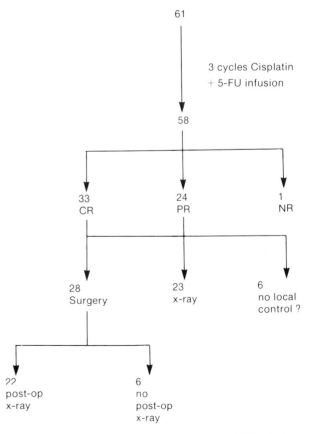

Figure 3 The incomplete "tree" for cis-platin + 5-FU infusion. (From Weaver et al[19])

form, with adequate follow-up, it will be difficult to fully evaluate this study.

It is hard to separate the 61 patients reported by Weaver et al[19] from the 26 patients with stage IV disease reported by Kish et al[17] or the 35 patients reported by Decker et al[18] in a later publication. The patients treated by Kish et al had only 96-hour infusions of 5-FU and so are presumably different. The 35 patients treated by Decker et al had 120-hour 5-FU infusions and appear similar to the earlier 61 pa-

tients reported by Weaver et al, except that all except one in the Decker et al study had stage IV disease. Since the three exclusions from completing three cycles are identical in both papers, it must be assumed that these 35 are part of the 61 reported one year earlier.

The Radiation Therapy Oncology Group has piloted cisplatin plus 120-hour infusions 5-FU in 23 evaluable patients with advanced lesions prior to surgery.[20] They saw nine (39%) complete and 12 (52%) partial responses, for a 91 percent overall response

TABLE 6   Neoadjuvant or Induction Regimens Reported at the 1984 ASCO Meeting

Investigators	Regimen	No. of Patients	% CR	% CR+PR	Local Control	Adjuvant Chemotherapy	Approx % RFS 2 yr
Perry et al[10] Walter Reed Army Medical Center	Sequential 5-FU MTX	18	22	79	x-ray	Yes Cisplatin Vinblastine Bleomycin	23
Hill and Price[21] Royal Marsden	Vincristine Bleomycin 5-FU MTX Hydrocortisone	200	—	66	"curative"	—	—
Jules Bordet Institut[22]	"CABO" Cisplatin MTX Bleomycin Vincristine	27	7	63	Surgery and/or x-ray	No	—
Frustaci et al[23] Pordenone General Hospital	IA Cisplatin	34	26	65	Surgery and/or x-ray	—	—
Mortimer et al[24] Univ Washington	IA Cisplatin	11	18	54	"Definitive local therapy"	No	—
Radiation Therapy Oncology Group[20]	Cisplatin + 5-FU Infusion	23	34	91	Surgery and postop x-ray	No	—
Cripps et al[25] Ottawa Civic Clinic and Hospital	5-FU MTX Cytoxan Bleo or Bleo Cisplatin MTX	29	7	50	Surgery and/or x-ray	No	—
NCI Head and Neck Contracts Program[26]	Cisplatin + Bleo (1 cycle)	282	3	37	Surgery and postop x-ray	Yes Cisplatin	57
Holoye et al[27] Medical College of Wisconsin	"Bleo-" CMF Cytoxan MTX 5-FU + Bleomycin (2 cycles)	43	2	67	X-ray	No	28
Levitan et al[28] Boston, VA	Cisplatin + Bleomycin or Bleomycin alone	101	14	51	Surgery and/or x-ray	No	—
Spaulding et al[29] SUNY, Buffalo	Cisplatin VCR Bleomycin (2 cycles)	46	24	88	Surgery and/or x-ray	No	61
	Cisplatin Vinblastine 5-FU Infusion (2 cycles)	25	4	80	Surgery and/or x-ray	No	36
Robinson et al[30] Israel	Cisplatin Bleomycin MTX (3 cycles)	20	10	55	X-ray	No	—
Laccourrey et al[31] Paris	Cisplatin 5-FU Bleomycin (3 cycles)	43	23	84	Surgery	—	—

rate. The complete responses were seen in 5/6 patients with T3N0 disease and in 3/4 with T4N0 lesions. Two of five who had surgery after CR had no tumor found in the specimen. There was no added morbidity after surgery and postoperative irradiation. The toxicities observed included nausea and vomiting (87%), leukopenia (52%), diarrhea (17%), and renal abnormalities (13%).

A demonstration of the popularity of neoadjuvant pilot studies is found in the 1984 ASCO proceedings. A total of 13 abstracts on this subject have been published (Table 6). These include two randomized studies (Table 7). Only three of the 13 studies include more than 50 patients, and seven include less than 30 patients. Both of the randomized studies are negative experiences. The NCI Head and Neck Contracts Program three-arm study is the largest. It can be criticized for utilizing only one cycle of cisplatin plus bleomycin, although, as was seen in Table 6, there was no apparent difference between one and two cycles in terms of response induction. The 282 patients tabulated in Table 6 are a combination of both induction arms in the three-arm study. In terms of response, the 57 percent 2-year RFS, however, is reflective only of the one arm with neoadjuvant cisplatin. Where approximate 2-year RFS data are available, the range is from 23 to 61 percent, the second highest being from the NCI study, which is not superior to local control therapy only.

RADIATION THERAPY PLUS CHEMOTHERAPY

There is an extensive literature on the combination of irradiation and chemotherapy which dates back many years. In the past, the three most commonly studied drugs were methotrexate, 5-FU, and hydroxyurea. This data base has been reviewed and can be viewed as essentially negative.[7] Nearly all of these early studies involved drugs given either just prior to x-ray therapy and/or concomitantly with it. These studies were designed to test the hypothesis that these drugs were acting as radiation sensitizers, which would improve both the local control incidence and duration. Although studies that used drug prior to x-ray therapy could be viewed as "neoadjuvant," the duration and intensity of the treatment could not be viewed as adequate by today's standard.

The two drugs now being studied most prominently with irradiation are bleomycin and cisplatin. Pilot studies of more complex combination regimens have been tried, but with toxicity limiting the enthusiasm for large-scale randomized trial follow-up. Bleomycin in combination with radiation therapy has been studied in Japan and Europe with results that appear positive, but are often difficult to interpret.[32,33] The difficulties with many of these studies include lack of randomization, small numbers, low doses of radiation therapy, and inadequate description of case selection factors. The Northern California Oncology Group is currently performing a prospective study comparing 7000 rads alone to 7000 rads plus bleomycin in patients with stage III–IV disease deemed to be inoperable.[34] The code has not been broken on this study, but one arm seems to be superior in preliminary literature reports.

The RTOG has studied cisplatin with irradiation simultaneously to test the potential of the drug as a radiation potentiation.[35] The drug was given at a dose of 100 mg/m^2 every 3 weeks simultaneously with 7000 rads. A total of 35 patients have finished therapy, and the complete response rate is 83 percent (29/35), with 5 additional patients achieving a partial response for a 97 percent overall response. Five of the six patients with less than CR had N3b disease. With the median follow-up time being 1 year, 23 patients are disease-free, four are alive with disease, and eight

TABLE 7   Randomized Trials of Induction Therapy in Head and Neck Cancer

Group	Local Control	Arms	% 2 year Survival	Induction Response	Stage of Disease
NCI Head and Neck Contract Program (462 patients)[26]	Surgery followed by x-ray	1. Cisplatin + Bleo 1 cycle	56	37%	Resectable Stage III–IV
		2. Cisplatin + Bleo (1 cycle) plus 8 cycles cisplatin after local control	58		
		3. Local control only	59		
Medical College of Wisconsin (83 patients)[27]	Irradiation	1. Bleomycin Cytoxan Methotrexate 5-FU (2 cycles)	28	67%	Stage III–IV
		2. Local control only	42		

have died. The toxicity has been acceptable, and the group deems this regimen appropriate for a randomized trial, which in ongoing.

REFERENCES

1. Strong EW. Sites of treatment failure in head and neck cancer. Cancer Treat Symposia 1983; 2:5–20.
2. Lindberg RD. Sites of first failure in head and neck cancer. Cancer Treat Symposia 1983; 2:21–31.
3. Dennington ML, Carter DR, Meyers AD. Distant metastases in head and neck epidermoid carcinoma. Laryngoscope 1980; 90:196–201.
4. Carter SK. The chemotherapy of head and neck cancer. Semin Oncol 1977; 4:413–424.
5. Carter SK, Livingstonj RB. The chemotherapy of head and neck cancer. In: Carter SK, Glatstein E, Livingston RB, eds. Principles of cancer treatment. New York: McGraw-Hill, 1982:408.
6. Hong WK, Schaeffer S, Issel B, et al. A prospective randomized trial of methotrexate versus cisplatin in the treatment of recurrent squamous cell carcinoma of the head and neck. Cancer 1983; 52:206–210.
7. Goldsmith MA, Carter SK. The integration of chemotherapy into a combined modality approach to cancer therapy V. Squamous cell cancer of the head and neck. Cancer Treat Rev 1975; 2:137.
8. Veronesi A, Tirelli V, Galligioni E, et al. No evidence of dose dependency of ciplatinum activity in advanced head and neck squamous carcinoma. Results of a randomized study. Proc ASCO 1984; 3:178.
9. Kish J, Ensley J, Weaver A, et al. Superior response rate with 96-hour 5-flourouracil infusion vs 5-FU bolus combined with cis-platinum in a randomized trial with recurrent and advanced squamous head and neck cancer. Proc ASCO 1984; 3:179.
10. Perry DJ, Davis RK, Duttenhaver JR, et al. Multimodality therapy for unreasonable squamous cell carcinoma of the head and neck. Proc ASCO 1984; 3:178.
11. Randolph VL, Vallejo A, Spiro RH, et al. Combination therapy of advanced head and neck cancer: Induction of remission with diamminedichloroplatinum (II), bleomycin and radiation therapy. Cancer 1978; 42:460–467.
12. Hong WK, Shapshay SM, Bhutani R, et al. Induction chemotherapy in advanced squamous head and neck carcinoma with high dose cis-platinum and bleomycin infusion. Cancer 1979; 44:19–25.
13. Glick JH, Marcial V, Richter M, et al. The adjuvant treatment of inoperable stage III–IV epidermoid carcinoma of the head and neck with platinum and bleomycin infusions prior to definite radiotherapy. Cancer 1980; 46:1919–1926.
14. Elias EG, Chretian PB, Monnard E, et al. Chemotherapy prior to local therapy in advanced squamous cell carcinoma of the head and neck. Cancer 1979; 43:1025–1031.
15. Spaulding MB, Kahn A, De Los Santos R, et al. Adjuvant chemotherapy in advanced head and neck cancer: An update. Am J Surg 1982; 144:432–436.
16. Peppard SB, Al-Sarraf M, Powers WE, et al. Combination of cis-platinum, oncovin, and bleomycin (COB) prior to surgery and/or radiotherapy in advanced untreated epidemoid cancer of the head and neck. Laryngoscope 1980; 90:1273–1280.
17. Kish J, Drelichman A, Jacobs J, et al. Clinical trials of cis-platin and 5-FU infusion as initial treatment of advanced squamous cell carcinoma of the head and neck. Cancer Treat Rep 1982; 66:471–474.
18. Decker DA, Drelichman A, Jacobs J, et al. Adjuvant chemotherapy with cis-diamminedicholorplatinum II and 120-hour infusion 5-flourourcil in stage III and IV squamous cell carcinoma of the head and neck. Cancer 1983; 51:1353–1355.
19. Weaver A, Flemming S, Kish J, et al. Cis-platinum and 5-flourouracil as induction therapy for advanced head and neck cancer. Am J Surg 1982; 144:445–448.
20. Jacobs JR, Kinzie J, Al-Sarraf M, et al. Combination of Cis-platinum and 5-flourouracil before surgery in patients with resectable head and neck cancer. Proc ASCO 1984; 3:180.
21. Hill BT, Price LA, MacRoe K. Importance of primary site in assessing 6 year survival data in advanced epidermoid head and neck cancer treated with initial combination chemotherapy without cisplatin. Proc Asco 1984; 3:178.
22. Van Rijmenant ME, Dor R, Balikdjian G, et al. Combined modality approach to T3–4 or N3 squamous cell carcinoma of the head and neck. Proc ASCO 1984; 3:179.
23. Frustaci S, Tumolo S, Veronesi A, et al. Intra-arterial cis-platin in head and neck cancer. Proc ASCO 1984; 3:179.
24. Mortimer J, Cummings C, Laramore G, et al. Selective intra-arterial cisplatin for localized (stage III and IV) unresectable head and neck cancer. Proc ASCO 1984; 3:179.
25. Cripps C, Danjoux E, Nichol J, et al. Pre-treatment with chemotherapy in patients with advanced head and neck cancer. Proc ASCO 1984; 3:181.
26. Jacobs C, Wolf GT, Makuch RW, et al. Adjuvant chemotherapy for head and neck squamous carcinomas. Proc ASCO 1984; 3:182.
27. Holoye PY, Kun L, Toohill R, et al. Prospective randomized trial of adjuvant chemotherapy in head and neck cancer. Proc ASCO 1984; 3:183.
28. Levitan N, Krueger S, Bromer R, et al. Predictive factors for tumor response to induction chemotherapy in advanced squamous cell carcinoma of the head and neck. Proc ASCO 1984; 3:183.
29. Spaulding MB, De Los Santos R, Klotch D, et al. Induction chemotherapy in head and neck cancer: Superiority of a bleomycin containing regimen. Proc ASCO 1984; 3:187.
30. Robinson E, Zidan G, Kuten A, et al. Progress report on the treatment of locally advanced head and neck cancer by bleomycin, methotrexate, and cisplatinum combined with radiotherapy. Proc ASCO 1984; 3:187.
31. Laccourrey H, Brasnau D, Lacau St. Guily J, et al. High response rate after induction chemotherapy in stage III head and neck cancers. Proc ASCO 1984; 3:187.
32. Inuyama Y. Bleomycin treatment of head and neck carcinoma in Japan. In: Carter SK, Crooke ST, Umezawa H, eds. Bleomycin: current status and new developments. New York: Academic press, 1982:267.
33. Berdol P. Head and neck carcinoma: Treatment with bleomycin and radiation. In: Carter SK, Ichikawa T, Mathe G, Umezawa H, eds. Fundamental and clinical studies of bleomycin. Gann monograph on cancer research No. 19. Tokyo: University of Tokyo Press, 1976:133.
34. Fu KK, Phillips TL, Silverberg IJ, et al. Adjuvant chemotherapy with bleomycin and methotrexate in patients irradiated for advanced inoperable head and neck cancer: preliminary results of an NCOG randomized trial. In: Salmon SE, Jones SE, eds. Adjuvant therapy of cancer III. New York: Grune and Stratton, 1981:175.
35. Al-Sarraf M, Kinzie J, Marcial U, et al. Combination of cis-platinum and radiotherapy in patients with advanced head and neck cancer: Radiation Therapy Oncology Group progress report. Proc ASCO 1984; 3:180.

9. Reconstruction: Yesterday, Today, and Tomorrow

IAN A. McGREGOR, Ch.M., F.R.C.S.

Reconstructive methods have greatly improved over the last fifteen years, and the entire picture has changed strikingly. However, it is still not possible to predict the future of reconstruction in intraoral cancer. There may be a considerable divergence between the direction which one feels reconstruction ought to take and the direction taken in the event. A new discovery in any of the fields relating to oral cancer and its surgery (in etiology, pathology, resection) might alter completely the direction that reconstruction takes. Advances in the other treatment methods currently in use, radiotherapy and chemotherapy, conceivably might revolutionize the surgical approach to both resection and reconstruction.

And yet, in reconstruction we have reached a situation of stability of a sort. The flood of new techniques is apparently receding, and we can now view the field dispassionately. The problem of assessing these methods has not been made any easier by the uncritical manner in which they have been presented in the journals, through the eyes of the enthusiast rather than the realist. And so it is by word of mouth, by finding a communal dissatisfaction with a technique for reasons that are clearly valid but went unmentioned in the original description, that ultimate judgments must be made and techniques properly discarded. The profession is ready for this process, and if the current disenchantment with the transfer of rib as a composite with the pectoralis major myocutaneous flap is taken as a sample, the process is already well under way. Such a sifting will do nothing but good.

In the quest for improvement in functional and cosmetic results, it becomes necessary to analyze in some detail the role played by the *tongue* and the *mandible* in producing these results.

THE TONGUE

The tongue was once regarded more as a source of tissue to close postexcisional defects than as a key structure in the mouth. No consideration was given to its subsequent function and to the effect that loss of that function would have in contributing to the creation of an oral cripple. This attitude has changed, but surgeons still do not take sufficient account of the tongue and its functional deficits as a factor in assessing postoperative results, sometimes even adding to the deficit in the course of reconstruction.

When one analyzes the deficits of the tongue in the varying combinations of resection-reconstruction as these have developed in the last thirty years, that is, over the period during which reconstruction of defects has replaced direct closure, it is possible to isolate the various effects of surgery on function.

If the tumor is to be resected, loss of muscle substance and denervation are unavoidable, but added to the resulting disabilities is the factor of tethering of the residual tongue. This factor, which is more significant than the others, has been created by the surgeon. It is the creation of tethering which one would hope to see increasingly avoided in the future.

With regard to tethering and its effect on function, the first consideration is the functional importance of the different parts of the tongue. There is no doubt that the anterior free segment of the tongue is its key element, in disposing of saliva and food and in speech. In the normal disposal of saliva, the tip of the tongue dips down to scoop up the bolus of saliva from the anterior floor, passing it back between the dorsum and the palate into the pharynx. Similarly, it is the free anterior segment which manipulates the food bolus in the mouth. In the normal enunciation of many consonants, the tip is brought into contact with the gingiva of the upper incisors and canines.

With a tethered tongue tip it is not possible to perform any of these functions properly, and the disability that results is one that can be recognized at a glance in the patient with a handkerchief constantly in his hand to help cope with his drooling of saliva. Tethering in this context must be considered to include the tongue tip which has been turned back on itself in order to close a defect, a practice regularly illustrated in textbooks of surgery. This practice I would hope to see cease altogether, replaced by reconstruction of the resected component of the tip, leaving a tongue of normal length. I would hope to see, as a cardinal principle of intraoral reconstruction, that *any segment of tongue remaining after a resection should be maintained in its preoperative position within the mouth and that tissue reconstructing the resected segment should replace it both in site and volume.* It is astonishing how effectively what at operation appears to be a remnant of the tongue tip is capable of providing the force to move a flap, itself devoid of muscle, into functional adequacy.

THE MANDIBLE

The mandible is so closely linked with so many aspects of surgical management that it is necessary to consider these aspects individually.

There was a time when management of the mandible was quite straightforward: it was simply resected. As recently as 1970 it was written that "in managing carcinoma of the tongue, resection of the mandible makes it easier to close the defect by suturing the cheek mucosa to the tongue"—not exactly a valid reason for resecting the mandible.

If each aspect of the influence of the mandible is

to be analyzed, the first aspect must concern the surgical approach to the oral cavity.

Surgical Approach. Most tumors occurring intraorally arise inside the horseshoe of the mandibular body, and it is the approach to this site that is therefore of most concern. The "pull-through" approach, though abandoned in enlightened centers, is still used in many places.[1] If the surgeon who persists in using the method is scrupulous in trying to clear the tumor locally, he must resect the tissues in an unselective manner because of the inadequacy of the exposure. If the major tumor of the tongue or the floor of the mouth is to be visualized properly, obviously an osteotomy of the mandible must be carried out, the mandibular "swing" approach.[2] One would hope to see this approach becoming standard practice. The spontaneous comment has been made to me by the pathologist who examines my resection specimens that since routine adoption of the "swing" approach, adequacy of resection of the tumor has not changed, but the amount of normal tissue removed in addition has dropped dramatically. The influence on the size of the defect is obvious, and the beneficial effect on reconstruction equally so. I would hope, however, to see a change in the routine osteotomy site used preparatory to the swing, from the symphysis to the site just anterior to the mental foramen (Fig. 1). The site anterior to the mental foramen gives equally good exposure and it avoids dividing the tongue muscles,[3]

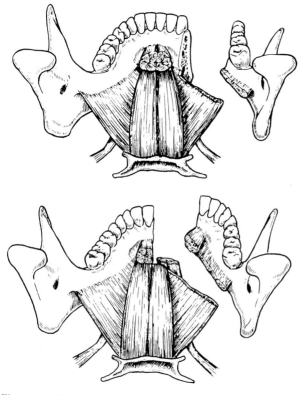

Figure 1 The osteotomy sites, symphyseal and anterior to the mental foramen, showing the structures divided to achieve the mandibular "swing."

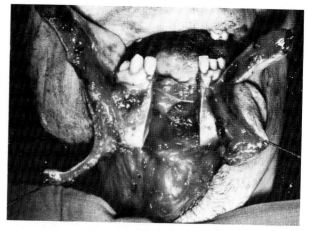

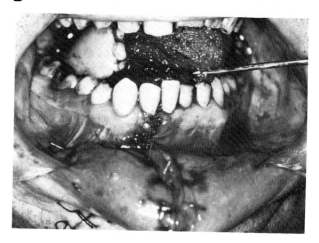

Figure 2 Symphyseal osteotomy, without extraction of teeth. *A*, The mandible divided. *B*, The mandible reconstituted.

which are attached to the genial tubercles. With the power-driven saws that are currently available, it should generally be possible to avoid extracting a single tooth in dividing the bone (Fig. 2).

In the recent past, the mandible was sacrificed, not for reasons of tumor involvement, but because its removal made exposure easier in such tumor sites as the posterior third of the tongue, the fauces, and the retromolar trigone, or because it made closure of the defect easier. Despite some resistance to a change in this routine, the development of mandibular swing has reduced resection to provide exposure (Fig. 3)

The Mandible and Tumor Spread. The use of mandibular resection for the purpose of exposing the tumor may no longer be defensible, but the question remains regarding resection of the mandible because of tumor involvement, suspected or actual. Too little is known about the mode of invasion of the mandible from the common tumor sites—floor of mouth, tongue, and retromolar trigone, in both the dentate and the edentulous bone. Despite the numbers of

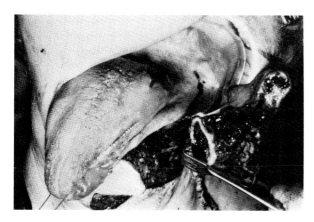

Figure 3 Exposure of the posterior tongue and fauces, using the mandibular swing approach with the osteotomy located anterior to the mental foramen.

A

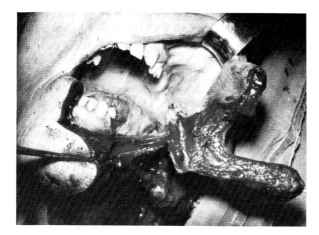

B

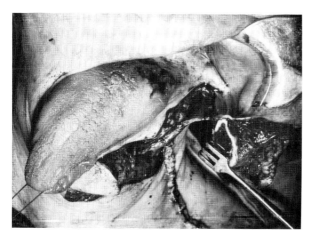

Figure 4 The site of attachment of mylohyoid to the mandible in *A*, The dentate bone, and *B*, The edentulous bone. Note the difference in height, the attachment in the edentulous bone being virtually on the occlusal ridge.

mandibles resected over the years, little has been published on the mechanisms of spread into and through the bone. This aspect of resection requires further investigation.

In the United Kingdom, dental conservation in the social category prone to oral cancer does not carry a high priority, and most patients are edentulous. On investigation of the mode of involvement of the mandible in this group, the findings, though unexpected, have conformed to a consistent pattern. On the basis of these findings, I have altered my surgical approach, and the results have validated the conclusions reached by the investigation.

Of the changes in the mandible that result from loss of the teeth, the important ones relate to tumor spread and concern the changes in the relative height of the attachment of mylohyoid to the bone and the anatomy of the occlusal ridge. The resorption of the alveolar process of the mandible which follows loss of the teeth leaves the mylohyoid attached much closer to the occlusal ridge, toward the retromolar trigone, almost on the ridge itself (Fig. 4). The occlusal ridge left after the healing process which follows dental clearance is also not exactly what one might expect.[4] Instead of a complete covering of cortical bone along the ridge, there are at best multiple foramina communicating with the medullary cavity, at worst an entire ridge consisting of medullary bone (Fig. 5). This

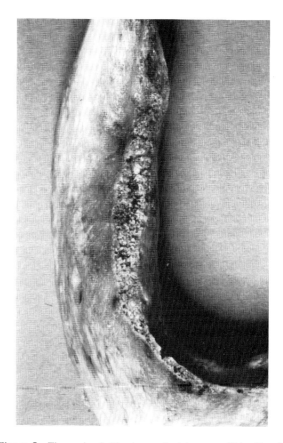

Figure 5 The occlusal ridge in an edentulous mandible. Note in this bone a total absence of cortical bone.

has the effect of leaving the mucoperiosteum overlying the occlusal ridge in direct continuity with the medullary cavity. The mandibular canal is lined equally with medullary bone, and this extends the direct continuity to the inferior dental nerve.

With these changes as a background, it has been found, contrary to what one might expect, that the way in which tumor extends onto and into the mandible is not usually through the lingual plate of the bone. The mylohyoid, with the overlying sublingual gland and the deep part of the submandibular gland, seems to have a considerable capacity for acting as a relatively effective, though temporary, tumor barrier, and involvement of the bone is by lateral spread above the mylohyoid. The effect is to carry tumor onto the occlusal ridge where the incomplete cortical covering allows ready access into the substance of the bone (Fig. 6).

Spread within the bone thereafter has taken two main forms, frequently distinct though sometimes mixed. The tumor has been found to spread downward into the bone on a relatively broad front (Fig. 7), or to pass selectively into the perineural spaces around the inferior dental nerve (Fig. 8), and then backward to and through the pterygoid muscles onto the trigeminal ganglion. In either event, the bone below the mandibular canal has been found to be involved at a comparatively late stage. In the light of these findings, if partial resection of the mandible is

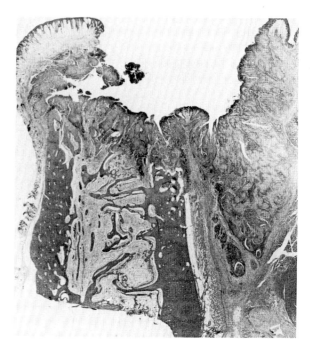

Figure 7 Spread of squamous carcinoma onto and into the edentulous mandible from the primary site, the floor of mouth. Note the absence of involvement of the lingual plate, tumor having entered through the occlusal surface, spreading on a broad front into the medulla of the bone.

feasible, a rim resection rather than a sagittal resection should be performed, removing in the process the canal with its contained nerve (Fig. 9).

The sequence in the dentate mandible remains to be examined. It may provide surprises comparable to those in the edentulous bone.

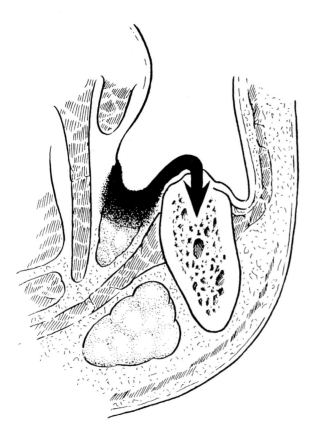

Figure 6 Diagram showing the predominant pattern of spread of tumor from the floor of mouth into the edentulous mandible.

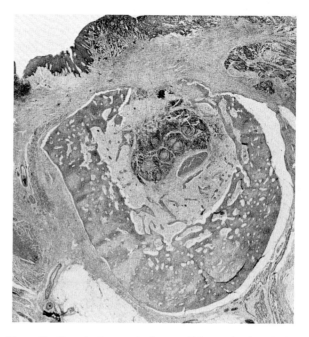

Figure 8 Spread of tumor in the mandible, predominantly in a perineural fashion along the inferior dental nerve, showing the absence of involvement of the surrounding mandible. Note complete absence of cortical bone over the occlusal surface.

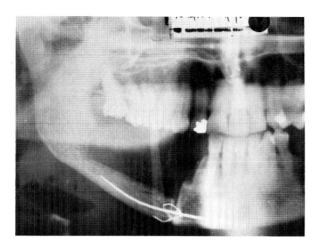

Figure 9 Mandibular osteotomy, used in conjunction with a rim resection, which included the mandibular canal with its contained inferior dental nerve. The nerve was found to be free of tumor.

Mandibular Resection and Reconstruction.

If mandible has to be resected, the nature of the future mandibular reconstruction must be considered. Does the bone invariably require to be replaced, and if it is to be replaced, what form should the replacement take, how much of the bone should be replaced, and at what stage in the reconstruction should it be replaced? At the outset, it must be acknowledged that, in the context of intraoral malignancy, bone grafting, early or late, with trays of all shapes and sizes, with and without bone chips have been failures. Over the years published papers have described techniques of bone replacement, but long-term failures have gone unreported. On biologic grounds these failures are not unexpected, and I do not see the situation changing in the future. The future in bone replacement clearly lies with the transfer of vascularized bone. The question that remains concerns when it is required, and the precise form it should take. To answer this question it is necessary to consider the disability that results from the various resections. To lose the ascending ramus carries a minimal disability. As the resection passes forward along the body of the bone, the bite loses strength, and the patient becomes increasingly unable to wear a lower denture. But if the symphysis is not crossed, the result has generally been regarded by many surgeons as acceptable.

If replacement is contemplated, however, the twisting shape of the mandible, curving horizontally in its body, turning sharply upward in its ramus, provides a real challenge, fortunately a challenge one is not invariably required to meet. Examination of resected bones has shown us that the posterior third of the ascending ramus, that is, the ramus behind the lingula, is rarely involved by tumor. The segment of bone at real risk is the segment that includes the inferior dental nerve. A vertical bony cut separating the posterior third of the ascending ramus from the anterior two-thirds, with its included inferior dental nerve, leaves a vertical segment of bone which includes the condyle with its attached external pterygoid muscle.

This segment is capable of providing a potential posterior attachment for bone transferred to replace the resected body. It becomes necessary then to replace only the horizontal segment of the body, and this is technically much simpler, regardless of the method of reconstruction selected.

If bone is only being partially resected, the preservation of the viability of the retained segment becomes relevant. If we consider the sources of blood supply of the mandible in relation to tumor site, along with the necessity, from a pathologic standpoint, of resecting the inferior dental nerve and blood vessels, it becomes apparent that the most important vascular source, and hence the one to be preserved, is that associated with the soft tissue attachment lateral to the mandible (Fig. 10), between the lower buccal sulcus and the lower border of the bone. It has been my ex-

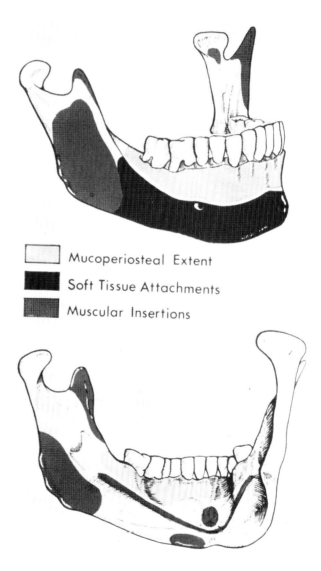

Figure 10 The sources of blood supply of the mandible. Note that the only significant source for the body of the bone likely to remain after rim resection, including the mandibular canal, is the soft tissue attachment of the buccolabial surface.

perience that if the bone segment left after any resection retains this attachment, it remains viable, as judged by its capacity to unite at an osteotomy site and produce a layer of cortical bone along a line of resection. This finding has obvious implications with regard to the form taken by any resection, but these are self-evident.

Surgery and Radiotherapy. Reconstruction, whether it is of soft tissue alone or along with bone replacement, does not exist in isolation. It is an element of overall tumor management, by radiotherapy as well as surgery, and as such it is liable to be influenced by changes in the other element. For example, in the patient whose neck has been irradiated as part of the treatment of the primary tumor site, the reconstruction chosen may be selected for advantages that relate only partly to its suitability for reconstructing the defect. Other considerations include the effect of the radiotherapy on the neck, whether the excision is part of a planned elective combination of treatments, or whether it is the more usual unplanned salvage procedure for tumor that has recurred at the primary site. These considerations determine to what extent the carotids are regarded as being at risk of "blow-out"[5,6] and whether the reconstruction should be selected to protect the vessels as well as to reconstruct the defect. It may also be that the state of the vessels in the neck after uncoordinated radiotherapy may be unsuitable for anastomosing to the free flap which might otherwise be suitable.

For these reasons one might choose a myocutaneous flap, whose protective muscle pedicle overlies the carotids, a flap which on other counts would be the less desirable of the alternatives. Taking the argument a stage further, the condition of the mandible after radiotherapy may influence whether resection is required irrespective of tumor clearance. This in turn may determine whether the reconstruction should include bone as part of the composite tissue transfer.

With regard to the relationship between radiotherapy and surgery, the coordinated elective use of both treatment methods in a single patient must be distinguished from the all too frequent uncoordinated use of either method in which the other is used only when tumor recurs. Fortunately, the trend in many of the more progressive centers is towards elective use of both methods seriatum. It is a trend that surgeons should encourage, just as they should stress the advantages of having the surgery precede the radiotherapy. Advantages of this sequence are (1) it allows the surgeon freedom to use the neck dissection incisions that are most convenient rather than those that add protection to the carotids; (2) it gives the surgeon greater freedom to exploit reconstructive techniques more effectively, in particular free flaps, (3) it allows the surgeon to manipulate the mandible with greater freedom, and to use the swing approach to the oral cavity without concern about adding to any reduction in the vascularity of the bone and contributing to osteoradionecrosis, (4) it makes conservative mandi-

bular surgery more a possibility, and (5) it virtually eliminates carotid blow-out as a hazard.

From the viewpoint of many radiotherapists, the surgeon is seen as the creator of deformity, as the creator of avascularity as a result of his surgical manipulations, an avascularity that reduces the effectiveness of radiotherapy and prevents the method from being exploited to the full. Surgeons explain that reconstructions bring a fresh blood supply to the area and, in short, that such fears regarding avascularity relate to the days before modern reconstructions. The radiotherapist's fears regarding deformity can be allayed only by the demonstrated effectiveness of reconstructions. The radiotherapist must be presented with a patient who to him is cosmetically and functionally acceptable. Only then is he likely to accept his role as a partner and not as the sole actor in the drama.

RECONSTRUCTIONS COMPARED

The practicing surgeon, who is faced with a defect that he has to fill, has to select from the available reconstructions the one that is appropriate in the circumstances. What are the trends in this field and what does the future hold? In reconstructive surgery, as in surgery generally, there are fashions, and the pendulum swings. But there is an onward movement, and the pendulum does not return quite to the same spot. It would be more accurate to say that it is attitudes and approaches to problems rather than details of method, which oscillate between extremes.

Methods of intraoral reconstruction have passed from direct suture, through skin flaps, to myocutaneous flaps, with the addition of free tissue transfer in each, using microvascular anastomosis, so that today the surgeon is faced with a veritable plethora of possible reconstructive techniques. Skin flaps are being relegated very much to a subsidiary role, to be used when other techniques have failed. For some of the flaps and in some of the roles, this is not altogether justified, but to be realistic one must accept the inevitability of the trend. The various flaps that use neck skin will be justifiably discarded. There are a sufficient number of techniques which allow a neck dissection, radical or functional, to be carried out unrestricted by considerations of modifying incisions to allow neck skin to be transferred as a flap. The deltopectoral flap seems likely to suffer the same fate. Most of the things it can do intraorally can be done equally well with one of the myocutaneous flaps, and in a single stage. I regret the discarding of the deltopectoral flap as it relates to the buccal mucosa, for in that site it still provides a highly effective reconstructing flap, large enough to replace the entire buccal mucosa, thin enough to replace it without too much bulk. In my personal view, it should remain the alternative to a free skin flap in this site, and one capable of giving as good an ultimate result.

With regret I see the forehead flap being reduced

to a back-up role. The skin that it transfers into the mouth still stands comparison with any of the newer flaps, and it has the desirable characteristic of safety and ease of use, but I would entirely accept the grafted forehead as a bar to its use.

Concerning the more recently described reconstructions, each flap, as already stated, has tended to be described in glowing terms, as a virtual panacea for all the problems of intraoral malignant tumors. What the future holds, it is hoped, is a more realistic recounting of the limitations and less desirable characteristics of these same flaps. This phase I might perhaps initiate now as my own contribution to creating the future which I would like to see in this respect.

The myocutaneous flaps and their extension, the osteomyocutaneous flaps, share certain features, while retaining individual characteristics in other respects. In general, they are bulky, and any trend which one sees in their use, increasingly or decreasingly, must of necessity take account of this fact. A desirable parallel trend is toward maintaining mandibular continuity whether by conservative resection or restoration by transfer of bone. The effect is to reduce the volume of the defect, and in such a situation the bulk of a myocutaneous flap may be highly undesirable, the mouth being unable to accommodate both the flap and the residual tongue without displacing the latter and disrupting its function, to the extent even of fixing it permanently in an abnormal position. With denervation of the muscle component of the flap, a proportion of the bulk is temporary, but even so it may still be highly undesirable, and it is a consideration in the selection of a reconstructive technique.

If we are assessing the comparative place of the various myocutaneous flaps, the currently accepted workhorse, the pectoralis major flap,[7] may be considered first. It is an extremely convenient method, but it has certain adverse and sometimes limiting features. Its use runs contrary to the use of a functional neck dissection in the form that retains sternomastoid. The neck containing sternomastoid is unlikely to tolerate the pedicle of a pectoralis major flap without compressing the pedicle to an unacceptable extent.

In some ways a much more serious deficiency of the method is the effect of gravity on the flap. Not surprisingly, it shares this deficiency with the deltopectoral flap. Unless its skin margins can be anchored to fixed points in the oral cavity, and that means mucoperiosteum of mandible or upper alveolus, the skin paddle is pulled down into the floor of the mouth. In certain sites this may be of no consequence, but when the flap is filling a defect of the tongue, the effect can be highly undesirable, tethering the tongue in the position most unsuited to effective functioning. In the posterior tongue the effect is less disastrous; in the anterior tongue, the free segment is liable to be totally anchored. This undesirable characteristic is well documented for the deltopectoral skin flap. Though less well documented to date, it applies equally to the pectoralis major myocutaneous flap.

The myocutaneous flap that provides the main alternative to the pectoralis major is the lateral trapezius flap of Demergasso,[8] and considered as a transfer of skin, it has adverse qualities compared with the pectoralis major flap. Its vascular basis is not altogether reliable. The artery is generally, though not always, present and standard; the vein is far from constant.[9] This means that as a first step the vascular pedicle must be identified as "present and correct" before the flap proper can be raised, and an alternative reconstruction must always be available in reserve in case the vessels are absent or unsuitable. The trapezius at the site of the pedicle is freqently bulky, and the dissection tends to be accompanied by considerable bleeding. The comparative slimness of the proximal element of the vascular pedicle, however, allows the flap to be accommodated in the neck along with a functional neck dissection preserving sternomastoid, although trapezius function cannot be preserved.

An adverse factor which is liable to weigh heavily with many surgeons, given a satisfactory alternative, is the alteration from the supine in the position of the patient, which is necessary to allow access to the flap site. To the surgeon used to operating with the patient supine, the alteration in the familiar landmarks can be most confusing.

In summary, the adverse factors make me feel that the trapezius flap is not likely to make significant inroads into the reconstructive territory now occupied by the pectoralis major flap.

The other myocutaneous flaps are unlikely to survive. Used in the context of intraoral malignant disease, the limitations of the sternomastoid myocutaneous flap[10] are crippling.[11] These limitations apart, the obvious absence of vascular connection between sternomastoid and the overlying skin, as judged during a neck dissection, would suggest that the ability of the muscle to perfuse an overlying skin paddle is more than a little dubious. The platysma myocutaneous flap has equally obvious undesirable qualities as a source of reconstruction in intraoral malignant disease.[12] In addition to the fact that its vascular sources are likely to be divided in the course of a neck dissection, it has the disadvantage, common to all reconstructions that use neck skin, of disrupting the standard practice of neck dissection without any compensating advantage.

The latissimus dorsi myocutaneous flap is used as a tissue source when a larger area defect requires reconstruction. It can be used in the standard intraoral defect, but is not the reconstructive procedure that first comes to mind. It seems more likely to be used exceptionally rather than routinely.

When one extends the reconstruction to include the transfer of bone, however, the virtues of the various flaps change somewhat. The pectoralis major with rib has had an extended trial, and although my personal experience is nil, a canvass of surgeons leads me to conclude that it is not sufficiently reliable to command universal approval. The spine of the scapula is an excellent piece of bone,[13] but it shares the uncertainty of its vascular pedicle with the lateral trapezius flap, its myocutaneous counterpart. It is also not really possible to make the transfer without turning the patient, and certainly in my mind this must be a strong minus point when deciding whether to use it.

FREE FLAPS

This technique of free flap transfer has progressed from using flaps originally designed as axial pattern skin flaps to using flaps designed at the outset as free flaps. One sees in this process a trend toward longer vascular pedicles using vessels of a larger caliber, thereby increasing both the convenience and reliability of the transfer. The flaps that are currently popular share a comparable degree of reliability. We know that skin settles well into the mouth, so that advocacy of mucosal replacement by mucosa in the form of a jejunal flap[14] as more appropriate is not a valid argument as far as the mouth is concerned, however valid the argument may be in favor of its role as a conduit to replace pharynx.

The criteria for selecting the free flap, given the usual patient's history as a heavy smoker with a considerable thirst for spirits, are such matters as ease of raising and transferring the flap, and its potential influence on postoperative management of the patient. The three flaps that have been described are the dorsalis pedis flap,[15] the jejunal flap,[14] and the radial forearm flap,[16] and they vary significantly from this point of view.

The dorsalis pedis flap can be difficult to raise, depending on the site of the take off point of its feeding vessel from the dorsalis pedis artery, and the donor site is liable to present problems. These problems frequently arise even in the young patient; in the older age group they must be considerably magnified. The addition of an abdominal operation to a major intraoral resection/reconstruction, which the use of a jejunal flap imposes on the type of patient already described, is also likely to restrict its use materially. The radial flap, with its use of the skin of the forearm, does not interefere with mobilization of the patient, and although 100 percent take of the graft applied to the donor site of the flap is not invariable, healing without loss of function has been the rule.

Viewed strictly in their role as a replacement for soft tissue defects, these three flaps are comparable in the role that they can fill and in the results obtained inside the mouth. When bone and soft tissue both require replacement, the radial flap has the considerable added virtue of allowing part of the thickness of the radius to be transferred as a composite along with the skin. Care is required postoperatively to protect the radius, but once the need for protection is recognized, the problem is not a serious one.

How then does one see the future in the relative use of the free and the myocutaneous flaps. It seems probable that for the standard large defects, particularly one that includes mandible, the pectoralis major flap is likely to remain the favorite for most surgeons. For the surgeon who is making a conscious and continuing effort to achieve the best results, in maintaining and restoring mandibular continuity, the free flaps are likely to be favored, and in this the radial flap would seem to have virtues compared with the alternatives.

PROBLEM OF THE SYMPHYSIS

Throughout this discussion the topic of symphyseal reconstruction has not been raised. There is no doubt that the major problems in intraoral reconstruction still relate to management of the tumor of the anterior floor where the symphysis of the mandible has been resected. We even still retain a specific name for the deformity—the Andy Gump (Fig. 11). To forecast advances in this field calls for a crystal ball, particularly since I do not see the problem being solved in the immediate future. However, one can at least define the problem, analyze its various components, and point to possible ways in which the deformity and the disabilities with which it is associated can be reduced.

It is significant that the phrase, Andy Gump deformity, was coined at a time when soft tissue reconstruction as we know it today was nonexistent, when defects were closed directly. Although the deficiency is of soft tissue and bone, attention has tended to be focused exclusively on the loss of the symphyseal bone to the exclusion of the soft tissue component. With the development of ways of reconstructing soft tissue, it has become possible to correct, at least in some measure, this aspect of the deformity. I would admit to remaining inadequate in reconstructing the entire defect, bony and soft tissue, but by reconstructing the soft tissue element, it has at least become possible to distinguish between the effect of the soft tissue loss and the effect of the bone loss.

Loss of bone is clearly responsible for the cosmetic disability. It would appear, however, that much

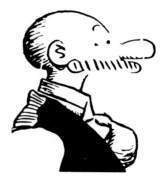

Figure 11 Andy Gump, the cartoon figure, epitomizing the post-symphyseal resection deformity. (With permission of Dr. Ralph Mullard.)

of the functional loss, that is, the inability to speak intelligibly and dispose of saliva, is very much the result of the soft tissue loss, most of all by the tethering of the free segment of the tongue. If the tongue can be retained in its proper position, free and mobile, a considerable proportion of the problem vanishes. Given adequate soft tissue replacement, the tongue totally detached from the symphysis, as part of the mandibular resection, seems to establish a fresh attachment, admittedly soft tissue rather than bony, but functionally effective for all that.

Even with current methods of reconstructing soft tissue, however, the effect, using flaps taken from the chest such as the pectoralis major flap, is to pull the tongue down into the floor, tethering it immobile in that position, with results that are just as functionally crippling as those that follow direct suture. The solution to such a problem may be to use a reconstructive method such as bilateral nasolabial flaps which, in addition to reconstructing the defect of the anterior floor site, have the incidental effect of holding the tongue suspended above the floor of the mouth. In the ordinary way, nasolabial flaps have their place in the small defect of the anterior floor or ventral tongue (Fig. 12), but there seems no reason why they could not be used in the extensive anterior floor–ventral tongue tumor to hold the tongue high in the mouth and prevent it from becoming anchored in the anterior floor. I have had occasion to use such flaps secondarily to hold in an elevated position a tongue that had become anchored as a result of the downward pull of a pectoralis major myocutaneous flap, and it proved unexpectedly effective. Faced with a comparable problem again, I would consider using the nasolabial flaps primarily, to resurface the ventral tongue and hold it up and free from the floor, while using the

pectoralis major flap to restore the anterior floor, in the hope of avoiding the tethering in the first place. In sum, there is strong evidence that the functional consequences which follow symphyseal resection may stem more from failure to reconstruct the soft tissue defect than from failure to restore bony continuity. The bony deficiency is responsible for the cosmetic element of the deformity, and ideally the bone should also be replaced.

One might properly state at this point that we require more information concerning bone invasion in the symphyseal segment of the mandible, its mechanism and extent, both in the dentate and edentulous bone, so that we can determine more accurately how much bone needs to be resected and, in particular, under what circumstances a rim can be left. I would suspect that retention of the lower rim of the bone is probably feasible more frequently than is often appreciated. In the symphysis, as in other parts of the mandible, maintenance of the attachment of the soft tissues of the chin to the bone is the key to survival of such a rim. It should not be forgotten that the improvement in appearance that results from such retention is as dramatic as the corresponding improvement in function which follows an adequate soft tissue reconstruction. In certain circumstances, it may still be possible to reconstruct soft tissue and bone simultaneously with a composite transfer incorporating vascularized bone.

At present, composite reconstructions are probably the exception rather than the rule. One would hope in forecasting that there would be an increase in their use where appropriate. Indeed if one is to be totally realistic, one might say that the most to hope for in reconstruction is that the future will at least see a more universal use of the methods that already exist but are used by far too few surgeons.

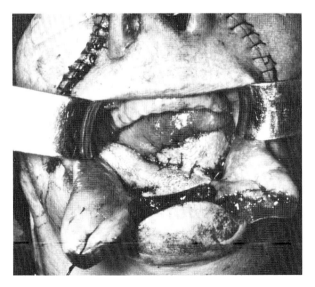

Figure 12 Bilateral nasolabial flaps used to reconstruct a defect of ventral tongue and anterior floor of mouth, showing the manner in which the flaps ''suspend'' the tongue high in the mouth.

REFERENCES

1. Ward G, Robben JO. The composite operation for radical neck dissection and removal of cancer of the mouth. 1951; Cancer 4:98.
2. Spiro RH, Gerold FP, Strong EW. Mandibular ''swing'' approach for oral and oropharyngeal tumors. Head Neck Surg 1981; 3:371.
3. McGregor IA, MacDonald DG. Mandibular osteotomy in the surgical approach to the oral cavity. Head Neck Surg 1983; 5:457.
4. Nakamoto RY. Bony defects on the crest of the residual alveolar ridge. J Prosthet Dent 1968; 8:685.
5. Marchetta FC, Sako K, Maxwell W. Complications after radical head and neck surgery performed through previously irradiated tissues. Am J Surg 1967; 114:835.
6. Briant TDR. Spontaneous pharyngeal fistula and wound infection following laryngectomy. Laryngoscope 1975; 85:829.
7. Ariyan S. The pectoralis major myocutaneous flap. Plast Reconstr Surg 1979; 63:73.
8. Guillamondegui OM, Larson DL. The lateral trapezius musculocutaneous flap. Plast Reconstr Surg 1981; 67:143.
9. Goodwin WJ, Rosenberg GJ. Venous drainage of the lateral trapezius musculocutaneous flap. Arch Otolaryngol 1982; 108:411.
10. Ariyan S. One stage reconstruction for defects of the mouth

using a sternocleidomastoid myocutaneous flap. Plast Reconstr Surg 1979; 63:618.

11. Larson DL, Geopfert H. Limitations of the sternomastoid musculocutaneous flap in head and neck reconstruction. Plast Reconstr Surg 1982; 70:328.

12. Futrell JW, Johns ME, Edgerton MT, Cantrell RW, Fitz-Hugh GS. Platysma myocutaneous flap for intra-oral reconstruction. Am J Surg 1978; 136:504.

13. Panje W, Cutting C. Trapezius osteomyocutaneous island flap for reconstruction of the anterior floor of mouth and the mandible. Head Neck Surg 1980; 3:66.

14. Reuther JR, Steinau H, Wagner R. Reconstruction of large defects in the oropharynx with a revascularized intestinal graft. Plast Reconstr Surg 1984; 73:345.

15. McCraw JB, Furlow LT. The dorsalis pedis arterialized flap. Plast Reconstr Surg 1975; 55:177.

16. Soutar DS, Scheker LS, Tanner NSB, McGregor IA. The radial forearm flap. Br J Plast Surg 1983; 36:1.

10. An Estimate of the Survival Benefit of Chemotherapy for Advanced Head and Neck Cancer and Its Implications to the Design of Clinical Trials

DAVID A. SCHOENFELD, Ph.D.

Since the late 1960s, chemotherapy has been used to treat advanced head and neck cancer. Early reports that head and neck cancer would respond to methotrexate led to nonrandomized studies of these agents[1,2] and comparative studies between different chemotherapeutic agents.[3] There has never been a study that compared the survival of patients treated with chemotherapy with a concurrent or even an historical control group. It has been assumed that these treatments improved survival because responders survived longer than nonresponders. Investigators have assumed that chemotherapy improves the survival of responders and leaves the survival of nonresponders unchanged. Making this assumption, I will use a simple mathematical model to estimate the survival of patients who received low-dose methotrexate or bleomycin, methotrexate, and platinum (BMP) as if they had not been treated. I will then compare this estimate with their actual survival to estimate the extent to which chemotherapy improves survival. These therapies were the best therapies in two consecutive Eastern Cooperative Oncology Group (ECOG) trials and can be used as a baseline with which to compare subsequent therapies.[3,4]

If the assumptions used to estimate the survival of untreated patients are correct, the effect of chemotherapy on survival is small. This would have implications for the design of clinical trials of treatments for advanced head and neck cancer. I will discuss the design of three types of trials; trials of aggressive new therapies, trials of new agents, and trials of alternative chemotherapies.

MATERIALS AND METHODS

Between 1973 and 1976, the Eastern Cooperative Oncology Group conducted a randomized trial (EST 1373) comparing low-dose methotrexate, high-dose methotrexate, and high-dose methotrexate plus cytoxin and cytosine arabinoside.[3] This trial established low-dose methotrexate as the best available agent for head and neck cancer for future ECOG studies. From 1977 to 1982, ECOG conducted a study (EST 1377) comparing low-dose methotrexate with or without *Corynebacterium parvum* to a combination of methotrexate, bleomycin, and platinum.[4] That trial found that the complete response rate was significantly higher with the combination. This chapter uses the data from patients receiving methotrexate in the first study and all patients in the second study.

In the first study, patients had to have had a histologic diagnosis of epidermoid carcinoma which was stage III or IV or was recurrent after radiation therapy or surgery. They had to have had a measurable lesion. Patients with prior chemotherapy, significant renal impairment, or ECOG performance status 4 (completely bedridden) were excluded. The eligibility criteria of the second study were somewhat more elaborate in that "advanced head and neck cancer" was rigorously defined as metastases below the clavicle or recurrent disease after 50 Gy. Furthermore, patients had to have had a serum creatinine <1.5 mg/dl, FEV_1 >60 percent of predicted, WBC > 4000/μl and platelets >100,000/μl. Patients with obstructive uropathy or prior immunotherapy were also excluded.

In both studies, MTX was given in a first dose of 40 mg/m² (intramuscularly), which was to have been increased to 60 mg/m² if the WBC >5000 and there was little or no mucositis on the eighth day; 60 mg/m² was to have been the weekly dose thereafter. The combination BMD consisted of MTX, 40 mg/m² on day 1 and 15; bleomycin, 10 units (intramuscularly) on days 1, 8, and 15; and cisplatin 50 mg/m² (intravenously) on day 4. The cisplatin was given 30 minutes after the institution of an intravenous infusion of D5 1/2 NS + 10 mEq KCl/L at the rate of one

This work was partially supported by grants from the National Cancer Institute CA-23415 and the ECOG grant CA-80086.

liter/hour for 2 hours. At the start of the infusion, 40 mg furosemide was given intravenously and 12.5 g mannitol was given intravenously immediately before the platinum. If the patient did not void at least 200 cc of urine in the first 30 minutes, the platinum was withheld. Dose modifications for both regimens are described elsewhere in publications reporting the results of the studies.[3,4]

The following discussion describes the method used to estimate the survival of untreated patients from data on patients who have received chemotherapy.

In order to estimate the survival curve of patients had they not been treated with chemotherapy, I make the assumption that at each time t the probability that a patient will die from disease in the next instant is the same for a patient who has not received chemotherapy as it is for a patient who has not yet responded to chemotherapy. Based on this assumption, the survival curve of patients who are not receiving chemotherapy is estimated by considering patients who died of toxicity at t and those who responded to treatment at time t as if they had been lost to follow-up at time t. Thus it is assumed that nonresponders do not derive any benefit from chemotherapy and that before they respond, a responder has the same chance of dying in the next instant as a nonresponder.

Notice that the assumption only makes sense for patients with approximately the same prognostic characteristics. Otherwise, suppose a characteristic predicts both a low response rate and poor survival. Then if a patient has not responded at time t, he is more likely to have the characteristic and hence has more chance of dying in the next instant than a randomly chosen patient who has not been treated. Thus, the procedure for estimating the survival curve for patients not treated with chemotherapy was to first determine which patient characteristics were prognostic for survival using a step-up Cox regression. Then these characteristics were used to stratify the patients. For each strata, the survival curve for patients had they not received chemotherapy was computed and finally these curves were averaged to give the survival curve for the entire study group had it not received chemotherapy. These curves were then compared to the actual survival curve of the study group to determine the effect of chemotherapy.

RESULTS

When ineligible patients are excluded, 201 patients have been treated by ECOG with low-dose methotrexate since 1973. This includes patients who also received *C. parvum*. The *C. parvum* group is included with the methotrexate group in the sequel since *C. parvum* had no effect on response or survival. An additional 81 patients were treated with a combination of bleomycin, cisplatin, and methotrexate. Table 1 shows the characteristics of these patients. The response rates were: methotrexate—CR 8 percent, PR 21 percent; BMP—CR 16 percent, PR 31 percent.

TABLE 1   Patient Characteristics

Characteristics	Treatment		
	MTX (201)	BMD (81)	Total (282)
Age			
30 - 40	3%	1%	3%
40 - 50	9%	14%	11%
50 - 60	45%	35%	42%
60 - 70	26%	40%	30%
> 70	16%	11%	15%
Time since first symptoms			
< 6 months	22%	17%	21%
7 - 12	29%	40%	32%
13 - 18	22%	19%	21%
19 - 24	8%	9%	9%
< 24	18%	16%	18%
Weight loss			
None	26%	21%	25%
> 5%	11%	10%	11%
5 - 10%	16%	14%	15%
Over 10%	38%	51%	42%
Unknown	8%	5%	7%
Performance status			
Ambulatory	69%	70%	69%
Nonambulatory	31%	30%	30%
Stage			
I, II, III	27%	22%	26%
IV	73%	78%	74%
Site			
Tongue	18%	12%	17%
Floor of mouth	13%	14%	13%
Tonsil	11%	14%	12%
Hypopharynx or larynx	32%	37%	33%
Other	25%	23%	25%
Sex			
Male	81%	83%	81%
Female	19%	17%	19%
Lung metastases			
No	69%	68%	68%
Yes	31%	32%	32%
Unknown			
Bone metastases			
No	90%	80%	87%
Yes	10%	20%	13%
Unknown			
Previous Surgery			
No	29%	26%	28%
Yes	71%	74%	72%
Previous Radiotherapy			
No	6%	2%	5%
Yes	94%	98%	95%

A step-wise Cox model was run using the characteristics on Table 1. Characteristics that were found to be significantly prognostic were: performance status, stage, weight loss, tongue primary, bone metastases, time since first symptoms, and protocol. Table 2 shows the results of this analysis.

For the purposes of comparing survival on methotrexate and BMD with the survival of patients with no treatment, patients were divided into three strata: nonambulatory, ambulatory stage IV, and ambulatory

TABLE 2 Favorable Prognostic Characteristics

Prognostic Characteristic	Beta	P-value
Ambulatory	-.53	<.001
Stage I, II, III	-.94	<.001
Weight loss <5%	-.34	.02
Site other than tongue	-.51	.07
No bone metastases	-.51	<.001
Time since first symptoms >2 years	-.45	.01
EST 1377	-.35	.04

stages I through III. These three groups were chosen because within each group the survival was roughly equal and a smaller number of strata yields a better estimate of the long-term survival in this type of analysis. Weight loss was not used because it appeared that it was coded differently in the two studies and thus was unreliable as a stratification factor. Table 3 shows median and one-year survival for patients receiving MTX, BMP, and no treatment. The latter estimates are calculated using the previously described mathematical model. Figure 1 shows the survival curves for these three treatment groups.

At present, there are no survivors of these studies. One patients was lost to follow-up at 14 months after treatment while all other patients are dead. The longest survival was 5 years. Only five patients lived longer than 3 years, and of these, three experienced partial responses and two had progressive disease.

DISCUSSION

Figure 1 shows that the effect of chemotherapy on patient survival is small. This analysis depends on the assumption that nonresponders were not benefited by chemotherapy nor were responders until they had responded. If the nonresponders were helped by chemotherapy, the procedure used in this paper would underestimate the benefit of chemotherapy. Similarly, if drug toxicity shortened the life of those who did not have a lethal toxicity, this analysis would overestimate the benefit of chemotherapy. Because this analysis depends on unverified (and unverifiable) assumptions, its conclusions cannot be taken as seriously as those of a randomized or even an historically controlled clinical trial. A randomized trial between

chemotherapy and no therapy would require no assumptions to ensure the validity of the estimate of the difference in survival. An historically controlled trial would require the assumption that the historical control group was similar to the treated group. However, this assumption could be verified or its effects minimized by comparing the patient groups or correcting for covariates. At the least, the analysis shows that the response rates of these treatments do not demonstrate that the treatments have a substantial survival benefit.

For the purposes of the following discussion, I will assume that the preceding analysis is valid. That is, that chemotherapy increases the one-year survival from 15 percent to 21 percent and does not produce any long-term survivors. I will also assume that the palliative benefit of chemotherapy is minimal. I will discuss the implications of these suppositions for present cancer therapy and for the design and conduct of future clinical trials.

The supposition that chemotherapy is only marginally effective for patients with head and neck cancer has different implications for cancer therapy in the United States and Europe than it does in most of the other nations of the world. In Europe and the United States, cancer therapy is not subject to triage. Any patients who desires chemotherapy can receive it. The results of the foregoing analysis show that refusal of chemotherapy is a reasonable choice for a patient with advanced head and neck cancer. For many patients, the small benefit of chemotherapy may not be worth the time and effort the treatment requires.

In the underdeveloped nations of the world, drugs are not available in sufficient quantities for treatment of every patient who might receive chemotherapy in the United States. In this situation, advanced head and neck cancer should not be treated with chemotherapy. What drugs are available should be reserved for diseases in which the benefit of chemotherapy has been demonstrated.

The supposition that our current chemotherapies for advanced head and neck cancer are ineffective has implications for how clinical trials should be conducted in the future. The supposition that chemotherapy is ineffective makes it ethically feasible to give experimental treatments to head and neck cancer patients who have not yet received chemotherapy. There

TABLE 3 Median and one-year Survival by Treatment and Strata

Strata	None*			Treatment MTX			BMD		
	Med	1 yr	#	Med	1 yr	#	Med	1 yr	#
Nonambulatory	3.4	6%	(87)	3.4	8%	(63)	3.8	17%	(24)
Ambulatory, Stage IV	5.9	16%	(145)	6.2	20%	(101)	6.4	20%	(44)
Ambulatory, Stage I, II, III	8.5	27%	(50)	8.4	30%	(37)	10.4	31%	(13)
Total+	5.2	15%	(282)	5.2	18%	(201)	6.0	21%	(81)

* Using mathematical model
+ Using a weighted average of the three survival curves

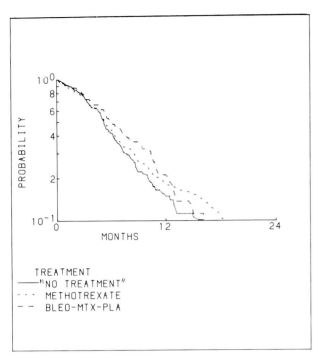

Figure 1 Survival by treatment.

are three types of clinical trials in which these patients can participate: clinical trials of aggressive therapeutic approaches, clinical trials of new agents, and clinical trials designed to determine the best therapy for use in an adjuvant setting. I will briefly describe each type of clinical trial and show how study size should be determined for each of them.

A clinical trial of an aggressive therapeutic approach is a trial of a new therapy that is significantly more toxic and more difficult to administer than standard chemotherapy, but which may have more potential for achieving a cure. An example of such a therapy is the high-dose alkylating agent therapy with autologous bone marrow transplantation which is under study at the Dana-Farber Cancer Institute for breast cancer and malignant melanoma.[7] The therapy requires bone marrow transplantation and 3 weeks of hospitalization. The statistical considerations for such a study are based on the following principles: (1) only a large improvement over standard therapy would be worthwhile since the new therapy is difficult to administer, and (2) any improvement will be confirmed by other studies.

There are two types of error that can be made in such a study. The study can show that the new therapy is better than the standard therapy when it is equivalent. This is called a type I or false-positive error, and the probability of such an error is denoted by α. On the other hand, the study can show that the new therapy is the same as the standard when it is really better. This called a type II or false-negative error, and the probability of such an error is denoted by β.

A study of an aggressive new therapy should be conducted as a nonrandomized study because (1) it may be impossible to find patients who will agree to be randomized between a very aggressive therapy and a standard therapy, and (2) a randomized study may have too much chance of achieving a false-negative result.

To illustrate this fact, suppose a study is done with 30 patients, and an increase in complete response rate from 20 percent to 45 percent would justify the increased expense and toxicity of the new treatment and would indicate that the new therapy is potentially curative. A nonrandomized study would claim a positive result if there were 11 or more complete responses. In this case, $\alpha = 0.026$ (10 or more CRs would give $\alpha = 0.06$) and $\beta = 0.24$. A randomized study with 30 patients would have $\beta = 0.73$ and would be more likely to give a negative result than a positive result even if the new treatment were actually superior.

A historically controlled trial may have a higher type I error (α) because the patients that are chosen for the trial may have a more favorable prognosis than the historical control group. For instance, if patients are chosen with a complete response rate of 25 percent under standard therapy and we falsely assume that the response rate was 20 percent, α increases to 11 percent. In this case, the sum of the error rates in the historically controlled trial is still superior to the sum of the error rates in the randomization trial. If small randomized trials are used to test aggressive new therapies, most superior therapies will not be detected.

Zelen has used the ratio of the probability of a true-positive result with the probability of positive result as a measure of the efficacy of a clinical trials strategy.[8] This ratio, which I will call the credibility, is given by $(1-\beta)\pi/\{(1-\beta)\pi + \alpha(1-\pi)\}$ where π is the proportion of trials which are testing an effective therapy. To be fair to randomized trials, I will assume that the historical control rate for a trial may be mis-estimated. Thus, the credibility of a randomized trial conducted at the 0.05 significance level depends on π and the credibility of a nonrandomized trial depends on π and the amount that the control response rate is mis-estimated denoted by Δ.

Table 4 indicates that the nonrandomized trial has less chance of error even if the historical control response rate is mis-estimated. However, a minor mis-estimation of the response rate will affect the credibility of a positive result. Thus, historically controlled trials of new aggressive therapies are preferable to randomized trials of the same size, but we should view positive results of such trials with skepticism until they are confirmed by randomized studies.

When planning a nonrandomized study of an aggressive new therapy for head and neck cancer, it is necessary to determine a sample size n_1 and a cut-off value I, so that a complete response rate I/n would indicate that the therapy should be tested further. Then α and β are computed by the formulas:

TABLE 4 Error Probabilities and Credibilities of Randomized and nonrandomized Trials with 50 Patients, Testing for a 20% Difference in Complete Response Rate with an Assumed Historical Rate of 20% and an Actual Rate of 20% + Δ

Type of Trial	Error Probabilities			Credibilities		
	Δ	α	β	Π = .1	Π = .2	Π = .3
Nonrandomized	0	.03	.10	.76	.88	.93
Randomized	0	.03	.65	.56	.74	.83
Nonrandomized	.025	.08	.05	.57	.75	.84
Randomized	.025	.03	.66	.56	.64	.83
Nonrandomized	.05	.16	.02	.40	.60	.72
Randomized	.05	.03	.66	.56	.74	.83
Nonrandomized	.1	.43	.00	.20	.37	.50
Randomized	.1	.03	.67	.55	.73	.84

$$\alpha = \sum_{j=I}^{n} \binom{n}{j} P_0^j (1 - P_0)^{n-j}$$

and

$$\beta = 1 - \sum_{j=I}^{n} \binom{n}{j} P_1^j (1 - P_1)^{n-j},$$

where P_0 is the historical control complete response rate and P_1 is the desired complete response rate for the new therapy. The numbers n and I can be adjusted by trial and error until α and β are acceptably small.

The second type of trial for patients with advanced head and neck cancer are phase II trials of new agents. After a patient has failed methotrexate or BMP therapy, his or her prognoses is very poor. Figure 2 shows survival for patients after treatment failure. The median survival is 3 months. It is difficult to decide what response rate for a new agent signifies that the agent is active when the patients in a study have previously failed methotrexate. In an ECOG study of advanced sarcoma,[9] Adriamycin, which is the best sin-

gle agent for sarcoma, had a response rate of only 12 percent when it was used after patients had failed actinomycin D. In an ECOG trial of melanoma with a crossover, methyl CCNU and DTIC only had a 2 percent response rate in patients who had failed the other therapy.[10] Thus, it may be best to test new agents on patients who have had no previous chemotherapy. Patients who did not respond to the new agents could then be given methotrexate if they wished. Although this sequence of therapies might not be optimal treatment, the uniformly poor results of methotrexate and BMD chemotherapy make this sequence ethical. A new agent which has activity as a single agent can then be combined with methotrexate, platinum, and other active drugs to form aggressive new therapies.

A study of a new agent in a group of patients who have not had prior chemotherapy must be designed so that it can be stopped early if the new agent is inactive. A rule that we have used in ECOG to detect a drug with a 30 percent response rate is to stop accrual on a study if we have seen two or less responses in the first 20 patients or four or less responses in the first 30 patients; the treatment is considered active if there are nine or more responses in 40 patients (Table 5).

Given the low effectieness of chemotherapy, phase III studies of a new treatment compared to a standard such as BMP should only be conducted if there is strong evidence that the new therapy will offer a substantial improvement or if the therapy is eventually intended to be used in the adjuvant setting where it might be more effective. However, even though the eventual goal of chemotherapy is to improve patient survival, response should be used as an end point since survival studies may require too many patients. As an example, consider the ECOG study comparing BMP to cisplatin and 5-FU infusion. The study calls for 110 patients per arm to show a difference in response rates from 15 percent (CR) and 35 percent (PR) to 25 percent (CR) and 40 percent (PR). Using the data in this paper, patients with complete, partial, and no responses have average survivals of 13.3, 11.6, and 6.5 months. If the survival for each of these groups where exponential, the hazard ratio for the two treatments

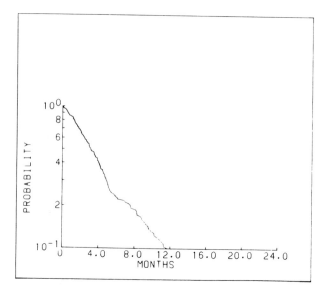

Figure 2 Survival after relapse or progression.

TABLE 5 Operating Characteristics of a Clinical Trial of a New Agent

Response Rate	Probability of Stopping at 20 (2 or less responses)	Probability of Stopping at 30 (4 or less)	Probability of Accepting New Treatment (9 or more)
5%	92%	.06%	<1%
10%	68%	.17%	1%
15%	40%	.17%	13%
20%	21%	.10%	39%
30%	4%	.01%	87%

would vary from 1.1 to 1.06, and the clinical trials would require 1500 patients per arm.

Use of response as an end point of a clinical trial allows us to detect small differences between treatments. Thus, they should be seen as a strategy of developing better therapies over time rather than a method ensuring that patients are given a superior therapy. If 5-FU + cisplatin has a better response rate, it may be more useful as an adjuvant to surgery in patients with early disease or it may be a better base for future combinations.

REFERENCES

1. Leone LA, Albala NM, Rege VB. Treatment of carcinoma of the head and neck with intravenous methotrexate. Cancer 1968; 21:828–37.
2. Mitchell MS, Wawro NW, DeConti RC, Kaplan SR, Papac R. Effectiveness of high-dose infusions of methotrexate followed by leucovorin in carcinoma of the head and neck. Cancer Res 1968; 28:1088–94.
3. DeConti RC, Schoenfeld D. A randomized prospective comparison of intermittent methotrexate, methotrexate with leucovorin, and a methotrexate combination in head and neck cancer. Cancer 1981; 48:1061–1072.
4. Vogl SE, Schoenfeld DA, Kaplan BH, Lerner JH, Creech RH, Horton J. A randomized prospective comparison of methotrexate with a combination of methotrexate, bleomycin and cis-platinum in head and neck cancer. Cancer, in press.
5. Vogl SE, Schoenfeld DA, Kaplan BH, Lerner HJ, Horton J, Paul AR, Barnes LE. Methotrexate alone or with regional subcutaneous *Corynebacterium parvum* in the treatment of recurrent and metastatic squamous cancer of the head and neck. Cancer 1982; 50:2293–2300.
6. Schoenfeld DA. Analysis of categorical data: logistic models. In: Mike V, Stanley K, eds. Statistics in medical research: methods and issues with applications of clinical oncology. New York: John Wiley, 1983; 432.
7. Peter WP, Eder S, Shrieler S, Henner WD, Bast R, Shnipper L, Frei E. High-dose combination alkylating agents and autologous bone marrow support: A phase I trial. Am Soc Clin Oncol C11D, 1984.
8. Zelen M. Problems and alternatives to classical implications or tumor radioresistance. New York: Masson, 1983; 401.
9. Schoenfeld D, Rosenbaum C, Horton J, Wolfer J, Falkson G, DeConti R. A comparison of Adriamycin versus vincristine, Adriamycin and cyclophosphamide versus vincristine, actinomycin-D and cyclophosphamide for advanced sarcoma. Cancer 1982; 50:2757–2762.
10. Costanza M, Nathanson L, Schoenfeld D, Wolfer J, Colsky J, Regelson W, Cunningham T, Sedrask N. Results with methyl-CCNU and DTIC in metastatic melanoma. Cancer 1977; 40:1010–1015.

PART TWO

CURRENT EVALUATION AND MANAGEMENT OF HEAD AND NECK CANCER

SECTION ONE / STAGING

11. Staging

INTRODUCTION

HARVEY W. BAKER, M.D.

Tables 1 through 6 in this section contain the TNM Staging Systems recommended by the American Joint Committee on Cancer (AJCC) for squamous cell carcinomas of the oral cavity, pharynx and larynx. The T categories represent an estimate of the extent of the primary tumor, the N categories describe regional lymph node spread, and the M category indicates distant metastasis. The various T, N, and M categories are combined into stage groupings; the stage of a given tumor is generally an accurate reflection of its prognosis.

The recommended staging systems have been based on difficulties encountered with previous staging systems, retrospective chart reviews, and the clinical experience of AJCC Task Force members. Current testing of the staging systems is being conducted in many institutions, and not unexpectedly, ambiguities in the rules and areas needing improvement are being discovered. A primary goal of the Task Forces preparing staging systems has been to keep them simple, reproducible, and scientifically valid.

The following four chapters present a critique of present-day staging of head and neck cancer by four experienced observers. They bring out areas of weakness in current staging, the influence of other factors on the prognosis, a detailed description of the process of staging, and its relation to treatment planning.

Dr. Keane presents a clear statement of the value and the importance of staging. He then examines the goal of reproducibility and brings out the problem of significant variation in observations by one or more examiners in regard to such factors as fixation and even the size of cervical nodes. He states that similar variations may result from the use of different radiologic examination techniques. He then gives an example of how ambiguities in the rules may lead to errors in clinical staging and he illustrates how such errors may affect the accuracy of end-result reporting.

Dr. Crissman describes the importance of histopathology in the prognosis and treatment of head and neck cancer. In addition to the familiar grading initiated by Broders, the more elaborate grading scheme proposed by Jacobsson is presented. This incorporates multiple histologic observations of both the tumor cell population and the host-tumor interface. Histologic changes in response to preoperative radiation therapy or chemotherapy which may be of prognostic importance are then reported. Finally, the newer technique of automated flow cytometry is discussed. Its ability to measure multiple cellular parameters may well be-

TABLE 1   Definition of T Categories of the Oral Cavity

T1	Greatest diameter of primary tumor 2 cm or less.
T2	Greatest diameter of primary tumor more than 2 cm but not more than 4 cm.
T3	Greatest diameter of primary tumor more than 4 cm.
T4	Massive tumor more than 4 cm in diameter, with deep invasion involving antrum, pterygoid muscles, base of tongue or skin of neck.

TABLE 2   Definition of T Categories of the Pharynx

	Nasopharynx (Includes Posterosuperior and Lateral Walls)	Oropharynx (Includes Faucial Arch, Tonsil, Base of Tongue, Pharyngeal Wall)	Hypopharynx (Includes Pyriform Sinus, Postcricoid area, Posterior Hypopharyngeal Wall)
T1	Tumor confined to one site of nasopharynx or no tumor visible (biopsy only).	Tumor 2 cm or less in greatest diameter.	Tumor confined to site of origin.
T2	Tumor involving two sites (both posterosuperior and lateral walls).	Tumor more than 2 cm but not more than 4 cm in greatest diameter.	Extension of tumor to adjacent region or site without fixation of hemilarynx.
T3	Extension of tumor into nasal cavity or oropharynx.	Tumor more than 4 cm in greatest diameter.	Extension to adjacent region or site with fixation of hemilarynx.
T4	Tumor involvement of skull or cranial nerve or both.	Massive tumor more than 4 cm in diameter, with invasion of bone, soft tissues of neck, or root (deep musculature) of tongue.	Massive tumor involving bone or soft tissues of neck.

TABLE 3 Definition of T Categories of the Larynx

	Supraglottis (Includes False Vocal Cords, Arytenoids, Epiglottis)	Glottis (Includes True Vocal Cords Including Anterior and Posterior, Commissures)	Subglottis
T1	Tumor confined to site of origin with normal mobility.	Tumor confined to glottis with normal mobility.	Tumor confined to the subglottic region.
T2	Tumor involves adjacent supraglottic site or glottis without fixation.	Supraglottic and/or subglottic extension of tumor with normal or impaired cord mobility.	Tumor extension to vocal cords with normal or impaired cord mobility.
T3	Tumor limited to larynx with fixation and/or extension to involve postcricoid area, medial wall of pyriform sinus or pre-epiglottic space.	Tumor confined to larynx with cord fixation.	Tumor confined to larynx with cord fixation.
T4	Massive tumor extending beyond the larynx to involve oropharynx, soft tissues of neck, or destruction of thyroid cartilage.	Massive tumor with thyroid cartilage destruction and/or extension beyond the confines of the larynx.	Massive tumor with cartilage destruction and/or extension beyond the confines of the larynx.

come an important tool in treatment planning and estimating the prognosis.

Dr. Chandler presents a detailed description of the process of staging cancer of the larynx which can well serve as a model for the staging of any other head and neck site. Although he describes newer instruments and evolving radiologic techniques in staging, he brings out the overriding importance of evaluation by a trained observer using the familiar laryngeal mirror and direct laryngoscope. He then illustrates the use of clinical staging in treatment planning and finally presents his end-results for cancer of the larynx according to stage grouping.

Dr. Johns describes the numerous factors that influence the prognosis in cancer of the major salivary glands including histologic type, grade, size, local extension, facial nerve involvement, cervical node metastasis, and distant spread. He illustrates how a number of these parameters are used to prepare a staging

TABLE 4 Definition of N Categories

The following regional lymph node classification is applicable to all cancers of the upper aerodigestive tract.

N0 No clinically positive nodes.
N1 Single clinically positive homolateral node 3 cm or less in diameter.
N2 Single clinically positive homolateral node more than 3 cm, but not more than 6 cm in diameter, or multiple clinically positive homolateral nodes, none more than 6 cm in diameter.
N2a Single clinically positive node more than 3 cm but not more than 6 cm in diameter.
N2b Multiple clinically positive homolateral nodes, none more than 6 cm in diameter.
N3 Massive homolateral node(s), bilateral nodes, or contralateral node(s).
N3a Clinically positive homolateral node(s), one of which is more than 6 cm in diameter.
N3b Bilateral clinically positive nodes.
N3c Contralateral clinically positive node(s) only.

TABLE 5 Definition of M Categories

M0 No (known) distant metastasis.
M1 Distance metastasis present — specify site(s).

system. He then makes recommendations for therapy, including postoperative radiation, based on staging and other important prognostic factors.

In addition to ambiguities in rules for staging and areas needing improvement, a major problem has been that staging systems recommended by the AJCC are different in some respects from those recommended by the International Union Against Cancer (UICC). These differences have interfered with international communication and cooperation, even between the United States and Canada.

The AJCC and the UICC have instituted a series of liaison meetings with the aim of making their recommended staging systems for all cancer sites identical by 1986, when both groups plan to publish new Manuals. There has been give and take on the part of both groups in the interest of reproducibility and scientific validity of staging of head and neck cancer. For example, in revising the N classification for cervical lymph nodes, the UICC has accepted the AJCC premise of a distinctly more favorable prognosis when only one small clinically positive node is involved (N1).

TABLE 6 Stage Grouping

The following stage groupings apply to all squamous cell carcinomas of the upper aerodigestive tract. The prognosis for a given tumor is closely related to its clinical stage.

Stage I	T1 N0 M0
Stage II	T2 N0 M0
Stage III	T3 N0 M0
	T1, T2, or T3 N1 M0
Stage IV	T4 N0 or N1 M0
	Any T N2 or N3 M0
	Any T Any N M1

The UICC has also recognized the difficulties in defining the term "fixed" and has accepted the AJCC classification of a node over 6 cm in diameter as N3. For its part, the AJCC has accepted the somewhat more favorable prognosis of bilateral and contralateral node involvement and has agreed that these parameters should be placed in the N2 rather than the N3 category. Both groups are aware of the reluctance of clinicians to accept changes in staging systems. After a 10-year trial, however, certain revisions seem important. If details of each patient's tumor are compiled on data collection forms (check lists), changing the clinical stage to comply with revised staging systems should present no great problem.

CLINICAL STAGING OF HEAD AND NECK CANCER

THOMAS J. KEANE, M.B., M.R.C.P.I., F.R.C.P.(C)

For the purpose of this discussion I have restricted my comments on staging of cancers of the head and neck to clinical staging. This is not meant to downgrade the important information that is available from postsurgical staging for cancers of this area, but to recognize the widespread use of clinical staging for head and neck cancer where primary treatment involves surgeons, radiation oncologists, and chemotherapists. Clinical staging is, therefore, the common language for all clinicians involved in the management of cancers in this area.

It is now 30 years since the UICC set up a special committee on Clinical Stage Classification and Applied Statistics, and 25 years since the inception of the American Joint Committee for Cancer Staging and End Results Reporting. It is not inappropriate, therefore, to consider what has been achieved in this time period.

I would like to start by reviewing the purposes of clinical staging. These have been summarized by the AJC and the UICC as follows.

1. To provide a way by which information regarding the state of a cancer can be communicated to others.
2. To assist in decisions regarding treatment.
3. To give some indication regarding prognosis.
4. To provide a mechanism for comparing the results of treatment.

It was hoped that these 4 stated goals of clinical staging could be achieved by the use of a tumor-node-metastasis (TNM) classification system based on disease extent. For the purposes of this discussion, this staging process is considered to involve four steps: (1) histologic confirmation, (2) clinical and radiologic examination, (3) recording of information, and (4) assigning TNM stage.

HISTOLOGIC CONFIRMATION

Histologic confirmation of malignancy is not a significant problem for the majority of carcinomas of the head and neck. The major area of difficulty emerges in the diagnosis of in situ carcinomas, particularly carcinoma in situ of the vocal cord. There appears to be no universally accepted criterion for the diagnosis of in situ carcinoma and what may be keratosis with atypia in the opinion of one pathologist may be carcinoma in situ in the opinion of another. As a result, a meaningful comparison of different methods of treatment of in situ carcinoma between different centers is not possible unless one can be certain that each center is describing the same entity.

CLINICAL AND RADIOLOGIC EXAMINATION

The problems regarding clinical examination and the use of radiologic information are separate and will be examined independently.

A great deal of discussion and debate has been focused on the degree with which clinical findings correlate with pathologic findings. Although good clinical pathologic correlation is desirable, more fundamental questions to be addressed pertain to which information should be used in a clinical staging system. In this regard I believe priority should be given to those clinical findings about which physicians agree most often and which are reproducible by the same observer and between different observers. Studies of observer variation have received surprisingly little attention in discussions regarding clinical staging. There is evidence, however, that observer variation is a significant source of error. This question has been studied at The Princess Margaret Hospital by Warr et al.[1] Their study addressed the question of measurement error using both large and small simulated nodules and malignant neck nodes. The findings from their study, shown in Table 1, demonstrate clearly that even with scrupulous measurement techniques in a study where the observers knew their skill in measurement was being assessed, a significant degree of error can exist in estimating size. Although this is only one example,

TABLE 1 False Categorization of Size Change from Comparision of All Pairs of Measurements of the Same Lesion

	Percent False Categorization as		
	(> 50% decrease in area)	*(> 25% decrease)*	*(> 25% increase)*
Simulated nodules (1.0–2.6 cm)	12.6	31.0	34.3
Simulated nodules (2.3–6.5 cm)	1.3	19.7	24.0
Neck nodes	13.1	32.1	33.4

I would suggest that anyone who has struggled to measure a lesion in the oropharynx, particularly when more than one anatomic area is involved, would support my contention that such measurements may contain a significant element of observer error.

In the context of neck nodes, using the UICC N3 category of fixity, there is, I suspect, an even greater problem. This would appear to be due to the absence of a universally accepted definition of fixation. In fact, when offered a choice from a number of criteria for fixation, 24 different physicians treating laryngeal carcinoma in 14 centers across Canada gave the responses shown in Table 2.

Radiologic examinations pose a similar problem. An example is the use of different techniques to assess cartilage involvement in larynx cancer. There is no uniform standard and physicians may use some or all of the following: plain film radiology, tomography, xeroradiography, CT scanning, and, for those who have access to it, NMR imaging. Each method claims a high degree of accuracy, but to my knowledge, no one has addressed the question of which is most applicable to a clinical staging sytem.

RECORDING OF INFORMATION

In the AJC system for recording information, the data form asks for the growth characteristics of the tumor to be recorded. For oral cavity carcinoma, the examiner is asked to choose between a number of descriptive terms as follows: exophytic, superficial, moderately infiltrating, deeply infiltrating, and ulcerated. Although this information is not used directly in assigning T stage, it is believed to be important

TABLE 2 Criteria for Fixity (N3)

	No. of responses
The node or nodes is absolutely immobile.	18
The node is relatively immobile and can only be moved together with the underlying tissue to which the node is adherent.	10
The node is fixed to skin only.	1
Any of the above findings.	4

More than one category could be chosen by each physician.

information concerning tumor behavior. I believe that these growth characteristics are valuable and worth recording. The difficulty in using these terms lies in the fact that they clearly mean different things to different observers. This is shown in a study at our center in which 14 surgeons and radiation oncologists were shown five examples of oral cavity carcinoma. The tumors chosen were all raised above the mucosal surface and nonulcerated. The physicians were asked to describe these lesions, using one of five choices. The descriptive categories available were as follows: verrucous, exophytic, polypoid, any of the above terms, none of the above terms. The results shown in Table 3 demonstrate that in the absence of agreed criteria, descriptive terms can have a very different meaning among observers. It is likely that the use of clearly defined criteria would solve this problem. This has been done in a clinical study of observer variation in the assessment of rectal carcinoma at our institution.[2] In this study the use of criteria for descriptive terms as applied to primary rectal carcinoma produced a high level of agreement among those using criteria compared to those using the same terms without agreed-upon criteria.

ASSIGNING TNM STAGE

Superficially, TNM staging would appear to be a simple process, but at least in some situations, this is not always the case. To test this, 24 physicians in 14 centers across Canada were asked to assign TNM stage according to the UICC 1978 TNM classification for cancer of the larynx. Physicians were provided with the following clinical information:

*T2*A patient presents with a squamous carcinoma confined to the anterior one-third of the right vocal cord and the anterior commissure. The mobility of the right cord is thought to be impaired, but is not fixed. The tumor does not have any supraglottic or subglottic extension on clinical or radiologic examination. There are no glands palpable in the neck. The chest roentgenogram and the remaining clinical examination are normal.

All physicians agreed that the N and M categories were N0M0. The T stage, however, was assigned as follows: T1, 1; T1a, 10; T1b, 3; T2, 9; and T3, 1. It would appear that the presence of impaired mobility led many to categorize the tumor as T2 despite the absence of supra- or subglottic extension.

TABLE 3 Choice of Descriptive Terms for Oral Cavity Carcinoma

Case	*Verrucous*	*Exophytic*	*Polypoid*	*None*	*Any*
I	5	5	0	4	0
II	2	7	4	0	2
III	2	6	0	6	0
IV	0	3	2	7	2
V	3	4	0	6	1

TABLE 4 Correct Stage Distribution

	T1	T2	T3	T4	Total
Proportion cured	36/40	16/20	10/20	5/20	67/100
% Cured	90	80	50	25	67

TABLE 5 Stage Distribution with Staging Error

	T1	T2	T3	T4	Total
Proportion cured	27/30	15/20	15/28	10/22	67/100
% Cured	90	75	53	45	67

This is due to the ambiguous manner in which the T2 category group is described in both the UICC and AJC staging manuals.[3,4]

One of the purposes of the TNM system, as originally outlined, was to allow the comparison of results between different methods of treatment. Although this is still a laudable goal, I do not believe that a clinical staging system based on anatomic disease extent can never fully accomplish this objective. Indeed, when one reviews the wide range of quoted survival rates for patients within individual TNM categories for head and neck cancer, even when the treatment methods applied are similar, one is forced to conclude that factors other than anatomic extent of disease have a major role in prognosis. Some of these nonanatomic prognostic factors are known, for example, the influence of the sex of the patient with larynx cancer on control with radiation.[5] Other factors, such as performance status, were undeniably important, though not often documented. Still others, which reflect host-tumor interactions, such as the antibody-dependent cellular cytotoxicity assay in nasopharyngeal carcinoma, are being evaluated and appear to be powerful independent prognosticators.[6]

As for the impact of staging error on results of therapy, staging error may falsely suggest a response to therapy when no such improvement exists. I will illustrate this with the following example. Suppose one takes a population of 100 patients with head and neck cancer whose true stage distribution and cure rate by stage is shown in Table 4. This group has been constructed to show a gradiant in cure rate of 90 percent for T1 to 25 percent for T4, with an overall cure rate of 67 percent. We now consider the effect which a staging error can have on this population. The redistribution of stage categories incorporating the staging error is shown in Table 5. There is still a significant gradiant in cure rate from T1 to the T4 category: however, the redistribution of patients would appear to indicate a 45 percent cure rate for the T4 category. It is important to note, however, that the overall cure rate remains at 67 percent. Without the availability of the cure rate for the whole population, the staging error showing such an apparent improvement in cure rate for T4 patients could not be detected.

In conclusion, I would like to suggest that the present TNM system has been very successful in a relatively short time period. It has achieved many of its objectives and has been an undoubted help in the development of communication between physicians. It is my hope that these considerable achievements will not be accompanied by a sense of complacency. I believe there is still considerable work to be done in addressing some of the persistent difficulties inherent in clinical staging.

REFERENCES

1. Warr D, McKinney S, Tannock I. Influence of measurement error on assessment of response to anti-cancer chemotherapy and a proposal for new criteria of tumor response. J Clin Oncol 1984; 2(9):1040–1041.
2. Boyd N, Cummings BJ, Harwood AR, Rider WD, Thomas GM. Observer variation in the assessment of patients with rectal cancer. Dis Colon Rectum 1982; 25:664–668.
3. American Joint Committee for Cancer Staging and End Results Reporting Manual for Staging of Cancer. 1978.
4. UICC TNM Classification of Malignant Tumors. 3rd ed, 1978.
5. Harwood AR. Cancer of the larynx - the Toronto experience. J Otolaryngol Suppl 11, 1982.
6. Neel HB III, Pearson GR. Prognostic value of antibody dependent cellular cyctotoxicity testing in North American patients with nasopharyngeal carcinoma. Americal Society of Head and Neck Surgery Meeting, Palm Beach, Florida, May, 1984. (Abstract)

HISTOPATHOLOGY AS A PROGNOSTIC FACTOR IN THE TREATMENT OF SQUAMOUS CELL CANCER OF THE HEAD AND NECK

JOHN D. CRISSMAN, M.D.,
JOHN ENSLEY, M.D.

The histologic grading of squamous cell carcinoma (SCC) represents an estimation by pathologists of the biologic behavior of the neoplasm. The primary purpose of such an assessment is to guide the clinician in deciding an individual patient's therapy. Quantitative grading of cancers was initiated by Broders,[1] who developed a comprehensive and semireproducible scheme for determining tumor differentiation. This classification was first applied to squamous cell carcinomas of the lip, and the grades of squamous cell carcinomas were divided into four categories, based on the proportion of the neoplasm resembling normal squamous epithelium. The greater the proportion of the tumor resembling the tissue of origin, the greater the degree of tumor differentiation. Additional histologic parameters such as degree and pattern of keratinization, intercellular relationships, nuclear pleomorphism, and frequency of mitotic figures have been integrated into the determination of SCC differentiation. Most pathologists have simplified the four grades proposed by Broders and divide squamous cell carcinomas into three grades (poorly, moderately, and well differentiated).

The criteria for determining grade of SCC have not changed substantially since Broders' early description. The pattern and degree of keratin formation and how closely a tumor resembles normal keratinizing epithelium are still the major parameters utilized in assessing tumor differentiation. As many clinicians have long suspected, the grading of SCC is a subjective exercise, and its contribution to patient management is variable. However, a number of histologic observations have been described that have been demonstrated to have prognostic value. The major issue is whether these factors have significant predictive value to be integrated into the determination of tumor grade and, in turn, aid the clinician in planning therapy.

A number of careful studies evaluating various clinical and pathologic factors for prognostic value have been performed for SCC of the head and neck. This chapter is not intended to be an extensive review of the literature, and only our interpretation of representative studies will be cited. The majority of studies suggest that conventional SCC grade has limited prognostic value, usually with less statistical power than the clinical parameters of tumor size and regional lymph node metastases, which define tumor stage. Because of the limited prognostic value assigned to tumor grade, it has not achieved status as a major determinant in planning patient therapy. The major issue is whether there are histopathologic parameters that are of significant value in predicting the biologic behavior of SCC and would be helpful in patient management.

Two representative studies of SCC of the larynx resulted in similar conclusions.[2,3] Division of the SCC into well and poorly differentiated groups was of significant prognostic value in predicting regional lymph node metastases in both studies.[2,3] Neither study found a correlation between tumor grade and size, although larger neoplasms were observed to have a higher frequency of regional lymph node metastases, which is consistent with the majority of the literature on tumor staging. Both studies reported that the pattern of tumor invasion into the host stroma was of major prognostic value. One series divided the SCC into tumors with pushing margins (Fig. 1) and neoplasms with infiltrating cancer[2] (Fig. 2). The second study identified five patterns of tumor invasion, but for statistical evaluation also grouped the patterns of invasion into pushing and infiltrating patterns of invasion of the host stroma. Both studies identified an infiltrative pattern of invasion that was statistically significant in predicting regional lymph node metastases with a power greater than[2] and equal to[3] the significance observed for the relationship of tumor grade and regional metastases. In addition, it was observed that nerve sheath invasion was a poor prognostic factor.[2] This observation is logical in that tumors with pushing borders would be unlikely to invade lymphatics, blood vessels, or nerve sheaths, and neoplasms with a pattern of invasion with single cells or small aggregates of cells would be more likely to penetrate into both perineural spaces and vascular spaces. However, in the small number of tumors in which vascular invasion (16%) was identified, no correlation with prognosis could be established.[2] This latter observation is surprising, but may reflect the low frequency of vascular space invasion identified in this study of laryngeal SCC. In a study of head and neck SCC from multiple sites, 33 of 54 patients (61%) had vascular space invasion identified in the initial biopsies.[4] All patients with regional lymph node metastases were in the group with vascular space invasion, and it was concluded in this study that identification of vascular space invasion was an important prognostic factor. A more recent study of SCC of the pyriform sinus also evaluated multiple parameters predicting patient outcome.[5] In 108 patients with pyriform sinus SCC and preoperative irradiation, the presence of keratinization was associated with higher frequency of local and regional failures (p = 0.11).[5] However, a greater proportion of the poorly differentiated tumors were in the nonkerati-

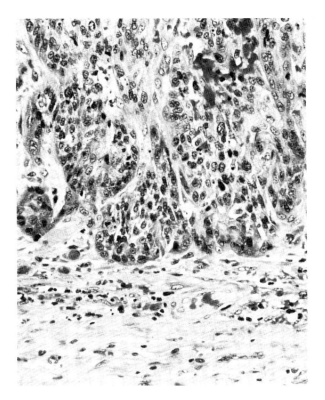

Figure 1 Photomicrograph of SCC demonstrating a relatively well-defined demarcation between the tumor and host stroma. This is representative of a "pushing pattern of invasion.

nized group and associated with a significant probability of distant metastases (p = 0.02).[5] Pattern of invasion or extent of inflammatory infiltrate at the tumor-host interface failed to be an important predictor in this study population.

Recently, Jakobsson proposed a semiquantitative grading scheme for squamous cell carcinoma which incorporates multiple observations describing histologic parameters of both the tumor cell population and the host-tumor interface.[6] The parameters describing tumor cell population include structure and growth of the neoplasm, degree of keratinization, nuclear pleomorphism, and the frequency of mitoses. The histologic parameters used to describe the tumor-host interface include mode of invasion, the degree or stage of invasion, identification of vascular invasion, and evaluation of the plasma/lymphocytic cellular response. The observations pertaining to the tumor cell population are similar to those utilized in Broders' classification, but Jakobsson's approach allows individual evaluation of each histopathologic parameter and incorporates the tumor-host interface parameters into the quantitative grade. Jakobsson's proposal appears to represent the most comprehensive grading scheme yet devised for evaluating squamous cell carcinoma. In addition, it represents a technique for evaluating the contribution of individual histologic parameters regarding tumor behavior. Selected histologic parameters have been evaluated regarding their

importance in predicting patient outcome in numerous studies, but all of the potential histologic factors have not been studied in such a comprehensive manner. However, the application of Jakobsson's histologic criteria is difficult and has required considerable modification.[7] In the original study by Jakobsson on laryngeal squamous cell carcinomas, he noted that the pattern of invasion predicted recurrences in early (T1) neoplasms, but that nuclear pleomorphism correlated better with the recurrence rate in the advanced cancers (T2-T4).

The initial suggestion by Jakobsson of a quantitative score to determine tumor grade was partially supported by his original data. Evaluation of a larger series of laryngeal carcinomas determined that a tumor score correlated better with survival than the current WHO grading format. Jakobsson stressed the value of multivariant analysis of individual histologic parameters in determining relative prognostic values, and the concept of a quantitative score to evaluate tumor grade continues to receive some support from the pathology community. This has been reinforced by a number of investigators who have demonstrated the value of Jakobsson's tumor scoring for squamous cell carcinomas from various other sites in the oral cavity.

A comprehensive study of SCC of the oropharynx, applying a modification of Jakobsson's histologic scoring system, failed to demonstrate significant

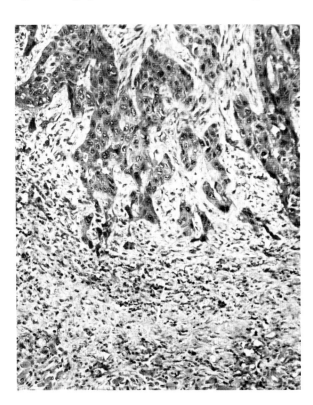

Figure 2 This photomicrograph is characteristic of an invasive pattern with small cords and aggregates of cells advancing into the host stroma. This type of pattern is associated with an aggressive course, often with a higher frequency of both lymph node and systemic metastases.

correlation for tumor scores.[8] Comparison of total tumor scores or subtotals of selected tumor- and host-related parameters failed to predict survival or occurrence of regional lymph node metastases. However, when regression analyses on the individual histopathologic parameters were performed, the infiltrating pattern of invasion was significant in predicting survival. This confirms previous studies documenting the importance of this observation as the most consistent histopathologic parameter in determining the biologic behavior of SCC of the upper aerodigestive tract. When the clinical features of these 77 patients with SCC of the oropharynx were excluded and only the histologic parameters were ranked for predicting survival, the frequency of mitoses achieved statistical significance. A similar evaluation limited to patients with T2 and T3 tumors (which had similar survivals in the study) demonstrated that both increased numbers of mitoses and an infiltrative pattern of host stroma invasion were associated with a poor prognosis. Similarly, it was demonstrated that vascular/lymphatic space invasion in the initial biopsy was predictive of regional neck lymph node metastases.

Reviewing these representative studies of head and neck SCC, it becomes clear that tumor grade can be helpful in predicting patient outcome in selected instances. However, in the studies evaluating multiple histologic parameters to determine a ''quantitative'' tumor score, the results are mixed. Some studies demonstrate that total scores of the individual parameters are of value, and other studies fail to support these attempts at deriving a quantitative tumor grade. More importantly, the studies evaluating individual histologic parameters demonstrate that the pattern of invasion is of significant importance in evaluating the biopsy and appears to approach the statistical power of conventional morphologic grade in predicting patient outcome in several studies. Although the pattern of tumor invasion is not traditionally incorporated into the determination of tumor grade, the majority of evidence suggests that it should be, as it not only adds to the predictive power of conventional tumor grade, but is probable equal to it.

RELATIONSHIP OF HISTOPATHOLOGY AND RESPONSE TO THERAPY

In a study of SCC of the base of the tongue,[9] survival correlated with the demonstration of radiation sterilization of tumor as evidenced by histologic identification of keratin granulomas. Patients with either a complete or a partial response to the preoperative irradiation had approximately six times better 5-year survival than patients without detectable tumor response (58% versus 10% 5-year survivals in responders and nonresponders, respectively). In a similar study of SCC of pyriform sinus,[5] there was a greater proportion of the nonkeratinizing tumor than keratinizing neoplasms eradicated by preoperative irradia-

tion. However, this observation did not translate to improved survival. The clinical factors that predicted better survival are all well-recognized parameters and included adequate excision with tumor-free margins, absence of regional lymph node metastases, and lack of extranodal extension (confinement of the node if present). The only histologic factor identified as predictive of improved survival was the identification of granulomatous inflammation, presumably an indicator of tumor sterilization to the preoperative irradiation.

The histologic parameters predicting response, relapse, metastases, or survival with preoperative chemotherapy have not been well studied. In one of the few studies in the literature evaluating histology and chemotherapy, 40 oral cavity SCC treated with bleomycin demonstrated some interesting observations.[10] Tumor differentiation (grade) and size did not appear to be helpful in determining tumor response to bleomycin. However, the study evaluated tumor pattern of invasion and determined that the SCC with well-defined or pushing tumor-stromal interfaces appeared more sensitive to the chemotherapy than tumors with an infiltrating pattern. This study lends additional support to the value of the pattern of invasion in determining tumor grade or degree of differentiation.

At Wayne State University we have evaluated a series of cis-platinum-containing combination multi-cycle chemotherapy regimens as adjuvant therapy in advanced-stage head and neck SCC. The complete and partial response rates have steadily improved using this approach.[11] Because of the marked improvement in response rates, a detailed evaluation of tumor grade multiparameter histologic observations was done. The overall clinical responses in 146 patients (complete and partial) were essentially the same for all tumor grades: 79 percent for well-differentiated, 86 percent for moderate, and 89 percent for poorly differentiated. The median survivals were 22, 16, and 12 months for well-, moderate, and poorly differentiated neoplasms respectively. Patients with complete responses (CR) and well- or moderately differentiated SCC had a 70 percent 3-year survival in comparison to 18 percent in the CR patients with poorly differentiated tumors.[12] Evaluation of multiple histologic parameters, both individually and in a cumulative score, did not identify any additional predictive parameters in this series of advanced cancers. None of the individual parameters of keratinization, nuclear grade, frequency of mitoses, inflammation, vascular invasion, or pattern of invasion resulted in predicting response to therapy or survival. The evaluation of cumulative scores was similar to the observations using conventional grading approaches. The 2-year survivals for tumor scores less than 12 (well-differentiated), 12 to 18 (moderately differentiated), and greater than 18 (poorly differentiated) were 84, 70, and 46 percent respectively.[12] This demonstrates that tumor grade has some value in predicting patient prognosis, especially in the CR groups.

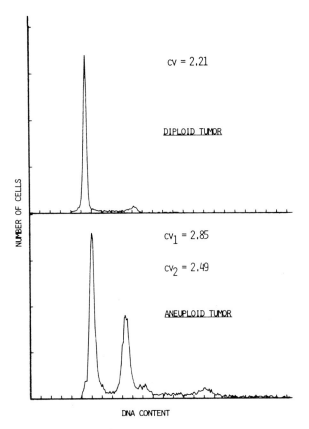

cv = 2.21

DIPLOID TUMOR

$cv_1 = 2.85$

$cv_2 = 2.49$

ANEUPLOID TUMOR

NUMBER OF CELLS

DNA CONTENT

Figure 3 Two DNA histograms of SCC of the head and neck. The upper curve demonstrates a normal complement of DNA or diploid histogram. The large peak is the nonreplicating fraction (G0 and G1) and the second smaller peak represents the cells in or near mitoses (G2 and M). The plateau between the peaks are the fraction of cells replicating DNA (S). In the lower diagram, two large peaks are evident. The left and higher peak is diploid (as determined by non-neoplastic lymphocytes as a control) and the second and slightly lower peak represents a portion of the tumor with abnormal aneuploid DNA content. Coefficient of variation (CV) is a measurement of the precision of the DNA distribution.

FLOW CYTOMETRY

Recently, automated cytometry has been employed in an attempt to quantitate certain cellular parameters such as cell size, DNA/RNA content, measures of cellular proliferative activity (S-phase fraction), cell surface markers, and cytochemical reactions on an individual cell basis. An extensive review of the technical aspects of flow cytometry and its application to diagnostic pathology and clinical oncology is beyond the scope of this chapter and has recently been elegantly reviewed.[13] This new technology promises to measure multiple cellular parameters, including nuclear chromosome ploidy and fractions of tumor cell population synthesizing DNA (S-phase fraction), many of which are incorporated in a semiquantitative manner into histologic grading.

Several recent reports and reviews have looked at the application of this technology to clinical samples of both solid and hematologic malignant disease.[14] To date, these data indicate the most significant correlations between flow cytometry-determined cellular parameters, and prognostically important clinical factors such as response to therapy, disease-free survival, and overall survival have been noted in the hematologic malignant disease. The data relevant to solid tumors is less concrete. The majority of the flow cytometry studies on solid tumors have reported on several histologic varieties and combined tumors from different sites. Flow cytometry studies on squamous cell carcinomas are uncommon owing to the great difficulty of achieving single cell suspensions. The application of flow cytometry requires single cells (or nuclei) and any clumps or debris may prevent accurate measurement.

A prospective study of patients with squamous cell carcinomas of the head and neck is in progress at Wayne State University in an attempt to identify flow cytometry-determined cellular parameters that may

TABLE 1   Comparision of DNA Index and Clinical Parameters

	DNA Index				Fraction Aneuploid	% Aneuploid
	1.0	1.1–1.5	1.6–1.9	2.0		
Stage						
I–II	3	0	0	1	1/4	25
III	6	3	3	2	8/14	57
IV	5	5	8	2	15/20	75
Primary						
T1–T2	5	2	1	2	5/10	50
T3	5	3	6	3	12/17	71
T4	4	3	4	0	7/11	64
Nodal Status						
N0	9	3	6	3	12/21	57
N1–N3	5	5	5	2	12/17	71
Grade						
WD	4	1	3	1	5/9	56
MD	5	5	4	2	11/16	69
PD	5	2	4	2	8/13	62

correlate with pertinent clinical features such as stage, size of primary, degrees of lymph node involvement, grade, response to therapy, and survival. Preliminary studies using a WD murine squamous cell carcinoma, LC12, were conducted in an attempt to optimize the techniques of tumor dissociation, fixation, and staining prior to their application to clinical tumor specimens.[15] Techniques derived from these studies have resulted in average cell yields of nearly 90×10^6 cells/ g tissue, dye exclusion viabilities of >90 percent, and improved in vitro stem cell clone growth when applied to clinical samples of squamous cell carcinomas.

To date, 36 specimens of squamous cell carcinomas of the head and neck have been analyzed with respect to cell size, DNA content, and S-phase fractions. Representative DNA histograms of both diploid and aneuploid tumors are shown in Figure 3. Preliminary data are shown in Table 1 comparing DNA index (ratio of cellular DNA content relative to diploid cells) and the clinical parameters of stage, size of primary, nodal status, and grade of tumor. The data involving S-phase fractions, clinical response to therapy, and survival are too premature for analysis at this time. Sixty-seven percent (24/36) of these tumors were aneuploidal, and approximately one-third had diploid histograms. An examination of the initial data displayed in Table 1 reveals that progressions in stage of tumor, size of primary, degree of nodal involvement, and grade of tumor are associated with overall increases in the percent of tumors with aneuploidal content. Whether cellular parameters determined by flow cytometry will prove to be a significant improvement or addition to histology in solid tumors is yet to be determined. However, the better quantitation and more specific evaluation of various parameters such as chromosomal ploidy and fraction of proliferating cells holds great promise for better subclassification of a histologically homgeneous but clinically heterogeneous group of neoplasms.

REFERENCES

1. Broders AC. Carcinoma. Grading and practical application. Arch Path 1926; 2:376–381.
2. McGavran MH, Bauer WC, Ogura JH. The incidence of cervical lymph node metastases from epidermoid carcinoma of the larynx and their relationship to certain characteristics of the primary tumor. Cancer 1961; 14:55–66.
3. Kashima HK. The characteristics of laryngeal cancer correlating with cervical lymph node metastasis, Workshop No. 14, In: Alberti PW, Bryce DP, eds. Centennial Conference on Laryngeal Cancer. New York: Appleton Century Crofts, 1976, pp 855–864.
4. Poleksic S, Kalwaic HJ. Prognostic value of vascular invasion in squamous cell carcinoma of the head and neck. Plast Recontr. Surg 1978; 61:234–240.
5. Martin SA, Marks JE, Lee JY, Bauer WL, Ogura JH. Carcinoma of the pyriform sinus; predictors of TNM relapse and survival. Cancer 1980; 46:1974–1981.
6. Jakobsson PA. Histologic grading of malignancy and prognosis in glottic carcinoma of the larynx, Workshop No. 14. In: Alberti PW, Bryce DP, eds. Centennial Conference on Laryngeal Cancer. New York: Appelton Century Crofts, 1976, pp 847–854.
7. Crissman JD, Gluckman JL, Whiteley J, Quenelle D. Squamous cell carcinoma of the floor of the mouth. Head Neck Surg 1980; 3:1–7.
8. Crissman JD, Liu WY, Gluckman JL, Cummings G. Prognostic value of histopathologic parameters in squamous cell carcinoma of the oropharynx. Cancer 1984; 54:2995–3001.
9. Rollo J, Rozenbom CV, Thawley S, Korba A, Ogura J, Perez CA, Powers WE, Bauer WC. Squamous cell carcinoma of the base of the tongue: A clinicopathologic study of 81 cases. Cancer 1981; 43:333–342.
10. Yamamoto E, Kohama G, Sunakawa H, Iwai M, Hiratsuka H. Mode of invasion, bleomycin sensitivity and clinical course in squamous cell carcinoma of the oral cavity. Cancer 1983; 51:2175–2180.
11. Decker DA, Drelichman A, Jacobs J, Hoschner J, Kinzie J, Loh J, Weaver A, Al-Sarraf M. Adjuvant chemotherapy with Cis-diaminedichloroplatinum II and 120 hour infusion 5-fluorouracil in stage III and stage IV squamous cell carcinoma of the head and neck. Cancer 1983; 51:1353–1355.
12. Ensley J, Crissman J, Weaver A, Stanley R, Reed M, Al-Sarraf M. The impact of tumor morphology on the complete response rate and overall survival in patients with head and neck cancer treated with cis-platinum containing combination chemotherapy. Proc ASCO 1983; 2:168.
13. Lovett EJ, Schnitzer B, Keren DF, Flint A, Hudson JL, McClatchey KD. Application of flow cytometry to diagnostic pathology. Lab Invest 1984; 50:115–140.
14. Frankfurt OS, Slocum HK, Rustum VM, Arbuck SG, Pavelic ZP, Petrelli N, Huben RP, Pontes EJ, Greco WR. Flow cytometric analysis of DNA aneuploidy in primary and metastatic solid tumors. Cytometry 5:71–80, 1984.
15. Ensley J, Maciorowski Z, Crissman J, Haas C, Sapareto S, Decker D, Corbett T, Kish J, Al-Sarraf M, Vaitkevicius V. Inferior cell yields and alterations in histograms produced by technical differences in tissue preparation employing a standard reference murine tumor. Proc AACR 1984; 25:129.

STAGING OF CANCER OF THE LARYNX

JAMES RYAN CHANDLER, M.D.

The value of staging a patient with cancer is self-evident to all readers. Owing to the efforts of the International Union Against Cancer and the American Joint Committee on Cancer (formerly the American Joint Committee for Cancer Staging and End Results Reporting), physicians responsible for diagnosing and managing patients with cancer of the head and neck in foreign countries as well as in the United States have become more aware of the value of staging. The essentials of the staging process are outlined in the TNM-Atlas,[1] available from the International Union Against Cancer and explained in even more detail in the Manual for Staging of Cancer,[2] published by the American Joint Committee for Cancer. A clear description of the staging procedure for patients with cancer of the larynx is provided in the latter manual, which should be available in the library of every head and neck surgeon as well as every radiation and medical oncologist. I refer you to this publication for a wealth of information and specific directions for staging each given patient. The specific information required for staging cancer of head and neck sites and of melanoma is summarized in a pamphlet,[3] which can be carried in the doctor's pocket or kept in each examining room. It is not possible for one to remember the specific details of staging all cancers for all sites in the head and neck, and one must of necessity refer to the manual or pamphlet except in clear-cut uncomplicated cases. I will not burden you with a recital of the material which can be found in these manuals, but rather will discuss with you some of my own personal thoughts about the ''why, when, and how'' of the staging process itself.

WHY

The best or proper treatment of a given patient with a cancer cannot be planned without full and accurate assessment of the type of malignant tumor: its origin and size, involvement of adjacent structures, whether or not regional or distant metastases are present, the age and occupation of the patient, his nutritional status, and many other factors. Staging is concerned with most of these parameters. Since prognosis depends largely on the site and size of the primary tumor and whether or not regional metastases are present, these considerations have received our greatest attention. Furthermore, they are relatively easily defined and can be analyzed for reporting and comparison with experience of other institutions. Proper staging of the disease should also enable the physician to counsel patients and their families appropriately with regard to the proposed treatment and prognosis.

WHEN

The staging process begins with the initial examination of the patient which includes, after the history, a visual inspection of the larynx. For this, I prefer reflected light from a head mirror. The larynx is scrutinized at rest, during quiet breathing, during phonation at different pitches, during rapid breathing, and occasionally on inspiratory phonation. This latter maneuver frequently brings the anterior commissure and full glottic surface of the epiglottis into view. Any impairment of motion as well as changes in color, texture, vascularity, and differences between the two cords can best be detected by indirect mirror laryngoscopy.

Following mirror laryngoscopy, the larynx should be palpated for any evidence of irregularity of the cartilaginous framework or its associated ligaments and membranes. The absence of laryngeal crepitation would indicate either extralaryngeal extension to a significant degree or extralaryngeal hypopharyngeal origin. Palpation should include the neck on each side for the detection of any palpable lymph nodes. Inherent in the staging process is the dependence on the judgment, skill, and experience of the examiner to stage as N-positive only those nodes that are felt to be clinically significant. The ubiquitous submanidbular nodes can practically always be disregarded as well as the small shotty posterior triangle nodes. The suspected neoplasm should be indicated on appropriate diagrams at the time of the first examination and first suspicion of a neoplasm. Inherent in this initial step of the staging process is the beginning of a formulation of a plan of treatment. The staging process may then be completed by a variety of other clinical and accessory clinical procedures.

HOW

History. The larynx is easily accessible to inspection and palpation, and historical data are of relatively little assistance. Nonetheless, in certain instances, a careful history can assist the clinician in the early steps of the staging process by suggesting that the lesion may be extralaryngeal in origin, perhaps multiple, or even possibly metastatic. The history of previous surgical procedures or other treatment to the larynx is important.

Mirror Laryngoscopy. This examination is by far the single most important means of not only making the diagnosis of cancer of the larynx, but of staging the disease in the vast majority of instances. The skilled clinician can stage properly a carcinoma of the larynx at the time of his initial examination. Mirror laryngoscopy, giving the examiner the ability to observe the larynx in its physiologic state and from a distance with magnification, provides an unparalleled opportunity for the skilled examiner to determine the full extent of almost any neoplasm in this region.

Telescopic Laryngoscopy. The Storz Hopkins Rod laryngoscope has been touted as a most excellent way of examining the larynx. Its primary virtue is said to be that it provides full access to the anterior commissure and lingual aspect of the epiglottis. However, I have found that its small inverted and, to me, distorted image is inferior to that seen in the mirror. Furthermore, in the very patients in whom its use would seem to be of advantage, the marked gag reflex, usually accompanied by aggresive salivation, presents the same obstacles to adequate viewing experienced with mirror examination.

Fiberoptic Laryngoscopy. The same comments pertaining to telescopic laryngoscopy are applicable here. The advantage of the fiberoptic instrument is that it can be passed through the patient's nose and permits the larynx to be viewed from a distance, even in patients with extremely hyperactive gag reflexes. However, the same disadvantages hold; furthermore, in such patients, when the instrument is advanced closer to the larynx in order to obtain a better view, gagging is inevitably the result. A major advantage of this instrument is that it does give the examiner access to the anterior commissure and lingual surface of the epiglottis, although its position along the posterior hypopharyngeal wall provides a less satisfactory view of the posterior commissure and arytenoids.

Direct Laryngoscopy. Sir Morell MacKenzie excelled in the indirect manipulation of the larynx, including the taking of tissue for microscopic examination. However, during the past thirty to forty years, direct laryngoscopy, first under local anesthesia and more recently under general anesthesia, including the use of the microscope, has become almost a sine qua non for the biopsy procedure. There is no question that general anesthesia with complete relaxation of the patient, which permits an unhurried examination of both the interior and exterior of the larynx as well as the hypopharyngeal structures and esophageal inlet, can provide useful information in the staging process. Binocular vision provided by the wider laryngoscopes and the addition of the microscope really adds very little. I have always marvelled and wondered at what information could be secured by "microscopic laryngoscopy" of a tumor so massive in bulk that a prior tracheotomy was required. Direct laryngoscopy is necessary to determine the lowermost extent of tumors originating in the hypopharynx and postcricoid region. In fact, some lesions cannot even be seen without this operative procedure. Particularly bulky tumors arising on the lingual aspect of the epiglottis, and occasionally those arising on its anterior surface, make direct laryngoscopic examination difficult because of the retrodisplacement of the epiglottis and the tendency of the lesion to bleed on manipulation. Of course, direct laryngoscopy also provides the clinician the opportunity of removing tissue for histo-

logic examination and confirmation of his clinical diagnosis. Consideration of intraoperative consultation by the pathologist and frozen section diagnosis may avoid a nondiagnostic surgical intervention.

Radiography. Routine or plain roentgenograms of the neck, even with specialized soft tissue techniques, are of little value. Plain tomograms of the larynx in the coronal plane, with and without phonation, do provide some information regarding cord mobility and irregularities of the vocal cords, particularly their subglottic configuration; they also delineate large supraglottic masses. However, they usually provide no more information to the clinician than his initial examination with the mirror. After all, the radiologist has only photographs of shadows with which to make his deductions and inferences as compared to the laryngologists's infinitely superior primary eyesight.

True, computerized tomography can be helpful in selected instances. For bulky tumors or those arising from supraglottic structures and when direct laryngoscopic evaluation is difficult or even hazardous, the advantage of noninvasive three-dimensional mapping of neoplasms in the larynx, as well as elsewhere, has truly been a remarkable advance in diagnostic technology. It should not be used indiscriminately because in most cases it provides little or no additional information to the studies already described. Nonetheless, in the bulky supraglottic lesion in a patient in whom a conservation procedure is being contemplated, or in the patient with a subglottic lesion possibly extending into and involving the trachea, it may be useful.

Laryngograms enjoyed great popularity in the past, but now should be reserved for special instances in which the air/soft tissue interface requires better delineation than can be secured by mirror laryngoscopy.

Radionuclide Scans. There are of no use at the present time.

Blood Chemistry Studies. These studies are useful on rare occasions in far-advanced cases in which distant metastases or synchronous other neoplasms are suspected.

Immunologic Studies. These have little use at present, but are expected to be more helpful in the future.

Pathology. The microscopic examination of removed tissue by the pathologist is essential for the specific diagnosis and is the basis upon which the staging rests. Without a positive pathologic diagnosis of cancer, there is no cancer, and therefore the staging process is moot. Ninety-five percent of malignant neoplasms of the larynx are squamous cell carcinomas, and the vast majority of the remainder arise from the glandular epithelium of the organ. The exceptions are those arising from other tissues of the larynx, including cartilage, blood vessels, and connective tissue. The occasional metastatic lesion from the lung, kidney, and pancreas must not be forgotten.

Host Performance Status. Although not usu-

TABLE 1 Survival Rates, 1973–1980

	Number of Patients	3 Years			5 Years			Survival	
		Alive	Dead	Unknown	Alive	Dead	Unknown	3	5
Stage I	156	100	26	30	56	35	65	81.6%	71.7%
Stage II	63	35	15	13	20	18	25	73.5	64.4
Stage III	88	38	32	18	21	35	32	59.5	51.4
Stage IV	64	17	40	7	14	41	9	33.9	31.1

ally taken into account in the staging process, this status certainly has a great deal to do with the planning of treatment and with prognosis. Perhaps in the future it will be included in the staging process.

Other Possible Considerations in the Staging Process. In addition to the aforementioned, it is possible in the future that special tumor markers, cell kinetics, and other immunologic studies will be useful in cancer staging.

Upon completion of the staging process, the diagram of the lesion, as noted at the initial examination, should be revised if necessary and all other pertinent information entered on the appropriate data forms. Those in the AJJC Manual are excellent.[2] It should be recognized that, although indispensable in our current state of the art of care for the patient with cancer, the staging of the disease is probably in its infancy. We owe a great debt of gratitude to the American College of Surgeons who, in 1959, with the collaboration and participation of the American Cancer Society, American College of Physicians, American College of Radiology, College of American Pathologists, and the National Cancer Institute, led to the widespread adoption of the TNM Cancer Staging System in the United States. It is hoped that the American Joint Committee on Cancer will become a permanent committee devoted to the dissemination of both old and new knowledge regarding the characteristics of cancer and its proper staging and treatment.

The staging system in present use is primarily a clinical diagnostic staging system (TNM). The surgical evaluative staging (sTNM) and postsurgical resection pathologic staging (pTNM) provide a constant check on our accuracy for the all-important initial clinical diagnostic staging. Unfortunately, this is not possible for patients treated with radiation therapy. Retreatment staging (rTNM) is helpful in evaluating and considering possible salvage surgical procedures or other treatment modalities. Autopsy staging (aTNM) is helpful in only a few isolated instances.

USEFULNESS

Once staging has been completed, a program of management can be formulated and presented to the patient. Knowing that the patient with stage I glottic cancer has a better than 90 percent chance of being completely cured of his disease enables the physician and the patient to choose an appropriate method of treatment which would involve either radiation ther-

apy or surgical excision. Neither chemotherapy nor combination therapy would be an option. A total laryngectomy, for example, would be totally inappropriate as would a neck dissection of any type. The age, sex, and occupation of the patient could be given greater consideration with the availability of two nearly equal options.

On the other hand, in a patient with stage IV carcinoma of the supraglottic larynx who is perhaps 74 years of age and with advanced cardiopulmonary disease, it would be quite inappropriate to plan a surgical procedure with a high morbidity rate and a mortality approaching 10 percent. In my own view, whenever the mortality rate of any given or contemplated surgical procedure approaches or is greater than the chance of cure, palliative therapy only is indicated.

As stated previously, group staging of patients with cancer of the larynx assists the surgeon in rendering a prognosis. The commonly accepted cure rate for the various stages of cancer of the larynx are in the range of better than 90 percent for stage I, about 65 percent for stage II, perhaps 35 percent for stage III, and somewhere around 10 or 15 percent for stage IV.

We have analyzed our experience over a period of $7\frac{1}{2}$ years from January, 1973 through June, 1980. The 3- and 5-year survival rates are as shown in Table 1 and indicate that in our own experience, the actual survival rate for stage I is somewhat less than that commonly accepted, and that for stage IV is somewhat better. These figures cannot stand careful scrutiny, of course, as they are too few for statistical validity and obviously include patients with a great variety of lesions at different sites within the larynx. Analysis of any one of the individual stages with regard to site and treatment, and with better follow-up information, would provide one with additional data. Nonetheless, these results and figures can be compared with those from other institutions, and with constant analysis and refinement in staging as well as treatment, control of the disease will eventually improve.

REFERENCES

1. Spiessl B, Scheibe O, Wagner G (eds). *TNM-Atlas: Illustrated Guide to the Classification of Malignant Tumors*. New York· Springer-Verlag, 1982.
2. Beahrs OH, Myers MH (eds). *Manual for Staging of Cancer*. 2nd ed. Philadelphia: JB Lippincott Co, 1983.
3. *Staging of Cancer of Head and Neck Sites and of Melanoma 1980*, American Joint Committee on Cancer pamphlet, 1980 (National Cancer Institute Grant CA 11606).

STAGING OF SALIVARY GLAND CANCERS

MICHAEL E. JOHNS, M.D.

The purpose of staging cancers is to provide a single quantitative system that gives estimates of tumor burden, thereby allowing the oncologist to estimate prognosis, to compare results of different treatments, to communicate about similar patients, and, it is hoped, to plan the best mangement strategy for each patient. Although staging systems were proposed as early as 1946 by Denoix, only recently have the salivary glands been subjected to a staging system. There are many reasons for this: (1) the variety of histopathologic types, each with its own biologic behavior; (2) its extreme infrequency, limiting the experience in any single institution or of any one surgeon; and (3) the need for long-term survival information (10 to 20 years). Since death from disease may occur at 10, 15, or 20 years, 5-year survival rates provide inadequate information.

In 1981 an ad hoc group of the AJCC proposed a staging system for salivary gland cancer. Whether this system will have long-term significance remains to be seen. At this time treatment planning must still be individualized and requires a knowledge of all the available information in the literature. There are a number of variables that potentially influence survival and thus stage of disease. This chapter will focus on these factors, discuss the role of radiation therapy of these tumors, and make recommendations for treatment based on the current TNM system and on factors that influence survival.

HISTOPATHOLOGY

The prerequisite for adequate treatment of parotid malignant tumors is an accurate histopathologic diagnosis since the biologic aggressiveness of these tumors appears to correlate with the histology. The correlation of histopathology with biologic behavior has allowed these tumors to be divided into two groups: low-grade and high-grade cancers. The low-grade cancers include acinous cell carcinoma and low-grade mucoepidermoid carcinoma. The high-grade cancers include adenoid cystic carcinoma, high-grade mucoepidermoid carcinoma, carcinoma ex mixed tumor, squamous-cell carcinoma, and adenocarcinoma.

As seen in Table 1, the survival rates continue to fall even at 10 years, with only the mucoepidermoid and acinous cell carcinomas having 10-year survival rates comparable to the 5-year survival rates. Ten-year or greater survivals have been reported by only a few authors,[1-4] but their data further demonstrate that deaths from the tumor continue to occur up to 20 years after diagnosis.

Until recently, the mucoepidermoid carcinoma was the only malignant parotid tumor that could be histologically classified as low- or high-grade. More recently, there have been attempts to correlate histologic features with survival in adenoid cystic carcinoma and acinous cell carcinoma.[5-9] Nevertheless, there still seems to be considerable controversy among pathologists regarding the histologic subclassification of adenoid cystic carcinoma and acinous cell carcinoma. It is not unusual for a single carcinoma to have all multiple histologic patterns present, making subclassification quite subjective. It seems then that histologic variants should not be used to establish management principles at this time.

Although retrospective subclassification of specific salivary gland carcinoma into high- and low-grade lesions based on histologic patterns may correlate with the ultimate biologic outcome, it is unlikely that such classifications will be helpful during the intraoperative procedure through the analysis of frozen sections. These factors should nevertheless be kept in mind, and the use of adjuvant radiation therapy or chemotherapy may be indicated when permanent section analysis demonstrates high-grade histologic patterns.

LYMPH NODE METASTASIS

Radical neck dissection has frequently been proposed as a concomitant part of the management of parotid cancer whether or not lymph node metastases are present. Today it is well accepted that if a patient has a clinically positive node, the prognosis is altered and surgical management is indicated. However, indications for a prophylactic neck dissection are controversial. Many head and neck surgeons might agree that if there is a 25 percent or greater likelihood of occult metastases, a neck dissection is indicated. Others might argue, however, that there is no evidence showing clearly that waiting for the occult metastasis to become clinically manifest adversely affects the ultimate outcome of the disease process.

In an effort to determine which of the histologic classes of tumors have a propensity for lymphatic metastasis, the pooled data available in the literature[2,4,10,11] and the experience at the University of Virginia were studied to determine the incidence of cervical metastases that develop at *any* time in the course of the disease (i.e., those present on initial examination, occult metastases discovered at neck dissection, or metastases occurring later). As shown in Table 2, only the high-grade mucoepidermoid and squamous cell carcinomas have any propensity for neck metastasis. The incidence of cervical node metastasis at the time of initial presentation in all parotid cancers is said to be 13 percent. Spiro and co-worker found the incidence of occult cervical nodes to be 16 percent or less for all parotid cancers except squamous-cell carcinoma, where they found a 40 percent incidence of

TABLE 1   5- and 10-year Survival Rates among Patients with Parotid Carcinoma

Histologic type of carcinoma	5-yr	10-yr	5-yr	10-yr	5-yr	10-yr	5-yr	10-yr
Mucoepidermoid					96%	95%		
Low-grade	97%	97%	92%	90%			94%	94%
High-grade	56%	54%	49%	42%			35%	28%
Acinous cell	90%	80%	—	—	80%	80%	86%	—
Adenoid cystic	75%	60%	45%	28%	65%	29%	82%	77%
Adenocarcinoma	75%	60%	—	—	72%	62%	49%	41%
Arising from mixed tumor	50%	30%	63%	39%	—	—	77%	—
Squamous cell	—	—	—	—	57%	57%	42%	—
Undifferentiated	30%	25%	—	—	44%	22%	30%	—

occult metastasis[2] (Table 3). In their series, only 10 (16%) of 64 high-grade mucoepidermoid carcinomas had occult metastasis. Using a modification of the current American Joint Committee (AJC) staging system for cancer of the parotid gland, Spiro et al. found that stage I tumors of the parotid had a 1 percent incidence of neck metastasis, stage II tumors a 14 percent incidence, and stage III tumors a 67 percent incidence.[2] Fu and co-workers found that stage I tumors have a 13 perent incidence, and stage III tumors a 33 percent incidence.[3]

In a review of the experience with adenoid cystic carcinoma of the parotid and submandibular glands seen at the University of Virginia, Marsh and Allen reported that regional spread occurs by continuous growth and rarely occurs by lymphatic extension.[12] The incidence of neck metastasis in acinous cell carcinoma is almost equally as rare.

Treatment planning can be modified when the first echelon of lymph nodes is exposed during parotidectomy; it is here that metastasis is most likely to occur first. Biopsy of any suspicious nodal tissue can be obtained at that time to help in determining the need for neck dissection. If postoperative irradiation is to be employed as an adjunct to surgery, this in itself may control any occult metastasis. The presence of facial nerve paralysis has also been associated with a high likelihood of lymph node metastasis. Eneroth reported a 77 percent incidence,[13] and Conley and Hamaker a 66 percent incidence[14] of lymph node metastasis in patients who presented with facial nerve paralysis.

The evidence suggests that in untreated parotid cancers the incidence of cervical metastasis is low. More important, occult metastasis is rare in all but squamous cell carcinoma. T3 parotid cancers and cancers associated with facial nerve paralysis have a high association with regional node metastasis, but there is no information to suggest that the N0 neck is best treated by a prophylactic radical neck dissection.

FACIAL NERVE PARALYSIS

Facial nerve paralysis associated with a parotid mass indicates malignancy, carries an adverse prognosis, and occurs with varying frequency, depending on the histologic type (Table 4). Eneroth found no cases of facial nerve paralysis in a series of 1,790 benign parotid tumors, but in 378 malignant parotid tumors he found 46 cases of facial nerve paralysis.[13] In the latter group the mortality rate was 100 percent at 5 years, and the average survival interval after onset of paralysis was 2.7 years. In a multi-institutional study published later, Eneroth and co-workers reviewed 1,029 cases of malignant parotid tumors and found an incidence of facial nerve paralysis of 14 percent and a 5-year survival rate of 9 percent for these patients.[15] Conley and Hamaker reviewed 279 malignant parotid tumors and did not find that facial nerve paralysis was quite as hopeless a prognostic indicator: nine of 34 patients were free of disease at 5 years, and four of 26 patients who were available for 10-year follow-up were free of disease at 10 years.[14] Spiro and co-workers found a 5-year survival rate of 14 percent in 43 patients with facial nerve paralysis.[2] It can be concluded, then, that facial nerve paralysis occur-

TABLE 2   Rates of Lymph Node Metastasis among Patients with Parotid Carcinoma

Histologic type of carcinoma	No. with metastasis/ Total No. of Cases	
Mucoepidermoid (high-grade)	62/140	(44%)
Acinous cell	8/60	(13%)
Adenoid cystic	3/58	(5%)
Adenocarcinoma	37/144	(25%)
Arising from mixed tumor	24/117	(21%)
Squamous cell	24/65	(37%)
Undifferentiated	15/64	(23%)
Total	78/637	(12%)

TABLE 3   Rates of Occult Lymph Node Metastasis among Patients with Parotid Carcinoma

Histologic type of carcinoma	No. with Metastasis/ Total No. of Cases	
Mucoepidermoid (high-grade)	10/64	(16%)
Malignant mixed	0/48	(0%)
Acinous cell	2/13	(6%)
Adenocarcinoma	2/23	(9%)
Adenoid cystic	0/19	(0%)
Squamous cell	4/10	(40%)

TABLE 4   Frequencies of Facial Nerve Paralysis among Patients with Malignant Parotid Carcinoma

Histologic type of carcinoma	Eneroth (1972)	Conley (1975)	Both Series Combined	
Mucoepidermoid	8%	11%	16/171	(9%)
Acinous cell	2%	0%	1/83	(1%)
Adenoid cystic	22%	11%	15/86	(17%)
Adenocarcinoma Arising from mixed tumor	8%	15%	10/92	(11%)
Squamous cell	—	5%	5/70	(7%)
Undifferentiated	24%	23%	4/21	(19%)
Total			78/637	(12%)

ring in the presence of a parotid mass indicates both malignancy and a poor prognosis.

SKIN AND OTHER LOCAL EXTENSION

There are no reports available on the significance of skin involvement by parotid tumors. An unusual occurrence today, it does indicate advanced malignancy and decreased survival. When seen, it is usually in a massive tumor and requires wide resection of the involved facial skin.

LOCATION

The parotid gland is not truly divided anatomically into two lobes, but the facial nerve divides the gland into two portions, the superficial portion and the deep portion. The deep portion of the parotid gland is less accessible surgically, and one might conclude that a malignant tumor of the deep lobe would have a less favorable prognosis than one in the superficial lobe. Nigro and Spiro studied 36 patients with malignant tumors of the deep lobe and found no difference in survival for those patients when compared to all patients with carcinoma of the parotid.[16] The 5-, 10-, and 15-year survival rates for deep lobe tumors were 61 percent, 52 percent and 48 percent, respectively. These figures compare favorably with survival rates for malignant tumors in all sites of the parotid. However, they did report that a decreased survival rate occurred if the mass presented in the oral cavity via the parapharyngeal space.

In planning therapy it might be kept in mind that after Warthin's tumor, the acinous cell carcinoma is the next most frequent tumor to occur bilaterally and multicentrically. Chong et al suggest the need for total parotidectomy with this tumor because of the potential for multicentricity, and they report improved rates of local control for total parotidectomy as compared with partial parotidectomy in this histologic group of tumors.[17]

STAGE

In the *Manual for Staging of Cancer* by the AJC,[18] the size of the mass is a prominent factor in staging parotid gland cancer (Table 5). Size is the major difference between the T1 (0 to 2 cm), T2 (2 to 4 cm), T3 (4 to 6 cm), and T4 (>6 cm) lesions. Although the staging system has not been fully evaluated, Spiro and co-workers have done a considerable amount of work correlating stage of disease with prognosis, incidence of lymph node metastasis, and distant metastasis.[2,19,20] Their staging system is somewhat different from the AJC system in that they use diameters of 0 to 3 cm for T1, 3 to 6 cm for T2, and 6 cm for T3 lesions. Spiro et al reported 5-year survival rates of 85 percent for T1 cancers, 67 percent for T2 cancers, and 14 percent for T3 cancers. Using the same staging system as Spiro, Fu and co-workers found a 5-year survival rate of 88 percent and a 10-year determinate survival rate of 83 percent for stage I cancers, a 5-year survival rate of 76 percent and a 10-year survival rate of 76 percent for stage II cancers, and a 5-year survival rate of 49 percent and a 10-year survival rate of 32 percent for stage III cancers.[23]

The correlation of stage with distant metastasis is quite notable in the studies of Spiro and co-workers.[2,21,19,20] They found that the stage I lesions had a 2 percent incidence of distant metastasis, whereas the stage III cancers had a 39 percent incidence of distant metastasis. Furthermore, they were able to correlate recurrence rates with the stage of disease and found that T1 lesions recurred in only 7 percent of cases, whereas T3 lesions had a 58 percent recurrence rate. In their study of mucoepidermoid carcinoma,[20] they found that lymph node metastasis, distant metastasis, recurrence, and overall survival correlated well with the stage of disease.

In 1981 a multi-institutional study of the staging system for cancer of the salivary glands was published and formed the basis for the 1980 AJC staging for major salivary gland cancers.[22] The results of this retrospective study of 861 patients with cancer of the salivary glands led to the proposal of a new TNM classification system for these tumors (see Table 5). This system involves the use of five clinical variables: size, local extension, palpability or suspicion of regional lymph nodes, and presence or absence of distant metastases. In this system it should be noted that the T classification is based solely on size and that T4 has two subdivisions, a and b, based on whether

**TABLE 5 Proposed Staging System for
Major Salivary Gland Cancer (AJC 1980)**

T0 No clinical evidence of primary tumor

T1 Tumor 0.1–2 cm in diamater without significant local extension

T2 Tumor 2.1–4 cm in diameter without significant local extension

T3 Tumor 4.1–6.0 cm in diameter without significant local extension

T4a Tumor >6 cm in diameter without significant local extension

T4b Tumor of any size with significant local extension

N0 No evidence of regional lymph node involvement (including palpable but not suspicious regional lymph nodes)

N1 Evidence of regional lymph node involvement (including palpable and suspicious regional lymph nodes)

NX Regional lymph nodes not assessed

M0 No distant metastases

M1 Distant metastases such as to bone, lung, etc.

Stage I	T1N0M0
	T2N0M0
Stage II	T3N0M0
Stage III	T1N1M0
	T2N1M0
	T4aN0M0
	T4bN0M0
Stage IV	T3N1M0
	T4aN1M0
	T4bN1M0
	Any T Any N and M1

or not there is significant local extension.

The initial evidence suggests that the staging of salivary gland cancers probably should play the most significant role in our treatment planning, particularly since prognosis seems dependent on size more than on histology.

DISTANT METASTASIS

Distant metastasis obviously indicates a poor prognosis. The incidence of distant metastasis in parotid cancer is 20 percent overall (Table 6) and is as high as 50 percent in adenoid cystic carcinomas.[2,3,23] The most frequent site of metastasis is the lung, and the next most frequent site is bone. The aggressive behavior of parotid cancers as manifested by this high incidence of distant metastasis (higher than that seen in squamous cell cancer of the head and neck) sug-

**TABLE 6 Incidence of Distant Metastasis among
Patients with Parotid Carcinoma**

Histologic type of carcinoma	No. with metastasis/total	(%)
Mucoepidermoid	14/183	(8%)
Acinous cell	2/14	(14%)
Adenoid cystic	22/53	(42%)
Arising from mixed tumor	3/14	(21%)
Squamous cell	2/13	(15%)
Adenocarcinoma	25/91	(27%)
Undifferentiated	10/28	(36%)
Total	78/396	(20%)

gests the need for adjuvant chemotherapy programs to decrease the chance of failure at the distant site. At present, little experience is available in this area.

RADIATION SENSITIVITY

There is a need for treatment adjunct to surgery. The use of irradiation in salivary gland cancers has been controversial. In the past, these tumors have been reported as being radiation-resistant.[24] There is mounting evidence, however, that radiation therapy is effective in the treatment of salivary gland carcinoma in certain clinical situations.

In 1971, King and Fletcher reported local control in 81 percent of their patients with recurrent or inoperable parotid cancers, although the follow-up time varied from 2 to 20 years.[25] Rossman reported similar findings in 11 patients treated with irradiation as the only modality.[26] Five of the 11 patients received a Nominal Standard Dose (NSD) of greater than 1800 rets, and local control was achieved in all five patients at 2 to 6 years. Six of the 11 patients received doses of less than 1800 rets, and local control was achieved in only one of them.

Elkon and co-workers irradiated 19 patients, most of them for advanced disease (base of skull or cervical node involvement).[27] They achieved control in only two of the 19 patients, one with adenoid cystic carcinoma and the other with squamous cell carcinoma.

Data such as these suggest that irradiation can affect some salivary gland cancers and may be more effective when there is only minimal disease. Combining this experience with experience reported for squamous cell cancer, one might hypothesize that irradiation may be effective in the treatment of patients who have minimal residual disease or have a high likelihood of recurrence.

Rossman found that recurrence in patients treated with a combination of surgery and irradiation was only 17 percent, whereas patients treated with surgery alone had a 65 percent recurrence rate.[26] Elkon et al found a recurrence rate of 6 percent in 17 patients treated with irradiation for microscopic residual diseases.[27] Tapley, in a review of the experience at the M.D. Anderson Hospital in Houston, reported a 30 percent local failure rate in 54 patients treated with surgery alone and a 9 percent incidence in 33 patients treated with surgery and irradiation.[28] Shidnia and co-workers have noted a 50 percent rate of treatment success with surgery alone and a 70 percent rate of freedom from disease when combination treatment was employed.[29] Fu and co-workers reported that in 35 patients known to have microscopic tumor at or close to the surgical margin, local control was achieved with postoperative irradiation in 86 percent of the cases, whereas in 13 patients with similar margins treated with surgery alone, control was achieved in only 46 percent of the cases.[3] An interesting retrospective study by Tu and colleagues from the Peoples Republic of China demonstrated the superiority of combined therapy, that is, surgery and postoperative irradiation, in the management of parotid cancer.[30] In their study, patients were treated by surgery alone or by surgery and postoperative radiation therapy. In this study, postoperative radiation therapy increased local control over that resulting from surgery alone when (1) there was evidence of locally advanced disease, (2) the tumor belonged to one of the aforementioned high-grade categories, (3) the tumor was recurrent, and/or (4) the facial nerve was involved by the tumor. In all of these series, however, the follow-up period was variable and rarely exceeded 5 years, which is a short follow-up interval for this group of cancers. Nevertheless, when compared to recurrence rates at 5 years in other series of patients receiving only surgical treatment, these results are more than just encouraging.

Such data, although not final, dispel the long-held theories that salivary gland cancer is radiation-resistant and that there is no role for radiation therapy in its treatment. Combining radiation therapy with surgery reduces the incidence of local and regional tumor recurrence in selected instances. I agree with and utilize the seven indications of Guillamondegui et al for postoperative irradiation:[31]

1. High-grade cancers
2. Recurrent cancers
3. Deep-lobe cancers
4. Gross or microscopic residual disease
5. Tumor adjacent to the facial nerve
6. Regional node metastasis
7. Invasion of muscle, bone, skin, nerves, or any extra parotid extension
8. Any T3 parotid cancer

All of these indications are indicators of a poor prognosis, and surgical management alone in these situations has not provided adequate local and regional control. Furthermore, I have added to this list an eighth indication, any T3 lesion, to indicate that even low-grade T3 lesions have a poor survival and should be treated aggressively.

TREATMENT PRINCIPLES

Based on the foregoing distillation of available data from the literature and the experience at the University of Virginia, a treatment plan comprising four categories has been formulated, based on the factors that influence survival (Table 7). Treatment becomes progressively more aggressive from group I to group IV.

Group I includes the T1 and T2N0 low-grade malignant tumors. For this group, removal of the tumor with a cuff of normal tissue (usually total parotidectomy) is adequate treatment. The digastric triangle lymph nodes should be evaluated at the time of surgery. Although some data suggest that T1 high-grade mucoepidermoid carcinomas and perhaps other T1 cancers may respond to this same treatment, we are currently placing these high-grade tumors in group II.

Group II includes T1 and T2N0 high-grade malignant tumors. Treatment here includes total parotidectomy with regional resection of digastric nodes and preservation of the facial nerve (except those branches involved by the tumor grossly). If the nerve is involved, it is resected back to clear margins (frozen section), and immediate nerve grafting is performed. If the nerve is not grossly involved by the tumor, it is preserved, since all patients in this group receive radiation therapy to a wide field, including the upper echelon nodes. The vital function of the facial nerve can be preserved in such situations without sacrificing the chance for cure.

TABLE 7   Principles of Treatment for Parotid Carcinoma

Treatment Group	I	II	III	IV
Tumor Type	T1 and T2 low-grade	T1 and T2 high-grade	T3N0 or N+	T4
	Mucoepidermoid low-grade	Adenocarcinoma Malignant mixed Undifferentiated Squamous cell	Any reccurent tumors not in group IV	
	Acinous cell			
Parotid	Superficial or total parotidectomy	Total parotidectomy with ressection of regional nodes	Radical parotidectomy	Radical parotidectomy with resection of skin, mandible, muscles, mastoid tip, as indicated
	Preservation of VII N		Sacrifice of VII N with immediate reconstruction	Sacrifice of VIIN with immediate reconstruction
		Neck dissection for N+ neck only	Neck dissection for N+ neck only	Neck dissection for N+ neck only
		Postoperative irradiation	Postoperative irradiation	Postoperative irradiation
Submandibular	Submandibular triangle resection	Wide excision of submandibular triangle	Radical neck dissection to include XII N and lingual N	Surgery to fit disease extent
		Preserve nerves unless involved		
		Postoperative irradiation		

Group III includes T3N0 or N+ high-grade cancers and recurrent cancers. For this group, a radical parotidectomy (sacrifice of facial nerve) and modified neck dissection for N0 or radical neck dissection for N+ neck metastasis is carried out. If there is evidence of facial nerve involvement into the mastoid, the surgeon should be prepared to follow the nerve into the mastoid until negative margins are achieved. Primary facial nerve grafting is carried out at the time of surgery. All patients receive postoperative irradiation to a wide field that includes the primary lesion and the same side of the neck from the skull base to the clavicle, including the masotid bone.

Group IV includes those tumors >6 cm and/or with extraparotid extension. For this group, aggressive radical surgery to achieve adequate margins is indicated. In addition to radical parotidectomy and neck dissection, surgery in this group *may* include resection of the masseter muscle, buccal fat pad, skin, mandible, ear canal mastoid, or other involved structures as indicated. Postoperative irradiation is used routinely. The facial nerve is reconstructed by grafting techniques, but in this situation, with a potentially avascular bed for the nerve graft, additive procedures such as dynamic muscle transfers utilizing the masseter or temporalis muscle performed at the time of primary surgery may provide important functional and cosmetic reconstruction. In this group the chances for long-term survival are low, and the treatment results in considerable morbidity.

REFERENCES

1. Eneroth CM, Hamberger CA. Principles of treatment of different types of parotid tumors. Laryngoscope, 1974; 84:1732.
2. Spiro RH, Huvos AG, Strong EQ. Cancer of parotid gland. Am J Surg 1975; 130:452.
3. Fu KK, Leibel SA, Levine ML, Friedlander LM, Boles R, Phillips TL. Carcinoma of the major and minor salivary glands. Cancer 1977; 40:2882.
4. Conley J. Salivary Glands and the Facial Nerve. New York: Grune & Stratton, 1975.
5. Eby LS, Johnson DS, Baker HW. Adenoid cystic carcinoma of the head and neck. Cancer 1972; 29:1160.
6. Spiro RH, Huvos AG, Strong EW. Adenoid cystic carcinoma of salivary origin: a clinicopathologic study of 242 cases. Am J Surg 1974; 128:512.
7. Perzin KH, Gullane P, Clairmont AC. Adenoid cystic carcinoma arising in salivary glands. A correlation of histologic features and clinical course. Cancer 1978; 42:265.
8. Bataskis JG, Chinn EK, Weimert TA. Acinic cell carcinoma: a clinicopathologic study of thirty-five cases. J Laryngol Otol 1979; 93:325.
9. Spiro RH, Huvos AG, Strong EW. Acinic cell carcinoma of salivary origin: a clinicopathologic study of 67 cases. Cancer 1978; 41:924.
10. Hollander L, Cunningham MP. Management of cancer of the parotid gland. Surg Clin North Am 1973; 53:113.
11. Rosenfeld L, Sessions DG, McSwain B, Graves H. Malignant tumors of salivary gland origin. Ann Surg 1966; 163:726.
12. Marsh WL, Allen MS. Adenoid cystic carcinoma, biologic behavior in 38 patients. Cancer 1979; 43:1463.
13. Eneroth CM. Facial nerve paralysis: a crition of malignancy in parotid tumors. Arch Otol 1972; 95:300.
14. Conley J, Hamaker RC. Prognosis of malignant tumors of the parotid gland with facial paralysis. Arch Otolaryngol 1975; 101:39.
15. Eneroth CM, Andreasson L, Veran M, Biorklund A, Carlsoo B, Modalski B, Olofssond J, Paabolainen M, Toll B. Preoperative facial paralysis in malignant parotid tumors. ORL, 1977; 39:272.
16. Nigro MF Jr, Spiro RH. Deep lobe parotid tumors. Am J Surg 1977; 134:523.
17. Chong GC, Beahrs OH, Woolner LB. Surgical managment of acinic cell carcinoma of the parotid gland. Surg Gynecol Obstet 1974; 138:65.
18. American Joint Committee for Cancer Staging and End Results Reporting: *Manual for Staging of Cancer*. Chicago: American Joint Commitee, 1980.
19. Spiro RH, Huvos AG, Strong EW. Acinic cell carcinoma of salivary origin: a clinicopathologic study of 67 cases. Cancer 1978; 41:924.
20. Spiro RH, Huvos AG, Birk R, Strong EW. Mucoepidermoid carcinoma of salivary gland origin: a clinicopathologic study of 367 cases. Am J Surg 1978; 136:461.
21. Spiro RH, Huvos AG, Birk R, Strong EW. Adenoid cystic carcinoma of the salivary origin: a clinicopathologic study of 242 cases. Am J Surg 1974; 128:512.
22. Levitt SH, McHugh RB, Gomez-Marin O et al. Clinical staging system for cancer of the salivary gland: a retrospective study. Cancer 1981; 47:2712.
22a. Levitt SH, McHugh RB, Gomez-Marin O et al. Parotid tumors. Acta Otolaryngol (Stockh) (Suppl) 1963; 191:1.
23. Rafla S. Malignant parotid tumors: natural history and treatment. Cancer 1977; 40:136.
24. Evans JC. Radiation therapy of salivary gland tumors. Radiol Clin Biol (Basel) 1966; 35:153.
25. King J, Fletcher G. Malignant tumors of the major salivary glands. Radiology 1971; 100:381.
26. Rossman KJ. The role of radiation therapy in the treatment of parotid carcinomas. Am J Roentgenol 1975; 123:492.
27. Elkon D, Colman M, Hendrickson FR. Radiation therapy in the treatment of malignant salivary gland tumors. Cancer 1978; 41:502.
28. Tapley ND. Irradiation treatment of malignant tumors of the salivary glands. Ear Nose Throat J 1977; 56:110.
29. Shidnia H, Hornback NB, Hamaker R, Lingeman R. Carcinoma of major salivary glands. Cancer 1980; 45:693.
30. Tu G, Hu Y, Jiang P, Qin D. The superiority of combined therapy (surgery and postoperative irradiation) in parotid cancer. Arch Otolaryngol 1982; 108:710.
31. Guillamondegui OM, Byers RM, Luna MA, Chiminazzo H, Jesse RH, Fletcher GH. Aggressive surgery in treatment for parotid cancer: the role of adjunctive postoperative radiotherapy. Am J Roentgenol 1975; 123:49.

SECTION TWO / DIAGNOSTIC IMAGING

12. Diagnostic Imaging

INTRODUCTION

WILLIAM N. HANAFEE, M.D.

Technologic advances in radiology have given a new meaning to the word "imaging". Nuclear magnetic resonance (MR or NMR), ultrasound, and thermography have all joined the field of imaging without the need of ionizing radiation. At present, magnetic resonance imaging (MRI) is the most exciting modality on the horizon because it offers the opportunity of in vivo chemistry as well as proton imaging.

CT will continue to contribute to the management of head and neck cancers for the forseeable future. Two of the following chapters concern imaging with CT. One is an emphasis on detection and staging of aerodigestive tract tumors; the other presents a rather thorough discussion of lymph node and other neck masses. The third chapter summarizes state of the art using radionuclide scanning. All imagers would agree that it is time to re-evaluate the use of our facilities to reduce the cost of medical care. No longer should one routinely perform all of the plain films, tomograms, angiograms, and scans when one procedure will give *all* the definitive answers even though it be more complex and expensive. The referring physician needs considerable assistance in reaching this decision. Close communication with the radiologist is absolutely essential in order to avoid all the redundant radiologic procedures. As indicated in the following chapters, many of the studies, such as diagnostic angiography, pluridirectional tomography, and some of the nuclear scans, may no longer be considered an integral part of diagnostic work-up unless they give *all* the information required for patient management.

MRI will definitely play a major role in the diagnosis and staging of head and neck cancers. A full description of the principles and techniques of magnetic resonance imaging is beyond the scope of this introduction. The reader is referred to several classic detailed articles in the literature.[1-3] My remarks will be based on rather limited experience over the past 2 years using a permanent magnet of 3000-gauss strength. Approximately 800 to 1000 scans have been performed with this system, of which 75 to 100 have been performed for head and neck tumors. Even with this limited experience, some conclusions would seem to be warranted. The ability of magnetic resonance imaging to provide axial, coronal, and sagittal planes without requiring the patient to move or assume uncomfortable positions is extremely helpful to determine the extent of tumor masses about the skull base.

With regard to the head and neck, I would like to evaluate MRI according to structure examined:

Better Than CT
  Intracranial extensions and skull base
  Cerebellopontine angles
    and internal auditory canals
  Nasopharynx
  Tongue
  Vascular structures
Equal to CT
  Lymph nodes
  Oropharynx
  Hypopharynx
  Larynx
Interesting Points
  Paranasal sinuses
  Inner ear structures
  Lateral neck masses
Definitely Inferior to CT
  Most paranasal sinuses
  Middle ear disease
  Mandible

The density relationships of various tissues are quite different on magnetic resonance imaging as compared to CT scanning. CT is based on x-rays being stopped by tissues of increasing density. The NMR signal encompasses the availability of hydrogen atoms, the presence or absence of flowing blood, and the water content of the tissues. Water may form bonds with protein, and these bonds also influence the amount of signal. In addition to chemical composition, the technical factors of performing the scan bear considerable relationship to the type of signal that is viewed. For example, multiple echos come from the resonance of hydrogen atoms in an NMR magnet. In the early echos, structures that closely simulate water have very little signal compared to the high signal coming from fat. On the film that records the image, fat would appear "white", whereas water would appear "black". Muscle and fascial planes are of intermediate gray scale, with muscle having more signal than gray fibrous tissue. Bone presents an interesting phenomenon, with the medullary cavity being white indicating bright signal because of its fat content, whereas compact cortical bone is black indicating no signal because of the sparsity of mobile hydrogen atoms.

If one listens for late echos, the density relation-

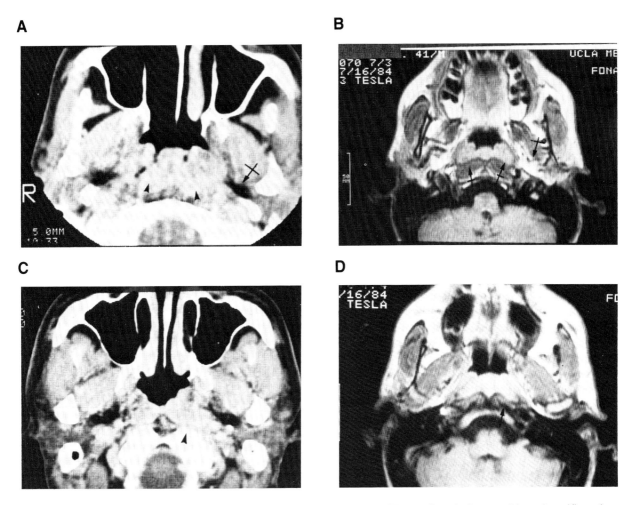

Figure 1 Prominent adenoidal pad in a patient suspected of having AIDS. *A*, CT scan through the eustachian tube orifices shows prominent adenoidal pad (▶). The paralaryngeal low density spaces (↔) are well preserved. *B*, MR scan through the eustachian tube orifices shows that the pharyngobasilar fascial planes are well preserved (↔) as are the paranasopharyngeal spaces more laterally placed (↔). *C*, CT scan through the vault of the nasopharynx shows that the asymmetry continues with some questionable fullness of the left side of the nasopharynx in the region of the paraspinal muscles. *D*, The shadow of the longus colli and rectus capitus muscles appear normal (↔). There is no evidence of infiltration from the mucosal surfaces and adenoidal paths.

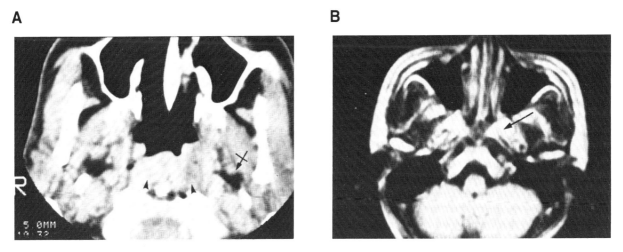

Figure 2   Continued on following page.

C

D

E

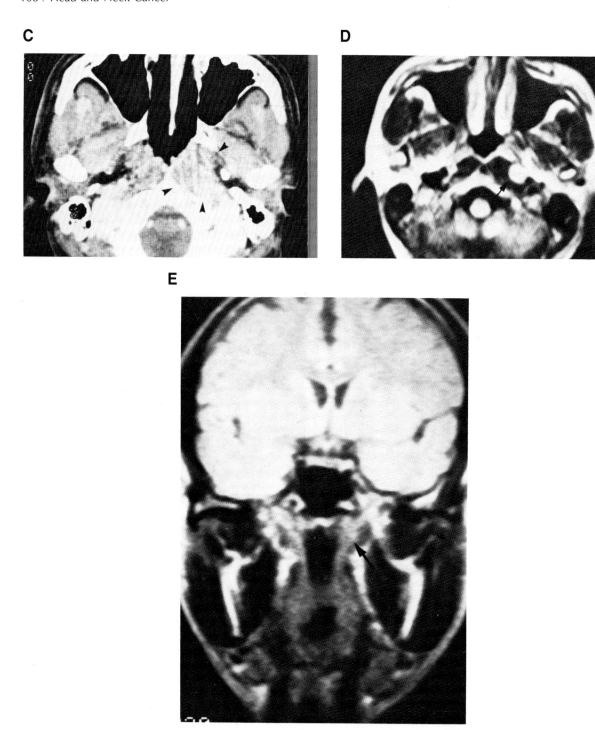

Figure 2 Carcinoma of the nasopharynx. The tumor arose from the posterior pharyngeal wall immediately medial to the eustachian tube orifice on the left. *A,* CT scan through the nasopharynx shows some fullness of the left side of the nasopharynx near the eustachian tube orifice (▶), but the paranasopharyngeal spaces are well preserved (↔). *B,* MR scan through the eustachian tube orifices and vault of the nasopharynx shows bright signal from the latter echos (→) infiltrating to the region of the longus colli and rectus capitis muscles. *C,* Scan just below the eustachian tube orifice shows increased bulk of the posterior nasopharyngeal wall (▶). *D,* MR image at this same level shows that the increased bulk is related to a large lymph node (→) and some infiltration adjacent to the eustachian tube orifice. *E,* Coronal scan through the nasopharynx showing the increased bulk and asymmetry of the nasopharyngeal wall (→).

ships begin to change. The signal from fat, which is bright on the early echos, begins to die out and fat becomes dark gray. Water has a very long persistent signal and becomes bright in relationship to the other structures present.

Early investigators showed that there is a tendency for malignant tumors to have a much longer signal related to water associated with proteins.[4] Overlap of prolonged signals occurs between some tumors and normal variations, so that prolonged signals cannot be used as absolutely diagnostic tools for identifying malignant tumors.

NASOPHARYNX

The nasopharynx and skull base region are ideal for magnetic resonance because of well-developed fascial planes that separate muscle bundles. The blood flow in arteries and veins is brisk and can easily be identified. At CT, separating structures that are immediately adjacent to the skull base is difficult because of partial voluming effects. This means that the scanner sees part of the bony skull base along with muscle bundles and cannot clearly separate the two. With magnetic resonance, coronal and sagittal views make identification of individual structures extremely easy. Superficial adenoid hypertrophy (Fig. 1) can be differentiated from deep infiltrating tumor (Fig. 2).

LARYNX

Larynx scanning with NMR offers all of the advantages of polytomography plus CT scanning. The coronal view permits accurate determination of the level of the ventricles, and the combination of coronal and sagittal scanning can tell if there is extension of a supraglottic tumor into the region of the glottis or if a true cord tumor has extended into the subglottic space. Magnetic resonance imaging also demonstrates a high signal coming from the paralaryngeal space because of the abundance of loose areolar tissue. Disruptions of the fascial planes can occur with inflammatory disease, so that further experimentation is necessary with various pulsing sequences to develop better tissue specificity.

SUMMARY

All of the imaging modalities are worthless unless there is good communication between clinician and the radiologist. The endoscopist's view is the only method for identifying mucosal lesions and physiologic disturbances. As will be seen in the ensuing chapters, significant contributions to the knowledge concerning deep structures is now possible by a variety of imaging techniques.

REFERENCES

1. Wehrli FW, MacFall JR, Glover GH, Grigsby N. The dependence of nuclear magnetic resonance (NMR) image contrast on intrinsic and pulse sequence timing parameters. Magnetic Resonance Imaging 1984; 2:3–16.
2. Edelstein WA, Bottomley PA, Hart HR, Smith LS. Signal, noise and contrast in nuclear magnetic resonance imaging. J Comput Assist Tomogr 1983; 7:391–401.
3. Alfidi RJ, Haaga JR, El Yousef SJ, Bryan PJ, Fletcher BD, LiPuma JP, Morrison SC, Kaufman B. Preliminary experimental results: Humans and animals with a superconducting, whole-body, nuclear magnetic resonance scanner. Radiology 1982; 143:175–181.
4. Damadian R. Tumor detection by nuclear magnetic resonance. In: Nuclear medicine, yearbook of cancer 1972. Chicago: Yearbook Medical Publishers, 1972:286.

COMPUTERIZED TOMOGRAPHY IN THE DIAGNOSIS OF HEAD AND NECK DISEASES: A CLINICAL APPROACH

MICHAEL FRIEDMAN, M.D.
VYTENIS T. GRYBAUSKAS, M.D.
MAHMOOD MAFEE, M.D.
EMANUEL SKOLNIK, M.D.
MARGARET MILLER, R.N., M.S.N.

The importance of radiology as a diagnostic aid in the treatment of head and neck disease has been clearly shown by many published reports. Our colleagues, the head and neck radiologists, continue to impress us with their ability to identify minute details of anatomy and disease processes. This ability to detect disease by radiologic techniques, whether conventional radiography, computerized tomography, or nuclear magnetic resonance, no matter how impressive to the radiologists, often means little to the clinician. The fact that a CT scan can clearly show a metastatic neck node with a necrotic center is a fascinating radiologic experience, but may add no information to what the experienced clinician could diagnose by palpation.

The purpose of this paper is to review the value of CT scanning and its effect on treatment in three specific areas: (1) metastatic neck disease, (2) primary hyperparathyroidism, and (3) parotid tumors.

The ability to improve our diagnostic accuracy in these areas sometimes creates more questions than it answers. Cantrell brought up the very important question of cost effectiveness with respect to CT scanning for metastatic disease. He estimated that the routine use of CT scanning for every new case of head and neck cancer would add $20 million to health care expenditures annually.[1] In discussion of CT scanning we would like to qualify its application into several categories. (1) those in which CT scanning is useful and cost-effective for all cases, (2) those that require CT scanning as part of a scientific study that relates to accuracy of diagnosis and treatment results, and (3) those that require CT scnning only for specific patients or situations.

METASTATIC NECK DISEASE

Currently, nodal disease is staged by clinical examination only. Reports in the literature on the accuracy of the clinical examination vary widely. Beahrs reported an accuracy of 88 percent with a very low incidence of false-negative findings.[2] Southwick, however, found a 30 percent rate of false-positive clinical examinations and a 39.9 percent rate of false-negative examinations.[3] A review of our patients indicates a clinical accuracy rate of 82 percent; our studies have shown that we can improve our accuracy with the use of CT scanning.[4]

Early reports on the use of CT scanning for cervical lymphadenopathy were encouraging. Mancuso et al found CT scanning to be accurate in 21 of 23 patients when CT was correlated with pathologic specimens.[5] In this study, some of the criteria for diagnosing metastatic cancer were developed. Reede and Bergeron believed that the CT scan was beneficial in detecting metastatic nodes, but provided no correlation with pathologic findings.[6]

The potential benefits in highly accurate CT scanning for cervical adenopathy are numerous. Treatment of the high-risk clinically negative neck has long been a source of confusion and controversy.[7-10] Since the incidence of occult metastases in advanced tumors is significant, treatment of the clinically negative neck, with either radiation therapy or neck dissection, has been advocated. Other clinicians, however, believe that treatment of the the neck should be delayed until disease is evident clinically, citing the number of unnecessary neck dissections performed for occult nodal disease. Positive CT scans in patients with occult metastases would certainly influence decision making in treatment and may alter clinical staging.

Methods

Patients with head and neck cancer treated at the University of Illinois and affiliated hospitals since 1981 have been evaluated with CT scanning. The findings in 50 consecutive patients who underwent radical neck dissection provide surgical confirmation of CT findings and form the basis of this study. All patients presented with advanced disease and were at high risk for regional metastases. Staging of nodal disease was performed by clinical examination only.

Scans were obtained with a GE CT-T 8800 scanner using the following operational factors: 9.6 seconds of scan time, 200 mamp, 576 pulses, 3.3-ms pulse width, and 120 kv (peak). The patient was placed in the supine position with the neck hyperextended. Axial scans 5 mm thick were obtained during quiet breathing, starting 2 cm below the inferior border of

TABLE 1 Summary of Results of Patients with Clinically Palpable Nodes

No of pts.	Clinical	CT	Pathology
30	+	+	+
0	+	−	+
1	+	−	−
1	+	+	−

TABLE 2 Summary of Results of Patients with Clinically Negative Neck Examinations

No. of pts.	Clinical	CT	Pathology
9	−	−	−
2	−	+	−
5	−	+	+
2	−	−	+

the cricoid cartilage and extending cephalad to the tip of the mastoid process. All scans were obtained during intravenous infusion of 120 ml of 60 percent Conray contrast material. An additional bolus of 30 ml of this contrast was injected at the onset of scanning to improve visualization of the vascular structures. The use of intravenous contrast is essential for evaluation of node-bearing areas.

All CT scans were re-evaluated retrospectively, without knowledge by the radiologist of clinical staging, to establish the following: (1) presence and size of enlarged nodes, (2) location of abnormal nodes, (3) central necrosis within an enlarged node, (4) vascular involvement by nodal disease, and (5) obliteration of fat and fascial planes. All nodes greater than 1 cm were considered to be positive. These findings were then correlated with the pathologic findings from the radical neck dissections. No patient who had both a CT scan and radical neck dissection was excluded from

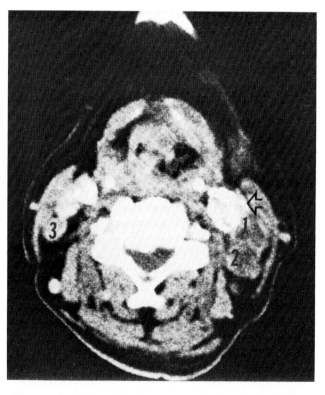

Figure 1 CT shows large necrotic nodes (*1,2*), clinically palpable on the left. A small contralateral node is noted on the patient's right (*3*), not clinically palpable. Note compressed left internal jugular vein (*arrow*).

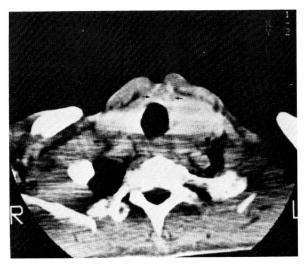

Figure 2 CT scan shows a round soft tissue mass (*arrows*) anterior to the trachea, with the same density as thyroid.

the study regardless of the quality of the CT scan. CT accuracy was then compared to clinical accuracy in this group of patients.

Results

The results of this study are summarized in Tables 1 and 2. The overall accuracy of CT diagnoses

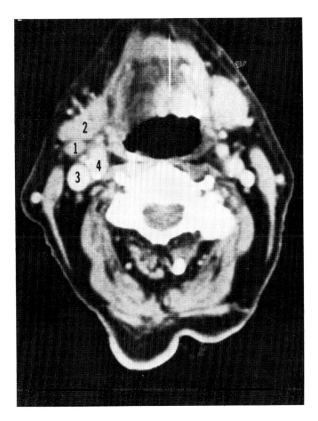

Figure 3 CT shows an ovoid density (*1*) posterior to the submandibular gland (*2*). Note the internal jugular vein (*3*) and carotid artery (*4*).

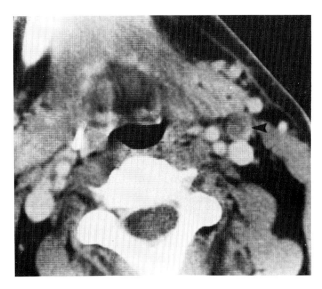

Figure 4 CT shows a 1.2-cm node with a central low density and peripheral enhancement (*arrow*).

was 90 percent. The majority of patients in this study had clinically positive nodes as well as positive CT and pathologic findings (Table 1; Fig. 1). All patients who had clinically positive nodes confirmed on pathology specimens were correctly diagnosed by CT. In one patient, an advanced laryngeal tumor, felt to be a metastatic node by clinical examination, was diagnosed as a thyroid mass by CT and confirmed as aberrant thyroid tissue on pathologic sectioning (Fig. 2). One patient who was clinically positive and CT positive, but pathologically negative, had a 2-cm hyperplastic node.

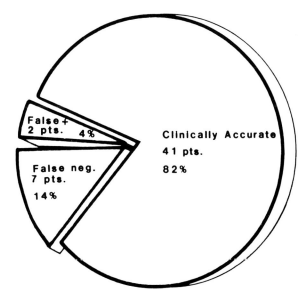

CLINICAL ACCURACY
50 PATIENTS

False +
2 pts. 4%

False neg.
7 pts.
14%

Clinically Accurate
41 pts.
82%

Figure 5 Overall accuracy of the clinical examination in 50 patients.

**CT ACCURACY
50 PATIENTS**

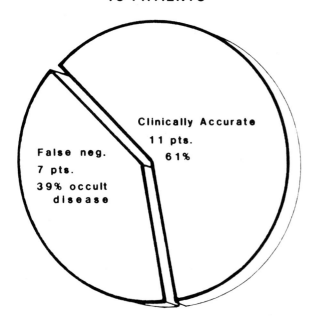

Figure 6   Overall accuracy of the CT scan in 50 patients.

A clinically negative neck, in patients at high risk for nodal metastases, was confirmed by both CT and pathologic study in nine patients. Two patients who were clinically and pathologically negative were CT-positive (false-positive) (Fig. 3). Both patients had hyperplastic nodes measuring greater than 2.5 cm. Two

**CT EVALUATION IN
THE CLINICALLY NEGATIVE NECK
18 PATIENTS**

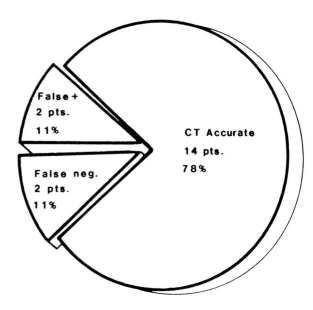

Figure 8   CT accuracy in 18 patients with a clinically negative neck examination.

patients were clinically and CT-negative, but pathologically positive (false-negative). In both cases the metastatic node was less than 1 cm, one being 3 mm.

The most significant group of patients were the

**THE CLINICALLY NEGATIVE NECK
18 PATIENTS**

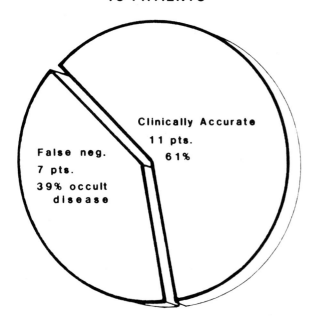

Figure 7   Clinical accuracy in 18 patients with a clinically negative neck examination.

**THE CLINICALLY POSITIVE NECK
32 PATIENTS**

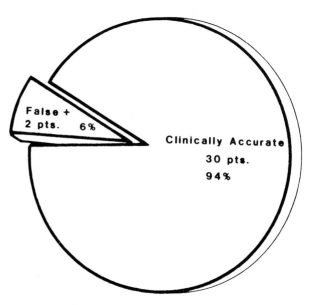

Figure 9   Clinical accuracy in 32 patients with a clinically positive neck examination.

THE CT POSITIVE NECK
38 PATIENTS

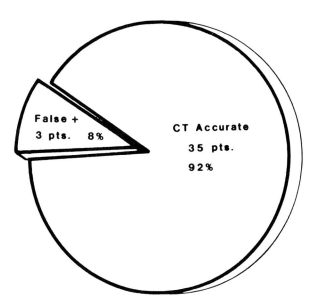

False +
3 pts.   8%

CT Accurate
35 pts.
92%

Figure 10 CT accuracy in 38 patients with a clinically positive neck examination.

five patients who were clinically negative, but CT-positive and pathologically positive. These patients had occult nodal metastases which were accurately diagnosed on CT scanning (Fig. 4). The smallest node that was positive pathologically and diagnosed by CT was 1 cm.

Comparison of clinical accuracy with CT accuracy indicates that the CT is superior in correctly evaluating nodal disease. In this study, the clinical examination was correct in 82 percent of patients (Fig. 5), whereas the CT was correct in 90 percent (Fig. 6).

In patients with a clinically negative neck examination, seven of 18 patients were found to have occult metastases (Fig. 7). CT increased the accuracy from 61 percent to 78 percent in these patients. More importantly, the incidence of undetected occult metastases decreased to 11 percent (Fig. 8).

The clinical accuracy in patients with palpable nodes in this study was 94 percent, with 6 percent false-positive (Fig. 9). The reliability of a positive CT scan was 92 percent, with 8 percent false-positive (Fig. 10).

Discussion

Although radiologic findings have been used as a diagnostic tool in tumor staging of the primary site and distant metastases, they have not been clearly shown to be valuable in the staging of nodal disease. The reliability of CT scanning in detecting metastatic cervical lymphadenopathy has been established with this study. It follows, therefore, that staging of nodal disease should be based on CT findings as well as clinical examination. A patient with a clinically negative neck examination and positive CT scan should be staged as N^+ disease. A patient with a clinically positive neck examination may not require CT if the contralateral neck is not at risk. In any event, if a clinically positive neck has a negative CT scan, it should remain staged as N^+ disease just as a T1 tumor of the larynx that could not be demonstrated by CT scan would be staged.

The value of improved diagnostic acumen in nodal disease would specifically benefit patients with occult metastases. In a high-risk group of patients, 39 percent had occult disease based on clinical staging. With the additional information supplied by CT scanning, this figure is decreased to only 11 percent. The question of elective treatment of the neck must now be re-evaluated in light of the increased accuracy of CT in the detection of occult nodal disease.

If treatment of the neck is based on CT findings only, the question arises as to the incidence of false-positive CT examinations. In comparison with the clinical examination, the incidence of treatment of the pathologically negative neck is not significantly increased. Based on clinical examination alone, two of 32 patients were incorrectly diagnosed as having positive nodes. Based on positive CT examinations, three of 38 patients were incorrectly diagnosed as having metastatic disease. Utilization of CT as the criterion for treatment of nodal disease increases the detection of occult metastases, but does not significantly increase the number of patients who undergo treatment of a pathologically negative neck.

Although positive CT scans in patients with clinically palpable nodes do not necessarily alter treatment of the diseased neck, additional clinical information can be obtained. Most importantly, CT provides evaluation of the contralateral neck (see Fig. 1). Detection of occult disease would alter therapy, staging, and possibly prognosis. In this study, three patients with unsuspected contralateral disease were correctly diagnosed by CT.

Other important information that may be obtained from CT studies of patients with clinically palpable nodes includes the integrity of the vasculature. Jugular vein thrombosis was correctly diagnosed in three patients (Fig. 11). Involvement of the carotid artery is more difficult to accurately assess. Although the finding of a normal carotid on CT eliminates arterial involvement by nodal disease, obliteration of the carotid artery is not reliable as a sole indication of carotid artery involvement. In two patients, the carotid artery could not be visualized by CT scan (Fig. 12). At surgery, the carotid was felt to be uninvolved, but surrounded by tumor. The finding of an abnormal carotid on CT scan should be further evaluated by dynamic CT or arteriogram.

CT also offers a modality to follow nodal response to radiation therapy. Figure 13 indicates a retrojugular node that could not be detected prior to

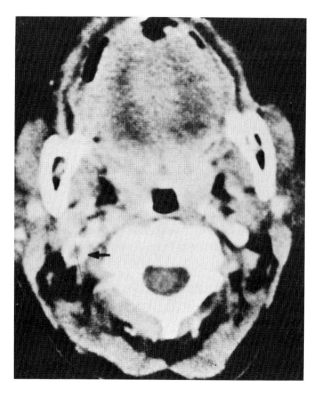

Figure 11 CT shows a lucent image in the central portion of the internal jugular vein, consistent with thrombosis (*arrow*).

treatment of a nasopharyngeal carcinoma. Following treatment, the CT scan illustrates an increase in nodal size (Fig. 14).

Our study correlated clinical, CT, and pathologic findings in a high-risk group of patients. Routine use of CT scanning in patients with a low incidence of nodal metastases must be further evaluated.

The current criterion for diagnosing nodal disease on CT is primarily based on size. This finding alone will not detect small tumor metastases or distinguish the large hyperplastic node from a tumor. Early studies suggest density may be a key factor in differentiating a tumor from hyperplastic nodes. Retrospective review of inaccurate diagnoses in this study indicates that nodes with a central low density are malignant. Density measurements will detect differences between the peripheral and central portion of the node before central necrosis can be seen. This difference is more evident after infusion.

In patients with a known primary, any enhanced or nonenhanced mass in the lymph-node-bearing area with a central low density, irrespective of size, should be considered nodal metastases (see Fig. 4). Although statistical evidence is insufficient, further studies are under way. Use of this criterion may further increase CT accuracy.

The effects of inclusion of subclinical CT positive nodes as N$^+$ disease leaves many questions unanswered. We need to determine whether the CT positive node alters the prognosis of the clinically based N0 and N$^+$ disease statistics. The behavior of the CT-

positive node compared to the clinically positive node is not known. Whether radiation therapy is as effective on the CT-positive node as it is in "occult metastases" needs to be determined. Further studies are necessary and could lead to significant improvements in the diagnosis and therapy of patients with head and neck cancer.

Based on these findings we are certainly not advocating that computerized tomography be part of the evaluation for all cases of head and neck cancer. On the other hand, we strongly believe that there is a place for CT scanning in specific areas. Treatment of the high-risk neck currently follows three different philosophies: (1) that which treats surgically, (2) that which treats with radiation, and (3) that which does not treat. For those who treat surgically, we are suggesting re-evaluation of the philosophy for the CT-negative neck and continuation of surgical treatment for the CT-positive neck. In this situation it should be part of the evaluation of all high-risk necks. This includes a midline lesion with one side of the neck positive and the other side at high risk. Those who treat the high-risk neck with radiation are faced with a greater dilemma. Perhaps only those patients with positive CT scans should be treated with radiation, and all CT-negative necks should not be treated, assuming the primary lesion itself does not warrant treatment with radiation. If radiation has been shown to be effective to improve control of the primary lesion, inclusion of the neck adds little to morbidity or cost of treatment. On the other hand, perhaps radiation is really not effective for the CT-positive neck, and those patients should

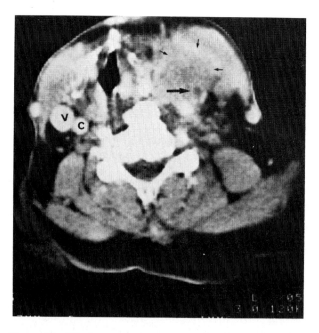

Figure 12 CT shows a large tumor mass (*small arrows*). The common carotid artery (*c*) and internal jugular vein (*v*) are seen on the patient's right side. On the patient's left side, there is thrombosis of the internal jugular vein (*big arrow*) and compression of the common carotid artery.

be treated with surgery, and radiation reserved for the CT-negative neck. Only future studies that include CT scans may possibly answer these questions. We definitely believe that all studies that deal with treatment and survival results should use the most accurate method of diagnosis, which includes CT scans. Those who do not treat the high-risk neck at all should definitely include CT scans for all patients at high risk. A positive scan should certainly alter their philosophy and lead to treatment of the CT-positive neck. The assumption that the patient with occult disease could be safely treated when the nodes became positive would be true if all patients had perfect follow-up. In the overall population of patients with head and neck cancer, close follow-up does not occur on a significant number of patients.

Finally, even if we do not accept routine scanning for any population of patients, there are certain patients who are more likely to benefit from the scan. When the possibility of muscular, carotid, or internal jugular vein invasion exists, CT scan has been shown to be of definite value. The patient with the short, fat, and muscular neck or the patient who has already had radiation is much more difficult to examine for the presence of nodes. CT scanning would certainly play a role in these situations.

Cost-effectiveness is an important question that must be answered. The cost of using routine CT scans for all cases of head and neck cancer at high risk for metastatic neck disease must be compared to the sav-

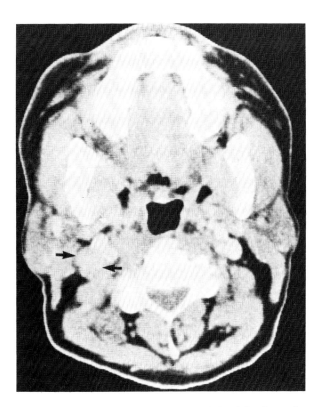

Figure 14 CT shows an increase in nodal size following radiation therapy (*arrows*).

ings of unnecessary neck dissections that can be avoided by CT scanning. In addition, the cost of unnecessary radiation treatment must be included as well. Finally, there are many situations that require CT scanning for evaluation of the primary tumor. Evaluation of cervical nodes with this scan adds nothing to cost or morbidity. It goes without saying that we must also evaluate the morbidity associated with more radiation and surgery.

PARATHYROID LOCALIZATION

Although the vast majority of patients with hyperparathyroidism have parathyroid adenomas, an appreciable number of patients have ectopic sites of a single adenoma or multiglandular disease. Many techniques have been used to localize parathyroid adenomas. Noninvasive methods include barium swallow with cineradiography, thyroid scan, selenomethionine scan, and ultrasound. Although these techniques have proved useful in individual cases of massive adenomas, none has been reliable and accurate in identifying small adenomas.

Arteriography with venous sampling of the parathyroid glands has been thought to be the most reliable study for preoperative localization of adenomas. Although an accuracy rate of 90 percent has been achieved,[11] other studies report a lower rate.[12] Because of the risk of complications with this technique, arteriography has been reserved for those patients with

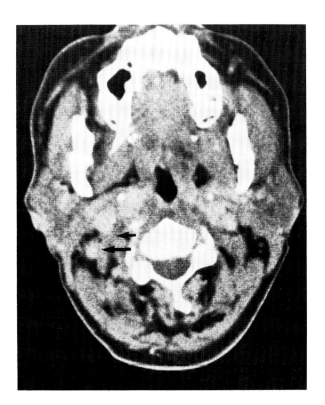

Figure 13 CT shows several nodes in retrojugular region prior to radiation therapy (*arrows*).

persistent hypercalcemia after an unrevealing neck exploration.

Recently, computed tomographic (CT) scanning has been suggested as a noninvasive modality to detect the location of parathyroid adenomas. Reports in the literature have mixed assessments of the value of the CT scan in preoperative localization of adenomas. Doppman et al, in a 1977 report of the cases of ten patients, localized a parathyroid adenoma in three patients.[13] Only one patient with a 19-g adenoma had a diagnostically accurate CT scan of the neck. However, they were successful in localizing two of three mediastinal adenomas, and believed that this was the primary importance of the CT scan. Adams et al, in a series of 18 patients, identified a discrete tumor mass in the neck by CT scan in only one patient.[14] Other reports,[15] including those of Shimshak et al[16] and Gouliamos and Carter,[17] have been more encouraging.

Technique

We have reported on our technique for scanning and diagnosis of parathyroid abnormalities that has a high degree of accuracy in preoperative identification of parathyroid abnormalities.[18] Eight consecutive patients were studied with preoperative CT scans.

Patients were scanned at 1-cm intervals from the angle of the mandible to the level of the aortic arch. If the scan would fail to identify a clinically suspected abnormality in the neck or superior mediastinum, the mediastinum below the arch would also be included. For the last three patients, the scan was initiated with a bolus injection of 30 to 40 ml of iodinated diatrizoate meglumine (renographic contrast medium), followed by an infusion of 300 ml of 30 percent diatrizoate meglumine. This bolus-infusion technique helped identify the vessels and enhance the thyroid tissue. Analysis of these structures on cross section enabled us to distinguish them from parathyroid tissue. The parathyroid adenoma or hyperplasia does absorb some contrast in its vascular bed. However, the differential enhancement of the thyroid tissue and vascular structures is so distinct that these structures can easily be recognized from parathyroid abnormalities.

An enlarged thyroid gland, at times, makes identification of small parathyroid adenomas difficult (Table 3, Case 1). In patients whom we strongly suspect of having a parathyroid adenoma, we now routinely scan the area of the thyroid gland and obtain 5-mm sections with a 3-mm space (overlapping sections). After reviewing the sections, additional 1.5-mm sections are obtained in any suspicious areas.

Results

This method has increased our diagnostic capability to assess accurately the size and exact level of the adenoma. In our series of eight patients, the preoperative diagnosis by CT scan was correct in seven,

TABLE 3 Summary of Patients with Primary Hyperparathyroidism Studied with CT Scans

Patient	CT	Surgical Findings	Pathology
No. 1	Diffuse hyperplasia vs Thyroid enlargement	Marked thyroid enlargement L superior parathyroid adenoma	285-mg adenoma
No. 2	R superior parathyroid adenoma	L superior parathyroid adenoma	669-mg adenoma
No. 3	Diffuse parathyroid hyperplasia	Multiglandular hyperplasia	Parathyroid hyperplasia
No. 4	L inferior parathyroid adenoma	L inferior parathyroid adenoma	4.0-g adenoma
No. 5	R inferior parathyroid adenoma Enlarged thyroid	R inferior adenoma Thyroid enlargement	2.0-g adenoma
No. 6	R inferior parathyroid adenoma	R inferior adenoma	6.2-g adenoma
No. 7	L inferior parathyroid adenoma	L inferior parathyroid adenoma	714-mg adenoma
No. 8	Enlarged thyroid R inferior parathyroid adenoma	Thyroid enlargement R inferior parathyroid adenoma	1.8-g adenoma

including one patient with multiglandular disease (see Table 3). The one patient whose adenoma could not be identified by CT had a markedly enlarged thyroid gland obscuring the adenoma. This was the first patient in the series; with the subsequent modification in the CT technique, particularly injection of contrast media and smaller sections through the thyroid gland, this lesion also could be identified preoperatively.

Discussion

Positive findings on CT scanning include three possibilities: a large mass identifiable as an adenoma, unilateral obliteration of the retrothyroid-paratracheal-esophageal space, or bilateral obliteration of this space. Although the identification of a distinct mass on CT is extremely reliable (Fig. 15), use of this criterion solely would result in a low accuracy rate for identification of smaller adenomas or hyperplasia.

The most important radiologic finding in our study was obliteration of the retrothyroid-paratracheal-esophageal space. This space is crucial in searching for parathyroid adenomas. By CT, it is usually symmetric and shows a low attenuation value because of fatty planes. Elimination of this space or effacement

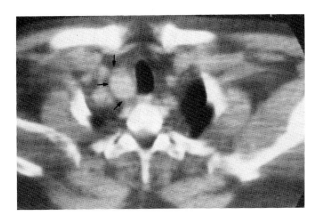

Figure 15 Large parathyroid adenoma (*arrowheads*).

of the fatty planes are the key signs to correctly diagnose small parathyroid adenomas. This finding was observed in four patients, all of whom had small adenomas, the smallest being 0.7 g (Fig. 16). With proper CT scanning, adenomas as small as 4 to 6 mm should be detected in this space.

The third possible CT finding is bilateral obliteration of the pratrachcal fatty planes, which is indicative of multiglandular disease (Fig. 17). This was the finding in one patient (see Case 3, Table 3), which was proved at surgery to be parathyroid hyperplasia.

Since completion of our study, we routinely scan our patients and have continued to accurately locate the abnormal parathyroid gland or glands.

The importance of preoperative localization of parathyroid adenomas is evident for several reasons, particularly detection of mediastinal adenomas. Mediastinal adenomas occur in approximately 10 percent of patients with hyperparathyroidism.[19] Although the incidence of low mediastinal adenomas requiring sternotomy is relatively low (3%),[20] by the identification of these cases we avoid the unrevealing neck exploration. Patients with high mediastinal adenomas can be treated successfully with a neck exploration. Early

exploration of the superior mediastinum allows prompt identification of the adenoma and avoids a prolonged cervical exploration with the possibility of many fruitless frozen sections, which would be routine prior to superior mediastinal dissection. Patients with a preoperative diagnosis of parathyroid hyperplasia still undergo a cervical exploration, but the procedure most likely will involve removal of portions of all four glands. Depending on the surgeon and institution, surgery for hyperplasia may also involve cryopreservation or autotransplantation. The combination of these factors results in planning differences for the procedure. The operative time, prognosis regarding the incidence of hypoparathyroidism, preparation of materials for cryopreservation, and donor sites can all be established with more accuracy if hyperplasia can be distinguished from adenoma based on preoperative scanning.

A completely normal cervical and mediastinal scan was not encountered in our series. If this does occur, it would suggest a parathyroid hormone-producing neoplasm as a cause of the hyperparathyroidism. A normal scan may indicate the need for further evaluation of a paraneoplastic syndrome prior to surgery.

One of the key factors for the increased accuracy in our study was the radiologic finding of obliteration of normal fatty planes. Previous neck surgery undoubtedly results in alteration of these key tissue planes and makes interpretation of the CT scan far more difficult and less accurate. Reserving CT scanning for patients who have had a nondiagnostic neck exploration diminishes the value of this reliable examination.

PAROTID TUMORS

Diagnosis of parotid tumors by computerized tomography is still in the experimental phase. Al-

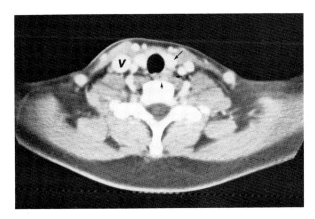

Figure 16 Large arrow indicates enhanced, enlarged thyroid gland. Small arrow indicates unilateral obliteration of paratracheal-retrothyroid-esophageal space. Note comparison with normal side. V denotes internal jugular vein.

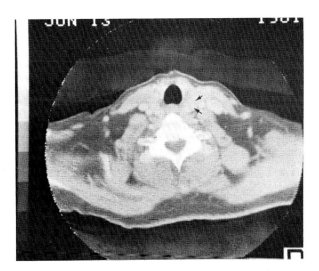

Figure 17 Bilateral obliteration of paratracheal-retrothyroid-esophageal space, consistent with multiglandular disease. Arrows indicate thyroid nodule, which is difficult to distinguish from parathyroid tissue without enhancement (see also Fig. 16).

though other authors have shown the ability to accurately diagnose the malignant or benign nature of parotid tumors by CT scanning, its clinical value has not been demonstrated.[21] Routine scanning for parotid tumors may never be of value, since preoperative diagnosis of a benign tumor would not negate the need for surgery in most cases. There are situations, however, in which surgery may be a significant risk for the patient, and the ability to diagnose a benign tumor may allow delay of surgery until a safer time. We are currently in the midst of a controlled study to assess accuracy of CT diagnosis of parotid masses and compare it to clinical accuracy. Since 80 percent of tumors are benign, and some malignant tumors have characteristic preoperative findings, the clinical accuracy of determining malignancy is greater than 80 percent.[22] To be proved highly dependable for preoperative assessment, CT diagnoses would have to approach 100 percent accuracy. This is unlikely to be the case in our study or any other.

Figure 18 represents the finding of a malignant mixed tumor with microinvasion of nerve fibers. Although the CT findings do demonstrate some irregularity in the posterior border of the tumor, many benign mixed tumors have similar findings.

Although the ability to detect displacement and invasion of the facial nerve by the CT scan has been demonstrated, this often adds little to the clinical plans.[21] Displacement of the nerve can be suspected by the clinical finding of a mass overlying the styloid process. The decision to do a retrograde dissection of the facial nerve is a personalized decision which is usually made only during surgical dissection and usu-

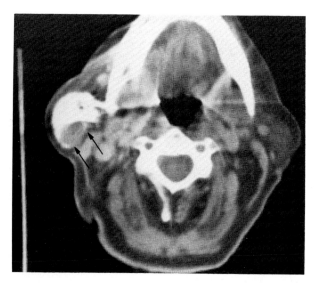

Figure 19 Axial CT sialogram showing a smoothly outlined filling defect (*arrows*) within the right parotid gland. This was a malignant lymphoma.

ally would not be affected by CT findings.

Figure 19 represents a malignant lymphoma presenting on an intraparotid mass. The CT findings show a well-defined mass with perfectly smooth borders characteristic of a benign tumor.

Figure 20 clearly demonstrates a cystic mass and indicates a benign process. Surgery, however, was recommended for this young patient, so that the CT had no effect on the treatment of the patient.

The value of CT sialography has clearly been shown in two specific areas. Som has reported on the characteristic appearance of sarcoidosis involving the parotid gland.[23] Figure 21 represents the CT sialogram of a patient who developed a left parotid mass

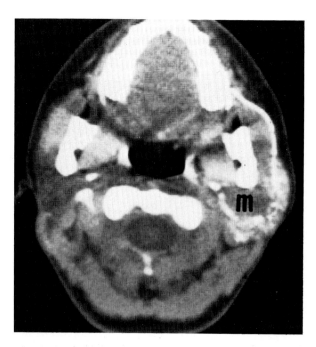

Figure 18 Axial CT sialogram showing a mass (*m*) in the left parotid gland. Note contrast in Stensen's duct and in complete filling of the left parotid gland. This was a malignant mixed tumor.

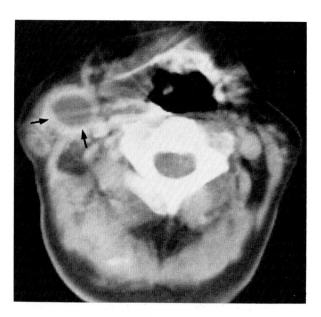

Figure 20 Axial CT sialogram showing a cystic mass (*arrows*).

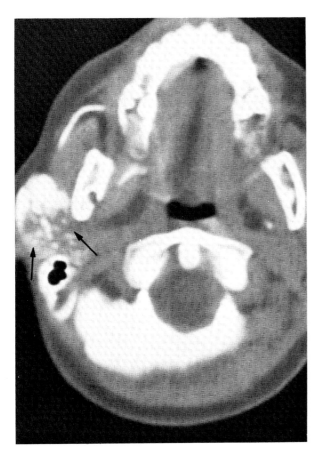

Figure 21 Axial CT sialogram with classic appearance of sarcoid involving parotid. Note irregular filling defect (*arrows*) indicative of infiltrative process.

one year after a right parotidectomy for a right parotid mass. The right parotid mass contained granulomas consistent with sarcoidosis. In view of the diagnosis, the second mass was treated with steroids, and complete resolution occurred within 3 weeks.

Som and Biller have also demonstrated the value of CT scanning in parapharyngeal space tumors.[24] The decision regarding the surgical approach depends on whether the tumor originates from the parotid or from minor salivary glands or other tissue adjacent to the parapharyngeal space. Although these tumors are rare, CT is of value in all cases.

CT has also been shown to be of value in differentiation of enlarged lymph nodes from a parotid tumor.[24] Although this may be of value in some rare situations, in most situations the lymph node that will require CT scanning will also require surgery for diagnosis.

Although young patients with parotid masses should have surgery regardless of CT findings, there are specific uses for preoperative scanning. Older patients, at higher risk for surgery, with a preoperative diagnosis of Wharton's tumor, may need observation only. Timing of surgery may be affected by preoperative identification of malignancy. In addition, the possibility of preoperative identification allows better preparation of the patient.

CONCLUSIONS

Computerized tomography has been clearly shown to be an accurate method of diagnosis in head and neck disease. However, we do not recommend it for all cases of head and neck tumors. We do believe that the diagnosis of metastatic cervical disease is more accurate by CT scanning than by clinical examination and that the results of a CT scan should be incorporated in clinical staging. A patient with a clinically negative neck examination and positive CT scan should be considered to have N$^+$ disease. A patient with a clinically positive neck examination and a negative CT scan should still be considered as having N$^+$ disease. We strongly believe that all centers studying progression and treatment of nodal disease should incorporate CT scanning into the study.

The clinical usefulness of CT scanning is restricted to patients with disease that has a high incidence of nodal metastasis; this includes T3 and T4 lesions of most areas and all lesions of the tongue. Patients with clinically positive neck examinations should have CT scans to evaluate the contralateral neck if the lesion has potential for bilateral metastases.

We have found CT scanning in the preoperative examination of patients with hyperparathyroidism to be highly accurate. Large cervical adenomas can easily be visualized. With a new generation scanner and the use of infusion techniques, even small adenomas and diffuse hyperplasia can be diagnosed accurately. The value of CT scanning for identification of mediastinal adenomas has been previously reported. Based on the results of correlation of CT diagnosis, surgical findings, and pathologic diagnosis in this series, we recommend preoperative scanning on all patients with the diagnosis of primary hyperparathyroidism.

CT sialography for evaluation of parotid tumors cannot be recommended on a routine basis, but may be of value in selected cases. For the patient who is at increased surgical risk, CT diagnosis may help in the decision whether to operate on a CT benign tumor. Preoperative information indicating a malignant tumor can often help in the preparation of the patient. Large tumors can cause displacement of the nerve and this can be recognized on CT scanning and help in surgical exploration. All patients with sarcoidosis who present with a parotid mass and patients with parapharyngeal masses should have CT sialography.

All of the applications of CT scans in head and neck disease are based on studies performed with meticulous attention to technique of scanning and interpretation by a head and neck radiologist with intimate knowledge of head and neck anatomy. Extrapolating our results to a situation in which head and neck surgery is performed only occasionally may not yield the same accuracy.

REFERENCES

1. Cantrell RN. Computed tomography for cervical adenopathy; does the cost justify the results? Arch Otolaryngol 1984; 110:441–442. (Editorial)
2. Beahrs OH, Barber KW. The value of radical dissection of structures of the neck in the management of carcinoma of the lip, mouth, and larynx. Arch Surg 1962; 85:49–56.
3. Southwick HW, Slaughter DP, Trevino ET. Elective neck dissection for intraoral cancer. Arch Surg 1960; 80:905–909.
4. Friedman M, et al. Metastatic neck disease evaluation by computed tomography. Arch Otolaryngol 1984; 110:443–447.
5. Mancuso AA, Maceri D, Rice D, et al. CT of cervical lymph node cancer. AJR 1981; 136:381–385.
6. Reed DL, Bergeron RT. CT of cervical lymph nodes. J Otolaryngol 1982; 11:411–418.
7. Nahum AM, Bone RC, Davidson TM. The case for prophylactic neck dissection. Laryngoscope 1977; 87:588–599.
8. Reed GF, Miller WA. Elective neck dissection. Laryngoscope 1970; 80:1292–1304.
9. Skolnik EM, Katz AH, Becker SP, et al. Evolution of the clinically negative neck. Ann Otol Rhinol Laryngol 1980; 89:551–555.
10. Ogura JH, Biller HF, Wette R. Elective neck dissection for pharyngeal and laryngeal cancers. Ann Otol Rhinol Laryngol 1971; 80:646–651.
11. Doppman JL. Parathyroid localization: Arteriography and venous sampling. Radiol Clin North Am 1976; 14:163–188.
12. Heller S. Parathyroid arteriography. Otolaryngol Clin North Am 1980; 13:161–167.
13. Doppman JL, Brennan MF, Koehler JO, et al. Computed tomography for parathyroid localization. J Comput Assist Tomogr 1977; 1:30–36.
14. Adams JE, Adams PH, Mamtora H, et al. Computed tomography and the localization of parathyroid tumors. Clin Radiol 1981; 32:251–254.
15. Kovarik J, Willvonseder R, Kuster W, et al. Localization of parathyroid tumors by computed tomography. N Engl J Med 1980; 303:885.
16. Shimshak RR, Schoenrock GJ, Taekman HP, et al. Preoperative localization of a parathyroid adenoma using computed tomography and thyroid scanning: Case report. J Comput Assist Tomogr 1979; 3:117–119.
17. Gouliamos AD, Carter BL. Parathyroid adenomas: Identified by CT scan. Comput Tomogr 1981; 5:59–63.
18. Friedman M, Mafee M, Shelton V, et al. Parathyroid localization by computed tomographic scanning. Arch Otolaryngol 1983; 109:95–97.
19. Colacchio T, LoGerfo P, Feind C. Surgical treatment of parathyroid disease. Head Neck Surg 1980; 2:487–493.
20. Kelly TR. Primary hyperthyroidism: A personal experience with 242 cases. Am J Surg 1980; 140:632–635.
21. Stone DN, Mancuso A, et al. Parotid CT sialography. Radiology 1981; 138:393.
22. Skolnik E, Friedman M, et al. Tumors of the major salivary glands. Laryngoscope 1977; 87:843–861.
23. Som PM, et al. Parotid gland sarcoidosis and the CT Sialogram. J Comput Assist Tomogr 1981; 5:677.
24. Som PM, Biller HF. The combined CT-Sialogram. Radiology 1980; 135:387–390.

COMPUTED TOMOGRAPHY AND MAGNETIC RESONANCE IMAGING IN THE DETECTION AND STAGING OF HEAD AND NECK CANCER

ANTHONY A. MANCUSO, M.D.

TECHNIQUE

Computed tomography (CT) or magnetic resonance (MRI) examination of the head and neck region, as anywhere else in the body, should be tailored to the specific complaint of the patient. Certain guidelines concerning positioning, section thickness, and use of intravenous contrasts are useful to ensure consistently high-quality examinations.

Since most of the regions of the head and neck are fairly compact, it is usually wise to use sections approximately 5 mm thick. Although sectioning at 1-cm increments might expedite some studies, "fill in" sections are often necessary, and it is probably better strategy just to do contiguous sections through the areas of interest. This is especially true if the sections are confined to one portion of the upper aerodigestive tract, such as the nasopharynx. When surveying the head and neck region for the possible presence of tumor,

it is still best to do thinner contiguous sections through areas of high yield such as the nasopharynx, tonsillar regions, and base of the tongue. When evaluating the neck for cervical lymphadenopathy, the sections may be done at 1-cm intervals with 5-mm thick sections and appropriate fill-in sections as indicated either by the survey scan or physical examination. Because of signal to noise considerations, section thickness is likely to be limited to 7 to 8 mm in magnetic resonance imaging systems operating at up to 0.5 tesla (T). Thinner sections are obtained on these units at the expense of prolonged imaging times. Thinner sections should be routinely available on higher field strength units at lower data acquisition times.

For CT studies other than those of the larynx and neck, the plane of section should be roughly parallel to the hard palate. For laryngeal scans and neck scans, the neck is slightly hyperextended and the gantry angled so that the central axis of the larynx is perpendicular to the scanning plane. Preliminary projection radiographs should be used for planning the number of sections and will ensure that the angle of the plane of section is as desired.

During CT examination the patient should not swallow, cough, or make any sudden movement during scanning. Scan should be done in suspended respiration as a routine. This virtually eliminates motion artifacts in all but the least cooperative patients. If the patient does a Valsalva maneuver during suspended respiration, repeat sections through the true and false cords of the larynx may be necessary since the Valsalva causes these structures to be pressed together in the midline. Phonation is not used, and modified Valsalva may rarely be necessary to distend the pyriform sinuses. Physiologic maneuvers to distend the upper airway are not necessary with newer scanners because of their ability to produce high-resolution images of the surrounding deep tissue planes.

We use the following specific technique for planning our studies and infusing iodinated contrast:

1. Start an IV using a three-way stopcock and hanging a 150 cc bottle of diatrizoate sodium 25 percent to keep open.
2. Obtain projection radiograph and plan study.
3. Inject 50 cc of diatrizoate meglumine or diatrizoate sodium 76 percent, and immediately after the bolus is in, start IV running at maximum flow rate. The bolus should be injected slowly to avoid incuding nausea in the patient.
4. Begin scanning immediately and continue to acquire data as rapidly as possible while monitoring the study for image quality, pathology, and possible changes in sectioning technique based on what is seen.

This technique ensures adequate opacification of vessels and vascular compartment of tumors for about 15 minutes. The low viscosity of the diatrizoate sodium 25 percent seems to be a key factor in maintaining adequate flow rate while the bolus brings us up to adequate IV concentration so that scanning can begin immediately.

Our indications for intravenous contrast injection include (1) staging cervical metastases, (2) defining the extent of a primary tumor, (3) looking for intracranial extension of tumors within the nasopharynx or infratemporal fossa, and (4) differential diagnosis of benign lesions in the parapharyngeal space, major salivary glands, and neck.

Magnetic resonance imaging, with its long acquisition times, requires that the patient be allowed to breathe and even swallow during the study. Swallowing and other movement is discouraged. MRI does not require the infusion of intravenous contrast since the "flow void" phenomenon results in little signal from the vascular structures; these appear black on most images, and contrast from surrounding tissues is excellent. We rely on different pulse sequences to provide the information about tumor margins relative to normal surrounding structures. It is necessary to do more than one pulse sequence in each patient. In general, we use only spin echo techniques and perform a sequence with a short repetition time (this is T1-weighted) and one with a longer repetition time (this provides T2-weighted information).

DETECTION OF AN OCCULT PRIMARY OF THE UPPER AERODIGESTIVE TRACT

Occasionally, patients present with an upper or mid cervical enlarged node with no apparent site of primary tumor in the nasopharynx, oropharynx, or larynx. Fine-needle aspiration of a node may show squamous cell carcinoma, in which case the overwhelming possibility is that the primary is within the upper aerodigestive tract but not visible at clinical examination, sometimes including panendoscopy under anesthesia.[1-5] In the past, CT scans of the nasopharynx and oropharynx have shown the primary carcinoma responsible for these metastases when there was no sign of tumor following endoscopic examination either in the office or under anesthesia.[1-5] However, this accounts for a very small percentage of patients presenting with head and neck carcinoma. Sometimes patients present with other evidence of primary tumor in the upper aerodigestive tract, such as atypical facial pain and distribution of the third division of the trigeminal nerve or otalgia. In some of these patients, CT has shown deeply infiltrating lesions in the absence of visible mucosal disease.[2,6] Both groups of patients are most likely to have primary sites in the nasopharynx, tongue base, or faucial tonsil, depending on the spectrum of clinical signs and symptoms. Since magnetic resonance imaging produces anatomic displays equal to or better than current CT studies, a yield of diagnostic information similar to CT may be expected from MRI though specific experience in this regard is yet to be accumulated.

The occurrence of tumors growing within the upper aerodigestive tract which are not visible at examination under anesthesia is a distinctly unusual circumstance, but has convined us that CT or magnetic resonance imaging should be an integral part of the search for head and neck neoplasm which is suspected but not clinically obvious, no matter what the presenting circumstance. The approach to the study is dictated by the clinical circumstances. The patients presenting with cervical nodes should undergo a thorough examination of the upper aerodigestive tract by an experienced examiner.[3,7] If no primary site is visible, a fine-needle aspiration of the nodal mass should be performed. If the pathologic diagnosis is squamous cell carcinoma, we proceed with a detailed examination of the nasopharynx, including coronal sections if the axial sections are suspicious or if there is a strong clinical suspicion that the primary tumor may be near the roof of the nasopharynx. If the nasopharynx is normal, sections are made through the regions of the tonsillar pillars and tongue base. If these are normal, the examination is carried through the remainder of the neck, which will allow for examination of the pyriform sinuses as well as complete CT staging of the neck disease.

Under other circumstances patients may present with atypical facial pain in the distribution of the trigeminal nerve.[6] This requires a detailed examination of the nasopharynx and skull base. A somewhat different approach is taken to patients with referred otalgia since primary tumors in this group are most likely to arise in the tongue base or pyriform sinus.[6]

The yield of positive studies depends both on

careful screening of the patient groups to be studied and on the careful use of imaging technique.[2-7] In approximately 20 to 30 percent of patients with cervical metastases of unknown etiology, the responsible lesion is demonstrated on CT.[3] The CT study serves as a guide to the endoscopist, who then performs endoscopy under anesthesia and obtains a biopsy from the area in question on CT. This basically eliminates the need for blind biopsy during panendoscopy, although some role for this in the tonsillar fossa or at the tongue base may remain. In the patients presenting with facial pain, the highest yield group are those with atypical pain which has been progressive.[6,8] Some lesions may be found in patients with typical trigeminal neuralgia; however, this is a relatively low-yield group for demonstrating a responsible structural lesion.[9] Patients with otalgia are a relatively high-yield group if they are not mixed in with that group of patients who have long-term complaints of temporal mandibular joint pain. This is especially true if there are other related symptoms such as dysphagia or odynophagia.[6]

STAGING OF PRIMARY CARCINOMA OF THE UPPER AERODIGESTIVE TRACT AND NECK

Nasopharynx

The hallmark of a malignant lesion on a CT or magnetic resonance image is infiltration of the deep planes, specifically, the parapharyngeal space which borders the airway throughout the upper aerodigestive tract. Such deep infiltration is usually obvious and asymmetric. The extent of the primary tumor usually correlates well with its extent as seen on physical examination; however, CT may show submucosal spread to contiguous anatomic sites. Extensions to the infratemporal fossa and to the pterygoid plate region, and caudal spread out of the nasopharynx deep to the tonsillar pillars may all occur in nasopharyngeal primaries and be detectable only on CT or MRI.

Involvement of the retropharyngeal lymph nodes is common in nasopharyngeal carcinoma, and such spread may account for cranial nerve deficits in that the nodal groups are immediately adjacent to the carotid sheath and cranial nerves IX through XII. Clinically occult lymph node metastases may be seen on CT in the retropharyngeal nodes, and even palpable jugulodigastric and posterior triangle nodes can be visualized on CT studies.[10,11] Nasopharyngeal tumors commonly spread to involve the base of the skull. If the spread is to the jugular bulb region, deficits of cranial nerves IX through XII may be present. Also, a partial Horner's syndrome is possible. Spread through the base of the skull in the region of the foramen lacerum may lead to cavernous sinus syndrome in more advanced lesions. Spread to the dura and brain are seen in advanced tumors. CT is reliable in the detection of tumor in all of these locations, and the involvement or lack of involvement at the skull base is critical in planning radiation ports. There is still some question about the ability of magnetic resonance imaging to detect subtle involvement of the skull base. It is likely that on high-resolution thin-section studies magnetic resonance imaging will prove accurate; however, this must be proved on studies comparing both CT and magnetic resonance images before magnetic resonance can replace CT in this regard.

Oropharynx

Tumors within the oropharynx show deep infiltration. In general, CT or MRI should be used to study lesions that are deeply infiltrating. Superficial T1 or T2 lesions usually produce normal-appearing scans, the only value of imaging being to exclude deep infiltration. The studies may sometimes be degraded by dental fillings; however, with careful patient positioning and angling of the gantries, the oropharynx can always be studied.[12] The oral cavity, however, may be difficult to study if many fillings are present. Oral cavity lesions are usually amenable to complete physical examination. However, advanced carcinoma of the gingival buccal sulci and retromolar trigone region may require CT or MRI for complete evaluation. The effects of dental fillings are less on MRI since they occur only if the amalgams are ferromagnetic.

CT or MRI can be especially valuable in certain areas. In tonsillar carcinoma, sometimes extensive spread into the nasopharynx may be detected and not be apparent on the clinical examination. Similarly, posterolateral spread to involve the internal carotid artery or even further direct spread into the neck may occur and be only detectable by CT or magnetic resonance. Lesions of the tongue base are well known for their tendency to deep infiltration. On CT and magnetic resonance images, the tissue planes of the floor of the mouth and within the tongue base itself are well defined, and the depth of tumors can be determined with great accuracy.[12] This may be extremely helpful in deciding whether hemiglossectomy will encompass the entire tumor while preserving at least one lingual artery and hypoglossal nerve. This is especially pertinent in that many surgeons do not accept total glossectomy as a mode of therapy due to its extreme morbidity.

Larynx and Hypopharynx

CT and MRI provide only limited information concerning the mucosal extent of tumors. High-resolution magnetic resonance may actually prove much more informative than computed tomography in this regard. However, the determination of the mucosal extent of disease and status of vocal cord function is best determined by laryngoscopy. The imaging techniques, however, provide information concerning deep extensions of tumor which is far beyond that possible from endoscopic examination.[1] The following list emphasizes the major contributions CT and magnetic resonance imaging can make in helping clinicians decide whether partial laryngectomy, total laryngectomy, radiation therapy, or combined therapy is the most appropriate means of treatment:

1. Subglottic extension of the tumor and especially the relationship of the tumor to the cricoid cartilage.
2. Status of the anterior commissure.
3. Deep extension of tumor to involve the paralaryngeal space which may not be apparent on clinical examination. This is especially true of tumors that may have begun in the laryngeal ventricle.
4. Pre-epiglottic space extension which cannot be evaluated critically by any other means and may be pivotal in determining whether radiation or surgery is the more appropriate therapy for supraglottic cancer.
5. Cartilage invasion. Although subtle cartilage invasion may be difficult to diagnose, CT remains the most sensitive radiographic tool for determining whether cartilage invasion is present. Magnetic resonance imaging may improve on CT in this regard since the signals from tumor should be vastly different from that of either cartilage or ossified portions of the laryngeal skeleton.
6. Exolaryngeal extension of endolaryngeal tumors. This usually occurs only in the most advanced lesions, and these are usually transglottic at the time of diagnosis. Such spread may be seen through the cricothyroid membrane in the subglottic space in less advanced lesions.
7. Extensions of pyriform sinus tumors through the cricothyroid space to involve the postcricoid region. Also, extension of pyriform sinus tumors through the laryngeal framework and into the soft tissues of the neck are easily recognized. Occasionaly, pyriform sinus tumors spread across the midline within the pre-epiglottic space entirely beneath intact mucosa.
8. CT can usually clearly differentiate marginal supraglottic lesions from pyriform sinus lesions which on some occasions is difficult to do on clinical examination.
9. CT or MRI can detect clinically occult spread of supraglottic cancer to the tongue base. Such spreads have been seen in the absence of palpable abnormality at the tongue base.
10. CT is more accurate than physical examination at staging cervical lymph node metastases and is especially useful in determining the precise extent of extranodal spread of this disease.

Computed tomograhy and magnetic resonance imaging do have their limitations. These studies are not tissue-specific and are not likely to be in the near future. Sometimes the bulk of tumor may be overestimated on these imaging studies because of associated edema. Areas of normal demineralization in the laryngeal skeleton can lead to overinterpretation of subtle cartilaginous invasion. With regard to staging lymph nodes, a false-positive may occur because of enlarged reactive nodes and false-negatives because of microscopic tumor deposits in normal-size nodes. These are difficult problems for which there does not appear to be any ready solution.

DETECTION OF RECURRENT MALIGNANT TUMORS OF THE UPPER AERODIGESTIVE TRACT AND NECK

The patient who has been treated by either surgery or radiation therapy for a malignant tumor in the head and neck region presents a special set of difficulties for the physician who is trying to detect early recurrent disease. Postoperative or postradiation scarring and induration certainly limit one's ability to palpate the neck. Similarly, there seems to be a tendency for tumors to be "driven" submucosally when they recur following radiation therapy. Patients may be symptomatic for 6 to 12 months without any definite physical signs of recurrent tumor, either by palpation or on inspection of the mucosa. Biopsies may be negative. We have found that CT is capable of detecting recurrent tumor in the absence of physical findings in a significant percentage of patients who are symptomatic.[13] Its potential for picking up early recurrences in asymptomatic patients is yet to be proved. Patients at high risk for recurrent tumor (e.g., advanced tumors, close surgical margins, deeply infiltrating tumors) may benefit from a baseline study approximately 12 weeks following the completion of therapy.[13,14] We suggest that a follow-up study be done approximately every 6 months to 2 years. After 2 years local recurrence is much less likely in upper aerodigestive tract squamous cell carcinoma; however, continued surveillance might be useful. Certainly restudy would be indicated if the patient were to become symptomatic.

Magnetic resonance imaging is particularly promising with regard to detecting early local recurrences before they become symptomatic. Preliminary investigation indicates that during and following radiation therapy the tumor bed signal tends to decrease and become much like that of surrounding muscle tissue. If the signal within this presumed area of fibrosis were then to begin to increase over a period of time, one might be suspicious of recurrent tumor.[15] At present, follow-up with CT studies requires that tumor spread to a contiguous anatomic site before a definite suggestion of recurrence can be made.[13,14] In particularly inaccessible areas, suspicious CT or MRI findings can be confirmed by CT guided-needle aspiration biopsy.[5]

One particular area of interest in recurrent tumors is the retropharyngeal nodes. These nodes are basically inaccessible to the clinician. They can be seen easily when pathologically enlarged, and even when normal, on CT or magnetic resonance images.[11,13] Patients with squamous cell carcinoma arising in the upper aerodigestive tract are at fairly high risk for involvement of these nodes. If these nodes are enlarged by squamous cell carcinoma metastases from primary tumors arising in locations other than then asopharynx, the prognosis is grave.[11] CT or MRI can sometimes help to prevent unnecessarily aggressive attempts at salvage therapy by showing recurrent disease in this region or in other relatively inaccessible regions, such as the infratemporal fossa, or very extensive recurrent masses which are fixed to the deep structures of the head and neck.[11,13,14]

REFERENCES

1. Mancuso AA, Hanafee WN. *Computed tomography of the head and neck.* Baltimore: Williams & Wilkins, 1982.
2. Mancuso AA, Hannafee WN. Elusive head and neck carcinomas beneath intact mucosa. Laryngoscope 1983; 93:133–139.
3. Muraki AS, Mancuso AA, Harnsberger RH. Metastatic cervical adenopathy from tumors of unknown origin: the role of CT. Radiology. Radiology 1984; 152:749–753.
4. Schaefer SD, Merkel M, Kiehl J, Maravilla K, Anderson R. Computed tomographic assessment of squamous cell carcinoma of oral and pharyngeal cavities. Arch Otolaryngol 1982; 108:688-692.
5. Gatenby RA, Mulhern CB, Richter MP, Moldofsky PJ. CT-guided biopsy for the detection and staging of tumors of the head and neck. Am J Neuroradiol 1984; 5:287–289.
6. Kalovidouris A, Mancuso AA, Dillon W. A CT-clinical approach to the V, VII, IX-XII cranial nerves and cervical sympathetics. Radiology 1984; 151:671–676.
7. Mancuso AA. Cervical lymph node metastases: oncologic imaging and diagnosis. Int J Radiat Oncol Biol Phys 1984; 10:411–423.
8. Noyek AM, Kassel EE, Jazrawy H. Wortzman G, Holgate RC. Clinically directed CT in occult disease of the skull base involving foramen ovale. Laryngoscope 1982; 92:1021–1027.
9. Sobel D, Norman D, Yorke CH, Newton TH. Radiography of trigeminal neuralgia and hemifacial spasm. AJR 1980; 135:93–95.
10. Mancuso AA, Harnsberger HR, Muraki AS, Stevens MH. Computed tomography of cervical and retropharyngeal lymph nodes: normal anatomy, variants of normal, and applications in staging head and neck cancer. Part I: normal anatomy. Radiology 1983; 148:709–714.
11. Mancuso AA, Harnsberger HR, Muraki AS, Stevens MH. Computed tomography of cervical and retropharyngeal lymph nodes: normal anatomy, variants of normal, and applications in staging head and neck cancer. Part II: Pathology. Radiology 1983; 148:715–723.
12. Muraki AS, Mancuso AA, Harnsberger HR, Johnson LP, Meads GB. CT of the oropharynx, tongue base, and floor of the mouth: normal anatomy and range of variations, and applications in staging carcinoma. Radiology 1983; 148:725–731.
13. Harnsberger HR, Mancuso AA, Muraki AS, Parkin JL. The upper aerodigestive tract and neck: CT evaluation of recurrent tumors. Radiology 1983; 149:503–509.
14. Som PM, Shugar JMA, Biller HF. The early detection of antral malignancy in the postmaxillectomy patient. Radiology 1982; 143:509–512.
15. Mancuso AA, Fitzsimmons J, Mareci T, Million R, Cassisi N. MRI of the upper pharynx and neck: variations of normal and possible applications in detecting and staging malignant tumors. Part II: pathology. Submitted for publication.

RADIONUCLIDE IMAGING

ARNOLD M. NOYEK, M.D., F.R.C.S.(C), F.A.C.S.
N. DAVID GREYSON, B.Sc., M.D., F.R.C.P.(C)
JOEL C. KIRSH, M.D., F.R.C.P.(C)
BERNARD J. SHAPIRO, M.D., F.R.C.P.(C)

The effective treatment of tumors and other disorders of the head and neck can only be predicated on a realistic working diagnosis and a valid pretreatment staging of the disease. The time-honored diagnostic approach of history-taking and physical examination has been augmented in recent years by diagnostic "hands on" technologic advances such as the use of fiberoptic telescopes. However, our inspecting eyes (even with our telescopes) and our palpating hands are often left with suspected disease still hidden from direct clinical assessment. In the past decade, the advent of computed tomography (CT) has quietly revolutionized *anatomic* head and neck diagnostic imaging. Magnetic resonance imaging (MRI) promises further refinements in morphologic assessment. Less dramatic and less well recognized, however, have been the progressive and selective advances in *physiologic* imaging provided by radionuclide scans.[1-3]

It is the purpose of this brief manuscript to (1) outline the recent professional and technologic advances in radionuclide imaging, and (2) summarize the basic principles, potentials, limitations, and current clinical applications of the major categorizations of radionuclide head and neck imaging.

Space limitations restrict descriptions to general and specific principles augmented by the use of tables. Illustrations are omitted, but the references cited have been selected as contemporary, comprehensive, and well illustrated. They are specific sources for descriptions of technique, dosage schedules, and further references.

EVOLUTION OF NUCLEAR MEDICINE (Table 1)

New, important, yet abstract, is the professional evolution of radionuclide imaging as an integral aspect of the radiologic sciences. The specialty has grown through the maturation of dedicated nuclear scientists including physicians (by specialty board), physicists, and technologists. The entire process reflects the evolution of a specialty with the capability of graduate and undergraduate teaching, research, and, above all, responsible clinical service. This evolution has been paralleled by maturation in the clinician-imager relationship. Astute clinicians have recognized that innovative radionuclide imagers can contribute much to

Supported by the Saul A. Silverman Family Foundation, Toronto, Ontario, Canada.

TABLE 1 Evolution of Nuclear Medicine

Professional evolution
　The specialty
　The clinician/imager relationship

Technologic development
　Imaging hardware (camera electronics): anatomic resolution of
　　the functional image
　Computer software: computer-quantification of the functional
　　image
　Improved scan agents (increased specificity, immunotracers)
　Positron emission tomography: "real metabolism"

the diagnostic process and the ultimate welfare of their patients. The enquiring clinician, instead of being overwhelmed by the range and technology of various diagnostic modalities available, has joined the responsible imager in pre-imaging consultation, mutual review of scintigraphic findings, disease correlations, and continued education and advancement. This approach maximizes diagnostic yield in a relatively safe, minimally invasive, cost-effective atmosphere. Radionuclide imaging has "come of age" and should now be a selective diagnostic weapon in the overall clinical armamentarium.

This technologic evolution has been fed by, and has itself nurtured, technologic development. The first major technologic advances related directly to improvements in the imaging hardware and the electronics of the gamma camera and image recording. Gamma cameras with a large field of view have evolved, and sophisticated technology for recording emission computed tomographic (ECT) images has developed. In essence, there has been improved anatomic resolution of the functional image, whether provided by the classic triphasic radionuclide scan or by other elements of dynamic imaging.

Technologic advances in imaging hardware have been matched by advances in computer software. Computer quantification of the functional image has made an impact on the clinical diagnostic process, whether through specific computer enhancement or through the use of time-radioactivity curves.

Improved radiopharmaceuticals have also been developed. Radionuclide scans generally give findings of high sensitivity but low specificity. The search has therefore been for radiotracers with a higher specificity. The recent capability of labeling monoclonal antibodies gives the possibility of specific imaging of tumors, such as malignant melanoma. This offers the possibility of the "magic bullet" concept of the im-

TABLE 2 Clinical Problems in Diagnosis

Qualitative diagnosis
　Specific
　Group discorder

Quantitative diagnosis
　Extent (3 dimensions)
　Extension
　Local or systemic
　Specific anatomic/physiologic abnormality

munotracer, not only for diagnosis but for treatment.

Finally, there has been the advent of positron emission tomography (PET). The positron emitters are the basic physiologic elements of our universe (carbon, nitrogen, oxygen) labeled with radioactive tags which allow the imaging of "real metabolism," as for example, through the labeling of glucose with carbon-11.

RADIONUCLIDE IMAGING: PRINCIPLES AND APPLICATIONS

Among the clinical problems of qualitative and quantitative diagnosis (Table 2), some lend themselves preferentially to solution by radionuclide imaging. Radionuclide scans provide predominantly physiologic imaging and augment other examinations (anatomic imaging with conventional x-ray examination and CT; pathologic examination by needle biopsy). This segment of the manuscript summarizes the basic principles and current clinical applications of the major radionuclide imaging studies applicable to head and neck disorders (thyroid, salivary, bone, gallium, parathyroid). Although radionuclide imaging makes a significant contribution to improved cancer management, it is also equally important in the diagnostic approaches to other head and neck disorders (Table 3).

The tracer principle underlies the premise that physiologic changes precede morphologic changes in disease. Relatively safe radioactive elements, such as the gamma photon emitters, allow the tagging of biologic substrates and the imaging of these radiopharmaceuticals by gamma cameras, as the tracer enters metabolic pathways and specific organ systems. The concept of the triphasic scan allows anatomic/physiologic correlation through flow phase ("first transit" vascularity), blood pool (relative hyperemia), and delayed-phase images (ultimate physiologic incorporation).

Thyroid Imaging[4,5]

Historically, the thyroid scan is well established in the management of focal and diffuse thyroid disease. Technetium-99m pertechnetate (Tc-99mO$_4^-$) and iodine-123 scans are currently in clinical use; both are safe gamma-photon emitters. [131]I, a beta emitter, should ideally be restricted to therapeutic use.

Pertechnetate anion mirrors iodide anion physiologically; however, pertechnetate is only *trapped* by the thyroid gland, whereas iodide is both *trapped* and ultimately *organified* in hormonogenesis. The favorable gamma emissions of pertechnetate and ^{123}I allow gamma camera recordings (with pinhole collimation for magnification and definition) of structural lesions within the thyroid parenchyma, with resolution approximating 1.0 cm (or perhaps even less).

The pertechnetate thyroid scan is the "first line" or preliminary physiologic examination; it is usually done in combination with a radioactive iodine uptake

TABLE 3 Common Applications of Radionuclide Imaging in Head and Neck Disorders

Clinical problem	Radionuclide imaging technique	Findings
Carcinoma (oral, perioral, other)	3-phase bone scan (^{99m}Tc methylene disphosphonate) (+ whole body scan)	T-staging — subclinical extension to bone; definition of known bone involvement
	Whole body bone scan	M-staging in high-risk patient
	Liver/spleen scan	M-staging in high-risk patient
Osteogenic sarcoma	3-phase bone scan	Tumor extent (T-staging)
	+ whole body scan	Tumor dissemination (M-staging)
Lymphoma	^{67}Ga citrate	Lymphoma staging (soft tissue/bone)
	Whole body bone scan	Lymphoma staging in bone
Vascular tumor	3-phase bone or pertechnetate scan	Flow/pool phase screening for vascular tumor
Thyroid mass	^{99m}Tc pertechnetate (preliminary examination)	Focal vs diffuse disease Functioning vs nonfunctioning nodule ? Occult disease in high-risk patient
	^{123}I scan	Confirm "hot" pertechnetate scan (when appropriate)
Ectopic thyroid	^{99m}Tc pertechnetate (or ^{123}I)	Ectopic thyroid (usually lingual) ? Presence normal thyroid
Thyroid tumor (benign or malignant)	^{99m}Tc pertechnetate	Screening for nonfunctioning nodule
	^{123}I	Functioning tumor
	^{131}I	Treatment modality Treatment follow-up, e.g., functioning metastases
Infection	3-phase bone scan	Soft tissue (cellulitis, abscess) vs bone infection
	^{67}Ga citrate (or Indium-111 labeled WBCs)	Osteomyelitis (biologic activity; treatment success/failure)
TM joint	3-phase bone scan (+ whole body scan)	Nonbony vs bony involvement Local vs systemic arthropathy
Larynx	3-phase bone scan	Arthropathy
	^{67}Ga citrate	Radionecrosis/perichondritis
Bone sclerosis or osteoblastosis	3-phase bone scan (+ whole body scan)	Paget's disease Fibrous dysplasia Eosinophilic granuloma
	3-phase bone scan + brain scan	Meningioma
Bone lysis	3-phase bone scan (whole body scan)	Myeloma
Bone graft or flap	3-phase bone scan	Assess viability
Salivary gland mass/lesion(s)	^{99m}Tc pertechnetate (sequential images + washout)	Focal vs diffuse disease Overall function (Sjögren's syndrome) Salivary obstruction Detection of functioning tumor (Warthin's tumor, oncocytoma)
	^{67}Ga citrate	Sarcoidosis; abscess; lymphoma
Parathyroid adenoma (or carcinoma)	Computer subtraction — ^{99m}Tc pertechnetate and Tl–201 thallous chloride	Parathyroid adenoma or carcinoma (not hyperplasia)

study. Its first application is in the detection of diffuse or focal (or multifocal) thyroid disease. Therefore, it allows physiologic qualification and quantification of the focal lesion, nodule, or mass. The thyroid gland trapping of pertechnetate mirrors, in first approximation, thyroid uptake of iodine. Pertechnetate thus has the capability of imaging as follows:

1. The nonfunctioning or "cold" nodule (no trapping of pertechnetate or, by inference, of iodine).
2. The functioning or "hot" intrathyroid nodule.

However, a "hot" nodule on pertechnetate scan might only indicate trapping, perhaps related to the intrinsic vascularity of the lesion. It is usually essential to confirm that this nodule is actually functioning in hormonogenesis by radioactive ^{123}I scan. A "hot" nodule has only a 0.002 percent chance of being malignant. "Warm," isofunctioning, or nondelineated (but palpable) nodules should be considered "cold" or nonfunctioning in terms of their biologic tumor implication; this concept is often misunderstood. Furthermore, a "hot" or warm nodule on early pertechnetate blood pool image may reflect only soft tissue vascularity, and there may be no consistent relationship with ultimate functional activity.

3. The pertechnetate scan is useful in demonstrating ectopic thyroid disease. Its most frequent application is in the definition of the lingual thyroid gland; equally important is its demonstration of an absent thyroid gland in normal anticipated anatomic position. The retrosternal thyroid gland, though not truly "ectopic," is less satisfactorily imaged by Tc-99mO_4^- because of background radioactivity in adjacent great vessels. Here, ^{123}I is preferable. Thyroglossal duct cysts are not usually visualized unless there is significant amount of functioning thyroid tissue in the cyst walls.

4. Finally, the pertechnetate thyroid scan plays a less predictable role in the search for occult focal thyroid disease in the at-risk patient, e.g., the patient who has had irradiation to the head and neck. A much better morphologic search for occult disease is now effected by real-time high-resolution ultrasound.

Radioactive iodine (^{123}I, ^{131}I) allows the imaging of "true" physiology. Iodine-131 has an 8.1-day physical half-life and several different beta and gamma modes of decay. The beta particulate emissions account for its therapeutic applications, and its use should be so restricted. Iodine-123 has a favorable dosimetry for thyroid imaging with a 159-Kev gamma photon emission. The absorbed dose varies with the patient's thyroid endocrine status and actual uptake of iodine as related to blood TSH levels. Iodine-123 has a physical half-life of just over 13 hours and is optimally imaged at 4 to 18 hours. It is cyclotron-produced, somewhat expensive, and not always widely available.

Iodine-123 clarifies the previously noted focal uptake of a thyroid nodule on preliminary pertechnetate scan. This can be either a true "hot" nodule (confirming genuine organification of iodine) or it may demonstrate the "false function" of such a nodule. Iodine-123 is rarely required to demonstrate an ectopic thyroid focus developing along the thyroglossal duct (such as a lingual thyroid); here the positive pertechnetate scan suffices, both for ectopic thyroid definition and for scrutiny of the normal anticipated thyroid location for functioning tissue.

The final role for radioiodine relates to thyroid cancer management. When there are clinical/pathologic indications for treatment with [131]I (100 to 150 mCi dosage orally), whole body scans are obtained between 4 and 7 days after therapy. Presuming prior thyroid ablation, these images optimally demonstrate residual thyroid gland and/or functioning thyroid tumor in the thyroid surgical bed and/or the presence of functioning metastases in the neck, lungs, bony skeleton, or elsewhere. The ^{131}I scan for metastatic survey utilizes 2 to 10 mCi of sodium iodide-131 orally. This dosage level of ^{131}I can be repeated whenever there is clinical or biochemical suspicion of thyroid carcinoma metastasis or recurrence.

The role of suppression and thyrotropin stimulation tests is beyond our discussion; bascially they are used to evaluate the "hot" nodule and possible pituitary axis control.

Salivary Imaging[6,7]

Salivary radionuclide imaging with pertechnetate has but few major clinical roles: the evaluation of diffuse disease (such as Sjögren's syndrome), the evaluation of obstructive ductal disease (both parotid and submandibular), and the demonstration of functioning salivary tumors (invariably parotid). Only this latter group merits discussion at this time.

Sodium pertechnetate is the salivary scan agent; the pertechnetate anion reflects iodide anion physiology in that it is trapped but not organified by the thyroid gland. The radiopharmaceutical is also accumulated by, distributed within and excreted from the salivary glands. Details concerning molecular physiology and transport mechanisms are reviewed by Greyson and Noyek.[7] The salivary scan visualizes blood flow, functional activity, and excretion. The "washout" technique enhances the excretory image. The radionuclide scan findings in a variety of salivary disorders are indicated in Table 4.

During the functional phase, gross salivary physiology may be compared to the thyroid gland on the same image. Focal intrinsic, nonfunctioning lesions may reflect a variety of benign and malignant tumors or cysts. However, focal intrinsic, hyperfunctioning lesions are invariably Warthin's tumors or the rare oncocytoma. The intense focal accumulation of pertechnetate, in Warthin's tumor, is enhanced in the post-sialogogue (washout) image. A focal accumulation of pertechnetate producing a "hot" scan should not be confused with a diffuse positive washout scan due to ductal obstruction. We have now had experience with 26 parotid Warthin's tumors, all of which were correctly diagnosed by salivary scan preoperatively or prior to fine-needle aspiration biopsy.

Bone Imaging

Some brief consideration is due the physiology of bone in the action of the radionuclide bone scan agent—^{99m}Tc methylene diphosphonate (^{99m}Tc MDP). Bone consists of calcium salts deposited within a matrix of organic polymers. The major bone mineral is hydroxyapatite, which forms crystals in a lattice-like frame. The mineral appears surrounded by a hydration shell, which is in contact with the extracellular fluid compartment. Thus ions, such as radionuclides, that are deposited on the surface of the crystals may pass through this hydration shell and enter into an exchange reaction within the lattice structure. At any time, only a small percentage of the total bone min-

TABLE 4 Salivary Scan Findings*

	Flow	Function	Washout
Sjögren's syndrome	↓	↓	↓
Obstruction	↓	±↓	↑
Warthin's tumor or oncocytoma	↑	↑	↑
Benign mixed tumor	±↑	↓	↓
Malignant tumor	±↑	↓	↓
Cyst	↓	↓	↓
Acute inflammation	↑	↓	↑

*Arrow direction depicts activity compared with normal.
From Greyson and Noyek.[3]

eral is available for such exchange reaction, which tends to take place primarily in areas of new bone formation. The delayed incorporation of bone-seeking radiopharmaceuticals in areas of osteogenesis, with the passage of time, appears more dependent on the movement of the tracer from the surface into the interior of the crystal than factors related to regional perfusion. Utilizing the tracer principle, it is possible to image the radioactively tagged phosphate anion and detect physiologic bone changes *in advance* of clear clinical, pathologic, and anatomic findings. The triphasic bone scan demonstrates not only the delayed phase incorporation of the phosphate anion into bone metabolism, but the soft tissue flow and blood pool phase physiology which underlies this response (Table 5).

Virtually all osteolytic bone disease (perhaps with the exception of multiple myeloma) incites a marginating osteoblastic response. It is this marginating osteoblastic response, and its sensitive but nonspecific detection by gamma cameras, which occasions the clinical importance of the bone scan. Bone must be

TABLE 5 Three-phase Bone Scanning of Facial Skeleton and Skull Base

Lesion	Flow and pool	Delayed scan
Neoplasm		
Soft tissue	+ or −	−
Bony infiltration	+ or −	+
Vascular	++	+/−
		(depending on site)
Inflammation		
Acute sinusitis/cellulitis	+	− or mild +
Acute osteomyelitis	+	++
Chronic osteomyelitis	+/−	+
Trauma		
Recent fracture	+	+
Delayed union	+	+
Non-union	−	− or mild +
Bone graft/flap		
Free (nonvascularized)	−	− early postop
		+ late
Vascularized (micro-	+	? + at 3 hrs
vascular anastomosis)		+ (with computer at
		18 hrs
Flap (e.g., pectoralis	+	? + at 3 hrs
major + rib)		++ computer image
		at 18 hrs

demineralized by 30 to 50 percent for detection by conventional radiographic studies. However, the osteoblastic response about such bone dissolution may be detected in the range of but 5 to 10 percent hypermineralization. This finding occurs in benign and malignant tumors, healing fractures, osteomyelitis, and a range of systemic bone disorders. The specificity of these scintigraphic findings must be augmented by other radiologic or surgical procedures. Similarly, primary osteoblastic disease such as osteoma, osteogenic sarcoma, or meningioma may be easily detected and quantified by the bone scan.

The bone scan has several major applications.[8] Its role in the pretreatment staging of oral, perioral, and other head and neck cancers relates to the detection of subclinical bone involvement by adjacent carcinoma. This is of critical importance in the election of treatment modalities. Furthermore, when bone involvement is recognized by clinical examination, conventional radiology, or CT, the bone scan provides a more realistic depiction of pretreatment tumor extension. It also plays a role in improved M-staging in the high-risk patient for skeletal metastases; carcinoma of the nasopharynx is one such entity in which the whole-body bone scan should be utilized in pretreatment evaluation. The triphasic bone scan has diagnostic value in osteogenic sarcoma, both in evaluation of the presenting lesion and the detection of systemic pulmonary and skeletal metastases. The bone scan plays a lesser role in the systemic staging of lymphoma and malignant melanoma. The bone scan also plays a variety of roles in the diagnosis of systemic bone disorders, meningioma, and bone graft viability. The reader is referred to the monograph by Noyek for further details. The critical role of the bone scan in the management of the patient with osetomyelitis is discussed below, as it is carried out in combination scan with gallium citrate.

Gallium Imaging[8-11]

Gallium-67 citrate (^{67}Ga) is a relatively safe agent with a half-life of 78 hours and a triple peak gamma photon emission which can be well recorded by gamma cameras. The typical adult gallium scan provides approximately five times the radiation hazard of the bone scan, in total body exposure, but is still considered well within safe limits. Gallium binds to albumin (transferrin) and is taken up in nonspecific binding by actively dividing cells in the lysozome component (tumor cells, white cells, bacteria). It also has osteogenic activity. It enters organelles in soft tissues and forms insoluble gallium-phosphate complexes in bone. It clears slowly and does not enter pus freely. Ideal imaging occurs within 48 to 78 hours, but useful images can be obtained within 24 to 96 hours.

Gallium scanning has a nonspecific role in the management of head and neck cancer. Gallium is taken up readily (but not exclusively) by melanoma and lymphoma; it therefore has some role in the staging of these disorders. Hodgkin's lymphoma is more readily imaged than non-Hodgkin's lymphoma. Many times, however, gallium scanning is simply part of the post-biopsy staging process, and other well-defined guidelines are laid out for other diagnostic modalities. Gallium citrate may or may not be taken up by squamous cell carcinoma, either at the primary site or in secondary disease; this is too unpredictable to be of real clinical value.

One area of real predictive value, however, lies in the diagnosis of osteomyelitis and in the assessment of the biologic activity of the disease and of treatment effectiveness. When acute osteomyelitis is suspect, the bone scan allows the preliminary diagnosis of osteomyelitis well in advance of established conventional and CT radiographic findings. When osteomyelitis is suspect, triphasic bone scanning is carried out. The blood pool phase of the bone scan reflects the hyperemia of the infective insult; the "hot" delayed phase demonstrates the marginating osteoblastic response about the infective insult itself.

Once the diagnosis of osteomyelitis is made on the bone scan, the patient receives an immediate intravenous injection of gallium citrate and is returned to the nuclear medicine unit in 48 hours (optimally) for imaging. A positive gallium scan actually reflects the infective focus and should match the photon-excess image on the blood pool phase of the MDP scan. When effective treatment has been carried out (intravenous antibiotics, hyperbaric oxygen, surgical debridement), the gallium scan should revert to normal. The bone scan, however, will remain "hot" for many months, as healing continues. In 25 cases of osteomyelitis of the head and neck studied over the past 4 years, all 25 were correctly diagnosed by bone scan (whereas conventional/CT imaging only suggested a preliminary diagnosis in 16 instances). The primary treatment response (either success or failure) was also accurately evaluated in all 25 patients. Details of this study have just been published in *Laryngoscope*.[11]

Parathyroid Imaging[6,12-15]

The search for improved management approaches to the patient with biochemical primary hyperparathyroidism continues. Encouraged by the occasional successful imaging of large parathyroid adenomas utilizing ^{75}Se selenomethionine (the parathyroids are a major site of amino acid synthesis), Robinson correctly predicted the site of parathyroid disease in 9 of 12 surgically confirmed cases, utilizing simultaneous parathyroid scanning and a computer-subtraction technique of overlying thyroid images.[12] In 1983, Ferlin et al, from the University of Padua in Italy, extended this experience by localizing enlarged parathyroids with technetium-thallium subtraction scans.[13] Double tracer scanning utilizing ^{99m}Tc as pertechnetate and Tl-201 as chloride and a computerized image subtraction technique demonstrated intra- or extra-thyroidal focal uptake of thallium in 37 of 61 patients with biochemical primary hyperparathyroidism. The results were very optimistic in that,

of 24 patients undergoing surgical exploration, 18 parathyroid adenomas, 5 carcinomas, and 1 hyperplastic parathyroid gland were found exactly in the anatomic site predicted by scintigraphy. In the two patients with negative scan who underwent surgery, hyperplastic parathyroid glands with a diameter of less than 0.5 were found in each instance. Young and co-workers described equally encouraging radionuclide imaging findings.[14] There have also been some discouraging clinical voices, however.[15]

The ingenious concept of computer-subtraction of two sets of radionuclide images may overcome critical diagnostic limitations imposed by the small size of the parathyroid gland and the low anatomic resolution of the gamma camera. Additionally, the adenomatous parathyroid may be "lost" in the high intrinsic vascularity of the thyroid gland (which itself takes up many radiopharmaceuticals) or behind the photon-attenuating sternum. Currently the best opportunity for parathyroid imaging utilizes synchronous scanning by a thyroid-parathyroid agent (Tl-201 Cl) and by a thyroid only agent (^{99m}Tc pertechnetate). Computer-subtraction allows the potential of imaging the parathyroid gland itself when it is involved by adenoma, but not by hyperplasia.

REFERENCES

1. Noyek AM, et al. Sophisticated radiology in otolaryngology. II. Diagnostic imaging: non-roentgenographic (non-x-ray) modalities. J Otolaryngol 1977; 6 (Suppl 3):95–117.
2. Greyson ND, Noyek AM. Nuclear medicine in otolaryngological diagnosis. Otolaryngol Clin North Am 1978; 11(2):541–560.
3. Greyson ND, Noeyk AM. Clinical otolaryngology. In: Maisey MN, Britton KE, Gilday DL (eds). Clinical nuclear medicine. London, England: Chapman and Hall, 1983:371.
4. Noyek AM, Greyson ND, et al. Thyroid tumor imaging. Arch Otolaryngol 1983; 109:205–225.
5. Blahd WH, Rose JG. Nuclear medicine in diagnosis and treatment of diseases of the head and neck. II. Head Neck Surg 1981; 4:213–223.
6. Blahd WH, Rose JG. Nuclear medicine in diagnosis and treatment of diseases of the head and neck. I. Head Neck Surg 1981; 4:129–138.
7. Greyson ND, Noyek AM. Radionuclide salivary scanning. J Otolaryngol 1982; 11(Suppl 10):1–47.
8. Noyek AM. Bone scanning in otolaryngology. Laryngoscope 1979; 89(Suppl 18):1–87.
9. Hoffer P. Status of gallium-67 in tumor detection. J Nucl Med 1980; 21:394-398.
10. Noyek AM, Zizmor J. Lymphoma and leukemia of the upper airway and orbit. Sem Roentgenol 1980; 15(3):251–260.
11. Noyek AM, Kirsh JC, Greyson ND, et al. The clinical significance of radionuclide bone and gallium scanning in osteomyelitis of the head and neck. Laryngoscope 1984; 94(Suppl 34):1–21.
12. Robinson PJ. Parathyroid scintigraphy revisited. Clin Radiol 1981; 33:37–41.
13. Ferlin G, Bursato N, et al. New perspectives in localizing enlarged parathyroids by technetium-thallium subtraction scan. J Nucl Med 1983; 24:438–41.
14. Young AE, Gaunt JI, et al. Location of parathyroid adenomas by thallium-201 and technetium 99m subtraction scanning. Br Med J 1983; 286:1384–1386.
15. Corcoran MO, et al. Correspondence. Br Med J 1983; 286:1751–1752.

SECTION THREE / SURGICAL MANAGEMENT

13. Diagnosis and Management of Early Cancer

INTRODUCTION

DONALD P. SHEDD, M.D.

The chapters that follow address the issue of early cancer of the upper aerodigestive tract (UADT), a subject of great importance in view of the modest cure rates achieved when one treats advanced disease. A definition of early cancer must be somewhat arbitrary. For purposes of the present coverage, early disease is defined as lesions under 1 cm in diameter or lesions that are superficial. Also included in the definition of early cancer are some of the dysplastic lesions and carcinoma in situ.

PATHOLOGY

To understand the pathology of early UADT cancer, it is essential to know the natural history of neoplasia in the UADT, for example, whether it evolves in orderly progression through a series of stages. The existence of dysplastic lesions, both of moderate and of severe degree, is well recognized, and carcinoma in situ is a clear-cut entity. What is difficult to know is whether an invasive carcinoma is preceded by changes of the following sequence: (1) dysplasia, moderate, (2) dysplasia, severe, (3) carcinoma in situ, and (4) invasive carcinoma.

Also of great interest is the question whether any of the stages in the evolution of an invasive carcinoma is reversible if the extrinsic cocarcinogen, such as tobacco, is eliminated.

DIAGNOSIS

To diagnose early cancer, it is important to know the earliest clinical manifestations of neoplastic change. More needs to be known about the long-term significance of white patches (leukoplakia) and red patches (erythroplasia) in oral, pharyngeal, and laryngeal mucosa. It is recommended that the word "leukoplakia" be used only as a clinical descriptive term and not as a term that carries any histologic implication. In my experience, velvety red patches (erythroplasia) are frequently the clinical expression of carcinoma in situ. Such lesions show an affinity for topically applied to-

luidine blue, a procedure that provides tentative confirmation of the suspected diagnosis.[1] Biopsy makes the final diagnosis. On some occasions, exfoliative cytology is useful as an approach to confirmation, in that a positive cytology is helpful. A negative cytology in the face of a strong clinical suspicion should lead one to carry out a proper biopsy.

There has been an increasing realization in recent years, of the multicentric nature of cancer in the UADT. The second primary tumors can occur at the same time as the initial primary (synchronous) or at a later time (metachronous). Awareness of multicentricity has led to an increasing tendency to carry out thorough endoscopic appraisal of the entire region, the so-called triple endosdcopy (laryngoscopy, bronchoscopy, and esophagoscopy) for a patient with a known primary tumor in the UADT.[2] There are varying opinions as to the validity of this approach at the time the initial primary tumor is diagnosed, and there is some question concerning how often such an examination should be repeated in long-term follow-up.

TREATMENT

Once one has reached some level of agreement concerning the pathology and diagnosis of early cancer of the head and neck, one is in a better position to address questions of treatment.

Oral Lesions

Localized. The majority of early lesions in the mouth are localized and circumscribed. For these lesions, adequate excision is the treatment of choice, and radiation therapy can be used in specific instances.

Nonlocalized. A number of patients are seen who have diffuse areas of neoplastic change involving wide areas for which the term "field cancerization" has been used. If the area is reasonably small, excision and coverage with a free skin graft or with a pedicle graft may be feasiable. In occasional patients, the area of involvement is so great that radiation therapy becomes the best option.

Pharyngeal Lesions

Early pharyngeal cancers are not often seen. It is not uncommon, however, when operating for an advanced laryngeal or pharyngeal cancer, to find small second primary lesions in the pharynx. These are usually amenable to excision as part of the planned operation. Occasionally an early pharyngeal cancer is discovered in the long-term follow-up of a previously treated patient. Such lesions can be excised or can be treated by radiation therapy. Multicentricity is not uncommon in the pharynx, particularly in the faucial area, and this can pose a difficult treatment problem.

Laryngeal Lesions

In the larynx, the wide spectrum encompassed by the term *chronic laryngitis* poses many diagnostic and treatment challenges. It is essential to have a high index of suspicion and a readiness to carry out biopsy procedures, usually by suspension laryngomicroscopy. When a definite diagnosis is reached, appropriate treatment may include the full range of modalities, both radiotherapeutic and surgical, with possible inclusion of cold steel excisions, laser, and electrocoagulation. Choice among the available options is governed by a number of factors, including the experience and preferences of the personnel available.

EPIDEMIOLOGY

Fascinating material is available on geographic patterns in head and neck cancer incidence. The fact that oral cancer has such a high incidence in India and its relationship to betel chewing and smoking habits

in the subcontinent are subjects of great interest. Available evidence suggests that the causative factor in the development of gingivobuccal cancer in India is the tobacco added to the quid. In the Bombay area, it is not uncommon to find a more posterior type of oral cancer (base of tongue), presumably related to the smoking of a type of native cigarette, the bidi. Extensive studies of the precancerous mucosal lesions seen in Indian villagers have been carried out by Pindborg and associates. Studies such as these carry considerable potential for increasing our understanding of the stages in development of neoplastic disease in the mucosa of the UADT.

CONCLUSION

The advanced stages of head and neck cancer cause severe degrees of human misery and, eventually, death. The potential is high for recognition of neoplasia of the UADT in its early stages. Early discovery carries the probability for high cure rates.

REFERENCES

1. Shedd D, Hukill P, Bahn S, Ferraro R. Further appraisal of in vivo staining properties of oral cancer. Arch Surg 1967; 96:16.
2. Atkinson D, Fleming S, Weaver A. Triple endoscopy, a valuable procedure in head and neck surgery. Am J Surg 1982; 144:416.
3. Pindborg JJ. Lesions of the oral mucosa to be considered premalignant and their epidemiology. In: Mackenzie I, Dabelsteen E, Squier C, eds. Oral Premalignancy. Proceedings of the First Dow Symposium. Iowa City: University of Iowa Press, 1980.

EARLY CANCER OF THE HEAD AND NECK: DIAGNOSTIC CONSIDERATIONS

ARTHUR WEAVER, M.D.

Squamous cell cancer of the head and neck is best understood as a local manifestation of a life style-induced systemic disorder affecting all of the mucous membranes of the upper aerodigestive tract. The concept that a single cell or a few cells suddenly change behavior and then run rampant, producing a cancer that grows from a single locus, is no longer an acceptable explanation of this disease. Accumulated evidences now indicate that all of the surface epithelial cells of the upper aerodigestive tract are slowly being modified by often identifiable carcinogens and are thus being progressively transformed into premalignant or malignant cells. Multiple tumors arising

synchronously or metachronously in this area now present one of the major dilemmas in successful management of cancers of the head and neck.

My personal experience indicates that approximately 10 percent of the patients with squamous cell cancer have another cancer in the head and neck area, lung, or esophagus, found synchronously at the initial work-up. Each year I see several patients with what I have chosen to call "bases loaded" carcinoma: malignant disease presenting simultaneously in the lung, esophagus, and head and neck region. In addition to those tumors that may present initially, new metachronous lesions occur in approximately 7 percent of my cancer patients each year thereafter. I inform my patients that a second head and neck cancer is likely if their life style does not change following successful therapy of their initial tumor. These individuals have already shown sensitivity to these tumor-inducing agents by developing their first cancer, and only death or life style changes will preclude the development of additional head and neck malignant disease. Dr. Joseph S. Incze of the Veterans Administration Medical Center in Boston has published fascinating evidence of these induced cellular changes.[1] He has shown that biopsy specimens of grossly and histologically normal mucous membrane taken from patients with known head and neck cancer and from heavy smokers without cancer demonstrate similar electron microscopic mucosal alterations. He has identified several gradations of cellular change, from normal to frankly malignant, induced by tobacco. Happily, he has also demonstrated that many of these changes are reversible for individuals who quit smoking. It seems appropriate then to view the mucosa of the heavy smoker and/or drinker as being in some stage of alteration on the road to maligancy.

Several years ago, after being repeatedly "burned" by having a second cancer show up in the head and neck area, or the esophagus, or the bronchus of patients for whom I had treated squamous cell cancer, I determined to do a triple endoscopy on all my patients before starting therapy.[2,3] I have found that these laryngoscopic, bronchoscopic, and esophagoscopic examinations can be safely and effectively performed under local anesthesia. The subsequent surprise of discovering unsuspected lesions readily viewable by endoscopy of the aerodigestive tract is thus usually avoided.

Head and neck cancer occurs infrequently in individuals who use neither tobacco nor alcohol, and heavy use of either of these substances should alert the physician to the possibility of head and neck malignant disease. I have suggested that mouthwash may serve as a weak mucosal carcinogen for some patients who use these substances compulsively[4] When we analyzed 200 consecutive patients with squamous cell cancer on our head and neck service, we found 11 patients who had no history of beverage alcohol and tobacco use, but used mouthwash compulsively. Most mouthwashes contain significant amounts of alcohol (average 15 to 28%). There was only one patient with head cancer in whom there no history of tobacco or alcohol (including mouthwash) use.

Early premalignant changes and T1 cancers are seldom symptomatic. Detection of these lesions therefore requires a careful plan and meticulous technique of examination. Early cancer and even carcinoma in situ are recognizable on gross examination. These changes, however, are subtle. The experienced examiner carries a significant advantage in the gross diagnosis of these lesions. Condict Moore, in analyzing the sites of origin for cancer in the oral cavity, has pointed out that the floor of the mouth, retromolar trigone, tonsilar fauces, and lateral tongue are the sites of most frequent occurrence.[5] Frequently, physicians other than those with special interest in these areas fail to do a thorough examination of the oral cavity, pharynx, and larynx when examining asymptomatic patients. I believe that physicians should take a lesson from our dental colleagues who are emphasizing a routine careful oral examination for cancer. This is most important for patients past 40 years of age who

use tobacco or alcohol. Appropriate examination of the oral cavity requires a relaxed patient, a good source of light, and appropriate equipment. Most examiners who are not thoroughly experienced with the use of a head mirror will find a good fiberoptic headlight a comfortable light source. Tongue blades, gauze, and laryngeal and nasopharyngeal mirrors are the only other necessities for a routine cancer examination of the head and neck area.

THE EXAMINATION

The examination begins with a careful observation of the anatomic landmarks and survey of the face and neck for any possible asymmetry or observable skin lesions. Palpation of the neck and thyroid area may reveal thyroid abnormality or significant enlarged neck nodes. Examination of the oral cavity, pharynx, and hypopharynx should systematically include all the visible mucous membranes of these areas. Palpation of any suspicious areas, particularly of the posterior tongue, can be important supplementation to visual examination. Use of laryngeal and nasopharyngeal mirrors is not difficult to learn if these examinations are made a routine part of the head and neck examination.

The Lips

The vermillion border of the lips is the most likely area to be involved with premalignant or early malignant changes. Fissures, ulcers, or patches of leukoplakia should be noted.

Buccal Mucosa

With the mouth open, the light source is focused on the buccal mucosa. Observe the parotid orifices and their secretion. Survey the mucous membrane of the entire inner cheek. This is a particularly common place for leukoplakia to be noted in smokers. Pipe and cigar smoke, snuff, or chewing tobacco use may also produce chronic inflammatory or malignant changes in this area. The snuff user may also have leukoplakia or malignant change in the sulcus between the lower lip and gum.

Floor of the Mouth

The anterior floor of the mouth is best observed by having the individual elevate the tip of the tongue to the palate. A careful examination with good light of this area reveals the submaxillary ducts and any evidences of ulceration or leukoplakia. It is important to compare the symmetry of both sides of the floor of the mouth and note any color or texture differences. Bimanual palpation of the floor of the mouth may also be valuable.

The Tongue

The patient is asked to stick out his tongue, and deviation or asymmetry is noted. The tongue is grasped with gauze and each side of the tongue is closely inspected back to the retromolar trigone. Palpation of the lateral and posterior tongue are particularly valuable, and a quick sweep of the examining finger may pick up carcinomas that might otherwise be missed.

Hard and Soft Palate

With the head titled back and the light focused, these areas should be examined for asymmetry, protrusions, and texture changes. One should be aware of the torus palatinus, which is a developmental change that has been mistaken for carcinoma of this region.

Faucial Arches and Tonsils

A tongue blade and light help to bring this region into focus. The anterior tonsilar pillar and tonsilar fauces are particularly frequent sites for malignant change. Palpation of the tonsil may also help to detect a carcinoma that might otherwise be missed.

Teeth and Gums

Although the aveolar ridges are not a particularly common site for oral cancer, tumors can occasionally be found here, and examination to note any associated dental problems is important.

Larynx and Nasopharynx

Techniques for indirect mirror examination of the larynx and nasopharynx are easily found in standard texts and will be omitted here. The base of the tongue, vallecula, epiglottis, larynx, and hypopharynx are each carefully inspected with the laryngeal mirror.

While examining the larynx, it is important to notice motion of the arytenoids and vocal cords as well as any asymmetry or pooling within the piriform sinuses. A good examination of the nasopharynx is more difficult to learn, but can be mastered with some practice. Fortunately, in this country, carcinoma of the nasopharynx is rather infrequent.

Early carcinoma of the mucous membranes of the head and neck may have various presentations:

1. *A white area (leukoplakia).* White patches in the oral cavity may vary from diffuse, barely perceptible changes in the mucous membrane to highly thickened plaques with heaped up or verrucose appearance. Ulcers, and indurated areas within leukoplakia may indicate malignant change. Leukoplakia found in areas other than the alveolar ridges should be considered suspect.

2. *Red areas (erythroplakia).* True erythroplakia presents as velvety, totally red patches of the mucous membrane and is an unusual presentation. Areas of ulceration in this lesion suggest invasive carcinoma.

3. *Mixed red and white patches (erythroleukoplakia).* More frequently, early carcinoma does not present as a purely white or purely red lesion, but has a variegated appearance of red, slightly ulcerated mucous membrane speckled with flecks of white hyperkeratosis. Carcinoma in situ frequently gives this variegated appearance, and when the area is wiped with gauze, petechial hemorrhages occur from this minor trauma.

Ulcers

Ulceration of the mucous membrane is associated with a number of benign and malignant conditions. Inflamatory ulcers are usually painful, and malignant ulcers may also on occasion be tender. Gentle palpation of the ulcer area may reveal induration, which suggests the possibility of malignancy.

Masses

Most carcinomas presenting as masses cannot be classified as early cancer. Carcinomas of the oral cavity, however, can have minimal surface erosion and considerable deep tumor proliferation. In such instances the lesion is more easily palpated than visualized.

ANCILLARY EXAMINATION TECHNIQUES

Some have suggested that magnification is of value in oral examination. It may not be practical for routine examination, but is best reserved for questionable areas of mucosal change. The magnification associated with the bronchoscope and the esophagoscope can be used with particular benefit for observing mucosal changes. Both of these instruments can also be used for magnified examination of the larynx.

Toluidine blue application to an area of suspected oral cancer stains the area of the carcinoma and any adjacent carcinoma in situ. Toluidine blue does not stain normal mucosa. It does, however, color many benign lesions and leukoplakia.

To perform this test, the patient should rinse his mouth and swallow several sips of water. Excess saliva should be suctioned from the mouth and 1 percent acetic acid solution should be applied to the suspected area. Excess fibrin or debris in an ulcer should be removed by suction or gauze, and a small amount of 1 percent toluidine blue should be applied to the lesion and surrounding mucosa. The patient then should rinse his mouth with water to flush out the excess dye. The abnormal mucus membrane is stained by this technique.

This technique seems more valuable for the physician who sees an occasional case of head and neck cancer. Subtle changes are more likely to be evident to the experienced examiner. Adjacent epithelium surrounding most cancers is undergoing significant cellular change, and if the tumor is to be appropriately treated, this area must be included in any treatment program.

Exfoliative cytology has been recommended as a method for diagnosis of oral cancer. Indeed, malignant cells are frequently shed from carcinoma in situ and invasive cancer of the oral cavity. However, there may be false-positive and false-negative results with this technique, and it is not a substitute for a good biopsy specimen.

Biopsy

Small lesions of the oral cavity can be adequately treated and diagnosed by excisional biopsy. Failure to get a positive biopsy in a suspected cancer requires tissue recuts or rebiopsy. Dr. Crissman, in his chapter, has emphasized the necessity for appropriate tissue specimen.

SUMMARY

The physician's best aid in the diagnosis of early head and neck cancer is a high index of suspicion. Every long-term smoker is suspect for this disease. The patient who also combines significant alcohol intake with his smoking habit becomes a prime suspect. Any patient who has had squamous cell cancer of the upper aerodigestive tract remains as a "red alert" suspect until he makes a complete life style change for several years. We recommend triple endoscopy for these patients with any sign or symptoms suggesting head and neck cancer.

REFERENCES

1. Incze J, Vaughan CW, Lui P, Strong MS, Kulapaditharom B. Malignant changes in normal appearing epithelium in patients with squamous cell carcinoma of the upper aerodigestive tract. Am J Surg 1982; 144:401–405.
2. Weaver A, Fleming SM, Knechtges TC, Smith DB. Triple endoscopy: A neglected essential in head and neck cancer. Surgery 1979; 86:493–496.
3. Atkinson D, Fleming SM, Weaver A. Triple endoscopy: A valuable procedure in head and neck surgery. Am J Surg 1982; 144:416–418.
4. Weaver A, Fleming SM, Smith DB. Mouthwash and oral cancer: carcinogen or coincidence? J Oral Surg 1979; 37:250–253.
5. Moore C, Catlin D. Anatomic origens of oral cancer. Am J Surg 1967; 114:510–513.

HISTOPATHOLOGIC DIAGNOSIS OF EARLY CANCER

JOHN D. CRISSMAN, M.D.

The pathologist's role in early cancer diagnosis is a complex and challenging responsibility. Clear definition of the histopathologic expression of intraepithelial neoplastic transformation in squamous mucosa of the upper aerodigestive tract is not well documented. This is in contradistinction to intraepithelial precursor changes in the uterine cervix, where the histopathologic definitions (and nomenclature) are well defined. It must be recognized by the head and neck surgeon that the histologic categorization of epithelial dysplasia represents an estimation by the pathologist of the probability of the epithelial alteration progressing to invasive cancer if left untreated or incompletely excised. With the increased use of endoscopic examination with multiple biopsies, it is anticipated that more detailed histopathologic criteria will eventually evolve that will better define the mucosal changes which represent true transformation to intraepithelial neoplasia.

This chapter reflects many of the observations that I have made in conjunction with my surgical colleagues over the past decade. It must be stressed that the pathologist cannot provide the best diagnosis without first understanding the clinicopathologic implications of the diagnosis. The latter demands a close working relationship between pathologist and head and neck surgeon to provide optimum patient care. It has been my pleasure to be associated with an inquisitive group of surgeons, initially at the University of Cincinnati and currently at Wayne State University. I appreciate the time they have taken to educate me about head and neck cancer and to stimulate my interest in this group of diseases.

MUCOSAL ALTERATIONS PRECEDING SQUAMOUS CELL CARCINOMA: LEUKOPLAKIA AND ERYTHROPLAKIA

The reaction of squamous mucosa to injury depends on the anatomic site involved. Even in the upper aerodigestive tract mucosa, preneoplastic and neoplastic hyperplasias have different morphologic expressions in different sites. The usual reaction of any squamous mucosa to injury includes cellular proliferation or hyperplasia, either of a reactive (reversible) or neoplastic (irreversible) type. The pathologist's objective is to identify which of these changes is neoplastic and likely to persist/progress or recur.

Mucosal hyperplasia is reflected by epithelial thickening (acanthosis) and varying degrees of accumulation of surface keratin (hyperkeratosis), regardless of the type of injury. These hyperplastic changes are most commonly encountered in the buccal mucosa, alveolar ridge, hard palate, dorsal tongue, and laryngeal glottis, resulting in a clinical appearance of leukoplakia. The histologic expression of leukoplakia is usually an orderly progression or maturation of the cells from the basilar layer to the anucleated surface keratin. In spite of this orderly histology, leukoplakia is often considered one of the precursor states of squamous cell carcinoma. Careful study of both the gross appearance and the histology of leukoplakia does not appear to support this concept (Table 1). Follow-up of patients with clinical leukoplakia results in an appreciable but low frequency of transformation to invasive squamous cell carcinomas (Table 2). The majority of homogeneous leukoplakia mucosal changes are usually found on the buccal mucosa, dorsal tongue, and alveolar ridges, anatomic sites in which invasive carcinomas are relatively infrequent (Table 3). However, it must be stressed that leukoplakia changes in the floor of the mouth, ventral tongue, and soft palate must be viewed with suspicion, as these anatomic sites are more commonly associated with malignant transformation.

Conversely, erythroplakic or red mucosal changes commonly represent carcinoma in situ (CIS) or invasive carcinomas and have a high risk of transformation to malignancy. Erythroplakia is the most common mucosal change in early asymptomatic squamous cell carcinoma, and therefore must always be viewed with suspicion. The mucosa is thin and consists of atypical cells with abnormal epithelial maturation. The most common sites of erythroplakia are the floor of the mouth, ventral tongue, soft palate-tonsil complex,

TABLE 2   Malignant Transformation of Clinical Oral Leukoplakias

	No. of Patients Observed	Observation periods/years range (mean)	Percentage of Subsequent Carcinomas
Pindborg (1968)[5]	248	1–9	4.4*
Silverman & Rozen (1968)[6]	117	1–11 (3.5)	5.9†
Einhorn & Wersall (1967)[7]	782	1–20 (12)	4‡
Banoczy (1977)[8]	670	1–30 (9.8)	6.0

*3.7 years to development of cancer; 7 patients had speckled appearance.

†3.4 years to development of cancer; 2 patients with speckled appearance.

‡Cumulative frequency for patients observed 20 years.

pyriform sinus, and other areas of the hypopharynx, corresponding to the common sites of squamous cell carcinomas (see Table 3). Mixed or speckled patterns of admixed white and red mucosal changes represent a variant of erythroplakia (see Table 1). It is possible that many of the early reports of the high association of leukoplakia with significant epithelial abnormalities represented leukoplakia with erythroplakia or speckled mucosal change and not pure leukoplakias.

EPITHELIAL ALTERATION PRECEDING CARCINOMA

It is well documented that erythroplakic mucosa represents major epithelial maturation abnormalities with associated cytologic atypia. These alterations are analogous to intraepithelial neoplasia of the female genital tract. One major histologic difference is that the upper aerodigestive tract is normally keratinized and often responds to injury by developing surface keratin. This keratinizing form of dysplasia is less common in the female genital tract.

In biopsies from thin mucosa with little maturation or surface keratinization, the neoplastic nature of the intraepithelial change is usually obvious. When there are attempts at epithelial maturation, a diagnosis of mild or moderate intraepithelial neoplasia or dysplasia is indicated. When there is total, or near-total, replacement of the mucosa by "uncommitted" basaloid-appearing cells, with little or no evidence of epithelial maturation or organization (differentiation), the intraepithelial changes are indicative of severe dysplasia or CIS. Admittedly, the separation of these four subgroups of epithelial changes (mild, moderate, severe dysplasia and CIS) are somewhat subjective, but this combination of maturation abnormalities of the epithelium and the cytologic atypias of individual cells define the current grading system.

In my experience, the most important criterion for diagnosing neoplastic transformation in upper aerodigestive tract mucosa is the loss of epithelial organization and abnormal maturation within the epi-

TABLE 1   Histopathologic Changes Associated with Mucosal Appearance

	Dysplasia		Carcinoma	
	Leukoplakia			
Mashberg (1978)[1]	3/43	(7%)	3/43	(7%)
Waldron & Shafter (1975)[2]	153/3256	(5%)	104/3256	(3%)
Silverman et al. (1984)[3]	2/107	(2%)	7/107	(7%)
	Speckled Leukoplakia and Erythroplakia			
Mashberg (1978)[1]	6/58	(10%)	33/58	(57%)
Silverman et al. (1984)[3]	20/128	(16%)	30/128	(23%)
	Erythroplakia			
Mashberg (1978)[1]	1/44	(2%)	28/44	(64%)*
Shafer & Waldron (1975)[4]	26/65	(40%)†	33/65	(51%)

*Includes both CIS and invasive cancer.

†65 biopsies in 58 patients from a series of 64,354 biopsy specimens.

TABLE 3   Distribution of Mucosal Changes in the Oral Cavity: Number of Patients (percent of total patients)

	Tonsil Retromolar Trigone	Floor of Mouth	Tongue	Palate	Buccal	Alveolar	Lip
Histopathology							
Oral Dysplasia/CIS Waldron & Shafer (1975)[2]	10 (3.3)	45 (15)	22 (7.3)	34 (11.3)	54 (17.9)	51 (16.9)	75 (25)
Oral CIS Shafer (1975)[9]	6 (7.3)	19 (23.2)	18 (22)	5 (6.1)	9 (11)	9 (11)	16 (19.5)
Oral Dysplasia Mincer et al (1972)[10]	3 (4.5)	11 (16.4)	8 (11.9)	4 (6.0)	9 (13.4)	18 (26.9)	14 (21)
Mucosal Appearance							
Erythroplakia Shafer & Waldron (1975)[4]	12 (18.8)	18 (28.1)	8 (12.5)	8 (12.5)	5 (7.8)	13 (20.3)	—
Leukoplakia Waldron & Shafer (1975)[2]	197 (5.9)	289 (8.6)	277 (6.8)	361 (10.7)	736 (21.9)	1204 (35.9)	346 (10.3)

thelium. Normally, the squamous mucosa matures in an organized fashion with a well-defined basal layer. The suprabasal cells are also small, but increase in size as they migrate to the surface. The nuclei are generally equidistant from each other, resulting in an orderly "mosaic" appearance. Near the surface, cytoplasmic keratinization develops and the cells alter their orientation. Loss of this orderly maturation with mosaic distribution of nuclei along with altered cytologic characteristics (e.g., N/C ratio, nuclear pleomorphisms) results in mucosal alterations diagnostic of intraepithelial neoplasia or dysplasia.

Cellular atypia is difficult to define, and assessment of cytologic alterations is partially dependent on the location of the cell within the epithelium. Cells with abundant cytoplasm are normal near the surface of squamous mucosa and distinctly abnormal near the basal layers. Likewise, cytoplasmic keratinization is normal near the mucosal surface and markedly abnormal in the depths of the epithelium. The proliferation of small "uncommitted" cells normally found near the basal layer are distinctly abnormal when they comprise a substantial portion of the mucosa. The distribution of mitotic figures is also helpful in assessing mucosal maturation. Normally, mitoses are only found in or near the basal layer in the morphologically uncommitted cell populations. Identification of mitoses in the upper layers of the mucosa is another indication of loss of normal maturation. Identification of abnormal mitoses is essentially found only in neoplastic transformed mucosa.

Nuclear alterations are also important parameters in evaluating cytologic atypia. The rationale of this observation is that changes in nuclear size, shape, and staining represent alterations in chromosomal content. Unfortunately, hematoxylin stains a number of nuclear proteins besides DNA. By the use of the Feulgen staining reaction specific for DNA, it has been demonstrated that increased DNA is present in intraepithelial neoplasia.[15,16] The increase in DNA over normal levels is referred to as hyperdiploid and represents an abnormal or aneuploid chromosomal population, a marker of neoplastic transformation. Figures 1 and 3 both represent examples of intraepithelial neoplasia as demonstrated by the accompanying DNA histograms in Figures 2 and 4. The histograms were performed by Dr. Y. S. Fu utilizing Feulgen DNA staining and microspectrophotometric analysis. The critical issue remains: at what point can we distinguish mild-to-moderate mucosal alterations that are truly neoplastic from those that are in response to some other reversible injury? In another chapter of this monograph, we have determined that DNA histograms of squamous cell carcinomas determined by flow cytometry correlate poorly with hematoxylin-stained nuclei. As a result, the classic cytologic observation of nuclear pleomorphism does not readily differentiate neoplastic aneuploidy from reactive tetraploidy or increases in nonchromosomal nuclear protein.

Most of the intraepithelial neoplasias of the upper aerodigestive tract have surface keratinization, and the agreement for evaluation of these forms of dysplasia/CIS is not well defined. As a result, the criteria for diagnosis and grading of intraepithelial neoplasia in the head and neck region is not uniform. It is my experience that the "classic" or nonkeratinizing form of intraepithelial neoplasia, which is common in the female genital tract, is uncommon in upper aerodigestive tract mucosa. The atypical cellular proliferations which commonly accompany neoplastic change are usually present in the lower portions of the epithelium and are manifested by either "premature" expression of keratin (dyskeratosis) or proliferation of morphologically uncommitted or "undifferentiated" cells. In many instances both features are present. Nuclear pleomorphism, reflected by variation in nuclear size, shape, and staining, is usually present, along with increased numbers of mitotic figures.

An anatomic site that is characteristic of this form

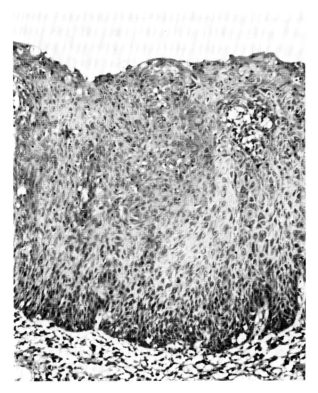

Figure 1 Photomicrograph of an intraepithelial neoplastic transformation in a hyperplastic epithelium. This tissue, which is representative of extensive intraepithelial proliferation, was taken from multiple sites in the larynx. Invasive neoplasm was not identified.

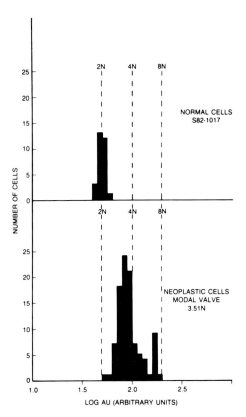

Figure 2 DNA histogram of the epithelial changes noted in Figure 1. All the nuclei demonstrate significant increases in DNA content, confirming the neoplastic nature of the hyperplasia.

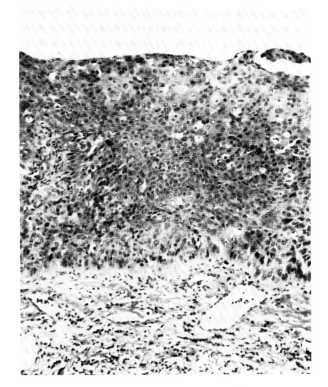

Figure 3 Photomicrograph of thickened hyperplastic laryngeal epithelium with a minimum of demonstrable squamous differentiation. The mucosa is hypercellular with varying degrees of organization. In most areas the nuclei are closely approximated with loss of tissue organization.

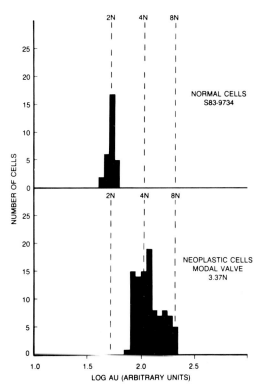

Figure 4 DNA histogram from the tissue demonstrated in Figure 3. There is a significant shift in the DNA histogram with an aneuploid distribution.

of thickened hyperkeratotic intraepithelial neoplasia is the laryngeal glottis. The glottis represents a special type of squamous mucosa possessing a high propensity for development of surface keratin. Instances of injury to the glottic mucosa usually cause marked proliferation of the epithelium, resulting in acanthosis and some accumulation of surface keratin, which may appear leukoplakic. Erythroplakic changes are seldom encountered in the glottis, but do occur in other sites in the laryngeal mucosa. In several series of carefully studied laryngeal glottic dysplasias or keratoses, between 3.26 percent and 4.31 percent developed subsequent invasive carcinomas (Table 4). The well differentiated nature of most epithelial proliferations of the laryngeal glottis usually do not demonstrate appreciable cytologic atypia, which is reflected by the low frequency of progression to invasive cancers. It should be noted that a select subgroup of these patients do not demonstrate severe maturation or cytologic abnormalities characteristic of severe intraepithelial neoplastic transformation. However, the mucosal alterations which persist or recur after vocal cord stripping, indicating neoplastic change, are the epithelial changes that bear close follow-up.[17]

GRADING OF INTRAEPITHELIAL NEOPLASIA

The diagnosis of severe or high-grade intraepithelial neoplasia is usually reproducible among experienced pathologists. When sufficient proliferation of small morphologically uncommitted cells comprises the majority of the mucosal thickness, or when marked maturation and cytologic abnormalities are found, severe grade of intraepithelial neoplasia is an appropriate diagnosis. It is generally agreed, but not well documented, that severe mucosal alterations have an appreciable frequency of either persistence or transformation to invasive carcinomas (Table 5). The division of severe intraepithelial neoplastic changes into severe dysplasia and CIS is not only difficult but highly subjective. Both changes are defined to represent degrees in the spectrum of intraepithelial neoplasia approaching invasive carcinoma. Their separation represents an estimation of the frequency of progression to invasive cancer, an estimation often difficult to derive on morphologic grounds. It is suggested that an alternative approach, similar to the scheme proposed for the female genital tract, is to classify the histologic criteria for severe dysplasia and

TABLE 4 Frquency of Subsequent Carcinoma in Laryngeal Keratoses/Dysplasia

	No. SCC/No. Patients	%
McGavran, Bauer, & Ogura (1960)[12]	3/84	3.57
Norris & Peale (1963)[13]	5/116	4.31
Crissman (1979)[14]	3/92	3/26

TABLE 5 Transformation of Oral Dysplasia to Carcinoma

		F/U Period (mean)
Silverman et al (1984)[3]	8/22 (36.4%)*	7.2 years
Banoczy and Csiba (1976)[11]	9/68 (13%)	6.3 years
Mincer et al (1972)[10]	5/45 (11%)	3.77 years†

*20/22 speckled pattern.
†Calculated from available data.

CIS as severe (grade III) squamous intraepithelial neoplasms (SIN III). This suggestion will undoubtedly provoke controversy, as does any suggested change in terminology. Nevertheless, it is extremely important for the surgeon to understand what disease the pathologist is attempting to define, regardless of the diagnostic terminology used. In order to maximize communication, the pathologist should be cognizant of the surgeon's findings prior to diagnosing mucosal biopsies, and conversely, the surgeon must understand the nature of the pathologist's definition of diagnostic terms used in the grading of intraepithelial neoplasia.

The major difficulties in classifying and diagnosing intraepithelial neoplasia exist in the moderate or intermediate group. This group displays clear epithelial maturation disturbances and cytologic abnormalities, but not to the extreme found in severe intraepithelial neoplasia. We know that intermediate forms of atypia represent a mixture of reversible hyperplasias and true neoplastic transformations. It is not possible to differentiate these two important subgroups and to accurately predict which patient will progress and which will regress. For this reason, I would suggest that they also be classified in an intermediate group, such as moderate dysplasia or SIN II. It is important for the pathologist and surgeon to understand that this group of epithelial changes are worrisome and need to be carefully monitored because their biologic behavior is unpredictable.

The final and least disturbing subgroup are those epithelial changes exhibiting only minor maturation and cytologic abnormalities. These mucosal injuries are highly unlikely to represent carcinogenic influences and invariably represent reversible hyperplasias that respond to conservative therapy. Because they are unlikely to represent intraepithelial neoplasia, the use of such terminology is inconsistent. A term descriptive of a reversible process, such as reactive hyperplasia or keratosis, would best inform the surgeon of the pathologist's assessment of the biologic potential of the excised mucosa.

EARLY INVASIVE OR MICROINVASIVE CARCINOMA

The differentiation between benign papillary ingrowth of hyperplastic mucosa and early neoplastic invasion of submucosal tissue is often difficult. In many situations, irregular poorly organized projections of squamous cells originating from an overlying neoplastic epithelium is easily diagnosed as early or microscopic invasion. When the mucosa is hyperplastic, without significant atypia or evidence of SIN, and projections extending into the submucosa are well organized, a diagnosis of pseudoepitheliomatous hyperplasia is appropriate. It is my impression that the key issues involved in this critical differential diagnosis are the status of the overlying epithelium (reactive versus neoplastic) and the pattern of the suspected foci of invasive epithelium. Figure 5 demonstrates an unequivocal focus of microinvasive carcinoma originating from an epithelium with neoplastic transformation confirmed by DNA analysis. When a well-defined basal layer with evidence of maturation is present, and the epithelium is sufficiently organized to appear capable of producing basement membrane at the epithelial-stromal interface, a diagnosis of papillary ingrowth or pseudoepitheliomatous change is indicated. When the suspected focus of invasion is poorly organized with appreciable cellular pleomorphism and irregular intercellular relationships, it is not a reactive process and a diagnosis of invasion is indicated. The interface of the epithelial and stromal demarcation is an important parameter in differentiating these two diagnoses. When the epithelium is sufficiently organized to cause suspicion that a basement membrane of normal thickness is present, the suspected epithelium is most likely to be reactive. These rules do not apply to verrucous neoplasms, which present a different spectrum of diagnostic problems.

Epithelial ingrowths which arise in a background of intraepithelial carcinoma and which have poorly demarcated borders with the host stroma represent invasive cancer. If the infiltration consists of single groups or cords of cells, it is invasive. When a broad band of epithelium extends into the submucosa, the differential between reactive and invasive neoplasm becomes more difficult. If there is sufficient cytologic atypia and lack of organization or orderly maturation, it is most likely to be invasive carcinoma. If there is a well-demarcated epithelial stromal interface and attempts at organization or maturation as if the epithelium is sufficiently organized to be producing basement membrane, I generally take a conservative posture and do not call them invasive. It is hoped that the use of immunohistochemistry to demonstrate the presence or absence of basement membrane (laminin or type IV collagen) will be helpful in this critical differential.[18] Lack of immunologically detectable basement membrane appears to represent a major step in differentiating malignant invasion from reactive ingrowths. This technique holds great promise and may represent a major contribution in helping the pathologists with this critical differential diagnosis. Examples of the use of this technique are demonstrated in Figures 6 and 7. Figure 6 demonstrates thickened epithelium with "reactive" papillary ingrowths with well-delineated basement membrane. Figure 7 represents carcinoma "pushing" into the underlying stroma without any demonstrable basement membrane, indicating true invasion.

The clinical significance of early or microinvasion is not clear, but in circumstances in which the pathologist is confident that the focus of early invasion is the most severe change present, i.e., in excisional biopsies or biopsies of small erythroplakic

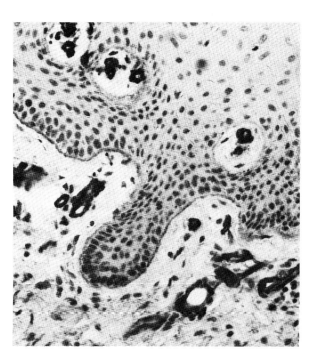

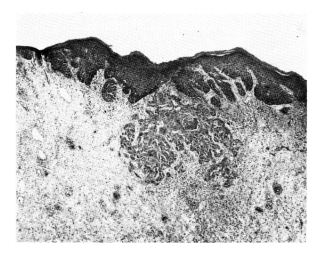

Figure 5 This is a lower magnification of laryngeal mucosa with extensive intraepithelial neoplastic transformation. DNA histograms confirmed the presence of aneuploid cell populations. This is an example of microinvasive squamous cell carcinoma arising in neoplastic epithelium. (× 81)

Figure 6 This photomicrograph demonstrates the distribution of basement membrane along the basal layer of hyperplastic epithelium. This is an immunoperoxsidase stain utilizing an antibody to type IV collagen, a component of basement membrane. (× 566)

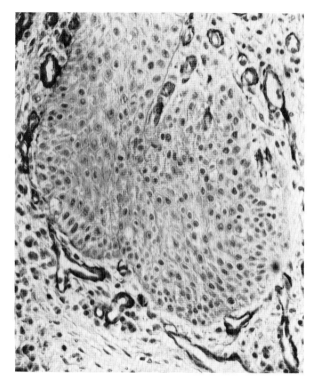

Figure 7 This photomicrograph demonstrates a papillary ingrowth from an abnormal-appearing epithelium which fails to demonstrate basement membrane. Note the strong reaction of type IV collagen in the basement membrane of the small blood vessels adjacent to the invading carcinoma. (× 566)

REFERENCES

1. Mashberg A. Erythroplasia: The earliest sign of asymptomatic oral cancer. J Am Dent Assoc 1978; 96:615–620.
2. Waldron CA, Shafer WG. Leukoplakia revisited. A clinicopathologic study of 3256 oral leukolplakias. Cancer 1975; 36:1386–1392.
3. Silverman S, Gorsky M, Lozada F. Oral leukoplakia and malignant transformation. Cancer 1984; 53:563–568.
4. Shafer WG, Waldron CA. Erythroplakia of the oral cavity. Cancer 1975; 36:1021–1028.
5. Pindborg JJ, Renstrup G, Poulsen HE, Silverman S. Studies in oral leukoplakias V. Clinical and histological signs of malignancy. Acta Odontol Scand 1963; 21:404–414.
6. Silverman S, Rozen RD. Observations on the clinical characteristics and natural history of oral leukoplakia. J Am Dent Assoc 1968; 76:772–777.
7. Einhorn J, Wersall J. Incidence of oral carcinoma in patients with leukoplakia of the oral mucosa. Cancer 1967; 20:2189–2193.
8. Banoczy J. Follow-up studies in oral leukoplakia. J Maxillofac Surg 1977; 5:69–75.
9. Shafer WG. Oral carcinoma in situ. Oral Surg 1975; 39:227–238.
10. Mincer H, Coleman SA, Hopkins KP. Observations on the clinical characteristics of oral lesions showing histologic epithelial dysplasia. Oral Surg 1972; 33:389–392.
11. Banoczy J, Csiba A. Occurrence of epithelial dysplasia in oral leukoplakia. Oral Surg 1976; 42:766–774.
12. McGavran MH, Bauer WC, Ogura JH. Isolated laryngeal keratosis: Its relation to carcinoma of the larynx based on a clinicopathologic study of 87 consecutive cases with long-term follow-up. Laryngoscope 1960; 70:932–950.
13. Norris CM, Peale AR. Keratosis of the larynx. J Laryngol Otol 1963; 77:635–647.
14. Crissman JD. Laryngeal keratosis and subsequent carcinoma. Head Neck Surg 1979; 1:386–391.
15. Giarelli L, Silverstri F, Antonutto G, Stanta G. Observations of the pathologist on precancerous lesions of the larynx. Acta Otolaryngol 1977; 84(Suppl 344):7–18.
16. Hellquist H, Olofsson J, Grontoft O. Carcinoma in situ and severe dysplasia of the vocal cords. Acta Otolaryngol 1981; 92:543–555.
17. Crissman JD. Laryngeal keratosis preceding laryngeal carcinoma. Arch Otolaryngol 1982; 108:445–448.
18. Barsky SH, Siegal GP, Jannotta F, Liotta LA. Loss of basement membrane components by invasive tumors but not their benign counterparts. Lab Invest 1983; 49:140–147.
19. Crissman JD, Gluckman J, Whiteley J, Quenelle D. Squamous cell carcinoma of the floor of the mouth. Head Neck Surg 1980; 3:2–7.

mucosal changes, a diagnosis of early or microinasive carcinoma is indicated. It appears that these foci of early invasion have a lower incidence of regional lymph node metastases and presumably distant spread. This allows the surgeon to modify the choice of treatment, possibly to a less radical procedure than commonly elected when an unqualified diagnosis of squamous cell carcinoma is rendered.[19]

TREATMENT OF EARLY LESIONS OF THE HEAD AND NECK

WILLARD E. FEE, Jr, M.D.
DON R. GOFFINET, M.D.

Few areas in medicine evoke as much controversy unsupported by scientific fact as this topic. As individuals, surgeons and radiotherapists may go to their graves defending their modality of treatment as better than the other, each having a spokesman claiming a higher chance of cure with less morbidity than the other. That person who speaks with the most authority and wins his way is certainly that person commanding the microphone, speaking with the loudest volume, being the most entertaining with beautiful slides, and falling unto defeat by the Aristotelian logical fallacy of *argumentum ad veracundium*.

There is little new that can be said about treatment of early lesions of the head and neck. Significant advances in treatment of early lesions may be on the horizon with the identification of tumor-associated antigens and/or tumor-specific antigens and resultant

Supported in part by the Jack Tang Fund.

production of monoclonal antibodies that prove to be clinically worthwhile in diagnosis and/or treatment directed against those antigens. If we are fortunate to discover the cause of head and neck cancer, surely more specific therapies will evolve, and this is not the subject of the remainder of this discussion. We choose to deal here with only those modalities which heretofore have been advocated for treatment of pathologic diagnoses that we now understand and to provide some thoughts on directions of treatment of early lesions. Even this disclaimer does not forecast a hopefully anticipated change in pathologic differentiation of disease processes of the head and neck as we know them today. Consider the breakthrough that immune typing might have on the future treatment of lymphomas. Let us hope that a similar breakthrough evolves in our area of interest.

LEUKOPLAKIA, DYSPLASIA, AND ATYPIA

If we assume that epithelial dysplasia and/or atypia reflects the epithelium's attempt to deal with some noxious stimulus, all one needs to do is eliminate the noxious stimulus and most of these aberrations will disappear. The problem is that we continue to see people with these epithelial changes who do not smoke, drink alcohol, or wear dentures, and so it becomes difficult or impossible to treat some patients by the process of elimination because the offending agent(s) cannot be identified. Disheartening is the fact that several studies document a similar rate of progression to invasive cancer in those patients who quit smoking compared to those who continued to smoke.[1,2] Certainly it is beneficial to the overall health of the patient to eliminate any noxious stimulus, and we encourage them to do so with such quotes as ''Smoking (or drinking) is good for our business'' or ''Smoking is a poison to the body; you need your body to live.'' Close observation of these patients with early liberal biopsies of suspicious areas is all that can be done at present. Certainly, no one would advocate the use of chemotherapy, radiation therapy, or radical surgery for simple leukoplakia or epithelial dysplasia.

Speckled leukoplakia and erythroplakia are best considered ''premalignant'' or ''malignant-associated'' diseases and require excisional biopsy and close follow-up of the patient because of their high association (28% to 91%) with either carcinoma in situ or frankly invasive carcinoma.[3,4] The use of toluidine blue staining may be helpful to those who do not see many early cancers, but we frankly have not yet found a patient with an area that stained positively with toluidine blue from whom we would not already have obtained a biopsy. Strong disagrees and advocates supravital staining for all patients with these early lesions, believing that in approximately 1 of 10 patients, an area will stain positively that would not otherwise have been detected.[5]

Excisional biopsy of only the mucosa is necessary to obtain tissue for a thorough pathologic examination to eliminate the possibility of carcinoma in situ or frank invasive cancer. If the pathologist has difficulty differentiating between in situ and early invasive cancer, re-biopsy (taking a thin layer of submucosal tissue or muscle, depending on the location) or treating the patient as if it were an invasive cancer is indicated. Hard data are lacking in this regard, but the work of Gillis et al suggests that almost 20 percent of patients with leukoplakia of the larynx progress to invasive squamous cell carcinoma regardless of the treatment modality.[1] Perhaps in this group of patients with speckled leukoplakia and/or erythroplakia there is a role for experimental therapies such as treatment with retinoic acid; these studies are already under way and within our lifetime some answers will be forthcoming. Personally, we favor surgical excision of these lesions and do not think it makes any difference whether or not it is done with cold steel, the laser, or the Shaw Hemostatic Scalpel. There is nothing more efficient and less expensive than cold steel excision. Although the laser may get the job done, it is at the expense of increased time and very costly instrumentation, and we are unable to advocate its use except when coupled to the microscope for use in laryngeal disease. Cryosurgery or electrodesiccation may be effective in achieving the desired end result of return to a normal mucosa, but without the ability to establish a firm diagnosis of carcinoma in situ and/or invasive squamous cell carcinoma. We mention them only to condemn their use in this setting.

An adequate specimen surgically removed must be properly handled by the surgeon and pathologist in order to obtain the correct diagnosis. Most of the specimens are small (1 cm × 1 cm × 0.2 cm) and should be placed in saline to prevent drying, placed on Gelfoam with the epithelial surface up, folded, and deposited in formalin to prevent coiling of the specimen. By alternate method, the tissue is fixed to dehydrated cucumber slices with glue and then the entire unit is processed as a block.[6]

CARCINOMA IN SITU

Carcinoma in situ is a pathologic diagnosis that has evoked considerable controversy as to the best form of treatment. Almost any form of treatment is adequate as long as it treats or removes all of the offending mucosa. By definition, nothing more than the mucosa need be treated or removed, and in all cases the result should be 100 percent cure.

Whatever the treatment modality, there is a recurrence rate and development of invasive squamous cell carcinoma due to unknown patient factors or the vagaries in surgical and/or radiation therapy skills. There is also the possibility that the diagnosis may have been incorrect and that what may have been interpreted as a carcinoma in situ may really have been an invasive carcinoma had the specimen been serially sectioned with review of every section, which is not only impractical but phenomenally expensive.

Theoretically, the radiation therapist would have an edge over the surgeon in treating a broader volume, but the facts remain that the treatment successes are essentially equal and no randomized prospective study has been performed. Thus, selection of treatment for carcinoma in situ would depend on the lesions's location, the skill of the surgeon and radiotherapist involved in the patient's treatment, and the psychosocial and medical needs of the patient. For example, carcinoma in situ of the anterior tongue, floor of mouth, buccal mucosa, or alveolar ridge can be easily treated under a local anesthetic in an outpatient setting by a qualified surgeon, efficiently and inexpensively, with only a minimal amount of discomfort to the patient. An excellent specimen can be obtained and oriented adequately for the pathologist in order to rule out the possibility of invasive squamous cell cancer. Lesions in the hypopharynx, on the other hand, present a more difficult challenge for the average surgeon in complete removal in one specimen without crush artifact for adequate pathologic interpretation. The average radiation therapist would have less difficulty treating a lesion in this area than would the average surgeon in our opinion.

EARLY INVASIVE CANCER

Invasive squamous cell cancers, when discovered early (stage 1), respond well to either modality of therapy at any site. In most cases there is little to recommend one modality of therapy over another when the skills of the treating physicians are equal and there are no supervening psychological factors. All that has been said regarding surgical techniques and instrumentation in the preceding section is applicable here as well.

Large T1 lesions of the anterior and posterior tongue, supraglottic larynx, and hypopharynx require treatment of the N0 neck by either radiation therapy or surgery, which is still another unresolved controversy. Even among surgeons there is disagreement whether a "functional" neck dissection (preserving the spinal accessory nerve, internal jugular vein, and sternocleidomastoid muscle) is the operation of choice in this setting. Our own preference is to utilize radiation therapy in most instances, as a 90 percent control rate has been demonstrated.[7]

FUTURE DIRECTIONS

The entire field of head and neck cancer treatment is plagued with the need for randomized, prospective studies. The inability of one physician (even one institution) to carry them out (owing to insufficient numbers of patients) makes this wanted scientific proof very difficult to obtain. Although frustrating from an intellectual point of view, the fact that there are few facts allows for ethical experimentation which provides excitement (and frequently disappointment) for the clinical investigator.

Hematoporphyrin-derivative (HpD) phototherapy for treatment of small localized lesions shows enough promise to warrant further experimentation.[8] HpD is a complex mixture of hematoporphyrin mono- and diacetate, vinyl porphyrins, proto- and deuteroporphyrins, and several additional porphyrin compounds. HpD has been shown to concentrate in the cytoplasm of normal and cancer cells within 3 hours after IV injection and begins to wash out of normal cells within 24 hours while it is retained in cancer cells and reticuloendothelial cells. When exposed to blue light, the HpD produces a salmon-red fluorescence in cancer cells. Precise cytotoxic mechanisms are poorly understood. An Argon laser is used to pump a dye laser, using Rhodamine B dye to produce an output wavelength of 630 nm, which can be focused into an optical fiber modified to produce a spot diameter of 5 to 10 mm. A "tuneable" wavelength laser has been developed by Coherent Radiation, Palo Alto, California, and should facilitate research in this area. Limitations of this technique are the size of lesion (<2 cm), skin photosensitivity, and availability of HpD. It may be possible to isolate purified porphyrins which will selectively be taken up and retained only by cancer cells, eliminating the photosensitivity problem and the need to keep patients in a reduced light environment after HpD injection. In terms of efficiency and efficacy, it is not likely that this technique will compete effectively for surgically accessible lesions. It shows promise for small tumors of the esophagus and tracheobronchial tree and will need to be compared to results of radiation therapy.

Sporadic research has been done on vitamin A and 13-cis-retinoic acid (13-C-RA) therapy for various keratoses of head and neck mucous membranes. Shah et al have not shown a lasting beneficial effect using 5 to 10 mg of 13-C-RA when applied topically in the form of oral lozenges;[9] however, Koch and Schettler reported a 57 percent remission of leukoplakia after oral administration of 60 mg/day of 13-C-RA.[10] Controlled, randomized, prospective, and double-blind clinical trials supported by Hoffman-La Roche are already under way to study its efficacy in patients with leukplakia/erythroplakia.

Hyperthermia combined with irradiation delivered by teletherapy or brachytherapy may prove more advantageous than irradiation therapy alone. Accessibility to currently available probes for heating is a significant limitation, although one of us (Goffinet) has developed a new catheter which can deliver both heat and brachytherapy to implanted areas.[11] Electron delivery by intraoral cones is also a likely technique to receive attention, but this technique will have difficulty competing with the efficiency of simple surgical excision.

The recent identification of tumor-associated and

tumor-specific antigens of squamous cell carcinoma by Carcinex (Burlingame, California) is the most exciting new development in our opinion, not only from a diagnostic viewpoint, allowing subidentification of squamous cell carcinoma, but also as a potential treatment with murine monoclonal antibodies. Phase II clinical trials may begin as early as 1985 and are likely to consume much of the clinical investigation in our center for the remainder of the decade.

Any new treatment modality for early lesions of the head and neck will need to be investigated with great care and with the realization that serious ethical considerations will need to be addressed. The fact remains that standard therapy (surgery or irradiation) produces such a high rate of cure for most areas that one could question the use of any other form of therapy. Fortunately, Human Investigation Committees at each center are empowered with the responsibility of fostering research and the protection of patients. We will have the burden of proof to show why new modalities should be tested at all. The need to develop new treatment modalities will continue until we are 100 percent successful in controlling every cancer or precancerous lesion, which is not likely in our lifetime.

REFERENCES

1. Gillis TM, Incze J, Strong MS, et al. Natural history and management of keratosis, atypia, carcinoma in situ, and microinvasive cancer of the larynx. Am J Surg 1983; 146:512–516.
2. Hellquist H, Lundergren J, Oloffson J. Hyperplasia, keratosis, dysplasia, and carcinoma in situ of the vocal cords. A follow-up study. Clin Otolaryngol 1982; 7:11–27.
3. Bancozy J, Csiba A. Occurrence of epithelial dysplasia in oral leukoplakia. Oral Surg 1976; 42:766–774.
4. Poswillo D. Evaluation, surveillance and treatment of panoral leukoplakia. J Maxillofac Surg 1975; 3:205–208.
5. Strong MS, Vaugh CW, Incze J. Toluidine blue in the diagnosis of cancer of the larynx. Arch Otolaryngol 1979; 91:515–519. (Reconfirmed by personal communication with MS Strong, July 14, 1984.)
6. Holinger LD, Miller AW. A specimen mount for small laryngeal biopsies. Laryngoscope 1982; 92:524–526.
7. Goffinet DR, Fee WE, Goode RL. Combined surgery and postoperative irradiation in the treatment of cervical lymph nodes. Arch Otolaryngol 1984; 110:736–738.
8. Cortese DA, Kinsey JH. Hematoporphyrin-derivative phototherapy for local treatment of cancer of the tracheobronchial tree. Ann Otol Rhinol Laryngol 1982; 91:652–655.
9. Shah JP, Strong EW, DeCosse JJ, et al. Effect of retinoids on oral leukoplakia. Am J Surg 1983; 146:466–470.
10. Koch H, Schettler D. Klinische Erfrahrungen mit Vitamin-A-saure-derivaten bei der Behandlung von Leukoplakien der Mundhschleimhaut. Dtsch Zahnaerztl Z 1973; 28:623.
11. Goffinet DR. US Patent Application No. PA 1009.

14. Management of the N0 Neck

INTRODUCTION

ELLIOT W. STRONG, M.D.

The status of the cervical lymph nodes in the patient with documented primary squamous cancer of the upper aerodigestive tract is of vital prognostic significance.[1] The management of the clinically negative (N0) neck in these patients is controversial. Alternatives include observation only, limited neck excision, modified neck dissection, radical neck dissection, or radiation therapy.

The error in clinical assessment of the N0 neck is variously reported from 10 to 50 percent. Dr. Cox addresses this in his presentation with further details. The likelihood of cervical nodal metastases from squamous cancer of the head and neck varies with the site and size (stage) of the primary cancer.[1] The ability to clinically detect metastases in lymph nodes depends on the extent of such nodal involvement, the configuration and muscular development of the neck,

and the expertise and experience of the examiner. There are few diagnostic aids beyond physical examination. Lymphangiography has little practical value,[2] radionuclide scanning is too imprecise and inaccurate, but computerized tomographic scanning holds some promise as a diagnostic tool,[3] at least in patients with more than microscopic disease. Minimal (subclinical) metastatic tumor continues to evade recognition by currently available diagnostic methods.

The various primary sites of tumor in the head and neck carry different risks of nodal metastases from very low (lip) to very high (nasopharynx).[1] It is generally agreed that the potential risk of nodal involvement of 15 percent or more justifies elective treatment of the cervical lymph nodes at risk. Dr. Schuller discusses the anatomic distribution of macroscopic and microscopic metastases. He points out that the distribution of metastatic tumor in lymph nodes is similar whether clinically apparent or occult and that, while most metastatic deposits are in the jugular lymph node chain, there are certainly metastases in the spinal accessory chain, particularly superiorly, in close proximity to the spinal accessory nerve. In rare instances tumor may be confined only to the spinal accessory lymph nodes. The risk of incomplete resection of such metastatic tumor while sparing the nerve is obvious, particularly if the tumor has penetrated the capsule of the involved lymph node.[4] If the primary tumor is to be treated by radiotherapy, the entire neck at risk should be electively irradiated. If the patient is to be treated surgically and if that excision demands exposure via the neck, the cervical lymph nodes should be electively removed as well. Although there has been no randomized study to document the validity of elective neck dissection, there has been more benefit derived from early than from delayed treatment of involved lymph nodes, those progressing from N0 to N+.[5,6]

Dr. Lingeman describes the fascial anatomy of the neck and the three choices of modified neck dissection to resect the lymph nodes. Although the modified neck dissection is a technically more demanding and time-consuming procedure if done adequately and carefully, it removes the same lymph nodes as are resected in the radical neck dissection. While there is no randomized controlled prospective study documenting the therapeutic superiority of modified over radical neck dissection,[7,8] our authors agree that the modified procedure is probably adequate in the N0 neck and results in significantly less postoperative shoulder morbidity. In general, the modified operation has as its keystone the preservation of the spinal accessory nerve.

Dr. Schuller addresses the subject of shoulder morbidity, which largely relates to trapezius muscle function. It is agreed that the anatomy of the nerve supply to the trapezius is variable and unpredictable, and while there are clinical studies comparing pre- and post-operative shoulder function in modified and radical neck dissections, they are clinical and lack precision and scientific documentation.[9] Some 40 percent of patients who undergo modified neck dissection preserving the spinal accessory nerve have postoperative shoulder disability, whereas only 60 percent of the patients who undergo classic radical neck dissection sacrificing the nerve have such postoperative dysfunction and disability. Further investigation of trapezius muscle innervation and scientific assessment of shoulder function following various modifications of neck dissection are necessary. Although modified neck dissection is an adequate procedure to provide a specimen for pathologic staging of cervical nodal disease, it is considered to be inadequate therapy for the clinically N+ neck. Any histologic evidence of metastatic tumor in the clinically N0 neck indicates the need for postoperative radiation therapy.

Dr. Cox believes that 5000 rads in 5 weeks with conventional fractionation is adequate for the eradication of subclinical disease, but that higher doses are necessary when microscopic metastases are recovered or gross tumor left behind. The increasing morbidity of such combined therapy related to radiation dose is recognized, and Dr. Schuller documents the extent of the functional sequelae in his presentation. It is generally agreed that radiation therapy should be delivered to all of both sides of the neck to prevent subsequent appearance of contralateral metastases, particularly in those primary sites approximating the midline, that is, the floor of the mouth, soft palate, nasopharynx, base of tongue, and supraglottic larynx. Although such combined therapy has not been shown to improve survival by randomized prospective studies, there does appear to be enhancement of local tumor control.

REFERENCES

1. Farr HW, Goldfarb PM, Farr CW. Epidermoid carcinoma of the mouth and pharynx at Memorial Sloan-Kettering Cancer Center, 1965 to 1969. Am J Surg 1980; 140:563–567.
2. Fisch UP, Siegel ME. Cervical lymphatic system as visualized by lymphography. Ann Otol 1964; 73:869–883.
3. Mancuso AA. Cervical lymph node metastases: oncologic imaging and diagnosis. Int J Rad Oncol Biol, Phys 1984; 10:411–423.
4. Johnson JT, Barnes EL, Myers EN, Schramm VL Jr, Borochovitz D, Siegler BA. The extracapsular spread of tumors in cervical node metastases. Arch Otolaryngol 1981; 107:725–729.
5. Spiro RH, Strong EW. Epidermoid carcinoma of the oral cavity and oropharynx: elective vs therapeutic radical neck dissection as treatment. Arch Surg 1973; 107:382–384.
6. Spiro RH, Strong, EW. Epidermoid carcinoma of the mobile tongue. Treatment by partial glossectomy alone. Am J Surg 1971; 122:707–710.
7. Lingeman RE, Helmus C, Stephens R, Ulm J. Neck dissection: radical or conservative. Ann Otol Rhinol Laryngol 1977; 86:737–744.
8. Jesse RH, Ballantyne AJ, Larsen D. Radical or modified neck dissection—a therapeutic dilemma. Am J Surg 1978; 136:516–519.
9. Leipzig B, Suen JY, English JL, Barnes J, Hooper M. Functional evaluation of the spinal accessory nerve after neck dissection. Am J Surg 1983; 146:526–530.

SURGICAL MANAGEMENT OF THE N0 NECK

RALEIGH E. LINGEMAN, M.D.

Surgery for management of the N0 neck has been done by a variety of operations. En bloc radical neck dissection has been accepted as the most effective method of surgical treatment of metastatic cancer of the neck, and the technique of this operation has become well standardized. It is done in a relatively short period of operating time and with an operative mortality for a unilateral procedure of less than 1 percent. This classic en bloc procedure has stood the test of time as the basic operation for control of metastatic cervical cancer and for the training of head and neck surgeons, but there are surgical schools of thought that favor a more conservative operation. These operations range from sparing of the spinal accessory nerve with radical neck dissection to modified neck dissection with preservation of the sternocleidomastoid muscle, internal jugular vein, spinal accessory nerve, and occasionally the cervical plexus.

HISTORICAL REVIEW

Credit for the first description of a well-structured anatomic dissection of the cervical lymphatics goes to George Crile, Sr. of Cleveland, who published his results with planned dissection of the cervical lymphatic of 132 operations in the Journal of the American Medical Association on December 1, 1906. Crile was a pioneer in surgery of the head and neck and for years had studied surgical anatomy of the neck aimed at clearing the cervical lymph nodes involved with metastasis from primary head and neck disease. Crile stated that the key to understanding thorough dissection of the neck was the need for excision of the internal jugular vein and its adnexal tissues in order to thoroughly remove the fibrofatty lymphatic tissue from the cervical region. For the next 60 years, it was accepted without question that the en bloc neck dissection needed to include the internal jugular vein, sternocleidomastoid muscle, and spinal accessory nerve in order to thoroughly remove the lymphatic system of the neck, and no serious objectives were raised concerning sacrifice of these structures. This procedure was well established as a safe and valuable ablative surgical technique by Hayes Martin, who published his results of this operation in 1951. Since that time, radical en bloc neck dissection has been a standard procedure for control of cervical metastasis from primary lesions of the head and neck region.

In 1960, John Conley modified the basic technique by introducing the posterior-cervical anatomic dissection, which without question is a superior anatomic technique of neck dissection. Beginning in 1966, a change in the philosophy of neck dissection for surgery of metastatic cervical cancer was initiated. Interest was stimulated in this country by Ballantyne and Jesse at MD Anderson Hospital in Houston, by Ettore Bocca in Italy, and by surgeons at Indiana University in Indianapolis. This was based on the question as to why certain important structures such as the carotid artery; vagus, phrenic, hypoglossal, and lingual nerves; and supraclavicular trunks of the brachial plexus could be spared, and yet others such as the sternocleidomastoid muscle and spinal accessory nerve should not be salvaged in order to obtain a greater degree of neck and shoulder girdle function. Since that time, modified neck dissection has been done in greater numbers and is simply a dissection of the cervical lymphatic system with sparing of the spinal accessory nerve, internal jugular vein, sternocleidomastoid muscle, and occasionally the cervical plexus. The rationale of doing this less-than-radical en bloc neck dissection for control of metastatic cancer to the neck is that one can attain the same control of neck disease in the N0 neck as with radical neck dissection and with much less morbidity.

SURGICAL ANATOMY

Neck dissection, whether it be radical or modified, is actually a surgical dissection of the anterior and lateral neck done for the purpose of removing metastatic tumor involving the cervical lymph-bearing tissues. The fascias and fascial spaces are important since these represent the basis for recognizing tissue planes in carrying out a proper dissection of the neck. Deep to the platysma muscle is a discrete fascial layer of the superficial layer of the deep cervical fascia which invests all structures in the neck much like a collar. This fascia attaches dorsally to the cervical spines and extends cranially to the occiput, mastoid, and inferior margin of the mandible. In attaching to the mandible, it invests the submandibular gland and thereby provides a distinct fascial compartment for the gland. As it relates to the sternocleidomastoid and trapezius muscles, this fascia assumes a bilaminar character as it invests each muscle in turn. Elsewhere the fascia is a single lamina, as in the region of the anterior cervical triangle and across the ventral midline covering the lateral triangle between the borders of the sternocleidomastoid and trapezius muscles. From the deep surfaces of the superficial layer of the deep fascia, extensions of connective tissue contribute to the formation of an investment for the carotid artery, internal jugular vein, and vagus nerve known as the carotid sheath.

Multiple laminae of deep fascia invest the supra- and infrahyoid strap muscles and can be identified as thin muscle fascia laminae. The deepest of such laminae associated with the thyrohyoid muscle, thyroid gland, and trachea invests the cervical parts of the airway and is referred to as pretracheal or middle layer of the deep cervical fascia. The deepest cervical fascia invests the prevertebral muscles. Aptly termed the prevertebral fascia, it extends from the base of the skull to the tubercles and transverse process of all cervical vertebrae, and is continuous along the ventral surface of the prevertebral column into the posterior mediastinum. Consequently, in the lateral region of the neck between the superficial layer of the deep cervical fascia or investing fascia forming a roof and the prevertebral fascia forming a floor, the contents of the lateral triangle are contained within a substantial but variable amount of fibrofatty and loose connective tissue. The contents are neurovascular structures including the spinal accessory nerve, peripheral branches of the cervical nerve plexus, numerous small arteries, veins, and lymphatic structures.

Since lymph nodes and lymphatics are embedded in the fibrofatty connective tissue lying between the anterior and posterior layers of the deep cervical fascia and are closely associated with the fascias of the carotid sheath, the connective tissue is removed from the anterior and lateral triangles of the neck as completely as possible during the course of a neck dissection and eradication of lymph-bearing tissue. Although the lymph nodes have a close relationship with the investing muscle fascias, they are never directly related to or intimate with the vessels or muscles covered by them. Invasion of the muscles and vessels by metastatic cancer of the lymph nodes in the neck may occur only by direct invasion after the capsule of the lymph node has been effaced. Radical neck dissection of the lymphatic system of the neck implies resection of all structures contained in the anterior and lateral triangles of the neck, and a modified neck dissection implies thorough removal of the fatty lymphatic connective tissue but with preservation of the sternocleidomastoid muscle, internal jugular vein, spinal accessory nerve, and the cervical plexus.

INDICATIONS

Indications for surgical management of the N0 neck must be regarded from the following basic principles:

1. The primary lesion is to be removed surgically and is accompanied by a high risk of metastasis to the cervical lymphatics and first-echelon nodes.
2. The neck will be entered as a part of the surgery for removal of the primary tumor.
3. There should be no clinical evidence of distant disease.

Surgical management of the N0 neck is contraindicated when primary disease is treatable with irradiation therapy which includes possible metastasis from the nasopharynx and selected tonsil lesions. The decision as to when to perform an en bloc radical neck dissection or modified neck dissection for a neck staged

at N0 is not difficult. If the primary tumor involving the oral cavity, oropharynx, or hypopharynx is staged at a level of II or III with high risk of metastasis and if it is decided that surgery is the treatment of choice for the primary tumor, a modified neck dissection should be carried out. In my opinion, there are few situations in which en bloc radical neck dissection for N0 disease could be recommended, and in practically all cases, N0-staged necks should be treated with modified neck dissection with the expectancy that salvage will be as effective as might be expected for a more radical procedure.

The basic objective of neck dissection for N0 neck disease, whether it be radical neck dissection or modified neck dissection, is to remove all cervical lymphatic tissue which may contain occult cancer, and no modification of the basic operation should change this. Of course, no one questions this rationale, but if all lymph-bearing tissue could be excised with sparing of certain anatomic structures, maintaining a greater degree of shoulder girdle function and yet not compromising control of cancer, this is the desire and objective of surgery of neck dissection for the N0 neck. The experience at the MD Anderson Hospital and that at Indiana University indicate that with the neck staged at N0, the chance of error from negative to positive is somewhere between 10 and 20 percent. Other investigators quote as high as 35 to 40 percent occult disease with the neck staged at N0. Based on this information, it is recognized that with management of N0 necks by radical neck dissection, 8 out of 10 patients will not have positive nodes, and that the price paid for sacrifice of an important structure such as the spinal accessory nerve is the incapacitating shoulder syndrome with persistent pain due to the strain placed on supporting shoulder muscles, with drooping of the shoulder and loss of shoulder girdle function related to the absence of trapezius function. If it is the decision of the surgeon to perform a radical neck dissection and the spinal accessory nerve is sacrificed, the accessory nerve should be reconstructed with a cable graft. The result has been satisfactory for partial or complete return of function over a period of many months.

SURGICAL PROCEDURE

The surgery of classic en bloc neck dissection is well known to everyone, and there is no need to discuss this operation other than to state that the dissection as described by John Conley is the best anatomic procedure that can be practiced by head and neck surgeons at this time. Conley carries his dissection from the anterior border of the trapezius muscle in a medial and anterior direction, identifying and displaying all anatomic structures before removing the metastatic disease.

There are three modified neck dissections to be discussed. The first is the standard neck dissection with sparing of the spinal accessory nerve. This is a modification of the en bloc radical neck dissection, but with the important feature of conservation of the spinal accessory nerve, and this is frequently the choice of many surgeons. After elevation of the skin flap, the spinal accessory nerve is identified in the anterior neck in its relation to the internal jugular vein and the posterior belly of the digastric muscle and is followed inferiorly to determine whether it enters the muscle or passes deep to the sternocleidomastoid muscle. In most cases, the nerve passes directly through the muscle, emerging at Erb's point along the posterior border of the sternocleidomastoid muscle at its upper and middle thirds. The accessory nerve is then followed in a downward direction until it passes under the anterior border of the trapezius muscle. With the nerve identified, it is carefully dissected away from the surrounding muscle fibers of the sternocleidomastoid muscle, and the muscle is separated from its attachment to the mastoid process and reflected downward.

After the sternocleidomastoid muscle is severed from its mastoid attachment, the internal jugular vein and relation of the nerve to this muscle are identified. The remainder of the dissection is along the anterior border of the trapezius muscle and carried in a careful dissection medially and upward, with clearing of the posterior cervical group of nodes together with the supraclavicular nodes. The omohyoid muscle is avulsed from beneath the clavicle; the sternal and clavicular attachments of the sternocleidomastoid muscle are cut; brachial plexus and phrenic nerve are identified and preserved. The internal jugular vein is dissected from the vagus nerve and common carotid artery, clamped, cut, ligated, and transfixed, and the dissection of the deep jugular nodes carried into the upper neck where the internal jugular vein is ligated, cut, and transfixed beneath the posterior belly of the digastric muscle after the accessory nerve is identified and preserved. Dissection is then carried into the submandibular area with clearing of the submandibular and submental groups of nodes.

There is a modification of the en bloc neck dissection that ablates all of the lymph-bearing tissue that is removed in the classic operation, but with the important feature of preserving the spinal accessory nerve and sternocleidomastoid muscle, with or without sparing of the internal jugular vein. If the dissection includes only the anterior triangle of the neck, the external jugular vein is ligated high and low and the superior fascia, which has been preserved, is interrupted along the upper border of the submandibular compartment and followed along the anterior border of the sternocleidomastoid muscle to the clavicle. The spinal accessory nerve is identified in the upper part of the anterior triangle of the neck in relation to the internal jugular vein, the posterior belly of the digastric muscle, and the bony prominence of the transverse process of the first cervical vertebra.

At this time it is necessary to dissect the group of lymph nodes beneath the posterior belly of the digastric muscle—the superior deep jugular nodes—which are the nodes most commonly involved in metastatic cancer of the head and neck. This is done by retracting the sternocleidomastoid muscle laterally, identifying the splenius capitis muscle, and carefully dissecting the fibrofatty lymphatic tissue in this area from beneath the sternocleidomastoid muscle and from the spinal accessory nerve. This is without question the *most important* part of the modified neck dissection. With the sternocleidomastoid muscle retracted laterally from the underlying fibrofatty lymphatic tissue, dissection is carried to the deep prevertebral muscles and their fascias, beginning in the mid and lower part of the neck. The omohyoid muscle is avulsed from beneath the clavicle and reflected medially and anteriorly with identification and preservation of the brachial plexus and the phrenic nerve.

The dissection is now similar to the posterior radical neck dissection; dissection is carried medially and anteriorly to the roots of nerves C3 and C4, which are cut. Dissection is carried to the carotid sheath, the internal jugular vein is identified, and the deep jugular nodes dissected in an upward direction from the lateral, posterior, and anterior aspects of the jugular vein. The upper nodes have already been cleared so that when the dissection reaches the upper part of the neck, the operator identifies and preserves the hypoglossal nerve descending between the jugular vein and the internal carotid artery. The contents of the submandibular triangle of the submental area are cleared of these nodes and the procedure completed.

If the decision is made to include the lateral cervical nodes in the dissection, the dissection is much the same as that just described, except that the spinal accessory nerve is identified not only in the anterior triangle, but also as it emerges in relation to Erb's point along the posterior border of the sternocleidomastoid muscle. From this point, dissection of the nerve is carried in a downward direction to its innervation of the trapezius muscle. The fascia enclosing the sternocleidomastoid muscle is cut anteriorly and posteriorly, and the sternocleidomastoid muscle elevated from underlying structures from the mastoid process to the clavicle. Careful dissection of the subdigastric or superior group of deep jugular nodes is done as mentioned previously, exposing the splenius capitis muscle, the accessory nerve, and the internal jugular vein, and dissection is carried forward and medially. Dissection is then started from the anterior border of the trapezius muscle and carried anteriorly and medially. The omohyoid muscle is avulsed beneath the clavicle, identifying and preserving the brachial plexus and phrenic nerve deep to the prevertebral fascia and carrying the dissection to the roots of the third and fourth cervical nerve roots. These roots are cut, the dissection is carried to the carotid sheath, and the lower and middle group of deep jugular nodes cleared from the lateral, posterior, and anterior aspects of the jugular vein. The dissection is carried into the upper neck, and again the submandibular and submental areas are cleared of this group of nodes. The procedure is now complete. The procedure just described is the most that is done in a conservative modified type of neck dissection and, at completion of the surgery, is the same picture one would see with an en block neck dissection, but with the perservation of the sterno-cleidomastoid muscle, spinal accessory nerve, and the internal jugular vein along with the brachial plexus, phrenic nerve, sympathetic trunk, carotid arterial system, and the hypoglossal nerve.

RESULTS

The results of surgical management of the N0 neck are presented not only with respect to control of metastatic cancer of the neck, but also with respect to the education of young surgeons who will be doing oncologic surgery of the head and neck. Although radical neck dissection is still the basic operation for control of metastatic neck cancer and should continue to be taught to young surgeons in training as a standard procedure, it is my opinion that the modified neck dissection should be an important part of their training. It should be recognized that the modified neck operation is more difficult and more time-consuming than the standard en bloc procedure. The radical en bloc neck dissection can be done more rapidly and technically is much easier to accomplish, but if the surgeon can master the technique of modified neck dissection, he is able to deal with any pathologic condition that may be treated by surgery of the neck. To perform a modified neck dissection effectively and safely, a surgeon must have a thorough working knowledge of the anatomy of the neck and, more specifically, the anatomy of the cervical connective tissues and lymphatics. As previously mentioned in this discussion, it is my opinion that there are few indications for the standard en bloc neck dissection as surgical management of the N0 neck. The incapacitating shoulder syndrome that results from sacrifice of the accessory nerve produces significant alteration of shoulder girdle function in at least 80 percent of patients who undergo the standard en bloc operation. Loss of the spinal accessory nerve causes persistent pain due to the strain placed on supporting shoulder muscles, with drooping of the shoulder and loss of shoulder girdle function related to the absence of trapezial activity. All patients who have had sparing of the accessory nerve, either with the standard radical neck dissection or with the modified operation, have some pain and limitation of shoulder function, but this is expected to be temporary. In my experience, the patients who have had sparing of the accessory nerve as part of their neck dissection ultimately have good function of the shoulder girdle.

TABLE 1 Experience with Radical Neck Dissection and Modified Neck Dissection for Management of the N0 Neck — 1966–1981

	Cases	Recurrence in Neck*	% Reccurrence
N0 disease			
Radical neck dissection	115	17	14
Modified neck dissection	235	27	11

*Disease present at primary site in all patients with recurrent neck disease.

Cosmetic deformity is of no great concern unless the patient has been subjected to a bilateral procedure. Patients who undergo bilateral en block neck dissection demonstrate progressive atrophy of the trapezius muscle on each side with increasingly more severe cosmetic disfigurement. Cutaneous anesthesia from either procedure is an annoying symptom, but it improves over the first 6 to 12 months following surgery. In the hands of many surgeons who practice modified neck operations with preservation of the cervical plexus, the prospect of postoperative cutaneous anesthesia is totally eliminated.

An analysis of the results of neck dissection for management of the N0 neck in the years 1966 to 1981, is presented in Table 1. The total number of cases during these years was 350, which were broken down into 115 patients having the en bloc neck dissection and 235 the modified neck dissection. Practically all of the radical neck dissections were done in the years between 1966 and 1976.

The current practice at Indiana University for surgical management of the N0 neck is as follows: If the primary tumor is to be treated surgically and the neck staged at N0, either modification of the standard neck dissection with sparing of the accessory nerve or one of the other two modified neck procedures, as already described, is performed. Radiation therapy is given 3 weeks postoperatively if positive nodes are present. Radiation therapy is not given for metastatic melanoma. If the primary lesion is treated with radiation therapy, 5000 rads are given to each side of the neck and surgery is not recommended.

In conclusion, the modified neck dissection is as effective in the treatment of the N0 neck as the en bloc radical neck dissection, but it is more difficult and more time-consuming. With the use of this operation and based on the review of our experience since 1966, it is my opinion that this is a procedure of choice.

MANAGEMENT OF THE N0 NECK

DAVID E. SCHULLER, M.D.

The management of the N0 neck is based on the current understanding of certain anatomic facts, the biologic behavior of neck nodes in head and neck cancer, the rationale of therapy, and its impact on quality of survival.

DESCRIPTION AND RATIONALE OF THERAPEUTIC ALTERNATIVES

Radiation therapy can be used to treat one or both sides of the N0 neck. It has an excellent chance of controlling microscopic nodal disease,[1] being a comprehensive means of treating all lymph nodes and lymphatic channels within the neck tissues.

Surgical approaches represent the alternative to radiation therapy. The traditional or radical neck dissection, originally described by Crile in 1906, involves an attempt at completely removing all the lymph nodes and lymphatic channels on one side of the neck by intentionally sacrificing certain structures, such as the internal jugular vein, sternocleidomastoid muscle, submandibular gland, and spinal accessory nerve. Although this procedure has been found to be an effective means of eradicating microscopic nodal disease, it results in pain and discomfort, primarily with shoulder movement.

The alternative is the modified neck dissection, in which the aforementioned structures are preserved, but the node-bearing tissue is resected. The failure rate with the modified neck dissection, which is usually coupled with radiation therapy, is reported to be comparable to the failure rate with radical neck dissection for the N0 neck.[2]

ANATOMIC DISTRIBUTION OF CERVICAL NODES

Of the 800 lymph nodes in the body, an estimated 300 of them are located within the soft tissue of the neck.[3] On either side of the neck, there are basically three major lymphatic drainage pathways—the internal jugular, the spinal accessory, and transverse cervical chains (Fig. 1). The internal jugular group of nodes drains the majority of sites within the head and neck region. The spinal accessory nodal group represents lymph nodes adjacent to the eleventh cranial nerve throughout its entire course from inferiorly in the posterior triangle to superiorly, where it lies adjacent to the internal jugular vein as it exits the jugular foramen at the skull base. The transverse cervical group of lymph nodes connects the spinal accessory with the internal jugular in the lower neck region.

RELATIONSHIPS OF METASTATIC NODES TO THE SPINAL ACCESSORY NERVE

One of the major considerations in choosing the appropriate type of neck dissection (traditional versus modified) is whether the spinal accessory nerve can justifiably be preserved. There is no question that the spinal accessory nerve does have nodes adjacent to it, but some reports in the literature have documented a relatively infrequent occurrence of involvement with nodal metastases.[4,5] However, these studies evaluated the portion of the spinal accessory nerve located only in the posterior triangle.

When the *entire* course of the spinal accessory nerve was prospectively studied,[6] it confirmed the previous reports that the nerve was infrequently associated with metastatic nodes in the posterior triangle. However, in its superior portion, where it is closely related to the internal jugular vein, there is a high frequency of involvement with metastases. In those patients with an N+ neck nodal status, the spinal accessory nodal chain was frequently involved with disease. The same report documented that the spinal accessory nodal chain could be involved with microscopic cancer in what was presumed to be a N0 neck (Table 1). It was formerly believed that the spinal accessory lymph nodes were not involved with cancer unless the jugular nodes had evidence of metastases. The previously mentioned report documented that in patients with clinically positive N> jugular nodes, the spinal accessory nodes were also involved, but it also demonstrated that the spinal accessory nodes could be microscopically positive in an N0 neck even in the absence of palpable jugular adenopathy. Therefore, it is apparent that the spinal accessory nodes can be involved with either clinically detectable or microscop-

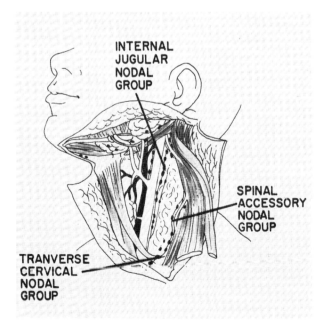

Figure 1 The three major lymphatic drainage pathways.

TABLE 1   Location of Metastases in Therapeutic and Prophylactic Radical Neck Dissections

| | No. of Specimens | No. with Negative Nodes | Number and Location of Metastatic Nodes | | |
			Jugular Accessory	Accessory Only	Accessory Normal
Therapeutic	27	4	12	6	5
Elective	23	18	2	1	2
Total	50	22	14	7	7

ically occult (N0) metastatic carcinoma independent of the disease status of the jugular nodes.

MORBIDITY OF TRADITIONAL VERSUS MODIFIED NECK DISSECTION

It is important to understand the impact of the various therapeutic alternatives on the quality of survival following completion of therapy. Most advocates of the modified neck dissection do not propose this as a therapeutic alternative to traditional neck dissection alone, but rather it is being advocated in the setting of a combined therapy approach in which radiation therapy is added to the modified dissection. There has been little in the literature to evelute the morbidity of these current total therapeutic programs.

A recent report evaluating patients from a number of institutions studied the morbidity of the total treatment programs that did include traditional and modified neck dissections.[7] The results of this evaluation showed that there was no difference in the proportion of patients returning to their pretreatment job status, irrespective of whether modified or traditional neck dissection was used (Table 2). There did appear to be a greater negative influence on the patients' social activities following traditional neck dissection, and the limiting factor was identified to be the problem with shoulder movement following this treatment. However, this study also implicated radiation therapy as having a significant adverse impact on patients' psychosocial traits following completion of therapy,

TABLE 2   Distribution of Reasons for not Returning to Usual Job (n = 99)

Reason	RND patients with a positive response (%)	MND patients with a positive response (%)	Significance
Limitation of shoulder movement	55.2	59.1	NS
Pain, limitation related to removal of tumor	62.1	76.2	P .05
Reasons other than treatment	53.3	50.0	NS

NS = not significant; RND = radical neck dissection; MND = modified neck dissection.

so that the patient who received radiation therapy, irrespective of the type of the surgical dissection, reported feeling more dependent on others than did patients who received no radiation therapy. This study demonstrates that no treatment program is free of morbidity, whether it be traditional neck dissection, modified neck dissection, or radiation therapy.

TREATMENT RECOMMENDATIONS

The most common primary tumor sites in the head and neck are the larynx, oral cavity, oropharynx, and hypopharynx. The overwhelmingly most common histologic type is squamous cell carcinoma. When one considers the treatment of the clinically negative neck according to disease stage for squamous cancer, there is little debate regarding treatment of the early or the advanced disease. However, there is room for disagreement regarding treatment of the N0 neck with middle-stage disease. In N0 necks with a T1 primary and no distant metastatic disease, it is unlikely that the neck nodes need to be treated, irrespective of the primary tumor site, because the incidence of microscopic disease is so low. However, patients with the T4N0M0 classification are uniformly advised to undergo treatment of the neck, irrespective of the primary tumor site. And despite the controversy surrounding treatment of the clinically negative neck with T2 or T3 lesions, involving any of the aforementioned primary sites, I recommend treatment because of the rather frequent presence of microscopic disease with this tumor stage.

Once the decision is made to treat the N0 neck, it then becomes imperative to decide *what* type of treatment is most appropriate—radiation therapy, modified neck dissection, traditional neck dissection, or some combination. As mentioned earlier, it has been clearly established that radiation therapy represents a curative modality for treating certain neck nodal disease, especially the N0 neck. Radiation therapy has the advantage of permitting simultaneous bilateral neck nodal treatment, and the morbidity of radiation therapy alone may be less than with either of the surgical alternatives.

Of the two surgical approaches, the modified neck dissection is often used as the only treatment for the N0 neck to eliminate some of the morbidity identified with the combined therapy approach. However, there is nothing in the literature to support the theory that the modified neck dissection is superior to either traditional dissection or radiation therapy alone in controlling neck nodal disease in the N0 neck. The advantage it has over radiation therapy is that it provides histologic information that may well be useful to subsequent treatment planning.

When one considers standard radical neck dissection for the N0 neck, there appears to be no particular advantage over the modified dissection. The intentional sacrifice of the spinal accessory nerve in this particular clinical situation may unnecessarily add to the morbidity of the procedure without providing any increase of disease control in exchange. However, the recent awareness of the significance of extracapsular spread of carcinoma, reported by Johnson and co-workers,[8] is of some concern when the matter of modified versus radical neck dissection is debated. It is possible that such unrecognized extracapsular nodal disease may be better treated with the traditional neck dissection, which involves a closer dissection to nodal-bearing tissue, than with the modified approach. This currently is a matter of theoretical concern rather than a documented observation.

SUMMARY

The management of the N0 neck demands an awareness of certain anatomic observations and an awareness of the biologic behavior of microscopically occult metastatic disease. It is also important to have an appreciation for the morbidity of the therapeutic options to aid one in the determination of the proper treatment. I recommend that the N0 neck be treated, for any disease stage beyond T1 lesions, for the major primary tumor sites involved with squamous cell carcinoma. The use of irradiation or surgery needs to be individualized, and each has its advantages and disadvantages.

REFERENCES

1. Wang CC. Radiation therapy in the management of oral malignant diseases. Otolaryngol Clin North Am 1979; 12:73–80.
2. Lingeman RE, Helmus C, Stephens R, Ulm J. Neck dissection: radical or conservative. Am Otol Rhinol Laryngol 1977; 86:737–741.
3. Hellstrom KE, Hellstrom I. Immunologic defenses against cancer. In: Good RA, Fisher DW (eds). *Immunobiology*. Stanford CT: Sinauer Associates, Inc., 1971.
4. Skolnik EM, et al. Preservation of XI cranial nerve in neck dissections. Laryngoscope 1967; 77:1304.
5. McGavran MH, Bauer WC, Ogura JH. The incidence of cervical lymph node metastases from epidermoid carcinoma of the larynx and their relationship to certain characteristics of the primary tumor. Cancer 1961; 14:55.
6. Schuller DE, Platz CE, Krause CJ. Spinal accessory lymph nodes: a prospective study of metastatic involvement. Laryngoscope 1978; 138:439–450.
7. Schuller DE, et al. Analysis of disability resulting from treatment including radical neck dissection or modified neck dissection. Head Neck Surg 1983; 6:551–558.
8. Johnson JT, et al. The extracapsular spread of tumors in cervical node metastasis. Arch Otolaryngol 1981; 107:725–729.

MANAGEMENT OF CLINICALLY OCCULT (N0) CERVICAL LYMPH NODE METASTASES BY RADIATION THERAPY

JAMES D. COX, M.D.

Metastases to the cervical lymph nodes constitute a problem second in importance only to the management of the primary tumor in patients with carcinomas of the upper respiratory and upper digestive tracts. In spite of the fact that many patients do not have cervical lymph node metastases at the time of presentation, in large surgical series,[1,2] as many patients fail in the cervical lymph nodes as fail at the primary site. Some of the cervical lymph node metastases may result from spread after recurrence of the primary tumor, but many occur as the result of untreated occult metastases, which eventually become clinically apparent.

The frequency with which patients present with clinical evidence of metastasis to cervical lymph nodes varies considerably with the site of the primary tumor. However, there is a direct relationship between the frequency of cervical lymph node metastasis at the initial presentation and the probability of metastatic adenopathy appearing in the untreated neck.

Prophylactic treatment of any site at risk for metastasis does not imply prevention of metastasis, but rather prevention of the clinical appearance of metastasis. Thus, it is appropriate to refer to "prophylactic neck dissection" or to "prophylactic irradiation" of the lymph nodes which drain a particular site. This use of the term "prophylactic" is similar to its use when discussing prophylactic antibiotics in patients with rheumatic heart disease or other valvular abnormalities: bacteremia is not prevented, but the antimicrobial presumably kills the organisms and thus prevents the occurrence of endocarditis.

The decisions to include prophylactic treatment of the cervical region in the initial management of patients with carcinomas of the upper aerodigestive tract rest on the risk of subclinical metastasis, the effectiveness of the treatment in preventing the development of overt metastasis, the success with which it is possible to treat clinically overt metastases when they become evident (discussed elsewhere in this book), and the acute and late morbidity of the prophylactic treatment. These considerations will be addressed in regard to the radiotherapeutic management of clinically occult cervical lymph node metastasis.

RISK OF CERVICAL LYMPH NODE METASTASIS BY SITE OF PRIMARY TUMOR

Nasal Cavity. Bosch et al reported 40 patients with cancer of the nasal cavity, five of whom presented with cervical lymph node metastases; two patients subsequently developed cervical lymph node metastases.[3] Robin and Powell described cervical lymphadenopathy in 10 percent of 90 patients with carcinomas of the nasal cavity.[4]

Paranasal Sinuses. Robin and Powell reported 17 percent (64 of 382) of patients with carcinomas of the paranasal sinuses with cervical lymphadenopathy at the time of presentation: clinically apparent nodes were described in 17 percent (50/298) of patients with antral carcinomas, 13 percent (10/78) of patients with primary tumors in the ethmoid, and two of six patients with primary tumors arising in the frontal sinus and sphenoid.[4] Lee and Ogura described seven patients with cervical adenopathy at presentation among 96 patients with carcinoma of the maxillary sinus; 16 percent (14/89) of patients with no evidence of cervical adenopathy subsequently failed in the neck.[5] Pezner et al found cervical node metastases in 13 (21%) of 63 patients with squamous carcinoma of the maxillary antrum; nine of the remaining patients subsequently developed cervical adenopathy.[6]

Oral Cavity. Modlin described cervical metastases on admission in 21 (12%) of 179 patients with carcinomas of the lower lip seen at the Ellis Fischel Cancer Hospital of Columbia, Missouri forty years ago; 15 (10%) of the remaining patients developed cervical metastases after treatment of the primary tumor.[7] A much more recent series from Memorial Sloan-Kettering Cancer Center showed only 3 percent (1/38) of patients with cancer of the lower lip presenting with cervical adenopathy; 8 percent (3/37) developed metastatic adenopathy after treatment of the primary tumor.[1]

Mendelson et al reported 45 patients with carcinomas of the anterior two-thirds of the tongue with metastatic adenopathy among 340 patients seen at the Mayo Clinic.[8] Over 60 percent of these favorably selected patients had tumors less than 2 cm in diameter, and only 6 percent had tumors 4 cm or larger. Of the remaining 295 patients, 32 of 169 who did not have a neck dissection subsequently developed cervical adenopathy, and 26 of 126 who underwent a prophylactic neck dissection had histologic evidence of metastases. Thus, 58 (20% of the 295 patients who could be classified as N0 at presentation) had subsequent evidence of cervical lymph node metastasis. Strong reported 49 patients (36%) with carcinoma of the oral tongue presenting with cervical node metastasis; 25

(28%) of the clinically N0 patients failed in the cervical region after treatment of the primary tumor.[1]

Harrold described cervical adenopathy in 295 (38%) of 785 patients with carcinoma of the floor of the mouth seen at Memorial Hospital in New York prior to 1965; 33 percent of the remaining patients developed metastatic adenopathy after treatment of the primary lesion.[9] A more recent series from the same institution revealed clinically positive nodes in 49 (43%) of 115 patients with carcinoma of the floor of the mouth; 11 (17%) of the N0 patients subsequently developed metastatic cervical adenopathy.[1]

Oropharynx. Strong reported metastatic adenopathy in 39 (66&) of 59 patients with carcinoma of the tonsillar fossa; four of the remaining patients subsequently developed metastatic adenopathy.[1] However, in radiotherapy series, the proportion presenting with positive nodes is even higher; Fletcher reported palpable lymph nodes in 76 percent of 140 patients with carcinoma of the tonsillar fossa.[10]

Whicker et al found histologically positive cervical lymph node metastases in 56 (55%) of 102 patients with carcinoma of the base of the tongue; 97 percent of the patients had undergone a unilateral or bilateral cervical lymphadenectomy.[11] Nonetheless, 22 (48%) of the remaining patients developed subsequent nodal metastases, most of which were in the contralateral cervical region. Strong reported a higher frequency of cervical node metastasis at the time of presentation; 70 percent of 87 patients with carcinoma of the base of the tongue had clinically positive nodes. Seven of the remaining patients eventually developed metastatic cervical adenopathy. Fletcher described clinically apparent nodes in 78 percent (144/185) of patients with carcinoma of the base of the tongue.[10]

Nasopharynx. Dixon reported that 149 (72%) of 209 patients with carcinoma of the nasopharynx had cervical lymphadenopathy at the time of diagnosis.[12] Messic et al described cervical lymphadenopathy in 213 (85%) of 251 patients with carcinoma of the nasopharynx seen at the M.D. Anderson Hospital in Houston.[13] Few data are available on the frequency with which untreated cervical nodes become manifest in patients with carcinoma of the nasopharynx. Ho described a series of 32 patients who had no cervical lymphadenopathy at presentation and who did not receive irradiation to the cervical regions; five of these patients had failure in the cervical lymph nodes and another six had failure at the primary site with accompanying cervical adenopathy.[14]

Piriform Sinus. Biller and Lucente found palpable lymph nodes which proved to contain metastases in 65 (59%) of 111 patients with carcinoma of the piriform sinus; 19 (41%) of the remaining patients had occult metastases.[15] Shah et al reported clinical cervical adenopathy in 65 percent of 301 patients seen at the Memorial Sloan-Kettering Cancer Center in New York.[16] Thirty-four (33%) of the N0 patients either had microscopically involved nodes at the time of radical neck dissection or developed metastases in the

TABLE 1   Frequency of Cervical Nodal Metastasis by Site of Primary Tumor

Site	Positive Nodes at Admission (%)	Positive Nodes after Treatment of Primary (%)	Total Positive Nodes (%)
Nasal cavity [3, 4]	10–13	6	15–18
Paranasal sinus [4–6]	7–21	14–18	21–32
Oral cavity			
Lower lip [1, 7]	3–12	8–10	11–20
Mobile tongue [1, 8]	13–36	20–28	44–54
Floor of mouth [1, 9]	37–43	17–33	57
Oropharynx			
Tonsillar fossa [1, 10]	66–76	20	73–76
Base of tongue [10, 11]	55–78	27–48	76–78
Nasopharynx [12–14]	72–85	34	85+
Piriform sinus [15, 16]	59–74	33–41	75–79
Larynx			
Supraglottic [1, 15]	28–49	25–30	46–65
Glottic [2, 17]	0–12	2–15	25

cervical region in the follow-up period.

Larynx.   Biller and Lucente found overt cervical metastases in 38 (28%) of 135 patients with carcinomas of the supraglottic larynx; 24 (25%) of the remaining patients had occult metastases determined at neck dissection. Strong reported 49 percent (42/85) of patients with supgralottic laryngeal carcinomas with clinically positive nodes at the time of presentation; 13 (30%) failed in the cervical region following treatment of the laryngeal tumor.[1]

Mittal et al reported only three (2%) failures in the cervical nodes among 177 patients with T1N0 carcinomas of the true vocal cord.[17] Lindberg described cervical adenopathy in 12 percent of 191 patients with glottic carcinomas, most of whom had advanced (T3 or T4) lesions; 25 (15%) of the N0 patients manifested cervical adenopathy as the first site of failure.[2]

Table 1 summarizes the frequencies of cervical lymph node metastases by the various primary sites within the upper aerodigestive tract. There is a correlation between the frequency with which nodes are positive at presentation and the frequency with which they become manifest clincially after treatment of the primary tumor if the cervical nodal regions remain untreated. Low-risk sites include the nasal cavity, lower lip, and glottis. Carcinomas of the paranasal sinuses slightly more frequently give rise to clinical and subclinical cervical lymph node metastases. Sites of intermediate risk for overt and occult cervical metastases are the mobile tongue, floor of the mouth, and supraglottic larynx. High-risk areas include the tonsillar fossa, base of tongue, nasopharynx, and piriform sinus.

METASTASES TO CONTRALATERAL CERVICAL NODES

Table 2 summarizes the data from the extensive review of the Memorial Sloan-Kettering Cancer Center experience by Strong.[1] As would be expected from the anatomic locations and the relative frequencies of ipsilateral cervical lymph node metastases, the pri-

mary sites with the highest risk of contralateral metastasis are the mobile tongue, floor of mouth, base of tongue, nasopharynx, piriform sinus, and supraglottic larynx.

FREQUENCY OF OCCULT CERVICAL METASTASIS BY SIZE OF PRIMARY TUMOR

A relationship between the frequency of cervical lymph node metastasis from carcinoma of the floor of the mouth and the size of the primary tumor was reported by Harrold, from the Memorial Hospital of New York.[9] The data suggest that there is a very modest increase in the combined frequencies of overt and subclinical metastases related to the size of the primary tumor (Table 3); tumors less than 4 cm in diameter result in metastases in approximately 55 percent of patients, whereas tumors 5 cm or greater produce metastases in two-thirds of patients. However, there is a much more striking increase in the frequency with which lymph nodes are clinically positive with increasing size of the tumor and a corre-

TABLE 2   Failure in Contralateral Cervical Lymph Nodes by Site of Primary Tumor

Site	Number Patients	Contralateral Nodal Failure	
		No.	%
Oral cavity			
Lip	38	1	3
Mobile tongue	137	18	13
Floor of mouth	115	13	11
Oropharynx			
Tonsillar fossa	59	5	8
Base of tongue	87	14	16.
Nasopharynx	43	11	26
Piriform sinus	69	13	19
Supraglottic larynx	85	18	21

Data from Strong.[1]

TABLE 3 Carcinoma of Floor of Mouth: Frequency of Cervical Nodal Metastasis* by Size of Primary Tumor

Size	No. Patients	Positive Nodes at Presentation (%)	Positive Nodes after Treatment of Primary† (%)	Total Positive Nodes (%)
< 2.0	128	19	43	54
2.0–2.9	212	28	36	55
3.0–3.9	204	37	30	56
4.0–4.9	122	52	20	62
> 5.0	119	61	17	68

*Proved by histopathologic examination.
†Percent of patients who were N0 at presentation.
Data from Harrold.[9]

sponding decrease in the frequency with which cervical nodes appear in a clinically negative neck following treatment only of the primary tumor. The implication from these data is that a relatively greater risk of occult metastases exists for smaller primary tumors; conversely, there is a greater probability that larger tumors will result in overt lymphadenopathy and have a lower frequency of subclinical metastasis. This inverse relationship of risk of occult cervical metastasis and size of the primary tumor cannot necessarily be generalized to other primary sites in the upper respiratory and digestive tracts. Spiro and Strong found a higher frequency of metastases appearing in cervical lymph nodes with larger tumors of the mobile (oral) tongue after treatment by partial glossectomy alone— 29 percent (28/95) for T1, 43 percent (33/77) for T2, and 77 percent (10/13) for T3 lesions.[18] However, these latter findings confirm the impression that sites that are associated with a high frequency of clinical cervical metastasis have a high risk of occult metastases, even with relatively small primary tumors.

PROPHYLACTIC IRRADIATION OF THE NECK

Fletcher recently summarized the radiobiologic foundation and a large body of clinical data pertaining to the radiotherapeutic management of "sub-clinical disease".[19] He observed that moderate doses of radiations (45 to 50 Gy) are sufficient to eradicate subclinical metastases from a variety of epithelial malignant tumors, including carcinomas of the upper aerodigestive tract. Indeed, total doses of 30 to 40 Gy eliminated occult metastases in two-thirds of patients, and a total dose of 50 Gy was sufficient to reduce subsequent metastases to 10 percent of the expected frequency. Million,[20] Barkley et al,[21] and Lehman et al[22] have provided corroborating data (Table 4).

The total dose required to control subclinical disease in the absence of a prior surgical procedure is sufficiently low that there is little morbidity. Fraction sizes of 1.8 to 2.0 Gy per day, weekly doses of 9.0 to 10.0 Gy, and total doses of 45 to 50 Gy result in a very mild dry desquamation and few late effects except epilation of the beard. Considerably higher doses are required if the radiation therapy is delivered for

TABLE 4 Frequency of Cervical Nodal Metastasis after Irradiation of the Clinically Uninvolved (N0) Neck

Site of Primary	Ref	No. of Patients	No. Cervical Node Mets
MOb T, FOM	19	9	0
MOb T, FOM	21	23	1
TON F, BOT	20	29	0
SUP L, HYP	20	84	3
		145	4 (3%)

MOB T = mobile (oral) tongue; FOM = floor of mouth; TON F = tonsillar fossa; BOT = base of tongue; SUP L = supraglottic larynx; HYP = hypopharynx.

control of microscopic disease within an operated field.[23,24] This presumably is related to hypoxia resulting from altered vasculature due to the operation. The necessity of a higher total dose increases the probability of complications. An even higher dose may be required for control if the interval from resection to postoperative irradiation is unusually long. Vickram et al found, for a given dose of postoperative irradiation, a higher frequency of recurrence following irradiation for subclinical disease if the delay was greater than 6 weeks following operation, as compared to less than 6 weeks.[25] This is best explained by an increased population of clonogenic cells, albeit still subclinical, with the passage of time after the operative procedure.

SUMMARY

Management of the cervical lymph nodes is a problem second only to the management of the primary tumor in patients with carcinomas of the upper aerodigestive tract. The frequency with which patients present with clinical evidence of metastasis to cervical lymph nodes varies considerably with the site of the primary tumor. The frequency is relatively low with carcinomas of the nasal cavity, lower lip, glottis, and paranasal sinuses. Significantly higher frequencies of clinical lymphadenopathy occur with carcinomas of the mobile tongue, floor of the mouth, and supraglottic larynx. Very high frequencies of clinical cervical node metastases are seen with carcinomas of the tonsillar fossa, base of tongue, nasopharynx, and piriform sinus. There is a direct correlation between the frequency of lymph node metastasis at the time of presentation and the risk of subsequent metastasis in the cervical region following treatment of the primary tumor. The frequency of initial clinical cervical metastasis increases with the size of the primary tumor. Conversely, the risk of subclinical metastasis decreases with the size of the primary tumor, so that the overall frequency of clinical and subclinical metastasis changes relatively little according to the size of the primary tumor. Thus, the risk of subclinical metastasis is highest with small tumors in sites that usually give rise to metastatic adenopathy. Prophylactic irradiation of the cervical lymph node-bearing regions is able to destroy micrometastases and prevent clinical adenopathy. This can consistently be accomplished with modest total doses (45 to 50 Gy in 5 weeks) if there has not been operative intervention. If an operative procedure precedes the irradiation, higher total doses are required owing to hypoxia from altered vascularity. If the interval from resection to irradiation is prolonged, higher doses are also required owing to an increased number of clonogenic cells in the operative bed. The morbidity from irradiation in the absence of an operative procedure is minimal, but late effects increase in frequency and severity as total doses increase. Prophylactic irradiation of the clinically negative (N0) cervical regions is rarely indicated in patients with a low risk of metastasis (when nasal cavity, paranasal sinuses, lower lip, or glottis is affected). Prophylactic cervical irradiation is indicated in virtually all patients who present without palpable adenopathy, but who have carcinomas of the oropharynx, nasopharynx, hypopharynx, and supraglottic larynx.

REFERENCES

1. Strong EW. Sites of treatment failure in head and neck cancer. Cancer Treat Symp 1983; 2:5–20.
2. Lindberg RD. Sites of first failure in head and neck cancer. Cancer Treat Symp 1983; 2:21–31.
3. Bosch A, Vallecillo L, Frias Z. Cancer of the nasal cavity. Cancer 1976; 37:1458–1463.
4. Robin PE, Powell DJ. Regional node involvement and distant metastases in carcinoma of the nasal cavity and paranasal sinuses. J Laryngol Otol 1980; 94:301–309.
5. Lee F, Ogura JH. Maxillary sinus carcinoma. Laryngoscope 1981; 91:133–139.
6. Pezner RD, Moss WT, Tong D, Blasko C, Griffin TW. Cervical lymph node metastases in patients with squamous cell carcinoma of the maxillary antrum: the role of elective irradiation of the clinically negative neck. Int J Radiat Oncol Biol Phys 1979; 5:1977–1980.
7. Modlin J. Neck dissections in cancer of the lower lip. Five-year results in 179 patients. Surgery 1950; 28:404–412.
8. Mendelson BC, Woods JE, Beahrs OH. Neck dissection in the treatment of carcinoma of the anterior two-thirds of the tongue. Surg Gynecol Obstet 1976; 143:75–80.
9. Harrold Jr CC. Management of cancer of the floor of the mouth. Am J Surg 1971; 122:487–493.
10. Fletcher GH. Squamous cell carcinomas of the oropharynx. Int J Radiat Oncol Biol Phys 1979; 5:2073–2090.
11. Whicker JH, DeSanto LW, Devine KD. Surgical treatment of squamous cell carcinoma of the base of the tongue. Laryngoscope 1972; 82:1853–1860.
12. Dickson RI. Nasopharyngeal carcinoma: an evaluation of 209 patients. Laryngoscope 1981; 91:333–354.
13. Mesic JB, Fletcher GH, Goepfert H. Megavoltage irradiation of epithelial tumors of the nasopharynx. Int J Radiat Oncol Biol Phys 1981; 7:447–453.
14. Ho JHC. An epidemiologic and clinical study of nasopharyngeal carcinoma. Int J Radiat Oncol Biol Phys 1978; 4:181–198.
15. Biller HF, Lucente FE. Conservation surgery of the head and neck. Semin Oncol 1977; 4:365–373.
16. Shah JP, Shaha AR, Spiro RH, Strong EW. Carcinoma of the hypopharynx. Am J Surg 1976; 132:439–443.
17. Mittal B, Rao DV, Marks JE, Perez CA. Role of radiation in the management of early vocal cord carcinoma. Int J Radiat Oncol Biol Phys 1983; 9:997–1002.
18. Spiro RH, Strong EW. Epidermoid carcinoma of the mobile tongue. Treatment by partial glossectomy alone. Am J Surg 1971; 122:707–710.
19. Fletcher GH. Lucy Wortham James Lecture. Subclinical disease. Cancer 1984; 53:1274–1284.
20. Million RR. Elective neck irradiation for TX N0 squamous carcinoma of the oral tongue and floor of mouth. Cancer 1974; 34:149–155.
21. Barkley Jr HT, Fletcher GH, Jesse RH, Lindberg RD. Management of cervical lymph node metastases in squamous cell carcinoma of the tonsillar base of tongue, supraglottic larynx, and hypopharynx. Am J Surg 1972; 124:461–467.
22. Lehman RH, Cox JD, Belson TP, Yale RS, Byhardt RW, Toohill RJ, Malin T. Recurrence patterns by treatment modality of carcinomas of the floor of the mouth and oral tongue. Am J Otolaryngol 1982; 3:174–181.
23. Marcus Jr RB, Million RR, Cassissi NJ. Postoperative irradiation for squamous cell carcinomas of the head and neck: analysis of time-dose factors related to control above the clavicles. Int J Radiat Oncol Biol Phys 1979; 5:1943–1949.
24. Arriagada R, Eschwege F, Cachin Y, Richard JM. The value of combining radiotherapy with surgery in the treatment of hypopharyngeal and laryngeal cancers. Cancer 1983; 51:1819–1825.
25. Vikram B, Strong EW, Shah J, Spiro RH. Elective postoperative irradiation therapy in stages III and IV epidermoid carcinoma of the head and neck. Am J Surg 1980; 140:580–584.

15. Management of the N3 Neck

INTRODUCTION

CHARLES J. KRAUSE, M.D.

Patients who present with clinically staged N3 metastatic squamous cell carcinoma offer a fascinating and challenging array of management problems for the head and neck surgeon. In recent years, it has become clear that the most effective single indicator of prognosis available today in patients with squamous cell carcinoma of the head and neck is the extent of disease in the neck, not only because of a potential for recurrence in the neck, but also as an indicator of the biologic aggressiveness of the tumor in relation to its host. Figure 1, illustrating the survival of patients in the Head and Neck Contracts Program, demonstrates a sharp decline in survival with advancing N stage.[1] The number and location of positive nodes is important, as are the size and bilaterality of affected nodes.

Extranodal extension of tumor, as implied by size greater than 3 cm in diameter and/or fixation to surrounding structures, suggests a poor prognosis for control regardless of the treatment regimen selected.[2,3] Careful search of the pathology specimen for evidence of such extension is warranted.

The N3 classification, as suggested in the Amer-

ican Joint Committee for Cancer Staging and End Results Reporting (AJC), is listed in Table 1.[4] Earlier AJC classification for N3 included fixation. This was removed from the 1978 classification, apparently in response to frequent difficulty in obtaining interexaminer agreement as to when fixation is present, and to which structures the nodes are fixed. Most, though not all, of the fixed nodes are large, and usually greater than 6 cm in diameter. Also included in the N3 classification are bilateral nodes (of any size) and contralateral nodes. The treatment implications and perhaps the prognosis in these N3b and N3c patients are very different than in those with one or more large nodes (N3a).

TABLE 1 N3 Classification (AJC)

N3 Massive homolateral node(s), bilateral nodes, or contralateral node(s).

  N3a Clinically positive homolateral node(s), none over 6 cm in diameter.

  N3b Bilateral clinically positive nodes (in this situation, each side of the neck should be staged separately: that is, N3b: right: N2a: left, NI).

  N3c Contralateral clinically positive node(s) only.

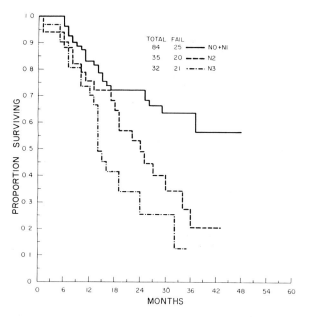

Figure 1 Survival of patients by N class in the Head and Neck Contracts Program. Note sharp decline in survival with advancing N stage.

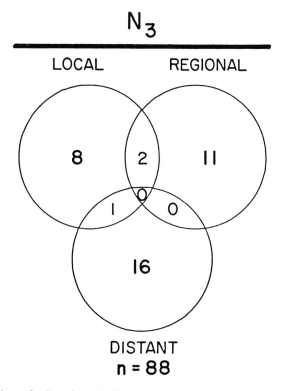

Figure 2 Data from the Head and Neck Contracts series illustrating the high incidence of first failure at distant sites in the N3 patient.

And finally, another important aspect of our search for improved methods of treating patients with N3 carcinoma is recognition of the high incidence of distant metastatic disease noted in these patients when local and regional control have been obtained. Figure 2 presents data from the Head and Neck Contracts series which illustrate clearly the high incidence of first failure at distant sites in the N3 patients. In 16 of 88 patients, the carcinoma recurred first as distant metastases, whereas in only 8, it recurred first locally, and in 11, it recurred first regionally. Clearly, as we search for improved methods of controlling the local and regional disease in these patients, we must not lose sight of our need to control distant disease as well. Indeed, to look at local/regional control without also assessing the impact of these treatment methods on distant disease is, I believe, short-sighted and ultimately against the interest of providing the best available patient care.

In the chapters that follow, some of the key issues associated with the management of these challenging patients are discussed.

REFERENCES

1. Wolf GT. Personal communication regarding Head and Neck Contracts Program data. 1984.
2. Santos V, Strong M, Vaughan C et al. Role of surgery in head and neck cancer with fixed nodes. Arch Otolaryngol 1975; 101:645–648.
3. Bartelink H, Boeur K, Hart G et al. The value of postoperative radiotherapy adjuvant to radical neck dissection. Cancer 1983; 52:1008–1013.
4. American Joint Committee for Cancer Staging and End Results Reporting: Manual for Staging of Cancer, 1977.

SELECTION CRITERIA FOR MODIFIED NECK DISSECTION WITH POSTOPERATIVE IRRADIATION FOR N3 STAGED CERVICAL METASTASIS

ROBERT M. BYERS, M.D.
ALANDO J. BALLANTYNE, M.D.

In any discussion concerning the treatment for metastatic squamous carcinoma to the neck, it is important to precisely define the stage of disease. There is a real difference in the biologic behavior and therapeutic implications among N3a, N3b and N3c staged neck disease. The neck containing metastatic squamous carcinoma measuring over 6 cm, invading the carotid artery or fixed to the bone of the mandible, mastoid, cervical vertebra, or base of skull, is a very different clinical situation from the neck containing a single bilateral, mobile, 2-cm midjugular node. In addition, one must be careful when suggesting various modifications of a standard radical neck dissection as treatment for N3 cervical metastasis so that there is no compromise in established cancer control.

The therapeutic objective is to eradicate all of the clinically known as well as any suspected subclinical disease in the neck. Sometimes this cannot be accomplished with surgery alone. Obviously it would be beneficial to the patient to preserve as much function as is possible when removing any metastatic cancer. Whether or not this can be accomplished is often dictated by the extent of the disease, but sometimes by the expertise of the surgeon. Depending on the location of the N3a cervical metastasis, certain structures may or may not have to be sacrificed in order for the surgeon to remove all of the gross disease. Occasionally it is necessary to actually resect more extensively than with the standard radical neck dissection. Fortunately, in selected instances, especially N3b and N3c stages, it may be possible to perform less than a standard classic radical neck dissection, preserving important structures.

The use of surgery and radiation in the treatment of cervical metastasis requires selectivity and cooperation between the surgeon and the radiotherapist. The control of the cancer appears to be equal with the use of either preoperative or postoperative radiation. Postoperative radiation, however, tends to give better results than preoperative radiation because the healing is accomplished and the radiation dose and fields can be better tailored to the specific areas where surgery has a high risk of failure. The postoperative radiation should be given within 6 weeks after surgery.

One of the most important considerations in deciding whether combined treatment is necessary is to first consider how the primary cancer should be treated. In many cases the primary and the nodal metastasis are not congruent, that is, the primary may be small and the nodal metastasis large or vice versa. If the small primary would be best treated with radiation therapy, but the advanced disease in the neck could not be sterilized with radiation alone, the treatment should be combined in the neck, and the sequence of the surgery and the radiation is determined by whether the disease in the neck is resectable. This is a crucial clinical decision because if the surgeon, when he attempts to remove the disease in the neck, cuts through gross disease or leaves the unresected but surgically disturbed disease behind, an unfavorable situation for successful treatment with postoperative radiation has been created. Therefore, it is important for the surgeon to properly assess whether he can completely remove all of the gross disease from the various important anatomic structures such as the internal carotid artery, the vertebral artery, the vagus nerve, and the brachial plexus. Most of the other structures of the neck can be removed, if necessary to eradicate the gross disease, without tragic alterations in function and increased mortality. Occasionally, a large unresectable metastatic deposit of squamous carcinoma in the neck can be treated with either chemotherapy or radiation therapy preoperatively to cause enough regression in its size to render the tumor resectable. Unfortunately, there is a problem with preoperative radiation. If the primary cancer would best be treated with radiation as the only modality of treatment, giving a lesser preoperative dose to the neck mass may be difficult because it sits right in the pathway of the necessary greater dose of radiation to the primary. Since the dose to the primary needs to be in the range of 6500 to 7000 rads in $6^{1}/_{2}$ to 7 weeks, the metastasis would also receive the same dose, which might make it difficult from a surgeon's standpoint to remove it with the expectation of good wound healing. Consequently, chemotherapy may be better used initially in this case. If the cervical mass regresses significantly, radiation therapy then could be given as definitive treatment for the primary as well as the metastasis. If only partial regression occurs, but enough to change an unresectable node to a resectable one, then a surgical excision followed by definitive radiation to the primary and postoperative radiation to the neck would seem appropriate.

Criteria which dictate the use of surgery after radiation for nodal metastasis include the size of the node, location of the node, dosage of radiation to the node, and response of the node to the given radiation. If a node is less than 3 cm, is in the first eschelon of lymphatic drainage from the primary, receives at least 6000 rads, and completely disappears, we would feel comfortable in not removing it surgically. In certain situations concerning the primary cancer, postoperative radiation is indicated even when the nodal metastasis is small. If there is submucosal lymphatic permeation or perineural invasion found after resection of the primary or if the adequacy of the margins of resection of the primary were suspect, the neck would be included in the postoperative radiation fields. Extracapsular invasion, regardless of whether the node is stage N3 or less, and the presence of multiple nodes are indications for postoperative radiation since there is a high incidence of regional recurrence following surgery alone. If there is suspected or proved retropharyngeal nodal involvement, we believe that postoperative radiation is indicated in order to eradicate potential disease at the base of the skull. If, at the time of resection of the primary or dissection of the ipsilateral neck, there is a good indication for postoperative radiation and there is a high potential for contralateral metastasis, but the contralateral neck is

stage N0, we would prefer not to dissect the opposite neck, but to treat the entire neck and primary area with postoperative radiation.

The most difficult clinical problem is the treatment of the unresectable nodal metastasis, particularly if it is high in the jugulodigastric, posterior cervical area, extending under the mandible toward the base of the skull. In many such cases the tumor is infiltrating around all of the branches of the external carotid and can be difficult to remove from the carotid bulb. Most masses that are in the midjugular region, even though they achieve a large size, can usually be peeled off the common carotid artery and grossly removed. However, sometimes they are intimately involved with the laryngeal structures. The surgical resection sometimes necessitates removal of a portion of the thyroid cartilage, hyoid bone, trachea, or even the entire larynx.

Resection of the common or internal carotid artery is not justified.[1] If the disease is invading the carotid artery or if microscopic disease is present within the adventitia, postoperative radiation should be given. In many cases, large masses in the upper jugulodigastric and lower posterior cervical areas in the neck completely encase the spinal accessory nerve; consequently, no effort should be made to save the nerve. Sometimes, however, the node or nodes are only adjacent to the nerve and can be dissected off, saving the intact nerve. Postoperative radiation preserves shoulder function without compromising the patient's cancer treatment. If a segment of the nerve needs to be removed, perhaps a nerve graft can be performed if there is a sufficient proximal and distal stump.

If the primary is unknown and the cervical metastasis is large, treatment of the primary takes a secondary role and a decision has to be made regarding the best treatment for the neck. If the node is resectable, postoperative radiation to the neck can be tailored to include areas suspected of harboring the occult primary, such as the nasopharynx, tonsil, pharyngeal walls, pyriform sinus, or base of tongue. Occasionally, if the cervical metastasis is secondary to a skin cancer, particularly from an area of the face or scalp where the drainage to the parotid nodes is likely, a superficial parotidectomy should be included with the resection of the cervical metastasis.

During the period from 1960 through 1974, 4038 previously untreated patients with squamous cell carcinoma of the oral cavity, oropharynx, hypopharynx, nasopharynx, paranasal sinus, and supraglottic and glottic larynx were treated at M.D. Anderson Hospital with either surgery, radiation, or a combination of both. The frequency of patients with necks staged N3 was 11 percent (459), of which 3 percent (131) were classified as N3a and 8 percent (328) as N3b. The overall first failure in the neck, regardless of the N stage or treatment modality, was 17 percent (706). Twenty-two percent of the patients with N3-staged necks treated with irradiation or surgery developed a recurrence in the neck, 25 percent with N3a and 21 percent with

N3b. Thirty-four patients with N-3 staged necks were treated with planned postoperative radiation, with a neck failure rate of 12 percent (4/34). Thirteen patients with N3 necks were treated with planned preoperative radiation, and 15 percent (2/11) failed in the neck. Thus, planned combined treatment for N3-staged neck disease was able to decrease the incidence of regional failure by almost 50 percent.

In addition, we have treated 28 patients who had primaries which were judged best treated with radiation alone, but had large neck metastasis. The size of the metastasis was at least greater than 3 cm, and it was expected to not be sterilized by radiation alone. Consequently, the mass was removed, and then definitive radiation was given to the primary and postoperatively to the neck. So far, after at least 2 years of follow-up, we have had no regional recurrence in the neck with this treatment concept. There have been radiation failures in the primary since many of these lesions were in the late T2 or T3 stage. However, the percentage of failure in the primary is not worse than would be expected with the same type of lesions treated in the conventional way.

REFERENCES

1. Kennedy JT, Krause C, Loevy S. The importance of tumor attachment to the carotid artery. Arch Otolaryngol 1977; 103:70–73.

MANAGEMENT OF PATIENTS WITH N3 CERVICAL LYMPHADENOPATHY AND/ OR CAROTID ARTERY INVOLVEMENT

DON R. GOFFINET, M.D.
SHYAM B. PARYANI, M.D.
WILLARD E. FEE, Jr., M.D.

When cervical lymph nodes involved by metastatic squamous cell carcinoma are larger than 6 cm, or when the neoplasm has extended through the nodal capsule and invaded the soft tissues of the neck, the carotid sheath, or cervical vertebrae, local control is difficult to achieve and cure is unlikely.[1–10] In this chapter, we present the treatment results in a group of patients with advanced (N3) cervical lymph node disease who underwent planned, combined resection of the primary site, radical neck dissection, and postoperative irradiation.[11] In addition, another group of patients with large cervical neoplasms attached to the carotid artery who were treated not only by resection, but also by intraoperative iodine-125 seed-Vicryl suture implants to the carotid region, will be discussed.[12]

MATERIALS AND METHODS

Combined Surgery and Postoperative Irradiation

Twenty-one patients underwent planned resection of the primary site and either bilateral radical neck dissections[4] or ipsilateral neck dissections[13] at Stanford between 1975 and 1982. The primary sites and N stages are listed in Table 1. There were two patients with oral cavity primary cancers, five with involvement of hypopharyngeal structures, eight with oropharyngeal primary neoplasms, and six with supraglottic laryngeal carcinomas. Seventeen of the 21 patients had stage N3b cervical lymphs nodes; four had N3a cervical lymphadenopathy (AJC Staging).[14] With the exception of two patients, all had advanced primary lesions. Seven of these patients also had introperative ^{125}I seed-Vicryl suture carrier implants at the time of the initial procedure.

After resection of the primary site and cervical

TABLE 1 Cases of N3 Cervical Lymph Nodes Treated by Surgery and Postoperative Radiation Therapy (21 patients)

Site	AJC Staging
Oral cavity (2)	
Tongue	T2N3b
Floor of mouth	T4N3b
Oropharynx (8)	
Tonsil	T3N3a
	T3N3a
	T3N3b
	T4N3b
Ant. pillar	T3N3b
Palate	T3N3b
Base of tongue	T2N3b
OP walls	T4N3b
Supraglottic larynx (6)	
Epiglottis	T1N3b
	T4N3b
	T4N3b
	T4N3b
	T4N3b
Ary. epig. fold	T4N3b
Hypopharynx (5)	
Pyriform sinus	T1N3a
	T2N3b
	T3N3a
	T3N3b
	T3N3b

lymph nodes, megavoltage radiation therapy was begun within 4 weeks of the surgical procedure. All fields were treated daily, at a dose rate of 200 rads per day, 5 days per week, for a total of 5000 to 5500 rads to the primary site and necks if the margins were uninvolved; total radiation doses of 6000 to 6600 rads were given to the contralateral cervical region if a radical neck dissection had not been performed for stage N1 involvement, or when the surgical margins were either involved by neoplasm or questionably free of cancer. The mediastinum was treated with a "T-shaped" anterior field, matched onto the opposed lateral primary portals, in all instances. The mediastinal dose of 5000 to 5500 rads was calculated at a depth of 5.0 cm. A 6-Mev linac was used exclusively, and these patients were treated in the sitting position, immobilized by a bite block.

^{125}I Vicryl Carotid Implants

Forty-three patients received intraoperative ^{125}I seed-Vicryl suture carotid implants at the time of cervical lymph node resection at Stanford between 1975 and 1982 (Table 2). Thirteen patients were previously untreated, whereas 30 had received prior radiation therapy and/or surgery and had, at the time of re-resection and implantation, no evidence of disease other than the cervical lymph node recurrence. The 13 previously untreated patients had involvement of the following primary sites: oropharynx—4 (tonsil, 2; base of tongue, 2); pyriform sinus—4; supraglottis—2 (aryepiglottic fold and epiglottis); nasopharynx—1; and unknown primary site—2. Six of the 13 patients had stage N3a cervical lymphadenopathy, five had stage N3b neoplasms, and the other two patients had stage N2a cervical lymph nodes. The mean values of millicuries per seed inserted, total millicuries implanted, total dose in one year (in rads), and implant volume in cubic centimeters are noted in Table 3 for patients with no prior therapy, and in Table 4 for those with cervical recurrences.

The ^{125}I seed-Vicryl carrier implant was preplanned by the use of a PDP-11/45 treatment planning computer, which determined both the end-to-end seed spacing in the suture and the distance between the Vicryl sutures according to the volume to be implanted and the seed strength available.[13,15] Planar implants were performed.[16] Approximately 5 days post-implantation, orthogonal localizing radiographs were taken, and by the use of a digitizing light pen, the ^{125}I seed coordinates were entered into a General Electric treatment planning computer so that the total radiation doses to the implant volumes could be calculated and displayed, as well as the isodose distributions.

TABLE 2　^{125}I Vicryl Carotid Implants
(Stanford, 1975–1982; 43 Patients)

No prior Rx	13
Prior Rx (Curative)	30

TABLE 3　^{125}I Vicryl Carotid Implants
(No prior Rx — 13 Patients)

Mean	
mCi/seed	0.45
Total mCi	19.5
Total dose (rads)	16,000
Implant volume	31.5 cc

TABLE 4　^{125}I Vicryl Carotid Implants
(Prior Rx — 30 Patients)

Mean	
mCi/seed	0.41
Total mCi	14.5
Total dose (rads)	15,600
Implant volume	25.4 cc

RESULTS

Combined Surgery and Postoperative Irradiation: 21 Patients

Ten of the 21 patients are without evidence of disease (48%), either alive (7 patients) or dead from intercurrent causes (3), with a mean follow-up of 20 months. Eight of the 21 patients relapsed in the resected and irradiated neck (38%), while a single patient failed only at the primary site and two (10%) developed only distant metastases (Table 5). The status of the cervical lymph nodes and the results of treatment according to lymph node size and the presence or absence of histopathologically proven soft tissue extension are listed in Table 6. When soft tissue extension was present, usually in combination with a large nodal mass, local control was not obtained in any of the five patients, whereas all those with large neck masses (but without soft tissue extension) were locally controlled in the neck by combined surgery

TABLE 5　Results of Treatment of N3 Cervical Lymph Nodes by Surgery and Postoperative Radiation Therapy (Stanford 1975–1982; 21 Patients)

No evidence of disease	10 (48%)
Neck relapse	8 (38%)
Primary relapse	only 1 (5%)
Metastases	only 2 (10%)

TABLE 6　Node Findings after Treatment of N3 Cervical Lymph Nodes by Surgery and Postoperative Radiation Therapy (Stanford 1975–1982; 21 Patients)

Node Finding	No. of Pts	Control in Necks
Soft tissue extension	5	0　(0%)
> 6 cm without soft tissue extension	5	5 (100%)
< 6 cm without soft tissue extension	11	8　(77%)

and radiation therapy. Local control was also achieved in 77 percent of the patients whose lymph nodes were smaller than 6 cm. Intraoperative ^{125}I seed Vicryl implants were performed in seven of these 21 patients. Local control was achieved in the implanted volume in five of the seven patients (71%), but recurrences were noted in head and neck sites outside of the implant volume in six of these seven patients, and none is without evidence of disease (Table 7).

[125]-I Carotid Implants and No Prior Treatment: 13 Patients

Local control was obtained in the implanted volume in 10 of the 13 patients (77%) with no prior treatment who underwent carotid area implantation of ^{125}I seed-containing sutures. No relapses were noted in any head and neck sites in seven of the 13 patients (54%); two (15%) remain alive, without evidence of disease (Table 8). The mean follow-up in this group is 13 months.

[125]-I Carotid Implants for Recurrences: 30 Patients

In the 30 previously treated patients with a cervical relapse, but no other apparent evidence of failure after surgery and/or irradiation, local control in the implant volume was obtained in 23 of 30 patients (77%) and in all head and neck sites in one-half (15 of 30). Three patients remain without evidence of disease (10%), with a mean follow-up of 7.9 months (Table 9).

[125]-I Carotid Implants—Complications: 43 Patients

The complications that occurred after [125]I Vicryl intraoperative implants were performed are listed in Table 10. Patients who had received prior treatment had a 20 percent incidence of complications, whereas patients who were previously untreated had an incidence of 54 percent. Superficial skin ulcers encountered in the group with no prior treatment occurred mainly during postoperative irradiation, approxi-

TABLE 7   Results of Intraoperative [125]I Implants During Treatment of N3 Cervical Lymph Nodes by Surgery and Postoperative Radiation Therapy (Stanford 1975–1982; 7/21 Patients)

Local control (implant volume)	5/7 (71%)
Local control (all head & neck sites)	1/7 (14%)
No evidence of disease	0/7

TABLE 8   Results of Treatment with [125]I Vicryl Carotid Implants (No prior Rx — 13 Patients)

Local control (implant volume)	10/13 (77%)
Local control (all head & neck sites)	7/13 (54%)
No evidence of disease	2/13 (15%)
Mean Follow-Up — 13 months	

TABLE 9   Results of Treatment with [125]I Vicryl Carotid Implants (Priox Rx — 30 Patients)

Local control (implant volume)	23/30 (77%)
Local control (all head & neck sites)	15/30 (50%)
No evidence of disease	3/30 (10%)
Mean Follow-Up — 7.9 months	

TABLE 10   Complications of Treatment with [125]I Vicryl Carotid Implants (43 Patients)

No Prior Rx (13 Patients)		Prior Rx (30 Patients)	
Skin ulcer	4	Wound dehisc.	3
Wound dehisc.	1	Flap necrosis	1
Flap necrosis	1	Fistula	1
Dysphagia	1	Facial n. palsy, (transient)*	1
	7/13 (54%)		6/30 (20%)

*The patient with a postoperative facial nerve palsy underwent extensive dissection for recurrent neoplasm in the cervical, carotid, and retromandibular regions. Nerve function returned slowly postoperatively.

mately 2 months after implantation, at the time of the first half-life of the isotope (60 days), when 50 percent of the radiation dose had been delivered. These ulcers were superficial and healed spontaneously, but this risk of cutaneous injury has been reduced by shielding the implant volume at a postimplant radiation dose of approximately 3600 rads.

DISCUSSION

The ^{125}I seed-Vicryl implants performed as intended, since the recurrence rate in the implanted volume was low, averaging 20 to 25 percent in these patients with large cervical metastases which involved the carotid sheath.[17,18] The complications of flap necrosis and skin ulceration in the implanted patients have become less frequent as more information about the late effects of ^{125}I on tissues has become available. When irradiating postoperatively after an I[125] seed-Vicryl suture implantation, we now shield the implant volume at approximately 3600 to 4000 rads, use ^{125}I seed strengths less than 0.49 mCi, and continue to carefully preplan the implants.[19] By the use of such a dose reduction to the implant volume during external beam radiation therapy and by closing defects with myocutaneous flaps, the risk of ulceration has been reduced. Although we were unable to correlate the volume implanted with either local control or the risk of complications in this study, we believe that total ^{125}I doses of approximately 15,000 rads in untreated patients and 10,000 to 11,000 rads in previously irradiated patients are the maximum that should be given (specific gamma ray constant of 1.7 used in these calculations).[19]

In patients with N3 cervical lymphadenopathy managed by combined radiation and surgery, there was a 38 percent incidence of local failures, despite resection and planned high-dose postoperative irradiation. All five patients with massive cervical lymph node involvement and histopathologic demonstration of soft tissue extension failed, despite all our efforts. These patients all had massive neoplasms, which although technically operable, were probably incurable. In patients with smaller lesions, high local control rates were achieved (13 of 16, 80%). Complications following these procedures were few.

For those with massive adenopathy and soft tissue extension, surgery, postoperative irradiation, and intraoperative implantation are often insufficient treatment to cure the cancer, although control in the implanted volume may be achieved. Therefore, the addition of other modalities such as chemotherapy, hyperthermia, or radiosensitizing drugs should be considered for such patients.

REFERENCES

1. Bartelink H, Breur K, Hart G, et al. The value of postoperative radiotherapy as an adjuvant to radical neck dissection. Cancer 1983; 52:1008–1013.
2. Deutsch M, Leen R, Parsons J, et al. Radiotherapy for postoperative recurrent squamous cell carcinoma in head and neck. Arch Neurol 1973; 29:316–318.
3. Fee WE, Steadman MG. Planned carotid artery resection in head and neck surgery. Trans AA00 1977; 84:814–815.
4. Jesse R, Fletcher G. Treatment of the neck in patients with squamous cell carcinoma of the head and neck. Cancer 1977; 39:878–882.
5. Kennedy J, Krause C, Loevy S. The importance of tumor attachment to the carotid artery. Arch Otolaryngol 1977; 103;70–73.
6. Olcott N, Fee WE, Enzmann WE, et al. Planned approach to the management of malignant invasion of the carotid artery. Am J Surg 1981; 142:123–127.
7. Pearlman N. Treatment outcome in recurrent head and neck cancer. Arch Surg 1979; 114:39–42.
8. Santos V, Strong M, Vaughan C, et al. Role of surgery in head and neck cancer with fixed nodes. Arch Otolaryngol 1975; 101:645–648.
9. Skolyszewski J, Korzeniowski S, Reinfuss M. The re-irradiation of recurrences of head and neck cancer. Br J Radiol 1980; 53:462–465.
10. Syed A, Feder B, George F, et al. ^{192}Ir afterloading implants in the retreatment of head and neck cancers. Br J Radiol 1978; 51:814–820.
11. Goffinet Dr, Fee WE, Goode RL. Combined surgery and postoperative irradiation in the treatment of cervical lymph nodes. Arch Otolaryngol 1984; 110:736–738.
12. Fee WE, Goffinet Dr, Paryani S, et al. Intraoperative iodine-125 implants: Their use in large tumors in the neck attached to the carotid artery. Arch Otolaryngol 1983; 109:727–730.
13. Martinez A, Goffinet DR, Palos B, et al. Sterilization of ^{125}I seeds encased in Vicryl sutures for permanent interstitial implantation. Int J Radiat Oncol Biol Phys 1979; 5:411–413.
14. Beahrs OH, Myers MH, eds. Manual for Staging Cancer. 2nd ed. Philadelphia: JB Lippincott Co, 1983; pp 25–43.
15. Sandor J, Palos B, Goffinet DR, et al. Dose calculations for planar arrays of ^{192}Ir and ^{125}I seeds for brachytherapy. Appl Radiol 1979; 8:41–44.
16. Palos B, Pooler D, Goffinet DR, et al. A method for inserting Iodine-125 seeds into Vicryl absorbable sutures in preparation for permanent implantation into tissues. Int J Radiat Oncol Biol Phys 1980; 6:381–835.
17. Goode R, Fee W, Goffinet DR, et al. Radioactive suture in the treatment of head and neck cancer. Laryngoscope 1979; 89:349–354.
18. Martinez A, Goffinet DR, Fee W, et al. Iodine-125 suture implants as an adjuvant to surgery and external beam radiotherapy in the management of locally advanced head and neck cancer. Cancer 1983; 51:973–979.
19. Goffinet DR, Martinez A, Fee WE. ^{125}I Vicryl suture implants as a surgical adjuvant in cancer of the head and neck. Int J Radiat Oncol Biol Phys. In press.

MANAGEMENT OF THE N3 NECK: INTRAOPERATIVE RADIATION

RONALD C. HAMAKER, M.D., F.A.C.S.
MARK I. SINGER, M.D., F.A.C.S.
NEWELL PUGH, M.D.
DAVID ROSS, M.D.
PETER GARRETT, M.D.

The definition and classification of fixed disease in the neck have been controversial. Clinical evaluation is often misleading in the classification of N3. The American Joint Committee for North America defined N3 disease as a massive homolateral node(s), bilateral nodes, or contralateral node(s).[1] The N3a represents clinically positive homolateral node(s), one greater than 6 cm in diameter. N3b consists of bilateral positive nodes with each side staged separately. N3c represents a contralateral node(s) only. It was felt that everyone could measure accurately and that nodes greater than 6 cm were beyond their capsule. This extranodal extension decreases the survival rate and increases local recurrence in the neck. The Union Internationale Centre Le Cancer (UICC) for Europe classified N3 disease as evidence of involvement by fixed regional lymph nodes.[2] Our surgical and radiation therapy groups have adopted the classification as set forth by the American Joint Committee. Fixation to associated structures in addition to size is noted for our own identification and prognostic acumen in each patient.

The N3 disease, which will be considered in this report, is evidenced by fixed nodes. Fixation occurs in many forms, each being a different therapeutic problem. Fixation to skin is easily recognized. However, fixation to the carotid artery may not be noted until surgical exposure. Similarly, a node less than 3 cm can be attached to the carotid adventitia. Fixation by extension into the sternomastoid muscle is much easier to remove in a radical neck dissection unless the disease has penetrated bone at the base of the skull or sternoclavicular joint. Invasion into deep muscles of the neck or into the brachial plexus creates major morbidity and incurability in most of the patients. Bilateral fixed disease does occur, and a new classification of N4 has been recommended by Stell.[3] This disease presents a twofold increase in the treatment problems of N3, and the prospects of curability are minimal.

N3 disease in most institutions is treated with a combination of radiation, surgery, and, more recently, chemotherapy. Major attempts by radiation oncologists with high doses of 7000 rads or greater have been combined with booster doses or radioactive implants in palliation. Surgeons have resected all of the cervical skin, claviculosternal joints, portions of the temporal bone, carotid and subclavian arteries, brachial plexus branches, and deep musculature to the spine in attempts at cure. These attempts to salvage and palliate patients with fixed disease demonstrate the morbidity of local recurrence.

Recent studies have shown an improvement in local control of extensive head and neck cancers. [125]I permanent implants have become popular and demonstrate good palliative efforts and potential curability. Martinez et al found that in patients treated with curative intent by surgery and ^{125}I, local control was 58 percent, while control in the implanted site was 100 percent.[4] The actuarial survival was 50 percent at 5 years. In recurrent cancers after surgery and/or external beam radiation, the local control was 50 percent. They had a complication rate of 7 percent related to the implant only. They found that total activity and the volume of tissue implanted were directly correlated to the complications. Volumes greater than 45 ml developed skin ulcers which healed slowly. They treated 15 carotid arteries without rupture. Vikram et al also utilized ^{125}I implants.[5] Their local failure in neck implants was 26.5 percent with disease recurring within 16 months after implantation. No difference in local control was noted with different histologic types.

Intraoperative radiation therapy (IORT) is a method that involves delivery of a large single dose of radiation to the tumor bed with preservation of the normal tissue while the patient is under anesthesia. Improved energy sources have enabled intraoperative radiation to evolve as a practical method in the 1970s. The Japanese reported the use of IORT for abdominal and cerebral tumors. Their experience exceeds that of all other investigators combined. Four institutions in the United States—Mayo Clinic, Massachusetts General Hospital, Howard University, and National Cancer Institute—have initiated clinical and laboratory evaluation of this method.

To date, no one has reported the utilization of intraoperative radiation therapy in the head and neck. In April 1982, Head and Neck Surgery Associates, in a combined effort with the Methodist Hospital of Indiana Radiation Oncology Department, began intraoperative radiation therapy of extensive head and neck cancer. A total of 31 patients have been treated by this method.

In this chapter we will present our early experience with intraoperative radiation therapy for N3 disease. Since the study began in 1982, 12 patients have received intraoperative radiation therapy to the neck for fixed disease. The majority of these cases have consisted of recurrent disease after radiation and/or surgery failure. Initially, during the feasibility study, the efforts were palliative in nature. Now, local control seems to be more feasible in microscopic and minimal gross residual disease.

INDICATIONS

The indications for intraoperative radiation therapy in neck disease are similar to those for head and neck in general. They are:

1. Tumor with extensive recurrence in the neck after resection and/or radiation.
2. Tumor fixation to the carotid or deep muscles.
3. Tumor extending from the neck with fixation to bone (clavicle, sternum, spine, or base of skull).
4. Close margins in attempt to preserve function or a vital structure.

Initially, the indications regarding close margins were applied primarily to recurrent cancer. Once the safety of the procedure had been determined, this indication was expanded to nonirradiated cases. These indications were adopted through the combined experiences of local failure by the radiation oncologist and the head and neck surgeons.

TECHNIQUE

Intraoperative radiation therapy is scheduled in the afternoon or on weekends to accommodate the daily schedule of patients undergoing conventional external beam radiation via the linear accelerator. The radiation therapy room is modified to meet the Indiana State Board of Health requirements for open wounds. The patient is transported under anesthesia, well monitored, through the halls and down an elevator to Radiation Therapy. The therapy requires approximately 15 to 20 minutes.

The energy source can be converted from 4 Mev to a 7 Mev or 11 Mev accelerator. The 80 percent depth dose is 1.1 cm, 2.2 cm, and 3.1 cm respectively. The Lucite cones constructed to direct the beam of irradiation are 4, 5, 6, and 9 cm in diameter. The volume of treatment can be rather large. A combined decision about cone size and positioning of the cone is done by the radiation oncologist and the head and neck surgeon in the operating room. Normal tissue within the cone area is shielded with lead or retracted from the area.

Intraoperative radiation therapy is a multidiscipline approach to cancer treatment. A team is required to make this method safe and successful. Twelve ancillary personnel in addition to surgeons, radiation oncologists, and anesthesiologists are required for the surgery, transportation, set-up, and radiation therapy.

PATIENT ANALYSIS

The average age of these 12 patients with N3 disease was 62 years, with ages ranging from 47 to 71 years (Table 1). There were only two females in the treatment group. Squamous cell carcinoma was the only histologic type. There were three patients with gross disease and an equal number with microscopic disease. Close margins on the carotid, where the adventitia or external carotid was resected for tumor

ablation, accounted for another six patients. Nine patients had previous treatment with radiation in combination with surgery or alone for cure.

The port sizes ranged from 4 to 9 cm. A 4 Mev energy source was the most common, but a 7 Mev was utilized twice. An 11 Mev was used in one case for gross disease when minimal debulking was accomplished. Cases 1 through 4, 6, and 12 were treated for palliation only. The other six were treated for cure, realizing that their disease was significant and the cure rate was extremely low.

DISCUSSION

The feasibility study of intraoperative radiation therapy in head and neck cancer reported elsewhere demonstrated the safety of the procedure despite the transfer of the patients to radiation therapy.[6] There were no deaths, cardiorespiratory problems, anes-

TABLE 1   Intraoperative Radiation Therapy (IORT) TO N₃ Disease

Case No.	Sex	Age	Pathology & Location	Disease for Intraop Rad Therapy	Previous Treatment	Intraop Rad Therapy Dose	Postop Radiation Therapy	Disease Control in · IORT Port	Status	Cause of Death
1	F	71	SCE tongue to necks	G-Clav. head M-Deep cerv. mm CM-BOT	Partial glossect	10 GY, 4 Mev to 4 ports		N/A	DOC 3 days	Mucous plug
2	M	57	SCE stoma	G-Innominate & vertebral	Laryng. & neck + 60 GY	20 GY, 4 Mev		Unknown	DUC 1 month	Innom art blowout
3	M	62	SCE neck from larynx	M-carotid bed	Laryng. & neck + 60 GY	20 GY, 4 Mev		C	DOD 6 months	Lung mets & TIA
4	M	61	SCE larynx BOT to neck & skin	CM-carotid BOT	Laryng. & neck + 60 GY	10 GY, 4 Mev 10 GY, 4 Mev	50 GY	C	DOD 7 months	Loc dis outside port
5	M	60	SCE to neck from max	CM-carotid	Maxillectomy	15 GY, 7 Mev	60 GY	A	DOD 9 months	Lung & rib mets
6	M	65	SCE FOM to neck	G-Neck & carotid	FOM & Mod neck + 50 GY to neck	20 GY, 11 Mev		C UNCONT	DOD 11 months	Loc dis
7	M	65	SCE Larynx	CM-Carotid	Neck & larynx, car graft + 66 GY	15 GY, 7 Mev		A	DOD 13 months	Bone mets
8	M	68	SCE larynx	M-Carotid	Laryngᴇ + 60 GY	20 GY, 4 Mev			NED 12 months	
9	M	68	SCE tongue	CM-Deep MM	68 GY	20 GY, 4 Mev			NED 5 months	
10	F	60	SCE BOT	CM-BOT CM-Carotid	45 GY	15 GY, 4 Mev 10 GY, 4 Mev			NED 2 months	
11	M	47	SCE larynx	CM-Carotid		20 GY, 4 Mev	At present		NED 1 month	
12	M	63	SCE Temporal Bone	CM-transverse process C2	Surg. + 50 GY	25 GY, 4 Mev	Pending		NED 1 week	

Abbreviations: MM = muscles; SCE = squamous cell carcinoma; GY = dose of 100 rads; G = gross; M = microscopic; CM = close margins; C = clinical; A = autopsy; UNCONT = uncontrolled; TIA = transient ischemic attacks; MAX = maxilla; BOT = base of tongue; FOM = floor of mouth; NED = no evidence of disease; DOC = dead of other causes; DUC = dead of unknown causes; LOC DIS = local disease.

thesia failures, serious difficulties, or infections.

The amount of intraoperative radiation therapy, 1000 to 2500 rads, has not created a problem in treatment about the carotid artery. Investigators at the National Cancer Institute have shown that there is little effect on the retroperitoneal vasculature of dogs at doses lower than 4000 rads.[7] The majority, or seven of the 12 patients, received 2000 or more rads. Cases 3 and 7 had carotid resection for gross disease. Case 7 had a blowout from disease, requiring resection and graft reconstruction. In both of these cases, the muscular bed medial to the carotid was treated with intraoperative radiation therapy.

The carotid artery that had resection of the external system or was stripped of adventitia is covered with muscle after intraoperative radiation therapy. The intention was to reinforce the suture line or carotid wall with a buttress of vascularized muscle, providing bulk between the carotid and the cervical skin. In this situation, our intraoperative therapy (IORT) dose was 1000 to 1500 rads. However, with time and experience, our dosage to the carotid has increased as in case 12.

The innominate artery in case 2 ruptured and was the cause of death. This artery had gross disease around it and was treated with 2000 rads by a 4 Mev source through a 6-cm cone. The patient developed a separation of the tracheostoma (not treated by IORT), and the resultant sinus tract penetrated into the intraoperative radiation therapy port. This innominate rupture could have been caused by tumor destruction, by tumor necrosis from intraoperative radiation therapy with arterial wall collapse, or by infection along the sinus tract to the heavily irradiated tissue with resultant necrosis. An autopsy was not obtained to determine the etiology. A pectoralis muscle flap had been placed over the irradiated artery, but the sinus tract seemed to be deep to the muscle buttress.

There were two other complications involving fistulas. Case 10 developed a hypopharyngeal cutaneous fistula well away from the intraoperative radiation therapy port. This fistula ultimately closed in 6 weeks. The second fistula (case 5) developed from the pyriform sinus to the skin 3 months after completion of 6000 rads of external beam postoperative radiation. The pyriform sinus had been protected during the intraoperative radiation therapy to the carotid artery. However, the necrosis from the fistula extended to the irradiated carotid and rupture resulted. No attempt was made to salvage this patient by ligation as distal disease was present in the ribs and lung. A review of the external radiation done elsewhere demonstrated overlapping ports with a heavy dose at the interface and site of necrosis. This case is indirectly a complication of intraoperative radiation therapy. The complication rate in intraoperative radiation therapy to the neck has been 25 percent, with 17 percent directly related to the procedure.

Autopsy information on two of these patients had demonstrated intraoperative radiation therapy to be cancericidal in its port of 1500 rads (cases 5 and 7). Clinical impression has suggested no control by intraoperative radiation therapy in one patient, case 6, and control of the irradiated disease in two others. Case 6 had extensive bulky disease in the neck. After the skin flaps were elevated, debulking was done, but to a small degree because of potential harm to the carotid artery. Intraoperative radiation therapy had absolutely no effect on this disease. Case 3 died of distal disease without evidence of tumor recurrence in the neck. Case 4 had extensive recurrence in the skin, and wide resection of the skin was performed prior to intraoperative radiation therapy. Intraoperative radiation therapy to the carotid and base of tongue for narrow margins was accomplished, but the disease recurred around the periphery in the unresected skin. Additional external beam radiation did not suffice.

Radiobiology of single large radiation doses suggests that 1500 rads will cause a 10^4 to a 10^5 cancer cell kill.[8] With microscopic disease or close margins, in which case a high potential for undiagnosed microscopic disease exists, intraoperative radiation therapy may be most effective. The intraoperative radiation therapy decreases the cancer cell population to an exceedingly small number. Treatment of these remaining cells with external-beam postoperative radiation should be highly successful. The gross disease in case 4 was too extensive to allow any impact by intraoperative radiation therapy. Small volumes of gross disease may be controlled, especially when intraoperative radiation therapy is used in conjunction with postoperative external-beam radiation.

The purpose of intraoperative radiation therapy is to provide a high dose of radiation to a selected tumor bed, sparing vital structures and normal tissue in a uniform and safe method. Knowing the depth of penetration allows for proper selection of the energy source. The routine concern for spinal cord and skin tolerance is totally eliminated.

In contrast, [125]I Vicryl therapy carries a potential danger to normal tissues, both medial and lateral to the seeds. Vikram et al provided lead-impregnated plastic shields to be worn over the implant area when indicated for protection to nursing personnel.[5] The radioactive threads present a slight potential risk to the surgeon and the radiation oncologist. Application of radioactive seeds or threads to a small tumor plaque on the bulb or internal carotid could be extremely difficult technically. The uniformity of dose in intraoperative radiation therapy is controlled by calculation and application of radiation principles and not by aligning suture material or implanting seeds. Tumor bulk can create difficulties along the carotid artery in knowing the exact location to avoid puncture by radioactive threaded seeds or seed implants. Radiobiologically, the large single doses cause a greater cell rate kill than the slower dose rates of [125]I. Despite these theoretic advantages of intraoperative radiation therapy, ^{125}I implants have obtained satisfactory results for 5-year follow-up.

The major disadvantage of intraoperative radiation therapy has been the surgical scheduling. Completion of the daily schedule in radiation therapy is essential. Miscalculation in resection time prior to intraoperative radiation therapy can delay transfer or cause waiting periods in the operating room. Cancelled intraoperative radiation therapy causes unnecessary preparation and expense. A radiation suite in the operating room would be ideal, but costly unless more surgical services find advantages to the technique.

SUMMARY

IORT for fixed disease in the neck is new, feasible, and safely performed in a general hospital. The advantages of large single-dose fractions in cell kill are well known in radiobiologic literature. Incorporating IORT with conventional external radiation in untreated N3 necks may prove to be highly successful in local control.

REFERENCES

1. Chandler JR, Guillamondegui OM, Sisson GA, Strong EW, Baker HW. Clinical staging of cancer of the head and neck: a new "new" system. Am J Surg 1976; 132:525–528.
2. UICC. TNM Classification of Malignant Tumours. Geneva, 1978.
3. Stell PM. Fixed, bilateral cervical nodes. J Laryngol Otol 1983; 97:851–856.
4. Martinez A, Goffinet DR, Fee W, Goode R, Cox RS. 125 Iodine implants as an adjuvant to surgery and external beam radiotherapy in the management of locally advanced head and neck cancer. Cancer 1983; 51-973–979.
5. Vikram B, Hilaris BS, Anderson L, Strong EW. Permanent iodine-125 implants in head and neck cancer. Cancer 1983; 51:1310–1314.
6. Hamaker RC, Singer MI, Pugh N, Ross D, Garrett P, Coffey G. Intraoperative radiation for head and neck cancer: A feasibility study. Presented to the International Conference on Head and Neck Cancer, Baltimore, July 26, 1984.
7. Sindelar WF, Tepper J, Travis EL, Terrill R. Tolerance of retroperitoneal structures to intraoperative radiation. Ann Surg 1982; 196:601–608.
8. Hall EJ. Radiobiology for the Radiologist. Hagerstown, Maryland: Harper & Row, 1978.

SIMULTANEOUS BILATERAL NECK DISSECTION

KUMAO SAKO, M.D.

When one speaks of an N3b neck category and the treatment by simultaneous bilateral radical neck dissection, it may immediately bring to mind a situation of inoperability, high morbidity, and a low or zero cure rate. Upon closer inspection and evaluation, the situation may not be quite so dismal and is deserving of some further consideration.

THE N3b NECK

The N3 neck has three subgroups[1] (Table 1). In the N3b subgroup there are bilateral clinically positive cervical nodes. However, neither side of the neck may have a node greater than 6 cm or even greater than 3 cm, or both sides of the neck may have one or more nodes greater than 6 cm in diameter. An appreciable number of patients being considered as possible candidates for simultaneous bilateral radical neck dissection, however, may have only an N1 or N2 staging of one side of the neck. With this in mind, a look at our own experience may be helpful in determining whether the indications for bilateral radical neck dissection are easily discernible and whether the results justify such an approach.

MATERIALS AND METHODS

From January 1960 through December 1978, 48 patients with clinical N3b neck underwent simultaneous bilateral (one-stage) neck dissection performed as part of an oral, laryngeal, oropharyngeal, or pharyngeal resection for squamous cell carcinoma. Forty-two patients underwent a classic bilateral radical neck dissection. In four patients, one of the internal jugular veins and spinal accessory nerves were preserved. In two patients, both of the veins and spinal accessory nerves were preserved.

The primary sites are shown in Table 2. The largest number were in the supraglottic larynx (18 cases) and oral cavity (14 cases). All of the surgical speci-

TABLE 1 Subgroups of the N3 Neck

N3a Clinically positive homolateral node(s), one more than 6 cm in diameter
N3b Bilateral clinically positive nodes
N3c Contralateral clinically positive node(s) only

TABLE 2 Simultaneous Bilateral Neck Dissection: Primary Sites

Larynx	
Supraglottic	18
Glottic	2
Pyriform sinus	7
Lateral pharynx	1
Oral	14
Oropharynx	6
Total	48

mens had lymph node clearance. No patients in this group received routine planned postoperative radiation or preoperative or postoperative chemotherapy. There were 45 males and 3 females, and the age ranged from 38 to 79 years.

RESULTS

In 39 patients the nodes in the neck were clinically less than 3 cm, in four patients between 3 and 6 cm, and in only five patients greater than 6 cm.

The histologically positive node distribution in the ipsilateral and contralateral neck dissections are shown in Table 3. Twenty-nine of 48 patients had at least three positive nodes in one or both sides of the neck.

Seven patients died of other causes within 9 months postoperatively and were free of disease at the time of death. Two other patients died of other causes at 52 and 58 months after surgery and were free of disease at the time of death. These two patients were included in the evaluable group as almost all relapses in head and neck cancer occur within 3 years.

There were five postoperative deaths within one month after surgery. Thus the evaluable group was comprised of 36 patients. Twenty (55%) patients survived 13 months or more (Fig. 1), 11 (30%) of the 20 patients for more than 2 years, and 7 (19%) were free of disease at 5 years. One of these patients, after a small local recurrence in the edge of the primary site at 6 months, was controlled with a full postoperative course of radiation therapy of 6000 rads.

In those patients with three or more positive nodes in at least one side of the neck, 3/29 (10%) were free of disease at 5 years. Almost all of the patients dying of their disease developed local as well as regional recurrences. The majority developed distant metastases as well. Morbidity was significant in the patients postoperatively and the three most common complications were facial edema and swelling (72%), wound infection (77%), and fistula formation (39%).

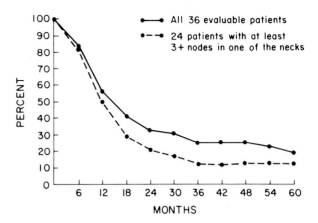

Figure 1 Survival curves in therapeutic simultaneous bilateral neck dissections.

DISCUSSION

In the majority of patients with squamous cell carcinoma of the head and neck area who undergo therapeutic simultaneous bilateral neck dissections at the time of resection of the primary lesion, the primary lesion is in the midline or crosses the midline, giving rise to early contralateral nodal spread, as can be seen by our findings and that of others.[2-5]

For patients presenting with clinically positive metastases, staging of the neck dissections has several disadvantages and risks. These are (1) the initial resection may require entering the contralateral neck, (2) there is risk of transecting lymphatics with tumor cells and seeding of the neck tissues, and (3) unforeseen complications may delay the second neck dissection, and during the delay a node in the contralateral neck may become fixed.

Our results and those of others demonstrate the feasibility of simultaneous neck dissections.[2-6]

Selection of patients with N3b necks for simultaneous neck dissections may be controversial if, after reviewing our statistics, one believes that survival rates of 55 percent for greater than 13 months, 30 percent for more than 2 years, and only 19 percent for 5 years do not justify a massive resection and bilateral dissection. However, the prognosis and survival of patients with three or more positive nodes in at least one side is no less favorable than in our previous study of prognosis in the study of nodal involvement of an ipsilateral neck alone in oral carcinoma.[7] In that study, three or more positive nodes gave a 13 percent 5-year survival. In only four patients were nodes measured to be between 3 and 6 cm, and in only five patients was there a node larger than 6 cm. In the majority of the patients, each side of the neck was individually assessed as less than an N3 neck.

Capsular invasion and perinodal spread have been

TABLE 3 Positive Node Distribution in the Ipsilateral and Contralateral Necks

Contralateral neck	Ipsilateral Neck				
	0+	1+	2+	3+	>3+
0+	4				2
1+		3	7	1	2
2+		2	3	1	3
3+		1	2		1
>3+	1	3	1	2	9
Total	5	9	13	4	17

shown to be associated with a decreased survival rate.[7-9] In our present review, complete data regarding extranodal spread were not available. Extranodal spread is seen more often with nodal involvement of large size. In an examination of 10 recent consecutive neck dissection specimens from patients with 3 cm or larger clinical nodes, all were positive nodes with capsular invasion or extension into perinodal soft tissues (Fig. 2).

The morbidity and incidence of complications are high following simultaneous bilateral neck dissection, but can be minimized somewhat by modifications of the standard radical neck dissections when feasible,[5] or by a rigorous program to control alterations of physiology when both internal jugular veins must be resected.[6]

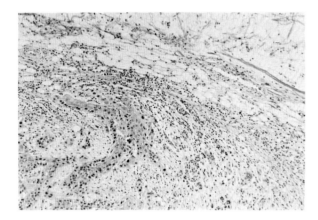

Figure 2 Photomicrograph showing extranodal spread of metastatic squamous cell carcinoma.

SUMMARY

The majority of patients with squamous cell carcinoma of the head and neck who present with N3b clinical necks (bilateral clinically positive nodes) are candidates for therapeutic bilateral neck dissections. The number of patients having a long-term disease-free interval and 5-year survival, although modest, appears to justify the procedure. No clear-cut guidelines for the selection of patients could be elucidated from our limited series of patients.

REFERENCES

1. American Joint Committee on Cancer. Staging of Cancer of Head and Neck Sites and of Melanoma. 1980.
2. Moore OS, Frazell EL. Simultaneous bilateral neck dissection. Am J Surg 1964; 107:565–568.
3. Rufino CD, McComb WS. Bilateral neck dissections; analysis of 180 cases. Cancer 1966; 19:1503–1508.
4. Razack MS, Baffi R, Sako K. Simultaneous bilateral neck dissection. J Surg Oncol 1980; 15:387–392.
5. Ballantyne AJ, Jackson GL. Synchronous bilateral neck dissection. Am J Surg 1982; 144:452–455.
6. McQuarrie DG, Mayberg M, Ferguson M, Shons AR. A physiologic approach to the problems of simultaneous bilateral neck dissection. Am J Surg 1977; 134:455–460.
7. Kalnins I, Leonard AG, Sako K, Razack MS, Shedd DP. Correlation between prognosis and degree of lymph node involvement in carcinoma of the oral cavity. Am J Surg 1977; 134:450–454.
8. Noone RB, Bonner Jr HB, Raymond S, Brown AS, Graham III WP, Lehr H. Lymph node metastases in oral carcinoma. Plast Reconstr Surg 1974; 53:158–166.
9. Johnson JT, Barnes EL, Myers EN, Schramm Jr VL, Borochovitz D, Sigler BA. The extracapsular spread of tumors in cervical node metastasis. Arch Otolaryngol 1981; 107:725–729.

16. Cancer of the Oral Cavity

INTRODUCTION

GEORGE A. SISSON, M.D.

It appears that there is general agreement that treatment management affects an optimistic progress for T1 lesions of the oral cavity.

Unfortunately, *late* diagnosis continues to be commonplace, and what could be a satisfactory experience for both physician and patient, in most instances, becomes one of patient misery and physician frustration, and culminates in high treatment costs for a poor result.

In the chapters that follow, the authors discuss some of the problems arising because of late diagnoses of cancers of the oral cavity and define contemporary management for these problems and look for possible solutions. For these discussions, we adhere to the 1980 AJC head and neck classification which includes the lip, buccal mucosa, mouth floor, oral tongue, hard palate, upper and lower gingiva, and the retromolar trigone. Late diagnosis of lesions found in these sites (with the exception of the lips) is frequent because early symptoms and signs are easily overlooked by the patient and doctor; even if noticed, they are not considered indicative. Although these areas are 100 percent visible for physical examination, poor examinations continue to be performed by general physicians and the busy specialist. A tongue depressor, an oral mirror, and good light source are all that is necessary for adequate primary examinations.

Cancer of the oral cavity comprises 5 percent of all body cancers; of these, most or 28 percent are cancers of the oral tongue and 26 percent of the floor of the mouth. The remaining 46 percent are equally divided among the other oral locations. Overall cures of cancers found in these sites (lip excluded) continue to be around 40 percent when they should be close to 80 percent. The reality is that most lesions, when presented for treatment, are stage III or IV! Difficult decisions now must be made since surgical procedures

must be recommended that often leave the patient disfigured or incapacitated.

Although the future of cancer treatment holds some promise of improvement because of current basic and clinical research, we must address the problems of today's patient and treat with combined or single techniques that have proved worthwhile.

In the chapters that follow, the authors (1) reexamine information previously accepted as fact, (2) discuss some of the more recent techniques, (3) reaffirm proved methods of treatment, and (4) provide an update as to the state of the art.

TONGUE FLAPS IN CANCER SURGERY OF THE ORAL CAVITY

VAHRAM Y. BAKAMJIAN, M.D.

Large, mobile, and centrally situated, the tongue is a most readily available source of local flaps for the repair of excisional defects in the oral cavity. Each symmetrical half, separated from the other by the fibrous midline raphe, is supplied by the lingual artery of its own side (Fig. 1), with no significant amount of cross circulation other than at the very tip of the organ and some at its base. A dorsal lingual branch from each artery posteriorly ascends to the base; the remaining main terminal branch, the deep lingual or ranine, follows the underside, giving at intervals vertical offshoots into the lingual substance as it proceeds foward and upward to the tip. Here it ramifies to anastomose with its counterpart from the opposite side. The pattern of this vascular distribution constitutes the basis for the interesting assortment of mus-

culomucosal flaps that are obtainable for reparative use from the tongue, without damaging its essential functions.

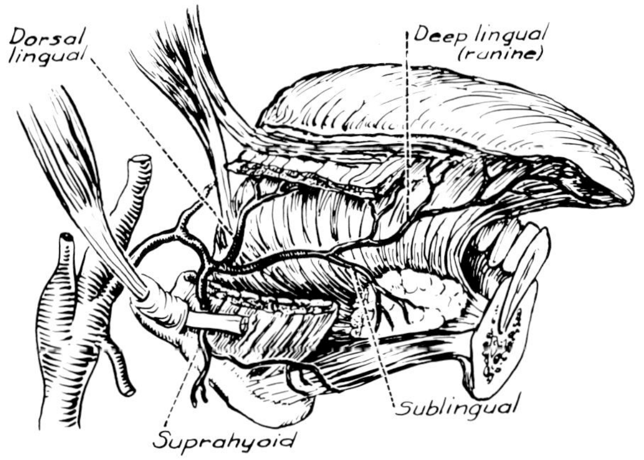

FLAPS FROM THE DORSAL SURFACE OF THE TONGUE

In the main, such a flap is derived longitudinally from one or the other side of the midline, with either a posterior or an anterior base (Fig. 2, *A* and *B*); if on rare occasion it is developed traversely, it may not

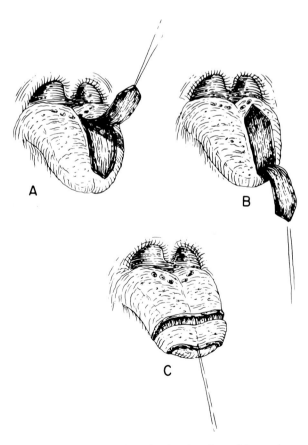

Figure 2 Flap forms from the dorsal surface of the tongue.

Figure 1 Vascular anatomy of the tongue.

cross the midline and succeed unless it is bipedicled (Fig. 2C). Approximately 7 mm in thickness, these flaps are raised with the mucosa to include the closely adhering corium, which is a dense submucous felt-work of connective tissue with elastic fibers and numerous penetrating vessels and nerves that supply the papillae, and the superior lingual muscle, which is the outermost stratum of intrinsic musculature of the tongue. Their donor wounds are easily closed by direct suture, but require scrupulous attention to hemostasis and to obliteration of dead space with one or more layers of buried sutures, lest a hematoma with gigantic swelling of the tongue ensue to embarrass not only viability of the flap, but also the airway to the lungs. This linear closure, in the case of a longitudinal donor wound, reduces the width, but not the functioning length of the remaining tongue, whereas in the case of a transverse wound, it shortens and blunts the lingual end to a degree that may not be warranted. Discretion, therefore, is important in using the transversely oriented bipedicle flap.

A longitudinal flap, based posteriorly at or a little past the circumvallate line and in length extending to near the tip of the tongue, when rotated laterally and backward, can neatly cover a faucial or a retromolar defect of moderate size (Fig. 3). With a lesser degree of rotation, this flap can provide covering for buccal defects in posterior areas of the cheek (Fig. 4). In the latter instance, however, an edentulous space may be

needed to admit the flap to its destination in the cheek without danger of the pedicle's being chewed by the molar teeth.

The same longitudinal flap based anteriorly on the freely mobile end of the tongue enjoys a wider range of usefulness in the anterior environs of the oral cavity. Here also, in the instances in which the flap needs to cross the line of the jaws with intact dentition, it will have to be protected by a specially prepared bite-block for the individual case, to be worn particularly in the postoperative early period of awakening from anesthesia, until the patient can cooperate fully to desist from biting the pedicle. Unlike the posteriorly based flap, this flap requires a second procedure to divide it from the site of the reconstruction.

By a rotation laterally and forward it can be applied to the repair of defects in the anterior portion of the cheek (Fig. 5). By a swing farther forward and a twist that brings its raw face to the front, it can be applied to a labial reconstruction (Fig. 6). With the same swing and more of a twist that turns its raw face down, it can be applied to repair of the anterior oral floor (Fig. 7). Through a window created in the median raphe, it can be made to pass to repair a contralateral defect of the anterior oral floor and undersurface of the tongue (Fig. 8). Or by a twist of 180° at the pedicle that turns its raw face upward, it can be used in the closure of an oroantral defect (Fig. 9).

And as for the transversely disposed bipedicle

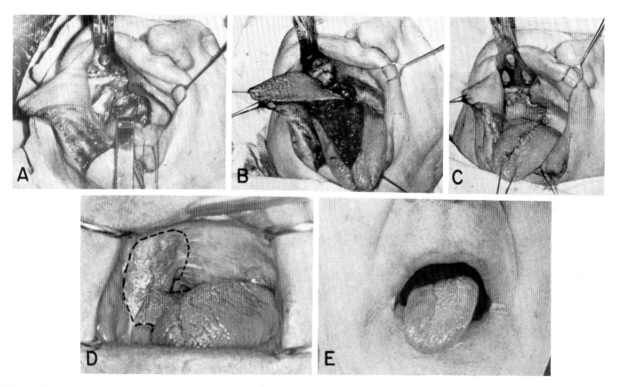

Figure 3 A wide retromolar and faucial resection for cancer in a 69-year-old male patient and immediate repair with a posteriorly based flap from the ipsilateral half of the dorsal surface of the tongue. *A*, The defect. *B*, The flap. *C*, Repair and direct suture closure of the donor wound. *D* and *E*, End result with satisfactory function of the tongue.

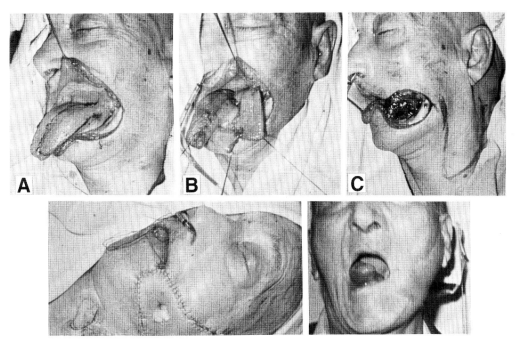

Figure 4 A full-thickness cheek resection for buccal cancer in an 88-year-old male patient and single-stage reconstruction with a posteriorly based flap from half of the dorsal surface of the tongue for lining, and a small sternomastoid musculocutaneous flap for outer cover. *A*, Full-thickness cheek defect and outline of the tongue flap. *B*, Raised tongue flap with directly closed donor wound. *C*, Lining repair completed with the tongue flap. *D*, External closure with musculocutaneous flap completed. *E*, End result with good protrusion of the tongue.

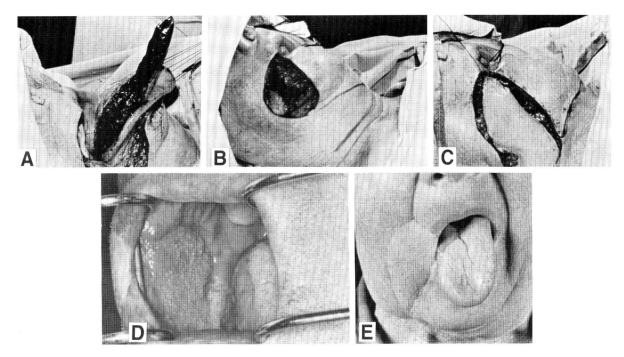

Figure 5 An anterior full-thickness resection of the cheek for cancer of the oral commissure in a 71-year-old male patient and reconstruction with an anteriorly based flap from the ipsilateral dorsal surface of the tongue for lining and a submental flap of skin for the outside. *A*, Full-thickness commissure-and-cheek defect and raised tongue flap. *B*, Lining restoration completed with the tongue flap, and outline of the skin flap. *C*, Skin flap rotated to cover the defect externally. *D* and *E*, Final result with satisfactory function of the tongue after division of both flaps in a second-stage procedure.

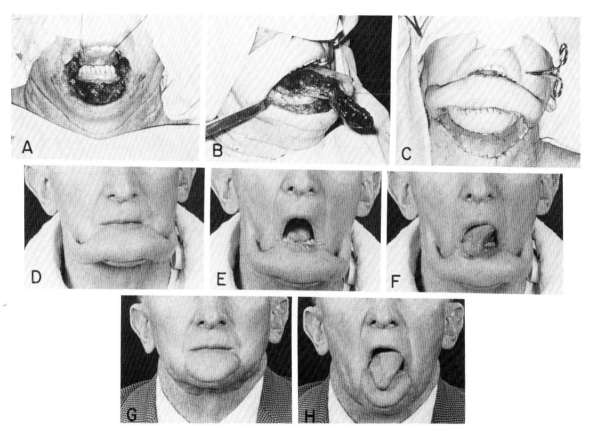

Figure 6 A total lower lip resection, including skin of the chin for recurrent cancer, in a 60-year-old male patient and reconstruction with an anteriorly based tongue flap for lining and vermilion, and a bipedicle flap of submental neck skin for external cover. *A*, Excisional defect. *B*, Tongue flap. *C*, The repair. *D* and *E*, Interim result, demonstrating action of the tongue before its division from the reconstructed lip. *G* and *H*, Final result after division of both flaps, with satisfactory function of the tongue.

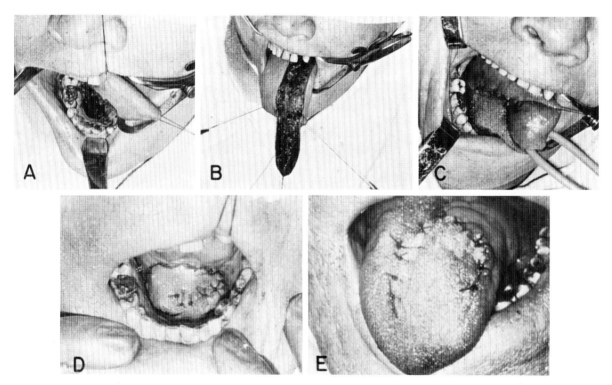

Figure 7 A pull-through resection of the anterior oral floor, in-continuity with radical neck dissection, for cancer persisting after radiotherapy in a 59-year-old male patient and reconstruction with an anteriorly based flap from the dorsal surface of the tongue. *A*, Excisional defect in the oral floor. *B*, Raised tongue flap. *C*, The repair. *D* and *E*, Final result at the time of division of the flap in a second-stage procedure.

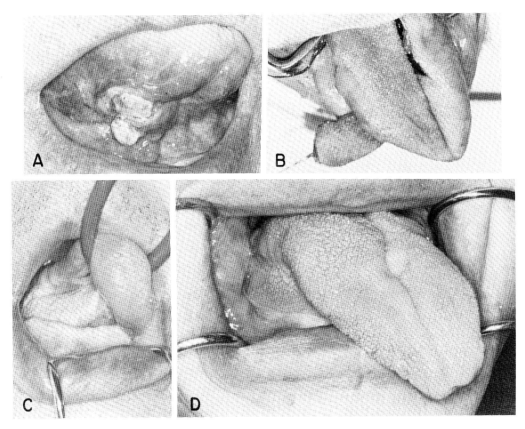

Figure 8 A pull-through resection of the right anterior floor of the mouth and undersurface of the tongue, in-continuity with radical neck dissection, for cancer in a 69-year-old male patient and reconstruction with an anteriorly based flap from the contralateral dorsal surface of the tongue, passing through a window created in the median raphe. *A*, The lesion. *B*, Flap in transit through the opening in the median raphe. *C*, Interim result. *D*, Final result with a functionally intact tongue.

tongue flap, despite the fact that its use will shorten and blunt the lingual tip, on occasion it can be used to advantage when obtained from a larger and longer tongue than of average size. Pulled forward and down from the anterior third of the dorsal surface, it can be applied to a defect in the anterior oral floor, or with a 90° twist forward, it can be applied to a reconstruction of the lip (Fig. 10).

FLAPS FROM THE FRONT END OF THE TONGUE

Meant specifically for use in labial reconstructions, the flaps in this category are derived by either a vertical or a horizontal slicing of the lingual tip. By means of a vertical cut, a bi-wing flap may be formed for vermilion reconstruction from the smooth perimeter of the tongue, centrally based either on the dorsal side of the lingual tip (Fig. 11*A*) or on its ventral side (Fig. 11*B*)—in appearance reminiscent of a hammerhead shark. By means of a horizontal cut, a variety of broad-based flaps, shorter than they are wide, may be formed for lining and vermilion repairs by reflection dorsally (Fig. 11*E*), ventrally (Fig. 11*D*), or fish-

mouth fashion in both directions (Fig. 11*C*). Durable and highly dependable, these flaps may have one disadvantage in that they tend to shorten the tongue. However, unless the tongue is smaller and shorter than average to begin with, this concern is more theoretical than it is practical, since no appreciable dysfunction seems to result from their judicious employment. The following are presented as examples.

The bi-wing flap, based centrally on the dorsal side of the lingual tip, is particularly well suited to restore vermilion in a lower lip reconstruction (Figs. 12 and 13), just as the ventrally based flap can be used for the upper lip.

Dorsally reflected, a broad posteriorly based flap serves for lining in an upper lip reconstruction, while the smooth tip margin of the tongue itself provides the vermilion (Fig. 14).

A double-flap formation by the fish-mouth type of splitting, if made through an incision placed a little on the dorsal side of the lingual edge, provides a dorsally reflected short flap for vermilion and a slightly longer ventrally reflected flap for lining in the reconstruction of a lower lip (Fig. 15). The somewhat papillary surface of the upper flap may not match ideally

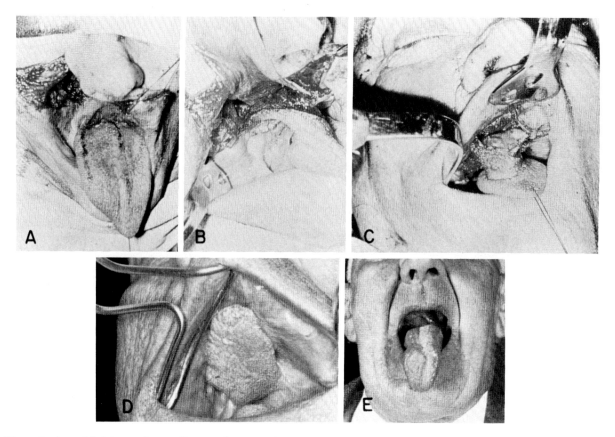

Figure 9 A partial right anterior maxillectomy for a recurring verrucous carcinoma in a 69-year-old male patient and reconstruction with an anteriorly based flap from the dorsal surface of the tongue. *A*, Excisional defect and outline of the tongue flap. *B*, Flap upturned with 180° twist of the pedicle, and skin grafting of its antrally oriented raw surface. *C*, First stage of repair completed. *D* and *E*, Final result with good function of the tongue remaining after division of the pedicle and closure of the oroantral fistula.

with the normal vermilion, but improves in time with atrophy.

FLAPS FROM THE VENTRAL SURFACE OF THE TONGUE

Thicker, papillary, and large in expanse on the dorsal surface, the investing mucous membrane of the tongue becomes thinner and smooth and much less extensive in area on the ventral surface. Thus, although flaps from the ventral surface would be better suited for vermilion restoration, they are not available for easy use as are the flaps obtained from the dorsal surface, since the deficiency resulting from the direct closure of a sizable donor wound at this restricted zone cannot but cause distortion and severely impair the mobility of the tongue. Nevertheless, in one instance it was possible to create two posteriorly based flaps, each taking half of almost the entire ventral surface mucosa of the tongue (Fig. 16) to use in the repair of an excisional defect of the anterior oral floor and alveolar margin (Fig. 17). By medial and forward rotation, the two flaps were brought into the excisional defect where, coming together, their lateral edges were

sutured in the midline, and the one large donor wound they left on the underside of the tongue was grafted with skin. Thus the graft was given a far better chance to take on the convex and more substantial base offered by the donor wound than would be the case were the graft applied to the alveolar and oral floor defect, and the problems of graft contraction and of impairment of mobility of the tongue were effectively avoided.

CONCLUSION

The age-old and elemental method of using the tongue by direct suture to close excisional defects in the oral cavity forces the entire organ (or what remains of it after a resection) into the role of a reparative flap, this usually with significant detriment to its functions. In contrast, a diverse variety of small true-flap methods are described that can equitably borrow from the relative abundance of lingual mucosa for transfer and advantageous use in different deficit areas in and around the oral cavity, without appreciably compromising the lingual functions.

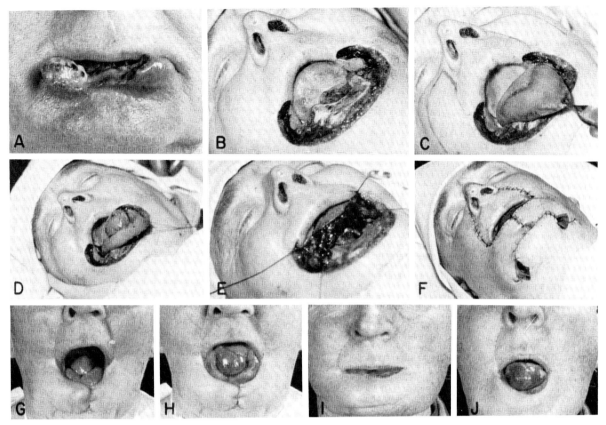

Figure 10 A more than commissure-to-commissure resection of the lower lip, including the front teeth and alveolus, with skin of the chin and outer bony table of the symphisis menti, for an infiltrating and destructive carcinoma, persisting after intensive radiotherapy, in a 56-year-old male patient and reconstruction with a transverse bipedicle flap from the anterior third of the dorsal surface of the tongue for lining and vermilion, and bilateral inferiorly based nasolabial skin flaps. *A*, The lesion. *B*, Surgical defect. *C*, Outline of the flaps. *D*, Bipedicle tongue flap pulled forward and its donor wound closed. *E*, Raw side of the flap turned to the front. *F*, Repair completed with the nasolabial flaps on the outside. *G* and *H*, Interim result, showing action of the tongue. *I* and *J*, Final result with blunted but well-functioning tongue after its division from the reconstructed lip.

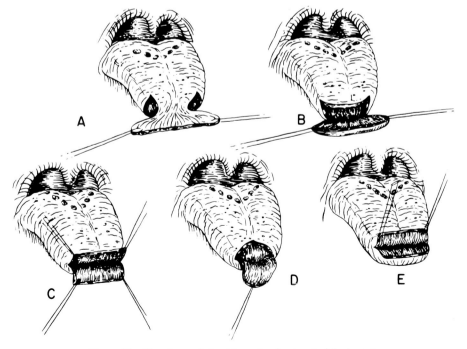

Figure 11 Flap-forms derived from the front end of the tongue.

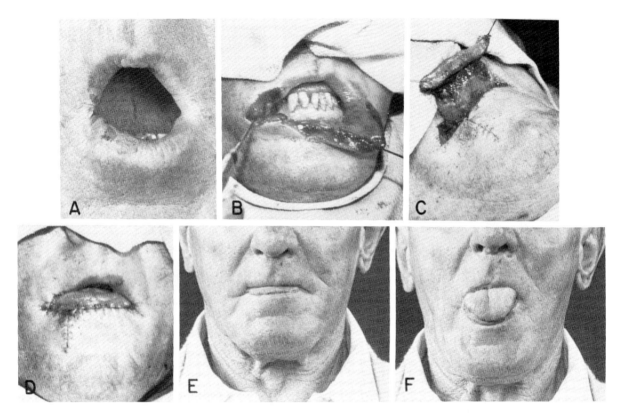

Figure 12 A wedge resection and full vermilionectomy of the lower lip for recurrent cancer in a 59-year-old male patient and reconstruction with a bi-wing, dorsally based flap from the smooth perimeter of the tongue for vermilion. *A*, The lesion. *B*, The resection. *C*, Tongue flap. *D*, Repair at first stage. *E* and *F*, Final result after division of the tongue from the reconstructed vermilion.

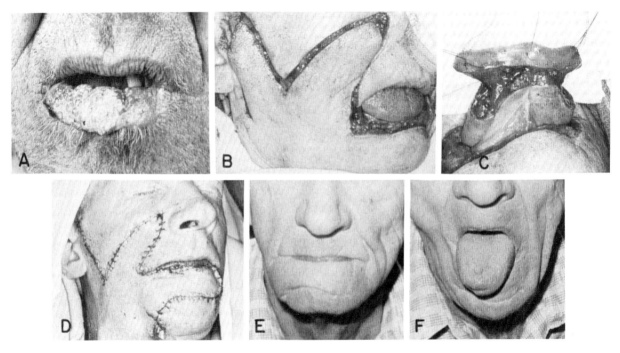

Figure 13 A total resection of the lower lip, including only half the height of its mucosal side, for a verrucous cancer in a 58-year-old male patient and reconstruction with a bi-wing flap from the smooth perimeter of the tongue and a bilobe skin flap from the cheek. *A*, The lesion. *B*, Bilobe skin flap and the excisional defect of the lower lip. *C*, Tongue flap. *D*, First stage of repair completed. *E* and *F*, Final result and good function after division of the tongue from the reconstructed lower lip.

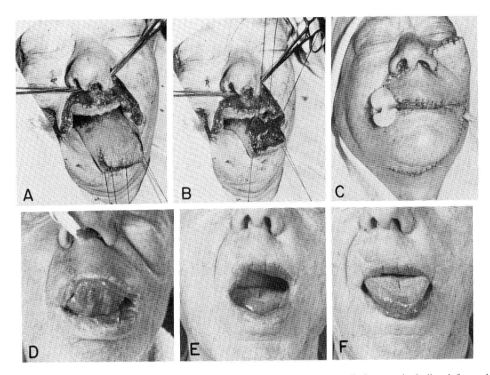

Figure 14 A near-total resection of the upper lip for basal cell recurrent cancer after radiotherapy, including left nasal vestibule and lower third of the columella in a 70-year-old male patient, and reconstruction with a broad and short posteriorly based flap from the tongue-end to provide lining, while the smooth free edge of the tongue provided vermilion and a large facial-submental skin flap provided the outer covering. *A*, Excisional defect and tongue flap. *B*, Upward reflection of the tongue flap. *C*, First stage of reconstruction completed. *D*, Interim appearance with the attached tongue. *E* and *F*, Final result and good function after division of the tongue and skin flaps.

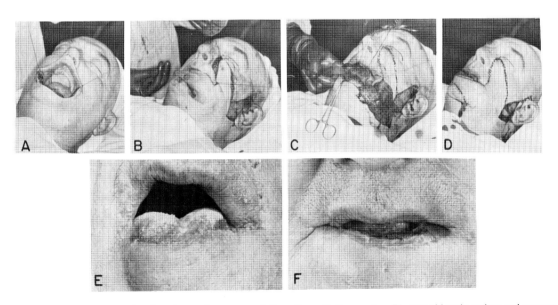

Figure 15 A total lower lip resection for advanced cancer persisting after radiotherapy in a 71-year-old male patient and reconstruction with two flaps obtained by a fish-mouth splitting of the lingual tip, a shorter one reflected dorsally for vermilion, the other reflected ventrally for lining, and a bilobe skin flap from the cheek for the outside. *A*, The defect. *B*, Bilobe skin flap. *C*, Fish-mouth splitting of the lingual tip. *D*, First stage of repair completed. *E*, Interim condition with the attached tongue. *F*, Final result after division of tongue from the reconstructed lip.

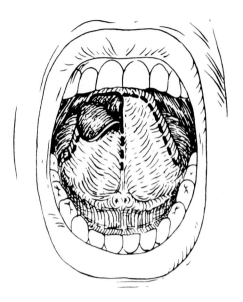

Figure 16 A pair of flaps from the ventral surface of the tongue for anterior use on the floor of the mouth.

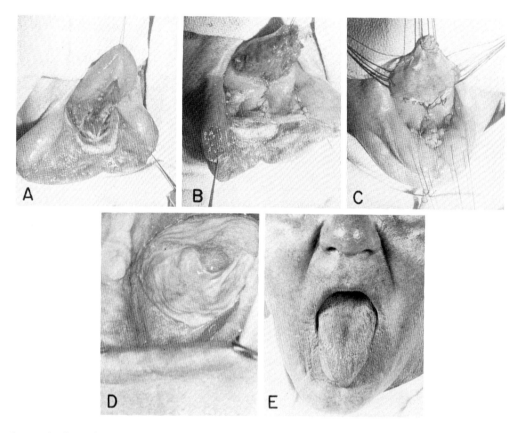

Figure 17 An anterior floor of mouth and alveolar margin resection for cancer in a 50-year-old male patient and reconstruction using a pair of posteriorly based flaps from the ventral surface of the tongue. *A*, Excisional defect. *B*, Two ventral flaps from the tongue rotated medially and forward into the floor of the mouth. *C*, Repair completed with a skin graft over the donor area on the undersurface of the lingual tip. *D*, Healed graft on the underside of the tongue. *E*, Normal protrusion of the tongue.

TOTAL GLOSSECTOMY: RECONSTRUCTION USING MYOCUTANEOUS FLAPS

JACK L. GLUCKMAN, M.D., F.C.S.(S.A.), F.A.C.S.

Total glossectomy is the most mutilating of all surgical procedures performed in the head and neck. The tremendous physical disability and the concomitant psychologic problems render this a most traumatic event for both the patient and the physician. By far, the most common indication is advanced cancer of the tongue which is, unfortunately, associated with an extremely poor prognosis regardless of the therapeutic regimen utilized. Because of this poor prognosis and the magnitude of surgery needed to excise the lesion, the oncologist may seek alternative forms of therapy, i.e., radiation alone or in combination with chemotherapy, in order to avoid glossectomy, with usually predictably poor results. Even if surgery is decided upon, knowledge of the resultant disability from total glossectomy may sway the surgeon to compromise his resection in an attempt to retain some functioning tongue. This course also is courting disaster and results in subsequent recurrence and further suffering.

It is certainly beyond the scope of this chapter to discuss the exact indications for total, as opposed to partial, glossectomy, but we are all familiar with the difficulties in adequately assessing large tumors of the tongue, as well as the alarming tendency for spread by local microembolization resulting in islands of tumor cells outside the obvious area of resection. A plea is therefore made for wide margins of resection, even if this should necessitate total glossectomy. In addition, this resection should be performed as early as possible rather than reserving the total glossectomy for postradiation salvage when all of these problems of evaluation are further compounded.

The possibility of performing total glossectomy purely for palliation when knowledge that cure is unlikely needs to be addressed. Patients with advanced cancer of the tongue are in extreme distress from pain, ulceration, and hemorrhage, and total glossectomy may afford excellent relief from this misery and should be considered in this situation.

Total glossectomy is extremely disabling and affects many vital functions including mastication, speech, and swallowing:

1. *Mastication*. The tongue plays an integral role in mastication. Its prime function in this process is to mix the food with the saliva and then direct the bolus to the teeth. Obviously, if this function is lost, the patient's diet may be reduced to soft foods and liquids.

2. *Speech*. The tongue is essential to articulation. Total glossectomy, therefore, severely compromises speech. Although a surprising number of patients are able to get themselves understood, others are totally unintelligible and may have to resort to electronic aids for communication.

3. *Swallowing*. The most important function of the tongue is its contribution to the oral phase of swallowing. The tongue molds the food into a bolus against the palate and then propels it posteriorly into the pharynx. Inability to perform this maneuver results in significant dysphagia. This takes the form of inability to activate swallowing as well as incoordination of the act of swallowing with secondary aspiration. The reasons for aspiration include the formation of a direct conduit from the oral cavity into the larynx after reconstruction and interference with both sensory and motor nerves essential to the act of swallowing.

These problems are frequently compounded by additional surgery that may be needed to ablate the tumor (e.g., mandibulectomy, palatectomy, and laryngectomy) usually together with neck dissection. Each of these associated ablative techniques has its own set of problems as regards rehabilitation, and combined with total glossectomy, the result may be devastating.

Reconstruction of so complex a structure is obviously a formidable task which has challenged surgeons for decades. The basic problem consists of replacing a dynamic sensitive structure which is intricately involved in many finely coordinated functions with an inert mass of tissue. The aim, therefore, is not only to close the defect and prevent fistula formation, but also to preserve as many of the functions of the tongue as possible. The ideal methods of reconstruction should utilize a flap that gives predictable results, is bulky, and can be re-innervated to replicate the movements of the tongue.

Speech is very difficult to restore, and rehabilitation is dependent on the speech therapist and the motivation of the patient to learn a new technique. It is frequently surprising to note how well total glossectomy patients can be understood with proper training.

Deglutition, however, is another problem entirely, chronic aspiration being a potentially lethal complication of the procedure. As has already been stated, the problems with deglutition are due to a multitude of factors, not least of which is the inability of the tethered reconstructed floor of mouth to compress the bolus of food against the palate to force it into the pharynx. In this situation, postoperative swallowing therapy is essential to train the patient in alternate swallowing techniques. Palatal prosthetics may be of help in lowering the palate, thereby facilitating this maneuver to allow commencement of the swallowing process.

In considering the prevention of aspiration, the role of total laryngectomy needs to be considered. There are two indications for total laryngectomy, i.e., oncologic indications and prevention of aspiration. In the pre- and intraoperative evaluation of these patients, great care should be taken to assess the root of the tongue and the pre-epiglottic space. If these areas are involved, a total laryngectomy is usually indicated, and the problem of aspiration therefore is not relevant. However, if a decision is made not to remove the larynx for oncologic reasons, the problem of whether it should be prophylactically removed to prevent aspiration needs to be considered.

In making this decision, the patient's emotional status, particularly with regard to motivation, and general physical condition with emphasis on pulmonary reserve and ability to withstand aspiration, need to be considered. Two courses are therefore available: (1) a prophylactic laryngectomy in patients who both physically and emotionally would not be able to tolerate aspiration, and (2) a trial of leaving the larynx in situ and a vigorous attempt at rehabilitation. The latter course is preferable in many patients, with the knowledge that if it is not successful after a period of time, an interval total laryngectomy may be performed. Alternatively, a gastrostomy combined with cuffed tracheostomy or other laryngeal or tracheal procedures to prevent chronic aspiration may suffice. Biller et al[1] recently described a prophylactic laryngoplasty performed at the time of the total glossectomy which allowed a good voice, but minimized the chances of aspiration.[1] This procedure may be a satisfactory compromise in these situations.

Many methods of reconstruction have been designed to close the defect resulting from total glossectomy. These include local and regional pedicle flaps, myocutaneous flaps, and revascularized free grafts. Although none is ideal, the myocutaneous flaps appear to offer many advantages over other techniques. These advantages include:

1. The design of the flap is facilitated because the excellent blood supply allows a variety of shapes without regard to the conventional length/width ratio.
2. Reconstruction is done as a single stage. This is in sharp contrast to many of the other regional flaps which require subsequent division and replacement of their pedicle.
3. These flaps are reliable, and excellent results have been reported by most authors.
4. Technically they are easy to harvest with no special skills or training required, as compared to the need for microvascular training if free flaps are to be used.
5. The bulk of the flap adequately replaces the mass of the tongue and floor of mouth. This has many advantages. It minimizes the pooling of food and saliva that occurs with other less bulky flaps (Fig. 1). In addition, it is postulated that the bulk helps to direct the food away from the larynx and into the lateral

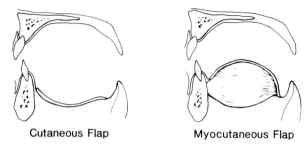

Cutaneous Flap   Myocutaneous Flap

Figure 1 This demonstrates the advantage of the bulky myocutaneous flaps over the conventional cutaneous flaps. The bulk prevents pooling of secretion on the reconstructed floor of mouth.

food channels during deglutition (Fig. 2).
6. The potential for innervation exists. This theoretic advantage remains controversial. Re-innervation of myocutaneous flaps using the severed hypoglossal nerve has been described using the sternocleidomastoid,[2] pectoralis major,[3] and the latissimus dorsi[4] flaps with various results. Neurotization has been demonstrated, but whether this can be translated into meaningful movement remains to be seen.

A wide variety of myocutaneous flaps are available for reconstruction of the tongue: (1) pectoralis major, (2) latissimus dorsi, (3) trapezius, (4) sternocleidomastoid, and (5) platysma. Details of these flaps, together with the techniques for harvesting, will not be discussed here, but descriptions are readily available in current literature. Individual preference usually dictates the flap of choice; in our experience, however, the pectoralis major myocutaneous flap remains the most popular, having proved to be simple to harvest and extremely reliable. The possibility of

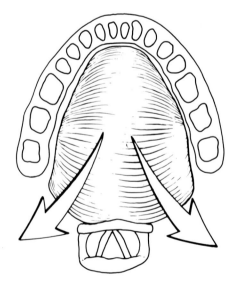

Figure 2 The bulk of the myocutaneous flap directs food laterally away from the larynx and therefore decreases the likelihood of aspiration.

designing double paddles and the potential for transferring rib or sternum with the flap as an osteomyocutaneous flap make this a most attractive flap to use.

The sternocleidomastoid myocutaneous flap has been described for reconstruction following total glossectomy. Although it is conveniently placed, its disadvantages include a limited cutaneous component, limited mobility, and a high incidence of cutaneous flap necrosis. Furthermore, its use in patients with potential neck metastasis is controversial. This flap probably has a limited role in the management of total glossectomy patients.

The trapezius myocutaneous flaps have been successfully used to reconstruct the oral cavity. The obvious advantage is the relative thinness of the muscle, which decreases the bulk somewhat. The disadvantages include the fact that the patient has to be repositioned during the procedure, and the relatively short length of the transverse cervical vein restricts the range of the flap.

The latissimus dorsi myocutaneous flap is an excellent flap which offers all the advantages of the pectoralis major myocutaneous flap. The choice of flap rests ultimately with the surgeon.

A platysma myocutaneous flap should be included in this group, but the thinness of the flap and its lack of reliability, particularly if previous radiation has been given which may compromise the blood supply, tend to limit its use.

In conclusion, total glossectomy is a mutilating procedure resulting in a significant functional disability. Reconstruction is difficult and should be geared not only to closing the defect, but aiding rehabilitation, particularly with regard to speech and swallowing. The myocutaneous flaps, particularly the pectoralis major flap, appear to fulfill many of these aims.

REFERENCES

1. Biller HF, Lawson W, Baek S. Total glossectomy—a technique of reconstruction eliminating laryngectomy. Arch Otolaryngol 1983; 109:69–73.
2. Mikaelian D. Reconstruction of the tongue. Laryngoscope 1984; 94:34–37.
3. Conley J, Sachs M, Parke R. The new tongue. Otolaryngol Head Neck Surg 1982; 90:58–68.
4. Carden ET. A re-animated neotongue. Am Acad Otolaryngol, Poster Presentation, Anaheim, CA, September, 1980.

ROLE OF THE REGIONAL MUSCLE FLAP IN HEAD AND NECK RECONSTRUCTION

STEPHEN J. MATHES, M.D.

INDICATIONS

In a recent review of indications for immediate head and neck reconstruction, Edgerton states, "The choice of the most suitable reconstructive procedure is usually more difficult than execution of the surgical maneuver required to excise a tumor."[1] Through the efforts of Edgerton,[2] MacGregor,[3] and Bakamjian,[4] the concept of early or immediate reconstruction is now well accepted in the management of head and neck cancer. Whether the cancer resection is palliative or curative, restoration of oral lining and facial skin allows healing without excessive scar contracture. A risk of oral cutaneous fistulas, carotid exposure, and infection in retained mandibular segments is minimized. A major step toward patient rehabilitation is accomplished by providing the foundation for restoration of form and function through primary wound closure.

Failure to achieve a healed wound after a major extirpative procedure delays adjunctive cancer treatment. The effectiveness of postoperative radiation therapy is well established. However, persistent communication of the oral cavity with the radical neck wound or local infection delays needed radiation therapy. Adjunctive chemotherapy for advanced intraoral cancer is also delayed when wound complications delay primary healing.

Immediate closure of the oral cavity prevents exposure of vital structures (i.e., carotid, dura, mandible) to the bacterial flora inherent to the mouth. Cicatricial contracture associated with delayed wound healing which may tether the tongue, larynx, mandibular segments, and oral stoma is avoided. Future operative procedures are not required until adjunctive therapy is completed. In the meantime, the deformity and its emotional impact on the cancer patient is reduced.

SAFETY

In his recent Hayes Martin Lecture, Conley stated, "A great advanced came about 5 years ago with the introduction of the regional myocutaneous flap. They are now the most important flaps in the armamentarium of the head and neck surgeon."[5] In order to benefit from immediate reconstruction, flap safety is essential. Furthermore, confidence in the ability to close the wound allows the head and neck surgeon to fully resect a tumor and to incorporate adjunctive therapy (i.e., pre- and postoperative radiation therapy) in cancer management. With the identification of skin fascial and musculocutaneous regional flaps, reliable flaps are now available to accomplish immediate reconstruction.

The temporal[3] and deltopectoral[4] flaps, based on vascular pedicles distant to the cancer site, initially provided the skin and soft tissue needed to apply the concept of immediate reconstruction after major extirpative procedures involving the oral cavity. With the identification of the vascular pedicles to muscle and their overlying skin territories, the musculocutaneous flap has greatly expanded the ability of the reconstructive surgeon to provide immediate wound coverage.[6,7]

Regional muscles with major vascular pedicles distant from the tumor site can be elevated with safety. The pattern of circulation and location of vascular pedicles is constant. Since a muscle provides circulation to the overlying skin via musculocutaneous perforators, a skin island can be precisely designed over the muscle to restore missing palatal and oral mucosa and skin. Since the flap dissection is between muscle planes, flap elevation is not complex and does not excessively prolong the operative procedure after the extirpative procedure is completed. Finally, since the skin island is located at the distal end of the flap, the skin will fill the extirpative defect while the intervening muscle covers vital structures (i.e., carotid) and fills the space resulting from mandibulectomy. Since immediate inset of the musculocutaneous flap is accomplished if the muscle base of the flap is located beneath neck skin (i.e., after radical neck dissection), the flap circulation does not depend on revascularization from the defect site. This assists wound healing, especially if radiation vasculitis is present, and provides a new source of wound circulation. Furthermore, the need for a controlled fistula associated with skin fascial flaps is generally eliminated.

In a recent survey of 105 reconstructive surgeons regarding muscle and musculocutaneous flap safety, 4244 flaps were utilized for reconstruction of defects in all body regions with a recipient site complication rate of 8 percent.[8] A major recipient site complication was complete or partial flap loss in which a further reconstructive procedure was required to accomplish wound coverage or satisfy the reconstructive goal. Four hundred and seventy-one (11%) of these muscles or musculocutaneous flaps were utilized for head and neck reconstruction with a complication rate of 15 percent. The slightly higher complication rate when the musculocutaneous flap is used for head and neck reconstruction reflects both the complexity of reconstruction in this area and the early use of less reliable muscle flaps. For instance, use of the sternocleidomastoid flap, with its less reliable pattern of circulation,[7] resulted in an unacceptable recipient site complication rate of 41 percent. The most frequently utilized muscle flap, the pectoralis major (39%), failed in only 7 percent of patients. Thus, reliable regional muscle flaps are now identified which will accomplish reconstruction after major head and neck surgery with safety.

RECONSTRUCTIVE LADDER

The reconstructive surgeon cognizant of the importance of the reconstructive ladder, ranging from simple to more complex techniques, will only select the muscle or musculocutaneous flap (a complex technique) when direct closure, skin graft, or local random flap (a simple technique) will not accomplish a successful, reliable reconstruction.[8] The skin graft and local tongue flap are useful after extirpation of small interoral tumors. The single or bilateral nasolabial flaps[9] or the platysmal musculocutaneous flap[10,11] (Fig. 1) also provide safe coverage when marginal or segmental mandibular resection is required without incontinuity neck dissection.

The use of local skin fascial or musculocutaneous flaps is less reliable after major intraoral extirpative procedures, especially if associated with a radical neck dissection. The vascular pedicles to the platysma[7] and sternocleidomastoid[12] are divided in order to accomplish an adequate lymphadenectomy. The pectoralis major[13] and the posterior trapezius[14,15] (Fig. 2) represent the two most useful regional musculocutaneous flaps when the extirpative defect warrants a distant flap for safe closure. Both muscles are large with a wide arc of rotation. A distally located skin island can be transposed to the lower face and turned either for intraoral or skin facial coverage. Direct closure of the donor defect is usually possible.

The major vascular pedicle to the pectoralis major, the thoracoacromial artery, is located beneath the clavicle, away from the intraoral cancer and prior or future effects of radiation therapy. Since the vascular pedicle of the trapezius muscle, the transverse cervical artery, is located in the base of the neck, this pedicle must be preserved during neck dissection or its patency confirmed by arteriogram if used in a secondary procedure after prior radical neck dissection. After major resection for intraoral cancer, the regional muscle flap, a complex technique in the reconstructive ladder, frequently represents the best method to restore mucosal and skin continuity and to provide well-vascularized soft tissue over bone and vital structures.

BACTERIAL RESISTANCE

In a recent review of 54 consecutive patients with chronic wounds with established infection, use of muscle or musculocutaneous flap for coverage after wound debridement provided stable wound coverage without recurrent infection in 93 percent of patients.[16] The resistance of the muscle or musculocutaneous flap is similarly observed in head and neck reconstructive procedures. Unlike random or even the skin fascial deltopectoral flap, the musculocutaneous flap resists the bacterial contamination inherent to the oral cavity after extirpative procedures.

This observation is supported by experimental studies in the canine models initially comparing musculocutaneous with random pattern flaps and most recently with skin facial flaps. The musculocutaneous flap demonstrates a superior resistance to bacterial inoculation on both its skin and deep surface when compared to the random pattern flap.[17] Although the skin surface of the musculocutaneous flap and that of the skin fascial flap are similarly resistant to necrosis after bacterial inoculation, the muscle surface of the musculocutaneous flap has significantly greater resistance to bacterial inoculation than does the fascial surface of the skin fascial flap.[18]

Current studies to ascertain the mechanism of this superior resistance of the musculocutaneous flap to

A

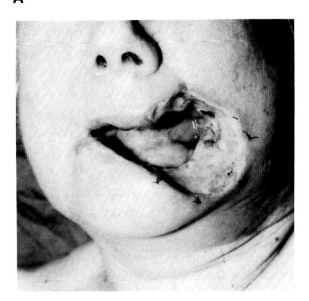

Figure 1 Platysma musculocutaneous flap. *A*, Defect after chemosurgical excision of lip commissure tumor. *B*, Skin island of platysma musculocutaneous flap (P) located in lower neck. Cervical flap (C) will be used to restore facial skin defect. *C*, Platysma musculocutaneous flap (P) will be transposed over mandible with skin island used to restore buccal sulcus. *D, Flap inset 3 years after operation. Oral competence and function are preserved. E*, Donor site for skin island in inferior neck closed with skin grafts. (From Mathes and Nahai.[19])

B

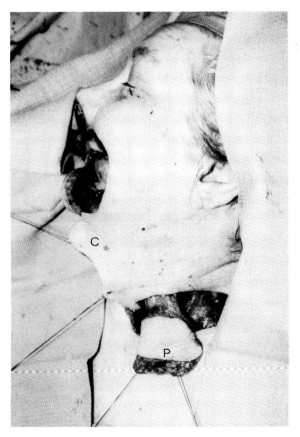

C

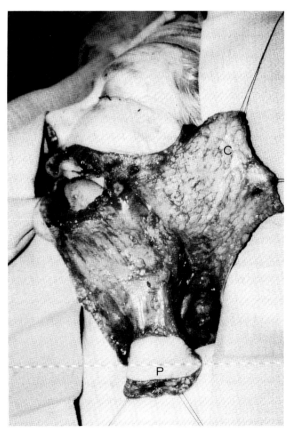

D

E

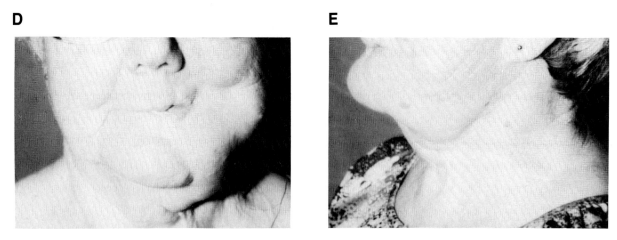

Figure 1 Continued.

A

B

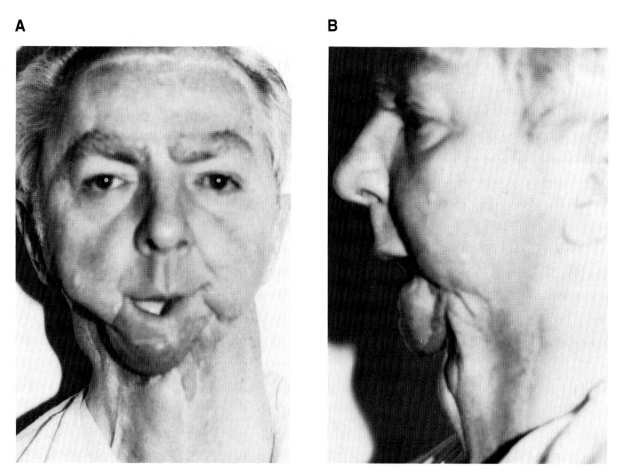

Figure 2 Posterior trapezius musculocutaneous flap for reconstruction of lower third of face. *A*, Patient shown, who has undergone mandibulectomy and radiation therapy for intraoral carcinoma and immediate reconstruction with temporal flap, now presents for staged lower face and mandibular reconstruction. *B*, Lateral view: inadequate skin and soft tissue for mandible reconstruction. *C*, Posterior trapezius flap design. Skin island extends from mid scapula to inferior edge of trapezius muscle origin. Patient is in lateral decubitus position to allow simultaneous access to face and back; s = scapular; m = posterior midline; T = skin island over trapezius muscle. *D*, Flap inset site extends from left neck to right mastoid area. *E*, Flap inset one year after operation. *Note:* Flap was divided and inset completed 8 weeks after initial flap elevation. *F*, Flap provided adequate coverage for mandibular reconstruction. *G*, Donor site closed directly. Anterior trapezius muscle fibers are intact and preserve function of shoulder elevation.

C

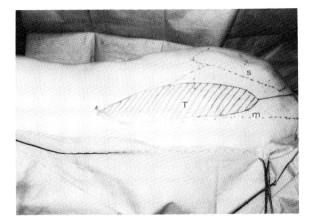

D

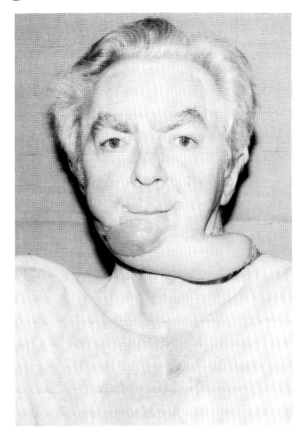

E

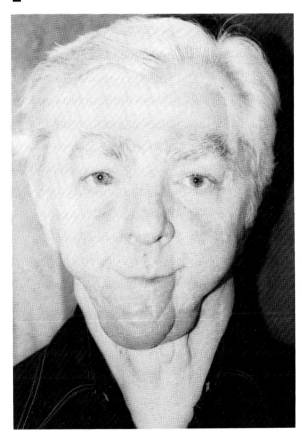

F

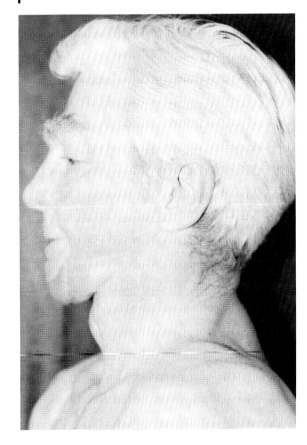

Figure 2 Continued.

G

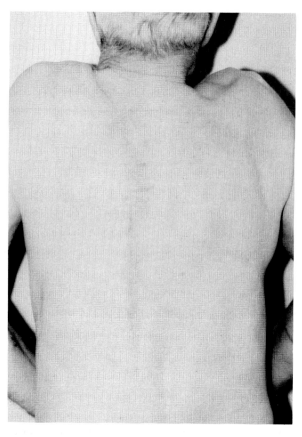

Figure 2 Continued.

infection, observed both clinically and experimentally, have identified significantly greater oxygen tensions in the distal musculocutaneous flap when compared to the random pattern flap. Although leukocyte mobilization appears adequate after bacterial inoculation of random and musculocutaneous flaps, the improved blood flow, oxygen delivery, and bacterial resistance observed in the musculocutaneous flap considerably improved the reliability of this flap type for use in head and neck extirpative surgery. The musculocutaneous flap provides an environment for primary wound healing and for later use as a bed for bone grafts for mandibular reconstruction or other secondary procedures.

FORM AND FUNCTION

Despite the overwhelming advantages of immediate reconstruction after extirpation of intraoral cancer, problems of drooling due to loss of lip sensibility, normal animation, and mastication persist. However, flap selection should preserve form and function with minimal donor site mobility. Although reliable, the temporal skin fascial flap results in a visible donor site defect (see Fig. 2a). Both the pectoralis major and posterior trapezius have donor sites located on the trunk. The posterior trapezius donor site is routinely closed directly and the flap is designed to

preserve the anterior muscle fibers necessary to avoid shoulder droop (see Fig. 2g). Fortunately, no significant functional deformity has been observed after use of the pectoralis major in reconstructive surgery. In general, the donor site is closed directly, although use of a large skin island may necessitate skin grafting the donor site. In the female patient, location of the skin island over the inferior edge of the muscle in the inframammary area avoids breast deformity after direct closure. When severe breast ptosis is noted, this low skin island would include excessive breast tissue bulk. In this situation, the posterior trapezius musculocutaneous flap is preferred. The bulk of the musculocutaneous flap is beneficial when mandibulectomy is performed. The muscle fills the space and assists in control of retained mandibular segments. However, control of both vertical rami by internal or external fixation devices is preferable when central mandibular resection is required.

As previously noted, the muscle provides a well-vascularized bed for later autogenous bone grafts. The use of vascularized bone accompanying the pectoralis major musculocutaneous flap (fifth or sixth rib) or trapezius musculocutaneous flap (scapula) has been successfully utilized. Although this eliminates one future reconstructive requirement, it is often difficult to satisfactorily position both skin island for mucosal or skin replacement and bone for immediate manidublar restoration. Wound closure is the major priority of immediate reconstruction and should not be jeopardized by vascularized bone positioning. If immediate bone reconstruction is a high priority in a curative resection, microvascular transplantation of vascularized bone (deep circumflex iliac osteocutaneous flap) is preferred. Furthermore, the donor site of the pectoralis major osseous musculocutaneous flap often requires closure with a secondary abdominal flap to cover exposed pleura and costal cartilages.

CONCLUSIONS

The regional muscle flap has a definite place in head and neck reconstructive surgery. Although its bulk may alter form, its safety and technical ease during transposition to the oral cavity defect allows reliable single-stage reconstruction after major extirpative procedures. The healed wound allows continuation of vital adjunctive cancer therapy. With satisfactory tumor control or cure and avoidance of wound complications, elective secondary procedures can be designed if needed to complete patient rehabilitation.

REFERENCES

1. Edgerton MT. General principles in the surgical treatment of patients with head and neck cancer. In: Converse JM, ed. Reconstructive Plastic Surgery. 2nd ed. Philadelphia: WB Saunders, 1977; 2511.
2. Edgerton MT. Replacement of lining to oral cavity following surgery. Cancer 1951; 4:110.
3. MacGregor IA. The temporal flap in intraoral cancer: Its use

in repairing the post-excisional defect. Br J Plast Surg 1963; 16:318.

4. Bakamjian VY. A two-stage method for pharyngoesophageal reconstruction with a primary pectoral skin flap. Plast Reconstr Surg 1965; 36:173.

5. Conley J. Changes in head and neck surgery. Am J Surg 1983; 146:425.

6. McCraw JB, Dibbell D, Carraway J. Clinical definition of independent myocutaneous vascular territories. Plast Reconstr Surg 1977; 60:341.

7. Mathes SJ, Nahai F. Classification of the vascular anatomy of muscles: experimental and clinical correlation. Plast Reconstr Surg 1981; 61:177.

8. Mathes SJ, Nahai F. Muscle and musculocutaneous flaps. In: Goldwyn R, ed. The unfavorable result in plastic surgery. 2nd ed. Boston: Little, Brown, 1984.

9. Cohen IK, Edgerton MT. Transbuccal flaps for reconstruction of the floor of the mouth. Plast Reconstr Surg 1971; 48:8.

10. Futrell JW, Johns ME, Cantrell RW, Fitz-Hugh GS. Platysmal myocutaneous flap for intraoral reconstruction. Am J Surg 1978; 136:504.

11. Coleman JJ, Nahai F, Mathes SJ. Platysmal musculocuta-

neous flap: Clinical and antomic considerations in head and neck reconstruction. Am J Surg 1982; 144:477.

12. Owens N. A compound neck pedicle designed for the repair of massive facial defects: formation, developments and application. Plast Reconstr Surg 1955; 15:369.

13. Ariyan S. The pectoralis major myocutaneous flap: a versatile flap for reconstruction in head and neck. Plast Reconstr Surg 1979; 63:73.

14. Mathes JS, Nahai F. Clinical atlas of muscle and musculocutaneous flaps. St. Louis: Mosby CV, 1979; 414.

15. Mathes SJ, Alpert BS. Advances in muscle and musculocutaneous flaps. Clin Plast Surg 1980; 7:15.

16. Mathes SJ, Feng LJ, Hunt TK. Coverage of the infected wound. Ann Surg 1983; 198:420.

17. Chang N, Mathes SJ. Comparison of the effect of bacterial inoculation in musculocutaneous and random pattern flaps. Plast Reconstr Surg 1982; 70:1.

18. Chang N, Calderon W, Price D, Mathes SJ. Comparison of the effect of bacteria inoculation in musculocutaneous and fasciocutaneous flaps. Surg Forum 1984; 35:587.

19. Mathes SJ, Nahai F. Clinical applications for muscle and musculocutaneous flaps. St. Louis: CV Mosby CV, 1981; 73.

COMPOSITE RESECTION AND RECONSTRUCTION WITH SKIN GRAFTS FOR ORAL CAVITY AND OROPHARYNX CANCER

DONALD G. SESSIONS, M.D.

Composite resection (CR), the so-called jaw neck dissection (JND) or commando operation, is the standard surgical method for treating cancer of the oral cavity and oropharynx. This operative approach allows for wide exposure and resection of extensive areas of tumor-involved tongue, floor of mouth, mandible, buccal area, tonsil, pharyngeal wall, and adjacent structures necessary to effect a cure for cancer of these areas. Modern reconstructive techniques allow closure of almost any resulting defect. The cosmetic and functional deficits that result can be considerable[1-3] and vary to a certain extent with the technique employed.

Cosmetic defects following composite resection may include cheek depression, lip and chin scars, and deviation of the chin toward the side of the resection. Cheek depression is due to loss of the mandible and adjacent soft tissue. Closure of the defect by suturing the tongue to remaining buccal mucosa frequently compounds the deformity.

The standard approach to composite resection has been the lip-splitting incision. Its continued use has been advocated,[4] but even the strictest adherence to technical detail in closure cannot eliminate the conspicuously placed scars.

Functional deficits following composite resection are generally related to difficulties in speaking, swallowing, and chewing. Decreased tongue mobility is due to both surgical excision of tongue and reconstructive techniques which tether the tongue to the cheek or use the remaining tongue as a flap. This results in difficulties with swallowing and articulation, especially the formation of speech fricatives (e.g., this, that) which require lingual-dental approximation. The unopposed pull of the pterygoid muscles on the side opposite the resection combined with wound contracture lead to chin deviation toward the side of resection and to mandibular retrusion. Severe malocclusion and subsequent inability to effectively masticate food often result.

The standard technique for reconstruction of composite resection defects include primary closure and the use of local or regional flaps. The use of distant free flaps has been suggested.[5] Primary closure, which requires approximation of the medial margin of resection, usually the tongue, to the lateral pharyngeal wall and cheek tissues, creates the greatest cosmetic and functional problems and should be reserved for closing small defects. The development of numerous local and regional pedicle flaps has eliminated some of the problems associated with primary closure. Local flaps borrow heavily from tissue nearby and can restrict function.[6] Regional flaps require several stages and considerable donor site morbidity. The use of free flaps requires the use of microvascular techniques and also results in donor site morbidity. The number of techniques attests to the fact that no one method is ideal.

In an attempt to minimize these problems, an alternate approach to standard composite resection and reconstruction was developed. The essentials of this procedure include the use of a non-lip-splitting visor flap for exposure and excision of the lesion, reconstruction with a skin graft formed into a three-dimensional pouch to fill the dead space created by the resection, and the routine use of intermaxillary fixation for immobilization of the reconstructed area.[7]

SURGICAL TECHNIQUE

Resection

A standard tracheostomy is performed through a separate vertical incision over a previously placed oral endotracheal tube, and anesthesia for the remainder of the procedure is supplied through the tracheostomy site. The horizontal visor incision is made, extending from the mastoid tip past the midline to approximately the midbody of the contralateral mandible, staying at least 4 cm below the inferior border of the mandible (Fig. 1). The flap is raised superiorly to the level of the mandible, taking care not to injure the marginal mandibular branch of the facial nerve. A standard S-shape vertical incision is dropped inferiorly, beginning well posterior to the carotid artery. Alternately, a McFee-type incision, employing a separate inferior parallel horizontal incision 3 cm above the clavicle, can be employed. A standard neck dissection is performed, basing the specimen on the inferomedial periosteum of the mandible, submandib-

ular triangle, floor of mouth, or tongue region, depending on the location of the primary lesion.

The visor flap of chin and cheek skin is elevated to provide exposure to the mandible and the primary lesion. This is accomplished by making an incision in the gingival-buccal sulcus from just anterior to the region of the mental foramen on the noninvolved side to the region of the mental foramen on the involved side (Fig. 2). This incision should be placed at least 2 cm from the alveolar ridge to facilitate later closure. The incision is then connected extraperiosteally over the mandible into the neck, creating the anterior portion of the visor. At the level just anterior to the mental foramen on the involved side, a vertical incision is made through the periosteum on the lateral aspect of the mandible, connecting the intraoral incision to the inferior border of the mandible. From this point, an incision through the periosteum is made posteriorly along the inferior border of the mandible to the angle. The lateral mandibular periosteum is then elevated along with the flap, as is done with the standard lip-splitting incision. At this point, the visor flap consisting of chin and cheek tissue can be elevated superiorly over the face (Fig. 3A), creating excellent exposure for the standard mandibular osteotomies and mucosal incision necessary for the extirpation of the primary lesion. The patient is paralyzed for relaxation, and the visor flap is elevated superiorly with large rubber drains. Initial mandibular osteotomy just anterior to the mental foramen is followed by superior osteotomy of the condyloid and coronoid processes. Oral cavity exposure is maintained with a side-biting mouth gag. Further exposure is obtained during the resection by traction on the tongue with a towel clip

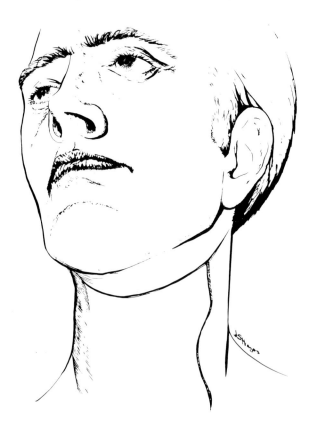

Figure 1 The horizontal limb of the incision extends from the mastoid tip to the contralateral mental foramen 3 cm below the mandible. The vertical limit of the incision is begun well posterior to the carotid artery.

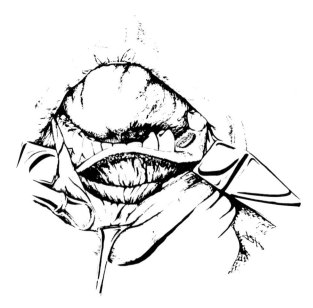

Figure 2 Mucosal incision. The gingival-labial and gingival-buccal incision is connected to the horizontal portion of the neck incision extraperiosteally, creating the anterior portion of the visor flap. The posterior or cheek portion of the visor flap is raised subperiosteally.

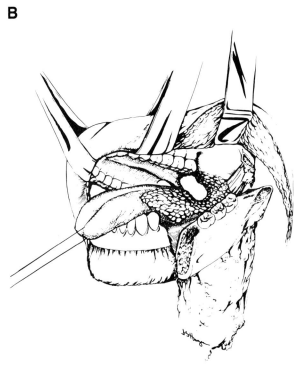

and medial depression of the tongue with a metal tongue blade (Fig. 3*B*). Following resection of the specimen, all suspicious margins are checked by frozen section.

Reconstruction

Skin to be used for the reconstruction is harvested from the anterolateral thigh. The size of the graft is dependent on the size of the defect to be reconstructed. Ordinarily the graft utilized for the pouch construction would be 12 cm in length and 5 cm in width, with a thickness of .0018 to .0020 inches.

Simultaneously, apparatus for intermaxillary fixation is applied. Standard arch bars are used when possible. If dentition is not present or adequate, previously modified dentures or Gunning splints with attached arch bars are wired in place.

If the base of tongue or lateral pharyngeal wall has been included in the resection, reconstruction begins at the posteroinferior aspect of the defect. The free margin of the tongue base is approximated to the free margin of the lateral pharyngeal wall only up to the level of the inferior pole of the tonsil on the uninvolved side. This portion of the closure is seldom more than 2 cm in length, even if the defect extends to the level of the vallecula.

The skin graft is sutured in place and a generous three-dimensional pouch created (Fig. 4). Interrupted 3-0 silk sutures are used to approximate the graft to the mucosal margin, and the ends are left long to secure the cotton bolus that will be inserted later. The graft and pouch can be fashioned from a single piece of skin starting anteromedially adjacent to the cut end

Figure 3 *A*, The visor flap consisting of chin and cheek tissue is elevated superiorly. Exposure is obtained with rubber drains, tongue retraction, and a side-biting mouth gag. *B*, Following mandibular osteotomy anterior to the mental foramen, superior osteotomies of the condyloid and coronoid processes are performed. Posterior exposure is obtained by retraction of the tongue and depression with a metal tongue blade.

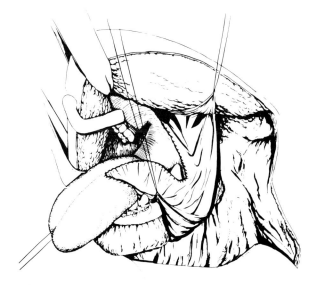

Figure 4 Skin or dermis is sutured circumferentially to the mucosal margin of the defect, starting anteriorly adjacent to the cut end of the mandible body and progressing posteriorly along the tongue, superiorly along the pharynx, palate, and maxilla, and laterally along the buccal mucosa.

of the body of the mandible, attaching one corner of the graft to this area. Proceeding posteriorly, the lateral margin of cut tongue is approximated to the edge of the skin graft lengthwise until the posterior extent of the defect is reached. This is usually the area where the tongue base margin is approximated to the lateral pharyngeal wall. At this point, the graft is progressively attached posterosuperiorly along the pharyngeal, palatal, and maxillary margins and then laterally and anteriorly along the buccal margin of the resection until the level of the cut end of the body of the mandible is again reached, this time from the anterobuccal side. The long intraoral sutures are arranged sequentially and brought out the mouth. The pouch is created using a running 3-0 chromic suture by closing the graft to itself and trimming the excess skin when the desired pouch depth has been achieved (Fig. 5). Ideally, the pouch should fill the void created by the excised portions of the tongue, floor of mouth, mandible, and submaxillary space contents down to the level of the digastric muscle.

The visor flap is repositioned. The inside of the skin graft is lined with Xeroform gauze, and cotton balls liberally impregnated with antibiotic ointment or Betadine are placed intraorally to create a three-dimensional pouch (Fig. 6). The long ends of the tacking sutures are firmly tied over the bolster packing, creating a saliva-tight closure for the graft pouch. When viewed through the neck incision, the pouch bulges into the submandibular area and extends toward the level of the hyoid bone and the digastric muscle. The gingival-buccal incision on the contralateral side is closed. The jaws are wired into occlusion (Fig. 7).

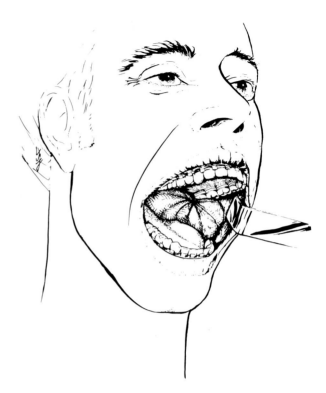

Figure 6 The inside of the pouch is lined with Xeroform gauze, and cotton balls liberally impregnated with antibiotic ointment are placed inside the pouch to create a bolus. The long ends of the tacking sutures are firmly tied over the bolster, creating a saliva-tight packing over the graft pouch. Note the arch bars in place.

A dermis graft is placed over the carotid artery, Hemovacs inserted, and the neck wound closed. An external pressure dressing is applied. Postoperatively, Hemovacs are removed when drainage decreases to less than 15 cc per day. This usually occurs about 4 days after surgery. The external pressure dressing is maintained for at least 7 days. The bolus is removed at 10 days, and the patient remains in intermaxillary fixation for 4 weeks. The tracheotomy is removed at 10 to 14 days, and nasogastric feedings are maintained until the arch bars are removed. The patient can be discharged home for several weeks on nasogastric feedings after the tracheotomy site is healed.

RESULTS

This procedure has been used for the last 8 years in over forty patients. The parameters evaluated have included operative and postoperative complications, cancer status, cosmesis, speech, occlusion, swallowing, oral hygiene, graft characteristics, general status, and ability to be gainfully employed.

Complications

There was one patient with major complications. This patient had wound infection, fistula formation, and carotid artery catastrophe and was salvaged. Mi-

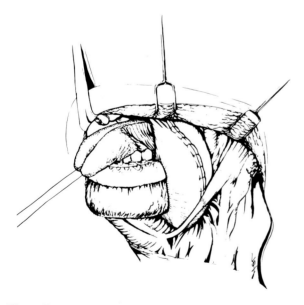

Figure 5 The pouch is formed by excising the excess skin or dermis and closing this on itself when the desired pouch depth has been achieved. The pouch fills the void created by the en bloc excision of the cancer and its surrounding tissue.

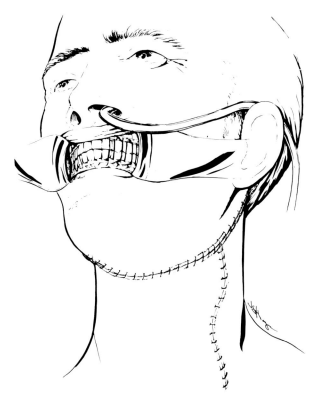

Figure 7 The jaws are wired into occlusion. Intermaxillary fixation is maintained for 4 weeks and results in full immobilization of the healing wound.

nor complications included partial graft slough, unexplained bleeding from the tracheostomy site, and, in one patient, transient bilateral vocal cord paralysis which resolved spontaneously over a 6-week period, resulting in delayed but successful decannulation. One patient had localized osteomyelitis of the cut end of the mandible, and this was successfully resected 7 months postoperatively.

Cancer Status

This surgical approach showed no adverse effect on long-term survival in these patients. The cure rate in this group was unchanged from that effected by the lip-splitting technique.

Cosmesis

The criteria for reporting cosmetic results centered on evaluation of the overall appearance of the lip and chin unit, the amount of cheek depression in the region of the resected mandible, and the amount of chin deviation and retrusion toward the side of the resection with the patient in repose. Although satisfactory appearance was achieved in all patients, over half were judged to be superior, based on the absence of the lip- and chin-splitting incision.

Cheek depression was not marked in any of these patients and seemed to correlate with the preoperative

prominence of the mandible angle and the amount of subcutaneous tissue present. Chin deviation toward the side of the resection and mandibular retrusion also were not significant.

Speech

Articulation, especially the fricatives, and overall intelligibility were considered satisfactory in all of the patients. Seventy-five percent were judged normal or near normal in voice and speech quality with occasional, barely detectable, difficulties with fricatives or hypernasality secondary to soft palate loss. Several patients had difficulties with fricatives significant enough to warrant speech therapy, even though their overall speech intelligibility was satisfactory. These patients had undergone extensive posterior tongue resection.

Occlusion

Both the anatomic and the functional aspects of occlusion were evaluated. Anatomic occlusion was satisfactory in 90 percent of patients. Although all of these patients deviated laterally toward the side of resection on opening, 60 percent were able to close within 2 mm or less of centric occlusion. Most patients were able to achieve the posterior occlusal contact necessary for mastication even if they were more than 2 mm off centric occlusion. One patient was unable to achieve occlusal contact posteriorly. He was the only patient in the series treated without intermaxillary fixation.

Function of the anterior dental arch was deemed adequate if the patient could bite solid foods such as an apple. Posterior function was adequate if solid foods could be effectively chewed to a consistency compatible with deglutition. Forty percent of patients had entirely normal anterior and posterior function and resumed a regular diet postoperatively. When correlated with the preoperative diet, all are eating their normal diets with the exception of the one patient with absent anatomic posterior occlusion who eats a mechanical soft diet.

Deglutition

Ninety percent of the patients have absolutely no swallowing difficulties. Several patients with extensive base of tongue resection have had occasional difficulty swallowing liquids. This has not led to problems with aspiration or weight loss.

Oral Hygiene

None of the patients had long-term difficulties with retained food or odorous desquamation in the region of the graft site. When correlated with the preoperative oral cleanliness, no significant changes have resulted.

Graft Characteristics

Appearance, amount of contraction, and durability were examined. Skin grafts retained the characteristics of skin whereas dermal grafts assumed an appearance more like that of mucosa.

The amount of graft contracture was difficult to estimate, but was not more than 50 percent in any instance, including the several patients in whom partial graft slough occurred in the immediate postoperative period. The graft contracture that occurred tended to obliterate much of the deep ''glossobuccal'' sulcus created at the time of the surgery. This was considered desirable as it prevented potential pooling of food and secretions in the suclus. In no instance did tethering of the tongue or distortion of the intraoral anatomy affect function.

General Status

When evaluated from a personal adjustment and social self-sufficiency standpoint, 75 percent of patients have approached their preoperative levels of function. The remainder have had varying social and personal adjustment problems that are expected following radical surgery and are adjusting slowly outside the hospital environment.

Gainful Employment

Ninety percent of patients were able to work from a functional standpoint, although only one-third of these patients have chosen to do so. This is not surprising when the average age of the group (62 years) is taken into consideration.

COMMENT

The central feature of this approach to repair following a composite resection for oral and oropharyngeal cancers is the one-stage skin graft reconstruction.[8] The routine use of the visor flap for exposure and the standard use of intermaxillary fixation during the postoperative period evolved as important features of this procedure.

The use of free split-thickness skin grafts in the oral and oropharyngeal cavity is certainly not new.[9] Edgerton and Desprez, in 1957,[10] reported the only large series of a single-stage skin graft reconstruction. Their technique involved application of the skin graft to the undersurface of the cheek and use of a tantalum gauze mold and stent dressing for immobilization. They reported 54 excellent graft takes in 73 patients, citing high radiation doses and inadequate graft immobilization for their failures. Slanetz and Rankow reported the use of skin for oropharynx and tonsil fossa coverage in ten patients with good results and advocated the use of a Xerofoam gauze bolster in place of a dental compound or tantalum gauze mold.[11]

The intent of this report has been to describe a procedure designed to minimize the cosmetic and functional problems frequently encountered in the surgical treatment of oral and oropharyngeal malignancies. Indications for this approach include advanced tumors of the tonsil, retromolar trigone, and base of tongue, particularly when mandibular alveolus must be resected. Review of the pathology specimens from these patients revealed adequate margins of resection, and no adverse effects on survival were noted when compared to larger series using similar treatment modalities.

The complication rate with skin graft reconstruction is acceptably low and compares favorably with primary closure or local or regional pedicle-flap reconstruction. One patient had wound infection, fistula formation, and carotid artery catastrophe and was salvaged. The procedure is appropriate for use with either pre- or postoperative radiation therapy, and these modalities did not appear to result in increased surgical morbidity.

The cosmetic improvement with this approach, when compared to the standard composite resection and primary closure, was gratifying. Absence of the lip- and chin-splitting incision, with its attendant scarring, was the most noticeable difference. The visor flap provided adequate exposure in every instance and is the standard incision currently used in approaching these lesions.

A reduction in the cheek depression in the region of the segmental mandible resection and lessening of chin drift and mandibular retrusion were also apparent. The use of the skin graft reconstruction, while not adding significant bulk to the defect, appears to lessen the cheek depression by avoiding the medial pull on the soft tissues of the cheek that results from primary closure of the buccal mucosa to the medial margin of resection. Combined with intermaxillary fixation, the reduced scar contracture creates less pull on the mandible.

Tethering of the tongue superolaterally, which is frequently seen with primary closure, was not observed in this series. This is the most important factor in the overall excellent speech and deglutition that resulted in these patients. In the cases in which tongue mobility was judged somewhat restricted, it was felt to be secondary to lack of tongue bulk from the primary resection, not to scarring or pulling of the tongue remnants by the lateral cheek tissues. Local or regional flap reconstruction in these instances would not have improved tongue mobility.

The creation of a ''glossobuccal'' sulcus by intentionally fashioning a deep skin graft pouch and allowing natural wound and graft contraction to lessen this depth was believed to aid in tongue mobility as well as handling of liquids and secretions. With previous resections, patients were noted to pool fluids on the operated side because of the lack of necessary tongue mobility to effectively clear the secretions and allow swallowing. Patients in this series were essentially free of drooling and swallowing problems.

While near-centric occlusion was achieved in less than 50 percent of the patients, functional occlusion was achieved in 90 percent overall and in 100 percent of the cases in which intermaxillary fixation was employed. This certainly justifies the routine case of intermaxillary fixation in these patients. It has the added advantage of assisting in graft immobilization during the early postoperative period and is believed to contribute significantly to the high rate of graft survival.

A comparison of the use of skin versus dermis as a graft material is difficult in this series because dermis was used only in a few patients and both graft materials yielded satisfactory results. Excessive contracture and desquamation were not noted with split-thickness skin grafts. We are currently using skin grafts almost exclusively.

The visor flap approach takes about 15 minutes longer during the exposure than the standard lip-splitting incision approach. This is well balanced by the time saved in not having to reconstruct the lip at the end of the procedure. The operating time of the skin graft reconstruction is prolonged for 60 to 90 minutes over that required for primary closure, but is significantly less than required for pedicle flap reconstruction. Forty minutes can be saved by presurgical application of the arch bars.

Large oral cavity and oropharyngeal lesions can be readily reconstructed by this method, as evidenced by the fact that over 60 percent of the lesions in the series were greater than 4 cm (T3). Patients with massive lesions involving more than one-half of the base of the tongue are not good candidates for this reconstruction and are better reconstructed by regional pedicle flaps or free flaps. Patients with extensive lesions of the anterior floor of the mouth should not have this closure because of the possibility of anterior pooling of secretions. These patients should have local flap reconstruction. The use of skin graft reconstruction is contraindicated in patients in whom immediate Kirschner wire stabilization is used or delayed bone grafting is contemplated. Pedicle flap closure is preferable in these patients. In our experience, bone grafting has seldom been necessary or desirable when dealing with posterior segmental mandible resection. The cosmetic and functional results achieved with the present approach have been considered very satisfactory by most patients concerned.

Recently, McConnel, Adler, and Teichgrabher reported functional results of various types of reconstructive procedures following surgical resection for oral cavity or oropharyngeal cancer. They compared results after reconstruction with skin grafts, tongue flaps, and myocutaneous flaps. Functions evaluated included speech intelligibility, articulation, tongue mobility, diadochokinesis, and oral phase swallowing. They found that split-thickness skin graft reconstruction resulted in the best scores for tongue mobility, diadochokinesis, articulation, and speech intelligibility. Tongue flaps had the lowest scores, whereas myocutaneous flaps were in the intermediate range for all of their tests. They noted that restoration of tongue mobility was the essential ingredient in restoring oral cavity function and noted that reconstruction with split-thickness skin grafts resulted in consistently better tongue mobility than the other two reconstructive procedures.

REFERENCES

1. Conley JJ. The crippled oral cavity. Plast Reconstr Surg 1962; 30:469–478.
2. Doberneck RC, Antoine JE. Deglutition after resection of oral, laryngeal and pharyngeal cancers. Surgery 1974; 75:87–90.
3. Marchetta FE. Function and appearance following surgery for oral cancer. Clin Plast Surg 1976; 3:471-479.
4. Babin R, Calcaterra TC. The lip-splitting approach to resection of oropharyngeal cancer. J Surg Oncol 1976; 8:433–436.
5. Panje WR, Krause CJ, Bardach J, Baker SR. Reconstruction of intraoral defects with the free groin flap. Arch Otolaryngol 1977; 103:78–83.
6. Sessions DG, Dedo DO, Ogura JH. Tongue flap reconstruction following resection for cancer of the oral cavity. Arch Otolaryngol 1975; 101:166–169.
7. Aramany MA, Myers EN. Intermaxillary fixation following mandibular resection. J Prosthet Dent 1977; 37:437–444.
8. LaFerriere KA, Sessions DG, Thawley SE, Wood BG, Ogura JH. Composite resection and reconstruction for oral cavity and oropharyngeal cancer. Arch Otolaryngol 1980; 106:103–110.
9. Conley JJ. Free skin grafting in the sinus, oral and pharyngeal areas in radical surgery of the head and neck. Cancer 1954; 7:444–454.
10. Edgerton MT, Desprez JD. Reconstruction of the oral cavity in the treatment of cancer. Plast Reconst Surg 1957; 19:89–113.
11. Slanetz CA, Rankow RM. The intra-oral use of split thickness skin grafts in head and neck surgery. Am J Surg 1962; 104:721–726.
12. McConnel FS, Adler RK, Teichgrabher JF. Speech and swallowing function series. Presented at "Head and Neck Cancer: Integration of Treatment and Rehabilitation. National Library of Medicine, Bethesda, MD. January 18, 1984 (In Press)

17. Cancer of the Larynx

INTRODUCTION

DOUGLAS P. BRYCE, M.D., F.R.C.S.(C),
F.R.C.S.(Ed.)Hon., F.A.C.S., ABot.

Cancer of the larynx presents different problems in the major centers in the world. Its management is dictated not so much by the expertise and knowledge of the physicians and surgeons and associates who deal with the disease, but by other factors. Perhaps the most significant factor is the socioeconomic one in that in the majority of the extremely heavily populated countries of this world, the management of laryngeal cancer is basically the management of far-advanced disease with facilities inadequate for the task. The problems to be resolved in these countries are those of overpopulation and education of the masses to seek appropriate medical attention at an early stage of the disease.

In addition to the socioeconomic factors of massive populations and poverty, there is the question of the organization of the health care system within the countries being studied. In those areas in which a socialized type of medicine is available to all people and the financial backing for the medical system is sufficient, an ideal arrangement exists for the care of malignant disease. Patients from all financial and social backgrounds can have access to specialized, centralized areas where the best equipment and personnel available can be congregated to study and care for their disease. In these areas, ideal opportunities exist for appropriate follow-up and for clinical studies that can only serve to improve the ultimate result of treatment. Thus standardized forms of treatment can be made available to all and the general level of care for the patient with serious disease, such as laryngeal cancer, can be satisfactorily high.

In countries where private enterprise is the predominant direction for the management of health problems, there is inevitably an unevenness in the quality of care throughout the country and an unavoidable selection of patient population for studies of clinical protocol.

The management of laryngeal cancer on an international scale therefore may differ from country to country and from health care system to health care system, depending on factors that are not strictly under the control of the medical profession. The effectiveness of radiotherapy, surgery, and chemotherapy in the treatment of cancer of the larynx and other areas depends on the facilities available in the area in which the patient lives. Nevertheless, assuming the happy coincidence of the social system which can afford the best medical care and the availability of equally expert clinicians, radiotherapists, and rehabilitationists, it is possible to discuss the treatment most likely to produce the best survival associated with the most effective conservation of function. Even at this level, however, we have difficulty in accepting a uniform international classification which would make our deliberations much more effective.

The chapters in this part cover in a general way the broad classifications of laryngeal cancer and the rationale for the various modalities of treatment which are being used today, particularly in North America and Europe.

Cancer of the larynx is the most commonly occurring malignant tumor in the head and neck area; fortunately it has the best prognosis. In the past twenty years the various types of management have been clearly outlined and the results of treatment by radiation therapy, surgery, and chemotherapy are known. However, because of some of the aforementioned factors, there is no general agreement as to the results of new methods of treatment when applied to the broad clinical divisions of laryngeal cancer.

Glottic carcinoma accounts for about 70 percent of laryngeal cancers in North America. The early T1, N0 lesions of the glottis may be treated by a multitude of modalities including, most recently, the laser. Because its prognosis is so favorable at this stage, the results for the various methods of treatment are all very similar. The treatment of choice in this area depends on the facility available and the individual preference of the surgeon. There is little doubt, however, that in the treatment of this disease, radiotherapy as a primary method of treatment expertly applied results in the most effective conservation of the voice. Such a result has to be balanced against the time involved in this treatment as opposed to the rapid and effective local and conservation surgical procedures.

In the other end of the spectrum, the large T4 glottic lesions with nodal metastases have a much poorer prognosis and the functional difference between radiotherapy and surgery is not so clearly defined. The prognosis in such patients is perhaps 45 percent 5-year survival, and conservation of function is less important than preservation of life.

It is in the T3 lesions with impaired mobility of the vocal cord or fixation of the cord in which the greatest difference of opinion as to appropriate therapy exists. It is generally recognized that conservation surgery has limited use in such lesions unless that surgery be specialized and extended. Such surgery requires considerable specialized expertise.

Radiotherapy as a primary modality is successful

in managing about 35 percent of patients with cure, but the application of surgical techniques, either conservation or radical, after the primary radiotherapy presents particular problems for the surgeon and the patient. The use of primary radiotherapy in such patients requires the optimum conditions of patient control, follow-up, and expertise in all disciplines of management. Nevertheless, if these conditions exist, about one-half of the survivors will have a normal larynx. The actual survival figure is somewhat better if surgery is a primary method of therapy, but the functional result is much poorer.

Cancer of the supraglottic larynx is a very different problem from that of the glottis. The prognosis in such tumors is not nearly so good, and the tendency to distal and regional metastases is much higher.

Once again, however, early T1 lesions have the best prognosis whether treated primarily by radiotherapy or by conservation surgery. In general, the more extensive lesions are managed by laryngectomy with appropriate neck dissection. It is interesting, but not yet explained, to note that the incidence of supraglottic malignant tumors is relatively much higher in some parts of the world than in North America; particularly in Scandinavia, Italy, and the Southeast Asian countries, the 70/30 ratio of glottic to supraglottic involvement by malignant disease is reversed.

There has been considerable pressure in the past 20 years for the surgical correction of the loss of voice following total laryngectomy. The traditional esophageal voice is often not attainable by the elderly patients, particularly those who have other unrelated diseases. A variety of tracheoesophageal or tracheopharyngeal fistulas have been developed over the years, but the multiplicity of the procedures indicates that all of these have their deficiencies. Which method of rehabilitation following laryngectomy is appropriate for the particular part of the world in which the patient lives is dependent on the social conditions of that country and the expertise and interest of the surgeons. All malignant tumors of the head and neck tend to occur in patients who have a high percentage of other associated heart, lung, or kidney diseases and all are associated with smoking, chewing, or drinking to a much higher extent than in the normal population. Cancer of the larynx is also affected by this etiologic factor, but this is more apparent in supraglottic than in glottic malignant tumors.

The other factor in common that laryngeal cancer has with head and neck cancers is the frequency of second primaries. Once again this is much higher in supraglottic cancers than in glottic. Nevertheless, the incidence of a second malignant lesion in the lung is very high, particularly among long survivors from their original management of the laryngeal cancer.

Cancer of the larynx is the most common malignant tumor in the head and neck area and has received the greatest concentrated attention of oncologic workers. It is a particularly attractive area because the prognosis is relatively good and the rewards of success in management are great and apparent, both for the patient and the physician and surgeon. An understanding of the basic causes of some of the differences of opinion among those who treat this disease and the varying results that occur will help to develop a more sympathetic attitude toward workers and can only ultimately reflect to the benefit of the patients suffering from this disease.

FAILURE ANALYSIS OF T1 GLOTTIC CARCINOMA TREATED WITH RADICAL RADIOTHERAPY FOR CURE WITH SURGERY IN RESERVE

GILEAD BERGER, M.D.
A.W. PETER Van NOSTRAND, M.D.
ANDREW R. HARWOOD, M.D., Ch.B., F.R.C.P.(C)
DOUGLAS P. BRYCE, M.D., F.R.C.S.(C), F.R.C.S.(Ed.)Hon., F.A.C.S., ABot.

Early squamous cell carcinoma of the true vocal cords is effectively treated by surgery or radiotherapy. High cure rates in the range of 85 to 90 percent have been reported with either modality.[1-9] In Toronto patients with early cancer of the larynx have been approached primarily with moderate doses of irradiation (5000 rads in 4 weeks in 20 fractions or equivalent). Surgery is used for patients who fail radiotherapy and are found to have residual or recurrent tumor. The advantages of this policy are (1) most patients with early glottic tumors are controlled and still retain their larynges and a natural voice; (2) occurrence of major radiotherapy complications such as laryngeal necrosis is infrequent; (3) early detection of recurrent tumors is possible since the incidence and extent of laryngeal edema is reduced; (4) a substantial proportion of patients with recurrent tumor are salvaged surgically; and (5) the incidence of severe postoperative complications is not increased.

This retrospective study was undertaken to analyze patients with T1N0M0 glottic squamous cell carcinoma who failed radiotherapy. Factors associated with tumor recurrence, salvage, mortality, and complications will be considered.

MATERIAL AND METHODS

In the 15-year period from 1965 to 1979 inclusive, 571 patients were originally staged as T1N0M0 squamous cell carcinoma of the vocal cords according to the 1978 TNM UICC classification[10] and underwent radical radiotherapy for cure at the Princess Margaret Hospital in Toronto. Their medical records were reviewed and the whole-organ serial-sectioning specimens of those who developed recurrent tumors and underwent salvage surgery were studied. These showed that of the 571 patients originally staged as T1N0M0, 34 patients should be excluded from the study for a variety of reasons. Fourteen patients were reclassified as T2N0M0. Of these, 10 patients had their tumor confined to the vocal cord, but the cord mobility was impaired. Previous publications from our institution had classified them as T1 tumors.[9,11] However, their outcome was significantly worse than those with normal mobility, and we felt that it would be more accurate to classify them as T2 tumors. Other investigators have also designated them T2 tumors.[12,13] The other four patients in this category had extension of their tumor beyond the confines of the glottic region, either supraglottically or subglottically. Twelve patients were found on review of the histology to have verrucous carcinoma; eight patients had primary subglottic tumor masquerading clinically as T1 glottic carcinoma. However, their surgical specimen disclosed that either the growth was confined entirely to the subglottic region or the major bulk of the tumor involved the subglottic region, and only the "tip of the iceberg" emerged above the level of the conus elasticus. Therefore the final series includes 537 patients with T1N0M0 glottic squamous carcinoma. There were 482 males and 55 females (9:1 ratio). All the patients except those treated in 1979 have been followed 5 years or more.

RESULTS

Forty-seven patients (8.8%) failed radiotherapy and were found to have residual or recurrent cancer within the first 5 years following treatment. Seven more patients developed recurrent cancer of the larynx after more than 5 years following radiotherapy; two of them appeared after more than 10 years. The contralateral vocal cord was involved in two of the seven late recurrences. These seven patients were excluded since it is most probable that these late recurrences represent second primary tumors of the larynx.[14]

Factors Influencing Success of Radiotherapy in T1 Glottic Cancer. A previous study showed that success or failure of radiotherapy were significantly influenced by the sex of the patient and by the size of the irradiation fields.[11] Thus increased incidence of failure was associated with the male sex and with smaller irradiation fields (<36 cm^2). The difference in local failure between T1a and T1b tumors was not statistically significant.

Time Interval Between Radiotherapy and Detection of Recurrent Tumor. Figure 1 shows the time distribution of recurrent tumor detection. In 85 percent of the cases, the recurrent cancer appeared within the first two years after completion of radiotherapy. The mean time interval between treatment and detection of recurrence was 14 months. Sometimes the diagnosis of recurrent cancer was not easy. Thus in eight patients, recurrence was suspected for some months before it was proved by biopsy. Seven of the eight patients underwent a negative direct laryngoscopy and biopsy, one patient had three negative biopsies before a positive biopsy was finally obtained.

Extent and Staging of Recurrent Tumor. Of the total 47 patients considered to have failed radiotherapy, 42 patients developed local recurrence and five patients presented with metastatic disease without evidence of local recurrence. Table 1 shows the classification and staging of the recurrent tumors. Only in 18 patients (38%) did the extent of recurrent tumor remain the same as that of the original disease. In 15 patients (32%), the tumor had reached the equivalent of stage II, seven patients (15%) had reached the equivalent of stage III, and six patients (13%) had reached the equivalent of stage IV. In one patient the stage of the recurrent tumor was not described. It is of interest that of the five patients who presented with metastatic disease, only one presented with nodal metastases confined to the ipsilateral neck. One presented with distant metastases only (pelvis and spine), and the other three had involvement of the contralateral neck (one patient), both sides of the neck (one patient), and contralateral neck and lungs (one patient).

Results of Salvage Surgery. Of the 47 patients who failed radiotherapy, 10 patients had no attempts at surgical management of the larynx. Five of these

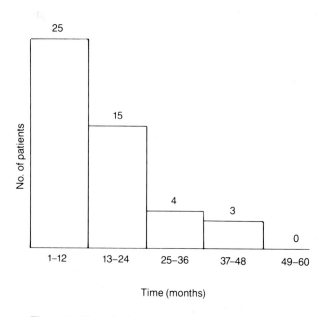

Figure 1 Time distribution of recurrent tumor detection.

TABLE 1   Staging of recurrences (rTNM) — 47 cases

Stage	rT	N	M	No.	%
I	rT1	N0	M0	18	38
II	rT2	N0	M0	15	32
III	rT3	N0	M0	6 } 7	15
	rT3	N1	M0	1	
IV	rT4	N0	M0	1	
	rT0	N3	M0	3 } 6	13
	rT0	N0	M1	1	
	rT0	N2	M1	1	
Unknown				1	2
Total				47	100

are the five patients who presented with metastatic disease and no evidence of local recurrence. The remaining five patients either refused surgery or were found to be unsuitable for surgery for a variety of reasons. Nine of these patients died of uncontrolled cancer, and one is alive with disease. Thirty-seven patients underwent salvage surgery; 32 of them were salvaged, and five patients died from uncontrolled disease. A detailed analysis of the surgical group shows that a partial laryngectomy procedure was performed on 15 patients, and a total laryngectomy with or without neck dissection was carried out on 22 patients. As shown in Table 2, 14 of the 15 patients who underwent partial laryngectomy were salvaged, and only one patient died from uncontrolled disease. However, two patients in this group subsequently required total laryngectomy. In one of these patients, the pathology specimen revealed that tumor was present at the inferior resection margin, and the second developed recurrence after hemilaryngectomy. Eighteen of the 22 patients who underwent total laryngectomy were salvaged, and four patients died from their disease.

Mortality. Fourteen of 537 patients with T1N0M0 died from uncontrolled cancer. This means that only 2.6 percent of the patients with stage I squamous cell carcinoma of the vocal cords who were treated with radical radiotherapy for cure and surgery in reserve died of their laryngeal malignancy.

In five of the fourteen patients who died, death was due to uncontrolled tumor at the primary site

TABLE 2   End Results (47 patients)

	No. of Patients	Controlled	Died
Partial laryngectomy (Vertical hemilaryngectomy, cordectomy, subtotal laryngectomy)	15	14*	1
Total laryngectomy ± neck dissection	22	18†	4
No surgery	10‡	0	9
Total	47	32	14

*Two patients underwent subsequent total laryngectomy.
†One patient underwent successful excision of stomal recurrence.
‡One patient alive with disease 3 years later.

without evidence of metastatic disease; four of these were in the group who refused surgery. Only one of the patients underwent an attempt at salvage surgery (total laryngectomy) with local failure only (stomal recurrence).

The remaining nine patients who died all had evidence of metastatic tumor; five of these patients were the group who developed metastatic disease without ever showing evidence of local (laryngeal) recurrence. Two additional patients died with neck metastases, having had their laryngeal disease controlled by surgical resection. The remaining two patients also had surgical resections, but died with extensive local disease and neck metastases. One of these patients also had distant metastases in liver and skin.

Postoperative Complications Following Radiotherapy. Fifteen patients (41%) of the 37 who underwent salvage surgery developed postoperative complications; 13 patients developed a single complication, two patients developed more than one. Infection and necrosis of neck flaps occurred in six patients, pharyngocutaneous fistulas in four patients, and pulmonary complications in three patients. Each of the following complications occurred once: neck abscess, pyogenic granuloma of the larynx, chyle leak, septicemia, hypocalcemia, and upper gastrointestinal bleeding. There were no postoperative deaths.

DISCUSSION

The TNM classification of malignant tumors (UICC or AJC) is designed to enable the investigator to evaluate the response of a homogeneous group of patients to various modalities of treatment. This classification is based on the clinical (preoperative or preradiation) assessment of the local, nodal, and distant extent of cancer. In centers where radiotherapy is used for the treatment of laryngeal carcinoma, this clinical (preradiation) assessment is usually the only means of tumor assessment, i.e., no specimen is obtained and no pathologic assessment is possible. In contrast, in centers where surgical resection is the principal modality of management, the surgeon has the opportunity for both a clinical (preoperative) and a pathologic (postoperative) assessment of the tumor. Recognizing that the clinical assessment of laryngeal tumors has an inaccuracy rate of 10 to 25 percent, even in the hands of experienced laryngologists (van Nostrand AWP, Olofsson J. Unpublished data), we must conclude that the staging provided from surgical centers is considerably more accurate than that from radiotherapy centers. This fact makes the evaluation and comparison of results of radiotherapy extremely difficult.

It is for these reasons that we made major efforts to produce as homogeneous a group of patients with T1 glottic carcinoma as we could, in order to be better able to compare our results with those from centers where surgery is the primary modality of therapy. Thus the patients whose charts revealed that they had T2 glottic carcinoma or verrucous carcinoma, as well as those whose surgical specimens indicated the existence of primary subglottic carcinoma, were excluded from this study.

Numerous reports have shown that most patients with early glottic cancer who fail radiotherapy are subsequently salvaged by surgery.[4,11,12,15,16] A partial laryngectomy is as effective as total laryngectomy if the recurrent tumor meets the established criteria for conservation surgical procedure.[17,18] It is evident therefore that partial laryngectomy in selected cases controls the growth and offers the patient a better quality of life with preservation of laryngeal speech. This analysis of the radiotherapy failure group lends support to this view. Salvation by surgery was achieved in 32 of the 47 patients who developed recurrent tumors. Of these, 12 patients were controlled by conservation surgery, and only 20 patients lost their larynx as a price for tumor control.

Neel et al stated that "laryngofissure and cordectomy for certain cancers of the larynx leads to a successful outcome in more than 95 percent of the patients".[8] The present study confirms that radical radiotherapy for cure with surgery in reserve is an effective method of eradicating T1 glottic tumors, resulting in a mortality rate of less than 3 percent.

The analysis of mortality shows that most of the deaths occurred in association with metastatic cancer to nodes and distant sites rather than local failure. The finding that metastatic disease accounted for most of the deaths is surprising since T1 glottic carcinoma had gained a reputation for its association with a very low incidence of metastatic spread.[13,19] This implies that no matter how low is the incidence of metastasis, its appearance always signifies a poor prognosis.

Finally, the unfavorable effects of ionizing radiation on laryngeal tissues may cause major complications or render the hypoxic tissues sensitive to any future intervention. Since the damage is proportional to the delivered dose, the complication rate is expected to increase in those receiving high doses of irradiation. This is supported by the study of Mintz et al, who reported a 30 percent incidence of perichondritis of the larynx when radiation exceeded 6500 rads, but was no higher than 14 percent in patients receiving less than 6400 rads.[20] Similarly, high morbidity is likely to occur in those undergoing operation following the delivery of high doses. Ballantyne and Fletcher reported that pharyngocutaneous fistulas developed in 10 patients out of 27, and there was one death from carotid rupture.[12] The present study demonstrates the advantage of using moderate doses of irradiation therapy. This policy is associated with fewer complications and does not appear to compromise the chances of tumor control. Thus, of the 537 patients included in the study, we have not seen a single case of clinical perichondritis or necrosis of the larynx, and of the 37 patients who underwent surgery following irradiation only four developed fistula and none had carotid rupture. Furthermore, the low incidence of

complications following treatment with moderate doses of irradiation was confirmed by Keene et al, who reported that pathologic chondronecrosis occurred in only one of 41 early tumors (pT1-pT2) of patients who failed radiotherapy and underwent laryngectomy.[21]

CONCLUSIONS

Of 537 patients with T1 glottic carcinoma treated by radical radiotherapy for cure with surgery in reserve, 97.2 percent are cured and 93.5 percent have their laryngeal speech preserved.

Radiotherapy cures more than 90 percent of T1 glottic tumors. Salvage surgery cures two-thirds of those who fail radiotherapy. Partial laryngectomy is effective in selected cases. In our hands, 2.6 percent of patients with T1 glottic carcinoma die of their tumor. Of those who die, most succumb to their metastases.

The complication rate of both radiotherapy and surgery following irradiation is low.

REFERENCES

1. Hibbs GG, Hendrickson FR. Telecobalt therapy of early malignant tumors of vocal cord. Radiology 1966; 86:447–449.
2. Perez CA, Holtz S, Ogura JH, Dedo HH, Powers WE. Radiation therapy of early carcinoma of the true vocal cords. Cancer 1968; 21:764–771.
3. Vermund H. Role of radiotherapy in cancer of the larynx as related to the TNM system of staging. Cancer 1970; 25:485–504.
4. Wang CC. Treatment of glottic carcinoma by megavoltage radiation therapy and results. Am J Roentgenol 1974; 120:157–163.
5. Miller D. Management of glottic carcinoma. Laryngoscope 1975; 85:1435–1439.
6. Skolnik EM, Yee KF, Wheatley MA, Martin LO. Carcinoma of the laryngeal glottis, therapy and end results. Laryngoscope 1975; 85:1453–1465.
7. Stewart JG, Brown JR, Palmer MK, Cooper A. The management of glottic carcinoma by primary irradiation with surgery in reserve. Laryngoscope 1975; 85:1477–1484.
8. Neel HB III, Devine KD, DeSanto LW. Laryngofissure and cordectomy for early cordal carcinoma: Outcome in 182 patients. Otolaryngol Head Neck Surg 1980; 88:79–84.
9. Harwood AR, Hawkins NV, Keane T, Cummings B, Beale FA, Rider WD, Bryce DP. Radiotherapy of early glottic cancer. Laryngoscope 1980; 90:465–470.
10. UICC TNM. Classification of malignant tumors. 3rd Ed. Harmer MH, ed. Geneva, 1978.
11. Harwood, AR. Cancer of the larynx—the Toronto experience. II. Glottic cancer. J Otolaryngol 1982; II (suppl. 11):5–9.
12. Ballantyne AJ, Fletcher GH. Surgical management of irradiation failures of nonfixed cancers of the glottic region. Am J Roentgenol 1974; 120:164–168.
13. DeSanto LW, Pearson WB. Initial treatment of laryngeal cancer. Minn Med 1981; 64:691–698.
14. Lawson W, Som M. Second primary cancer after irradiation of laryngeal cancer. Ann Otol Rhinol Laryngol 1975; 84:771–775.
15. Hawkins NV. The treatment of glottic carcinoma: An analysis of 800 cases. Laryngoscope 1975; 85:1485–1493.
16. Horiot JC, Fletcher GH, Ballantyne AJ, Lindberg RD. Analysis of failures of early vocal cord cancer. Radiology 1972; 103:663–665.

17. Biller HF, Barnhill FR, Ogura JH, Perez CA. Hemilaryngec-tomy following radiation failure for carcinoma of the vocal cords. Laryngoscope 1970; 80:249–253.
18. Burns H, Bryce DP, van Nostrand AWP. Conservation sur-gery in laryngeal cancer and its role following failed radio-therapy. Arch Otolaryngol 1979; 105:234–239.
19. McGavran MH, Bauer WC, Ogura JH. The incidence of cer-vical lymph node metastases from epidermoid carcinoma of the larynx and their relationship to certain characteristics of the primary tumor. Cancer 1961; 14:55–66.
20. Mintz DR, Gullane PJ, Thomson DH, Ruby RRF. Perichon-dritis of the larynx following radiation. Otolaryngol Head Neck Surg 1981; 89:550–554.
21. Keene M, Harwood AR, Bryce DP, van Nostrand AWP. His-topathological study of radionecrosis in laryngeal carcinoma. Laryngoscope 1982; 92:173–180.

TREATMENT OF LARYNGEAL CANCER

JOHN A. KIRCHNER, M.D.

If one employs radiotherapy as the primary treat-ment for every type of laryngeal cancer and reserves surgery for failures, it makes little or no difference whether the laryngeal framework has been invaded when the lesion is first examined because the external perichondrium is rarely involved except by very ex-tensive growths. The same is true if total laryngec-tomy is the standard form of treatment for all laryn-geal cancer, regardless of the size and location of the primary lesion. But if conservation (or partial) lar-yngectomy is part of the surgeon's practice, he must know how extensively the primary lesion has invaded the submucosal soft tissues or infiltrated the laryngeal framework before he makes an incision or a saw-cut into these structures.

The ideal method of predicting the extent of such invasion should be pretreatment CT scanning, and this has provided some degree of useful information in many cases. However, it has its limitations because the vagaries of ossification within the thyroid and cri-coid cartilages make it difficult, in some cases, to dis-tinguish between areas of destruction and regions of nonossification within the laryngeal framework.

Other methods, including laryngography, cine-laryngography, lateral xerography, and conventional tomography, provide indirect evidence of deep inva-sion. However, in assessing any particular primary le-sion for partial laryngectomy, direct laryngoscopic examination often provides information that cannot be obtained by any of these methods. One example is the glottic lesion that extends laterally along the su-perior surface of the true cord. Displacing the ven-tricular band laterally with the bevel of the laryngo-scope may reveal the tumor's lateral margin and its suitability for laser excision or partial laryngectomy (Fig. 1).

Supported by PHS Grant 5-RO11-CA22101-07 awarded by the National Cancer Institute, DHHS.

Similarly, the inferior extent of a bulky growth in the ventricular band may be difficult to determine by indirect laryngoscopy or by examination with the flexible fiberscope. The tumor may displace the true cord downward without crossing the ventricle, so that it is still suitable for horizontal supraglottic laryngec-tomy. However, this fact may not be apparent until the tumor is displaced laterally by the bevel of the laryngoscope, or until the lower part of the mass is pulled upward on a hook, revealing an uninvolved true cord below (Fig. 2).

On the basis of observations made on 355 sur-gical specimens obtained at partial or total laryngec-tomy and studied by serial section, the following guidelines have been established in our practice.

GLOTTIC CANCER

The T1 lesion usually remains superficial to the vocal ligament and conus elasticus. Control rates are equally good by radiotherapy or by local excision. The resultant voice is usually better after successful radio-therapy and is our treatment of choice.

For the T2 lesion, hemilaryngectomy is our treat-ment of choice because our cure rates are better than with radiotherapy (71% vs 35%).[1] Cure rates reported from other major centers show less discrepancy be-tween these modalities (73% vs 61% in Cocke's re-view of reports from 15 major treatment centers).[2] The reason for this disparity is not clear, but it is probably due to the difficulties of precise staging, particularly if pretreatment assessment is made purely on the basis of indirect laryngoscopy and radiographic studies.

Total laryngectomy is recommended for most T3 glottic lesions, with functional neck dissection in N0 or some N1 cases. If one or more positive nodes are found, adjuvant irradiation is administered.

Hemilaryngectomy is suitable for the occasional fixed-cord lesion that extends downward less than 1 cm below the glottic level in the anterior and midlar-ynx. Posteriorly, the inferior margin of safety is much less.

For T4 lesions, total laryngectomy with radical neck dissection is recommended. Postoperative irra-diation is used in most cases, particularly when there is extensive infiltrating subglottic growth, one or more positive nodes, or other evidence of aggressive be-havior such as perineural invasion or extranodal in-vasion of adjacent soft tissues.

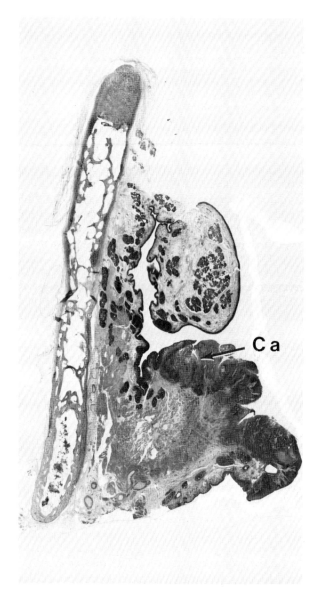

Figure 1 Coronal section of T2 glottic cancer removed by hemilaryngectomy. Limitation of motion in this case was due to extension of the growth along the superior surface of the true cord, without invasion of the thyro-arytenoid muscle. The lateral extent of this kind of lesion can sometimes be identified by displacing the ventricular band laterally on the bevel of the laryngoscope, a technique useful when resecting smaller glottic lesions by laser microlaryngoscopy.

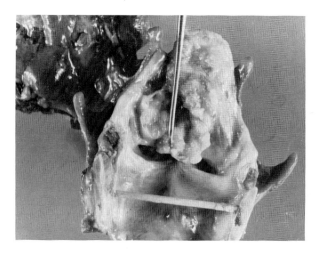

Figure 2 Bulky supraglottic cancer overhanging the true cords and concealing them during preoperative examination by indirect laryngoscopy. The ventricle and true cords are completely free of tumor. The specimen illustrates one of the difficulties in staging large supraglottic growths by clinical methods. Except for its proximity to the left arytenoid cartilage, this lesion might have been resectable by horizontal supraglottic partial laryngectomy.

ANTERIOR COMMISSURE

The dense mass of connective tissue at the level of the true cords at their insertion into the thyroid cartilage acts as a barrier to the forward spread of cancer until late in the disease.[3,4] The T1b lesion, therefore, is usually curable by radiotherapy or by partial laryngectomy.

T2 lesions that extend downward in the anterior larynx are usually curable by partial laryngectomy if the inferior edge of the tumor lies at or above the lower edge of the thyroid cartilage (approximately 1 cm below the anterior commissure).

The anterior glottic lesion tht extends upward onto the base of the epiglottis is a much more aggressive form of cancer and frequently invades the adjacent thyroid cartilage. It is not a suitable candidate for partial laryngectomy.

SUBGLOTTIC CANCER

Tumor extending more than 1 cm below the level of the glottis may (1) escape from the larynx via the cricothyroid membrane, and (2) infiltrate the cancellous interior of the thyroid or cricoid portions of the laryngeal framework under an intact mucosa some distance from the visible margin of the primary lesion. The value of conventional neck dissection for subglottic cancer is doubtful since the regional lymphatics are paratracheal rather than deep jugular in location.

SUPRAGLOTTIC CANCER

In contrast to subglottic cancer, which is often undertreated when managed surgically, supraglottic cancer is frequently overtreated. Horizontal supraglottic partial laryngectomy is adequate treatment for the majority of lesions involving the infrahyoid part of the epiglottis and for cancer of the ventricular band that does not extend downward across the ventricle. Gross examination of the inferior extent of a lesion after pharyngotomy is sufficient to define its limits of infiltration. In not a single instance among the 63 surgical specimens examined histologically has the line of resection been violated inferiorly by cancer when subtotal horizontal laryngectomy was performed after adequate exposure.

Invasion of the thyroid ala has not been found in any of the 63 specimens studied by serial section. The saw-cut made at horizontal supraglottic laryngectomy is therefore oncologically safe.

Invasion of the pre-epiglottic space renders the lesion unsuitable for radiotherapy.[5] The area can be resected as completely by horizontal supraglottic laryngectomy as by total extirpation of the larynx. Removal of the hyoid bone is rarely necessary because a safe margin usually exists between the advancing edge of the tumor and the inner surface of the hyoid bone.[6]

Cancer of the epiglottis or ventricular band that extends downward below the anterior commissure or ventricle can no longer be classed as "supraglottic" because it no longer follows the general principles just outlined. Such extension relegates the lesion to the "transglottic" category, with a high incidence of invasion into the thyroid cartilage.[7] This type of lesion is usually unsuitable for anything less than total laryngectomy.

Horizontal supraglottic laryngectomy after unsuccessful radiation therapy is oncologically unsafe because of unidentifiable margins and because of the unacceptably high rate of complications. Total laryngectomy must be employed in these cases.

Radiotherapy is indicated for early T1 supraglottic lesions and for those extending posteriorly onto the arytenoid cartilage. In the latter lesion, cervical node metastasis is more frequent than with lesion in the anterior supraglottic larynx. The N0 neck should be controllable by external beam therapy. The problem becomes more complex when enlarged cervical nodes are associated with the posterior supraglottic lesion. Our practice in these cases has been to treat the primary lesion and neck with external beam therapy and to follow this with functional or radical neck dissection. Healing in these cases is not a problem since the pharynx is not entered at operation.

Horizontal supraglottic laryngectomy with resection of the arytenoid cartilage usually results in some degree of aspiration postoperatively, even when the posterior end of the true cord is sutured into the midline against the cricoid plate. Some patients, especially those with compromised pulmonary function, cannot tolerate even occasional aspiration, and are better served by total laryngectomy if radiotherapy has been unsuccessful.

PYRIFORM SINUS CANCER

Early lesion of the pyriform sinus are rarely encountered in our practice. Partial laryngectomy is contraindicated if the apex of the pyriform sinus is involved by tumor at direct laryngoscopy or on barium swallow. The posterior and inferior margins of the thyroid cartilage and the upper edge of the cricoid are invaded in over half of such lesions, thus precluding a safe cut in the thyroid cartilage.[8]

DISCUSSION

It is equally short-sighted to employ routine radiotherapy or total laryngectomy as the primary form of treatment for all types of laryngeal cancer. The choice of treatment should be based on the location and size of the primary lesion, and on the status of the regional lymph nodes.

Partial laryngectomy with conservation of both the phonatory and protective functions of the larynx can achieve cure rates that equal or surpass those of radiotherapy in most types of supraglottic cancer and in T2 glottic lesions. Partial laryngectomy demands that every effort be made to determine the exact location and extent of the primary lesion, since safe margins are measured in millimeters, a concept difficult for the average pathologist to accept, but true, nevertheless, as shown by survival rates. If a lesion originally suitable for partial laryngectomy is treated unsuccessfully by irradiation, total laryngectomy is usually the only recourse.

Much of the controversy between surgeons and radiotherapists arises from the difficulty in staging the primary tumor by indirect laryngoscopy or by radiographic methods. One examiner's T2 glottic lesion may be another's T1, or still another's T3, with "fixation" being due merely to tumor bulk, or to extension along the superior surface of the vocal cord, with no invasion of the underlying muscle.[9] Treatment results reported by various centers are therefore difficult to interpret and to apply to one's own practice. Preoperative appearance of primary lesions, as compared with gross and microscopic features of the surgical specimens, promises to provide the most reliable information on the intralaryngeal spread of cancer and on the most appropriate forms of treatment.

REFERENCES

1. Kirchner JA, Owen JR. Five hundred cancers of the larynx and pyriform sinus. Laryngoscope 1977; 87:1288–1303.
2. Cocke EW Jr. Management of malignant neoplasms of the larynx. In: English GM, ed. Otolaryngology. Rev ed. vol. 5. Philadelphia: Harper & Row, 1981, Chapter 34.
3. Kirchner JA, Fischer JJ. Anterior commissure cancer—a clinical and laboratory study of 39 cases. Can J Otolaryngol 1975; 4:637–643.
4. Bagatella F, Bignardi L. Behavior of cancer at the anterior commissure of the larynx. Laryngoscope 1983; 93:353–356.
5. Fletcher GH, Lindberg RD, Hamberger A, Horiot J-C. Reasons for irradiation failure in squamous cell cancer of the larynx. Laryngoscope 1975; 85:987–1003.
6. Kirchner JA. Closure after supraglottic laryngectomy. Laryngoscope 1979; 89:1343–1344.
7. Kirchner JA, Cornog JL, Holmes RE. Transglottic cancer. Arch Otolaryngol 1974; 99:247–251.
8. Kirchner JA. Pyriform sinus cancer: a clinical and laboratory study. Ann Otol Rhinol Laryngol 1975; 84:793–804.
9. Kirchner JA, Som ML. Clinical significance of fixed vocal cord. Laryngoscope 1971; 81:1029–1044.

TREATMENT OPTIONS IN EARLY CANCERS OF THE LARYNX

LAWRENCE W. DeSANTO, M.D.

Early cancer of the larynx, particularly at the cordal (glottic) level, are a common problem to the otolaryngologist. Early diagnosis is possible because symptoms are undeniable, the larynx is easily examined, and the population is alert to the significance of voice alteration as a sign of serious disease.

Death as a consequence of early cancer is unlikely. Because few patients die of their disease, the consequences of treatment become the real issue in selecting from the options of treatment.

DEFINITION

An early cancer of the larynx is defined as one that is limited to a single site within the voice box and has not fixed a vocal cord. The significance of vocal cord fixation has survived over time as a key indicator that a cancer cannot be considered an early cancer. The scientific basis for understanding cordal fixation has been a later discovery through whole laryngeal section studies.

Early cancers come from the two major sites within the larynx: the glottis and the supraglottis.

Glottic cancers are the most common. They cause symptoms early because they affect the phonating surfaces of a vocal fold. Early glottic cancers are stage I or II, depending on their size (stage III implies cordal fixation). It is not fully appreciated that the staging system oversimplifies the range of early glottic cancers. There are very small, small, medium-sized, and larger cancers within each stage. Some stage I cancers are no bigger than the biopsy specimen taken to identify them. An understanding of the concept of a spectrum of severity within a single stage is important to treatment planning, which considers all treatment options. If only one option is considered, this substaging process is not important.

Early glottic cancers are curable. Actually, nobody should die from early glottic cancer. Because death as a consequence of the early growths is unlikely, the usual statistical methods of comparing treatment effectiveness (5-year "cure," determinant survival, or even actual probability of survival) are not very useful. With disease control anticipated, the consequences of treatment, treatment cost, and time of treatment become the important variables in selection of the appropriate treatment option.

Other important considerations in treatment planning are the patient's age, occupation, general health, reliability to follow-up, distance from treatment facility, and, most important, the patient's preference.

IN SITU CANCER

Intraepithelial, noninvasive, or so-called in situ cancer of the glottic larynx is a concept of controversy. In situ cancer implies an intraepithelial process that has not exited the thickness of the epithelium. Grossly, these lesions are similar to the white thickening that is called leukoplakia, keratosis, or the epithelial hyperplasia. These latter are all benign conditions that cause symptoms, indicate an unhealthy epithelial field, and, if removed, do not return. (New lesions may develop, but the ones removed do not.) In reality then, the diagnosis of carcinoma in situ represents more the words on a pathology report than a diagnosis of certain prognostic significance. The words on the paper do not predict biologic behavior.

My concept of "in situ cancer" is based on clinical experience with more than 200 cases. I consider this diagnosis as representing an epithelial change that probably is serious, but is not immediately so. I believe that is a sign of an unhealthy epithelial field. The lesion can be multicentric, is not rare, can be present for a long time (months to years) without threat to life or larynx, may progress to invasive cancer, is not particularly radiosensitive, and is easily overtreated.

In practice, what I often see is a patient whose vocal cord is biopsied or "stripped," and a few days later, the diagnosis of "carcinoma in situ" is delivered by a pathology report. I often see the patient and perform indirect laryngoscopy weeks later, after the biopsy reaction settles down, and can see no abnormality. In such patients, who are followed up for months or years, the lesion can reform on the cord or the cord can remain healthy-appearing.

The other scenario is that of the patient I see before biopsy. There is no certain way the diagnosis can be made with a high accuracy at indirect or direct examination. Lesions I call "leukoplakia" turn out to be called in situ cancer by the pathologist at frozen-section examination. When that diagnosis is delivered while the patient is still in the operating room and the laryngoscope is at hand, I simply remove the lesion and judiciously treat the base with laser pulse or electrocautery. Few lesions so treated reappear. Those that do are retreated at laryngoscopy. The controversy in the literature suggests that the two options for treating in situ cancer are "stripping" or radiation. In fact, neither seems the best treatment. "Stripping" implies simply a biopsy. I think a little more than stripping is appropriate. A few millimeters of the underlying cord surface should be treated with some physical agent such as electrocautery, profound cold, or laser pulse. Radiation is an attractive option when the patient is off the operating table or even at home when the diagnosis is made. No doubt radiation destroys some in situ cancers, but many patients also are treated for this condition who do not have any disease when they begin their radiation treatments—the lesion was removed by biopsy. It seems more appropriate to allow the biopsy reaction to settle down, to reappraise the cord at indirect laryngoscopy a month or 6 weeks later, and then to decide whether to repeat laryngoscopy or to radiate.

The suggestion that radiation to in situ cancer may result in an invasive cancer may or may not be true. If one acknowledges that a diagnosis of intraepithelial cancer represents an unhealthy epithelial field, perhaps what occurs in those who develop invasive cancer at a later date are simply manifesting the field's destiny, which may or may not have been stimulated by the ionizing radiation.

The question whether radiation makes in situ cancer better or worse is a moot one. The time and cost of external radiation as compared with those of simple endoscopic treatment places external radiation in a position of profound overkill. These practical considerations (of time and cost) seem more important than whether radiation makes a sick larynx sicker or destroys more cancer. The issue of voice quality is not pertinent in the in situ treatment controversies. Most voices are not significantly altered by judicious endoscopic therapy. Currently, most patients with in situ cancers are treated definitively at laryngoscopy.

An actual, unequivocal diagnosis of invasive squamous cancer at biopsy is a different problem. As this diagnosis is not difficult for the pathologist to make with a high degree of accuracy, the actual threat to the larynx is more certain than it is with in situ cancer. Treatment options exist, and none exists to the exclusion of the other. As already noted, the best option is selected on the basis of the other variables mentioned and not on the basis of the concept of cure only. In my practice, there are three treatment alternatives for early glottic cancer: endoscopic treatment, partial vertical laryngectomy meaning laryngofissure and cordectomy, and external fractionated radiation.

Endoscopic treatment for carefully selected early cordal lesions is an alternative that is poorly understood, unappreciated, or rejected as invalid. It is an old idea. Lynch,[1] New,[2] and Lillie[3] have reported on its value. Vaughan[4] endorses the concept in properly selected patients. The principle rests on the premise that there is a range of severity of the early growths, and some very early ones that can be properly exposed can be destroyed or removed at laryngoscopy.

The concept is supported by my experience and that of others, such as Stutsman and McGavran,[5] that in about 20 percent of patients in whom laryngofissure occurs after cordal biopsy, no cancer is found in the laryngofissure surgical specimen. A similar percentage of patients probably are subjected to external radiation who likewise do not have cancer at the beginning of the treatment program.

Selection is the key to endoscopic removal or destruction. The suitable lesions are small, discrete, and midcordal and must be completely exposed at laryngoscopy. Currently, excision by laser is my preferred method of removal because of its simplicity. In the past, the cutting electrocautery was just as effective. It is the concept and not the laser that permits endoscopic treatment for small glottic cancers.[6]

Of 200 patients with lesions, half in situ and half early invasive, six have had local recurrences, all of whom were retreated endoscopically. Two patients lost their larynx years after treatment through the laryngoscope. No patient died. No tracheostomies were required, and usually only 1 day of hospitalization was required.

PARTIAL LARYNGECTOMY FOR EARLY GLOTTIC CANCER

Some confusion exists concerning the partial operation options for early glottic cancers. For clarity, the following definitions will be used: laryngofissure-thyrotomy is the act of opening the larynx, usually in a vertical direction; cordectomy is the removal of a vocal cord and at times of appropriate adjacent subglottic and supraglottic tissue; and hemilaryngectomy is the removal of half of the larynx above the cricoid. Using these terms it should be apparent that a cordectomy can be accomplished through a laryngofissure or by means of a hemilaryngectomy. A hemilaryngectomy then is a more extensive operation than a cordectomy via a laryngofissure (thyrotomy). Cordectomies also can be accomplished through the mouth via appropriate laryngoscopy. Hemilaryngectomies can be vertical or horizontal operations. For glottic cancer, vertical operations are appropriate, and for supraglottic cancers, horizontal operations are needed. A laryngofissure is not a hemilaryngectomy.

In my practice, the basic open operations for early cordal cancers limited to a mobile vocal cord are the laryngofissure and the cordectomy. Although these operations were the first operations used for cancer of the larynx, they are not obsolete. They are options that are appropriate in properly selected patients. The proper lesion is the cancer localized to a mobile vocal cord. Likewise, either procedure is useful for those limited lesions that are suitable for endoscopic removal, but cannot be completely exposed. Different variations are described to manage anterior lesions that involve the anterior commissure and portion of the opposite cord. These variations are not different operations, but are simple technical adjustments to accommodate the cancer. In other words, the operations are flexible enough to be used for more than one situation. The key to selection is cordal mobility. If the involved cord or cords are mobile, removal through laryngofissure and its technical variation should be safe. The reason that cordal mobility is such an important concept is explained by the whole laryngeal section studies that explain cordal fixation by cancer. A cancer on a mobile cord simply cannot be too extensive because of subglottic, lateral, posterior, or superior spread to preclude removal through laryngofissure. Conversely, cords that are fixed or nearly fixed by cancer harbor cancers that have extended up, down, or out to a degree where removal at laryngofissure is not safe. The concept of cordal mobility as it relates to glottic cancer has stood the test of time and should not be ignored.[7]

The amount of tissue that can be removed at laryngofissure depends on the cancer. The amount of excision ranges from as little as the true cord back to the vocal process or as much as the true and false cords, 10 mm or more of subglottic mucosa to the top of the cricoid ring, and most of the arytenoid. The usual amount of excision for cordal cancer involves the cord plus half of the ventricle and a few millimeters of subglottic mucosa.

RECONSTRUCTION AFTER CORDECTOMY

After simple cordectomy via laryngofissure, no reconstruction is necessary. The raw area fills in and epithelializes, and follow-up is easier if there is nothing in the space left at cordectomy. The voice is altered. The degree of alteration varies from a breathy soft voice to a near normal voice. All of my patients do not demand an unaltered voice in the presence of cancer, and I continue to perform laryngofissure and cordectomy in 60 to 70 percent of my patients with early glottic cancer. This is so because those patients prefer the extirpative alternative when presented with the options in spite of voice alteration. In other words, I encourage patient participation in choice of therapy in situations in which options exist.

RESULTS OF LARYNGOFISSURE AND CORDECTOMY

My recent experience with laryngofissure and cordectomy was reported in 1980. Of 182 patients treated, seven had recurrences after treatment (four in the larynx and three in the neck after radiation failure). The mean hospital stay was 6 days. There were three deaths from cancer.[7]

HEMILARYNGECTOMY

A vertical hemilaryngectomy operation has very little to offer in the treatment of early cancer as just described. There is little oncologic benefit added by removal of the thyroid cartilage in patients with cancer on a mobile vocal cord. The hemilaryngectomy seems more appropriate for more advanced stages of glottic cancer in *carefully selected* situations.

A rare technical role for hemilaryngectomy for cancer on mobile cords is the situation in which mucosal spread extends posterior to the body of the arytenoid, that is, a few millimeters beyond the vocal process. By making the posterior vertical cuts through the thyroid cartilage prior to excision of the cancer and adjacent tissue, one causes the arytenoid to "pop" forward, flattening out the pyriform sinus and allowing a safer mucosal cut to be made behind the involved arytenoid.

The problem with the classic hemilaryngectomy for cancers on mobile cords is that it gives an extra margin of tissue laterally (the internal perichondrium and thyroid cartilage) at precisely the place (laterally) where it is least likely to be needed if selection is proper. Cancer simply cannot extend to the thyroid cartilage perichondrium if the cord is mobile. In other words, the removal of the thyroid cartilage is oncologically unnecessary and creates problems of voice and airway which are preventable by using the proper operation (laryngofissure and cordectomy).

EARLY SUPRAGLOTTIC CANCER

Early supraglottic cancer can be defined in the same way as early glottic cancer, that is, cancer that has not caused cordal fixation. Beyond this definition, the similarities between the two common cancers and the larynx end.

Early supraglottic cancer is a much different problem in several ways: (1) the diagnosis is more difficult; early glottic cancer changes the voice, but early supraglottic cancer is less obvious and may merely cause a vague throat discomfort or otalgia, symptoms common to many other less serious problems; (2) early supraglottic cancers metastasize to the cervical lymph nodes; a nodal metastasis manifested as a lump in the neck may be the first or only symptom; (3) supraglottic cancers can have metastasis early.

The third dimension is invisible so that what appears at indirect or direct laryngoscopy to be a relatively localized growth may not necessarily be so. The third dimension is anterior.

There exists in the epiglotic cartilage membranous foramina containing blood vessels and lymphatic vessels that provide a direct route for cancer to spread into the pre-epiglottic space. The pre-epiglottic space is that region anterior to the epiglottic cartilage between the hyoid bone above, thyroid ala below, and thyrohyoid membrane in front. This space can be filled with cancer that is not visible or palpable without cordal fixation. The significance of the pre-epiglottic space in supraglottic cancer as the invisible third dimension cannot be understated.[8]

There are four options to treat early supraglottic cancers: (1) supraglottic partial laryngectomy, (2) total laryngectomy and radiation therapy for cure, with surgery (usually laryngectomy) reserved for those tumors that cannot be controlled by the radiation (the radiate and watch concept), and (3) the near-total laryngectomy, an operation that can be sited between the supraglottic resection and the total laryngectomy.

Supraglottic partial laryngectomy is an oncologically valid approach to supraglottic cancers that have not extended to the glottic level. It is supported by results of whole-section studies. The recurrence rates are comparable to those after total laryngectomy, and the validity of the procedure has been time-tested.[9] The tissue bloc includes the hidden third dimension of the pre-epiglottic space. Voice quality is usually good after supraglottic resection. The operation seems to be ideal for supraglottic cancer. Unfortunately, not every patient can tolerate the procedure. Elderly, debilitated patients and patients with irreversible extensive chronic obstructive pulmonary disease, serious heart disease, and diabetes may be oncologically suitable for the operation, yet be physiologically incapable of recovering from the procedure. Then another alternative is appropriate.

The total laryngectomy is better tolerated by sick patients. The inherent separation of the respiratory system from the upper digestive system makes recovery more likely.

There appears to be a place for the so-called near-total laryngectomy as a compromise when the patient is oncologically suited for the supraglottic partial laryngectomy, but is physiologically incapable of tolerating it.

The compromise accepts a permanent tracheostomy, but keeps a small internal, lung-powered shunt between the pulmonary air source and the gullet for phonation. The precise place for this option is not a settled issue.[10]

The radiation option for early supraglottic cancer is controversial. No doubt some patients are cured and keep their larynx. The big problem is that unlike glottic cancer, for which staging can be precise, the anterior, invisible third dimension of the epiglottic cartilage, foramen, and pre-epiglottic space make staging less certain with supraglottic cancer. What appears to be a small early cancer at laryngoscopy may not be because the tumor has grown anteriorly. Cancer within the cartilage may be protected from otherwise lethal radiation.

Statistics have shown that patients with early supraglottic cancers do worse with radiation than patients with early glottic cancer. It becomes a philosophic issue as to the propriety of trying to save three, four, or five of 10 larynges by radiation with the realization that the other four, five, six or even seven people that do not get well must be treated again or will die.[11]

It might be more attractive to seriously endorse the radiate-and-watch concept if the salvage efforts could still be a supraglottic resection or even the near-total operation. Unfortunately, the reality of the problem in recurrence is difficult to detect in the radiated supraglottic cancer. There are clues, such as a swollen epiglottis and otalgia, but confirmation of residual disease deep to the epiglottis is not easy. In many cases, only when the cancer advances to fix the glottis by way of paraglottic space exterior is the recurrence confirmed, and then the cancer is no longer early. Also, supraglottic resection after radiation failure is never as safe as primary supraglottic resection.

Patients who accept the option of radiate-and-watch for supraglottic cancer in an effort to save their voices are substituting hope of an improbable event for reality. More larynges and perhaps more lives are lost than should be by this approach.

THE NECK AND EARLY LARYNX CANCER

With early glottic cancer, the concern about neck metastasis is small, and the need to treat the neck is infrequent. The few early glottic cancers that metastasize are probably best treated as the situation arises. The probability of neck metastasis for stage I and II glottic cancers is probably less than 10 percent, and so elective or "prophylactic" treatment to the neck is overkill.

In contrast, neck metastasis in early supraglottic cancer is real and is perhaps the major unresolved issue in the management of the disease. The problem is compounded because both sides of the neck are at risk.[9,11] Four possibilities are noted in patients with early supraglottic cancer: (1) both sides of the neck are clinically uninvolved by palpation, (2) one side of the neck has palpable nodes suspicious for metastatic cancer and the suspected neck disease is on the side of the supraglottic primary if there is a prominent side, (3) both sides of the neck have palpable nodes that are suspicious for cancer, and (4) the side opposite the primary lesion has a palpable node or has nodes that are suspect for cancer.

The scenarios determine the options. In scenario 1 the options are: (1) do nothing to either side of the neck, (2) do something to both sides of the neck, or (3) do something to one side of the neck (but which side?).

Elective therapy, whether radiation or neck dissection, delivered to the clinically negative neck that is also pathologically negative, is of no benefit. I do appreciate the information acquired from the specimen, consider it as a diagnostic staging test, and do not feel bad if the specimen is negative. Then I usually elect a neck dissection on one side when operating on supraglottic cancer. I ask the pathologist to screen the nodes when doing the supraglottic resection and then make a decision about the other side of the neck. If pathologic screening shows no metastasis, I stop. If screening is positive and the lesion is in the midline, I may perform a neck dissection on the opposite side. In most of the patients, the first side is negative for metastasis and nothing is done to the second side. (The issue of what kind of neck dissection is pertinent, but is a major controversy not appropriate to this chapter.)

REFERENCES

1. DeSanto LW, Devine KD, Lillie JC. Cancers of the larynx: glottic cancers. Surg Clin North Am 1977; 57:611–620.
2. DeSanto LW, Pearson BW. Initial treatment of laryngeal cancer: principles of selection. Minn Med 1981; 64:691–698.
3. Stutsman AC, McGavran MH. Ultraconservative management of superficially invasive epidermoid carcinoma of the true vocal cord. Ann Otol Rhinol Laryngol 1971; 80:507–512.
4. DeSanto LW. Selection of treatment for in situ and early invasive carcinoma of the glottis. Can J Otolaryngol 1974; 3:552–556.

5. Lillie JC, DeSanto LW. Transoral surgery of early cordal carcinoma. Trans Am Acad Ophthalmol Otolaryngol 1973; 77:192–196.
6. Miller D. Management of glottic carcinoma. Laryngoscope 1975; 85:1435–1439.
7. Neel HB, Devine KD, DeSanto LW. Laryngofissure and cordectomy for early cordal carcinoma: outcome in 1982 patients. Otolaryngol Head Neck Surg 1980; 88:79–84.

8. Coates HL, DeSanto LW, Devine KD, Elveback LR. Carcinoma of the supraglottic larynx: a review of 221 cases. Arch Otolaryngol 1976; 102:686–689.
9. McDonald TJ, DeSanto LW, Weiland LH. Supraglottic larynx and its pathology as studied by whole laryngeal sections. Laryngoscope 1976; 86:635–648.
10. Devine KD. Laryngectomy: vicissitudes in the development of a good operation. Arch Otolaryngol 1963; 78:816–825.

CONSERVATION SURGERY OF THE LARYNX

HUGH F. BILLER, M.D.

The term conservation surgery implies partial laryngectomy with preservation of the respiratory, protective, and phonatory functions of the larynx without sacrificing curability as compared to total laryngectomy.

The limits of tumor resection by partial laryngectomy require a knowledge of the biologic behavior of that particular tumor and the ability to reconstruct the larynx. The former determines the area to be resected. The reconstruction of the larynx remains the most difficult to accomplish, and most decisions for total laryngectomy are related to the inability to reconstruct the larynx. Since the ability to reconstruct continues to improve, the limitations of partial laryngectomy remain in a state of flux. As our reconstructive techniques become more sophisticated, the limits of partial laryngectomy will be extended.

GLOTTIC CANCERS

Tumors of the vocal cord that extend beyond the confines of the membranous cord to involve anterior commissure, subglottis, or arytenoid have the best chance of cure with surgery. These tumors are treated by the classic vertical partial laryngectomy (hemilaryngectomy).

Glottic tumors with fixation of the vocal cord respond poorly to radiotherapy and are best treated by surgery. The procedure utilized has been total laryngectomy. The classic vertical partial laryngectomy gives inadequate results. The hemilaryngectomy procedure does not allow for adequate margins subglottically. An oncologic partial procedure would require resection of the upper border of the cricoid cartilage. Adequate tumor control is obtained when this extended partial laryngectomy is performed. Reconstruction of the cricoid is mandatory if aspiration is to be avoided. The reconstruction is with the posterior border of the thyroid cartilage pedicled on the inferior constrictor muscle.[1] This technique allows for deglutition without aspiration at 2 weeks. Decannulation may require 2 to 3 months because of edema of the mucosal flap used to cover the cartilaginous graft.

SUPRAGLOTTIC CANCERS

Cancers involving the infrahyoid portion of the epiglottis rapidly invade the pre-epiglottic space and therefore respond poorly to radiotherapy as compared to surgery. Supraglottic tumors that remain superior to the anterior commissure rarely invade cartilage and are amenable to the classic horizontal partial laryngectomy (supraglottic resection). The rehabilitation is enhanced by the performance of a cricopharyngeal myotomy. Inability to decannulate is rare, and persistent aspiration is unusual. Perfect glottic closure is required for adequate rehabilitation of deglutition. This necessitates arytenoid replacement and midline cord fixation in cases of arytenoid removal. It also requires accurate postoperative evaluation and the institution of procedures to obtain glottic closure if postoperative glottic closure is absent.[2]

Select supraglottic tumors that extend inferiorly to cross the ventricle and involve the true vocal cord can also be treated by a partial laryngectomy. These tumors should not exhibit vocal cord fixation. The resection combines a hemilaryngectomy with a supraglottic resection (three-quarter partial laryngectomy). The larynx is reconstructed by utilizing the posterior portion of the thyroid cartilage pedicled on the inferior constrictor muscle.[3] This type of reconstruction results in glottic closure. Since the cartilage is covered by a pedicled mucosal flap, persistent edema and delay of decannulation for 3 to 4 months is common.

The performance of partial laryngectomy requires a thorough understanding of the anatomy and physiology of the larynx. As reconstruction methods improve, larger resections of the larynx will be possible. Theoretically, the only unit that is required to remain after partial laryngectomy is a singular mobile arytenoid. The extended resection would therefore include the epiglottis, both false cords, the entire thyroid cartilage, both vocal cords, one arytenoid, and one-half of the cricoid cartilage. A reconstructive procedure for this extended resection has not yet been devised, but there is no reason to suggest that a successful reconstructive procedure should not be anticipated in the future.

REFERENCES

1. Biller HF, Som ML. Vertical partial laryngectomy for glottic carcinoma with posterior subglottic extension. Ann Otol 1977; 86:715–721.

2. Biller HF, Lawson W, Sacks S. Correction of posterior glottic incompetence following horizontal partial laryngectomy. Ann Otol 1982; 91:448–449.
3. Biller HF, Lawson W. Partial laryngectomy for transglottic cancer. Ann Otoloaryngol Accepted for publication.

SURGICAL MANAGEMENT OF ADVANCED LARYNGEAL CANCER

BYRON J. BAILEY, M.D., F.A.C.S.
CHARLES M. STIERNBERG, M.D.

During the past two decades there has been a heightened interest in the surgical techniques employed in the management of advanced laryngeal cancer owing to (1) a better understanding of nodal metastases and their effect on prognosis, and (2) a greatly expanded armamentarium of reconstructive techniques after extensive neck surgery.

It is generally agreed that advanced laryngeal cancer includes stage III and stage IV carcinoma of the larynx. According to the *Manual for Staging of Cancer,* Second Edition, published by the American Joint Committee on Cancer in 1983, stage III carcinoma consists of any laryngeal lesion that is staged as T3 without nodal involvement (N) or distant metastasis (M) or any laryngeal lesion that is staged at T1, T2, or T3 with a single clinically positive homolateral node 3 cm or less in diameter and no distant metastasis. A lesion is classified as stage IV if the primary is a T4 with either N0 or N1 and M0; if the primary is any T with N2 or N3 and M0; or if the primary is any T1, the nodal involvement is any M1, and there is evidence of a distant metastasis.

The laryngeal primary assessment is defined in terms of the supraglottic, glottic, and subglottic regions, and the nodal involvement is characterized in terms of the number of nodes, size of nodes, and homolateral/contralateral/bilateral features that are clinically apparent preoperatively.

The specific requirements for staging are outlined in Tables 1, 2, and 3.[1]

The most frequent site of origin for carcinoma of the larynx is the vocal fold, and the most commonly encountered patient with advanced laryngeal carcinoma is a male smoker in his late 50s with a fixed vocal cord and a high probability of homolateral nodal involvement at the time he is first seen by the surgeon. The second most frequently encountered lesions is, in a similar patient, a translottic carcinoma (involving the vocal fold, ventricle, and true vocal fold), also with a high probability of homolateral nodal

TABLE 1 Classification of Primary Tumor (T)

Supraglottis

Tis	Carcinoma in situ
T1	Tumor confined to region of origin with normal mobility
T2	Tumor involving adjacent supraglottic site(s) or glottis without fixation
T3	Tumor limited to larynx with fixation or extension to involve postcricoid area, medial wall of pyriform sinus, or pre-epiglottic space
T4	Massive tumor extending beyond the larynx to involve oropharynx, soft tissues of neck, or destruction of thyroid cartilage

Glottis

Tis	Carcinoma in situ
T1	Tumor confined to vocal cord(s) with normal mobility (includes involvement of anterior or posterior commissures)
T2	Supraglottic or subglottic extension of tumor with normal or impaired cord mobility, or both
T3	Tumor confined to the larynx with cord fixation
T4	Massive tumor with thyroid cartilage destruction or extension beyond the confines of the larynx, or both

Subglottis

Tis	Carcinoma in situ
T1	Tumor confined to the subglottic region
T2	Tumor extension to vocal cords with normal or impaired cord mobility
T3	Tumor confined to larynx with cord fixation
T4	Massive tumor with cartilage destruction or extension beyond the confines of the larynx, or both

TABLE 2 Classification of Nodal Involvement (N)

NX	Minimum requirements to assess the regional node cannot be met
N0	No clinically positive node
N1	Single clinically positive homolateral node 3 cm or less in diameter
N2	Single clinically positive homolateral node more than 3 cm but not more than 6 cm in diameter or multiple clinically positive homolateal nodes, none more than 6 cm in diameter
N2A	Single clinically positive homolateal node more than 3 cm but not more than 6 cm in diameter
N2b	Multiple clinically positive homolateral nodes, none more than 6 cm in diameter
N3	Massive homolateral node(s), bilateral nodes, or contralateral node(s)
N3a	Clinically positive homolateral node(s), one more than 6 cm in diameter
N3b	Bilateral clinically positive nodes (in this situation, each side of the neck should be staged separately, i.e., N3b: right, N2a: left, N1)
N3c	Contralateral clinically positive node(s) only

TABLE 3   Stage Grouping

Stage I	T1, N0, M0
Stage II	T2, N0, M0
State III	T3, N0, M0
	T1 or T2 or T3, N1, M0
Stage IV	T4, N0 or N1, M0
	Any T, N2 or N3, M0
	Any T, any N, M1

involvement. In rare instances, conservation procedures can be employed for superficial transglottic lesions, but these lesions usually require aggressive management with either preoperative or postoerative radiation therapy in combination with total laryngectomy and neck dissection. As a generalization, it appears that there has been sufficient documentation of the equivalence of preoperative and postoperative radiation therapy from a therapeutic perspective, and there appears to be a worthwhile reduction in postoperative complications when postoperative radiation therapy is selected. The promise of the additional modality of chemotherapy, given either preoperatively or immediately postoperatively, awaits further scientific clarification by means of controlled prospective randomized clinical trials. Recently there has been a resurgence of activity in regard to the clinical application of immunologic therpy. Theoretically, immunologic therapy holds the greatest hope for the future, but its current practical role in the management of advanced laryngeal cancer has yet to be demonstrated.

The work of McGavran et al was extremely important in providing histopathologic correlates for the treatment of advanced laryngeal cancer. They expanded the scientific base of the early 1960s by utilizing precise pathologic techniques to illuminate our understanding of supraglottic, glottic, and transglottic carcinoma.[2] Their investigations revealed the high incidence of occult cervical node metastasis associated with advanced glottic and supraglottic carcinoma, and form the basis for much of our current practice of anticipating nodal involvement with these "high risk" primary lesions, even in the absence of palpable nodal metastasis. Our understanding of the natural history of laryngeal carcinoma and much of our rationale for selection of the most appropriate therapy are based on information gained by serial section of total laryngectomy specimens. This work was pioneered by LeRoux-Robert of France in the 1930s,[3] was introduced into this country by Tucker in the 1960s,[4] and was expanded significantly by Kirchner during the past decade.[5] From these studies, we have learned a great deal about the potential pitfalls of the surgical approach, we have modified various operative procedures, and we have increased our understanding of where to look for possible direct local spread and when to employ adjuvant therapeutic modalities. In brief, we have learned to manage advanced laryngeal cancer

on the basis of anticipation of aggressive tumor spread and have come to regard the intralaryngeal primary as only the "tip of the iceberg".

Patients with advanced glottic/supraglottic/transglottic carcinoma are very likely to develop cervical nodal metastasis. McGavran et al noted the presence of cervical node involvement in 13 of 25 patients with transglottic carcinoma, but even more significantly, almost one-third of the patients with clinically negative necks were found to have positive nodes when elective neck dissection was performed.[2] Additionally, he noted a rather high incidence of contralateral nodal metastasis in patients with advanced supraglottic and transglottic carcinoma. Later studies by Krischner confirmed these observations in a series of patients with advanced transglottic carcinoma.[5] In a related study of 500 patients with cancer of the larynx and pyriform sinus, Kirchner and Owens noted only a 20 percent incidence of palpable cervical lymph node involvement in patients with transglottic carcinoma, but there was a 46 percent incidence of occult cervical nodes in a group of 26 patients who underwent elective neck dissection.[6]

The incidence of delayed contralateral nodal metastasis from advanced laryngeal cancer was also studied by Biller et al, who noted that 21 of 67 ptients (31%) with transglottic carcinoma developed ipsilateral nodal metastasis and 4 of 67 patients (6%) developed contralateral nodal involvement.[7] The frequency of contralateral spread is increased by the discovery of either palpable or occult homolateral nodal involvement, and contralateral nodes are found even more frequently in patients with supraglottic carcinoma.

PREOPERATIVE ASSESSMENT

History and Physical Examination. Precision and thoroughness in the preoperative assessment of each patient is the first step toward successful management in the case of advanced laryngeal cancer, as it is in so many other fields of medicine. The most common chief complaint of patients in this category is hoarseness of several months' duration. If the lesion is extensive and bulky, dyspnea and shortness of breath on exertion are usually reported by the patient. When the true vocal cord is fixed or when there is extensive fixation and ulceration of the epiglottis, aspiration and dysphagia are sometimes the major complaints. Dysphagia and odynophagia are also associated with advanced laryngeal cancer that has spread to involve the base of the tongue or the pharynx.

Referred pain to the ear, tongue, or angle of the mandible is a particularly ominous sign. Referred otalgia is often associated with advanced laryngeal carcinoma, and it is probably secondary to invasion or distortion of the sensory fibers or the vagus nerve as proposed by Pittman and Carter.[8] They observed that referred otalgia correlated with tumor invasion of the cartilaginous laryngeal framework in 11 of 12 patients in their particular series. Transglottic carcinoma was more commonly associated with referred otalgia than all of the other varieities of advanced laryngeal cancer combined. A thorough physical examination is of the greatest importance, not only because of the need for information regarding the suspected laryngeal carcinoma, but also because of the very high incidence of associated malignant disease in other locations and other serious medical conditions. Indirect laryngoscopy is the keystone of the physical examination, and mastery of all of the refinements and nuances of this technique is a fundamental requirement for the laryngeal surgeon, who must document the precise extent of the lesion and degree of cord mobility at this first step. Palpation of the oral cavity, tongue base, and neck must be done carefully and repeatedly until the examiner is convinced of the correctness of the assessment.

At this point, a careful drawing is made of the lesion and a written statement of the staging is entered into the patient's medical record.

Radiographic Assessment. There is considerable diversity of opinion regarding the value of preoperative radiographic techniques, and different surgeons stress the value of information they feel can be derived from each of many studies. The techniques that are available range from the simple to the sophisticated and from the inexpensive to the expensive.

A soft tissue radiograph of the neck may help to outline the extent of a supraglottic carcinoma. Conventional tomography while the paient is voicing an inspiratory "E" may give valuable information regarding the presence or absence of tumor in the laryngeal ventricle. This same study is also helpful in assessing the degree of infraglottic extension of tumor or obilteration of one pyriform sinus region. The CT scan provides information regarding both the surface spread and the deep infiltration of carcinoma and has recently been popularized as the ideal technique for assessing the degree of invasion of the laryngeal cartilaginous framework.

Endoscopic Assessment. The final step in the preoperative assessment of each patient is the endoscopic examination of the upper aerodigestive tract. Direct laryngoscopy provides the most valuable information and the most precise determination of the superficial and deep extent of the primary lesion. In addition to the biopsies of the obvious primary, it is important to sample any other mucosal areas adjacent to the larynx that show any sign of change from a normal appearance. The base of the tongue, pyriform sinus, or cervical esophagus may show areas of severe dysplasia, carcinoma in situ, or microinvasive carcinoma that will alter the overall treatment plan.

We perform bronchoscopy and esophagoscopy at the same time that the direct laryngoscopic examination is done. Although some have criticized this practice as being difficult to defend on the basis of a low yield of other important information, we believe that there is not enough information at present to be certain of the best plan of action. It is our position that even if important additional information is gained from bronchoscopy and esophagoscopy in only 5 to 10 percent of patients, this yield is sufficient to continue the practice until it has truly been shown to be "unnecessary".

Direct laryngoscopy provides important information concerning the spread of tumor into regions that cannot be visualized by the indirect examination. The laryngeal ventricles and the infraglottic regions can be visualized by manipulating the tip of the anterior commissure laryngoscope carefully around the obstructing tumor and normal anatomic structures. It is important to keep in mind that bulky lesions, particularly transglottic tumors, increase the difficulty of direct laryngoscopy and frequently result in diagnostic errors. Pillsbury reported a 50 percent error in the staging of 114 laryngeal cancer specimens that were serially sectioned.[9] Understaging can lead to undertreatment, and this in turn may result in a lower cure rate than could have been achieved.

SURGICAL MANAGEMENT

Advanced laryngeal cancer that appears to be limited to the larynx itself, with or without cervical nodal involvement, is usually treated by performing total laryngectomy and neck dissection.

However, this chapter would be incomplete without a brief comment concerning the reports of successful management of T3 glottic carcinoma when extended frontolateral vertical partial laryngectomy is performed. It appears that a selected subset of patients with T3 glottic carcinoma can be managed almost as effectively by partial laryngectomy (with the associated preservation of laryngeal function) as by total laryngectomy, and with better survival rates than can be achieved using radiation therapy. The four leading proponents of this approach have reported the following survival rates in patients with T3 glottic carcinoma who were treated by extended frontolateral vertical partial laryngectomy: (1) Som—15/26 (58%) at 3-years follow-up;[10] (2) Skolnik—2/5 (40%) at 5-year follow-up;[11] (3) LeRoux-Robert—55/95 (58%) at 5-year follow-up;[12] and (4) Lesinski—12/18 (67%) at 5-year follow-up.[13]

It must be emphasized that these results were obtained in the hands of very experienced surgical innovators who have stressed a variety of modifications from standard partial laryngectomy techniques. It is also important to note that when conservation surgical procedures are pushed to their limits, one may expect a higher incidence of complications such as stenosis, aspiration, and tumor recurrence. It is fair to say that this topic remains controversial and unresolved at this time. We hope that future reports will provide even more information regarding the role of conservation surgery in these patients.

Extended supraglottic subtotal laryngectomy has also been recommended for T3 and T4 supraglottic carcinoma. Ogura et al report survival in seven of 10 patients with T3N0 supraglottic carcinoma and two of three patients with T3, N1–3 supraglottic carcinoma.[14] The results with selected T4 lesions were even better in that survival was noted in nine of 12 patients (75%) with T4N0 supraglottic carcinoma and in eight of 13 patients (73%) with T4N1–3 supraglottic carcinoma. These observations are confirmed by comparable reports by Bocca[15] and Som.[16] Again, great emphasis must be placed on the caveats regarding the extensive experience of these surgeons and the highly selected patient subpopulation that was chosen for management by subtotal supraglottic partial laryngectomy.

Another recent development that deserves mention here is the concept of "near-total laryngectomy" that has been investigated by Pearson.[17] Advanced laryngeal carcinoma can be managed by surgical resection of most of the larynx with preservation of sufficient tissue to permit the reconstruction of a "voice" shunt. The patient requires a tracheostomy for respiratory function, but is able to phonate without the need for a prosthesis and without postoperative aspiration.

At the University of Texas Medical Branch in Galveston, we have observed that most patients with advanced laryngeal cancer require total laryngectomy and neck dissection for surgical management. In many cases it is possible to spare the spinal accessory nerve without compromising the patient's chances for survival. This surgical procedure is almost always associated with postoperative radiation therapy.

TOTAL LARYNGECTOMY AND NECK DISSECTION

The first total laryngectomy reported to have been performed successfully for cancer was accomplished in 1873 by Theodor Billroth.[18] The procedure was very slow to gain widespread usage until refinements were added by other surgeons. Patients with advanced laryngeal cancer who were fortunate enough to survive the dangerous postoperative recovery period often succumbed to residual disease in the cervical lymph nodes.

A major advance in regard to the control of involved cervical nodes came with the publication of Crile's landmark article concerning "neck dissection".[19] This provided a standardized, systematic approach to the removal of metastatic carcinoma from the larynx and other head and neck primary sites.

Surgical Technique

A detailed description of the technique of total laryngectomy and neck dissection is beyond the scope of this chapter. However, a brief summary of this procedure is provided along with some references for those who wish to read further on the topic. The skin incision of preference is a low apron flap with the tracheostoma incorporated in the midline of the incision. If there has been previous irradiation of the neck, a

McFee incision is employed.[20] The skin flaps are elevated by means of a thermal knife, which serves to reduce blood loss during this stage of the operation.[21]

After the flaps have been elevated, the neck dissection is begun inferiorly and continued upward to the level of the larynx. The posterior region is developed along the anterior border of the trapezius muscle, and in many instances, it is possible to spare the spinal accessory nerve as this dissection is extended. The superior resection line is developed from the mastoid tip along the inferior margin of the mandible until the next specimen has been freed except for its attachment in the region in the larynx.

The laryngectomy portion is initiated with transection of the strap muscles just superior to the sternum. The ipsilateral lobe of the thyroid gland and the isthmus are left attached to the specimen in the case of a laterally-situated primary lesion.

An incision is made just superior to the hyoid bone, and the epiglottis is exposed and retracted forward to permit inspection of the upper portion of the endolarynx. With the primary lesion in view, the pharynx is exposed along the less involved side, and the decision is made regarding the level of tracheal transection as the larynx is dissected free.

Frozen section margins are obtained from all appropriate sites, and when reassurance of adequate clearance has been received, the pharynx is closed, a dermal graft is applied to protect the carotid, and the final closure of the skin flaps and fashioning of the tracheostoma is completed.

Treatment Results

Variability in the reporting of surgical management of carcinoma of the larynx is an obstacle to the comparison of one patient series with another. Unfortunately, many authors report their findings on the basis of the T stage only, whereas others include the N stage information as well. The duration of follow-up has varied from as short as 2 years to a more proper follow-up of 5 years. Changes in the staging systems over the last two decades have also introduced some problems with interpretation. The most fundamental problem encountered in the assessment of postoperative results is the retrospective, rather than the prospective, nature of the design and reporting of these series.

In spite of these problems, it is possible to draw valuable trend information from most of the published reports.

Advanced Supraglottic Carcinoma. Review of the literature indicates that advanced carcinoma of the supraglottic larynx is currently being treated by surgery alone with a success rate that ranges from 45 percent[22] to 69 percent[23] for stage III carcinoma and T3 primary tumors and from 35 percent[24] to 56 percent[25] for patients with stage IV disease and T4 primary tumors. The reports include primarily data based on the experience of surgeons employing total laryngectomy and neck dissection. This compares with treatment success rates in a similar population managed with radiation therapy for stage III disease and T3 primaries with survival from 21 percent[26] to 36 percent[22] after 5 years.

Surgery combined with radiation therapy accounts for the highest reported survival in patients with advanced supraglottic carcinoma. Wang reports 3-year survival of 24/28 patients (86%) with T3N0 and 7/22 patients (32%) with T3N1–3 supraglottic carcinoma.[27] His success with T4 lesions, with or without nodal involvement, ranges from 32 to 36 percent when combined surgery and radiation therapy are utilized. Goldman and Roffman have also shown that higher survival rates can be achieved utilizing combined preoperative radiation and surgery for advanced cancer of the larynx and laryngopharynx, including supraglottic carcinoma.[28] Other reports of interest to those seeking more information on this topic include the publications by Hendricksen,[29] Ogura et al,[30] and MacComb and Fletcher.[31] Some of the highlights of this information are summarized in Table 4.

A similar comparison of the results of these different treatment modalities in patients with advanced carcinoma of the glottic larynx is shown in Table 5. The management of T3 primary lesions of the glottic larynx by surgery alone results in 5-year survival with no evidence of disease in 56 percent[36] to 85 percent[13] of the patients treated. The range for T4 primary lesions of the glottis is from 26 percent[36] to 54 percent.[38] The surgical management of stage III disease of the glottic larynx is successful in 40 percent[11] to 90 percent[41] of the patients reported. Stage IV disease of the glottic larynx is generally associated with a very low degree of curability, as reflected in the absence of any survivors in the only series reporting their experience with this group.[39] Overall, it appears that surgery alone is successful in controlling advanced carcinoma of the glottic larynx in about 60 percent of the patients treated in this manner.

Radiation therapy is reported to be effective in obtaining 5-year survival with no evidence of disease in approximately 37 percent[33] to 60 percent[29] of the patients with T3 primary lesions at the glottic level.

TABLE 4 Comparison of Treatment Modalities in Advance Carcinoma of the Supraglottic Larynx

	T3	T4	Stage III	Stage IV
Surgery 55%	45%	56%[22]	51%[32]	
	53%	52%[25]	69%	50%[23]
	57%	35%[24]		
	68%[23]			
Radiation Therapy 30%	21%	23%[26]	35%	10%[35]
	26%[33]			
	27%	47%[34]		
	36%	14%[22]		
Combined radiotherapy and surgery	63%	33%[27]		

TABLE 5 Comparision of Treatment Modalities in Advanced Carcinoma of the Glottic Larynx

	T3	T4	Stage III	Stage IV
Surgery	56%	26%[36]	40–50%[11]	
	58%[37]		50%	0%[39]
	61%	32%[22]	62%[40]	
	72%	38%[25]	68–90%[41]	
	85%[13]	54%[38]		
	37%[33]			
Radiation therapy 50%	41%	25%[42]		
	55%	8%[22]		
	57%	30%[43]		
	60%	28%[29]		
Combined radiotherapy and surgery 65%	58–90%	66–74%[28]		
	62%[44]			

The 5-year survival of patients with T4 lesions of the glottis ranges from approximately 8 percent[22] to 30 percent.[43]

The use of combined radiotherapy in surgery for T3 and T4 glottic primary lesions of the larynx has produced 5-year survival ranging from 58 percent to 90 percent.[28] In other words, it appears that approximately 65 percent of the patients with advanced glottic cancer who are treated by combined modalities and observed for five years will remain free of cancer.

Carcinoma of the Subglottic Region. Carcinoma of the subglottic region occurs much less commonly than does laryngeal cancer arising at other sites, according to Sessions.[45] Carcinoma that originates from a point more than 5 mm below the free margin of the true vocal cord is classified as a primary subglottic tumor. More commonly, tumors originate at the glottic level and extend into the subglottic region in which case they are designated as secondary subglottic tumors. Primary subglottic carcinoma is particularly dangerous in view of the absence of early symptoms, but fortunately it is quite rare. Secondary subglottic carcinoma is observed as a condition associated with approximately one of every five patients with glottic carcinoma.

The treatment of subglottic carcinoma consists primarily of wide, total laryngectomy and ipsilateral neck dissection in most cases. The ipsilateral lobe and isthmus of the thyroid gland are included with the specimen, and a careful dissection of paratracheal nodes is recommended. Local recurrence due to inadequate excision is a major cause of management failure in this patient group. The trachea is transected at a point that is as low as possible without the need for resecting a portion of the manubrium sterni. Postoperative radiation therapy is advised by most who have experience with the management of this problem.

In a small number of highly selected patients with subglottic extension of a glottic carcinoma, a vertical subtotal laryngectomy is possible. These patients are characterized by a very superficial lesion and excellent cord mobility. Conservatism is advised in the selection of patients with subglottic carcinoma who are treated by subtotal laryngectomy procedures.

Treatment results in cases of subglottic carcinoma are related to the aggressiveness of therapy and the extent of subglottic invasion by the tumor. Sessions reports that patients with stage II and stage III lesions who have subglottic extension of more than 10 mm have survival rates in the range of 50 to 73 percent when they are treated by surgery plus radiation therapy. Patients with tumor extension in excess of 26 mm have been observed to have a recurrence rate of 92 percent regardless of the treatment modality. These results emphasize the treacherous nature of subglottic carcinoma and the necessity for careful follow-up of these patients.

Laryngopharyngeal Carcinoma. Advanced laryngeal carcinoma in which the primary tumor either arises or extends outside the larynx poses a separate and more challenging set of problems. These laryngeal lesions, which involve the vallecula, base of the tongue, pyriform sinus, and postcricoid region, are associated with a different set of symptoms, a typically prolonged interval prior to diagnosis, and a lower degree of curability.

The concept that a few of these patients might be managed by conservation surgery was introduced by Alonso from Uruguay.[46] Later, Ogura popularized these concepts by demonstrating the validity of conservation surgery as a sound oncologic approach and further refined the techniques into a more standard and reliable one-stage procedure.[47] It is in the area of reconstruction of patients who have undergone removal of laryngopharyngeal tumors that the surgeon is pressed to the limit to achieve adequate postoperative rehabilitation of speech, respiration, and deglutition while adhering to safe principles of adequate tumor excision.

PARTIAL LARYNGOPHARYNGECTOMY PROCEDURE

Muntz and Sessions have described the general indications for partial laryngopharyngectomy as the following: (1) the contralateral vocal cord must be tumor free and mobile, (2) the ipsilateral arytenoid may be involved, (3) the ipsilateral vocal cord should be mobile but may be superficially involved, (4) the apex of the pyriform sinus, the cricopharyngeus sphincter, and the postcricoid area must be tumor-free, and (5) there must be no thyroid cartilage invasion by tumor.[48]

These authors recommend neck dissection for all patients who satisfy the foregoing criteria. The technique of partial laryngopharyngectomy, including the details of various reconstructive options, is beyond the scope of this chapter, but as a general statement, it is noted that with careful patient selection, results equivalent to those of total laryngopharyngectomy can be achieved with preservation of important physiologic functions.

TOTAL LARYNGOPHARYNGECTOMY

In the presence of more advanced laryngopharyngeal tumors, total laryngopharyngectomy is required. This involves removing all of the larynx and either part or all of the pharynx in order to adequately excise the region of cancer involvement. Patients who present with laryngopharyngeal carcinoma require total laryngectomy when it has been determined that there is tumor involvement of the thyroid cartilage, the postcricoid area, the pyriform apex, or the cricopharyngeus sphincter, or when there is vocal cord fixation. The extent of the pharyngeal resection is modified according to the region involved and the size of the primary tumor. In most cases, it is possible to preserve sufficient local tissue to accomplish a primary closure. For patients with very extensive lesions, it is necessary to perform reconstruction using such options as a deltopectoral flap, a pectoralis major myocutaneous flap, or a gastric transposition. In the case of a postcricoid cancer, the option exists to employ a laryngotracheal autograft in which the anterior, uninvolved portion of the larynx is preserved and utilized to reconstruct the anterior pharyngeal defect.

The results of therapy provided to patients with laryngopharyngeal cancer correlates closely with the site and extent of the primary tumor and the incidence of cervical lymph node involvement. For example, small (T1 or T2) tumors involving the pyriform sinus and larynx can be managed with a 3-year survival rate of approximately 50 percent, and treatment of larger tumor (T3 or T4) of the pyriform sinus region provides a 3-year survival in the range of 16 to 40 percent. The presence of lymph node metastasis decreases the survival by one-third to one-half.

It has been demonstrated that partial laryngopharyngectomy provides survival rates that are as high as those following total laryngopharyngectomy when the patient population is carefully selected. PLP controls for local recurrence as well as TLP when the aforementioned indications are followed. When the tumor is larger or other unfavorable conditions are present, the failure rate locally, in the neck, and at distant sites is increased.

It has been noted by Inoue[49] and by Jesse[50] that the combination of adequate surgery and radiation therapy increases the survival beyond the capability of either modality when it is used alone. The major impact of combination therapy is seen in the reduction of local and cervical node recurrence of carcinoma.

REFERENCES

1. American Joint Committee on Cancer: Manual for Staging of Cancer. 2nd ed. Beahrs H, Myers MH, eds. Philadelphia: JB Lipincott Company, 1983.
2. McGavran MH, et al. The incidence of cervical lymph node metastases from epidermoid carcinoma of the larynx and their relationship to certain characteristics of the primary tumor. Cancer 1961; 14:55–66.
3. LeRoux-Robert J. Les epitheliomes intra-larynges. Thesis,

Gaston Doin and Cie, Paris, 1936.

4. Tucker GF Jr. A histological method for the study of spread of carcinoma within the larynx. Ann Otol Rhinol Laryngol 1961; 70:910–915.

5. Kirchner JA, Cornog JL, Holmes RE. Transglottic carcinoma—its growth and spread within the larynx. Arch Otol 1974; 99:247–251.

6. Kirchner JA, Owen JR. Five hundred cancers of the larynx and pyriform sinus—results of treatment by radiation and surgery. Laryngoscope 1977; 87:1288–1303.

7. Biller HF, Davis WH, Ogura JH. Delayed contralateral cervical metastases with laryngeal and laryngopharyngeal cancers. Laryngoscope 1971; 81:1499–1502.

8. Pittman MR, Carter RL. Framework invasion by laryngeal carcinomas. Head Neck Surg 1982; 4:200–208.

9. Pillsbury HRC, Krichner JA. Clinical versus histopathologic staging in laryngeal cancer. Arch Otol 1979; 105:157–159.

10. Som ML. Cordal cancer with extension to vocal process. Laryngoscope 1975; 85:1298–1307.

11. Skolnik EM, Yee KF, Wheatley MA, et al. Carcinoma of the laryngeal glottis: therapy and end results. Laryngoscope 1975; 85:1453–1466.

12. LeRoux-Robert J. A statistical study of 620 laryngeal carcinomas of the glottic region personally operated upon more than five years ago. Laryngoscope 1975; 85:1440–1452.

13. Lesinski SG, Bauer WC, Ogura JH. Hemilaryngectomy for T3 (fixed cord) epidermoid carcinoma of the larynx. Laryngoscope 1976; 86:1563–1571.

14. Ogura JH, Sessions DG, Spector GJ. Conservation surgery for epidermoid carcinoma of the supraglottic larynx. Laryngoscope 1975; 85:1808–1815.

15. Bocca E. Supraglottic cancer. Laryngoscope 1975; 84:1318.

16. Som ML. Conservation Surgery for carcinoma of the supraglottis. J Laryngol Otol 1970; 84:655–678.

17. Pearson BW. Subtotal laryngectomy. Laryngoscope 1981; 91:1904–1911.

18. Billroth T, Gussenbauer C. Ulber die erste durch T Billroth am Menschen ausgefuhrte Kehldopf-Extirpation und die Auswendig einges Kunstlichen Kehlkopfes. Arch Klin Chir 1874; 17:343–354.

19. Crile G. Excision of cancer of the head and neck with special reference to the plan of dissection based on 132 operations. JAMA 1906; 47:1780–1786.

20. MacFee W. Transverse incisions for neck dissections. Ann Surg 1960; 151:279–284.

21. Fee WE. Use of the Shaw scalpel in head and neck surgery. Otolaryngol Head Neck Surg 1981; 89:515–519.

22. Vermund H. Role of radiotherapy in cancer of the larynx as related to the TNM system of staging. Cancer 1977; 25:485–504.

23. Ogura JH, et al. Conservation surgery for epidermoid carcinoma of the supraglottic larynx. Laryngoscope 1975; 85:1808–1815.

24. Fletcher GH, et al. The place of radiotherapy in the management of the squamous cell carcinoma of the supraglottic larynx. Am J Roentgenol 1970; 108:19–26.

25. Alajmo E, et al. Five-year results of 1000 patients operated on for cancer of the larynx. Acta Otolaryngol 1976; 82:437–439.

26. Wang CC. Magavoltage radiation therapy for supraglottic carcinoma. Radiology 1973; 109:183–186.

27. Wang CC, Schulz MD, Miller D. Combined radiation therapy and surgery for carcinoma of the supraglottis and pyriform sinus. Laryngoscope 1972; 82:1883.

28. Goldman JL, Roffman JD. Combined preoperative irradiation and surgery for advanced cancer of the larynx and laryngopharynx. Canad J Otolaryngol 1975; 4:251–264.

29. Hendrickson FR, Kline TC, Hibbs GG. Primary squamous cell carcinoma of the larynx. Laryngoscope 1975; 85:1650–1666.

30. Ogura JH, Sessions DC, Spector GJ. Conservative surgery for epidermoid carcinoma of the supraglottic larynx. Laryngoscope 1975; 85:1808–1815.

31. MacCombs WS, Fletcher GH. Cancer of the Head and Neck. Baltimore: Williams & Wilkins, 1967.

32. Coates HL, et al. Carcinoma of the supraglottic larynx: a review of 221 cases. Arch Otolaryngol 1976; 102:686–689.

33. Jankovic I, Merkas Z. Radiotherapy as the Primary Approach in the Treatment of Laryngeal Cancer. Workshop 15. New York: Appleton-Century-Crofts, 1976; 881–888.

34. Henry J, et al. Radiotherapy in the treatment of T3-T4 supraglottic tumors. Laryngoscope 1975; 85:1682–1688.

35. Hansen HS. Supraglottic carcinoma of the aryepiglottic fold. Laryngoscope 1975; 85:1667–1681.

36. LeRoux-Robert J. Panel discussion on glottic tumors. IV. A statistical study of 620 laryngeal carcinomas of the glottic region personally operated upon more than five years ago. Laryngoscope 1975; 85:1440–1452.

37. Som ML. Cordal cancer with extension to vocal process. Laryngoscope 1975; 85:1298–1307.

38. Jesse RH. Panel discussion on glottic tumors. I. The evaluation of treatment of patients with extensive squamous cancer of the vocal cords. Laryngoscope 1975; 85:1424–1429.

39. Daley CJ, Strong EW. Carcinoma of the glottic larynx. Am J Surg 1975; 130:489–492.

40. Sessions DG, et al. The anterior commissure in glottic carcinoma. Laryngoscope 1975; 85:1624–1632.

41. Ogura JH, et al. Analysis of surgical therapy for epidermoid carcinoma of the laryngeal glottis. Laryngoscope 1975; 85:1522–1530.

42. Hawkins NV. Panel discussion on glottic tumors. VIII. The treatment of glottic carcinoma: an analysis of 800 cases. Laryngoscope 1975; 85:1485–1493.

43. Stewart JG, et al. Panel discussion on glottic tumors. VII. The management of glottic carcinoma by primary irradiation with surgery in reserve. Laryngoscope 1975; 85:1477–1484.

44. Constable WC, et al. Panel discussions on glottic tumors. IX. Radiotherapeutic management of cancer of the glottis. Univ Virginia 1956–1971. Laryngoscope 1975; 85:1494–1503.

45. Sessions DG, Ogura JH, Fried MP. Carcinoma of the subglottic area. Laryngoscope 1975; 85:1417–1423.

46. Alonso JM. Conservative surgery of cancer of the larynx. Trans Am Acad Ophthalmol Otolaryngol 1947; 51:633–642.

47. Ogura JH, et al. Conservation surgery for epidermoid carcinoma of the supraglottic larynx. Laryngoscope 1975; 85:1808–1815.

48. Muntz H, Sessions DG. Surgery of the laryngopharyngeal and subglottic cancer. In: Bailey BJ, ed. Surgery of the Larynx. Philadelpha: WB Saunders, 1985:293–316.

49. Inoue T, et al. Treatment of carcinoma of the hypopharynx. Cancer. 1973; 31:649–655.

50. Jesse RH, et al. The efficacy of combining radiation therapy with a surgical procedure in patients with cervical metastasis from squamous cancer of the oropharynx and hypopharynx. Cancer 1975; 35:1163–1166.

18. Management of Salivary Gland Tumors

INTRODUCTION

JOHN CONLEY, M.D.

Although many problems remain to be solved regarding tumors of the salivary glands, we have made significant advances in the understanding of their biologic behavior and management. The overall concepts are understandably still evolving.

In the incipient stages of the work there were three major deterrents to the management of these tumors. Specifically, there was no well-accepted histopathologic classification, there was no organized position regarding the best type of treatment, and there was a prohibitive fear regarding what to do with the facial nerve. These problems have been clarified by an interdisciplinary thrust incorporating pathologists, roentgenologists, and clinicians. Their efforts have been greatly aided by the introduction of new discoveries in medical science and advanced technology.

The chapters that follow are written by Peter Som, roentgenologist, Robert Fechner, pathologist, Roger Boles, otolaryngologist-head and neck surgeon, and Ronald Spiro, head and neck surgeon. They are all experts in their particular fields and their presentations elucidate the problems, the pitfalls, the advances, and the suggestions for management in each of their specialties.

In his chapter, Som discusses the roentgenographic diagnosis, the new advances in CT scanning, the use of isotopes, and sialography, and projects all of this imaging into the possible advances in the immediate future.

Fechner presents a workable histologic classification of salivary gland tumors and its application to the clinical management. He evaluates pleomorphism, aspiration biopsy, frozen section, and formal incisional biopsy. He also touches on the vagaries of certain specific salivary gland tumors, such as adenoid cystic carcinoma.

Spiro s chapter deals with tumors of the parotid gland, beginning with the basic aspects involved with diagnosis and treatment in the lateral lobe, the isthmus, and the deep lobe, modulating this according to the size of the tumor and the histopathology. The author also makes a statement concerning the complementary use of irradiation, discusses the critical criteria that relate specifically to prognosis, and describes some of the techniques used in reconstruction of this area by facial nerve grafts and regional flaps.

Boles discusses the diagnosis and treatment of submandibular and minor salivary gland tumors. This is a rather broad field, but an exceptionally interesting one as far as the histopathology, regional anatomy, clinical behavior, prognosis, and varieties of management are concerned. In his chapter, Boles emphasizes new trends in the criteria for conservative surgery and takes a position on the use of postoperative radiotherapy.

IMAGING OF SALIVARY GLAND TUMORS

PETER M. SOM, M.D.

The preoperative evaluation of salivary gland tumors is a great challenge to both the clinician and the radiologist. If sufficient tumor mapping can be provided, the surgeon can make the most informed decision as to the best operative approach, if the patient is an operable candidate. Accurate tumor mapping is also necessary if optimal radiation fields are to be planned.

The development and refinement of CT scanning have allowed significant progress to be made in this

area, so that angiography and sialography, which were the main diagnostic radiologic procedures in the pre-CT era, are no longer employed diagnostically. The use of contrast-enhanced CT scanning and Dynamic Scanning has obviated the need for diagnostic angiograms.[1] If the lesion is vascular by CT evaluation, then a therapeutic angiogram can be performed for definitive or preoperative embolization. Similarly, the high resolution scanners of today have eliminated the need for sialography. Only in rare cases, where the parotid gland tissue is very dense on CT, so that a small mass may not be easily identified within its margins, is sialography employed with the CT study.

Although contrast sialographic criteria are well established to make a diagnosis of an aggressive parotid or submandibular malignancy, this procedure gives no information about tumor spread outside of the gland capsule. This mapping is routinely seen on CT, and in the appropriate clinical setting, this soft tissue extension around the gland is one of the few CT findings that allows the radiologist to diagnose the presence of a malignancy.

Aggressive carcinomas also have poorly demarcated tumor margins that merge with the adjacent salivary tissue. It is the poorly defined mass margins and, when present, the soft tissue tumor extension outside of the gland, that are the new CT criteria of frank carcinoma. For those tumors that are confined to the gland, their position relative to the plane of the facial nerve can be accurately mapped.[2,3]

By comparison, benign tumors and most malignant salivary gland tumors appear as well demarcated, minimally enhancing masses on CT scans. Unfortunately, neoplasms such as low-grade mucoepidermoid carcinomas, acinic cell carcinomas, and adenoid cystic carcinomas can all look exactly like benign mixed tumors. It is only when a lesion is poorly marginated and appears to merge with the adjacent gland that a malignant tumor can be diagnosed on CT. Certain tumors can be suggestively diagnosed because they have mucoid density components on CT. These lesions include Warthin's tumors, mucoepidermoid carcinomas, and large mixed tumors. However, necrotic nodes or tumors occasionally can have a similar appearance, which illustrates the difficulty inherent in trying to establish a histologic diagnosis based upon the CT appearance of a neoplasm.

CT is also the method of choice for evaluating tumor extension to the skull base and cervical node metastases. In the case of the parotid gland, metastatic disease to nodes within the gland may be impossible to differentiate from a primary salivary mass. However, disease that has spread to the parapharyngeal space nodes and osseous metastases are well seen on CT, allowing for a diagnosis of metastases or lymphoma to be made.

It is now possible to preoperatively distinguish minor salivary gland tumors that arise in the parapharyngeal space or from the pharyngeal wall from deep-lobe parotid tumors. The parapharyngeal spaces are difficult regions to examine clinically. Each is buried deep in the upper neck beneath the ramus of the mandible, the parotid gland, and the sternocleidomastoid muscle. It is only after a mass has attained a considerable size that a bulge of the lateral pharyngeal wall can be clinically detected, or that a mass can be palpated under the angle of the mandible. Even then, the further clinical diagnosis of the mass is almost impossible unless a specific history suggests a particular entity. In 1981, we presented our initial radiographic and clinical experience in evaluating 30 parapharyngeal space masses.[4] A protocol was developed which allowed us to preoperatively diagnose nearly 75 percent of the cases. By comparison, it is estimated that prior to this time, a preoperative diagnosis was made in only 20 to 50 percent of the cases. Our initial interest in 1979 and 1980 was directed toward developing a method of differentiating deep-lobe parotid tumors from extraparotid parapharyngeal space masses. This distinction had great practical importance because surgical techniques had recently advanced to the point where the approach to such a case was dramatically different, depending on whether the mass was intraparotid or extraparotid in origin.

Following this work, our interest was directed to the further preoperative differentiation of the various extraparotid tumors that were encountered. We found that angiography, which was the major radiographic method used to evaluate these masses prior to the CT era, needed only to be done on patients whose parapharyngeal space masses enhanced on CT. No diagnostically or surgically useful information was gained by doing angiography on masses that did not enhance. This meant that an invasive study needed only to be performed on less than 40 percent of patients with parapharyngeal space masses.

Since our initial publication, further refinements in CT scanners, including increased spatial resolution and faster scan times, have obviated the need for a combined CT sialogram in order to differentiate an intraparotid from an extraparotid parapharyngeal space mass. In addition, the work of other investigators interested in this region,[5-8] combined with our experience with 104 patients, have led to a new modified protocol. One of the foremost changes is the utilization of the GE Dynamic Scan mode. We believe that this technique will obviate diagnostic angiograms on virtually all patients with parapharyngeal space tumors.

MATERIALS AND METHODS

The protocol developed was based upon the radiograhic and clinical experience gained with 104 consecutive patients presenting with parapharyngeal space masses. The distribution of the varied pathology is shown in Table 1. The current protocol performs 4 to 6 noncontrast, 5 mm thick contiguous scans in the inferior orbitomeatal (IOM) plane through the region of the tumor. The level that best shows the maximal diameter of the lesion is chosen as the reference plane for the Dynamic Scan study. We use a 3-second initial delay and then the standard GE 1.4-second delay for a total of 10 scans. The examination is begun with a bolus injection of 50 cc of contrast material through either an 18- to 20-gauge Angiocath

The greatest diagnostic difficulty encountered was distinguishing extraparotid benign mixed tumors from the nonenhancing-type neuromas. Their similar CT appearance and Dynamic Scan findings did not allow a confident distinction to be made in most cases. There was also one case of a large aggressive malignant lymphoma that could not be differentiated from a deep-lobe parotid mass. Although a specific diagnosis in each of the fifteen lymphoma and metastatic squamous cell carcinoma cases could not be made on CT, a diagnosis of malignant nodal disease was made in all cases. In the early development of the protocol, two neuromas were misdiagnosed as small glomus tu-

TABLE 1 Distribution of Pathology in Salivary Tumors

Parotid tumors			
Benign:	Pleomorphic adenoma		
	(benign mixed)	19 (4 large)	
Malignant:	Mucoepidermoid	4	
	Adenocarcinoma	2	
	Oncocytoma	1	
	Adenoid cystic	1	
	Acinic cell	1	
	Anaplastic	1	
	Malignant mixed	1	28.8%
Minor salivary gland tumors			
Benign mixed		10 (2 large)	
Malignant mixed		1	10.6%
Neuromas		12 (3 large)	
Neurofibromas		3	14.4%
Glomus tumors		9	8.0%
Lymphomas		8 (1 large)	
Metastatic nodes		9	
Branchial cleft cysts		8	
Abscesses		2	
Jugular vein thrombosis		2	
Aberrant carotid arteries		3	
Meningiomas		4	
Lipoma		2	
Liposarcoma		1	
Total		104	

mors; however, these patients did not have angiograms, and their CT scans were performed on an older generation (Delta 50) scanner. In all, twelve cases (11.8%) presented difficulties in establishing a precise preoperative diagnosis. Of these, the most significant group were the very large tumors which comprised ten of the twelve cases. By utilizing both the clinical and CT findings, there was no diagnosis that led to an inappropriate surgical approach. If only the CT findings had been relied upon, one very large neuroma would have been operated on via a parotid incision; however, in this case, history suggested the diagnosis. Of the remaining nine large masses, in-

cluding five extraparotid tumors, all were surgically treated as parotid deep-lobe lesions in order to provide better identification of the facial nerve trunk. In point of fact, seven of these nine cases were either in the parotid deep lobe or adherent to the deep surface of the parotid capsule. Some specific details of the four most common tumors are shown in Table 2. or a Butterfly set. At the conclusion of this part of the study, a contrast drip is connected to the intravenous line, and a complete series of 5-mm thick contiguous scans is obtained running from above the tumor to below it. If the mass extends through the skull base, direct coronal scans are obtained. Finally, graphs of attentuation versus time are made. The primary parameters that we graph include: the tumor bed, the carotid artery, the jugular vein, and a reference muscle.

Alternatively, a complete contrast-enhanced CT scan can be obtained with the intravenous line kept open with a slow drip of normal saline. The Dynamic Scan can then be performed after several minutes of the saline infusion.

RESULTS

We considered that a correct diagnosis had been made if a deep-lobe parotid mass was called intraparotid on the CT scans. The specific histology in virtually all of these cases cannot be confidently obtained from the CT scans and it is ultimately the parotid location of the tumor alone that determines the surgical approach. Twenty-six of the 30 cases of parotid tumors were confidently diagnosed as being intraparotid in origin. However, there were four very large parotid benign mixed tumors, two large minor salivary gland lesions, and three large neuromas that could not be reliably diagnosed as being either intraparotid or extraparotid in origin. This difficulty is attributable to the fact that these large tumors compressed and effaced the fat planes necessary to make this distinction.

TABLE 2 Details of the Four Most Common Tumors

	Range of Tumor Size (cms)	Vessels	ICA = internal carotid artery IJV = internal jugular vein		Average Tumor Density	
Neural Tumors	2×2 – 7×6 Average diameter 3.4	60% 20% 13% 7%	ICA Anteromedially displaced ICA + IJV normal position ICA + IJV posteriorly displaced ICA anterolaterally displaced IJV posterior displaced	66.7%	{ 40% > muscle 26.7% = muscle 33.3% < muscle	
Glomus Tumors	1×2 – 2×4 Average diameter 2.6	33.3% 22.2% 44.4%	ICA + IJV normal position ICA + IJV not well seen ICA anteriorly displaced IJV posteriorly displaced		88.9% > muscle 11.1% = muscle	
Minor Salivary Gland Tumors	2×2 – 3×5 Average diameter 3.2	90.19% 9.9%	ICA + IJV posteriorly displaced ICA + IJV normal position	81.8%	{ 18.2% > muscle 63.6% = muscle 18.2% < muscle	
Parotid Benign Mixed Tumors	1×2 – 3×5 Average diameter 2.6	57.9% 42.2%	ICA + IJV normal position ICA + IJV posteriorly displaced	89.5%	{ 31.6% > muscle 57.9% = muscle 10.5% < muscle	

DISCUSSION: NONENHANCING OR MINIMALLY ENHANCING ISODENSE LESIONS (SIMILAR TO MUSCLE TISSUE)

The clinical detection of a parapharyngeal space mass can be a difficult task because these lesions cause few if any early symptoms. It is only after the lesion has grown to 2.5 to 3.0 cm in diameter that a medial bulge of the lateral pharyngeal wall can be clinically appreciated. There is no consistent physical finding that can allow a clinician to confidently differentiate a deep-lobe parotid mass from an extraparotid lesion. The best method for making this distinction is still the visualization of a fat plane between the deep lobe and the posterolateral aspect of the mass. This fat plane represents the compressed fibrofatty supporting matrix of the parapharyngeal space. When it is seen, 100 percent of the time it means that the mass is extraparotid in origin. When the fat plane is not seen between the mass and the parotid gland, it probably means that the lesion is a parotid tumor. There were six cases of very large extraparotid masses in which the fat plane was either compressed or invaded and could not be identified on CT. Thus, an absent fat plane sign correctly identified a tumor as being intraparotid in 30 of 36 (80%) cases. If, based on the clinical and CT findings, the final assessment of a very large tumor is that it most likely is a parotid lesion, our experience indicates that it should be surgically treated as one, in order to gain the maximal operative control of the facial nerve trunk.[9]

We had approximately the same percentage of malignant deep-lobe tumors (36.7%) as other published series (24 to 35%). Overall, approximately two-thirds of the cases were pleomorphic adenomas. In only five of the eleven malignant cases was there obvious CT evidence of invasion of the parotid capsule and infiltration of the adjacent soft tissues, allowing a CT diagnosis of malignancy to be made.

The smaller benign mixed tumors usually are fairly homogenous in appearance and only demonstrate a minimal enhancement similar to that of muscle. The larger lesions have a more nonhomogeneous appearance with irregular areas of minimal enhancement intermixed with regions of lower attenuation, which represent areas of necrosis and cystic mucoid collection. This CT appearance is similar to that seen in many neuromas that have areas of hemorrhage, cystic necrosis, and fatty deposition within them.

The minor salivary gland tumors were all benign pleomorphic adenomas, except for one malignant mixed tumor. This ratio of benign (91%) to malignant tumors is far greater than the previously published figures for minor salivary gland lesions (45 to 50% benign), but is closer to the published figures for the parotid gland (65 to 76% benign). In addition, the medial tumor margin in 8 of these 11 cases was partially or totally separated from the superior pharyngeal constrictor by a fat plane seen on CT. This combination of findings suggests that these minor salivary gland tumors may arise within previously described salivary rests lying in the parapharyngeal space fat.[10] This concept is consistent with the fact that at surgery the superior pharyngeal constrictor was found to be intact and easily separable from the laterally lying tumor. This should not be the case if the lesion arose within the minor salivary glands of the pharyngeal mucosa. It is possible that the malignant, aggressive tumors arise within the mucosal glands, whereas the majority of the benign tumors arise within salivary rests.

The smaller extraparotid benign mixed tumors were consistently diagnosed preoperatively on CT. They were similar in appearance to the parotid lesions; however, they were clearly extraparotid in origin. In all of the intraparotid and extraparotid benign mixed tumors, both the internal carotid artery (ICA) and the internal jugular vein (IJV) were either normal in position or posteriorly displaced. By comparison, the ICA was anteromedially displaced in two-thirds of the neuroma cases. However, in the remaining one-third of the neuroma patients, these vessels were similar in appearance to those of the mixed tumor cases and thus could not be used as a differential finding (see Table 2). Dynamic Scan graphs show the mixed tumors to have flat or very mild increasing slopes in the range of 40 to 65 Houndsfeld units (HUs). The graphs of the larger neuromas and the nonenhancing type of smaller neuromas are similar in shape, but in the 30 to 60 HUs range. Unfortunately, lesions lying in the overlap area do not allow for a precise diagnosis to be established.

The remaining aspects of the protocol are directed toward the differentiation of the low-density and enhancing lesions that occur in the parapharyngeal space (Fig. 1). Although not germain to this present dicussion on salivary gland tumors, in the appropriate case this system has allowed the radiologist to provide the clinician with more precise information than at any previous time. Tumor mapping is more accurate on CT than by pure clinical assessment, and in many instances a specific diagnosis can be made without resorting to invasive techniques.

The precise role that magnetic resonance imaging (MRI) will play in establishing a more specific histologic diagnosis is unclear at this time. However, the future promises the clinicians even more diagnostic information upon which to base their approach to management.

The same precise tumor mapping described in the parotid and parapharyngeal space regions also applies to minor salivary gland tumors that occur in the palate, larynx, and trachea. In the region of the palate, direct coronal CT scans may provide a clearer picture of tumor extension into the lower nasal vault and antrum. Unfortunately, metallic tooth fillings which degrade the CT image, may prevent good quality coronal scans from being obtained. In these instances, reconstructed directed coronal or sagittal scans can be made from the data obtained in the axial scans. MRI

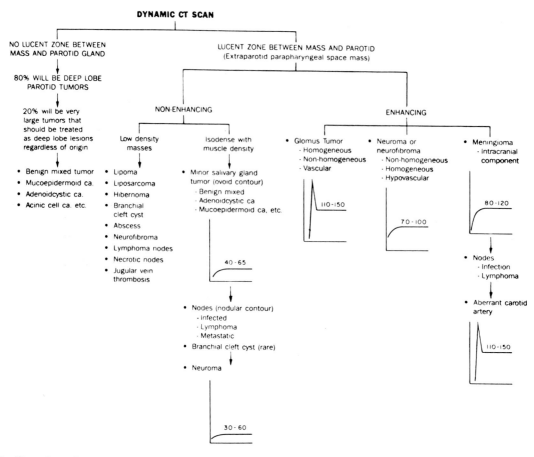

Figure 1 Flow chart of parapharyngeal space protocol. The graphs represent typical attenuation versus time curves for the various lesions.

scans are not degraded by the metallic fillings, and direct sagittal and coronal scans can be obtained easily. At the present time, MRI offers greater ease in imaging in planes other than the axial, while avoiding exposure to ionizing radiation. However diagnostically, little if any effect on the diagnosis or mapping of the lesion has so far been demonstrated. It is hoped that as more experience is gained with this new modality, a more dramatic impact on diagnosis and tumor mapping can be achieved.

REFERENCES

1. Som PM, Biller HF, Lawson W, Sacher M, Lanzieri CF. Parapharyngeal space masses: An updated protocol based upon 104 cases. Radiology 1984; 153:149–156.
2. Sone S, Higashihara T, Morimoto S, Ikezoe J, Nakatsukasa M, Arisawa J, Tamaki H. CT of parotid tumors. AJNR 1982; 3:143–147.
3. Bryan RN, Miller RH, Ferreyro RI, Sessions RB. Computed tomography of the major salivary glands. AJR 1982; 139:547–554.
4. Som PM, Biller HF, Lawson W. Tumors of the Parapharyngeal space: Preoperative evaluation, diagnosis and surgical approaches. Ann Otolaryngol 1981; 90:Suppl 80.
5. Unger JM, Chintapalli KN. Computed tomography of the parapharyngeal space. J Comput Assist Tomogr 1983; 7:605–609.
6. Bass RM. Approaches to the diagnosis and treatment of tumors of the parapharyngeal space. Head Neck Surg 1982; 4:281–289.
7. Mafee M. Dynamic CT and its application to otolaryngology. Head Neck Surg J Otolaryngol 1982; 11:307–318.
8. Shugar MA, Mafee MF. Diagnosis of carotid body tumors by dynamic computerized tomography. Head Neck Surg 1982; 4:518–521.
9. Batsakis JG. Tumors of the Head and Neck. Clinical and Pathological Considerations. 2nd edition. Baltimore: Williams & Wilkins, 1979.
10. Pesavento G, Ferlito A. Benign mixed tumors of heterotopic salivary gland tissue in upper neck: Report of a case with a review of the literature on heterotopic salivary gland tissue. J Laryngol Otol 1976; 90:577–584.

DIAGNOSIS OF SALIVARY GLAND NEOPLASMS

ROBERT E. FECHNER, M.D.

Neoplasms of the salivary gland began to be classified with some accuracy in the early 1950s. Since then, a great deal of long-term follow-up information has become available and has brought a solid clinicopathologic understanding to many of the tumors. Pathologists continue to recognize "new" neoplasms of major and minor salivary glands. The surgeon must accept the fact that there is a certain proportion of salivary gland neoplasms that are still poorly characterized, can cause difficulty for the most experienced head and neck pathologist, and will leave most pathologists diagnostically destitute.

There are several inherent problems in the diagnosis of salivary gland neoplasms including some of the most common tumors. The salivary gland ranks near the top of any organ in the number of different tumors that it is capable of generating. More than 20 categories of epithelial tumors exist, and there are numerous variations within some of these categories. For example, the monomorphic adenomas have at least five variants, none of which bears much resemblance to any other. "Look alike" tumors often cause confusion. For instance, the completely benign membranous monomorphic adenoma is similar to adenoid cystic carcinoma. Two other lesions that may be confused with each other are the low-grade papillary carcinoma and the highly lethal salivary duct carcinoma.[1] Parenthetically, the low-grade papillary carcinoma is also frequently diagnosed as one of several benign tumors.[2]

Mixture of cell types in a single tumor is epitomized by the mixed tumor with its uncommitted cells capable of differentiation into epithelial cells as well as cartilage.[3] Other mixtures include sebaceous cells that can be found in mixed tumors, mucoepidermoid carcinoma, monomorphic adenomas, and adenoid cystic carcinomas.[4]

Another problem is the variation in the appearance of tumors within a single histologic category, such as acinic cell tumors. Differences in the appearance of the individual cells and a broad spectrum of architectural arrangements complicate the diagnosis of this tumor. It is not an overstatement to say that no two acinic cell tumors ever look quite the same. The resolution of the diagnosis often requires histochemical or ultrastructural confirmation of the appropriate secretory granules. These studies cannot be carried out at the time of frozen section, and this fact contributes to the difficulties of frozen section (to be discussed). Similarly, mucoepidermoid carcinomas are on a cytologic continuum. Some tumors are clearly benign histologically, and others are blatantly malignant, but an intermediate group is difficult to judge regarding its metastatic potential. Both acinic cell and mucoepidermoid carcinoma can be totally cystic. The diagnostic cells may not evenform a continuous lining, and the tumor is easily passed off as a benign cyst.

One final example of variation within a single tumor is exemplified by adenoid cystic carcinoma. Its broad spectrum of patterns is acknowledged by the attempts to attach prognostic importance to tumors having one or another of the patterns.

Finally, there are reactive lesions that resemble neoplasms both clinically and microscopically. The most confusing is necrotizing sialometaplasia.[5] The majority of cases occur on the palate as spontaneous, ulcerated areas with a raised margin. A biopsy shows squamous metaplasia, often with nuclear atypia, and therefore mimics squamous carcinoma. In other foci, acinar cells are retained and are intermixed with squamous epithelium or are seen adjacent to squamous epithelium, raising the possibility of mucoepidermoid carcinoma. Necrotizing sialometaplasia has been reported in many sites following surgical trauma, and only the clinical information can avert a misinterpretation of carcinoma. Traumatized sites resulting in sialometaplasia include the nasal cavity, lip, gingiva, hypopharynx, paranasal sinuses, and parotid gland. In addition, there is one case in the larynx secondary to atheromatous embolization.[6]

Another reactive process that produces major alterations in a salivary gland epithelium is radiation therapy.[7] Nuclear abnormalities are prominent, and sometimes squamous metaplasia raises problems similar to those of sialometaplasia. Both radiation atypia and necrotizing sialometaplasia usually retain enough architecture to the lobules to distinguish them from carcinoma, but this necessitates a generous biopsy to assess.

The role of special techniques in the diagnosis of salivary gland tumors is limited. The identification of acinic cell tumors is sometimes facilitated by the demonstration of granules that are periodic acid–Shiff-positive resistant to diastase digestion. A poorly differentiated mucoepidermoid cancer consisting mainly of squamous cells and lacking glandular formation can be stained for mucin in order to confirm that it is a mucoepidermoid tumor. If no mucin is found, consideration must be given to the possibility of a metastatic squamous carcinoma from an undiscovered primary site.

Electron microscopy is occasionally useful for demonstrating the characteristic secretory droplets of acinic cell carcinoma or confirming the mitochondrial hyperplasia of an oncocytoma (or the rare oncocytic carcinoma). Clear cell tumors may prove to be glycogen-rich adenomas by electron microscopy or myoepitheliomas with innumerable cytoplasmic filaments. Ultrastructural examination has nothing to offer in distinguishing benign from malignant tumors.

219

Immunohistochemistry, usually employing the immunoperoxidase method, can be crucial in the diagnosis of undifferentiated tumors that could be large cell lymphoma or a carcinoma. For instance, leukocyte-specific antigen stains lymphocytes, but not epithelium. Conversely, stains for keratin, if positive, indicate an epithelial tumor. A variety of other antibodies to several other constituents of different tumor cells are being developed, and they may be useful in the future.[8,9]

Immunochemistry is sometimes helpful in deciding whether a lymphoid infiltrate is reactive or neoplastic. If the cells are polyclonal, as evidenced by staining for different globulins, the process is likely to be reactive. A monoclonal lymphoid infiltrate generally means that the lesion is a lymphoma.

Intraparotid lymph nodes sometimes cause problems. They are subject to conditions that may involve lymph nodes at any site, and these are usually readily diagnosed (sarcoid, toxoplasmosis, or cat scratch disease). Lymph nodes, however, may be the site of metastatic carcinoma, and sometimes this is the initial manifestation of the tumor. The intimate association of the node with the salivary gland parenchyma, coupled with the normal presence of acini within the node, often make it difficult to decide whether the tumor is metastatic to the lymph node or has arisen as a primary tumor within the parenchyma and secondarily involved the node.

FINE-NEEDLE ASPIRATION

The fine-needle aspiration technique has been used for more than 30 years in Scandinavia, and its use is rapidly increasing in the United States, where it is available in most departments of pathology. Recent monographs and a large periodical literature attest to the widespread interest in this procedure.[10]

Briefly, the method consists of inserting a 22-gauge needle into the lesion and applying gentle negative pressure on the syringe. The needle is moved back and forth in the mass so that it covers a broad volume, which increases the yield sampled compared to an ordinary large-gauge needle biopsy. Prior to removal of the fine needle, the pressure is equalized so that there is no loss of cells in the needle track as the needle is withdrawn. The aspirated material is smeared on a slide, immediately fixed, and stained. Unstained slides can be kept for special stains if later found to be indicated. Material can be appropriately fixed for electron microscopy,[11] and material can be used for flow cytometry. The procedure is surprisingly painless, and most patients readily agree to second aspirations if the first one is not diagnostic.

The value of fine-needle aspiration in verifying metastases of squamous carcinoma to cervical lymph nodes is incontrovertible.[12] The complications of fine-needle aspiration of salivary gland lesions are virtually nonexistent. Mavec et al noted an occasional small hematoma after 652 aspirations of salivary gland masses.[13] The concern expressed about seeding tumor is allayed by Engzell et al, who followed 157 cases of benign mixed tumor that had been aspirated prior to surgery.[14] After 10 years, there were three recurrences, but none of the recurrences involved the skin or the site of the aspiration. Two of the patients were specifically judged to have had incomplete excision of the original tumor. Furthermore, serial sections of needle tracks have failed to demonstrate tumor remnants.[12]

There are a few clinical settings in which fine-needle aspiration seems especially appropriate. For instance, a patient known to have a malignant tumor in another organ develops a mass in the region of the parotid gland. Material obtained by the fine needle can be compared with the primary cancer, either proving that it is metastatic or showing that it is a new and unrelated primary tumor. Another situation is the patient who has a fixed mass that is probably inflammatory either in the parotid lymph nodes or in the parotid gland itself. Aspiration can confirm the diagnosis of inflammation.[10] Other scenarios include an elderly patient in poor general health who has a clinically benign mass. If the aspiration shows a Warthin's tumor, observation of the patient may be wiser than operating on a harmless lesion.

It is not particularly meaningful to provide overall data regarding the accuracy of aspiration in salivary gland lesions because of the diversity of tumors, the selection biases of patients who undergo aspiration, and, above all, the differences in the skills of the pathologists. Most of the series reported in the literature emanate from institutions where both the pathologists and the surgeons are enthusiastic about the technique. This ideal relationship leads to careful clinical correlation and mutual recognition of the advantages and limitations. In this atmosphere, the accuracy of the technique is high. For example, Frable reported a sensitivity of diagnosing neoplasm in 75 of 81 patients (93%) in whom a neoplasm was subsequently found.[10] Sensitivity for the *absence* of neoplasms was in excess of 99 percent (109 of 110 cases). The single case thought to be a neoplasm (benign mixed tumor) on the aspirate turned out to be an inflammatory process with reactive epithelial alterations. Thus, out of 191 patients there were 6 false-negatives and this one false-"positive"

Sismanis et al had similar results.[15] Twenty-two of 23 aspirates (96%) of histologically proved benign lesions were interpreted as benign on the aspirate. The one false-positive was considered "suggestive of malignancy", but was only atypia (presumably secondary to inflammation) at the time of surgery. Of the malignant neoplasms, 17 of 20 (85%) were properly diagnosed as malignant.

In experienced hands, fine-needle aspiration accurately discriminates between benign and malignant lesions in excess of 95 percent of the cases. Admittedly, there is a small residue of malignant tumors that are either physically missed by the aspiration or

TABLE 1 Accuracy of Frozen Section of Parotid Tumors

	UCLA*	Stanford†	Mason‡
Benign Lesions	100/107 (94%)	58/61 (92%)	200/204 (98%)
False-positive	None	None	4/204 (2%)
Defer	7/107 (6%)	3/61 (8%)	0/204 —
Malignant lesions	9/25 (36%)	6/14 (43%)	46/52 (87%)
False-negative	6/25 (24%)	4/14 (29%)	6/52 (13%)
Defer	10/25 (40%)	4/14 (29%)	0/52 —

*Miller et al.[16]
†Hillel and Fee.[17]
‡Wheelis and Yarington.[18]

underinterpreted (false-negative), and very rare benign lesions that are overinterpreted as malignant (false-positive).

Whether all salivary gland lesions should be aspirated is debatable. Some surgeons believe that it will not alter their approach, and that aspiration is an unnecessary step. At our institution all minor and major salivary gland tumors undergo fine-needle aspiration. In the case of malignant tumors, it allows detailed counseling with the patients if the facial nerve may be resected or a neck dissection is planned. From the pathologist's viewpoint, we have found that the aspirations that are not fully diagnostic alert us to potential difficulties if a frozen section is to be done. At least a differential diagnosis will be generated preoperatively, and some advance thought can be given to the possibilities that may be encountered.

FROZEN SECTION

There are two detailed studies on the use of frozen section on parotid gland lesions from university hospitals.[16,17] After an analysis of these studies, I believe that comparable results would be obtained in large community hospitals with well-trained pathologists. This assumption was recently confirmed in a brief summary from the Mason Clinic.[18]

The two university series are remarkably similar in their results. In one study, 132 of 201 (66%) parotid tumors were examined by frozen section,[16] and in the other study, 75 of 108 (69%) tumors were examined by frozen section.[17] In the latter study, 81 percent of tumors examined by frozen section were benign lesions and 19 percent were malignant on permanent section diagnosis. A comparable proportion of benign and malignant lesions (88% and 12% respectively) was found in the cases that did not have a frozen section.

The accuracy of frozen section is much higher in benign lesions than in malignant lesions (Table 1). Ninety-two to 98 percent of benign lesions were correctly diagnosed, whereas the remainder had the diagnosis deferred.[16–18] In two series, none of 168 benign tumors was called malignant.[16,17] In the third series, 4 of 204 (2%) benign tumors were called malignant. There is no statement as to whether this altered the therapy in these four patients.

The accuracy of an intraoperative frozen section diagnosis of malignant tumor ranged from 36 to 87 percent. The diagnosis was deferred in 29 percent and 40 percent of the university cases, and specific but false-negative diagnoses were made in 24 percent and 29 percent respectively. This is presumably due to the natural reluctance of a pathologist to diagnose carcinoma unless he feels completely certain that it is the proper diagnosis. In the study by Hillel and Fee, four lesions were mistakenly diagnosed as benign at the time of frozen section.[17] One of these was eventually shown to be squamous carcinoma, one was a lymphoma, and two were low-grade mucoepidermoid tumors. One of the latter was the cystic variety, which has very little tissue. The diagnosis of malignant lymphoma is always difficult to make on frozen section. The lesions with a deferred diagnosis included an additional lymphoma and a mixed tumor of questionable malignant potential. Thus, one of the lesions that had a deferred diagnosis remained in a category of uncertain biologic potential even when multiple permanent sections were available for prolonged study. A summary of erroneous benign diagnoses (false-negatives) on frozen section and the subsequent final diagnosis of malignancy is given in Table 2.

The errors of diagnosis have been emphasized in this discussion, but one should keep a proper perspective because some patients do benefit from frozen section examination. In the group that did not have a frozen section, on the clinical assumption that they were all benign, four cases of malignant tumor were

TABLE 2 False-negative Frozen Diagnosis on Parotid Gland

Frozen Section Diagnosis	Permanent Section Diagnosis
Chronic inflammation	Mucoepidermoid carcinoma
Chronic scarring	Mucoepidermoid carcinoma
Inflammation	Mucoepidermoid carcinoma
Fibrosis	Mucoepidermoid carcinoma
Benign mixed tumor	Mucoepidermoid carcinoma
Oncocytoma	Acinic cell carcinoma
Adenoma	Acinic cell carcinoma
Mixed tumor	Adenoid cystic carcinoma
Lymphoid infiltrate	Lymphoma
Not carcinoma	Lymphoma
No tumor seen	Squamous carcinoma

Cases from Miller et al.[16] and Hillel and Fee.[17]

found.[17] Had the correct diagnosis been known, two of these cases would have had additional surgery. In the other two, a correct frozen section diagnosis would not have altered the surgical approach. Similarly, four of the patients who had a correct frozen section diagnosis of malignancy benefited from further surgery at the initial procedure.[17]

From the foregoing discussion, it is obvious that the frozen section diagnosis of salivary gland tumors does not attain the accuracy rate that it does in other sites. This does not nullify its value, but is a fact that must be kept in mind by the surgeon. A frozen section diagnosis must be used in the context of the clinical and operative findings. I think that Gates has summarized the situation nicely. "We cannot blame the pathologist if there is no tumor in the specimen, nor should we be concerned about subtle interpretative inaccuracies. Most of us would not do a radical operation or sacrifice the facial nerve solely on the basis of a frozen section diagnosis. Yet many of us would do this on the basis of our clinical acumen. The question then resolves to whether we do the extended operation now or at a later date after review of permanent sections. The answer depends on your relationship with your pathologist and your clinical intuition."[19]

SUMMARY

The numerous salivary neoplasms are a group of tumors notoriously heterogeneous and often difficult to diagnose. There continues to be progress in the pathologic recognition of "new" tumors. There is also continual refinement of pathologic criteria to predict the behavior of neoplasms.[20] Progress in the study of salivary gland tumors is slow, but it *is* steady.

REFERENCES

1. Garland TA, Innes DJ, Fechner RE. Salivary duct carcinoma: An analysis of four cases with review of literature. Am J Clin Path 1984; 81:436–441.
2. Mills SE, Garland TA, Allen MS, Jr. Low grade papillary adenocarcinoma of salivary gland origin. Am J Surg Path 1984; 8:367–374.
3. Mills SE, Cooper PH. An ultrastructural study of cartilaginous zones and surrounding epithelium in mixed tumors of salivary glands and skin. Lab Invest 1981; 44:6–12.
4. Cramer SF, Gnepp DR, Kiehn CL, Levitan J. Sebaceous differentiation in adenoid cystic carcinoma of the parotid gland. Cancer 1980; 46:1405–1410.
5. Fechner RE. Necrotizing sialometaplasia. A source of confusion with carcinoma of the palate. Am J Clin Path 1977; 67:315–317.
6. Walker GK, Fechner RE, Johns ME, Teja K. Necrotizing sialometaplasia of larynx secondary to atheromatous embolization. Am J Clin Path 1982; 77:221–224.
7. Harwood TR, Staley CJ, Yokoo H. Histopathology of irradiated and obstructed submandibular salivary glands. Arch Pathol 1973; 96:189–191.
8. Seo I-S, Zarling T, Hafez GR, et al. Immunocytochemistry of acinic cell and mixed tumors of salivary gland. Lab Invest 1984; 50:53-A; (Abstract).
9. Nadji M, Moskowitz LB. Antigenic expression in salivary gland tumors: A clue to histogenesis. Lab Invest 1984; 50:42A. (Abstract).
10. Frable WJ. Thin-needle aspiration biopsy. Philadelphia: WB Saunders, 1983:119–151.
11. Woyke S, Olszewski W, Domagala W, et al. Cytodiagnosis of acinic cell carcinoma. Ultrastructural study of material obtained by fine needle aspiration biopsy. Acta Cytol 1975; 19:110–116.
12. Feldman PS, Kaplan MJ, Johns ME, Cantrell RW. Fine-needle aspiration in squamous cell carcinoma of the head and neck. Arch Otolaryngol 1983; 109:735–742.
13. Mavec P, Eneroth C-M, Franzen S, et al. Aspiration biopsy of salivary gland tumours. I. Correlation of cytologic reports from 652 aspiration biopsies with clinical and histologic findings. Acta Otolaryngol 1964; 58:472–484.
14. Engzell U, Esposti PL, Rubio A, et al. Investigation on tumour spread in connection with aspiration biopsy. Acta Radiol Ther Phys Biol 1971; 10:385–398.
15. Sismanis A, Merriam JM, Kline TS, et al. Diagnosis of salivary gland tumors by fine needle aspiration biopsy. Head Neck Surg 1981; 3:482–489.
16. Miller RH, Calcaterra TC, Paglia DE. Accuracy of frozen section diagnosis of parotid lesions. Ann Otol Rhinol Laryngol 1979; 88:573–576.
17. Hillel AD, Fee WE, Jr. Evaluation of frozen section in parotid gland surgery. Arch Otolaryngol 1983; 109:230–232.
18. Wheelis RF, Yarington CT, Jr. Tumors of the salivary glands. Comparison of frozen-section diagnosis with final pathologic diagnosis. Arch Otolaryngol 1984; 110:76–77.
19. Gates GA. To freeze, or not to ... Arch Otolaryngol 1983; 109:229.
20. Tortoledo E, Luna MA, Batsakis JG. Carcinoma ex pleomorphic adenoma and malignant mixed tumors. Arch Otolaryngol 1984; 110:172–176.

TUMORS OF THE PAROTID GLAND

RONALD H. SPIRO, M.D.

The term "parotid" is derived from the Greek and means "near the ear." Although the typical presentation of parotid tumors anterior to the auricle overlying the ramus of the mandible is obvious, clinicians are occasionally misled when a neoplasm arising in the tail of the gland presents as a neck mass or, more rarely, as a lump behind the ear. Almost 10 percent of our patients have had parotid tumors which arise deep to the plane of the facial nerve in the so-called deep "lobe," but in only 2 or 3 percent was this deep origin clearly indicated by a swelling in the palate.[1] Accessory parotid tissue anterior to the gland in relation to Stensen's duct was the source of the tumor in 1 percent of our patients.[2] Parotid tumors may occasionally present as a nodule within the auditory canal, but this is rare in the absence of prior therapy.

Review of a 35-year experience with 1965 patients treated in our hospital for tumors of parotid gland origin confirms the usual ratio of 75 percent benign to 25 percent malignant. Tumors arising in accessory parotid tissue or presenting as palate swellings were more often malignant (50%). The distribution of our patients according to the histologic diagnosis is listed in Table 1, using a classification modified from that originally described by Foote and Frazell.[3]

DIAGNOSIS

Any swelling near the ear is best considered a parotid tumor until proved otherwise. In the patient who has a typical, asymptomatic, preauricular mass, additional studies are seldom required. Hyperplastic lymph nodes or focal inflammatory processes can mimic parotid tumors. Fine-needle aspiration biopsy can yield useful information, but we have not found parotid gland sialography helpful in this setting. When in doubt, it is preferable to admit the patient and perform an exploration under general anesthesia through a parotidectomy incision with the patient prepared for a gland resection, rather than attempt an outpatient biopsy under local anesthesia. If the patient proves to have a parotid tumor, the latter approach usually complicates subsequent definitive treatment.

In our experience, about 90 percent of patients with benign tumors and 70 percent with malignant lesions seek medical attention for a painless parotid mass. Consistent with the slow growth of benign parotid neoplasms, symptoms were present for more than 5 years in at least one-third. It is worth noting that a mass had been present for at least 5 years in 17 percent of patients with malignant tumors. Pain, reported

TABLE 1   Parotid Tumors Treated at Memorial Sloan Kettering Cancer Center: 1939 through 1983

	No. Patients	%
Benign		
Pleomorphic adenoma	1,093	81
Monomorphic adenoma	6	
Warthin's tumor	182	14
Benign cyst	28	2
Lymphoepithelial lesion	17	1
Oncocytoma	16	1
Total	1,342	100
Malignant		
Mucoepidermoid	272	44
Malignant mixed	107	17
Acinic cell	75	12
Adenocarcinoma	62	10
Adenoid cystic	54	9
Epidermoid	45	7
Other	8	1
Total	623	100

by 10 percent of patients with parotid cancers, was also noted in some patients with benign tumors (4%).

Small, benign parotid tumors are indistinguishable from their malignant counterparts, but larger parotid tumors tend more often to be malignant. Enlarged ipsilateral neck nodes or facial nerve dysfunction almost invariably indicates a malignant diagnosis, although we have observed facial nerve weakness in a few patients who had benign tumors.

Deep-lobe origin of a tumor is obvious when a palate swelling is associated with a parotid mass. On occasion, no external swelling may be apparent and differentiation from a parapharyngeal tumor may be facilitated by a CT scan performed in conjunction with a parotid sialogram.[4] Open biopsy through the mouth is undesirable as it will complicate definitive treatment.

TREATMENT

Surgery has long been our treatment of choice for parotid neoplasms. Although a significant number of our patients were successfully treated years ago by limited local excision, our minimal procedure now is a lateral or subtotal parotidectomy. The main trunk of the facial nerve is exposed posteriorly shortly after its exit from the stylomastoid foramen, and all branches are preserved as dissection is carried anteriorly.

When the tumor is located deep to the facial nerve, a lateral parotidectomy is first performed. Every effort is then made to retract and spare the nerve as the tumor is resected. Access to the retromandibular portion of the gland can be enhanced by excision of the adjacent submandibular gland and retraction of the mandible anteriorly. In rare circumstances, a mandibulotomy, or even a mandibulectomy, may be required for excision of a bulky or adherent "deep" lobe neoplasm.

Exposure of accessory parotid tumors is usually best accomplished by extending the conventional par-

223

otidectomy incision and raising a larger flap rather than incising the skin of the cheek directly over the tumor. Depending on the findings, the mass can either be resected by an extended subtotal parotidectomy or locally excised with preservation of Stensen's duct and the adjacent buccal branch of the facial nerve when possible.

In our experience, the extent of any parotid operation is primarily determined by the size of the tumor and the presence or absence of local extension. It was for this reason that we proposed a clinical staging system in 1979 which has since been adopted with modification by the American Joint Committee on Staging.[5,6] Regardless of histology, we believe that most tumors that are less than 4 cm in size can be adequately encompassed by a subtotal parotidectomy, which preserves the facial nerve.

We have found it necessary to resect the facial nerve trunk or some of its branches in only 50 percent of our patients with malignant tumors. In practice, we always try to preserve the nerve unless it is adherent to or involved by the tumor. When feasible, resected portions of the facial nerve should be replaced by free grafts taken from the ansa hypoglossae or other available cervical nerves. We have achieved satisfactory results without the use of microsurgical techniques.

Large tumors with significant local extension to deep tissues and/or skin (stage III) usually require a radical total parotidectomy with facial nerve sacrifice. Portions of the ear, mandible, and temporal bone may have to be excised in order to encompass the tumor. Regional or distant flaps may be necessary to replace resected skin. Our enthusiasm for extended parotid surgery has waned as it has become evident that survival is usually limited in patients with extensive tumors, especially if they are of high histologic grade, regardless how radical the extirpation.

Radical neck dissection has been reserved for patients with malignant tumors who present with clinical evidence of nodal metastasis on admission (20%). On occasion, we have performed lymphadenectomy electively in order to facilitate resection of large tumors which extend into the neck. Modifications of neck dissection may be appropriate in those with N0 disease, but would seem ill-advised in others, considering the poor prognosis in patients with palpable metastases.

Postoperative external radiation therapy is now routine for most of our patients with malignant parotid tumors. Although our experience is still small and the follow-up is insufficient, it confirms other reports that loco-regional recurrence can be significantly reduced in patients with stage II and stage III tumors.[7] Our treatment plan specifies a dose of 5000 to 6000 rads to the parotid bed and the neck using conventional fractionation. Every effort is made to initiate teletherapy within 6 weeks of surgery. We have no indication that this treatment hinders recovery of function in patients who have nerve grafts. Adjunctive radiation therapy is probably unnecessary in patients with small or low-grade tumors which have been adequately resected as their prognosis is usually excellent with surgery alone.

We have observed objective responses with cisplatin- or Adriamycin-based chemotherapy in some patients with inoperable or metastatic parotid cancer. Considering the unpredictability of current drug regimens, adjunctive chemotherapy is hard to justify in patients with resectable disease unless it is given during a carefully controlled clinical trial.

RESULTS

Our local recurrence rate in patients treated for benign tumors is 7 percent. This is probably a low estimate as decades of observation are required and our median follow-up was only 7 years. As a matter of fact, the disease-free interval exceeded 10 years in 34 percent of our patients who had adequate follow-up.

In patients with malignant tumors, the 5-, 10-, 15-, and 20-year "cure" rate was 55, 47, 40, and 33 percent, respectively, using the direct method. This excludes as indeterminate those patients who died postoperatively as well as those who had no evidence of recurrence when either they died of other causes or were lost to follow-up.

Survival curves based on histologic diagnosis alone show a trend toward better results in patients with acinic cell carcinoma and a less favorable outcome in those with adenocarcinoma, squamous carcinoma, and adenoid cystic carcinoma, but the differences are not significant. When the pathologist described the tumor as "low-grade," which was possible only in certain patients with mucoepidermoid, acinic cell, or adenocarcinomas, survival rates were high (96% at 5 years; 94% at 10 years) regardless of the precise histology, and the difference was highly significant when compared to the patients with "high-grade" tumors (51% at 5 years; 45% at 10 years).

Clinical staging was also significantly predictive of treatment results. Five-year survival was 96, 81, and 23 percent for patients with stage I, II, and III disease, respectively, whereas the 10-year survival was 95, 77, and 17 percent.

Results were significantly better in previously untreated patients when compared to those who received prior treatment elsewhere. Prolonged survival was unusual when either facial nerve palsy or cervical node metastasis was evident on admission.

Relatively few of the patients included in our most recent study (ending in 1973) had adjunctive treatment as this antedates our current commitment to postoperative radiation therapy. Although loco-regional control is likely to improve with adjunctive radiation therapy, it remains to be seen whether this will lead to increased survival. Moreover, if survival does indeed improve, we can anticipate an increase in distant metastasis, which currently occurs in at least 17 percent of patients, unless an effective chemotherapy regimen can be developed.

REFERENCES

1. Nigro MF Jr, Spiro RH. Deep-lobe parotid tumors. Am J Surg 1977; 134:523–527.
2. Johnson FE, Spiro RH. Tumors arising in accessory parotid tissue. Am J Surg 1979; 138:576–578.
3. Foote FW Jr, Frazell EL. Tumors of the major salivary glands. Cancer 1953; 6:1065–1133.
4. Som PM, Biller HF. The combined computerized tomography-sialogram, a technique to differentiate deep lobe parotid tumors from extraparotid pharyngomaxillary space tumors. Ann Otol Rhinol Laryngol 1979; 88:590–595.
5. Spiro RH, Huvos AH, Strong EW. Cancer of the parotid gland, a clinicopathologic study of 288 primry cases. Am J Surg 1975; 130:452–459.
6. American Joint Committee for Cancer Staging and End Results Reporting: Manual for Staging of Cancer. Chicago, 1977, p 27.
7. McNaney D, McNeese M, Guillamondegui OM, Fletcher GH, Oswald MJ. Postoperative irradiation in malignant epithelial tumors of the parotid. Radiol Oncol 1983; 9:1289–1295.

CARCINOMA OF THE SUBMANDIBULAR MINOR SALIVARY GLANDS

ROGER BOLES, M.D.

It has been most people's experience that the rate of malignancy among tumors of the submandibular and minor salivary glands exceeds that in the parotid gland.[1,2] In general, the rate of malignancy in the submandibular gland is about 50 percent and in the minor salivary glands over 80 percent.[3] Whatever the specific numbers, it can be said that the smaller the salivary gland, the higher the expectancy one can have for a tumor involving the gland to be malignant. Fortunately, tumors in general of the submandibular and minor salivary glands are much less frequent than tumors of the parotid gland.

Except for variations in frequency of occurrence in the submandibular and minor salivary glands, the histologic types of tumors that occur in these glands are essentially the same as those occurring in the parotid gland. Whereas mucoepidermoid carcinomas tend to be more common than other types of cancers in the parotid gland, adenoid cystic and adenocarcinomas tend to occur with greater frequency than mucoepidermoid cancers in the submandibular and minor salivary glands.[2,4]

In our experience at the University of California San Francisco, there have been no significant survival differences between patients with carcinoma of the major salivary glands and those with carcinomas of the minor salivary glands, with each group having around 70 percent survival for 5 years and 50 percent survival for 10 years.[4] Stage of the disease at presentation, histologic type, and anatomic location correlate much more closely, in most people's experience, with survival than with the particular subset of glands involved.[5] The submandibular gland may be the one exception to this rule. The primary difference between tumors of the major and minor salivary glands of greatest clinical importance is the higher frequency of inaccessibility and the difficulties of generous resectability of many minor salivary gland tumors. For this reason, we have had to depend a bit more heavily on radiation therapy to fully eradicate local and regional disease with minor salivary gland cancers. With major salivary gland cancers, we have made greater contributions surgically toward ultimate eradication of disease.

DIAGNOSIS

The clinical presentation of submandibular and minor salivary gland cancers is, for the most part, that of an enlarging, asymptomatic mass. Occasionally the mass may be painful or tender. Associated functional problems are determined by the anatomic location of the tumor, particularly as it grows and locally invades. For instance, cancer of the submandibular gland may cause a loss of sensation as well as hemiparesis and clumsiness of the tongue when it invades the lingual and hypoglossal nerves in the submandibular triangle. Tumors involving the larynx cause dysphonia and, eventually, breathing problems, whereas minor salivary gland cancers of the base of the tongue cause referred otalgia by involvement of the IX nerve and occasional hemiparesis of the tongue by involvement of XII.

Histologic Diagnosis. In our experience, treatment planning for these cancers has been greatly facilitated by fine-needle aspiration (FNA) biopsies. If the exact cell type cannot always be determined by this technique, at least a strong notion of whether the tumor is benign or malignant can be achieved.[6] Open biopsy may be done on minor salivary gland tumors when the tumor is ulcerating the overlying epithelium, when it is inaccessible for fine-needle aspiration, when the FNA technique is not locally available, or when there is great uncertainty about the cytologic picture of the FNA. Open partial biopsy of submandibular tumors is *not* a good practice unless the tumor has clearly ulcerated through the skin or floor of the mouth. The preferred approach for smaller tumors confined to the submandibular gland is total excision of the gland and the tumor along with the adjacent lymphatic, areolar, and connective tissue surrounding the gland, similar to the submandibular dissection done as part of a classic neck dissection.

Computerized Tomography (CT) and Magnetic Resonance Imaging (MRI). These studies have been helpful in determining the size and extent of minor salivary gland and submandibular tumors, especially when local invasion has taken place. These techniques have even been helpful in identifying regional cervical lymph node metastases, which may then be separately examined by biopsy by FNA if desired. We consider CT scanning (MRI, when available) essential in the diagnosis and treatment planning in all such circumstances before major surgical tissue disruption takes place. In this same vein, we consider the multidisciplinary team approach to diagnosis and treatment planning essential to achieve the best possible results and essential to the conduct of valid and reliable clinical studies in head and neck cancer. In our view, this objective is best achieved by having all new or recurrent head and neck cancer patients seen by a regularly scheduled, interdisciplinary head and neck tumor panel before any definitive treatment is initiated.

TREATMENT

For the most part, our treatment approach at the University of California San Francisco for the truly aggressive salivary gland malignant tumors has been a combination of surgery and irradiation therapy.

Surgery. The primary objective of surgery has been to achieve as near-total removal of all tumor as possible within the constraints of the patient's wishes and permission, the patient's general medical condition, the need to preserve critical vascular and central nervous system structures, and the objective of achieving reasonable postoperative function. To achieve a gross total removal of all tumor, surrounding tissues that are clearly involved may have to be removed, including the mandible, the palate, the orbit and its contents, the floor of the cranial fossa, and certain cranial nerves. In general, however, we tend to spare such structures if we possibly can, even though in so doing we achieve only minimal surgical margins by previous standards when irradiation therapy was not widely considered a routine part of the definitive treatment, and surgery *alone* was the recognized definitive treatment for these tumors. We have yet to statistically fully confirm the appropriateness of this lesser surgical approach because of the length of time it takes to confirm any valid data regarding malignant salivary gland tumors, and also because we have not done the broad *versus* the more limited surgical approaches in any sort of randomized way. Clearly, the local control rates have been greatly improved by combined surgery and irradiation therapy over radical surgery alone, and the resulting improved quality of life achieved by minimizing surgical cosmetic and functional defects has seemed to be worthwhile. We have noticed that this same approach has been adopted by other head and neck tumor centers.[5,7,8]

Radical neck dissection is most strongly indicated when palpable cervical metastases are present and particularly when they are demonstrated histologically to be tumor by FNA. Neck dissection is usually elected, particularly with cancers of the submandibular gland, when preoperatively nonpalpable nodes are found in the surgical field and demonstrated on frozen section to contain tumor. It is also usually elected for large tumors, especially those that have broken through the gland's capsule into the surrounding tissues. Some might elect to perform a neck dissection for the more histologically aggressive tumors, such as high-grade mucoepidermoids, adenoid cystic carcinomas, adenocarcinomas, squamous carcinomas, high-grade acinic cell carcinomas, undifferentiated tumors, and malignant mixed tumors, particularly when the primary tumor site is in continuity with the neck.[9] Under many of these conditions, modifications of the classic neck dissection are applicable.

Radiation Therapy. Irradiation therapy is given in combination with surgery for (1) all tumors considered to have unfavorable histologies (adenoid cystic carcinoma, high-grade mucoepidermoid carcinomas, adenocarcinomas, high-grade acinic cell carcinomas, malignant mixed tumors, squamous carcinomas, and undifferentiated carcinomas), (2) tumors that are large, (3) tumors identified at or near the surgical margin, which is often the case with minor salivary gland and submandibular gland tumors, (4) tumors with regional lymph node metastases, and (5) tumors that are recurrent. Radiation therapy remains an option for inoperable tumors, when patients refuse surgery, and for distant metastases. The irradiation field usually encompasses the entire neck on the same side as the primary lesion.

Adjuvant chemotherapy trials are being introduced widely on a pilot basis with a variety of agents in a variety of regimens. Our regional cooperative group in Northern California has agreed on such a pilot study of induction chemotherapy for tumors with poor prognosis (i.e., stages III and IV, poor prognosis histologies, regional or distant metstases, and recurrent tumors). The agents we have chosen to use are Adriamycin, 5-FU, and cisplatin.

DISCUSSION

Minor Salivary Gland Cancers. Because of the highly varied locations and histologic types of malignant tumors of minor salivary glands, it is difficult to be specific about prognosis and appropriate treatment programs for these tumors as a group. The emergence of radiation therapy as an efficacious modality of treatment for salivary gland cancers has given clinicians and patients greater options for management, particularly for minor salivary gland tumors in difficult or inaccessible locations, such as the larynx, nasopharynx, and trachea. Just exactly how these various options sort out over the long term for cure, survival, and palliation is still not entirely clear. Several points of view do seem to be emerging, however, on the basis of the recognition of the radiosensitivity of these lesions:

1. Surgery and radiation therapy, as planned and combined initial treatment, are probably most generally preferred for the majority, and certainly for the worst, of these tumors which are still considered operable.
2. Surgery of a more limited or conservative type when combined with aggressive radiotherapy may give as satisfactory tumor control as more radical and aggressive surgical procedures. Until the question is fully clarified, the more conservative surgical approaches do, perhaps, offer some trade-off for an improved quality of life.
3. Both salvage surgery and salvage radiation therapy, and combinations of both, have demonstrated their effectiveness in raising the overall control rates for these tumors and have given some patients a second chance who initially chose less than optimum treatment or who had unfortunate local recurrences.
4. The increasing recognition of the role of elective radiation therapy in the control of microscopic metastatic disease in the cervical lymph nodes in these and other tumors of the head and neck may reduce even further the already low incidence of manifest regional metastases of the minor salivary gland tumors as well as of smaller tumors of the submandibular gland.

Submandibular Salivary Gland Cancers. Because of the relatively low overall incidence of malignant tumors of the submandibular salivary glands, very few individuals, and even fewer institutions, can speak with great authority about all aspects of this particular problem. Probably most people and most institutions lump cancers in this gland, for purposes of management and statistical review, into the protocols for parotid tumors. Spiro and his group at Memorial suggest that stage-for-stage, cancers in the submandibular gland behave more aggressively than in the parotid and that therefore their group approaches submandibular tumors more aggressively surgically.[9] The principle of wide surgical margins for cancers is always hard to argue with and particularly so in the submandibular triangle, where the sacrifice of structures adjacent to the submandibular gland is not, in general, particularly devastating to the postoperative function of the patient. To add an incontinuity neck dissection to the submandibular procedure, modified when possible to preserve at least cranial nerve XI, is probably also quite justifiable for these aggressive tumors and should facilitate the achievement of more generous posterior and inferior margins.[9,10]

SUMMARY

Fine needle aspiration has become an exceedingly helpful biopsy technique for all salivary gland tumors as it has for other tumors and masses throughout the body.

Clinical staging of minor and submandibular salivary gland cancers is the most reliable criterion for prognostication and for treatment planning. CT scanning and magnetic resonance imaging have become essential for accurate staging of the vast majority of these cancers.

Surgery, whenever possible, is still generally accepted as the preferred initial treatment. The surgical goal for most of these cancers is total removal of all grossly identifiable tumor with as generous a surgical margin as can be achieved without excessive mutilation or functional impairment. Submandibular gland cancers may deserve a somewhat more aggressive surgical approach because of the unusually aggressive behavior of these cancers.

The radiosensitivity, and even radiocurability, of salivary gland cancers are now quite well established and have placed radiation therapy quite firmly into the primary treatment regimen in most institutions as an adjunct to surgery for the tumors carrying the worst prognoses. It is, of course, the only treatment available for small tumors located in structures which, if surgically sacrificed, would cause unacceptable deformity or disability.

Further cooperative clinical trials with chemotherapy and immunotherapy are clearly needed.

REFERENCES

1. Barwil JM, Reynold CT, Ibanez MI, et al. Report of one hundred tumors of the minor salivary glands. Am J Surg 1966; 112:493.
2. Batsakis JG. Tumors of the head and neck. Baltimore: Williams and Wilkins, 1979.
3. Conley J, Myers E, Cole R. Analysis of 115 patients with tumors of the submandibular salivary gland. Ann Otol 1972; 8:323–330.
4. Fu KK, Leibel SA, Levine ML, et al. Carcinoma of the major and minor salivary glands. Cancer 1977; 40:2882–2890.
5. Spiro RH, Koss LG, Hajdu SI, Strong EW. Tumors of the minor salivary gland origin. Cancer 1973; 31:117–130.
6. Frable WJ, Frable MA. Thin needle aspiration biopsy in the diagnosis of head and neck tumors. Laryngoscope 1974; 84:1069.
7. Guillamondegui OM, Byers RM, Luna MA, et al. Aggressive surgery in treatment for parotid cancer: Role of adjuvant postoperative radiotherapy. Am J Roentgenol 1974; 123:49–54.
8. Spiro RH, Havos AG, Strong EW. Cancer of the parotid gland. Am J Surg 1975; 130:452–459.
9. Spiro RH, Havos AG, Strong EW. Tumors of submandibular gland. Am J Surg 1976; 132:463
10. Byers RM, Jesse RH, Guillamondegui OM, Luna MA. Malignant tumors of submandibular gland. Am J Surg 1973; 126:459.

19. Cancer of the Thyroid Gland

INTRODUCTION

BLAKE CADY, M.D.

The chapters in this part, *Selected Topics in Thyroid Cancer*, address numerous controversies in contemporary management of thyroid cancer. In differentiated thyroid cancer, how much of the thyroid gland needs to be removed, and what type of lymph node resection should be done? Is the extent of surgery modified by the particular risk group of the patient or are all patients submitted to a standard procedure? Are microscopic foci of papillary carcinoma pathologic curiosities or clinical imperatives? How is surgical and radioiodine therapy adjusted for this histologic finding? Does radioactive iodine (RAI) used as an adjuvant change survival rates in differentiated thyroid cancer, particularly in young patients? Is radiation therapy in some form the cause of conversions of papillary carcinoma to anaplastic thyroid cancer, as repeatedly proposed by Crile? How should the endocrinologist adjust for the fact that young patients respond so well to RAI, but seldom really need it for the unusual case of metastatic disease they manifest, whereas older patients who need it because of fairly frequent metastases do not respond well in terms of cure?

How should we eliminate the complications of thyroid surgery? Should this occur by limiting the number of operations performed by more careful case selection, for instance, by use of needle biopsy? Should this occur by limiting the extent of surgery to avoid operations known to be associated with a high complication rate? Should we try to reduce complication rates by limiting the numbers or types of surgeons actually performing thyroid operations? For a disease with extremely high cure rates, complication rates should be at an absolute minimum.

Needle biopsy of the thyroid is now widely practiced, but controversy still surrounds the selection of the type of needles to be utilized. Fine-needle aspiration, large-needle aspiration, and cutting-core needle biopsy all have their advocates, but clear guidelines have not been agreed on. The real impact of needle biopsy on thyroid surgery is as yet unknown, but clearly fewer operations are being performed. This leads one to speculate that operative series reported in the literature that yield 80 percent incidence of cancer may indicate far too selective a screening of patients; these authors may not be removing enough benign tissue to eliminate future cosmetic, functional, and pathologic problems, including unsuspected carcinomas. Needle biopsies of lesions that need surgery anyway because of obvious carcinoma or major cosmetic problems really do not provide useful supporting data regarding the value of needle biopsy. Analytic reports of needle biopsy of 1-cm nodules would really provide the test of practical estimations about accuracy of the technique.

It is clear that the vast majority of thyroid nodules and thyroid cancers will continue to be operated on by general surgeons in community hospitals, and no program of specialty centers or cost-effective medicine will change this fact. The real question then remains: What is the most successful, least complicated, and most widely applicable type of thyroid surgery to be utilized and taught to the general surgical community of this country? Programs of total thyroidectomy for thyroid cancer probably do not meet these criteria. Reports in the literature of series with a relatively conservative surgical philosophy record just as much success in terms of cure as reports of total thyroidectomy, but with greatly reduced numbers of complications. Technical procedures can be done by highly trained and experienced super-specialists, but it does not necessarily follow that they should be done in that fashion generally, especially when data about increased efficiency, while theoretically possible, has not been practically acquired. There is no question that we are seeing a flood of iatrogenic injuries to recurrent laryngeal nerves and parathyroid glands as the doctrine of total thyroidectomy is disseminated into our communities where general surgeons perform relatively few thyroid operations. It behooves the surgical community to develop practical teaching for surgeons at large and not to focus on total thyroidectomy as the standard treatment, since specialists may thereby be accused of soliciting business for themselves while ignoring the needs of the vast majority of the population of the United States, who will continue to be operated on by general surgeons in community hospitals.

In the five excellent chapters that follow, the authors present their approach to contemporary aspects of thyroid cancer.

The use of radioactive iodine is discussed by Beierwaltes, one of the foremost advocates and reporters of the technique and its results. While RAI meets the ideal goal of an agent for treatment of metastatic cancer through its ability to "home-in" on specific cells by virtue of their iodine avidity and to carry a lethal form of treatment (radiation) that spares essentially all nonthyroid tissue, it does not produce uniform cures. Data regarding the meticulous formal approach of Beierwaltes to RAI use is presented and, while impressive, needs the advantages of a controlled trial to substantiate its widespread application as an adjunct therapy in a disease that is so highly curable with conservative surgery. Clearly, the use of RAI for metastatic disease is highly but not entirely successful, and controversy exists about the relative value of thyroid hormone administration and RAI. This approach has the advantage of careful documentation and long-term use and can be safely and effectively followed by all practitioners.

In his chapter, Block presents a comprehensive and practical analysis of medullary thyroid carcinoma and its management. His approach addresses all the major biologic and therapeutic possibilities and is recommended as a guide to management. He notes the problems that exist in following the progress of patients after adequate neck surgery by means of the extraordinarily sensitive tumor marker, calcitonin, since all therapy of metastatic disease is directed by symptoms rather than by calcitonin elevation per se.

The entire contemporary area of needle aspiration of thyroid nodules is beautifully described by Frable, who is a pathologist and cytologist and thus brings a unique perspective to this sometimes confusing field. He notes, as is emphasized by many, that we should not focus on exact diagnostic accuracy, but on the help this technique can bring to practical decision making regarding operations for thyroid nodules. Since many follicular lesions are difficult to distinguish as benign or malignant, even when the entire specimen is available in the pathology laboratory with multiple sections, one can hardly expect complete accuracy from needle aspiration cytology. However, decisions to operate or not to operate *can* be made based on this level of accuracy, though imperfect. Problems arise when pathologists are unfamiliar with thyroid cytology and when endocrinologists and physicians do not understand the limitations of the technique and the cytologic interpretation of thyroid aspirates, and thus may seek more specific diagnoses when only basic therapeutic judgments are available. It needs to be re-emphasized that needle aspiration cytology of the thyroid gland is just one more laboratory test to bring to bear in decision making and cannot be viewed as infallible; many clinical decisions to operate may be necessary for cosmetic and functional and even oncologic purposes, despite negative needle aspiration.

The problems in surgical management of locally advanced thyroid cancer are addressed in a thorough and practical manner by Guillamondegui of M.D. Anderson Hospital. He reports 47 cases of thyroid cancer that involved trachea, laryngeal cartilages, recurrent laryngeal nerve, muscles, esophagus, or other structures surrounding the thyroid. Thirteen of these cases were poorly differentiated carcinomas or sarcomas and all died, with a single exception. Thirty-four cases were well-differentiated cancers, and of these, 18 lived free of disease. Twenty of the 47 total cases and, by inference, 20 of the 34 differentiated cases were in the low-risk young age group. I calculated that 16 or 17 of these 20 low-risk patients lived free of disease for long periods of time. The median age of surviving patients was 27 years, while that of nonsurviving patients was 69 years, re-emphasizing the overwhelming impact of age on prognosis. Even though young patients appear with evidence of extensive involvement of the tissues about the thyroid gland, extremely high cure rates can be expected by following Guillamondegui's guidelines in management. Rarely is laryngectomy required for treatment of thyroid carcinoma, and only three patients were so treated in this series. Indications for laryngectomy would be intratracheal involvement with impending airway obstruction in a well-differentiated carcinoma that failed to respond to radiation therapy. In addition, patients with a useless larynx because of a bilateral recurrent laryngeal nerve paralysis and local tumor growth would be candidates for laryngectomy. Preservation of functionally important structures such as trachea, larynx, and recurrent laryngeal nerves is important, and they are sacrificed only if functionally useless. Radioactive iodine therapy is effective, judging from the fact that 82 percent of patients with advanced local disease in whom RAI was used are alive. This again emphasizes the efficiency of radioactive iodine therapy in young patients with differentiated thyroid carcinomas.

Complications in thyroid surgery are addressed by Ward, who describes the various nerve palsies that may occur in the vocal cords and arytenoids. He emphasizes the often-ignored aspects of trauma to the internal and external branches of the superior laryngeal nerves, which are in constant jeopardy during dissections about the superior thyroid vessels and the upper pole of the thyroid lobes. Discussion of other complications of thyroid surgery is complete, but a generally conservative approach is advocated, exemplified by the use of drains, pressure dressings around the neck, and use of calcium supplements whenever perioral tingling was noted postoperatively. These latter suggestions are at variance with my own practice—and that of many others—which advocates no drains, no dressings (so that careful inspection of the neck can be easily and repeatedly done), and calcium supplements only for persistently and significantly low calcium values so as to define the nature of the hypocalcemia and to stimulate parathyroid recovery. Bone avidity for calcium after surgery for Graves' disease, for instance, frequently produces hypocalcemia which, while of little physiologic consequence, is often productive of symptoms after bilateral subtotal thyroidectomy. Patients with this condition may display perioral tingling and a Chvostek sign without the need for calcium supplements.

RADIOIODINE THERAPY

WILLIAM H. BEIERWALTES, M.D.

INDICATIONS

Radioactive iodine therapy is only effective in the treatment of well-differentiated thyroid cancer (papillary and follicular). It is of no use in undifferentiated thyroid cancer (spindle, giant cell, and small cell).

In spite of earlier publications suggesting that it might be helpful in the treatment of medullary thyroid cancer, a recent publication proves that it is ineffective in the treatment of this lesion.[1] Hurthle cell carcinoma is a variant of follicular carcinoma and usually shows less uptake and less response to radioiodine therapy. Hurthle cell carcinoma of the thyroid also has a worse prognosis than follicular carcinoma.

PREPARATIONS FOR RADIOACTIVE IODINE THERAPY[2,3]

Radioactive iodine therapy should only be used in the patient with thyroid cancer who has had (1) a histopathologic diagnosis of well-differentiated thyroid cancer, (2) a "total" thyroidectomy, (3) residual uptake of radioactive iodine in the thyroidal bed (usually greater than 1% of the administered dose at 24 hours), (4) residual uptake in the cervical or mediastinal node areas after extensive lymph node plucking to remove all palpable nodes and all visibly involved nodes, or (5) uptake of radioiodine in lungs and/or in bone as evidence of thyroid carcinoma outside the neck.

Surgery

The first and most important step toward cure of the patient with thyroid cancer is adequate surgery at the time of the first operation. Lobectomy and isthmusectomy are done as the primary surgery for the initial lump. If the frozen section is positive, a second lobectomy is done immediately.

During these procedures, the cervical lymph nodes are examined. If they appear to be involved, numerous nodes are submitted for frozen section. If they are positive, I believe that extensive lymph node plucking should be done through a collar incision. Radical neck dissections are no longer necessary nor have they been proved to be of advantage in the prognosis. Generally speaking, if all of the palpably enlarged nodes are removed, radioactive iodine can obliterate cancer in any remaining nodes.

The total thyroidectomy has a low morbidity in the hands of experienced thyroid surgeons. It is used almost routinely in the treatment of children with Graves' disease. It is difficult to understand why the surgeon should be reluctant to perform a total thyroidectomy for histopathologically proved carcinoma of thyroid in an adult when the only argument among endocrine surgeons in the surgical treatment of Graves' disease in children is whether to perform a 95 percent thyroidectomy or a 100 percent thyroidectomy. Other reasons for favoring a total thyroidectomy are (1) when it is complete and there is no residual uptake of radioiodine, it allows avoidance of radioiodine therapy, (2) if the uptake is decreased to less than 2 percent, the thyroidectomy allows staging with radioactive iodine, (3) it also allows treatment of the primary and the metastases with one dose of radioactive iodine, (4) microscopic foci are present in the contralateral lobe in 38 to 87 percent of patients, (5) in some cases, a total thyroidectomy removes a focus of anaplastic carcinoma that could never be obliterated with radioiodine therapy, and (6) a total thyroidectomy is the most important device in preventing recurrence. The recurrence rate following unilateral lobectomy is 2 to 40 percent.

Mazziferi has shown that the recurrence rate after a subtotal thyroidectomy is twice that after a total thyroidectomy. Mazziferi has shown that in a 10-year follow-up of 575 patients, there were 84 recurrences with six deaths from the carcinoma.[4] Nineteen percent of the recurrences could not be eradicated by any means. Patients who died were over 30 years of age. The presence of cervical metastases was associated with increased recurrence rates. He found that external radiation therapy adversely affected the outcome in his patients.

Similarly, Haynie et al from M.D. Anderson reported on total thyroidectomy in 352 patients.[5] Ninety-seven of these patients developed recurrent disease. One-fourth of these patients failed to concentrate radioactive iodine. Forty-four patients died of progressive thyroid cancer. All of these patients were more than 40 years of age.

The most common cause of death from thyroid carcinoma is invasion of the structures of the superior thoracic inlet. Adequate primary surgery markedly decreases the risk of death from invasion of the structures of the superior thoracic inlet.

The patient should undergo a scan after having been "off" all thyroxine (T_4) and/or triiodothyronine (T_3) for 6 weeks after surgery. A delay of this scan may allow recurrence or metastases. Having the scan and treatment 6 weeks after surgery allows treatment to ablate the remnant and treatment of micrometastases without delay. It also allows immediate staging. Scheduling the scan for 6 weeks after surgery ensures better compliance than would scheduling for some indefinite later date.

Withdrawal of Thyroid Hormone

A common practice today is to withdraw T_4 for 6 weeks before the ^{131}I scan and therapy dose, but to withdraw T_3 for only 2 weeks. I am opposed to this because occasional patients with metastatic carcinoma show no uptake in the lung metastases at 2 weeks off T_3, but do show adequate uptake ater 6 weeks off T_3. An argument given for withdrawing T_3 for only 2 weeks is that the patient is more comfortable. Generally, patients off all thyroid hormone for 6 weeks after surgery have far less discomfort than patients who have had a total ablation of all uptake with radioactive iodine. If they do develop discomfort, it is usually during the last 2 of the 6 weeks. My patients have found that taking Dexatrim gives them pep and does not make them nervous during this last 2-week period.

Another argument for not withdrawing T_3 for longer than 2 weeks is that longer periods of withdrawal of thyroid hormone cause acceleration of tumor growth, but no references are ever given to support this. However, I have found three publications of controlled studies in animals that show that not only well-differentiated thyroid cancer, but also breast cancer and a sarcoma grow least rapidly in the presence of hypothyroidism and most rapidly in the presence of the euthyroid state.

Another argument used is that higher uptakes of radioactive iodine have been found at 2 weeks off T_3 than after 4 weeks off T_3. These articles generally are speaking about the thyroid remnant and only rarely, if at all, about uptake in lung or bone metastases. Another argument is that no new areas of uptake are detected at 4 weeks. Again, these are articles on patients with sizable thyroid remnants without distant metastases.

Most importantly, there are excellent publications documenting that "Following prolonged thyroid therapy in euthyroid patients, basal serum TSH may be used to differentiate euthyroid from hypothyroid patients *35 days after withdrawal of thyroid hormone.* The response to TSH does not improve this differentiation."[6] Thus, there are instances in which the pituitary does not recover for 35 days after the administration of thyroid hormone has been stopped.

Thyroid-Stimulating Hormone (TSH) Injections

I discontinue thyroid hormone and do not give TSH injections because TSH injections produce a high incidence of allergic reactions, the formation of neutralizing antibodies, and TSH resistance. TSH injections do not produce as high a level or as continuous a level of serum TSH as the effects of a total thyroidectomy with the patient off thyroid hormone. Under these circumstances, the patient produces his/her own TSH 24 hours a day.

Thallium-201 Tracers

An attempt has been made to use the radioactive isotope thallium-201 to image thyroid carcinoma while a patient is on thyroid hormone. Occasionally thallium-201 has detected metastases that have not concentrated radioiodine. It has also occasionally detected metastases while the patient is on thyroid hormone. Unfortunately, it also occasionally demonstrates normal lymph nodes and may commonly show no uptake in carcinoma that will show uptake with radioactive iodine.

Serum Thyroglobulin (HTG)

Some investigators have advocated the use of the serum thyroglobulin in place of taking the patient off thyroid hormone and using radioiodine scans. Unfortunately, the serum HTG is TSH-dependent, that is, the longer the patient is off thyroid hormone after a total thyroidectomy, the more sensitive the serum thyroglobulin in detecting carcinoma and the higher the HTG levels in patients who are known to have residual carcinoma. The conclusion, therefore, is that thyroglobulin levels should not replace radioactive iodine scans. The two methods complement each other, however, and should be used together to achieve the maximum sensitivity and reliability. That is, the serum thyroglobulin level may be strikingly elevated in patients with lung metastases or bone metastases who have no uptake of radioactive iodine because of anaplastic changes in their thyroid carcionoma.

Ablating Doses of Less Than 30 mCi of ^{131}I

Many people today argue that a dose of radioactive iodine less than 30 mCi should be given for "ablation" of uptake of the thyroid remnant rather than giving a treatment dose of 150 mCi. I do not use this procedure because when I first evaluated it from 1947 to 1950, I found that less than 30 mCi rarely ablates the uptake in the remnant, as judged by a 2-year follow-up. I have also found that the radiation delivered to micrometastases from a 150-mCi dose decreases the biologic half-life and the effective half-life of the radioiodine in the metastases. The second dose required to ablate the residual uptake in the thyroid increases the radiation dose and costs the patient time and money that could have been avoided if the patient had been given 150 mCi initially.

TREATMENT WITH RADIOACTIVE IODINE

Methodology

If the patient has no significant uptake in the thyroidal bed, cervical nodes, mediastinal nodes, or lungs or bones, I do not treat with radioactive iodine, but usually prescribe 0.15 to 0.2 mg of sodium-1-thyroxine (T_4) a day and ask the patient to return in 2 months for a serum TSH and a serum T_4 and T_3 resin uptake. If the serum T_4 and T_3 resin uptake are normal or slightly elevated and the serum TSH is less than 1.5, these values indicate that the patient is on an adequate suppressive dose of thyroid hormone.

For a clear-cut uptake in thyroidal remnant, a 150-

mCi ablation dose is given; for uptake in cervical nodes, 175 mCi; and for uptake in metastases outside the neck, a 200-mCi treatment dose.

The patient is followed by measurement of the radioactivity in his body at a distance of one meter with a cutie-pie radiation dosimeter. When the radioactivity falls below 4 mr/hour at a distance of one meter, the patient has less than 30 mCi of radioactive iodine in his body and is started on thyroid hormone and allowed to go home. This decrease of total body radioactivity to less than 30 mCi almost inevitably occurs at 3 days after the treatment dose, but may rarely occur on the second day or after the third day.

The patient returns in one year (having been off all thyroid hormone for 6 weeks) for a repeat chest roentgenogram, complete blood count, serum thyroglobulin, and a 2-mCi tracer dose of radioactive iodine for a pinhole view of his neck and chest. It has been argued that perhaps the sensitivity of detection of thyroid cancer would be greater with a larger tracer dose. The 2-mCi tracer dose with the pinhold with modern cameras represents by far the most sensitive method with the highest resolution of any method I have used since 1947. I also make it a routine to perform pinhold imaging of the neck and chest routinely when the patient's content of radioactivity drops below 30 mCi before discharge from the hospital. This practice allows me to perform a repeat scan without a repeat tracer dose with a total dose of 29 mCi. In my experience, only one of every 20 or 30 patients ever shows convincing evidence of foci of carcinoma that I have not detected with 2 mCi.

The patient returns one year after the treatment dose (having been off all thyroid hormone for 6 weeks and on a low iodine diet for one week, for a repeat interval history, physical examination, complete blood count, chest roentgenogram, serum T_4, T_3 resin test, serum TSH, and a repeat pinhole imaging of the neck and chest 24 hours after a 2-mCi tracer dose of Na ^{131}I. If the scan at one year is negative, I re-institute treatment with 0.2 mg of thyroxin and have the patient return in 2 years for a repetition of the studies that were performed at one year. If this imaging at 3 years after the treatment dose shows no evidence of residual thyroid carcinoma, the patient is asked to return every 5 years thereafter for repetition of the aforementioned studies. If a recurrence is found, I retreat with 200 mCi of radioactive iodine and begin the cycle again.

Recurrences

I have had patients (6%) develop recurrences up to 15 years after apparent cure. These patients had very extensive disease at the time of their original treatment. Thus, having treated and followed 1000 patients for up to 35 years, I can give strong assurance to the patient with nonextensive disease who has followed the foregoing protocol that he will have no recurrences as judged by our data to date.

Effectiveness of Therapy

In our study of 103 patients with metastases outside the neck, ^{131}I ablation of uptake and distant metastases was found to be with a threefold increase in survival over patients whose uptake is not ablated with radioactive iodine.[2]

Harmful Effects of ^{131}I Therapy

None of these patients died from or with leukemia, and there was no increased incidence of second cancers.[2] These results are in striking contrast to the results from x-ray therapy and cancer chemotherapy published in a review editorial by Chabner from the National Cancer Institute.[7] He found that cancer chemotherapy at its best, namely, in the treatment of carcinoma of the ovary, was associated with a 67- to 171-fold increased risk of acute leukemia at 2 years after the onset of treatment. He also published that x-ray therapy with chemotherapy at its best, namely, in the treatment of Hodgkin's disease, was associated with a 20-fold increased risk of second cancers at 4 years after the onset of treatment.

The Place of X-Ray Therapy

I do use x-ray treatment when the carcinomas of the thyroid fails to show significant uptake and is localized to some critical area. X-ray therapy (or chemotherapy) used before ^{131}I therapy has produced decreased effectiveness of subsequent ^{131}I therapy by decreasing the percent uptake and biologic half-life of ^{131}I in the thyroid carcinoma.

Place of Chemotherapy

I use chemotherapy when ^{131}I therapy and/or x-ray therapy are not indicated or have failed.

Treatment of Well-Differentiated Thyroid Cancer in Children

We have treated a total of 120 children with well-differentiated thyroid carcinoma 3 to 18 years of age at our institution from 1947 to 1982. The preparation for and the methods of treating children are the same as for adults. These treatments have resulted in a strikingly lower death rate than has been reported previously, 6 percent in patients referred to us for tertiary care.

We have published a follow-up on 40 children treated for thyroid cancer with a mean total dose of 196 mCi and a maximum total dose of 690 mCi and followed for periods of up to 25 years. There was no decreased fertility or increased incidence of abnormal birth history. None of these children had developed leukemia.[8]

Failure to Treat Young People With Lung Metastases With ^{131}I Because of Fear of Causing Pulmonary Fibrosis

Rall answered this question in an article in 1957. He showed that when he achieved less than 100 millicuries uptake of radioiodine in the lungs there was no subsequent pulmonary fibrosis. He achieved that unfavorable result only when there was more than 100 millicuries of uptake in the lungs with patients with diffuse bilateral metastases.[9] The highest percent uptake we have ever had in the lungs is 35 percent. Since we never give over 200 millicuries in a dose, it has been impossible for us to achieve a 100-millicurie treatment dose in the lungs, and we have never had a result of pulmonary fibrosis and deteriorating lung function.

Most Common Problems in Patients Referred to Our Tertiary Care Center

The most difficult problems that characterize patients referred to us for the treatment of thyroid carcinoma are (1) inadequate initial surgery, (2) reluctance on the part of the referring physician to treat the person who is young and curable aggressively, and (3) reluctance of the referring physician to stop treating an old patient with rapid and extensively growing carcinoma of the thyroid who is incurable by any method.

The most common problem we have faced in referrals from otolaryngologists is the initial use of a truly radical neck dissection in the treatment of carcinoma of the thyroid with metastases to the lymph nodes. There is general agreement that the truly radical neck dissection for well-differentiated thyroid cancer does not result in a decreased mortality, but does result in an increased morbidity. In the case of well-differentiated thyroid cancer, a radical neck resection is not necessary because of our ability to ablate this cancer in residual lymph nodes with radioactive iodine after initial surgery.

REFERENCES

1. Saad MF, Guido JJ, Samaan NA. Radioactive iodine in the treatment of medullary carcinoma of the thyroid. J Clin Endocrinol Metab 1983; 57:124.
2. Beierwaltes WH, Nishiyama RH, Thompson NW, Copp JE, Kubo A. Survival time and cure in papillary and follicular thyroid carcinoma with distant metastases: Statistics following University of Michigan therapy. J Nucl Med 1982; 23:561–568.
3. Beierwaltes WH. Controversies in the treatment of thyroid cancer: The University of Michigan approach. Thyroid Today 1983; 6(5):1–5.
4. Mazzaferri EL, Young RL. Papillary thyroid carcinoma: A 10-year follow-up report of the impact of therapy in 576 patients. Am J Med 1981; 70:511.
5. Maheshwaro TK, Hill CS Jr, Haynie TP III, et al. ^{131}I therapy in differentiated thyroid carcinoma: M.D. Anderson Hospital experience. Cancer 1981; 47:664.
6. Singer PA, Nicoloff JT, Stein RB, Joravillo J. Transient TRH deficiency after prolonged thyroid hormone therapy. Clin Endocrinol Metab 1978; 47:512.
7. Chabner BA. Second neoplasm—a complication of cancer chemotherapy. N Engl J Med (Editorial) 1977; 297:212.
8. Sarkar SD, Beierwaltes WH, Gill SR, Cowley BJ. Subsequent fertility and birth histories of children treated with ^{131}I for thyroid cancer. J Nucl Med 1976; 17:460–464.
9. Rall JE, Alpers JB, LeWallen CG. Radiation pneumonitis and fibrosis: A complication of radioiodine treatment of pulmonary metastases from cancer of the thyroid. J Clin Endocrinol 1957; 17:1263.

MEDULLARY THYROID CANCER: SURGICAL ASPECTS

MELVIN A. BLOCK, M.D., Ph.D.

Medullary thyroid carcinoma, though diagnosed in only 3 to 7 percent of thyroid carcinomas, possesses unique characteristics important in its management. These features, particularly its production of the humoral agent, calcitonin, as a marker, have made medullary thyroid carcinoma a tool in the understanding of certain basic characteristics of cancer.

BASIC CLINICAL FEATURES

The radioimmunoassay of serum calcitonin levels permits diagnosis, even before medullary thyroid carcinoma is manifest clinically, as well as an indication of persistent carcinoma in follow-up studies.[1] The clinical behavior of medullary thyroid carcinoma has been intermediate between the well-differentiated and the anaplastic thyroid carcinoma. This cancer originates from parafollicular cells, or C-cells, of the thyroid.

Medullary thyroid carcinoma is manifest in two major patterns, a sporadic variety and a hereditary form. The sporadic variety is characteristically unilateral, whereas the hereditary form is uniformly bilateral and associated with C-cell hyperplasia throughout all of the thyroid gland (Table 1).[2] Both forms have a predisposition to regional (cervical) lymph node metastases as well as distant metastases. Our experience indicates that when medullary thyroid carcinoma is palpable, cervical lymph node metastases are always present in the hereditary variety and in at least 50 percent of the sporadic cases.[2]

HEREDITARY MEDULLARY THYROID CARCINOMA

The hereditary form of medullary thyroid carcinoma occurs in families as an autosomal dominant inheritance. Jackson and associates have demonstrated a deletion within the short arm of chromosome 20 in patients with the multiple endocrine neoplasia (MEN)IIA and IIB types.[3] Screening of family members for elevation of serum calcitonin after provocative testing with pentagastrin, or a combina-

TABLE 1 Comparison of Essential Features of Hereditary and Sporadic Medullary Thyroid Carcinoma

Factor	Hereditary	Sporadic
Thyroid gland involvement	Uniformly bilateral	Unilateral
Diffuse C-cell hyperplasia	Present	Absent
Other endocrine disease	Present (MEN-II)	Absent or rare

tion of pentagastrin and calcium administration, permits detection of C-cell hyperplasia before the occurrence of medullary thyroid carcinoma. However, it is difficult to identify precisely the transition from C-cell hyperplasia to medullary thyroid cancer. It should be emphasized that recognition of medullary thyroid carcinoma can be achieved by screening tests before it is clinically evident or even evident by gross examination of the thyroid gland. It is only at this stage that operation has resulted in normal levels of serum calcitonin in our experience.[2]

C-cell hyperplasia may be the only finding in one or both thyroid lobes of a few patients in whom provocative testing by screening family members shows elevated levels of serum calcitonin. The concentration of C-cell hyperplasia or early medullary thyroid carcinoma characteristically is located in the central portion of the thyroid lobe, between the upper one-third and lower two-thirds of the lobe.

The hereditary form of medullary thyroid carcinoma really is a component of the multiple endocrine neoplasia-II (MEN-II) syndrome. Every patient in whom the diagnosis of medullary thyroid carcinoma is considered should be surveyed for the possibility of the multiple endocrine neoplasia syndrome.

The Multiple Endocrine Neoplasia-II (MEN-II) Syndrome. This familial syndrome comprises medullary thyroid carcinoma as its basic and uniform constituent with, in addition, pheochromocytoma and parathyroid hyperplasia occurring in some family members. The MEN-II syndrome appears to differ from the MEN-I syndrome in that all elements of the syndrome are not present in all affected individuals, whereas in the MEN-I syndrome, it appears that islet cell tumors of the pancreas, hyperparathyroidism, and pituitary tumors are present in all affected members. In the MEN-II syndrome, some families and some individuals of a given family do not demonstrate pheochromocytomas or other features of the syndrome other than medullary thyroid carcinoma.

The MEN-II syndrome is divided into two syndromes as follows: (1) *MEN-IIA syndrome*, which includes hyperparathyroidism in some individuals, but no mucosal neuromas, and (2) *MEN-IIB syndrome*, which does not include hyperparathyroidism, but uniformly includes features of mucosal neuromas. Both MEN-IIA and MEN-IIB patients uniformly have medullary thyroid carcinomas and some have pheochromocytomas as well.

Individuals with the MEN-IIB syndrome characteristically show facial and other features of mucosal neuromas at birth and manifestations of medullary thyroid carcinoma earlier in life than those with MEN-IIA. The doubling time of the medullary thyroid carcinoma appears to be more rapid in the MEN-IIA than the MEN-IIB syndrome. The more aggressive behavior of the MEN-IIB syndrome justifies early and extensive surgery for these patients, including those recognized in childhood.[4] There seems to be justification for performing total thyroidectomy solely on the basis of phenotype physical characteristics or of phenotype mapping of chromosome abnormalities for MEN-IIB without confirmatory elevation of a stimulated serum calcitonin level.[5]

The life-endangering manifestations of *pheochromocytoma* justify a search for this entity in patients with the MEN-II syndrome before thyroid operation is performed. Although evidence is not conclusive, it appears that pheochromocytoma or adrenal medullary hyperplasia is bilateral in these patients.

Hyperparathyroidism occurs in the MEN-IIA, but not the MEN-IIB.[6] Furthermore, it occurs unpredictably and only in some families. The hyperparathyroidism is usually mild. At operation for medullary thyroid carcinoma, an enlarged and hyperplastic parathyroid may be found in the absence of clinical evidence of hyperparathyroidism. Multiple parathyroid glands frequently are hyperplastic when hyperparathyroidism is present, but this is not uniformly true. In view of the mild manifestations of hyperparathyroidism, the parathyroid glands are preserved at the time of total thyroidectomy for medullary thyroid carcinoma unless they are grossly enlarged. If clinical manifestations of hyperparathyroidism are evident, a subtotal parathyroidectomy or total parathyroidectomy with autotransplantation of parathyroid tissue should be performed.

Policies for Operation. For patients with medullary thyroid carcinoma associated with the MEN syndromes, a total thyroidectomy is indicated in view of the uniform bilateral presence of carcinoma and/or C-cell hyperplasia and the diffuse presence of C-cell hyperplasia throughout the thyroid gland. Lymph nodes adjacent to the thyroid gland are removed, particularly if enlarged.

The indications for removal of cervical and anterior superior mediastinal lymph nodes in patients with medullary thyroid carcinoma of the MEN-II variety are not final, but a degree of selection appears to be justified. In my experience, the only patients of the MEN-II category who have had normal levels of serum calcitonin postoperatively have been those for whom the diagnosis was made early, by screening with provocative testing before any clinical evidence of thyroid cancer developed.[2] Thus, in this category of patients, it has been a policy to perform a total thyroidectomy and, at the time of operation, to remove midjugular lymph nodes on each side of the neck for frozen section study. If no microscopic evidence of metastatic carcinoma is found in these lymph nodes, a cervical and anterior superior mediastinal lymph node dissection is not performed. If metastatic carcinoma is present in these lymph nodes, an appropriate modified lateral cervical lymph node dissection and anterior superior mediastinal lymph node dissection are performed. Serum calcitonin levels can elevate many (10 or more) years later to indicate possible growth of minute amounts of metastatic carcinoma, not sufficient to produce elevations of serum

A

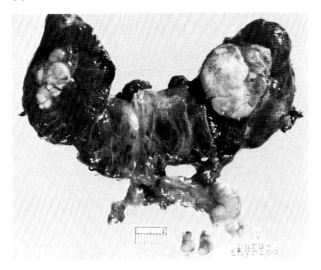

B

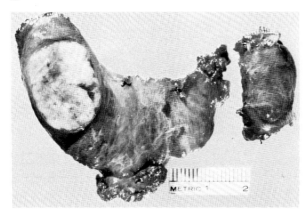

Figure 1 *A*, Thyroid gland involved by hereditary medullary thyroid carcinoma. Note bilateral lesions. An enlarged parathyroid gland was also removed. *B*, Thyroid gland involved by sporadic medullary thyroid carcinoma—unilateral lesions.

calcitonin earlier. If late elevation of serum calcitonin occurs, or if cervical lymphadenopathy develops, cervical lymph node dissections can then be performed. For patients with palpable medullary thyroid carcinoma, metastases to cervical lymph nodes have been uniformly present, justifying appropriate lateral cervical and anterior superior mediastinal lymph node dissections. In deciding whether or not to modify lateral cervical lymph node dissections from the classic radical procedure, the gross extent of metastatic disease in the neck, particularly with respect to invasion of structures outside the thyroid gland or cervical lymph nodes, provides a determining factor. Bilateral cervical lymph node dissection is performed when medullary thyroid carcinoma is bilaterally palpable or there is evidence of metastases to both sides of the neck. If a bilateral cervical lymph node dissection is performed, preservation of the internal jugular vein on one side of the neck is emphasized.

As previously noted, during thyroid operations for medullary thyroid carcinoma, care is given to evaluate parathyroid glands for gross enlargement. Enlarged parathyroid glands are removed, but emphasis is given to preservation of sufficient parathyroid tissue to ensure normal function. If clinical evidence of hyperparathyroidism is present, the high frequency of multiple gland involvement justifies subtotal parathyroidectomy.

SPORADIC MEDULLARY THYROID CARCINOMA

Sporadic medullary thyroid carcinoma is recognized now only after a palpable thyroid abnormality is present. Fine-needle aspiration biopsy permits recognition of this entity although difficulties in this specific diagnosis can be encountered.[7] An elevation of serum calcitonin can confirm a suspicion of medullary thyroid carcinoma on the basis of needle biopsy, diarrhea, or other manifestations of medullary thyroid carcinoma.

Once medullary thyroid carcinoma is identified, a reasonable attempt is made to determine whether a familial occurrence is present (screen family members) or whether the patient has manifestations of other endocrine disease consistent with the MEN-II syndrome.

In our experience, the sporadic variety of medullary thyroid carcinoma is unilateral, is not associated with diffuse C-cell hyperplasia in the thyroid outside the carcinoma, and is not associated with other endocrine disease (see Table 1). It may spread to regional lymph nodes with a lesser degree of frequency than the hereditary variety in view of our experience that approximately 50 percent of patients had normal serum calcitonin levels postoperatively even in the presence of palpable thyroid carcinomas preoperatively.[2]

Policies for Operations. If sporadic medullary thyroid carcinoma is recognized preoperatively or at the time of operation, a total or near-total thyroidectomy appears reasonable to ensure adequate removal of the neoplasm and provide adequate treatment if the patient should prove subsequently to have the hereditary variety. There is evidence that the hereditary type of medullary thyroid carcinoma, especially the MEN-IIB type, originates in a single individual.[5] Rossi and associates reported that nonfamilial medullary thyroid carcinoma appeared in one and C-cell hyperplasia appeared in the other of identical twins.[8] The high frequency of lymph node metastases justifies an appropriate lateral cervical lymph node dissection on the side of the thyroid carcinoma as well as a removal of lymph nodes in the anterior superior mediastinum. Bilateral cervical node dissections are considered unnecessary, except in the unusual case in which contralateral lymph node metastases occur.

If the diagnosis of medullary thyroid carcinoma is made in retrospect postoperatively, the level of serum calcitonin should be determined. In addition, the thyroid tissue removed should be studied for diffuse C-cell hyperplasia which, if present, indicates the hereditary variety. If the serum calcitonin is elevated, consideration should be given to performance of total thyroidectomy and removal of lymph nodes in the neck if this was not performed at the initial operation.

POSTOPERATIVE CARE

In cases of medullary thyroid carcinoma, serum calcitonin levels provide an extremely sensitive indicator

A

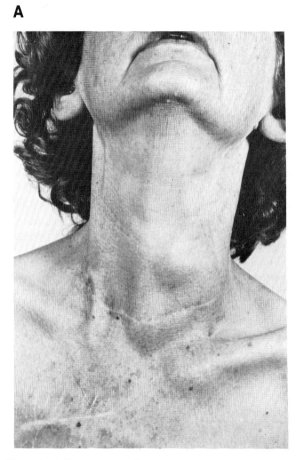

B

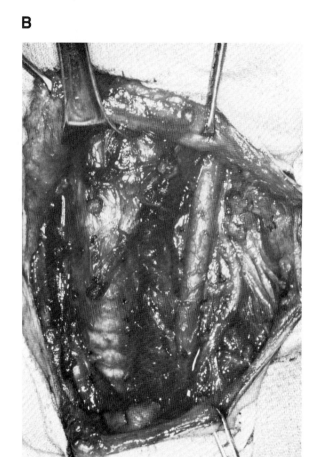

Figure 2 *A*, Recurrent sporadic medullary thyroid carcinoma in left neck, appearing 10 years after total thyroidectomy. *B*, Operative appearance of the neck following dissection of the recurrent carcinoma in left cervical lymph nodes.

of the presence of residual carcinoma after operation. Experience has demonstrated that occult metastases are common in medullary thyroid carcinoma and may never become clinically significant.[9] This is probably true for many malignant tumors for which a similar marker is not available.

For the hereditary variety of medullary thyroid carcinoma, normal levels of serum calcitonin following appropriate neck surgery have been obtained, for the most part, only in those patients with preclinical lesions identified by screening studies. Even in these cases, elevation of serum calcitonin may occur more than 10 years postoperatively.[4] Thus, prolonged follow-up is needed including periodic determination of serum calcitonin levels, performed at varying intervals on the basis of existing levels and evidence of interval change.

In the sporadic form of medullary thyroid carcinoma, appropriate neck operation is more likely than in the hereditary variety to result in normal serum calcitonin levels in our experience. These patients, of course, all had palpable thyroid lesions preoperatively. Periodic determination of serum calcitonin levels, along with physical examination of the neck, are justified for this group of patients.

The question arises as to what action is needed for pa-

tients in whom serum calcitonin levels remain elevated postoperatively. We have elected to treat recurrent medullary thyroid carcinoma only if it becomes symptomatic. For the majority of patients, the residual metastatic medullary thyroid carcinoma remains occult for the remainder of the patient's life. In some patients who complete their life expectancy and ultimately die from other causes, autopsy studies have shown only microscopic metastases to lymph nodes in the mediastinum and in residual cervical lymph nodes.[10] Thus reoperation or extensive studies to search for occult metastatic medullary thyroid carcinoma have not been cost-effective; these metastases seem to have no clinical significance in a large percentage of patients.

The only effective treatment for residual or recurrent medullary thyroid carcinoma is surgery. Thus it is important to examine the neck periodically for clinically recurrent medullary thyroid carcinoma and to reoperate if this is the only, or the dominant, recurrence. It is possible that the only, or dominant, recurrence is in the neck. Even though removal of recurrent disease in the neck may not provide cure on the basis of a return to normal serum calcitonin levels, the life-endangering potential of this recurrence is removed. With initial neck operations for medullary thyroid carcinoma now being more adequate, recurrence in the neck is becoming less frequent.[10] The critical surgical treatment for medullary thyroid carcinoma is early and thorough eradication from the neck.

In our experience, operation for distant metastases has not been justified in any significant frequency because, when they are clinically evident, removal is not feasible from the standpoint of local technical factors and/or presence of significant multiple metastases. As noted previously, a search for and removal of occult metastases has not been of real value on the basis of cost-benefit, multiplicity of metastases, technical difficulties, and evidence that many patients survive long periods of time without significant growth of these metastases.[10]

If during the postoperative follow-up period the levels of serum calcitonin elevate progressively, a search for recurrence, especially in the neck, is justified. If an operable metastasis is identified, an attempt to remove it is justified. It has been reported that ^{99mtc}(V) dimercaptosuccinic acid concentrates in medullary thyroid carcinoma and its metastases.[11] Metastases with a volume less than 10 cm^3 have been detected using axial transverse tomoscintigraphy in patients injected with ^{131}I-labeled monoclonal antibodies against carcinoembryonic antigen.[12]

Although surgery remains the only curative therapy for medullary thyroid carcinoma, external radiation therapy and radioactive iodine have been reported to be of benefit occasionally.[13,14] This is not entirely understandable in view of the recognized parafollicular cell origin of the neoplasm. However, there may be variants of medullary thyroid carcinoma which, for reasons not now understood, may have characteristics resembling carcinoma arising from follicular cells of the thyroid. Furthermore, some thyroid carcinoma may demonstrate characteristics of both follicular and parafollicular variations.[15] Thus we have encountered a patient with typical sporadic medullary thyroid carcinoma identified postoperatively on the basis of microscopic studies of slides prepared with haemotoxylin and eosin, but for whom immunocytochemical studies of the tissue failed to identify the presence of calcitonin.

Postoperative follow-up should also include periodic serum calcium determinations to check for possible hyperparathyroidism. Patients require thyroid hormone therapy after total thyroidectomy.

The results of treatment are improving as a better understanding of medullary thyroid carcinoma leads to earlier diagnosis and treatment. With early employment of treatment modalities, control of the disease appears possible for most patients. Medullary thyroid carcinoma having histologic features of an anaplastic carcinoma has a poorer prognosis than that with a more differentiated pattern.

REFERENCES

1. Block MA, Jackson CE, Tashjian AH Jr. Medullary thyroid carcinoma detected by serum calcitonin assay. Arch Surg 1972; 104:579–586.
2. Block MA, Jackson CE, Greenawald KA, Yott JB, Tashjian AH Jr. Clinical characteristics distinguishing hereditary from sporadic medullary thyroid carcinoma. Arch Surg 1980; 115:142–148.
3. Babu VR, VanDyke DL, Jackson CE, Miyeda K. Absence of increased chromosome instability in multiple endocrine neoplasia type 2 syndrome. Am J Hum Genet 1983; 35:59A.
4. Jackson CE, Talpos GB, Block MA, Norum RA, Lloyd RV, Tashjian AH Jr. Clinical value of tumor doubling estimations in multiple endocrine neoplasia type II (MEN-II). Surgery 1984; 96:981–986.
5. Jones BA, Sisson JC. Early diagnosis and thyroidectomy in multiple endocrine neoplasia, type 2b. J Pediatr 1983; 102:617–724.
6. Block MA, Jackson CE, Tashjian AH Jr. Management of parathyroid glands in surgery for medullary thyroid carcinoma. Arch Surg 1975; 110:617–624.
7. Kini SR, Miller JM, Hamburger JI, Smith MJ. Cytopathologic features of medullary carcinoma of the thyroid. Arch Pathol Lab Med 1984; 108:156–159.
8. Rossi RL, Cady B, Meissner WA, Wool MS, Sedwich CE, Werber J. Non familial medullary thyroid carcinoma. Am J Surg 1980; 139:554–560.
9. Block MA, Jackson CE, Tashjian AH Jr. Management of occult medullary thyroid carcinoma: Evidenced only by serum calcitonin level elevations after apparently adequate neck operation. Arch Surg 1978; 113:368–372.
10. Jackson CE, Talpos GB, Kambouris A, Yott JB, Tashjian AH Jr, Block MA. The clinical course after definitive operation for medullary thyroid carcinoma. Surgery 1983; 94:995–1001.
11. Ohta H, Yamamoto K, Endo K, Mori T, Hamanaka D, Shimazo A, Ikekubo K, Mahimoto K, Iida Y, Konishi J, Moritu R, Hata N, Horiuchi K, Yokoyama A, Torizoka K, Koma K. A new imaging agent for medullary carcinoma of the thyroid. J Nuclear Med 1984; 25:323–325.
12. Berche C, Mach JP, Lumbroso JD, Langlais C, Aubry F, Buchegger F, Carrel S, Rougier P, Parmentier C, Tubiana M. Tomoscintigraphy for detecting gastrointestinal and medullary thyroid cancers: First clinical results using radio labeled monoclonal antibodies against carcinoembryonic antigen. Clin Res 1982; 285:1447–1451.
13. Deftos LJ, Stein MF. Radioiodine as an adjunct to the surgical treatment of medullary thyroid carcinoma. J Clin Endocrinol Metab 1980; 50:967–968.
14. Simpson WJ, Palmer JA, Rosen IB, Mustard RA. Management of medullary carcinoma of the thyroid. Am J Surg 1982; 144:420–422.
15. Simonton SC, Sibley RK. Immunohistochemical analysis of follicular and papillary thyroid tumors. Lab Invest 1984; 50:55A.

ASPIRATION BIOPSY OF THE THYROID

WILLIAM J. FRABLE, M.D.

HISTORY

During the Battle of Cerisoles in 1544, a young Swiss soldier, Philip von Hohendax, was struck in the neck with a pick. Fortunately, Philip had a large goiter which was cystic. As reported by Crotti, the cyst drained and Philip survived.[1] Ashcraft et al have noted the episode as perhaps the first recorded treatment of a thyroid cyst by aspiration.[2]

Needle biopsy of the thyroid gland has had a few enthusiasts for some time. However, core or tissue needle biopsy has never become the general practice in the diagnosis of thyroid disease.[3-5] Why this is not a generally accepted procedure is still unclear. Complications, as reported by its proponents, have been few, with only two documented cases in which malignant tumor was implanted in the needle tract.[3,5]

Since the 1950s Europeans have embraced wholeheartedly the fine-needle aspiration biopsy technique for thyroid lesions, particularly cold nodules. In the past several years, the fine-needle aspiration biopsy method has enjoyed remarkable popularity within the United States. Several large series have been reported.[6-10] Since publication of my experience in 1980, there have been at least thirty citations concerning this procedure and its result within the American literature, including a comprehensive review by Ashcraft et al.[2,11] Some of these investigators employed both fine-needle aspiration biopsy and tissue needle biopsy, depending on the clinical situation and suspected lesion.[12,13]

INDICATIONS

Any enlargement of the thyroid may be examined by biopsy, but the major indication is a solitary nodule. Usually the solitary thyroid mass is cold, but recent reports suggest that aspiration before radioisotope uptake is the most cost-effective plan of management.[14] Multiple aspirations may be made of diffusely enlarged glands or multinodular thyroids, but it is the determination of the presence of a neoplasm in a patient with a solitary thyroid mass that is the raison d'etre for aspiration biopsy of the thyroid.

TECHNIQUE

I have used a 22-gauge $1^{1}/_{2}$-inch needle attached to a 20-ml syringe with a commercially available syringe pistol to perform aspiration biopsy of the thyroid. The details of the technique have been described elsewhere.[15] The patient should be correctly positioned so as to maximize the prominence of the mass to be examined. The best way to accomplish this is to place the patient in a supine position with a small pillow beneath the shoulders and upper back so that the neck is fully extended. Glass slides and all other necessary equipment should be readily at hand before the procedure is begun.

Some thyroid nodules may actually be more prominent with the patient in the sitting position. Fine-needle aspiration can be performed with the patient sitting up if there is a headrest on the back of the examining chair. Occasionally I have used a small skin-marking pencil to outline the area of the lesion so that the needle will traverse as little soft tissue as possible before entering the nodule. The sternocleidomastoid muscle should be avoided and can be pushed laterally with extension of the neck.[11]

Since the majority of thyroid nodules, even single cold masses, are areas of goiter, the aspirate is likely to demonstrate blood in the hub of the syringe quite quickly. It is important to terminate the aspiration at that point so as not to dilute the cells present with large amounts of blood. If several milliliters of blood are obtained, that portion of the specimen should be set aside for a cell block and the material within the needle used to prepare smears. The somewhat firm lesion of Hashimoto's thyroiditis may require vigorous aspiration to obtain a specimen, and true neoplasms themselves usually have a more solid feel at aspiration. This information is of value in making a final cytologic interpretation and is probably a contributing factor to the successful results of some European and American investigators.[16]

Fluid aspirated from a cyst should be processed by means of standard cytologic methods. My current preference is a cytospin preparation of cyst fluid as it provides excellent cytologic detail and a small area within which the cells will be displayed for convenient review. When a cyst is encountered, every attempt is made to aspirate it completely, following which the patient should be carefully re-examined for any residual mass. It is quite important to make a second aspiration of any residual mass to reduce further the possibility of missing a small neoplasm near or within a thyroid cyst.

My personal series encompasses 670 aspirations during the period from 1973 through 1983. There were 46 unsatisfactory aspirations of which nine were repeated and suitable material obtained. An additional ten aspirates were judged to have low cellularity and therefore not considered completely satisfactory. The usual reason for failure of an aspiration is missing the lesion. From the clinical follow-up to date, no neoplasm went undiagnosed in the remaining patients who did not have repeat aspirations.

COLLOID AND ADENOMATOUS GOITER

The common non-neoplastic lesions which make up the majority of thyroid aspirations fall into the categories of nodular goiter, toxic hyperplasia, thyroiditis, and cysts.[11]

Multiple or single masses of colloid and/or adenomatous goiter are the most commonly encountered thyroid enlargement that is aspirated. Because of the abundant colloid they are relatively acellular, and they do not lend themselve to core needle biopsy. In a recent report by Wang and Vickery, 50 percent of colloid nodules failed to provide a diagnostic biopsy. To overcome this, those authors now aspirate colloid nodules through the core needle.[17]

The aspiration smears are composed of a mixture of colloid and sheets and/or single or small groups of thyroid epithelial cells. The colloid is present in clumps that will stain a deep blue with Romanowsky stains (May-Grunwald-Giemsa) or appear as a variable pink-to-blue background covering most of the smear. The individual thyroid cells are quite uniform. As Zajicek and Franzen have pointed out, if colloid is easily seen on a thyroid aspiration smear, the presumption is that it is benign and not a true neoplasm. This rule proves exceedingly useful, though not absolute.[18] Colloid material stains variably orange, green, or yellow with Papanicolaou stain. Occasionally whole thyroid acini are found to contain a central mass of colloid.

Frequent histiocytes, some with hemosiderin pigment, will be found in aspirates from goiter and reflect areas of degeneration with old hemorrhage. Sheets of fibroblasts may also be found along with some enlarged and bizarre looking cells that are said by Broese to represent degenerating cells seen with goiters. These can be extremely atypical, but are present in only very small numbers.[19]

Because toxic hyperplasia is clinically quite evident, there is usually no need to aspirate such cases. In my few examples, the thyroid epithelium has been uniform, but with some variation in nuclear size. There may be some colloid, but it is rather thin and scanty. The cytoplasm of thyroid cells in Graves' disease has been described as finely vacuolated, the vacuoles being small and nearly invisible.[18]

THYROIDITIS

Cytologic features of Hashimoto's thyroiditis reveal abundant lymphocytes with focal collections of degenerating thyroid cells. In some areas the lymphocytes appear to be attached to the thyroid cells. The cellular infiltrate is mixed, composed of both lymphocytes and plasma cells. There are large pale lightly metachromatic cells with a lobulated nucleus and abundant cytoplasm. They occur in sheets or as single cells, representing the oncocytic or Askanazy cells, which are usually found as the histologic hallmark of Hashimoto's thyroiditis. It is rare to find colloid present on these smears. If both thyroid lobes are enlarged, the bilaterality of the disease can be confirmed by performing several aspiration biopsies.

Localized areas of chronic lymphocytic thyroiditis may present clinically as a solitary mass. Usually some lymphocytic and plasma cell infiltrate is found in the smear, but the typical oncocytes may not be present, while large sheets of thyroid epithelial cells and some reactive atypical but degenerated cells are found. These regressive cell changes that occur in some cases of thyroiditis as well as adenomatous goiter have also been described by Droese.[19]

Aspirations of giant cell thyroiditis have been rare in my series. The patients presented with multiple and/or single nodules. The smears have a composition of spindle-shaped histiocytic or epitheloid cells forming recognizable granulomas accompanied by a variable inflammatory infiltrate and the presence of multinucleated giant cells. The clustering of the spindle-shaped epithelial cells and their overlapping arrangement may suggest cell fragments of papillary carcinoma (Fig. 1). Since both papillary carcinoma and giant cell thyroiditis may have multinucleated giant cells, the cytologic pattern can occasionally be difficult to interpret. One aspirate of this type led to a false-positive diagnosis of papillary carcinoma of the thyroid.

In all cases of thyroiditis, the basic usefulness of the aspiration biopsy is to establish, on a firmer basis, the clinical diagnosis. Thus, an open biopsy or more extensive surgery is avoided, and the patient is reassured.

CYSTS

Perhaps the most immediate beneficial effect of aspiration biopsy is the removal of cyst fluid. Morphologically, however, aspiration of cysts is the least rewarding procedure. Surgical excision of thyroid cysts is often avoided when they are aspirated successfully. This has occurred in two out of three cases in my experience.

The composition of the contents of cysts results from old hemorrhage and degeneration within colloid and adenomatous goiter, leaving a turbid brown fluid or, occasionally, fluid that is clear, cloudy, or yellow in color. Most of the cells found in cyst fluid are histiocytes (macrophages) containing cytoplasmic deposits of hemosiderin. If thyroid epithelium is found, it should be studied carefully for any indication of

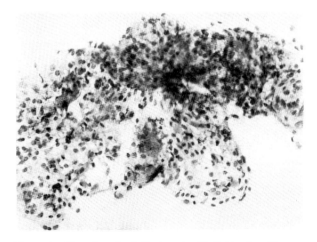

Figure 1 Clustering of spindle-shaped epithelioid cells with some nuclear clearing evident in the peripheral cells. Pattern suggested a possible papillary carcinoma from the aspirate of this solitary thyroid nodule. Histologic diagnosis was giant cell thyroiditis. Papanicolaou stain, × 300.

neoplastic alterations, specifically intranuclear inclusion bodies that might indicate papillary carcinoma. Papillary carcinoma of the thyroid may in part be cystic.[20,21]

NEOPLASMS

Hamburger et al have succinctly summarized the problem of the thyroid nodule by stating:

> Many patients have thyroid nodules; some nodules are malignant but not many; some patients die of thyroid cancer but not many; some patients with thyroid cancer are saved from death by surgical treatment but not many; some patients with thyroid nodules experience important complications from surgical treatment, in some instances even death. Therefore, the excision of all thyroid nodules to prevent death from thyroid cancer is not only impractical, but may do more harm than good.[13]

A simple diagnostic technique such as fine-needle aspiration biopsy is effective in detecting those patients who truly need surgical excision of their thyroid nodule. This has been the major thrust of needle biopsy of either tissue or aspiration type.[22,23]

The close resemblance between follicular adenomas and low-grade follicular carcinoma of the thyroid contributes to some inaccuracy with thin-needle aspiration biopsy. This differential diagnosis is also difficult from a histologic point of view, depending almost exclusively on the demonstration of vascular invasion for the diagnosis of carcinoma. The majority of authors agree that it is not possible to differentiate these two lesions on the basis of the aspiration biopsy smear alone,[6,18,24,25] but there is not complete agreement on this point. The reports of Krisch, who used morphometric diameter of the nuclei as an indicator of malignancy in follicular neoplasms,[26] and Lang et al, who used very fine cytologic criteria,[9] successfully made the separation.

Luck and Frable were not able to make a distinction between follicular adenoma and low-grade follicular carcinoma on the basis of nuclear area measurements in a small series of cases,[27] but Beyer Boon and her colleagues did show a statistically significant difference in a larger series of cases. As discussed with Dr. Boon, the contrasting results may be based on the use of different fixation methods. The Diff-Quick stain employed by Luck and Frable has as its fixative methyl alcohol in a concentration of nearly 100 percent, whereas the concentration of alcohol in the traditional formulation of the May-Grunwald-Giemsa stain, as used by Boon, is only 50 percent. Alcohol is known to cause cell shrinkage and, in the study of Luck and Frable, may have narrowed the nuclear size measurements between follicular adenoma and low-grade follicular carcinoma to the point that no significant difference could be detected.[29] Because of this difficulty, even with the most sophisticated cytologic methods, the preferred reporting when confronted with a follicular adenoma versus follicular carcinoma is "follicular neoplasm, adenoma versus low-grade follicular carcinoma." Figure 2 compares follicular adenoma with low-grade follicular carcinoma.

Thin-needle aspiration biopsies from adenomas, low-grade follicular carcinomas, or other definite thyroid cancers are usually highly cellular with a complete or nearly complete absence of colloid. With follicular adenoma the nuclei are slightly larger than those of normal thyroid epithelium. Uniform nucleoli are noted, but not in every cell. Chromatin structure tends to be finely granular and similar for follicular adenoma and low-grade follicular carcinoma. It is not surprising, therefore, that the measurements of the nuclear DNA have failed to reveal any significant difference.[30]

The other malignant neoplasms of the thyroid are usually easily recognized. I have had experience with at least one case of all of the various varieties, including two malignant lymphomas.

Papillary carcinomas of the thyroid are probably one of the easiest tumors to identify by aspiration biopsy because the smear may contain three-dimensional papillary fragments and some cells that have the characteristic intranuclear inclusions.[31] Four additional features of aspiration biopsy smears important to the cytologic diagnosis were found by Kini et al: monolayered sheets, tissue fragments, psammoma bodies, and multinucleated giant cells.[32]

The general composition of the smear reveals a total absence of colloid and many sheets or actual clusters of thyroid cells. The cells may not always appear in papillary formation and depth of focus is required to view them. The consistent appearance of some cells with glassy intranuclear inclusions is extremely important. I have found them in all my cases of papillary thyroid carcinoma.

Two cases of Hürthle cell carcinoma were diagnosed by biopsy and did not differ significantly from Hürthle cell adenoma. Clinically, both appeared to be malignant. It is not to be expected that on pure cytologic grounds Hürthle cell tumors would be predictable since they are also unpredictable histologically. Kini et al has had a similar experience with a series of 70 cases of Hürthle cell tumors diagnosed by aspiration biopsy.[33]

Aspirates from medullary carcinoma are quite cellular with either a spindle cell pattern or a predominance of round cells in sheets. Irregular acellular clumps of amorphous material may indicate the presence of amyloid, but must be distinguished from colloid. A characteristic red granularity of the cytoplasm is seen in many of the tumor cells. Several authors have correctly diagnosed medullary carcinoma on aspiration biopsy from both the cell pattern and the presence of the amyloid material.[24,25,34,35]

The giant cell and anaplastic thyroid carcinomas are quite obvious clinically, and aspiration provides a simple way to confirm the diagnosis. Smears reveal both the marked cellularity and pleomorphism that characterize giant cell thyroid cancer.[36] Anaplastic

A

B

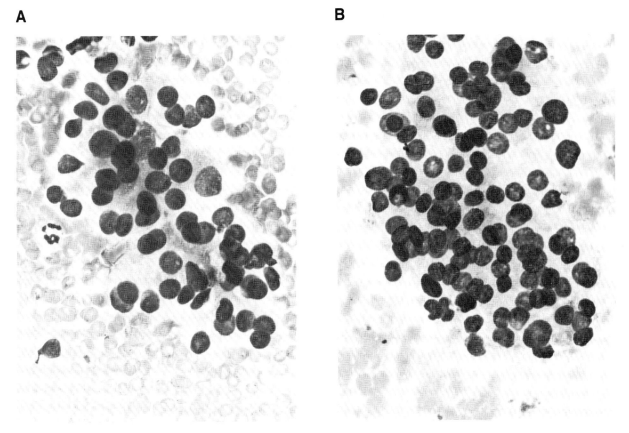

Figure 2 Comparison of cells aspirated from follicular adenoma, *A*, and low-grade follicular carcinoma, *B*. The nuclei actually appear larger and more variable in size in the aspirate from the adenoma than they do in the smear from the low-grade follicular carcinoma. Diff-Quick stain, × 600.

carcinomas of the small cell type, however, may be mistaken for lymphomas, and one must be careful to look for cellular cohesion.[19,25,37]

RESULTS

My personal experience is summarized in Tables 1 through 4. Sensitivity for the presence of a thyroid neoplasm, specificity for its absence, the predictive value of a positive diagnosis for a thyroid neoplasm, and diagnostic efficiency are all over 90 percent (Table 2).

Seven percent of the aspirates were unsatisfactory. There has been one false-negative for a follicular carcinoma in this group, a case in which metastatic carcinoma was diagnosed from an aspirate of the ileum, but the thyroid carcinoma producing that metastasis could not be aspirated because of an unusual degree of calcification of the capsule. Slightly less than 14 percent of the total aspirates were actually proved to be neoplasms (see Tables 1 and 3).

One incidental occult carcinoma occurred in the same lobe in which a nodular goiter had been successfully aspirated. This carcinoma was not clinically detected either. Because this patient was a child, surgery was undertaken. Beahrs and McConahey of the Mayo Clinic believe that aspiration biopsy of a soli-

TABLE 1 Thyroid Aspiration Biopsy

	Cytologic Diagnosis	False–Positive	False–Negative
Neoplasms			
Benign	(46)		
Follicular adenoma	38	(5)	
Hürthle cell adenoma	7		(1)
Schwannoma	1		
Malignant	(47)		
Follicular carcinoma vs. adenoma	8		
Papillary carcinoma	20	(1)	
Hürthle cell carcinoma	2		
Medullary carcinoma	1		
Giant cell and anaplastic carcinoma	13		
Metastatic carcinoma	2		
Lymphoma	1		
Goiter	316		(4)
Hyperplasia	7		
Normal Thyroid	59		
Cysts	57		
Thyroiditis	(85)		
Lymphocytic (Hashimoto's)	39		(1)
Acute	2		
Chronic nonspecific	40		
Granulomatous	4	(1)	
Unsatisfactory aspirations	46		(1)
Total aspirations	(670)		

TABLE 2   Thyroid Aspiration Biopsy: Predictive Value for a Thyroid Neoplasm

	True-Positive	False-Negative	Total
Number with neoplasm			
92	86	6	92
	False-Positive	True-Negative	
Number without neoplasm			
524	7	517	524
	True-Positive + False-Positive	False-Negative + True-Negative	
Totals 616	93	523	616

Sensitivity for a thyroid neoplasm	86/92	93%
Specificity for absence of thyroid neoplasm	517/524	98%
Predictive value of a positive aspirate	86/93	92%
Efficiency of diagnosis for neoplasm	606/616	97%

tary nodule of the thyroid in a child aged 15 years or younger is not indicated. Because they find that at least 50 percent of thyroid nodules in children are neoplasms, they prefer to proceed directly to surgical excision.[38]

Table 4 is a summary of false-negative and false-positive reports of thyroid aspiration biopsies in this series in respect to the diagnosis of a neoplasm (12 cases) or an exact classification of a thyroid tumor (2 cases). The most common problem was either overdiagnosis of adenomatous goiter as follicular neo-

TABLE 3   Thyroid Aspiration Biopsy: Actual Thyroid Neoplasms Confirmed Histologically

Follicular type	(45)
Adenoma	37
Carcinoma	8
Hürthle cell type	(10)
Adenoma	8
Carcinoma	2
Papillary carcinoma	18
Giant cell carcinoma	13
Other malignant neoplasms	5
Benign schwannoma	1

TABLE 4   Thyroid Aspiration Biopsy: Summary of False-Negative and False-Positive Diagnoses

	Cytologic Diagnosis	Histologic Diagnosis
False-positive reports		
	Follicular adenoma–5	Adenomatous goiter–5
	Suspect papillary carcinoma–2	Follicular adenoma–1
		Giant cell thyroiditis–1
False-negative reports	Adenomatous goiter–4	Follicular adenoma–4
	Hürthle cell adenoma–1	Hürthle cell carcinoma–1
	Hashimoto's thyroiditis–1	NonHodgkin's lymphoma–1
	unsatisfactory–1	Follicular carcinoma–1

plasms (false-positive, 5 cases) or underdiagnosis of an adenoma as adenomatous goiter (false-negative, 4 cases). The first error is the result of smears with high cellularity and a microfollicular pattern with small amounts of colloid; the second, the result of hemorrhage and degeneration in adenomas that may provide heterogeneous cell population and colloid as seen in typical smears from adenomatous goiter. Since less than 10 percent of the patients with nodules having an aspirate not reported as a neoplasm have been operated on, there may be other false-negative cases. To date, however, thyroid suppression has stabilized these lesions or caused them to regress, suggesting that the remaining number of potentially missed adenomas is likely to be small.

Not surprisingly, one case of a Hürthle cell neoplasm was classified as probably only adenoma and histologically was considered a carcinoma, whereas two cases of suspected papillary carcinoma, based on the aspiration smear, were histologically found to be a follicular adenoma and a case of giant cell thyroiditis. The latter is of interest because of the highly localized nature of the process and the large cellular fragments seen on the aspiration smear suggesting an epithelial neoplasm. In one patient a large thyroid mass was misdiagnosed as Hashimoto's thyroiditis. The smear was quite cellular, but the severe atypia of the lymphocyte population went unrecognized as lymphoma in this case. Because of the patient's severe dyspnea, an open biopsy of the thyroid was promptly performed, resulting in a correct diagnosis of thyroid lymphoma.

I have previously summarized the results of several series of thin-needle aspiration biopsies. False-negative and false-positive rates were compared along with the percentage of unsatisfactory smears. False-negatives ranged from 0.3 to 6.0 percent, whereas false-positives were 0 to 2.5 percent. These percentages are based on the total number of cases in each series.[11]

In a comprehensive review, Ashcraft et al have reviewed and compared the accuracy of needle aspiration with a fine needle, aspiration using a large needle, Vim-Silverman core biopsy, and drill biopsy of the thyroid. They divided the aspiration biopsy reports into those in which all patients subsequently had surgery and those in which patients were selected for surgery based on results of the aspiration biopsy and on other clinical and laboratory findings. In the first group of eight series, 848 cases had a benign aspiration report; 2.6 percent of this group were found on surgical excision to have malignant tumor of the thyroid. From these same series, 482 patients had an aspirate reported as either malignant or suspicious for malignancy; 1.5 percent of these were not confirmed as malignant histologically. Fifty-one aspirates were insufficient, and no malignancy was found in this group following surgery. The second group (surgery on a selective basis) comprised 20 reports with similar results, 2.4 percent false-negative among benign aspirates, 2.6 percent false-positives from the group of malignant and suspicious reports, and 1.1 percent malignant disease from the insufficient group of cases. There were 9161 benign aspirates, of which 2368 actually underwent operation; 1711 cases were reported in these combined series as malignant or suspicious and 1271 underwent operation. Six hundred and ninety two did not show malignancy, but only 33 showed no neoplasm at all. The false-positive rate is based on the failure to find *any* neoplasm in the thyroid.[2]

Among reports of large-needle aspiration biopsy, the eight reports were considered together with the following results: 3.3 percent false-negative biopsies among 553 cases, of which 184 were operated on; 4.0 percent false-positive rate for malignant thyroid tumor among 183 cases, of which 174 were operated on; and no malignancy in 138 cases with insufficient biopsy material, of which 23 were operated on.[2]

Vim-Silverman core needle biopsy (seven reports) resulted in a false-negative rate of 6.0 percent among 1586 cases, of which 168 were operated on; and 1.1 percent false-positive rate from 180 cases, of which 119 were operated on; and 7.4 percent rate of malignancy found at surgery from the insufficient biopsy group of 297 cases, of which 40 were operated on.[2]

With drill biopsy (three series), 56 of 85 cases operated on were reported benign with a 1.8 percent false-negative rate; there were no false-positives in four of four cases operated on.[2]

The authors concluded that no biopsy technique was clearly superior to any other; fine-needle aspiration had a lower yield of insufficient cases and is essentially free of complications in comparison to core needle biopsies.[2]

Since this very extensive review, a number of additional series using fine-needle aspiration[39-42] or comparing aspiration and core biopsy have appeared.[44-46] The results have been equally good.

COST AND IMPACT ON THYROID SURGERY

Recent concerns over the rapidly increasing costs of medical care have placed new emphasis on changes in the way medical problems are handled. Kaminsky compared the cost of evaluating the thyroid nodule by outpatient fine-needle aspiration with that for inpatient surgical therapy. He compared costs of thyroid aspiration biopsy ($100.00), scan ($215.00), ultrasound ($120.00), T_3 and T_4 uptake ($35.00), and physician's office charge for full medical evaluation ($100.00) with in-hospital surgical management of a thyroid nodule if it were found to be benign ($2700.00) or malignant ($4300.00). Clearly, from a cursory glance at these individual costs, considerable sums could be saved if aspiration could effectively select those patients most in need of thyroid surgery for a true neoplasms.[47]

Miller et al and Hamburger have provided more specific data from their large combined experience. They found that the use of needle aspiration or needle biopsy has decreased the number of patients needing surgery of their thyroid and doubled the percentage of cancers found in those patients operated on. Translated into specific figures, 1075 patients were saved $150.00 each by elimination of blood studies, ultrasound, or imaging with radionucleotides; $2500.00 was saved for 258 patients who were spared operation on the basis of needle aspiration or tissue needle biopsy results. This was a total of $806,250.00 or $750.00 per patient studied.[22]

In a similar evaluation, the Mayo Clinic found that thyroid aspiration biopsy reduced the nonsurgical patient cost by $400.00.[23]

COMPLICATIONS

Aspiration biopsy of the thyroid is virtually complication-free. I have seen one case of hematoma, which developed several hours after aspiration and delayed surgery for 2 weeks while it resolved. The patient had a correct aspiration biopsy diagnosis of papillary carcinoma from a cold nodule lying on the medial border of the left lobe of the thyroid. A few other patients have experienced transient light-headedness. Low pulse rates of 40 per minute have confirmed the suspicion that this is a result of vagus nerve stimulation.

Complications have been more frequent with Vim-Silverman needle biopsy, but still relatively few. Wang and Vickery reported four cases of hematoma, two of tracheal compression, two of transient laryngeal palsy, and one of implantation of a renal cell carcinoma, which had metastasized to the thyroid, within the needle tract folllowing core biopsy. This series numbers more than 1200 biopsies.[5] Crile reported one tumor implant in the skin following biopsy of a papillary carcinoma of the thyroid, one hematoma, and one transient paralysis of a vocal cord; Hamburger et al noted an occasional minor hematoma among 1023 needle biopsies of the thyroid.[3,13]

I believe that Ashcraft et al are quite correct when they state: "To continue to scorn the usefulness of fine-needle aspiration must reflect either unwarranted conservatism or ignorance of the data." I share their belief that fine-needle aspiration is the initial diagnostic test to be applied to the evaluation of a thyroid nodule.[2]

REFERENCES

1. Crotti A. Diseases of the thyroid, parathyroids and thymus. Philadelphia: Lea & Febiger, 1938:350.
2. Ashcraft MW, Van Herle AJ. Management of thyroid nodules. II.Scanning techniques, thyroid suppressive therapy, and fine needle aspiration. Head Neck Surg 1981; 3:297–322.
3. Crile G Jr. Struma lymphomatosa and carcinoma of the thyroid. Surg Gynecol Obstet 1978; 147:350–352.
4. Hawk WA Jr, Crile G Jr, Hazard JB, et al. Needle biopsy of the thyroid gland. Surg Gynecol Obstet 1966; 122:1053–1065.
5. Wang C, Vickery AL Jr, Maloof F. Needle biopsy of the thyroid. Surg Gynecol Obstet 1976; 143:365–368.
6. Einhorn J, Franzen S. Thin-needle biopsy in the diagnosis of thyroid disease. Acta Radiol Stockh 1962; 58:321–328.
7. Galvan G. Fine-needle biopsy of cold goiter nodules (author's translation). Munch Med Wochenschr 1977; 119:229–232.
8. Heikkinen J, Lehtinen M, Poyhonen L. Gamma imaging and thin needle biopsy in diagnosis of thyroid cancer. Duodecim 1979; 95:192–197.
9. Lang W, Atay Z, Georgii A. The cytological classification of follicular tumors in the thyroid gland (author's translation). Virchows Arch Pathol Anat 1978; 378:199–211.
10. Stavric GD, Karanfilski BT, Kalamaras AK, et al. Early diagnosis and detection of clinically non-suspected thyroid neoplasia by the cytologic method. Cancer 1980; 45:340–344.
11. Frable WJ, Frable MA. Fine-needle aspiration biopsy of the thyroid. Histopathologic and clinical correlations. In: Fenoglio CM, Wolff M, eds. Progress in surgical pathology. Vol 1. New York: Masson, 1980:105.
12. Miller JM, Hamburger JI, Kini S. Diagnosis of thyroid nodules. Use of the needle aspiration and needle biopsy. JAMA 1979; 24:481–484.
13. Hamburger JI, Miller JM, Kini S. Preoperative clinical-pathological diagnosis of thyroid nodules. Handbook and Atlas. Associated Endocrinologists—Northland Thyroid Laboratory, Southfield, MI 48075, 1979.
14. Van Herle AJ, Rich P, Ljung BE, et al. The thyroid nodule. Ann Intern Med 1982; 96:221–232.
15. Frable WJ. Thin-needle aspiration biopsy. Philadelphia: WB Saunders, 1983:7.
16. Frable WJ. Thin-needle aspiration biopsy. A personal experience with 469 cases. Am J Clin Pathol 1976; 65:168–182.
17. Wang C, Vickery AL Jr. A further note on the large needle biopsy of the thyroid gland. Surg Gynecol Obstet 1983; 156:508–510.
18. Zajicek J. Aspiration biopsy cytology. Part I. Cytology of Supradiaphragmatic Organs. New York: S Karger, 1974:67.
19. Droese M. Cytological aspiration biopsy of thyroid gland. Stuttgart: F. K. Schattauer Verlag:1980.
20. Jensen F, Rasmussen SN. The treatment of thyroid cysts by ultrasonically guided fine needle aspiration. Acta Chir Scand 1976; 142:209–211.
21. Walfish PG, Hazani E, Strawbridge HT, et al. A prospective study of combined ultrasonography and needle aspiration biopsy in the assessment of the hypofunctioning thyroid nodule. Surgery 1977; 82:474–482.
22. Miller JM, Hamburger JI, Kini SR. The impact of needle biopsy on the preoperative diagnosis of thyroid nodules. Henry Ford Hosp Med J 1980; 28:145–148.
23. Hamberger B, Gharib H, Melton J, et al. Fine-needle aspiration biopsy of thyroid nodules. Impact on thyroid practice and cost of care. Am J Med 1982; 73:381–384.
24. Kini W, Miller JM, Hamburger JI. The cytopathology of the thyroid nodule by fine needle aspiration. Acta Cytol 1978; 22:605–606.
25. Loewhagen T, Sprenger E. Cytologic presentation of thyroid tumors in aspiration smear. Acta Cytol 1974; 18:192–197.
26. Krisch K, Jakesz R, Erd W, et al. Punctate cytology of benign and malignant changes in the thyroid gland (author's translation). Munch Med Wochenschr 1976; 118:1383–1386.
27. Luck JB, Mumaw VR, Frable WJ. Fine-needle aspiration biopsy of the thyroid: Differential diagnosis by "Videoplan" image analysis. Acta Cytol 1982; 26:793–796.
28. Boon ME, Lowhagen T, Willems J. Planimetric studies on fine needle aspirates from follicular adenoma and follicular carcinoma of the thyroid. Acta Cytol 1980; 24:145–148.
29. Boon ME. Personal communication.
30. Sprenger E, Loewhagen T, Vogt-Schaden M. Differential diagnosis between follicular adenoma and follicular carcinoma of the thyroid by nuclear DNA determination. Acta Cytol 1977; 21:528–530.
31. Hapke MR, Dehner LP. The optically clear nucleus. A reliable sign of papillary carcinoma of the thyroid? Am J Surg Pathol 1979; 3:31–38.
32. Kini S, Miller JM, Hamburger JI, et al. Cytopathology of papillary carcinoma of the thyroid by fine needle aspiration. Acta Cytol 1980; 24:511–521.
33. Kini SR, Miller JM, Hamburger JI. Cytopathologay of Hürthle cell lesions of the thyroid gland by fine needle aspiration. Acta Cytol 1981; 25:647–652.
34. Ljungberg O. Cytologic diagnosis of medullary carcinoma of the thyroid gland. Acta Cytol 1972; 16:253–255.
35. Soderstrom N, Telenius-Berg M, Akerman M. Diagnosis of medullary carcinoma of the thyroid by fine needle aspiration biopsy. Acta Med Scand 1975; 197:71–76.
36. Schneider V, Frable WJ. Spindle and giant cell carcinoma of the thyroid. Cytologic diagnosis by fine needle aspiration. Acta Cytol 1980; 24:184–189.
37. Atay Z, Lang W, Georgii A. Classification of thyroid carcinoma by cytology. Zentralbl Allg Pathol 1978; 122:160–161.
38. Baehrs OH, McConahey WM Jr. Presented at Seventh Annual Cancer Symposium, Boca Raton Community Hospital, Boca Raton Florida, Feb.10, 1983.
39. Lowhagen T, Granberg P, Lundell G, et al. Aspiration biopsy cytology (ABC) in nodules of the thyroid gland suspected to be malignant. Surg Clin North Am 1979; 59:3–18.
40. Bodo M, Dobrossy L, Sinkovics I, et al. Fine-needle biopsy of thyroid gland. J Surg Oncol 1979; 12:288–297.
41. Brauer RJ, Silver CE. Needle aspiration biopsy of thyroid nodules. Laryngoscope 1984; 94:38–42.
42. Rosen IB, Palmer JA, Bain J, et al. Efficacy of needle biopsy in post radiation thyroid disease. Surgery 1983; 94:1002–1007.
43. Gerfo PL, Feind C, Weber C, et al. Encapsulated follicular thyroid lesions diagnosed by large needle biopsy. Surgery 1983; 94:1008–1010.
44. Miller JM, Hamburger JI, Kini SR. The needle biopsy diagnosis of papillary thyroid carcinoma. Cancer 1981; 48:989–993.
45. Goldfarb WB, Bigos TS, Eastman RC, et al. Needle biopsy in the assessment and management of hypofunctioning thyroid nodules. Am J Surg 1982; 143:409–412.
46. Block MA, Dailey GE, Robb JA. Thyroid nodules indeterminant by needle biopsy. Am J Surg 1983; 146:72–78.
47. Kaminsky DB. Aspiration biopsy for the community hospital. New York: Masson, 1981:5.

TREATMENT OF ADVANCED THYROID CANCER

OSCAR M. GUILLAMONDEGUI, M.D.

More than 90 percent of thyroid carcinomas belong to the so-called well-differentiated varieties. They include the predominantly papillary (papillary and mixed papillary-follicular types), the pure follicular, and the medullary carcinoma. Pure papillary and mixed papillary-follicular carcinoma have essentially the same clinical behavior.

The spindle- and giant-cell (anaplastic) carcinomas are a rare type of thyroid cancer (7% at the M.D. Anderson Hospital) and are characterized by a rapid growth and an early tendency to massively invade the tissues of the neck.

Most differentiated carcinomas of the thyroid have a long, slow course and a good prognosis, but some tumors are particularly aggressive. Of the patients with well-differentiated thyroid carcinoma, more than 80 percent survive and remain free of recurrence after adequate surgical treatment; of those who die of their disease, the majority have recurrent tumor in the tissues of the neck, sometimes accompanied by distant metastases.

Direct invasion of local tissues of the neck occurs in 15 percent of previously untreated patients with well-differentiated thyroid cancer.[1] This important feature must be recognized at the time of the initial, definitive surgical treatment, because it has an important prognostic significance: the treatment of these patients is less successful, and their survival definitely shorter than the rest of the patients in the series. In addition, the adequacy of the surgical resection also has a direct relationship to the eventual outcome of this group of patients.

The histologic appearance of well-differentiated thyroid cancers usually does not identify those that exhibit invasive tendencies or a more aggressive biologic behavior.[2-6] Patients with anaplastic tumors have an extremely poor survival rate, and the diagnosis clearly establishes certain predictions of local and regional invasion.

In an attempt to determine the biologic behavior of these tumors and to determine the most appropriate method of treatment, an analysis of the records of patients with locally invasive thyroid cancer at The University of Texas System Cancer Center M.D. Anderson Hospital and Tumor Institute was undertaken. During the decade of 1964 to 1974, 47 patients had clinical or histopathologic evidence of direct extension of tumor outside the thyroid capsule, invading surrounding anatomic structures. Of the 47 patients, 34 (72%) had well-differentiated tumors and 13 had poorly differentiated or anaplastic carcinomas. Thirty-three patients had proven lymph node metastases, bi-

lateral in 11. These 47 patients represented 21 percent of those patients with thyroid cancer treated at M.D. Anderson Hospital during the 10-year period. Six of the patients had had previous irradiation to the head and neck. A histologic diagnosis of thyroid carcinoma had been made earlier in 25 patients, eight of whom were referred with recurrence after partial thyroidectomy. In the remaining 17 patients, the diagnosis was obtained from an open biopsy of a cervical node or the thyroid. Most of the patients had evidence of invasion of structures in the neck at the time of their first observation. Forty patients had palpable enlargement of the thyroid, and in 10 the gland was clinically fixed to other cervical structures. Unilateral paralysis of a vocal cord was noted in 14 patients, suggesting direct involvement of a recurrent laryngeal nerve or the laryngeal structures. Sixteen patients had tracheal deviation and dysphagia. Twenty-eight patients had clinical cervical node metastases, five had pulmonary metastases, and one patient had osseous metastases in the thoracic spine. The trachea and recurrent laryngeal nerves were invaded most often since these organs are close to the thyroid gland. The laryngeal cartilage was involved in 16 patients. Many other structures of the neck were found to be invaded by tumor in the remaining patients (Fig. 1). The carotid sheath was penetrated in only a few cases; the tumor usually surrounded the vessels, but rarely actually invaded them. The size of the primary lesion was directly related to the degree of local invasion. Only one patient had a lesion less than 2 cm in diameter, and 68 percent of the patients had lesions larger than 4 cm in diameter.

TREATMENT

All patients were initially treated with a surgical resection. Total thyroidectomy was performed in 39 of 47 patients (Table 1). Twenty-three patients also underwent unilateral or bilateral neck dissection (Table 2). In the majority of cases, the tumor was removed from the involved structures without an at-

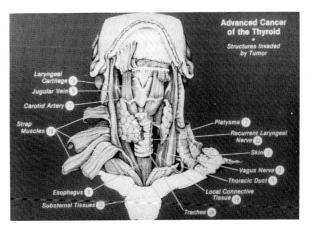

Figure 1 Structures invaded by tumor in patients with advanced cancer of the thyroid. The circled numbers indicate the number of patients with invasion of each structure.[1]

TABLE 1 Surgical Treatment of 47 Patients With Invasive Thyroid Carcinoma

Procedure	No. of Patients
Total thyroidectomy	39
Subtotal thyroidectomy	2
Thyroidectomy-lobectomy	4
Thyroid biopsy	2

TABLE 2 Surgical Procedures on 39 Patients With Invasive Thyroid Carcinoma Treated by Total Thyroidectomy

Procedure(s)	No. of Patients
Thyroidectomy alone	11
+Neck dissection	11
+Tracheostomy	4
+Neck dissection & trach	5
+Resection recurrent nerve	1
+Neck dissection & other Extensive resection (laryngectomy, etc.)	7

tempt to obtain wide surgical margins. Microscopic tumor was believed to be present at the conclusion of the procedure in 66 percent of the patients. A total laryngectomy was performed in only three patients, although the laryngeal cartilage was believed to be invaded in 16. Partial resection of the trachea was performed in only two patients, even though the tumor appeared to invade the trachea in 28. Of the 47 patients, 35 received additional treatment in the postoperative period. Radioactive iodine was used alone or in combination with other forms of therapy in 23 patients; 20 were given a single treatment (dose range 25 to 168 mCi) while three received multiple treatment (dose range from 233 to 434 mCi) over an extended period. Irradiation therapy, additional surgery or chemotherapy was given to the other 12 patients.

RESULTS

Twenty-two patients were alive at the time of this review: 19 were free of disease, one was alive with local recurrence 7 years after treatment, and two were alive with distant metastases 5.5 and 7 years postoperatively. Twenty-five patients were dead, 14 as a consequence of cancer, six from intercurrent disease or a second primary tumor, and five from surgical complications. The absolute survival was 46.8 percent (22 of 47), the determinate survival was 53.6 percent (22 of 41), and the final disease-free survival was 46.3 percent (19 of 41).

Twenty-eight patients with invasion of the larynx or trachea who underwent curative resections without removal of these structures were analyzed as a separate group. The determinate 10-year survival for these patients was 62 percent and disease-free survival was 50 percent. Three patients underwent laryngectomy as part of the treatment; two died within one year of un-

controlled local disease, and the third was alive and well 12 years later.

COMMENTS

The histologic type was the most important factor affecting the prognosis of locally advanced cancers. Ninety-five percent of the patients who survived had well-differentiated thyroid tumors, and only one patient with poorly differentiated carcinoma survived 5 years.

Several additional factors adversely affected the patients with locally invasive thyroid cancer. Advanced age and male sex played a statistically significant role in short survival (this correlates with the factors affecting the rest of the patients with thyroid cancer). The median age of the survivors in this series was 27 years; the median age in the nonsurvivors was 69 years. Males accounted for 44 percent of the patients who died and only 18 percent of those who were alive at the end of the study. The incidence of anaplastic carcinoma, as expected, also increased with advanced age. The size of the primary lesion and the number of adjacent structures involved were also of prognostic significance. In 84 percent of the patients who died of cancer, the primary lesion was larger than 4 cm. When more than four adjacent structures in the neck were involved by tumor, the result was uniformly fatal.

Most of the patients with thyroid cancer have been treated at the M.D. Anderson Hospital with total thyroidectomies. In addition, when lymph node metastases are present or suspected, a neck dissection, usually modified, is also indicated.[2-5,8] Less clear, however, is the role of extensive surgical procedures in treating patients with locally aggressive disease. Clark et al, in an early report from our institution, stated that the larynx should be preserved whenever possible, and reported only five laryngectomies in 218 patients with thyroid carcinoma treated from 1944 to 1964.[9] Intraluminal involvement of the larynx or impending airway obstruction is an indication for removal of the larynx or the trachea in well-differentiated tumors.[10] Extensive ablative procedures should not be performed on patients with anaplastic or spindle- and giant-cell carcinomas; survival is uniformly poor. In patients with well-differentiated locally advanced carcinomas, the role of surgical therapy should be the removal of all gross tumor with preservation of function whenever possible. Functionally important structures such as the trachea, the larynx, and the recurrent laryngeal nerves should be preserved. Only if intraluminal invasion is present and these structures are rendered functionless by extensive tumor invasion, should they be removed. Radioactive iodine used in the postoperative period has been proved effective in the treatment of patients with well-differentiated thyroid cancer.[11-13] Eighty-two percent of the patients treated with radioactive iodine in this series were alive 5 to 15 years after treatment. Adequate surgical excision, leaving only small foci of residual tumor, allows the most effective use of radioactive iodine while preserving vital function.

SUMMARY

The factors that adversely affected the survival of this group of patients included age, male sex, spindle- and giant-cell histology, and extensive involvement of adjacent structures in the neck. Surgical treatment aimed at removal of all gross tumor with preservation of vital structures whenever possible offers a reasonable chance of cure in locally aggressive well-differentiated thyroid cancer. Radioactive iodine is beneficial in the treatment of well-differentiated lesions.

REFERENCES

1. Breaux EP, Guillamondegui OM. Treatment of invasive carcinoma of the thyroid: How radical? Am J Surg 1980; 140:514–517.
2. Ibanez ML, Russell WC, Albores-Saavedra J, Lampertico P, White EC, Clark RL. Thyroid carcinoma-biologic behavior and mortality. Cancer 1966; 19:1039–1052.
3. Silverberg SG, Hutter RVP, Foote FW. Fatal carcinoma of the thyroid: histology, metastases, and causes of death. Cancer 1970; 25:792–802.
4. McKenzie AD. The natural history of thyroid cancer. Arch Surg 1971; 102:274–277.
5. Russell MA, Gilbert EF, Jaeschke WF. Prognostic features of thyroid cancer: A long-term follow-up of 68 cases. Cancer 1975; 36:553–559.
6. Franssila DO. Prognosis in thyroid carcinoma. Cancer 1975; 36:1138–1146.
7. Thomas CG, Buckwalter JA. Poorly differentiated neoplasms of the thyroid gland. Ann Surg 1973; 17:632–642.
8. Attie JN, Moskowitz GW, Margouleff D, Levy LM. Feasibility of total thyroidectomy in the treatment of thyroid carcinoma. Postoperative radioactive iodine evaluation of 140 cases. Am J Surg 1979; 138:555–560.
9. Clark RL, Ibanez ML, White EC. What constitutes an adequate operation for carcinoma of the thyroid? Arch Surg 1966; 92:23–26.
10. Djalilian M, Beahrs OH, Devine KD, Weiland L, DeSanto LW. Intraluminal involvement of the larynx and trachea by thyroid cancer. Am J Surg 1974; 128:500–504.
11. Thompson NW, Nishiyama RH, Harness JK. Thyroid carcinoma: Current controversies. Curr Probl Surg 1978; 15:11.
12. Block MA. Well-differentiated carcinomas of the thyroid. Curr Probl Cancer 1979; 3:8.
13. Beierwaltes WH. The treatment of thyroid carcinoma with radioactive iodine. Semin Nucl Med 1978; 8:79–94.

COMPLICATIONS OF THYROID SURGERY: THEIR PREVENTION, RECOGNITION, AND MANAGEMENT

PAUL H. WARD, M.D., F.A.C.S.

The complications of thyroid surgery are wound hematoma, unilateral and bilateral recurrent laryngeal nerve paralysis, unilateral and bilateral injury to the external branch of the superior laryngeal nerves, hypocalcemia, hypothyroidism, and thyroid storm. Awareness of the possible complications, prevention when possible, and early recognition lead to optimal management and patient care.

Every surgeon who operates on the thyroid gland is likely to experience these complications if a sufficient number of operations are performed. Prevention, recognition, and management of each of these complications are discussed in this chapter, with particular emphasis on the isolated and combined laryngeal nerve paresis and paralysis.

WOUND HEMATOMA

The incidence of wound hematoma can be markedly diminished by careful attention to hemostasis and wound drainage. Early recognition of the accumulation of blood in the wound is critical since tracheal compression and airway obstruction can present a life-threatening emergency. Should it occur, the wound should be reopened, under sterile conditions if possible, and the hematoma evacuated. Irrigation of the wound facilitates achievement of hemostasis by careful search, recognition, and ligation of bleeding vessels. Wound drainage and a compression dressing assist in prevention of recurrence.

INJURY TO RECURRENT LARYNGEAL NERVE

The incidence of recurrent laryngeal nerve injury is difficult to determine. It is certainly not rare and is most often secondary to trauma. In a series of cases of bilateral abductor vocal cord paralysis, Holinger et al found that 138 of 240 (58%) had thyroid surgery as the cause of their paralysis.[1] Most series include a variety of operative approaches by different surgeons for a variable group of diseases. Injury to the recurrent laryngeal nerve may be intentional (resection of tumor) or may result from inadequate knowledge of the anatomy, poor exposure, and/or hemostasis. Mere exposure of the nerves and minimal trauma can lead to paresis or paralysis. Different operative procedures (i.e., subtotal versus total thyroidectomy) place different numbers and combinations of nerves at risk.

In a series of cases operated on for carcinoma of the thyroid, Beahrs and Vandertoll reported a 17 percent incidence of bilateral vocal cord paralysis.[2] In a series of 356 thyroidectomies for carcinoma, Attie and Khafif reported 13 cases of unilateral injury and no bilateral nerve injury.[3] Clark et al resected the recurrent nerve in three cases and reported no bilateral injuries in a total of 120 thyroidectomies.[4] In a series of 400 total thyroidectomies, Thompson et al reported no bilateral recurrent nerve palsy.[5] The inconsistency in the complications in these series are obvious.

In the radical total thyroidectomy, both recurrent and both superior laryngeal nerves are at risk, making a total of 4×4 or 16 possible combinations of pure paralysis (Fig. 1). Different degrees of injury regeneration and misregeneration of abductor, adductor, and tensing fibers make innumerable combinations of paresis and paralysis possible.[6] In addition, lack of awareness of the importance of the external branches and the failure to look for an inability to diagnose a paralysis of one or both of these nerves explain the widespread confusion regarding vocal cord position that is prevalent in the literature.

Of major concern to the thyroid surgeon is acute bilateral recurrent nerve paralysis, since both cords may be positioned near the midline. As the patient awakens from anesthesia, the voice may be good (since the cords approximate); however, a failure to abduct results in airway obstruction that may be life-threatening, requiring a tracheostomy. If cut, or after trauma, the nerves undergo complete neurolysis, then, over time, there will be significant muscle atrophy with limited lateralization of the cords and some increase in the airway. When bilateral recurrent laryngeal nerve paralysis is permanent, the patient becomes respiratory- and voice-crippled for life. Permanent tracheostomy, arytenoidectomy, and reinnervation procedures offer moderate rehabilitation with a compromised voice and marginal airway. Prevention of the morbidity and mortality of unilateral or bilateral recurrent laryngeal nerve paralysis is primarily dependent on knowledge of the anatomy and meticulous dissection. The medial approach to the thyroid described by Rush et al[7] and the thoracic inlet approach to the recurrent nerves utilized by Loré et al[8] allow identification of the recurrent nerves and decreased bleeding with better visualization and preservation of the blood supply to the inferior parathyroid glands. Subtotal thyroidectomy and intracapsular removal described by some authors may decrease the incidence of bilateral recurrent nerve paralysis, but leave foci of tumor.[9,10]

Unless the larynx of every patient is examined with indirect laryngoscopy postoperatively, many unilateral recurrent laryngeal nerve paralyses will go unrecognized. The paralyzed cord is in the paramedian position, but shows some tensing motion with slight adduction due to contraction of the cricothyroid muscles (Fig. 2). Most of us can remember, as medical students, seeing patients on rounds who were hoarse the morning following surgery. The operating surgeon ascribed the hoarse voice to traumatic intubation. Fortunately, the majority of patients with uni-

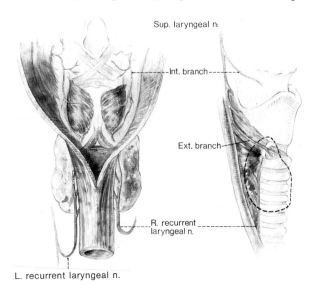

Figure 1 The muscles of the larynx are supplied by two pairs of motor nerves arising from the vagus trunk. The relationships of the recurrent laryngeal nerves to the trachea and the thyroid gland and their entrance into the larynx are shown in this posterior view of the laryngopharynx (*left*). The superior laryngeal nerve supplies motor fibers only to the cricothyroid muscles on each side through its external branch. The internal branch contains secretory and sensory fibers for the supraglottic portion of the ipsilateral larynx (*right*). Note the relationship of the upper pole of the thyroid gland to the external branches of the superior laryngeal nerves.

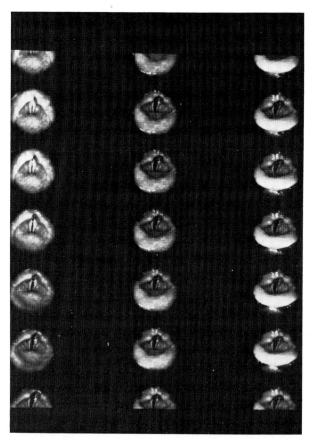

Figure 2 Serial photographs from a 16-mm motion film of a patient with pure recurrent nerve paralysis secondary to surgical division of the nerve. The vocal cord is in the paramedial (median) position. During inspiration it retains this position while the opposite cord abducts, producing a marginally adequate airway. During phonation, there is tensing and lengthening of both cords produced by the contraction of both cricothyroid muscles, which tilt the thyroid on the cricoid cartilage. In addition to the tensing and lengthening of the paralyzed cord, there is also a slight amount of adduction secondary to the contractions of the bilaterally innervated interarytenoid muscle.

lateral recurrent laryngeal nerve paralysis compensate even if function fails to return. The opposite cord is able to achieve glottic closure by crossing the midline to approximate the paralyzed cord. The patient with a compensated unilateral recurrent laryngeal nerve paralysis may have limited morbidity unless he or she is a singer, an actor, or a heavy voice user. Any type or combination of paralysis severely affects modulation of pitch and voice projection. The heavy voice user with a paresis or paralysis experienced vocal fatigue, hoarseness, and weakness of the voice after several hours of continuous voice use. These patients may come in for examination of the larynx months or years after the thyroid surgery. A history of loss of singing ability dating from the time of thyroid surgery is easily elicited.

The limited documentation in the literature of the morbidity of paralysis of the external branch of the superior laryngeal nerve indicates the minimal concern that most thyroid surgeons show for injury of this nerve.[6,8,11,12]

INJURY TO THE SUPERIOR LARYNGEAL NERVES

The two superior laryngeal nerves leave the vagus trunks on each side of the neck just below the nodose ganglion. They pass downward and behind the carotid artery and curve forward toward the larynx. Each superior laryngeal nerve divides into the internal and external branches. The internal branches penetrate the thyrohyoid membrane and supply the supraglottic portion of the larynx with secretory and sensory fibers. The motor fibers of the superior laryngeal nerve are contained within the external branch, which accompanies the superior thyroid artery as it progresses caudally, inferiorly and medially, to supply the cricothyroid muscle on each side. (see Fig. 1). Paralysis of the external branch of the superior laryngeal nerve must occur in a significant number of patients undergoing total thyroidectomy even when performed by the careful surgeon. The nerve passes in the visceral fascia initially behind the superior thyroid artery at the hyoid level, becoming anterior before entering the constrictor in three-fourths of the patients. In the remaining patients, the nerve passes between the anterior and posterior branches of the superior thyroid artery and descends within the pretracheal fascia on the anterior superior surface of the upper pole of the thyroid or descends parallel to the superior thyroid artery.[13] Dissection and division of the superior pole vessels imediately adjacent to the capsule of the upper pole of the thyroid gland will lessen the chances of damage. Because of the close relationship of the upper pole of the thyroid lobe and the entrance of the nerve intracapsularly in 7 percent of the cases, even the knowledgeable surgeon may occasionally damage the external branch of the superior laryngeal nerve. Proper informed consent regarding this risk and extreme care are important, particularly in professional singers, since damage to this or any of the motor nerves to the larynx will terminate their careers.

The unilateral loss of ability to contract the ip-

silateral cricothyroid muscle prevents the tilting of the thyroid on the cricoid cartilage with resulting absence of homolateral tensing of the cord. The larynx has an asymmetrical tilt with a shifting of the posterior portion of the larynx toward the paralyzed side. The paretic cord moves because of the action of the intact recurrent laryngeal nerve, but is at a different level and is hyperemic because of failure to tense. The speaking voice may be normal, but there is an inability to perform the fine coordinative efforts necessary for accurate pitch control.[6] When combined with a homolateral recurrent paralysis, the cord fails to move, does not tense, is at a different level than the opposite cord, and is hyperemic (Fig. 3). Isolated bilateral external branch superior laryngeal nerve paralysis is even more difficult to recognize. There is a bowing of the vocal cords secondary to a bilateral failure of the cricothyroid muscle to tilt the thyroid on the cricoid cartilage. The failure of movement of the epiglottic vallecular complex results in an overhang of the epiglottis and makes visualization of the anterior commissure difficult. The voice may be weak

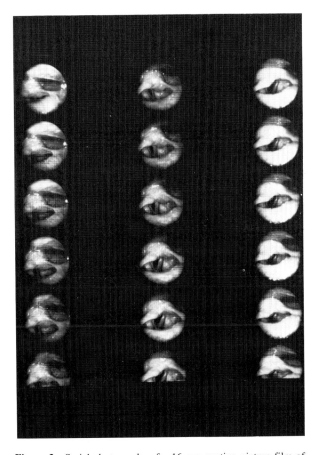

Figure 3 Serial photographs of a 16-mm motion picture film of a patient with right superior and recurrent laryngeal nerve paralysis. During phonation, the contraction of the opposite intact cricothyroid muscle produces an asymmetry of the thyroid-cricoid cartilage tilt with lengthening and tensing of the innervated cord. The tensed normal cord is thus at a different level than the flaccid paralyzed cord, which may have an injected appearance due to hyperemia. There is an asymmetrical shift of the posterior larynx toward the paralyzed side during phonation.

and breathy because of an air leak through the bowed cords. These patients are often sent to the speech therapist and psychiatrist for functional voice disorder. If there is a scar in the lower neck, this condition is much more likely to be an unrecognized traumatic bilateral external branch superior laryngeal nerve paralysis.

HYPOPARATHYROIDISM

The serious life-threatening complication of hypoparathyroidism, hypocalcemia, and tetany is also probably more frequent than generally reported. Again the type and extent of the thyroid surgery as well as the technical capabilities of the surgeons explain the disparity in the reported series. Transient versus permanent hypoparathyroidism is also an important consideration. Katz and Bronson reported only 1.6 percent of 630 cases,[14] Perzik reported 2.8 percent of 216 cases,[15] Attie and Khafif reported 3.2 percent of 249 cases,[16] and Thompson et al reported 4.1 percent of 123 cases.[5] An incidence as high as 29 percent at Memorial Hospital was reported by Tollefsen et al.[17] Attempts have been made to dissect the parathyroid glands from the specimen and reimplant them into the neck or arm muscles.[18,19] It is agreed that preservation of the parathyroid glands with their blood supply from the inferior thyroid vessels is preferable to dissection and transplantation.[20] When there is doubt about the status of the in situ parathyroid glands, identification of any parathyroid tissue attached to the specimen away from the tumor can be removed, sliced, and reimplanted into muscle as a safety measure. The division of the isthmus and medial approach, early identification of the recurrent nerves, inferior thyroid vessels, and sometimes the inferior parathyroid glands have proved most successful in our experience.

All patients undergoing total thyroidectomy must be watched for hypoparathyroidism and hypocalcemia. The presence of increased neuromuscular excitability accompanied by a decreased ionized serum calcium heralds the diagnosis. Muscle cramps, chest pains, laryngeal stridor, and cardiac irregularities may progress to death unless there is appropriate intervention. Positive clinical signs include facial irritability on tapping the finger over the parotid and masseter muscle (Chvostek's sign). The decreased serum calcium is accompanied by an increased serum phosphorus level and a positive Sulkowitch test (decreased or absent urinary calcium). The acute phase is treated with immediate, slow intravenous infusion of 10 ml of 10% calcium gluconate. The patient is followed closely clinically and with serum calcium determinations. Any perioral tingling, a positive Chvostek's or Trousseau's sign, or muscle cramping calls for repeated administration of calcium gluconate or calcium chloride. Emphasis is placed on the slow intravenous administration, since rapid infusion of calcium in patients taking digitalis preparations can result in cardiac arrest. The patient can gradually be converted to oral calcium in the form of calcium gluconate or calcium carbonate. A total daily intake of 1800 to 2400 mg is usually required. Intestinal absorption can be enhanced by administration of rapid-acting dihydrotachysterol (1 mg per day) and later 50,000 to 100,000 units of vitamin D. It is wise to follow the 24-hour urinary calcium excretion until it approaches normal in order to avoid the long-term effects of hypo- or hypercalcemia. Preservation and protection from devascularization of one or more of the parathyroid glands is the secret to prevention of this unpleasant complication, which may result in a life-long disability and dependency on daily ingestion of calcium and vitamin D.

HYPOTHYROIDISM

Hypothyroidism is an expected and accepted result of total thyroidectomy, but also occurs as a complication of subtotal thyroidectomy. The development of dry, scaly skin, coarse hair, a dull, flat facial expression, weight gain, edematous eyelids, and generalized myxedema call for thyroid screening and TSH tests. Fortunately, hypothyroidism can be easily corrected by daily oral ingestion of thyroid extract (2 to 4 grains), thyroxine (T_4) (200 to 250 μg), or triiodothyronine (T_3) (60 to 80 μg). Short-acting T_3 may be preferred initially for maintenance, then discontinued 4 to 6 days prior to postoperative radioactive iodine scanning; however, T_4 is preferred for long-term maintenance because of its longer, smoother action. TSH can be utilized to monitor adequate replacement levels of thyroid hormone.

Thyroid storm fortunately is now a rarely observed complication that presents during anesthesia or after surgery for hyperthyroidism. Tachycardia and hyperpyrexia are the signs noted during anesthesia and surgery. When noted, all manipulation of the thyroid gland should be stopped and the operation terminated. Sodium iodide, 1 to 2.5 g, is administered intravenously along with hydrocortisone (100 mg). Other measures include the administration of adrenergic blocking agents and glucose, and the utilization of hypothermia if indicated.

In the postoperative period, additional recognizable manifestations of thyroid storm include progressive disorientation and severe agitation. Loré and Perry admonish that survival is dependent on early diagnosis and treatment.[12] Treatment is directed toward management of the underlying illness, provision of supportive measures directed toward associated multiple system decompensation, reduction of secretion and production of thyroid hormones, and reduction of the effect of the thyroid hormone.

High doses of antithyroid drugs such as Propylthyiouracil (300 mg *q6h*) and intravenous sodium iodide (1 g *q8h*) are administered to reduce thyroid hormone output. Reserpine, to deplete catecholamines, or propranolol, a beta adrenergic blocking agent, can be given in an effort to decrease the peripheral effects of thyroid hormone. Prevention of thyroid storm is accomplished by achieving a euthyroid state preoperatively in patients with recognized hyperthyroidism. This is achieved by administration of Lugol's solution and antithyroid drugs, and the blocking of peripheral sympathetic effects with propranolol.

Despite all of the technology and treatment that serve to diminish these complications, the most important development has been accurate fine-needle aspiration. Obtaining a diagnosis via fine-needle aspiration prevents unnecessary surgery and eliminates the risks for many who might have sustained one or more of these complications.

REFERENCES

1. Holinger LD, Holinger PC, Holinger PH. Etiology of bilateral abductor vocal cord paralysis. Ann Otol Rhinol Laryngol 1976; 85:428–436.
2. Beahrs OH, Vandertoll DJ. Complications of secondary thyroidectomy. Surg Gynecol Obstet 1963; 117:535–539.
3. Attie JN, Khafif RA. Preservation of parathyroid glands during total thyroidectomy. Improved technic utilizing microsurgery. Am J Surg 1975; 130:399–404.
4. Clark RL Jr, White EC, Russell WO. Total thyroidectomy for cancer of the thyroid: significance of intraglandular dissemination. Ann Surg 1959; 149:858–866.
5. Thompson NW, Nishiyama RH, Harness JK. Thyroid carcinoma: current controversies. Curr Probl Surg 1978; 15:1–67.
6. Ward PW, Berci G, Calcaterra TC. Superior laryngeal nerve paralysis: an often overlooked entity. Trans Amer Acad Ophthal Otolaryngol 1977; 84:124–128.
7. Rush BF, Swaminathan AP, Patel R. A medial approach to thyroidectomy. Am J Surg 1975; 130:430–432.
8. Loré JM Jr, Kim DJ, Elias S. Preservation of the laryngeal nerves during total thyroidectomy lobectomy. Ann Otol Rhinol Laryngol 1977; 86:777–778.
9. Hardin WJ, Hardy JD. Carcinoma of the thyroid gland. Surg Gynecol Obstet 1971; 132:450–456.
10. Harrold CC, Wright J. Management of surgical hypoparathyroidism. Am J Surg 1966; 112:482–487.
11. Moosman DA, DeWeese MS. The external laryngeal nerve as related to thyroidectomy. Surg Gynecol Obstet 1968; 127:1011–1016.
12. Loré JM Jr, Perry RJ. The diagnosis and management of thyroid disease. Parts III and IV. J Contin Educ ORL and Allergy 1979; 41(4):13–25.
13. Hollinshead WH. Anatomy for surgeons. Vol I. The head and neck. New York: Hoeber-Harper, 1954:425.
14. Katz AD, Bronson D. Total thyroidectomy. The indications and results in 630 cases. Am J Surg 1978; 136:450–454.
15. Perzik SL. The place of total thyroidectomy in the management of 909 patients with thyroid disease. Am J Surg 1976; 132:480–483.
16. Attie JN, Khafif RA, Steckler RM. Elective neck dissection in papillary carcinoma of the thyroid. Am J Surg 1971; 122:464–471.
17. Tollefsen HR, Shah JP, Huvos AG. Papillary carcinoma of the thyroid. Recurrence in the thyroid gland after initial surgical treatment. Am J Surg 1972; 124:468–472.
18. Block MA. Surgery of the irradiated thyroid gland for possible carcinoma. Criteria, technique, results. In: DeGroot LJ, ed. Radiation-associated thyroid carcinoma. New York: Grune and Stratton, 1976:353.
19. Paloyan E. Operation for the irradiated gland for possible thyroid carcinoma. Criteria, technique, results. In: DeGroot LJ, ed. Radiation-associated thyroid carcinoma. New York: Grune and Stratton, 1976:883–894.
20. Lawson W, Biller HF. The solitary thyroid nodule: Diagnosis and management of thyroid disease. Am J Otolaryngol 1983; 4:43–73.

20. Skull Base Surgery

INTRODUCTION

UGO P. FISCH, M.D.

In the past decade surgery of the skull base underwent a spectacular and fascinating evolution. For years the skull base remained a solid no-man's land separating the surgical specialties working above it (neurosurgeons) and below it (head and neck, ENT, and plastic surgeons). This compartmental hierarchy was upset in the sixties by revolutionary surgical concepts based on a more comprehensive, multidisciplinary view of the problems. Two different lines of approach, anterior and lateral, developed from this situation. The *anterior or craniofacial* approach to the skull base derived from surgical techniques first used for the correction of congenital deformities of the face.[1] The *lateral or infratemporal* approach evolved from *otologic microsurgical* techniques introduced to reach the internal auditory canal through the supralabyrinthine and retrolabyrinthine compartments of the temporal bone.[2,3] The development of two different approaches to the skull base is a reflection of the diversity in architecture and complexity of the involved anatomic structures. The coronal flap and the variety of osteotomies are the main features of the anterior craniofacial approach. The delicate microsurgical exposure through the bony skull base of important structures such as the internal carotid artery, cranial nerves III to XII, and the cavernous sinus characterizes the lateral infratemporal approach.

The chapters that follow present the state of the art of each of the new approaches to the skull base. But before going into the heart of the matter, we should pay high credit to our neurosurgical colleagues for their generous and essential help in spite of our intrusion into their specialty. With this neurosurgical support, lesions previously considered inaccessible can now be removed from the deepest regions of the skull with minimal mortality and morbidity.

REFERENCES

1. Tessier P. Osteotomie totale de la face. Ann Chir Plast 1967; 12:273.
2. House WF. Surgical exposure of the internal auditory canal and its contents through the middle cranial fossa. Laryngoscope 1961; 71:1363.
3. Fisch U. Otoneurosurgical operations. In: Yasargil MG (ed). Microsurgery. Stuttgart: Georg Thieme, 1969.

LATERAL (INFRATEMPORAL FOSSA) APPROACH TO THE SKULL BASE

UGO P. FISCH, M.D.

The lateral or infratemporal approach to the skull base can be divided in two subgroups.

The one that we have called *type A* is in essence a *temporocervical approach* (Fig. 1). Its main features are the permanent anterior rerouting of the facial nerve distal to the geniculate ganglion, the temporary anterolateral dislocation of the ascending mandibular ramus, and the permanent obliteration of the middle ear cleft.[1-4] The type A infratemporal approach gives optimal exposure of the internal carotid artery from the carotid foramen to the foramen lacerum and is particularly suitable for the removal of lesions involving the infralabyrinthine and apical compartments of the temporal bone (e.g., chemodectomas or glomus temporale tumors).

The second subgroup of infratemporal ap-proaches to the skull base consists of *type B* and *type C* (Fig. 2). These two latter approaches can be qualified as *temporosphenoidal*. Their main features are the temporary dislocation of the zygomatic arch, temporalis muscle, and mandibular condyle; the microsurgical removal of the bone at the base of the middle cranial fossa including the pterygoid process; the division of the middle meningeal artery and of the mandibular nerve as well as the obliteration of the middle ear cleft.[1,2,4,5,6]

With type B and C approaches, the internal carotid artery is exposed from the carotid foramen to the cavernous sinus. The type B approach gives access to lesions involving the pyramid tip and clivus,[5] the type C approach to those situated in the infratemporal fossa, pterygopalatine fossa, nasopharynx, and parasellar region.[4,5] The principle of the B and C approaches resides in the microsurgical removal of the bone at the lateral skull base along the internal carotid artery, utilizing the space gained between the middle cranial fossa dura and the inferiorly displaced mandibular condyle (Fig. 3).

Of 264 operations performed at the lateral skull base between 1977 and 1983 in our institution, 219 (83%) required one of the aforementioned infratemporal approaches (Table 1). Although most of these

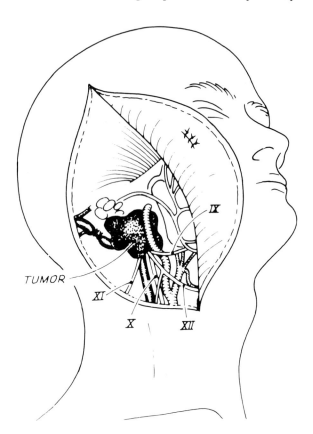

Figure 1 Tumor exposure achieved by type A infratemporal approach. Note the anterior rerouting of the facial nerve, permitting exposure of the intratemporal course of the internal carotid artery lateral to the tumor.

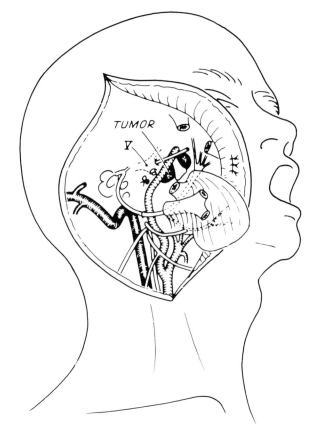

Figure 2 Exposure achieved by the type C infratemporal approach to skull base. Note the inferior displacement of the zygomatic arch and temporalis muscle, and the exposure of the internal carotid artery from the mesotympanum to the cavernous sinus.

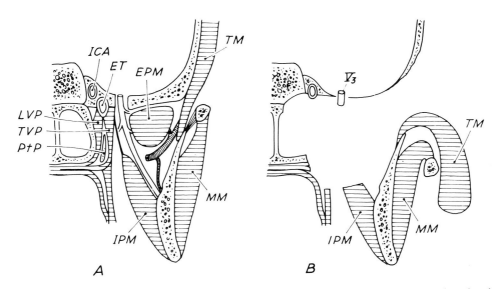

Figure 3 Principle of the infratemporal fossa approach type C to the skull base. *A*, Normal anatomy: coronal section through the left infratemporal fossa, clivus, sphenoid sinus, and nasopharynx. ICA = internal carotid artery; ET = eustachian tube; LFP = levator veli palatini muscle; TVP = tensor veli palatini muscle; PTP = pterygoid process; IPM = internal pterygoid muscle; EPM = external pterygoid muscle; TM = temporalis muscle; MM = masseter muscle. *B*, Access obtained by the inferior displacement of the zygomatic arch and temporalis muscle as well as by the removal of the bone at the base of the middle cranial fossa along the internal carotid artery. Note that the mandibular nerve (V3) has been sectioned at the foramen ovale. Further exposure of the parasellar region can be obtained by the extradural elevation of the temporal lobe.

surgical procedures involved lesions extending outside the skull base into the upper neck, the present review will remain confined to the type C approach, which presents the greatest interest to the head and neck surgeon because it involves lesions often originating from the soft tissues of the upper neck. Indications for the type C approach are shown in Table 2. The single surgical steps and the results will be analyzed separately, depending on the particular anatomic region involved by the tumor.

TABLE 1   Surgical Approaches to the Lateral Skull Base (N = 264)*

Infratemporal	219	
Type A (Temporocervical)		144
Types B + C (Temporosphenoid)		75
Petrosectomy for radical dissection of retromandibular Fossa (temporocervicofacial)	45	

*Performed from 1977 to 1983 at the University of Zurich.

TABLE 2   Surgical Indications for Type C Infratemporal Approach to Skull Base (N = 40)

Diagnosis	N
Nasopharyngeal CA	15
Juvenile nasopharyngeal angiofibroma	7
Adenoid cystic CA	7
Ameloblastoma, melanoma, meningioma, infratemporal paraganglioma, parapharyngeal pleomorphic adenoma, rhabdomyosarcoma, teratoma	11
Total	40

INFRATEMPORAL FOSSA

The most common infratemporal fossa tumor reaching the skull base is the adenoid cystic carcinoma. This tumor usually originates from the lateral wall of the eustachian tube (Fig. 4A). The underlying cause of the resulting unilateral tubal dysfunction remains undiagnosed for a long time until the appearance of a further neural involvement, most commonly a sixth nerve lesion (Fig. 4B). The skin incision used for the tumor removal is retroauricular, with extension into the temporal region (Fig. 5A). The external auditory canal is transected and closed as a blind sac. The temporozygomatic division of the facial nerve is exposed in the parotid region, and the frontal ramus is freed throughout its length for inferior displacement. The zygomatic arch is sectioned between the temporomandibular joint and the lateral rim of the orbit. The mobilized zygomatic bone with attached masseter muscle and the temporalis muscle freed from its bony origin are displaced inferiorly.

Under the magnification afforded by the operating microscope, the skin of the external auditory canal is removed with the drum and the malleus handle. By means of a drill, and under suction irrigation, the complete petrous air cell system is exenterated, skeletonizing the sigmoid sinus, the middle and posterior fossa dura, and the fallopian canal from the geniculate ganglion to the stylomastoid foramen. During this procedure the malleus head, the incus, and the stapes arch are removed. The bone of the glenoid fossa is drilled away to expose the temporomandibular joint, which is disarticulated (Figs. 5B, 6A). The infratemporal retractor is then inserted in such a way that the

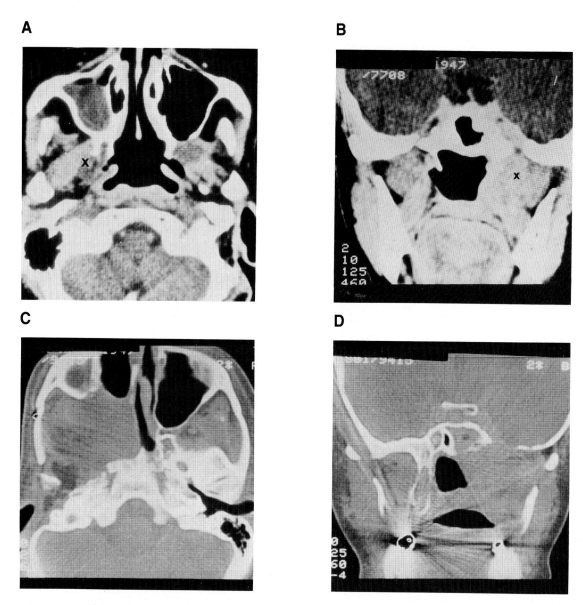

Figure 4   Adenoid cystic carcinoma of the left infratemporal fossa. *A*, Axial CT scan showing the tumor along the lateral wall of the eustachian tube (x). *B*, Coronal CT scan showing the tumor invasion at the base of the skull along the mandibular division of the trigeminal nerve in the foramen ovale (x). *C*, Postoperative axial CT scan. Note that bone has been removed lateral to the internal carotid artery at the base of the middle cranial fossa. The left middle ear cleft has been obliterated with abdominal fat. The external auditory canal is closed like a blind sac. The mandibular condyle is intact. The zygomatic arch has been wired in place anteriorly. The operative defect in the infratemporal fossa has been filled with the temporalis muscle. *D*, Postoperative coronal CT scan. Note that bone has been removed at the base of the left middle cranial fossa including the lateral wall of the sphenoid sinus. The parasellar extradural tumor extension has been removed after extradural superior retraction of the temporal lobe. The operative defect in the infratemporal fossa has been filled with the inferiorly pedicled temporalis muscle.

Figure 5   Surgical steps of the infratemporal fossa approach (right side). *A*, Retroauricular skin incision with extension into the temporal region. *B*, Surgical site following inferior displacement of the zygomatic arch and temporalis muscle. The pneumatic cell system of the middle ear cleft has been exenterated skeletonizing the middle cranial fossa dura (mcf) the sigmoid sinus (s) and the tympanic and mastoid segment of the fallopian canal. The stapes arch, incus, and malleus are removed. The internal carotid artery is identified in the mesotympanum. The glenoid fossa and articular tubercle have been removed, exposing the mandibular condyle (c) with the infratemporal retractor. *C*, Access obtained through the infratemporal approach following inferior displacement of the mandibular condyle seen between both retractors. *C*, Access obtained through the infratemporal approach following inferior displacement of the mandibular condyle with the infratemporal retractor. *D*, Closer view of the infratemporal fossa access to the nasopharynx. The lateral and superior walls of the nasopharynx as well as the eustachian tube with the surrounding soft tissues have been removed. Along the base of the middle cranial fossa one can see the contralateral pharyngeal ostium of the eustachian tube. Note the nasotracheal tube used for ventilation of the patient passing through the left choanal opening lateral to the vomer (v).

A

B

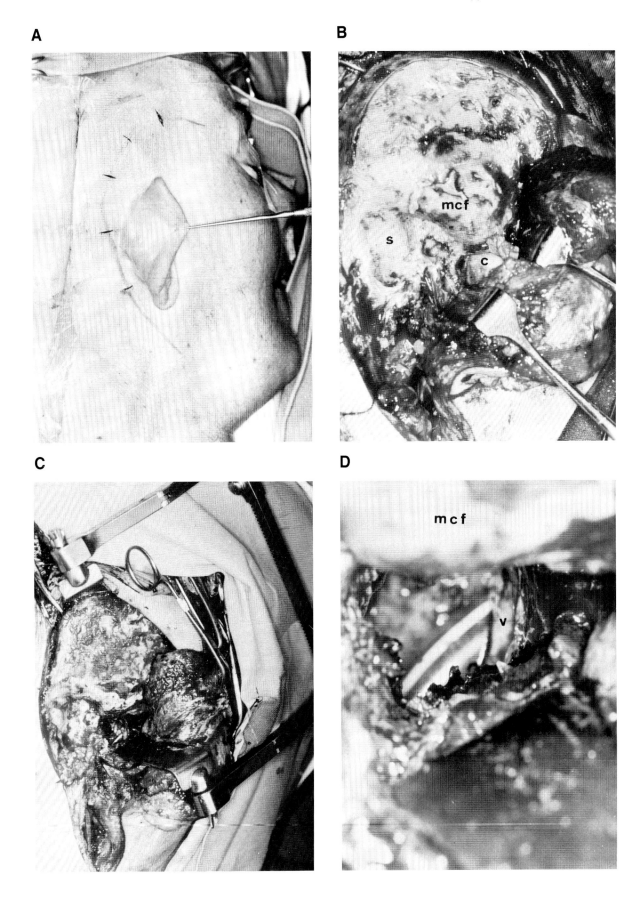

C

D

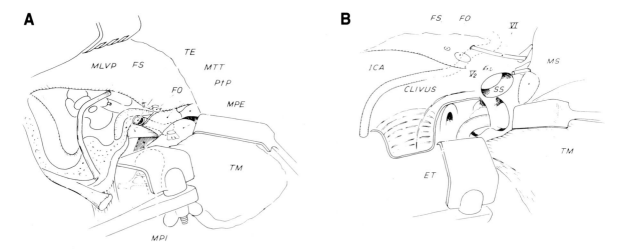

Figure 6 Surgical steps of type C infratemporal approach. *A*, Schematic representation of the surgical site following exenteration of the pneumatic air system of the temporal bone, exposure of the internal carotid artery from the carotid foramen to the foramen lacerum, and section of the middle meningeal artery and of the mandibular nerve. The infratemporal fossa retractor is inserted for inferior displacement of the mandibular condyle. FS = foramen spinosum; FO = foramen ovale; TE = eustachian tube; MLVP = musculus levator veli palatini; MTT = musculus tensor tympani; PTP = pterygoid process; MPE = musculus pterygoideus externus; MPI = musculus pterygoideus internus; TM = temporal muscle. *B*, Schematic view of the surgical site after removal of the right eustachian tube with surrounding soft tissues and laterosuperior wall of the nasopharynx. Access was obtained through the pterygopalatine fossa to the cavernous sinus after section of the maxillary nerve (V₂) and extradural elevation of the temporal lobe. ET = pharyngeal ostium of the left eustachian tube; ICA = internal carotid artery; FS = foramen spinosum; FO = forman ovale; VI = abducens nerve; SS = sphenoid sinus; MS = maxillary sinus; TM = temporalis muscle. (See also Fig. 5D).

lower blade displaces the head of the mandible inferiorly (Figs. 5*C*, 6*A*). The internal carotid artery is identified in the mesotypanum by removing the surrounding tympanic bone with the diamond drill. The posterior origin of the zygomatic arch and the articular tubercle are removed with the drill, leaving only a thin shell of bone over the middle cranial fossa dura lateral to the foramen spinosum and foramen ovale. The middle meningeal artery and the mandibular nerve are sectioned, allowing separation of the soft tissues from the base of the middle cranial fossa. The carotid artery is exposed as far as the foramen lacerum by detaching from it the medial cartilaginous portion of the eustachian tube (Fig. 6*A*). The pterygoid process is exposed and its base drilled away along the dura, giving access to the pterygopalatine fossa. If necessary, the maxillary nerve is identified at the foramen rotundum and severed at this level. The nasal cavity is entered through the medial wall of the pterygopalatine fossa (Figs. 5*C*, 6*B*). The soft tissues at the base of the skull are separated from the exposed horizontal segment of the internal carotid artery and from the inferior surface of the clivus. The lateral and medial pterygoid muscles are cut posteriorly along the exposed intratemporal vertical segment of the internal carotid artery. The maxillary artery is identified and coagulated bipolarly along the inferior edge of the dissection. The eustachian tube is then removed en bloc with the surrounding soft tissues and the laterosuperior wall of the nasopharynx, leaving a sufficient margin of normal tissue around the tumor (See

If the bone of the skull base is infiltrated by tumor, the eroded bone is drilled away with a diamond

bur until firm bone or dura mater is reached. Parasellar tumor extensions may be removed after extradural elevation of the base of the temporal lobe (See Figs. 3, 4*B*, 4*D*). When the cavernous sinus is infiltrated, total tumor removal is not attempted. In these cases, palliative irradiation is used after extirpation of the extradural portion of the lesion. Figures 4*C* and 4*D* show the extensive bone removal at the skull base necessary for adequate exposure of the tumor. The operative defect is filled out by the temporalis muscle, which is swung medially as an axial vascularized pedicle flap. The zygomatic arch is wired in its original place at its anterior end. Abdominal fat is used to fill out the temporal bone defect resulting from the exenteration of the pneumatic air cell system (subtotal petrosectomy). The wound is closed in two layers after introduction of two negative suction drains. The excellent cosmetic appearance of the wound and the absence of an appreciable deformity of facial contours are demonstrated in Figure 7.

NASOPHARYNX

Carcinoma

Recurrent or persisting carcinoma of the nasopharynx after irradiation is often localized in Rosenmueller's groove and infiltrates the base of the skull along the eustachian tube (Fig. 8*A*). These tumors may be resected by the same approach as that used for lesions originating in the infratemporal fossa. The soft tissues surrounding the eustachian tube are removed en bloc with the laterosuperior and posterior wall of

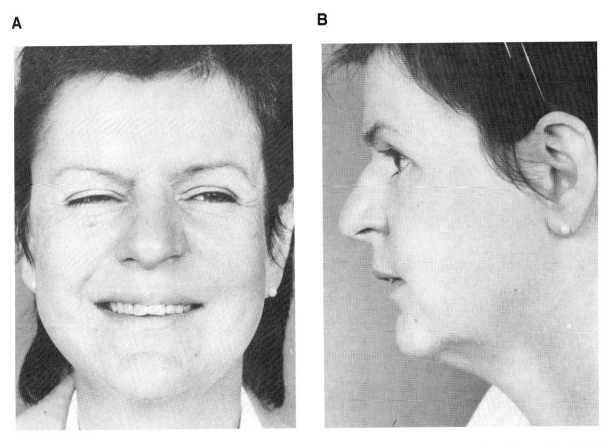

Figure 7 Patient whose scans are shown in Figure 4 six months following removal of the adenoid cystic carcinoma of the left infra-temporal fossa. *A*, Note the absence of scar and intact function of the facial muscles. *B*, The blind sac closure of the left external auditory canal as well as the retroauricular surgical scar are hardly visible.

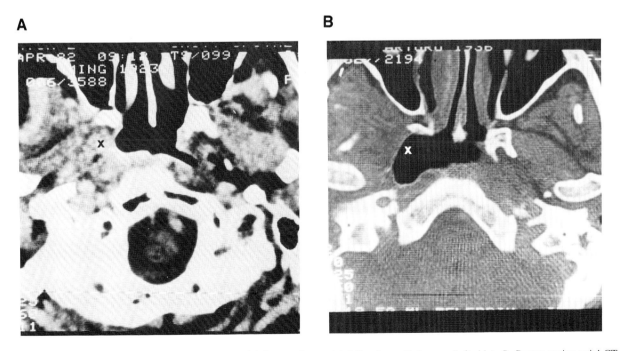

Figure 8 *A*, Axial CT scan showing a residual keratinizing carcinoma (x) following radiotherapy (left side). *B*, Postoperative axial CT scan showing radical tumor removal (x) through the infratemporal fossa.

the nasopharynx (Figs. 8B, 9A). On completion of the operation, only the opposite lateral wall of the nasopharynx with the contralateral pharyngeal ostium of the eustachian tube remains in situ (see Figs. 5D, 6B). The long-term results obtained in 13 patients with recurrent carcinoma of the nasopharynx after irradiation have been published elsewhere.[5] Radical removal was possible in all instances of recurrent T1 and T2 nonkeratinizing carcinoma. The radical removal of T3 and T4 recurrent tumors was impossible because of infiltration of the atlanto-occipital ligaments, cavernous sinus, and surrounding cranial nerves. In these instances, however, excellent palliation, particularly in regard to trigeminal pain, could be achieved. In view of the encouraging results obtained in limited recurring carcinoma, our follow-up of patients with a nasopharyngeal tumor following irradiation includes repeated biopsies, and as soon as there is histologic

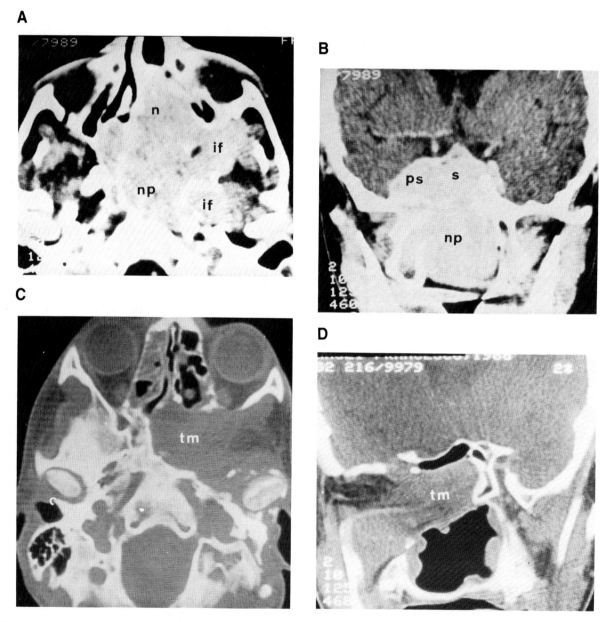

Figure 9 Juvenile nasopharyngeal angiofibroma class III. A, Axial CT scan showing tumor invasion of the nasopharynx (np), nasal cavity (n) and infratemporal fossa (if), with corresponding bone destruction. B, Coronal CT scan showing the tumor at the roof of the nasopharynx (np), infiltrating the base of the skull, sphenoid sinus (s) and right parasellar region (ps). The right cavernous sinus was compressed but not infiltrated by the tumor. C, Axial CT scan after radical removal. Note the extensive bony defect lateral to the internal carotid artery at the base of the middle cranial fossa. The mandibular condyle is intact. The temporalis muscle (tm) has been swung into the operative defect. D, Postoperative coronal CT scan showing the complete removal of the right pterygoid process and the extradural elevation of the right temporal lobe. The parasellar extension of the tumor was completely removed. The temporalis muscle (tm) is filling the operative defect up to the sphenoid sinus. The defect in the temporal bone area was filled out with a superiorly based sternocleidomastoid flap.

evidence of tumor persistence, we proceed to the surgical extirpation of the lesion via the infratemporal approach.

Juvenile angiofibroma

In 1983 I proposed the following classification of the juvenile angiofibroma of the nasopharynx:[5]

Class I: Tumor limited to the nasopharynx and nasal cavity with no bone destruction.

Class II: Tumor invading the pterygopalatine fossa, and the maxillary, ethmoid, and sphenoid sinuses with bone destruction.

Class III: Tumor invading the infratemporal fossa, orbit, and parasellar region, remaining lateral to the cavernous sinus.

Class IV: Tumors with massive invasion of the cavernous sinus, the optic chiasma, and/or pituitary fossa.

Class I and II tumors are curable by standard rhinologic and transpalatal procedures. In patients with class III tumors, radical removal is achieved through the type C infratemporal approach.[5] The surgical steps are the same as those described for the excision of infratemporal fossa tumors. The angiofibroma is separated first from the exposed internal carotid artery up to the foramen lacerum. In this way, life-threatening bleeding from this vessel can be avoided. After extradural elevation of the temporal lobe, the parasellar extension of the tumor can be separated from the lateral wall of the cavernous sinus, medial to the transected mandibular division of the trigeminal nerve, by means of bipolar coagulation and a modified septal raspatory (Fig. 9). The mobilized temporalis muscle is used as an axial vascularized pedicle flap to fill out the bony and soft tissue defect at the skull base (Figs. 9C, D). Preoperative embolization of the tumor via the internal maxillary artery facilitates its surgical extirpation from a lateral approach. Blunt dissection provides excellent exposure of the tumor portions lying within the nasal cavity and surrounding paranasal sinuses Fig. 9). The procedure can be carried out without major blood loss. The elegance of the lateral approach for extensive nasopharyngeal angiofibromas is documented in Figure 10, which shows no evidence of postoperative facial deformity.

In type IV tumors, only that part lateral to the internal carotid artery and cavernous sinus is removed in order to avoid lesions to cranial nerves III and IV. In such situations, radiation therapy is given if further tumor growth is demonstrated by computerized tomography.

PARAPHARYNGEAL SPACE

The infratemporal fossa approach type C can be used to remove tumors involving the parapharyngeal space from the base of the skull to the soft palate (Fig. 11). If the parapharyngeal space is involved down to the mesopharynx and tonsillar region, a combined retromandibular-infratemporal approach—leaving intact the continuity of the mandible—is employed. In such a case the facial nerve is mobilized from the geniculate ganglion to the parotid region in order to enlarge the surgical access by pushing it superiorly or inferiorly during tumor removal. A deltopectoral or pectoralis major myocutaneous flap may be necessary to reconstruct the excised lateral pharyngeal wall. The remaining operative cavity is filled out with the mobilized temporalis and sternocleidomastoid muscles (Fig. 12).

COMPLICATIONS

The complications of the infratemporal approach, types B and C, are shown in Table 3. There were no deaths in this group of 75 patients. The morbidity was limited to the unilateral conductive hearing loss secondary to the removal of the ossicular chain and obliteration of the middle ear cleft, as well as to the hypesthesia resulting from the section of the mandibular division of the trigeminal nerve. The postoperative conductive hearing loss is a relative complication since the eustachian tube function is usually already compromised by the underlying disease. In those rare instances of benign tumors situated lateral to the eustachian tube (2 patients out of 75), the eustachian tube and hearing function could be preserved. In all remaining instances, the exposure of the internal carotid artery throughout the temporal bone required the sacrifice of the eustachian tube; this is considered to be an acceptable price in view of the safety afforded by the direct visual control of the main arterial blood supply to the brain. The hyposensitivity of the face resulting from the section of the mandibular (and in some instances also from the maxillary) nerve is partially reversible after 3 to 6 months and not of primary concern to the patients. A noticeable masticatory dysfunction was observed in only two patients, in whom resection of the condylar process was necessary to gain access to large tumors extending into the upper neck. It appears, therefore, that preservation of the integrity of the mandibular condyle—which has been made possible in nearly all instances by the use of a special infratemporal retractor—prevents postoperative malocclusion in spite of the missing articular disc, articular fossa, and articular tubercle.

A most gratifying aspect of the lateral (infratemporal) approach to the skull base is also the avoidance of visible facial scars as well as of any noticeable disfigurement of facial contours. The only visible defect related to the intervention is the temporal depression due to the use of the temporalis muscle as an axial vascularized pedicle flap to obliterate the operative defect. A frontal muscle paresis, probably the result of undue inferior traction of the corresponding nerve, occurred only in two of 57 patients.

A

B

C

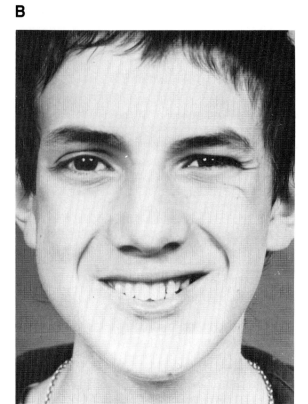

Figure 10 Juvenile nasopharyngeal angiofibroma class III. Patient whose scans are shown in Figure 9 six months following surgery. *A*, Lateral view showing the prolongation of the retroauricular incision in the neck as well as the supraclavicular horizontal incision used to mobilize the sternocleidomastoid muscle. *B and C*, Note the absence of visible scars in the face and the intact function of the facial muscles.

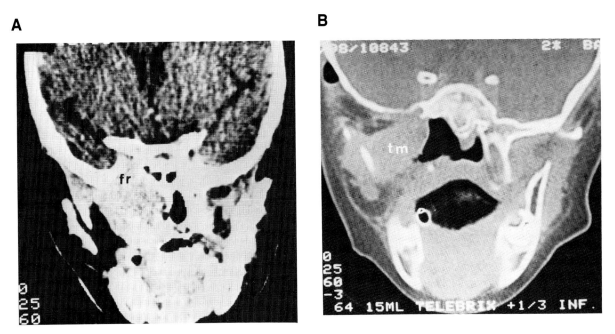

Figure 11 Rhabdomyosarcoma of the right parapharyngeal space in a 3-year-old child. Tumor persistence following chemotherapy and irradiation. *A*, Preoperative coronal CT scan showing invasion of the base of the skull up to the foramen rotundum (fr). *B*, Postoperative coronal CT scan showing radical removal of the tumor through a right infratemporal approach type C. The surgical defect has been filled out with the mobilized temporalis muscle (tm).

DISCUSSION

All three infratemporal fossa approaches (type A, type B, and type C) usually involve tumors infiltrating the bony base of the skull and the superior region of the neck. The type C approach is of particular interest to the head and neck surgeons because it is utilized for tumors originating from the infratemporal

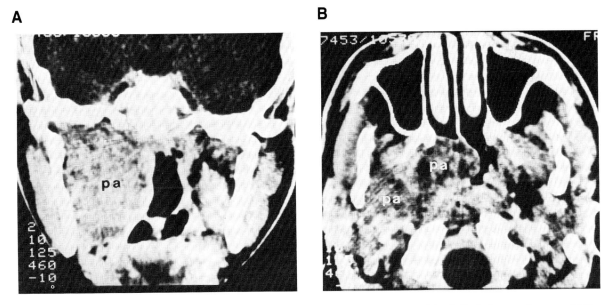

Figure 12 Recurrent pleomorphic adenoma of the right parapharangeal space reaching the base of the skull. *A*, Preoperative coronal CT scan showing the extension of the tumor (pa) in the right infratemporal fossa and base of the skull. *B*, Preoperative axial CT scan showing the tumor (pd) in the infratemporal fossa and nasopharynx. The left choanal opening is completely occluded by the tumor. *C*, Postoperative axial CT scan after radical tumor removal through a combined infratemporal-retromandibular approach. The defect in the left nasopharynx was closed with the temporalis muscle (tm). A superiorly based pedicle flap from the sternocleidomastoid muscle (scm) was used to fill out the retromandibular surgical defect.

C

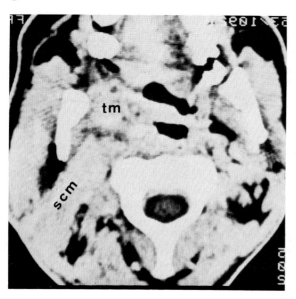

Figure 12 Continued.

TABLE 3 Complications of Types B and C Infratemporal Approach to Skull Base (N = 75)*

Complications	N	(%)
Mortality	—	—
Morbidity		
Conductive hearing loss	74	(98)
Hypesthesia V₃	69	(92)
Mandibular dysfunction	2	(2)
Paresis of frontal branch of VII	2	(2)
Disfigurement	—	—

fossa, the nasopharynx, and the parapharyngeal space. The described lateral approach to the skull base is, in essence, microsurgical and extradural. The principle of the approach is to gain surgical access by removing the bony base of the middle cranial fossa, displacing the mandibular condyle inferiorly, and exposing the internal carotid artery throughout the temporal bone up to the cavernous sinus. The short working distance, the ideal illumination and magnification afforded by the operating microscope, the utilization of a primarily aseptic operative field, and the absence of conspicuous scars and modifications of facial contours are the main advantages of the procedure. The disadvantages are the unilateral conductive hearing loss and hyposensitivity of the face resulting from the obliteration of the middle ear cleft and section of the mandibular division of the trigeminal nerve.

The lateral (infratemporal) approach to the skull base has opened new perspectives in the surgical management of skull base tumors. If the dream of the radical removal of tumors developing in the most hidden portions of the skull base is beginning to take real form, one has not to forget the still existing limitations imposed by malignant tumors infiltrating the cavernous sinus, the supraclinoid area, and the intradural portion of the cranial nerves. Further progress in the management of cancer at the base of the skull still requires, as in other head and neck areas, not only special surgical skills that have to accommodate the intricate anatomy of vital structures, but also the multidisciplinary help from specialists in radiology, chemotherapy, and immunotherapy.

REFERENCES

1. Fisch U. Infratemporal fossa approach for extensive tumors of the temporal bone and base of the skull. In: Silverstein H, Norrell H, (eds). Neurological Surgery of the Ear. Birmingham: Aesculapius Co, 1977.
2. Fisch U. Infratemporal fossa approach to tumors of the temporal bone and base of the skull. J Laryngol Otol 1978; 92:943–967.
3. Fisch U. Infratemporal fossa approach for glomus tumors of the temporal bone. Ann Otol Rhinol Laryngol 1982; 91:474–479.
4. Fisch U, Fagan P, Valavanis A. The infratemporal fossa approach to the lateral skull base. Otolaryngol Clin North Am 1984; 17:275.
5. Fisch U. Infratemporal fossa approach for nasopharyngeal tumors. Laryngoscope 1983; 93:36–44.
6. Fisch U, Pillsburgy HC. Infratemporal fossa approach to lesions in the temporal bone and base of skull. Arch Otolaryngol 1979; 105:999–1007.

CRANIOFACIAL SURGERY FOR CONGENITAL DEFORMITIES: ITS CONTRIBUTION TO SURGERY OF THE SKULL

IAN T. JACKSON, M.D., F.R.C.S., F.A.C.S.

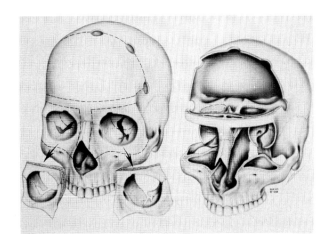

Figure 1 Approach and osteotomies for hypertelorism correction.

The traditional methods of approach to the anterior cranial fossa and the reconstruction of this area have been considerably modified by the addition of techniques developed for the treatment of congenital craniofacial deformity. The coronal flap has become the entrée to all areas above the horizontal mid area of the maxilla.[1-7] Magnificent exposure is obtained without obvious scarring. In malignant tumors, this latter feature is of less importance; additional facial resection and inevitable mutilation may be necessary for adequate tumor removal. There is less reluctance to remove large segments of orbit or maxilla for exposure; using standard osteotomy cuts, these segments are later replaced. In nonmalignant tumors and conditions such as fibrous dysplasia, immediate bony reconstruction is performed. Even the donor site for bone grafts has changed. In the past, iliac crest and split ribs held sway; now the most frequently used donor site is the skull. Split skull grafts provide abundant membranous bone, which seems to show less resorption with little or no donor site morbidity. The importance of communication between the extradural space and the nasopharynx is better understood, and methods for prevention of this hazardous situation have been developed.[5,8] Perhaps most important of all, plastic surgeon and neurosurgeon work together as a team.

CORRECTION OF ORBITAL HYPERTELORISM[4]

This procedure serves to illustrate many of the aforementioned points (Fig. 1). In hypertelorism, the orbits are spread apart by enlarged ethmoid sinuses, vertical facial clefts, or a midline encephalocele. The nose frequently shows considerable deformity. To obtain adequate correction of the deformity, the midline bony block is removed. The orbits are moved medially, and the nose is reconstructed.

A coronal flap is used, and this may be the sole approach unless a soft-tissue nasal procedure is required. A frontal bone flap is removed by the neurosurgeon, and the frontal lobes are retracted for anterior cranial base exposure.

A subperiosteal dissection exposes the skeleton of the nose, the orbits, and zygomatic arches, and the upper half of the maxilla.

The central bony block is removed; half its width is resected on either side of the cribriform plate, maintaining an intact dura. Every effort is made to preserve the nasal mucosa and to leave the nasopharynx inviolate. Osteotomies are made around the orbits, and the latter are moved medially. All resultant bony defects are grafted, usually with split skull. This is also used to provide support for the nasal dorsum. All mobilized bone and bone grafts are wired securely in place. The scalp is sutured back in position with suction drainage under the flap. In this sequence of events, there should be few, if any, complications.

Where there is a dural tear requiring repair with a graft and connection with an open nasopharynx, this is a different situation. The complications resulting from this can be meningitis or extradural abscess formation. In order to securely prevent this from happening, the nasopharynx must be separated from the extradural space with well-vascularized tissue. This purpose is best served with a flap of galea with the overlying frontalis muscle: the galeal frontalis flap. This can be introduced into the anterior cranial fossa base and proves to be an effective seal.

ANTERIOR CRANIAL BASE TUMORS

The approach outlined for hypertelorism can be applied to remove tumors of the anterior cranial base. This has resulted in fewer complications and a better success rate in tumor extirpation.

FIBROUS DYSPLASIA[9-1] (Fig. 2)

Although not strictly a tumor, this condition behaves like one and must be treated as such to prevent recurrence. This has been noted especially when it involves the fronto-orbital region.

A coronal flap approach is utilized, and a frontal bone flap is raised. Any involved frontal bone is removed. The affected orbital, nasal, and temporal areas are widely resected until normal bone margins are obtained. The bony defect is reconstructed immediately with split skull grafts if possible, or in combination with split rib grafts. Resorption of the grafts may eventually occur, causing bony irregularities that will require contour grafting.

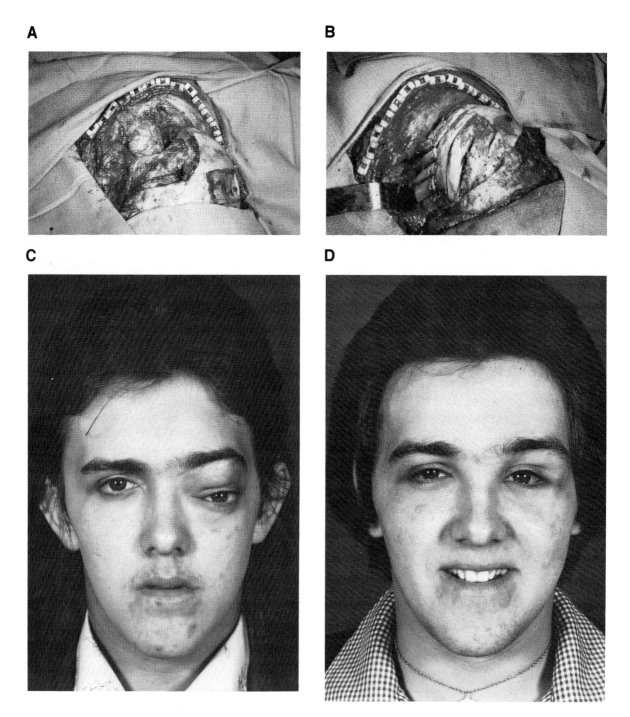

Figure 2 *A*, Resection of left temporal fronto-orbital fibrous dysplasia from coronal approach. *B*, Reconstruction with split rib grafts. *C*, Preoperative. *D*, Postoperative result.

There have been no complications in these cases and no recurrence of fibrous dysplasia.

PENETRATING MIDFACE CANCERS[5,12–19] (Fig. 3)

These are usually basal cell carcinoma, squamous cell carcinoma, adenocystic carcinoma, or mucoepidermoid carcinoma. There may have been multiple excisions in the past, augmented with radiotherapy and chemotherapy. Many will be considered inoperable on presentation by the referring doctors. A CT scan with contrast will give an indication of tumor extent, although sometimes this can be misleading, either exaggerating or minimizing apparent tumor size.

Surgery should be performed under frozen section control, and it should be radical. The main cause for concern is a communication between the extradural space and the nasopharynx.

A

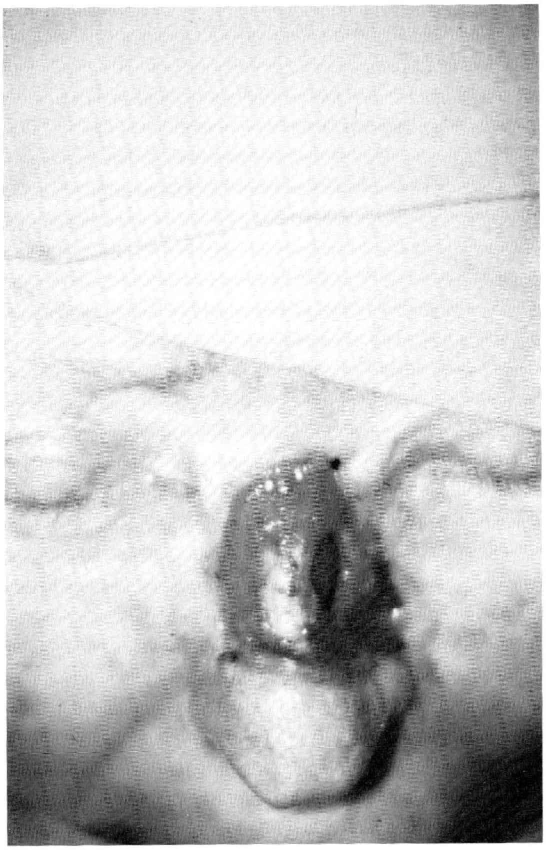

B

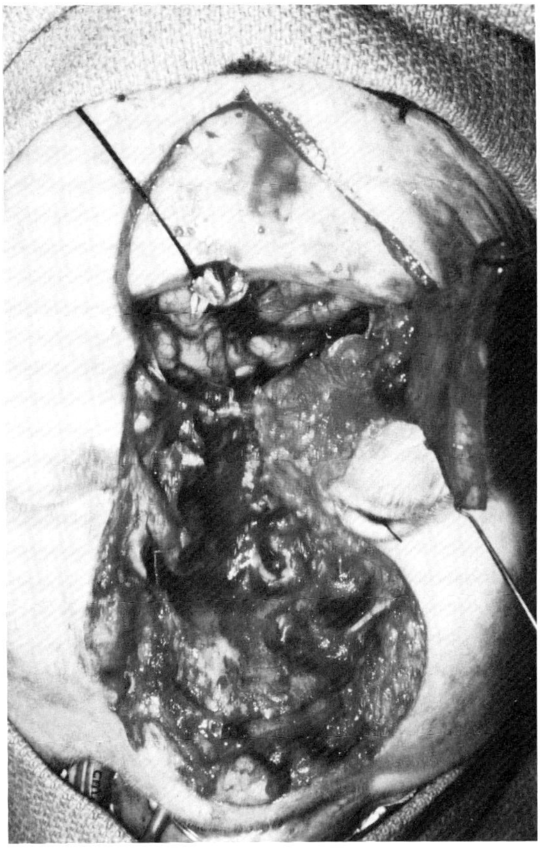

C

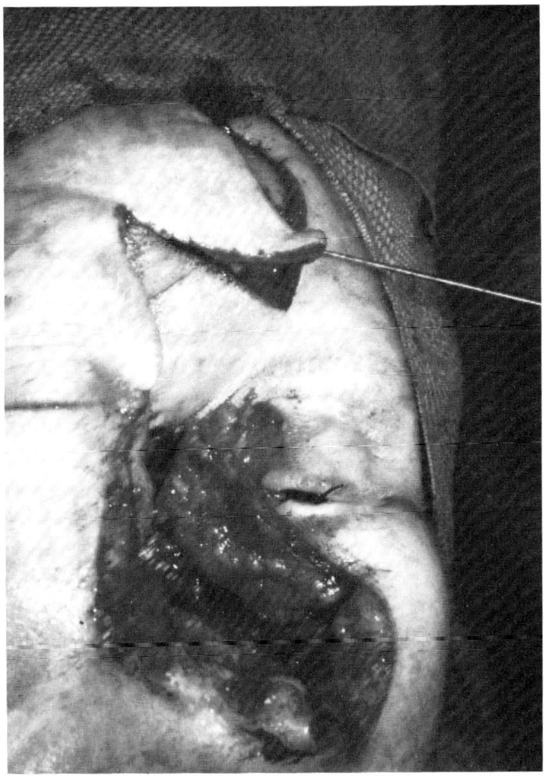

Figure 3   *A*, Penetrating basal cell carcinoma of nose. *B*, Resection. *C*, Cover with extended glabellar flap. *D*, Postoperative result at 4-year follow-up. E, With prosthesis.

D

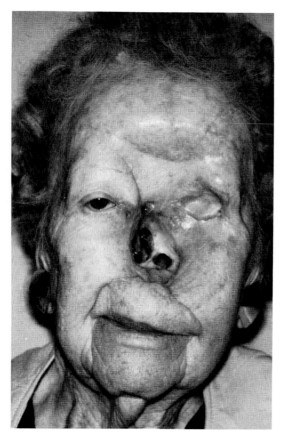

E

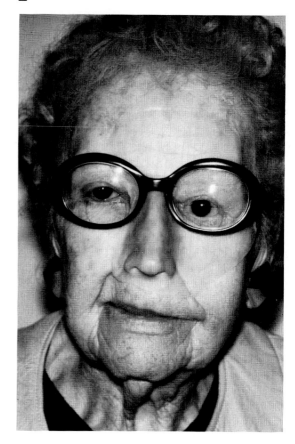

Figure 3 Continued.

The approach may be direct, or a coronal flap may be used, depending on tumor position and extent. The central cranial base to the posterior wall of the sphenoid sinus, the cribriform plate, and frequently the overlying dura are resected en bloc with the medial orbital walls and as much of the nasal cavity, nasopharynx, palate, and cheeks as indicated. An orbital exenteration may be indicated in some patients.

The dura is repaired, and the skull base is reconstructed with an extended glabellar flap based on the medial end of an eyebrow. This flap can be swung downward and backward to be sutured to drill holes in the skull base. The forehead defect is closed either directly or with a Z-plasty. The remainder of the nasal cavity is split skin grafted.

In 16 patients treated in this way, there has been one small extradural abscess, from which the patient recovered. There have been no deaths, and all patients are alive without local recurrence, the longest follow-up being $4^1/_2$ years. One patient has liver metastases.

SARCOMAS

These may occur in any position in the skull base area; those involving the anterior area occur around the orbit or in the nasal septal area. Rhabdomyosarcoma is most commonly seen, but those in and around the orbit are now treated with biopsy, chemotherapy, and radiotherapy.

CHONDROSARCOMA OF THE NASAL SEPTUM[7] (Fig. 4)

The greatest challenge in these cases is exposure. This has been greatly facilitated by the coronal flap combined with the face-splitting incision. The latter is an extension of the Weber-Ferguson incision. A frontal bone flap is elevated and removed. An osteotomy is performed bilaterally in the glabellar area and through the medial orbital walls; this is extended along the orbital floor unilaterally or bilaterally. As much maxilla or maxillae as required is included; the lower osteotomy is transverse above the tooth roots. This single large bony segment is now removed, following which the tumor is well exposed. It is now possible to perform a total en bloc tumor resection, including dura if necessary. The dura is repaired and the block of bone replaced. Since the area is now open into the nasopharynx, a flap of galea and frontalis muscles based on the supratrochlear vessels is swung down and used to cover the bone exposed to the nasopharynx. The

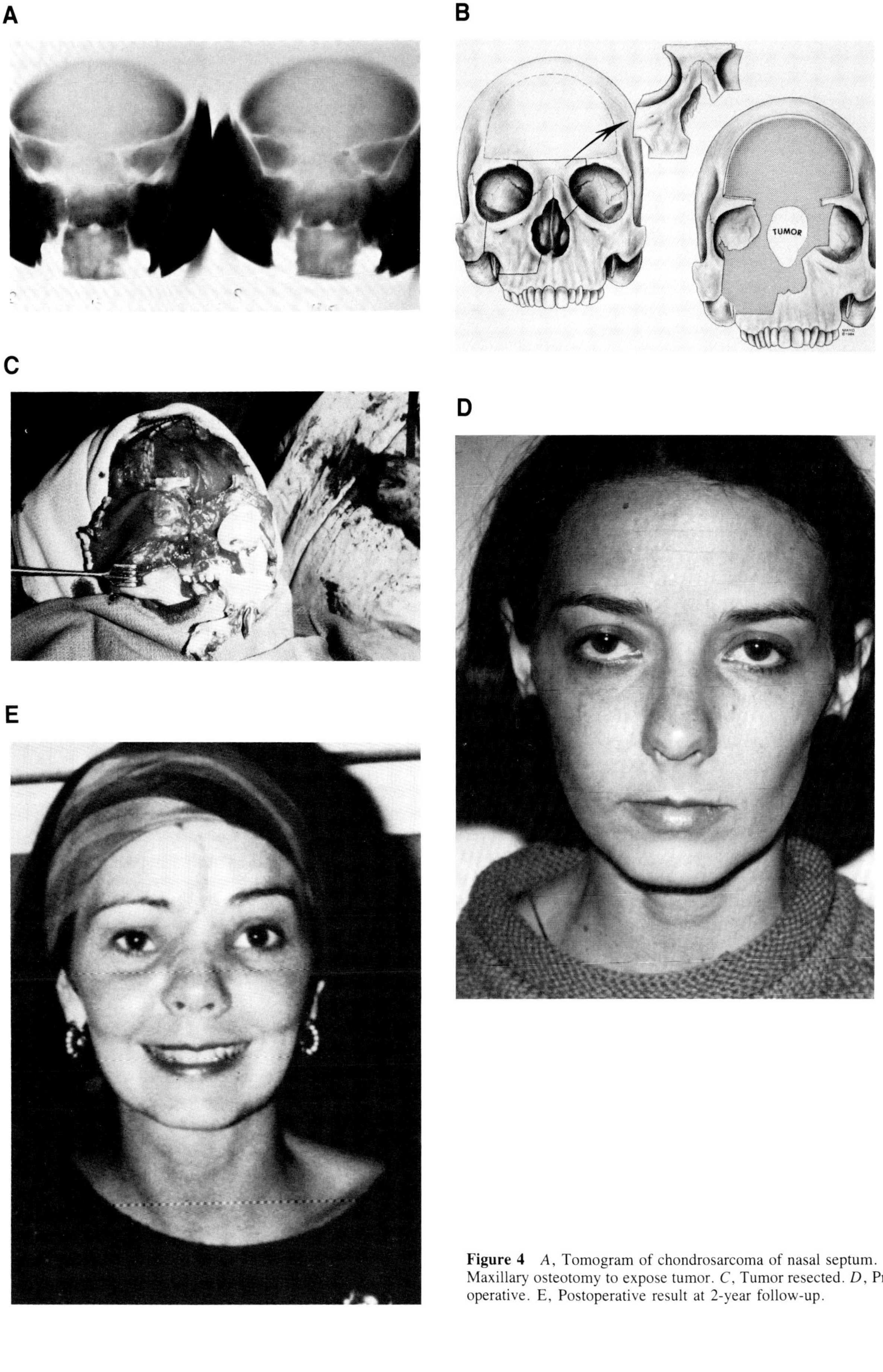

A

B

C

D

E

Figure 4 *A*, Tomogram of chondrosarcoma of nasal septum. *B*, Maxillary osteotomy to expose tumor. *C*, Tumor resected. *D*, Preoperative. *E*, Postoperative result at 2-year follow-up.

A

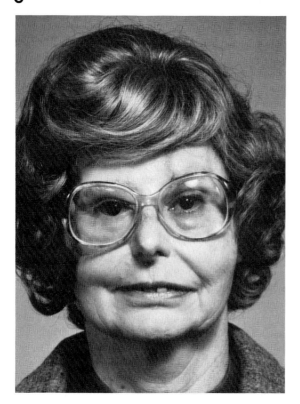

B

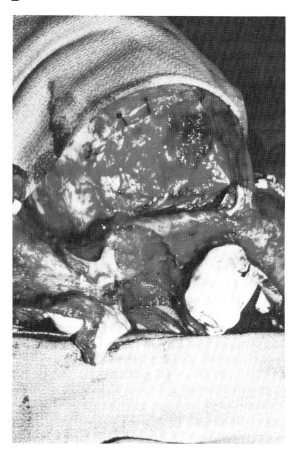

C

Figure 5 *A*, Recurrent esthesioneuroblastoma, right orbit and base of skull. *B*, Tumor resected with right maxilla. *C*, Postoperative result at 2-year follow-up.

A

B

C

D

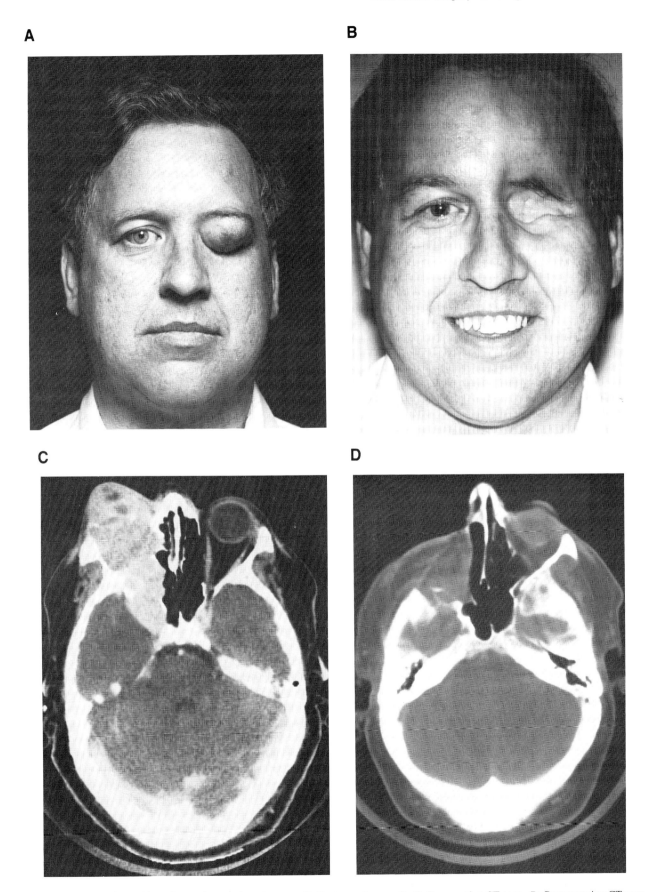

Figure 6 *A*, Patient with malignant hemangiopericytoma. *B*, Postoperative result. *C*, Preoperative CT scan. *D*, Postoperative CT scan.

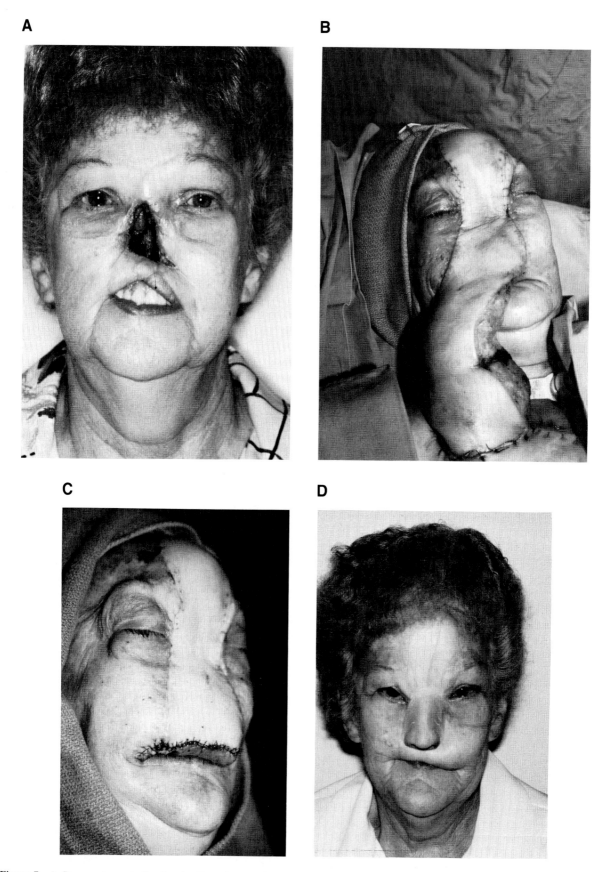

Figure 7 *A*, Recurrent penetrating basal cell carcinoma of mid face; forehead already used in previous reconstruction. *B, C*, Reconstruction with pectoralis major myocutaneous flap. *D*, Postoperative result at 4-year follow-up.

area is then resurfaced with a split skin graft. Of the three patients with this problem, one had an extradural abscess requiring removal of frontal bone. All are alive and well without recurrence, the longest follow-up being $2^1/_2$ years.

ORBITAL TUMORS[2,20,21] (Fig. 5)

Many varieties of tumor arise in and around the orbit. In many cases, total excision is possible only with a transcranial approach. A good example is a recurrent esthesioneuroblastoma involving the orbit, maxilla, and anterior skull base. The approach is by a coronal flap and a face-splitting incision. The floor of the anterior cranial fossa, the orbit and its contents, the nasal cavity, the contralateral medial orbital wall, and the maxilla are excised. The eyelid skin is preserved.

There is a very significant connection between the extradural space (with dural repair in situ) and the nasal and oral cavities. The cranial base is closed off laterally with a temporalis muscle flap and medially with a galeal frontalis flap. The orbital area is resurfaced by suturing the eyelid skin together. The mouth and nose are resurfaced with a split skin graft. Two years after the procedure, the patient is alive and well without recurrence.

RECONSTRUCTION

Although total reconstruction should be performed for nonmalignant conditions, only the minimal reconstruction required for prosthetic rehabilitation should be carried out in malignant tumors, especially if they are recurrent. A case that serves to illustrate this point is a man with a left orbital malignant hemangiopericytoma. This was resected, removing the frontal bone and the left orbit and its contents. Closure was obtained using the eyelid skin. Eighteen months later, he was explored to reconstruct the fronto-orbital area, and a small focus of tumor was discovered at the apex of the old resection. This was widely excised, and the reconstruction was left in abeyance. Had this ''second look'' not been necessary, this man would have died of his recurrence, which would have grown, obscured by the overlying reconstruction. He is alive and well without recurrence $3^1/_2$ years later. It is hoped that reconstruction can be performed in the near future (Fig. 6).

Another reason for delayed reconstruction is the utilization of an area that could be vital should a recurrence develop. This was seen in a patient with a penetrating midface squamous cell carcinoma. After many minor procedures, the nose was resected, and an immediate reconstruction was performed using the forehead. Once again, the tumor recurred under the nasal reconstruction, and this had to be resected. When she presented, there was a penetrating midface tumor that required the resection outlined earlier. It was not possible to use the forehead to reconstruct the floor of the anterior cranial fossa, and thus the more extensive and much more hazardous pectoralis major myocutaneous flap was used (Fig. 7). Because of the bulk of this flap, it is difficult to suture into the posterior edge of the resection. There is a greater possibility of extension of infection from the nasopharynx to the extradural space with this reconstruction.

DISCUSSION

Using accepted techniques for the correction of congenital craniofacial defects, it is possible to obtain wider exposure of craniofacial tumors. Having achieved this, resection can be accomplished under direct vision in an en bloc fashion.[1,6,7,21-24] When indicated, immediate reconstruction is performed; in the majority of malignant cases, it is delayed. More recent spin-offs from craniofacial surgery for congenital anomalies have been the use of split skull grafts, the galeal frontalis flap, and osteotomies for exposure and subsequent replacement. Tumor excision is now safer and more complete and, it is hoped, will result in an improved prognosis in these difficult cases.

REFERENCES

1. Derome PJ. The transbasal approach to tumors invading the base of the skull. In: Schmidek HH, Sweet WW, eds. Current techniques in operative neurosurgery. New York: Grune & Stratton, 1977:223.
2. Jackson IT, Hide TAH. Further extensions of craniofacial surgery. In: Jackson IT, ed. Recent advances in plastic surgery—2. New York: Churchill Livingstone, 1981:241.
3. Jackson IT, Hide TAH. A systemic approach to tumors of the base of the skull. J Maxillofac Surg 1982; 10:92.
4. Jackson IT, Munro IR, Salyer KE, et al. Atlas of craniomaxillofacial surgery. St. Louis: CV Mosby, 1982.
5. Jackson IT, Laws ER Jr, Martin R. A craniofacial approach to advanced recurrent cancer of the center face. J Head Neck Surg 1983; 5:474.
6. Jackosn IT, Marsh WR. Anterior cranial fossa tumors. Ann Plast Surg 1983; 11:479.
7. Jackson IT, Marsh WR, Hide TAH. Treatment of tumors involving the anterior cranial fossa. J Head Neck Surg 1984; 6:901–913.
8. Ousterhout DK, Tessier P. Closure of large cribriform defects with a forehead flap. J Maxillofac Surg 1981; 9:7.
9. Jackson IT. Fibrous dysplasia. In: Stark R, ed. Plastic surgery of the head and neck. New York: Churchill Livingstone, in press.
10. Jackson IT, Hide TAH, Gomuwka PK, Laws ER Jr, Langford K. Treatment of cranio-orbital fibrous dysplasia. J Maxillofac Surg 1982; 10:138.
11. Munro IR, Chen YR. Radical treatment of fronto-orbital fibrous dysplasia: the chain-link fence. Plast Reconstr Surg 1981; 67:719.
12. Clifford P. Transcranial approach for cancer of the antroethmoidal area. Clin Otolaryngol 1977; 2:115.
13. Ketcham AS, Hoye RC, VanBuren JM, et al. Complications of intracranial facial resection for tumors of the paranasal sinuses. Am J Surg 1966; 112:591.
14. Ketcham AS, Wilkins RH, VanBuren JM, Smith RR. A combined intracranial facial approach to the paranasal sinuses. Am J Surg 1963; 106:698.
15. Millar HS, Petty PG, Wilson WF, Hueston JT. A combined intracranial and facial approach for excision and repair of cancer of the ethmoid sinuses. Aust NZ J Surg 1973; 43:179.
16. Shah JP, Galicich JH. Craniofacial resection for malignant

tumors of ethmoid and anterior skull base. Arch Otolaryngol 1977; 103:514.

17. Sisson GA, Bytell DE, Becker SP, Ruge D. Carcinoma of the paranasal sinuses and cranial-facial resection. J Laryngol Otol 1976; 90:59.

18. Smith RR, Klopp CT, Williams JM. Surgical treatment of cancer of the frontal sinus and adjacent areas. Cancer 1954; 7:991.

19. VanBuren JM, Ommaya AK, Ketcham AS. Ten years' experience with radical combined craniofacial resection of malignant tumors of the paranasal sinuses. J Neurosurg 1968; 28:341.

20. Ray BS, McLean JM. Combined intracranial and orbital operation for retinoblastoma. Arch Ophthalmol 1943; 30:437.

21. Westbury G, Wilson JSP, Richardson A. Combined craniofacial resection for malignant disease. Am J Surg 1975; 130:463.

22. Derome PJ. Les tumeurs sphéno-ethmoïdales: possibilités d'exérèse et de réparation chirurgicales. Neurochirurgie 1972; 18(Suppl 1):1.

23. Edgerton MT. Discussion. Plast Reconstr Surg 1981; 67:730.

24. Schramm VL Jr, Myers EN, Maroon JC. Anterior skull base surgery for benign and malignant disease. Laryngoscope 1979; 89:1077.

SUPRAORBITAL RIM APPROACH TO LESIONS OF THE CRANIOFACIAL JUNCTION

JOHN A. JANE, M.D.
MICHAEL E. JOHNS, M.D.
ROBERT W. CANTRELL, M.D.
AUSTIN COLOHAN, M.D.
MICHAEL KAPLAN, M.D.

Improved visualization of the anterior skull base has resulted in better treatment of tumors involving this area. For example, the addition of frontal craniotomy to the facial approach to esthesioneuroblastoma has made en bloc removal feasible. The frontal

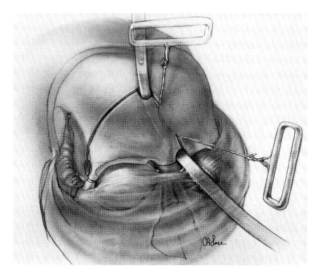

Figure 2 The Gigli saw is being used to complete the cut between the two frontal burr holes. The superior cut has already been performed.

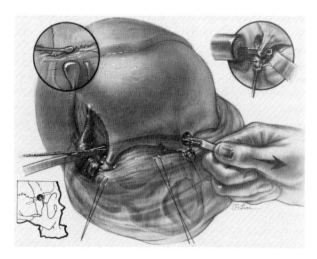

Figure 1 The Gigli saw is passed between the midline frontal burr hole and the burr hole behind the zygomatic process of the frontal bone, the position of the latter shown in the lower left inset. The periorbita is carefully stripped as shown in the upper left inset. A sagittal saw is used to cut through the zygomatic process of the frontal bone to facilitate the passage of the Gigli saw (upper right inset). The supraorbital cut is then made with good visualization, after inferior retraction and protection of the orbital contents.

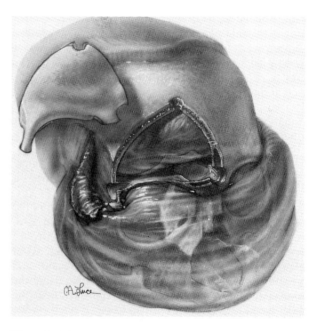

Figure 3 The free frontal flap has been removed, in which is incorporated part of the orbital roof.

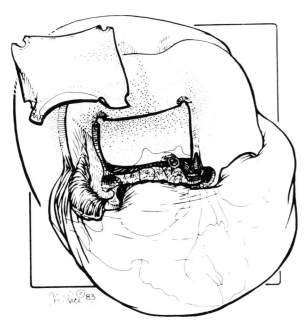

Figure 4 A diagrammatic representation of the exposure obtained.

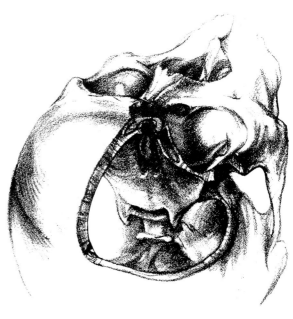

Figure 6 Operative view showing the excellent exposure back to the anterior clinoid and extending forward to the cribiform plate.

craniotomy itself can be modified, as will be described, for even better access to these lesions and indeed to any tumor involving the junction between the intracranial contents and the face.

TECHNIQUES

After placement of spinal drains, a standard hairline coronal scalp incision is turned down. The pericranium is left in place on the skull so that it, along with variable amounts of temporalis fascia, can be used in the repair of the defect in the floor of the frontal fossa. The pericranium is sharply incised just above the orbital rim, and the periorbita is dissected carefully from the orbital roof. Bur holes are placed in the midline just above the nasal frontal suture, behind the zygomatic process of the frontal bone, and superiorly just off the midline (Figs. 1 and 2). The Gigli saw guide is passed as shown (Fig. 2) and the flap turned (Fig. 3). We prefer using the Gigli rather than the craniotome because the beveled edges make the bone sit more securely. Figure 4 shows the resulting exposure. The orbital contents are visualized, thus making the subsequent medial cut in the orbit easier and

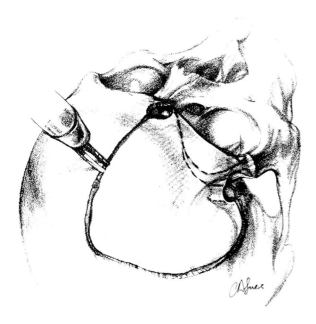

Figure 5 Operative view using the craniotome to turn the superior and lateral parts of the flap. The supraorbital cut is always made with the Gigli saw.

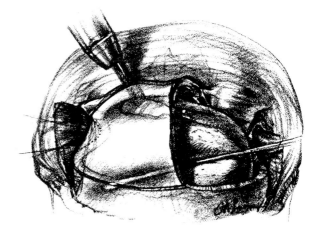

Figure 7 For bilateral exposure, the superior saggital sinus and dura overlying the opposite frontal lobe are detaced under direct visualization and the craniotome used to turn the contralateral osteoplastic bone flap.

more accurate. The cribiform plate is also seen, and the olfactory fibers can be dissected from it and clipped and cut. Figure 5 shows the actual operative view, this time the flap being turned with a craniotome. Figure 6 shows the operative view of the cribiform plate. If a bilateral exposure is necessary, the dura and sagittal sinus are separated from the skull, and the craniotome used to turn a second flap based on the opposite temporalis (Fig. 7). The result is seen in Figure 8.

The olfactory fibers are carefully removed from the cribiform plate. We often place a suture through the dura, place a clip behind it, and then cut the nerve with its dural investment (Fig. 9, *inset*). The subsequent chisel cuts are made under direct visualization,

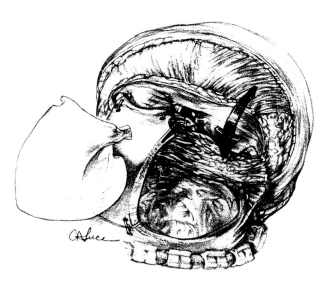

Figure 10 At the completion of the procedure a skin graft is placed from below and the pericranium and temporalis are used to cover the defect in the floor of the anterior fossa.

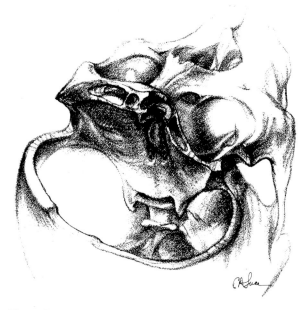

Figure 8 The bifrontal exposure afforded by this approach is shown.

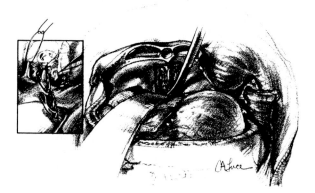

Figure 9 After retraction of the frontal lobe extradurally the olfactory fibers are carefully disected from the cribiform plate. The inset shows a ligature placed around the olfactory nerve and then secured in place with a clip before transection of the nerve to reduce the possibility of a CSF leak. The chisel cuts around the cribiform plate are then made.

as seen in Figure 9. Precise repair of the floor of the frontal fossa is essential. A skin graft is placed from the outside; then a flap of pericranium and temporalis is used to cover the floor (Fig. 10).

DISCUSSION

The techniques just described are designed to provide a better exposure of the floor of the frontal fossa. Olfactory groove and tuberculum sellae meningiomas are nicely handled from this approach, and the increased angulation of the view of the surgeon is particularly suitable for craniopharyngiomas.

We believe it is the procedure of choice for all orbital tumors except inferior lesions.[1]

The Otolaryngology-Head and Neck Service at the University of Virginia has had extensive experience with esthesioneuroblastomas. The surgical therapy for these lesions has slowly evolved and, at present, the superior visualization provided by either the unilateral or bilateral flap is our preferred approach.[2]

Undoubtedly, our approach and techniques will change. One essential feature should remain: the active collaboration between the intracranial and extracranial surgeon in dealing with lesions involving the junction of the skull and face.

REFERENCES

1. Jane JA, Park TS, Pobereskin LH, Winn HR, Butler AB. The supraorbital approach: Technical note. Neurosurgery 1982; 11:537–542.
2. Cantrell RW, Ghorayeb BY, Fitz-Hugh GS. Esthesioneuroblastoma: diagnosis and treatment. Ann Otol Rhinol Laryngol 1977; 86(6):760–765.

ANTERIOR CRANIOFACIAL SURGERY

VICTOR L. SCHRAMM Jr., M.D., F.A.C.S.

Craniofacial surgery for tumor resection is one of the most challenging areas in head and neck surgery. Until recently, patients with diseases at the junction of the cranial and facial skeleton were considered to be in a hopeless situation. Gradually, the dangers of surgical intervention in this area have been reduced so that the pessimistic outlook of the past has evolved to one of cautious optimism. Critical to the success of craniofacial surgery is the teamwork approach to the evaluation, anesthetic, and surgery. This report describes the application of surgical techniques currently in use for anterior craniofacial surgery.

The craniofacial approach is used for removal of benign tumors of the meninges that may extend through the anterior or middle fossa skull base, as well as benign or malignant neoplasms of the anterior facial structures, nose, and paranasal sinuses that approach the dura. Combined craniofacial resection is ideally suited to obtain a superior margin in the surgical management of tumors of the nose and paranasal sinuses, but may also be applied to a wide variety of other tumors as well. Tumors that arise in this area tend to be rare or uncommon, and only a small proportion of patients who are candidates for craniofacial resection have squamous cell carcinoma. It is difficult to define absolute indications and contraindications for craniofacial surgery because of the range of biologic behavior in the benign and malignant tumors that occur in this area. Relative contraindications for malignant disease include cavernous sinus involvement, a direct extension into frontal lobes of the brain, and tumors surrounding both optic nerves. Benign tumors, however, can be dissected from the optic nerves, and if the anterior approach is combined with an infratemporal fossa dissection, tumor can be removed from along the sixth nerve within the cavernous sinus. Except under unusual circumstances, patients with distant metastatic disease are not candidates for craniofacial surgery. Though not a definite contraindication, neck metastases from undifferentiated tumors in this region are associated with survivals of 6 months of less, and craniofacial resection may not be indicated.

EVALUATION

Precise determination of the location and extent of disease is perhaps more important in this region than in any other in the head and neck because of the frequent narrow margins of resection in craniofacial surgery. Physical examination remains the best technique for determining extension of disease near or into

facial skin. The ultimate planning of the surgical procedure, however, depends primarily on the location of tumor as documented by axial and coronal computerized tomography (Fig. 1). The neurosurgeon, head and neck surgeon, and radiologist should confer simultaneously so that any questions regarding the location of the tumor as it relates to possible resecta-

A

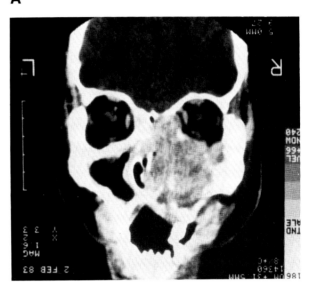

B

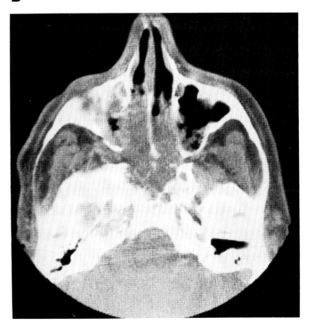

Figure 1 *A,* Coronal computerized tomogram of patient with maxillary, ethmoid and nasal squamous carcinoma involving roof of ethmoid and cribriform areas. *B,* Angled axial CT in patient with chondrosarcoma of maxilla and nasal cavity with posterior extension to involve sphenoid and clivus. Combined transfrontal cranial, infratemporal fossa, and lateral rhinotomy approaches provided exposure for gross tumor removal.

bility can be answered. Angiography is no longer routinely done, but may be indicated in special circumstances such as when preoperative tumor embolization is desired. Whenever possible, a tissue diagnosis should be obtained. A transnasal biopsy is usually possible when dealing with tumors of the nose and paranasal sinuses, but for other tumors, a biopsy should be done in a way that does not interfere with subsequent resection. A biopsy may not always be possible prior to surgery, but a likely diagnosis may be suspected from the location, CT scan appearance, and history of the tumor growth.

OPERATIVE TECHNIQUE

Although a standard operative technique is described here, modifications in the facial as well as the frontal approach are frequently necessary, depending on the type and location of the disease. The technique described is designed to prevent surgically related complications. Preoperatively, if palatal resection is required, a surgical obturator should be constructed. Antibiotic coverage, beginning at least 2 hours prior to surgery, is indicated for all patients. Either high doses of penicillin and chloramphenicol or a third-generation cephalosporin are given intravenously. Oral endotracheal anesthesia is administered and tracheostomy has not been found necessary. Although the anterior scalp may be shaved, no complications have arisen when the hair has just been parted along the incision line. To avoid complications of brain retraction, a lumbar subarachnoid catheter is used for spinal fluid drainage. After removal of 75 to 100 cc of spinal fluid, mannitol is given (50 to 75 g), and slight hyperventilation is instituted to lower the PCO_2.

The transfrontal craniotomy is usually done first. The coronal flap is outlined so that it falls approximately 2 cm behind the hairline and is extended above the ear to include both temporal arteries, as well as the supraorbital vessels. If a galeal pericranial flap is to be used, periosteum is elevated with the bicoronal flap. Periosteum is left over the frontal bone if an osteoplastic frontal sinus flap is chosen. The margins of the frontal sinus are outlined from a template traced from a Caldwell radiograph (6-ft film-to-tube exposure distance) (Fig. 2). An oscillating saw is used to incise the margins of the frontal sinus with a beveled cut to support the bone when it is replaced. All mucosa is removed from the frontal sinus, and then, by means of a cutting bur, the bone of the posterior table is removed on either side of the midline (Fig. 3). Once dura is exposed, it can be elevated away from the posterior table bone to protect it while the bone is removed. The dura is tightly attached in the midline and can be elevated most easily by approaching this area from both sides. Elevation is then carried lateral to the crista galli and olfactory nerves, and subsequently the crista is removed with a needle-nosed rongeur and the olfactory nerves transected with a No. 11 scalpel

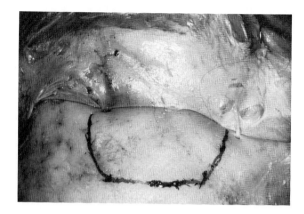

Figure 2 Coronal flap with periosteum retracted to level of supraorbital rims. Outline of frontal sinus marked on bone.

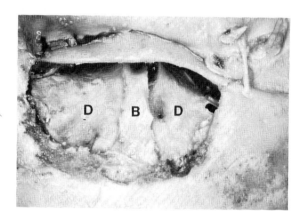

Figure 3 Anterior table of frontal sinus removed with beveled saw cut and posterior table partially removed, exposing dura (D) prior to removal of bone (B) from midline dura.

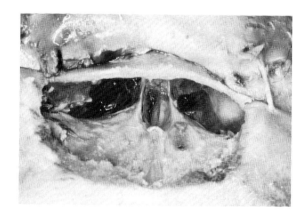

Figure 4 Posterior table of frontal sinus removed and dura elevated, exposing olfactory nerves in the midline.

blade (Fig. 4). Spinal fluid leak after transection of the olfactory nerves is inevitable. During the remainder of the dissection, the area of the olfactory bulb is protected by cottonoids. Closure of dura can be done as far as possible, but frequently the dura is most ef-

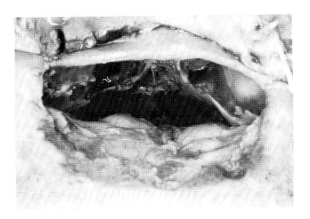

Figure 5 Olfactory nerves transected, crista galli removed, and dura elevated over orbits and posteriorly to optic chiasm.

ficiently closed following tumor resection through the facial exposure (Fig. 5).

The coronal flap is temporarily replaced while the anterior facial approach is carried out. Unless tumor resection requires otherwise, the facial approach is done through a lateral rhinotomy (Fig. 6). Addi-

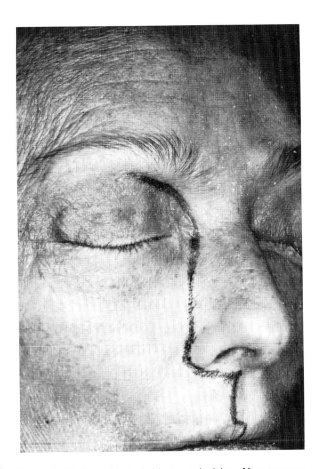

Figure 6 Outline of lateral rhinotomy incision. Note preservation of nostril margins and lip incision along edge of philtrum and stepped to midline at vermilion border.

tional exposure to the opposite orbital roof may be obtained through an external ethmoid-type incision. If the orbital contents are to be preserved, the periorbita is elevated around the lacrimal sac and along the superior medial and inferior orbit. The lacrimal sac and the anterior and posterior ethmoid vessels are divided. A precise lateral nasal osteotomy can be done with a reciprocating saw. The exact location of further facial bone cuts is dictated by the extent of resection. The superior bone cuts are done either from below, with the brain being retracted and protected by cottonoids and malleable retractors, or transcranially. The cut across the sphenoid into the sphenoid sinus is always done transcranially; the bone is scored with a drill and subsequently transected with a curved osteotome. After the bone cuts have been completed, the specimen is mobilized and soft tissue attachments removed or divided by scissors. All bone margins are smoothed with a double-action rongeur, and all exposed sinus mucosa is removed.

A watertight dural repair is critical if postoperative spinal fluid leak and meningitis are to be avoided. Direct suturing of dural tears is usually possible except in the midline. Often a temporalis fascia graft is necessary in the olfactory area. If no dura has been resected and if the dural closure is watertight, a skin graft may be placed directly on the dura to complete the anterior fossa reconstruction (Fig. 7). This is a satisfactory reconstruction if a maxillectomy or orbital exenteration has been done. If there is no direct access to the skin graft, crusting and postoperative cavity care problems are immense.

When dura has been previously irradiated, when dura has been resected and grafted, or when there is not direct access for cavity cleaning, a galeal pericranial flap reconstruction of the skull base is used. The galeal pericranial flap is outlined on the coronal flap to include a width adequate to incorporate the supratrochlear vessels. The length of the flap must be sufficient to reach the planum of the sphenoid (Fig. 8). The flap is elevated just superficial to the galea (Fig. 9), and then is turned over the frontal bone edge and positioned between dura and the nasal cavity (Fig. 10). The galeal pericranial flap can be made large enough so that it can fill the space left by cranialization of the frontal sinus. Before the anterior table bone is replaced, careful hemostasis must be ensured to avoid postoperative intracranial hematoma. The dura is secured to the edges of the bone and to the bone flap with tack-up sutures. The anterior table bone is then replaced (Fig. 11) and secured along the superior margins, leaving sufficient space for the galeal pericranial flap below. If postoperative radiation therapy is contemplated, wire sutures should be avoided so that local electron scatter and osteoradionecrosis do not subsequently develop. Skin grafting of the nasal side of the galeal pericranial flap is not necessary, and secondary healing leaves a mucosa-like wettable surface which requires little postoperative care by the pa-

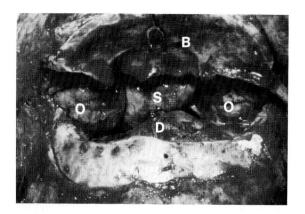

Figure 7 Osteoplastic frontal sinus approach showing attached bone flap (B), repaired dura (D), orbital contents (O), and nasal cavity skin graft (S).

tient. Postoperatively, a lumbar drain is left in place for 24 to 48 hours and a low-normal spinal fluid pressure is maintained. Intravenous antibiotics are continued as long as packing remains in the nose.

Variation from this technique may be necessary, depending on the extent of resection required. Al-

though bone grafting of the skull base has not proved necessary, immediate reconstruction of a resected frontal bone by split iliac crest or rib is advised.

The concept of wide en bloc resection is of necessity modified in the performance of craniofacial surgery. The goal is to have an adequate margin for the disease process, but this may not always be done with a single en bloc specimen. The pathologist examining the specimen needs to be advised as to the technique used and the resection margins obtained because grossly, particularly after tissue fixation, it may appear that multiple positive margins are present.

Because of the variety of benign and malignant diseases that are treated by craniofacial resection, the efficacy of the surgical technique can be stated in only general terms. In a personal series of over thirty patients, none treated by the technique described developed a major complication. Patients treated for benign disease or low-grade malignant disease, such as the esthesioneuroblastoma or chondrosarcoma, have remained free of local disease. Since half the patients with high-grade malignant disease have remained free of disease 3 or more years following resection, craniofacial resection may be considered for such patients in selected circumstances.

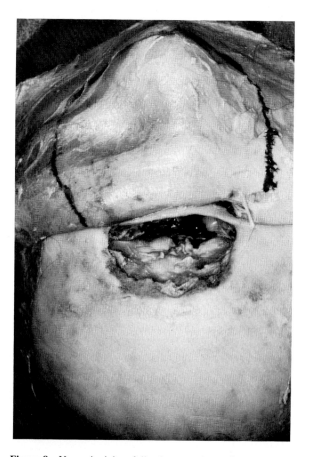

Figure 8 Unrepaired dura following resection and outline of galeal-pericranial flap on forehead coronal flap.

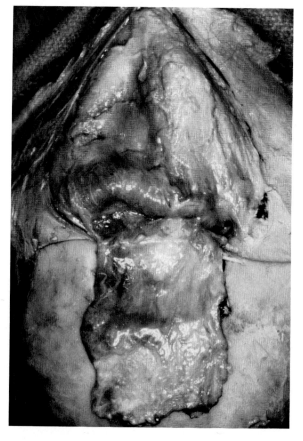

Figure 9 Galeal-pericranial flap elevated from coronal flap as arterialized flap based on supratrochlear vessels.

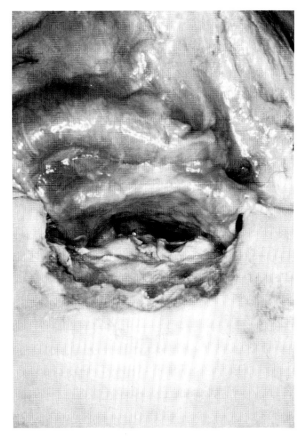

Figure 10 Galeal-pericranial flap rotated over margin of frontal bone between dura and nasal cavity, isolating all bone edges and dura from nasal cavity.

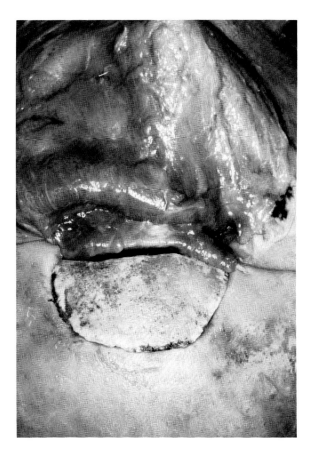

Figure 11 Anterior table bone flap replaced in a superior position, leaving space for the interposed flap.

21. Management of the Unknown Primary Tumor

INTRODUCTION

DARRELL A. JAQUES, M.D., F.A.C.S.

One of the most challenging problems in medical or surgical practice is the presentation of a patient with a mass in the neck. After what may be a very cursory evaluation, the most tempting next course of action, particularly to the surgeon, is to move directly to an open biopsy of the neck mass. This very strong temptation to do an immediate open biopsy must be resisted in favor of an orderly evaluation of the patient. Why should we be so arbitrary and adamant in our recommendation of this course of action? Why teach something which seems to be quite the opposite of "what comes naturally" to pathologists, internists, and surgeons alike? Carry the logic of our recommendation to a set of undesirable circumstances in which an open biopsy is done; the pathologic diagnosis is metastatic carcinoma, and the surgeon moves directly to radical neck dissection. Then, about 2 weeks llater, the patient complains of a sore throat. At that point, he is evaluated more thoroughly and, lo and behold, a large mass is seen in the hypopharynx/base of tongue region. Upon biopsy this proves to be squamous carcinoma and is, of course, the source for the metastasis in the neck. If you think this is a ridiculous set of circumstances, please be advised that it happens all too frequently. It also is totally avoidable if a methodical approach to the patient with the lump in the neck is carried out. That unfortunate patient whom we have just described has just had a therapeutic maneuver, namely radical neck dissection, as treatment for regional metastases before the primary malignant tumor was found, in spite of the fact it was most likely discoverable either by the same surgeon or by somebody more experienced in the proper evaluation. Certainly, if any surgeon were to take his boards and respond with that type of answer, he would probably fail. Who ever heard of treating the metastases without discovering or treating the primary first or at the same time? And then you say: "Well, my reason for doing the open biopsy of the mass in the neck is to get a clue as to where to look for the primary." My answer to that is that the primary might well be discovered as you set about the orderly evaluation without the necessity of an open biopsy of the mass in the neck. It is a fact that the incidence of the "unknown primary" diminishes as the experience and expertise of the head and neck surgeon increases. A bit of induration of one tonsil or slight excoriation and thickening of an area at the junction of the soft palate with nasopharynx, or a very tiny, erythematous, friable zone in the pyriform sinus, or an edematous, thickened area high in the nasopharynx, or an edematous, indurated, thickened zone in the soft palate palpable only under general anesthesia—all are subtle sources of metastases to the neck. Furthermore, when a patient undergoes a biopsy of the lymph node in the neck and is sent to me for further management, I discover the primary in most instances. It can be expected that no more than 5 percent of metastases to the neck present with an undiscoverable primary. Additional reasons for not launching into direct biopsy without complete evaluation include the fact that time is often lost with such an approach, the placement of the biopsy incision may compromise the ultimate radical neck dissection incision, and most importantly, the prognosis may be adversely affected because of the untimely node biopsy.

The examiner should bear in mind a classification of cervical lymphadenopathy as a basis for determining the ultimate source of the mass. Such a classification would include both benign and malignant sources and permit the development of a diagnostic profile of the patient.[1-3] The multiple characteristics of a diagnostic profile may typify benign or malignant disease. Variations tat preclude such a clear-cut distinction are not uncommon, but this system of organized thinking helps one to determine exactly which steps to take next and under what circumstances certain steps can be bypassed.

Included in this evaluation in the clinical setting is the use of the fine-needle aspiration biopsy of the mass. Present evidence would indicate that this is probably a safe technique. It is, however, fraught with great variation in success until extensive experience is gained by both the individual doing the fine-needle aspiration and the cytologist who makes the interpretation. This technique is not universally available, but perhaps in the future will be as common as H & E staining of fixed material from biopsies. Its rightful place in the management of the patient with the un-

known primary is yet to be fully determined, but it can never replace the orderly evaluation and assessment of the patient.

Assuming that a diagnosis was not obtained by all of the aforementioned steps, we then recommend a movement toward the search for the primary, which must include palpation of the oral cavity, pharynx, nasopharynx and palate, as well as the neck. In addition, panendoscopy is performed, to include nasopharyngoscopy, laryngoscopy, bronchoscopy, and esophagoscopy; if sinus films are abnormal, a Caldwell-Luc procedure is done to assess the sinuses and obtain material for pathologic examination. Consideration also must be given to the so-called "blind biopsy". This represents a blind biopsy of the nasopharynx and/or hypopharynx on the side of the metastasis. If absolutely no abnormality is found, as is usually the case, I recommend that an open biopsy be made on the mass in the neck and that this be an incisional biopsy if the mass is an extensive and large tumor, but otherwise an excisional biopsy, particularly if deep tissue planes will not be contaminated with tumor. Frozen section examination of the specimen can be performed and, if metastatic malignant disease is found, I recommend a neck dissection.

For several reasons, I recommend a neck dissection over primary radiotherapy: (1) 75 to 85 percent of the patients with an unknown primary will never manifest their primary, and those who argue that radiation will control the unsuspected primary are radiating 75 to 85 out of 100 cases unnecessarily; (2)uring the treatment of the neck metastases; (3) radiotherapy generally can be given only once to a particular region of the body, and if the primary were to manifest itself at a later date and at a site not accessible or amenable to surgery, there would be no reasonable therapeutic alternative at that point; and (4) the probability of cure of metastatic lymph nodes, particularly in larger clustered involvement, is less with radiotherapy than with surgery. There are radiotherapists who maintain that their modality will control the disease in the neck as easily as the primary, but even if that were true, the larger metastases in the neck would be less readily controlled since the larger primaries are not frequently cured by radiotherapy either. The main disability of a neck dissection is the loss of the spinal accessory nerve, and that can generally be corrected by a cable nerve graft. The disability from radiotherapy includes dryness of the mouth and pharynx, hoarseness, a degree of loss of taste, deleterious dental effects, and ligneous or indurated changes of tissues in the neck associated with edema of the anterior submental region of the neck as well as the hypopharynx and supraglottic laryngeal structures. The dreaded complication of transverse cervical myelitis secondary to radiation effects on the vasculature of the spinal cord would be prevented if only surgery were used. If a lymphoma is a possibility, a neck dissection usually is not indicated. Irradiation as primary treatment is a possibility, and the case for the use of radiation as the sole management is made by Fitzpatrick in another chapter. Postoperative radiotherapy should be considered in advanced cases.

The prognosis depends on the stage of the disease on presentation and varies from 15 percent to 80 percent with an overall survival of 45 percent.[1] Follow-up must include evaluation of the neck as well as continued search for the primary, since approximately 25 percent will eventually manifest the primary.

REFERENCES

1. Coker DD, Casterline PF, Chambers RG, Jaques DA. Metastases to lymph nodes of the head and neck from an unknown primary site. Am J Surg 1977; 134:517.
2. Jaques DA. Management of metastatic nodes in the neck from an unknown primary. In: Paparella MM, Shumrick DA, eds. Otolaryngology. Vol 3, 2nd Ed. Philadelphia: WB Saunders 1980: 2998.
3. Jaques DA. Solitary neck mass. In: Cameron JL, ed. Current surgical therapy 1984-1985. Philadelphia and Toronto: BC Decker 1984:547.

PATHOLOGIC AND CYTOLOGIC DIAGNOSIS OF A LUMP IN THE NECK

PHILIP S. FELDMAN, M.D.

Neck masses present a labyrinth of diagnostic possibilities. Before discussing the pathology of the unknown primary it is first helpful to review the differential diagnosis of a lump in the neck (Table 1). Time does not permit a detailed discussion of all these entities, and therefore only representative cases will be described, with emphasis on the pathology and corresponding cytology from material obtained by fine-needle aspiration (FNA).

FNA is essentially a "mini biopsy" whereby a palpable or roentgenographically visible mass is sampled by means of a fine needle (22-gauge) with negative pressure supplied by an attached syringe. The FNA obtains cellular material for cytologic studies in contrast to the larger cutting needle (14-G), which obtains a core of tissue for histologic examination. Martin pointed out that it was unwise to excise a lymph node for diagnostic purposes, but that the foregoing admonition did not apply to needle aspiration biopsies.[1] He recommended that "aspiration biopsy should always precede any consideration of open biopsy".[1] Today it is widely held that these recommendations should be followed.[2-4] In his chapter, Young elaborates on FNA and therefore I will not discuss FNA technique. At the University of Virginia Medical Center we average five FNA each day, and FNA of neck masses are essentially a daily occurrence. Both surgeons and pathologists perform FNA in our hospital. Pathology residents and fellows are currently instructed on how to perform and interpret FNA. The major consideration in deciding who should perform the aspiration is the adequacy of the person's training in all aspects of sampling the lesion and preparing the cell smears. A high degree of accuracy can be maintained regardless of who performs the FNA if that person has the necessary training and experience. If the aspirations are done by surgeons, close communication with the pathologist as to the clinical aspects of the case is essential.

NECK MASSES IN CHILDREN

The majority of neck masses in children result from inflammatory processes. Congenital cysts such as cystic hygroma, branchial cleft cyst, and thyroglossal duct cysts are common. Hemangiomas are the most common benign tumors of childhood and may produce a neck mass. The most frequent malignant tumors of childhood producing neck masses are malignant lymphomas, carcinoma of the thyroid, and rhabdomyosarcoma.

NECK MASSES IN ADULTS

Inflammatory lesions resulting in neck masses are infrequent in adults, whereas malignant neoplasms comprise the vast majority of neck lesions. Benign neoplasms are less frequent and consist of a variety of tumors. Twenty percent of the malignant tumors are primary in the neck and arise from thyroid, salivary gland, and soft tissue. However, in 80 percent of cases the malignant tumor represents a metastasis. In 85 percent of these patients the primary malignant tumor originates above the clavicle, in 10 percent from a distant primary, and in approximately 5 percent the primary is unknown.

Squamous cell carcinoma is the most common type of metastatic carcinoma in cervical lymph nodes, and the upper aerodigestive tract is the main source for these tumors.[3,5] Knowledge of the topographic distribution of lymph node metastases from squamous cell carcinomas of the head and neck assists surgeons in identifying the source of the metastasis.[6] However, the pathologist cannot ascertain the origin of the squamous carcinoma from the histology or cytology. There is one exception, the lymphoepithelioma, which is an undifferentiated squamous cell carcinoma. The pathologic and cytologic features are sufficiently distinct to enable the pathologist to suggest a nasopharyngeal origin. This is helpful since patients with lymphoepithelioma may consult their physician with a swelling

TABLE 1   Differential Diagnosis of a Lump in the Neck

Cervical Masses in Children
I. Congenital:
    1. Branchial cleft cyst
    2. Cystic hygroma (lymphangioma)
    3. Hemangioma
    4. Thyroglossal duct cyst
    5. Laryngocele
    6. Teratoma
II. Inflammation:
    1. Nonspecific lymphadenitis with lymphoid hyperplasia (overwhelming majority)
III. Neoplasms:
    A. Benign (see above)
    B. Malignant
        1. Lymphoma/leukemia
        2. Rhabdomyosarcoma
        3. Neuroblastoma

Cervical Masses in Adults
I. Congenital:
    1. Branchial cleft cyst
    2. Thyroglossal duct cyst
II. Inflammation:
    A. Lymph nodes
        1. Nonspecific lymphadenitis with lymphoid hyperplasia
        2. Specific lymphadenitis — cat scratch disease, toxoplasmosis
        3. Granulomatous lymphadenitis — tuberculosis, sarcoidosis, fungal disease
    B. Thyroid
        1. Thyroiditis
III. Neoplasms
    A. Benign
        1. Thyroid — follicular adenoma, Hurthle cell adenoma
        2. Salivary glands — benign mixed tumor (pleomorphic adenoma), papillary cystadenoma lymphomatosum (Warthin's tumor), monomorphic adenoma, benign lymphoepithelial lesion
        3. Soft tissue — lipoma, neurilemoma, carotid body tumor
    B. Malignant, primary (Approx 20%)
        1. Lymph nodes — malignant lymphoma
        2. Thyroid — papillary carcinoma, follicular carcinoma, medullary carcinoma, undifferentiated (small cell, giant cell, spindle cell) carcinoma
        3. Salivary glands — mucoepidermoid carcinoma, malignant mixed tumors, acinic cell carcinoma, adenoid cystic carcinoma
        4. Soft tissue — Rare
    C. Malignant, secondary (80% plus): histologic type and origin
        1. Squamous cell carcinoma — upper aerodigestive tract (most frequent source), lung, larynx, skin, esophagus, uterine cervix, salivary gland
        2. Adenocarcinoma — lung, breast, thyroid, salivary glands, gastrointestinal tract including pancreas, genitourinary tract (kidney, prostate), uterus, ovary
        3. Malignant lymphoma — any lymph node or extranodal site
        4. Small cell undifferentiated carcinoma — lung, esophagus, larynx
        5. Melanoma — skin, mucous membranes (oral cavity, upper respiratory tract) ear, eye
        7. Seminoma — testis

in the neck due to a lymph node metastasis.

Adenocarcinoma metastatic to cervical lymph nodes may arise from multiple sites: lungs, breast, thyroid, salivary glands, genitourinary tract (prostate, kidney), pancreas, uterus, and ovary. If the metastasis is located in the left supraclavicular region, the source of the metastasis is most likely located below the diaphragm. Butler et al reported 19 cases in which enlargement of supraclavicular lymph nodes was the initial manifestation of previously unrecognized prostatic carcinoma.[7] We have similarly seen several cases of prostate carcinoma in which the neck metastasis was the first evidence of the carcinoma. The FNA demonstrated an adenocarcinoma, and immunoperoxidase stain with prostate specific antigen was positive.[8] Subsequent biopsy of the prostate confirmed this diagnosis. Similarly carcinoma of the lung, thyroid, and kidney may also present with a neck mass as the initial manifestation of carcinoma.

Small cell undifferentiated (oat cell) carcinoma of the lung frequently metastasizes to cervical lymph nodes. It is important to realize that (1) the neck metastasis may be the initial manifestation of the lung cancer, and (2) the neck metastasis may not be confined to the supraclavicular area. This type of carcinoma may arise from an extrapulmonary site (e.g., esophagus and larynx).

Patients with malignant melanoma may develop metastases in cervical lymph nodes, and in approximately 4 percent, the site of primary origin is unknown.[9] The primary usually arises in the skin, but rarely arises from mucous membranes (oral cavity, upper respiratory tract), ear, and eye.

Metastatic esthesioneuroblastoma and seminoma may produce neck masses, but in these cancers the primary is usually known.

Since Young discusses the advantages of FNA, I will not review them here except to make a few brief comments on accuracy.

The most significant advantage of FNA is the high degree of accuracy possible with this procedure. Numerous reported series and our experience have documented that excellent results can be achieved from multiple body sites (e.g., breast, lung, lymph nodes, thyroid). The degree of accuracy is variable and depends on the site of the aspirate; the size, location, and nature of lesion; the experience and skill of the person performing and interpreting the FNA. During the developmental years of FNA, errors in technique and interpretation were not infrequent and contributed significantly to false-positive and false-negative diagnoses. However, as experience with FNA increased, the percentage of false-positive and false-negative diagnoses decreased concomitantly. False-positive diagnoses are a rarity today in FNA of the head and neck, breast, and lungs.[4,10-12] False-negative diagnoses range from less than 1 percent to approximately 7.0 percent.[4,10-12] If the FNA result is at variance with the clinical impression further investigation such as a repeat FNA or open biopsy is warranted.

In summary, FNA is a safe, inexpensive, and rapid procedure that accurately distinguishes between benign and malignant disease of the neck. For the cytopathologist, it is essential that (1) there is close communication with the surgeon, (2) correct technique is employed, and (3) cytologic criteria are carefully applied for interpretation of the cellular material. For the surgeon, it is essential to understand what the FNA diagnoses mean. An unsatisfactory FNA diagnosis provides no clinical information. A negative FNA diagnosis, though carrying considerable weight, does not exclude malignancy. A suspicious FNA diagnosis requires open biopsy. A positive FNA diagnosis has been regarded in many institutions as being as definitive as a tissue biopsy specimen. FNA is a procedure of the present, and its use will only increase in the future. It is fortunate that the renewed interest in FNA coincided with the development of newer techniques (e.g., immunoperoxidase and electron microscopy). The morphologic criteria currently used in pathology and cytology at times fail to identify the origin of the neoplasm. Histochemical stains are often nonspecific. Combining the FNA with immunoperoxidase methods enables the cytopathologist to more specifically identify the origin of the tumor (e.g., calcitonin for medullary carcinoma of the thyroid, prostate specific antigen for prostate carcinoma).

REFERENCES

1. Martin H. Untimely lymph node biopsy. Am J Surg 1969; 102:17–18.
2. McGuirt WF, McCabe WF. Significance of node biopsy before definitive treatment of cervical metastatic carcinoma. Laryngoscope 1978; 88:594–597.
3. Spiro RH, DeRose G, Strong EW. Cervical node metastasis of occult origin. Am J Surg 1983; 146:441–446.
4. Young JEM, Archibald SD, Shier KJ. Needle aspiration cytologic biopsy in head and neck masses. Am J Surg 1981; 142:484–489.
5. Batsakis JG, McBurney TA. Metastatic neoplasms to the head and neck. Surg Gynecol Obstet 1971; 133:673–677.
6. Lindberg R. Distribution of cervical lymph node metastases from squamous cell carcinoma of the upper respiratory and digestive tracts. Cancer 1972; 29:1446–1449.
7. Butler JJ, Howe CD, Johnson DE. Enlargement of the supraclavicular lymph nodes as the initial sign of prostatic carcinoma. Cancer 1971; 27:1055–1063.
8. Nadji M, Taylow SZ, Castro A, Chu TM, Morales AR. Prostatic origin of tumors: An immunohistochemical study. Am J Clin Pathol 1980; 73:735–739.
9. Baab GH, McBride CM. Malignant melanoma. The patient with an unknown site of primary origin. Arch Surg 1975; 110:896–900.
10. Frable WJ, Frable MAS. Thin-needle aspiration biopsy: The diagnosis of head and neck tumors revisited. Cancer 1979; 43:1541–1548.
11. Wanebo HJ, Feldman PS, Wilhelm MC, et al. Fine-needle aspiration cytology in lieu of open biopsy in management of primary breast cancer. Ann Surg 1984; 199:79–89.
12. Feldman PS, Kaplan MJ, Johns ME, et al. Fine-needle aspiration in squamous cell carcinoma of the head and neck. Arch Otolaryngol 1983; 109:735–741.

THE UNKNOWN PRIMARY: EVALUATION OF THE PATIENT

JATIN P. SHAH, M.D., M.S.(Surg), F.A.C.S.

The basic question regarding a palpable mass in the neck is whether this mass is benign or malignant. The patient with a mass in the neck should be assessed systematically, beginning with a detailed history and continuing with a thorough head and neck and general physical examination.

Points of significance in the patient's history are as follows:

1. *Age.* An enlarged cervical lymph node in patients over the age of 40 is in all probability metastatic disease of the lymph node, whereas in a younger patient it is likely to be benign enlargement or possibly lymphoma.
2. *Sex.* The incidence of carcinoma of the upper aerodigestive tract is significantly higher in men than in women. However, with the increasing smoking and drinking habits of women, the ratio of distribution between the two sexes is getting smaller and smaller.
3. *Race.* Metastatic lymph node disease from a primary skin tumor such as melanoma and squamous cell carcinoma of the skin is more common in the Caucasian patient. The possibility of such skin cancers in the Oriental or Black patient is very small.
4. *Smoking and Drinking.* A history of excessive smoking and alcohol ingestion significantly increases the likelihood that a palpable lymph node in the neck is a metastatic lesion with its primary source in the head and neck area.
5. *Other Symptoms.* A history of hoarseness, hemoptysis, epistaxis, shortness of breath, discomfort in the throat, or difficulty in swallowing is indicative of a potential primary source in the upper aerodigestive tract. A history of previous radiation exposure would raise the possibility of an occult carcinoma in the thyroid gland or skin within the portals of irradiation.

The physical characteristics of the enlarged lymph

node may be suggestive of a benign or malignant lesion, as follows:

1. *Duration*. The longer the enlargement has been present without any other symptoms, the more likely is the enlargement to be benign. There are certain exceptions to this, such as well-differentiated thyroid carcinoma, in which case metastatic disease to the lymph node may remain quiescent for many years. In the case of metastatic squamous cell carcinoma of the lymph node, the patient usually gives a history of having noted an enlargement for approximately 1 to 3 months.

2. *Change in Size*. Progressive increase in the size of the lymph node is a strong indication of malignancy. On the other hand, fluctuation in the size of the lymph node from large to small and large again would suggest either reactive hyperplasia or inflammatory origin.

3. *Pain*. Malignant lymph nodes are not likely to be painful unless they become large enough and cause pressure on cervical roots. On the other hand, inflamed lymph nodes are likely to be tender.

4. *Size of the Lymph Node*. Generally, lymph nodes smaller than 1 cm in diameter are less likely to be malignant, particularly if such nodes are present in more than one location and on both sides of the neck.

5. *Number of Lymph Nodes*. Multiple lymph nodes, particularly on both sides of the neck, are more likely to be benign in nature if they are less than 1 cm in size. However, one must exercise caution since some patients with lymphoma may present with bilateral lymph nodes which may be smaller in size.

6. *Consistency*. A soft flat lymph node is likely to be benign in contrast to a firm-to-hard mass, which is usually malignant. Fleshy mobile lymph nodes are characteristic for lymphoma.

7. *Location of Lymph Nodes*. The anatomic location of a palpable lymph node can suggest whether it is benign or malignant as well as a potential primary source. For example, in a young child, upper jugular lymph nodes near the angle of the mandible are commonly enlarged by reactive hyperplasia or by an inflammatory process secondary to upper respiratory infection. Similarly, submental lymph nodes are usually benign secondary to an inflammatory process. The most common site of lymph nodes metastatic from an unknown primary or from a primary in the head and neck area consists of the upper deep jugular lymph nodes lying anterior and deep to the sternomastoid muscle. Supraclavicular lymph nodes, particularly behind the clavicular head of the sternomastoid muscle, may be metastatic from a primary tumor below the clavicle—in the lung or esophagus or below the diaphragm. Metastatic lymph nodes along the accessory chain would draw one's attention to a possible primary in the nasopharynx. Midjugular lymph

nodes may represent metastases from a possible primary in the larynx or thyroid. It is therefore extremely important for the clinician to be aware of the anatomic relation of the location of the lymph nodes and their draining primary sites.

DEVELOPING A DIAGNOSTIC PROFILE

Once the history and physical examination have been completed, one can immediately draw a profile that will point toward the additional work-up.

A typical profile for a patient with a high probability of a benign enlargement of a lymph node is as follows: Female under the age of 20 who is a nonsmoker and nondrinker presents with many soft nodes which are smaller than 1 cm in size and are present bilaterally in several node chains. There is no history of increase in the size of these nodes and they have been present for weeks or months.

The profile that suggests malignant disease in a patient presenting with an enlarged lymph node in the neck is as follows: the high probability of a metastatic lymph node is characterized by a male aged 40 or over who is a heavy smoker and heavy alcohol drinker and presents with a node larger than 2 cm in diameter along the jugular chain or the supraclavicular fossa. The node may be of recent onset or has shown significant increase in its size, is painless, and has firm to hard consistency.

SEARCH FOR THE PRIMARY

After an appropriate history is obtained from the patient, the systematic physical examination should begin with a thorough examination of the head and neck area. Examination of the head and neck area should include inspection of the scalp, skin of the face, and neck. The scalp should be carefully examined since small primary tumors of the scalp can be easily missed in a patient with hair. Next the cervical lymph nodes should be examined, beginning with the contralateral negative side of the neck. Lymph nodes in the submental and submandibular triangles, the upper, middle and deep jugular chain, the posterior triangle, and accessory chain should be carefully palpated, as should occipital lymph nodes and lymph nodes along the trapezius muscle. Following this, the side of the involvement is carefully assessed. The palpable lymph nodes should be examined for size, number, consistency, mobility, and location; adherence of the overlying skin or fixation to deeper tissues should be recorded. The thyroid gland is then examined.

Examination of cranial nerve function begins with the extraocular muscles; then the sense of smell, the sensations of the skin of the chin and cheek, and function of the facial nerve are assessed. Examination of the external auditory canal is important and so is the palpation of both parotid glands and preauricular lymph nodes. Anterior rhinoscopy is then performed, and thereafter examination of the oral cavity, oropharynx, nasopharynx, hypopharynx, and larynx is performed in a systematic fashion. Mirror examination may be satisfactory; however, if that is not adequate, a fiberoptic light source may be used along with approprite telescopes for adequate assessment of the nasopharynx, hypopharynx, and larynx. Soft tissues in the oral cavity should be palpated carefully for small primary lesions which can be easily missed by inspection alone. The majority of the patients who present with a palpable node with metastatic disease in the neck have the primary tumor identified at initial careful head and neck examination. If a primary tumor is found, a biopsy is performed, the tumor is appropriately staged, and treatment recommendations are made. However, if no primary lesion is found, the palpated lymph nodes are staged according to the N staging recommended by the American Joint Committee.

If a palpable lymph node appears to be fleshy and mobile and the clinical suspicion is that of a lymphoma, peripheral lymph nodes in the axilla and groin are palpated, and the abdomen is examined for enlargement of the spleen and liver. On completion of the physical examination just described, the clinician usually is able to make a tentative clinical diagnosis of a benign or malignant mass.

LABORATORY TESTS

A battery of laboratory tests can be ordered which may provide clues to the possible cause for the lymphadenopathy. However, no specific diagnostic tests are available which will make a definitive histologic diagnosis. An exception to this rule may be estimation of serum calcitonin in a patient who presents with a palpable lymph node in the neck and a mass in the thyroid gland, a laboratory test that may establish the diagnosis of medullary carcinoma of the thyroid gland. Barring this, the routine blood tests that one may order include a complete blood count, mono test, serologic tests for syphylis, and a complete SMA-12.

RADIOGRAPHIC STUDIES

A chest roentgenogram is mandatory in all patients who present with a palpable mass in the neck that is suspected to be malignant. This may reveal pulmonary primary tumor and may also show hilar lymphadenopathy. X-ray films of paranasal sinuses may be ordered and may bring to light a small primary tumor in the maxillary antrum or ethmoid. It must be noted, however, that it is extremely rare for a small primary tumor of the paranasal sinus to cause palpable metastatic disease in the lymph nodes in the neck. For paranasal sinus tumors, metastases usually occur late in the course of the disease. A barium swallow may help to identify a primary tumor in the postcricoid area or esophagus itself or displacement of the esophagus by a potential primary lesion in the thyroid. Computerized tomography of the neck may provide additional assessment of lymph nodes in the neck, particularly in the obese patient.

RADIOISOTOPE SCANS

Thyroid scan may be of help in identifying abnormalities in the thyroid gland that is not palpable. This may be of particular help in the obese patient in whom palpation of the thyroid gland is not very easy. In many cases, however, a thyroid scan does not detect nodules under 1 m in diameter.

SKIN TESTS

A variety of skin tests are available for the diagnosis of infectious disease. Skin tests are available for tuberculosis, coccidioidomycosis, blastomycosis, and histoplasmosis. However, histologic diagnosis of the lymph node cannot be made without a biopsy in spite of a positive skin test.

Additional work-up in search of a primary in the lungs, esophagus, GI tract, or kidneys is not recommended at this point in the patient's evaluation. All such tests may be requested after accurate histologic diagnosis is made from the enlarged cervical lymph node.

In summary, if a detailed history and a thorough examination of the head and neck area and general physical examination suggest that the lymph node is benign, the laboratory tests just described are considered appropriate. However, if the palpable lymph node clearly appears to be metastatic in nature by virtue of its hard consistency and the classic malignant profile of the patient, a needle aspiration biopsy is performed at the initial evaluation of the patient to expedite establishment of histologic diagnosis and further work-up and treatment. On the other hand, if the palpable lymph node is soft and fleshy in nature and the profile of the patient points toward the possibility of lymphoma, the patient is subjected to an excisional biopsy of the entire lymph node for appropriate histologic interpretation and processing of fresh tissue for cell surface markers.

THE UNKNOWN PRIMARY: OPERATIVE EVALUATION

JAMES E. M. YOUNG, B.Sc., M.D., F.R.C.S.(C), F.A.C.S.

NEEDLE BIOPSY

One of the keys to planning surgery on a mass in the neck is having maximal information before submitting the patient to operation. Needle aspiration cytologic biopsy is the single most valuable investigative procedure for a patient presenting with a suspected malignant mass in the neck. Needle aspiration biopsy of neck masses was done by Hayes Martin in the 1930s using an 18-gauge needle.[1] This extensive Memorial Hospital experience remained unique because most pathologists were reluctant to interpret cytologic samples, and surgeons were concerned that tumor cells would be implanted along the needle tract. The recent use of the 22-gauge needle has repopularized needle aspiration cytologic biopsy because it simplifies the technique and the concern regarding tumor implant has not been realized.[2]

The technique of needle aspiration biopsy involves mounting a needle on the tip of a syringe and inserting the needle through the unanesthetized skin into the lesion. Suction is applied to the syringe while the tip of the needle is moved within the confines of the mass. Suction is released before the needle is withdrawn from the patient so that the tissue sample remains within the needle. Needle and syringe are disconnected, and the sample in the needle is subsequently expressed onto a slide by filling the syringe with air and using the air to force the sample from the needle. A second slide is dipped in 95 percent alcohol, placed on the specimen, and the two slides separated, both smearing and fixing the specimen at the same time. An alternative method is to rinse needle and syringe immediately with 50 percent alcohol sending the resulting solution to the cytology laboratory for slide preparation. The slides are stained by the Papanicolaou method.

As with any procedure, there are potential problems with needle aspiration biopsy. These include problems related to the aspiration and the technique of making the slide, the interpretation of the material obtained, and the nature of the lesion itself. An occasional false-negative can occur if the tip of the needle misses the lesion. Similarly, it is essential that the material obtained be smeared and fixed immediately or the sample is unreadable.[3] Some lesions can pose a diagnostic dilemma to the inexperienced cytopathologist. For example, inflamed branchial cleft cysts and chemodectomas can occasionally resemble poorly differentiated carcinoma,[4] and experience on the part of cytopathologist and clinician, with appropriate communication between them, can avoid problems in these areas. Follicular cell carcinoma, not only at the primary site but also when metastatic in lymph nodes, can be difficult to distinguish from normal thyroid tissue or a benign follicular adenoma on a cytologic basis alone, since a final diagnosis of malignancy almost always depends on the demonstration of vascular or capsular invasion which cannot be seen on needle aspiration biopsy. However, benign-appearing follicular tissue aspirated from a mass laterally or superiorly in the neck is almost always diagnostic of thyroid cancer, and cooperation between clinician and pathologist usually prevents a diagnostic dilemma in this situation.

The accuracy of needle aspiration technique in lymphoma is only about 75 percent,[3] and lymphomas require subsequent excisional nodal biopsy in almost all cases anyway. However, if the initial needle aspirate is suspect for lymphoma or at least rules out squamous cell carcinoma, considerable saving in time and money has been afforded both the patient and the clinician.

Most problems associated with the use of needle aspiration biopsy are averted if surgeon and cytopathologist are experienced and cooperate closely. When the cytologist is unable to give a definite diagnosis because of "inadequate" material, the needle aspiration should be repeated. When a cytologic diagnosis does not point to malignancy but malignancy is clinically suspected, the cytologic result must be evaluated in the light of the clinical situation and repeat aspiration, core biopsy, or open biopsy undertaken.

A core needle biopsy (originally with a Vim-Silverman needle and now usually using the Tru-cut needle) is occasionally of value if needle aspiration cytologic biopsy does not yield diagnostic material preoperatively. It can assist in the evaluation of scarcoma or benign soft tissue lesions or in differentiating squamous from adenocarcinoma if this has been difficult to do cytologically. Its disadvantages are the trauma it causes and the increased risk of tumor implant. Core biopsy in fact is less accurate than needle aspiration biopsy,[3] probably because with an aspiration technique, the tip of the needle is moved through several planes within the confines of the lesion and thereby samples different areas.

In the past, it has been suggested that a patient with an undiagnosed mass in the neck should be subjected to surgery for excisional biopsy and prepared for the possibility that his surgery may include any or all of the following: radical neck dissection, total thyroidectomy, mediastinal node dissection, parotidectomy, and possible tracheostomy.[5] The increasing difficulty in booking operating time makes it impractical to schedule a patient for an operation that may take from 1 to 6 or more hours. Certainly, considering the present problems of patient acceptance, limiting surgical uncertainty is indicated and needle aspiration biopsy almost invariably resolves this diagnostic dilemma before the patient ever gets to the operating room. Thus, needle aspiration biopsy allows the surgeon to plan appropriate surgery and to inform the patient of the exact nature of that surgery. It is a simple office procedure, requiring no anesthesia or incision, and can be done rapidly within a few minutes. It is inexpensive for both clinician and patient and is quite safe with no major complications.[3]

The specific diagnosis of cell type obtained at needle aspiration can suggest the likely primary site and indicate the direction of further investigation. If the aspiration is positive for squamous cell carcinoma, appropriate multiple endoscopic procedures can be scheduled and a variety of studies (e.g., thyroid scans) can be avoided. If the aspiration yields uniform or abnormal lymphocytes, appropriate excisional biopsy for a suspected diagnosis of lymphoma can be undertaken, obviating endoscopic procedures and inappropriate random biopsies.

Given the simplicity of needle aspiration biopsy and the present availability of expert cytologists, no patient suspected of having a malignant mass in the neck should undergo general anesthesia without an initial needle aspiration cytologic biopsy. Needle aspiration provides more information faster and less expensively than any combination of laboratory and radiologic investigations. It usually obtains a definite diagnosis and indicates the nature of further investigation and treatment. Thus most patients can avoid an inappropriate and exhaustive workup, which can unnecessarily delay appropriate treatment. Accordingly, a 22-gauge needle aspiration cytologic biopsy should be used at the time of the initial evaluation in every patient suspected of having a malignant mass in the head and neck area.

EXAMINATION UNDER ANESTHESIA

In most patients with a clinically malignant mass in the neck, the diagnosis of malignancy is established by needle aspiration before a general anesthetic is administered. If the preoperative work-up has failed to detect a primary site of malignant tumor in a patient whose needle aspiration was positive for squamous cell or poorly differentiated carcinoma, a careful examination under anaesthesia is performed. "Multiple endoscopy" of the upper aerodigestive tract (quadroscopy, panendoscopy) is performed, including direct laryngopharyngoscopy, fiberoptic bronchoscopy with tracheobronchial washings, and fiberoptic esophagogastroscopy. Careful examination of the nasopharynx is done using the headlight, mirror, and palate retraction. Complete palpation of the floor of the mouth, tongue, oropharynx, nasopharynx, upper surface of the soft palate, and hypopharynx is essential. It is important to emphasize that the examination described is done not only to find the as yet undetected primary that has presumably metastasized to the neck, but also to search for a second upper aerodigestive tract primary since the incidence of simultaneous primaries in the upper aerodigestive tract is considera-

ble.[6] It is for this latter reason that the esophagobronchoscopy done with rigid instruments alone is no longer adequate given the availability and the improved diagnostic yield of the fiberoptic instruments. A considerable number of unknown primary patients are found to have a primary in the lung, esophagus, or stomach (33 of 168 detected primaries, Tables 1 and 3), and as complete an examination of these areas as possible is indicated.

If a primary tumor is not found on visualization or palpation of the tissues in the upper aerodigestive tract, "directed" rather than "blind" biopsies are indicated. Obviously, any slightly abnormal or irregular mucosa is biopsied, and most authors recommend sampling of the ipsilateral base of tongue, piriform fossa, tonsil, postcricoid area, and nasopharynx. "Directed" biopsies should certainly be done at the areas most likely to be the site of the primary, depending on the position of the node in the neck and the likely

TABLE 1 Primary Identification Following Treatment for Unknown Primary: Total Number of Patients in Nine Series = 879*

Primary subsequently detected	168 (19%)
Head and neck	103 (61%)
Below clavicle	60 (36%)
Lymphoma	5 (3%)

*References 9 through 17.

TABLE 2 Identified Primary Sites in Head and Neck: 103/879 (11.7%)

Nasopharynx	26
Hypopharynx	17
Supraglottic region	13
Base of tongue	13
Tonsil	13
Oral cavity	8
Soft palate	2
Larynx	2
Antrum	2
Nasal cavity	2
Thyroid	2
Skin — SCC	1
Skin — melanoma	1
Ear canal	1

TABLE 3 Identified Primary Sites Below Clavicle: 60/879 (6.8%)

Lung	19
Esophagus	8
Stomach	6
Pancreas	8
Colon	1
Appendix	1
Ovary	4
Bladder	1
Prostate	1
Breast	2
Unspecified	9

site of undetected primary as described in large series (Tables 1 through 3). The differentiation of the tumor may act as a guide to the site of a primary, with poorly differentiated tumors and lymphoepithelial lesions arising more commonly in nasopharynx, tongue, and tonsil. Some authors have recommended a Caldwell-Luc operation under the same anesthetic if abnormality was detected on preoperative sinus films.[7] However, in the absence of symptoms or radiographic changes indicative of sinus abnormality, metastatic tumor in the neck from a primary in the sinuses is rare, and routine sinus exploration is not indicated (see Table 2).

OPEN BIOPSY OF A NECK MASS

Unfortunately, open biopsy is all too frequently the first step used to investigate nodal neck disease. MacComb reported that 77.5 percent of patients had already had an excisional or incisional biopsy at the time of referral,[8] and Barrie reported an incidence of 42 percent.[9] Inappropriate nodal biopsy spills tumor cells into adjacent tissues, rendering them relatively anoxic and therefore more resistant to radiotherapy, as well as impossible to detect at the time of subsequent surgery. This problem with open biopsy is one of the reasons that needle aspiration biopsy has gained in popularity during the past decade. If needle aspiration biopsy is used, it is exceedingly rare for the surgeon to have to do an open biopsy in a carcinomatous lesion, reserving this procedure for suspected or probable lymphomas, or rarer soft tissue tumors. In a patient with a suspected lymphoma it is preferable, if possible, that one node be completely excised and the specimen separated into a portion for routine, fungal, and tubercular culture and the greater portion for submission to the pathologist for imprint (touch-preparation) and appropriate frozen section examination.

If a definite diagnosis of malignancy has been established by needle aspiration biopsy preoperatively and endoscopy fails to reveal a primary tumor, direct open biopsy of the mass can be done under the same anesthesia used for endoscopy and palpation. It is important to place the incision in an appropriate position for excision at the time of subsequent neck dissection. On many surgical services, neck node biopsy is an operation awarded to the most junior member of the service, implying that it is easy, without complications, and of minimal importance. However, in patients with possible neck node metastases from an upper aerodigestive tract primary, open biopsy should not be undertaken unless the surgeon is prepared and able to proceed with neck dissection in those cases in which it is clearly indicated. The inexperienced surgeon treating these patients often attempts a nodal biopsy under local anesthesia, risks damage to sensory and motor nerves, occasionally causes air embolus, frequently obtains inadequate diagnostic material, and unfortunately spreads malignant cells through tissue planes where they are difficult to eradicate at subsequent definitive therapy. Several generations of head and neck surgeons have noted that when head and neck carcinoma recurs following an original ill-advised early node biopsy, it all too frequently occurs at the site of the original nodal biopsy, whether the patient is treated by radical surgery, radical radiotheray, or both. Therefore, open biopsy of neck masses should be done by surgeons who are prepared to completely evaluate the upper aerodigestive tract prior to biopsy, and who are familiar with needle aspiration techniques. They should also be prepared to proceed with definitive surgery at the time of open biopsy.

REFERENCES

1. Martin HE, Ellis EB. Biopsy by needle puncture and aspiration. Ann Surg 1930; 92:169–181.
2. Deeley TJ. Dissemination of malignancy. In: Needle Biopsy. London: Butterworths, 1974:40.
3. Young JEM, Archibald SD, Shier KJ. Needle aspiration ctyologic biopsy in head and neck masses. Am J Surg 1981; 142:484–489.
4. Hood IC, Qizilbash AH, Young JEM, Archibald SD. Fine needle aspiration biopsy cytology of paragangliomas. Acta Cytol 1983; 27:6:651–657.
5. Simpson GT. The evaluation and management of neck masses of unknown etiology. Otolaryngol Clin North Am 1980; 13:489–497.
6. Weaver A, Fleming SM, Knechtges TC, et al. Triple endoscopy: A neglected essential in head and neck cancer. Surgery 1979; 86:493–496.
7. Jaques DA. Management of metastatic nodes in the neck from an unknown primary. In: Paparella MM, Shumrick DA, eds. Otolaryngology. Vol 3, 2nd Ed. Philadelphia: WB Saunders 1980: 2998.
8. MacComb WS. Diagnosis and treatment of metastatic cervical canceorus nodes from an unknown primary site. Am J Surg 1972; 124:441–449.
9. Barrie JR, Knapper WH, Strong EW. Cervical nodal metastases of unknown origin. Am J Surg 1970; 120;466–470.
10. Spiro RH, DeRose G, Strong EW. Cervical node metastasis of occult origin. Am J Surg 1983; 146:441:–445.
11. Fried MP, Diehl WH Jr, Brownson RJ, Sessions DG, Ogura JH. Cervical metastasis from an unknown primary. Ann Otol 1975; 84:152–157.
12. Coker DD, Casterline PF, Chambers RG, Jaques DA. Metastases to lymph nodes of the head and neck from an unknown primary site. Am J Surg 1977; 134:517–522.
13. Jesse RH, Perez CA, Fletcher GH. Cervical lymph node metastasis: unknown primary cancer. Cancer 1973; 31:4:854–859.
14. Jose B, Bosch A, Caldwell WL, Frias Z. Metastasis to neck from unknown primary tumor. Acta Radiol Oncol 1979; 18:161–170.
15. Pacini P, Olmi P, Cellai E, Chiavacci A. Cervical lymph node metastases from an unknown primary tumor. Acta Radiol Oncol 1981; 20:311–314.
16. Yan ZY, Hu YH, Yan JH, Cai WM, Qin DX, Xu GZ, Wu XL. Lymph node metastases in the neck from an unknown primary. Acta Radiol Oncol 1982; 22:17–22.
17. Comess MS, Beahrs OH, Dockerty MB. Cervical metastasis from occult carcinoma. Surg Gynecol Obstet 1957: 607–617.

THE UNKNOWN PRIMARY: SURGICAL TREATMENT

JATIN P. SHAH, M.D., M.S.(Surg), F.A.C.S.

It has long been known that cervical lymph node metastases may be the first manifestation of an upper aerodigestive tract carcinoma. Years ago, Martin and Morfit estimated that approximately one-third of such patients had primary tumors that were obvious to the referring physician, and another third had primary tumors that were found after referral.[1] In the remaining patients, identification of the primary tumor became apparent within months or years during follow-up examination following treatment of neck node metastases, but in most such patients the primary source remained inapparent.

The importance of adequate evaluation by clinical examination and thorough examination of head and neck area cannot be overemphasized before an open lymph node biopsy is performed. However, this approach can lead to another problem. It is my impression that some patients with metastatic carcinoma in cervical lymph nodes and an apparent unknown primary tumor are unnecessarily subjected to an exhaustive work-up which often delays treatment significantly. I believe that the value of fine-needle aspiration biopsy deserves re-emphasis in this setting. When employed soon after complete head and neck examination during the initial patient visit, it can often rule out lymphoma and frequently provide a specific tissue diagnosis of epidermoid carcinoma. With such information in hand, the clinician can then proceed with multiple endoscopies and definitive treatment of metastatic nodes in the neck. The yield from bronchoscopy, esophagoscopy, washings, and multiple blind biopsies is usually very small, but it is advisable to perform these investigations prior to embarking on radical neck dissection as definitive treatment for metastatic disease of lymph nodes.

When a needle aspiration biopsy is not diagnostic, an open—preferably excisional—biopsy is indicated to establish accurate histologic diagnosis. Depending on the histologic nature and the location of the lymph node, additional work-up and/or treatment is indicated. If the diagnosis of squamous cell carcinoma or metastatic melanoma is rendered, additional radiographic work-up of the gastrointestinal tract, genitourinary tract, and chest is rarely worthwhile. On the other hand, if the diagnosis of adenocarcinoma is rendered, and the possibility of thyroid or salivary gland origin is ruled out, the work-up should include investigations of the alimentary tract, genitourinary tract, and lungs. Surgical treatment in that setting is rarely advocated.

Radical neck dissection generally is not recommended for a patient who presents with metastatic carcinoma in supraclavicular lymph nodes since the possibility of a primary source below the clavicle is high. When metastatic carcinoma to cervical lymph nodes is located in other parts of the neck, radical neck dissection is usually recommended regardless of the histology of metastatic lymph nodes in the absence of a primary tumor. Thus a radical neck dissection can be justified for metastatic epidermoid carcinoma, metastatic melanoma, metastatic undifferentiated or anaplastic carcinoma, and metastatic adenocarcinoma presenting in the upper half of the neck, presumably from a potential primary tumor in salivary glands. Spiro et al reported that 74 percent of patients with N1 disease survived after radical neck dissection alone.[2] On the other hand, patients with N2 and N3 disease offer a 5-year survival rate of only 41 percent, with treatment failure usually manifested in the dissected neck. These observations clearly indicate the need for combined therapy in patients who have bulky metastatic nodes in one location or multiple metastatic nodes in different locations in the same side of the neck. Local control exceeding 80 percent has been reported after treatment with the combination of surgery and postoperative radiation therapy.[3] The efficacy of radical neck dissection for various histologic types of carcinomas are of interest: for anaplastic or undifferentiated carcinoma, the 5-year survival rate is 53 percent; for epidermoid carcinoma, 48 percent; and for metastatic melanoma, only 20 percent; but no survivors were identified in patients who presented with metastatic adenocarcinoma (Fig. 1).

When a neck dissection is performed for patients who present with metastatic carcinoma to cervical lymph nodes with an unknown primary, a classic radical neck dissection is performed in nearly all instances, except for patients who present with a single metastatic lymph node less than 2 cm in diameter situated in the anterior triangle of the neck. In that clinical setting, perhaps one may consider preservation of the accessory nerve. All other patients with larger lymph nodes at one location or multiple metastatic lymph nodes or those who manifest extracapsular extension of disease from metastatic cancer should have a classic radical neck dissection.

The current philosophy on the head and neck service at Memorial Sloan-Kettering Cancer Center is to proceed with the classic radical neck dissection in patients who present with metastatic squamous cell carcinoma with an unknown primary. The radical neck dissection is followed by postoperative radiation therapy in any patient who has N2 or N3 disease as well as in patients with N1 disease who have ominous pathologic findings such as extension of disease beyond the capsule of the lymph node. A dose of 5000 rads is delivered to the entire neck in 5 weeks. Since the majority of the occult primary lesions originate in the hypopharynx, the presumed primary site is automatically included within the portal of irradiation of

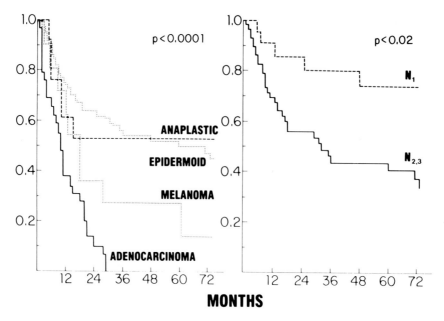

Figure 1 Cumulative survival according to histology of the involved nodes and nodal status in patients with squamous cell carcinoma. (From Spiro et al. Am J Surg 146:443. Reproduced with permission from the author and Am J Surg.)

the neck. However, if the patient presents with metastatic lymph nodes in the posterior triangle of the neck, the radiation portals are extended to include the nasopharynx.

The survival rates reported by Spiro et al and others indicate that aggressive treatment of the neck can yield long-term survival in patients with epidermoid, anaplastic, or undifferentiated carcinoma of occult origin.[2] In contrast, irradiation and chemotherapy are the preferred modalities of treatment for the patient who has metastatic adenocarcinoma, particularly presenting in the lower half of the neck with an inapparent primary tumor. Radical neck dissection is indicated in highly selective situations when the nodal disease is limited to the middle or upper part of the neck and salivary or thyroid origin cannot be ex-

cluded with certainty. Radical neck dissection continues to be the treatment of choice for occult metastatic melanoma in cervical lymph nodes despite the fact that long-term survival is achieved only in a very small number of patients.

REFERENCES

1. Martin H, Morfit HM. Cervical lymph node metastasis as the first symptom of cancer. Surg. Gynecol. Obstet. 1944; 78:133–159.
2. Spiro RH, DeRose G, Strong EW. Cervical node metastasis of occult origin. Am J of Surg 1983; 146:441–446.
3. Schwarz D, Hamberger AD, Jesse RH. The management of squamous cell carcinoma in cervical lymph nodes in the clinical absence of a primary lesion by combined surgery and irradiation. Cancer 1981; 48:1746–1748.

CERVICAL LYMPH NODE METASTASES FROM AN UNKNOWN PRIMARY TUMOR: THE PLACE OF RADIOTHERAPY

PETER J. FITZPATRICK, M.B., B.S., F.R.C.P.(C), F.R.C.R.
THOMAS J. KEANE, M.B., M.R.C.P.I., F.R.C.P.(C)

Malignant disease in the neck is common in clinical practice and is often the first sign of cancer. The majority of these patients have a primary cancer within the head and neck, but in about 5 percent, the primary is occult and undetectable. In 1974 we reported 233 patients with metastatic cancer in the neck and an unknown primary tumor from among 43,664 patients with malignant disease seen between 1958 and 1970.[1] This study led to a more thorough investigation of such patients, and many were submitted to a second quadroscopy when the first was negative. The advent of CT scanning also enhanced our diagnostic ability, and in the years between 1971 and 1982, although 64,489 new patients with malignant disease were seen, only 144 were classified as having metastatic cancer in the neck with an unknown primary tumor.

The Princess Margaret Hospital is a tertiary referral center and primary radiotherapy institute. Accordingly, most patients were preselected for this form of treatment, although a few had been initially treated by surgery. This clinical experience is reported in order to clarify a number of inconsistencies in the literature and to try to determine optimum care.

The lymphatic system on either side of the neck extends in chains from the base of the skull to the clavicle (Fig. 1). The lymph nodes in superficial and deep groups are located below the ramus of the mandible in the submental and submaxillary regions, and in close approximation to the carotid sheath, just deep to the anterior border of the sternomastoid extending from the base of the skull to the clavicle. Others are located in the supraclavicular fossa and the posterior triangle of the neck. These lymph nodes drain superficial tissues and deep structures of the head and neck. Because of the limited number of patients and in order to obtain meaningful information, it was necessary to establish two main clinical groups, cervical node involvement and supraclavicular node involvement. These groups differ in clinical behavior, prognosis, and response to treatment. The cervical nodes include the submental and submaxillary nodes and the upper and middle cervical nodes—groups 1, 2, and 3; the supraclavicular nodes include those in the supraclavicular fossa, the lower cervical chain and the posterior triangle—groups 4 and 5. If more than one group was involved, the tumor was classified according to the predominant site. When tumors metastasize through the lymphatics, not all of the nodes trap cancer cells and develop into regional metastases. This accounts for the variable clinical patterns.

MATERIALS AND METHODS

In all cases a careful history was taken and a complete physical examination performed. Investigations varied according to the histology, the clinical presentation, and the patient's general condition. Radiologic investigations, including CT scans (in recent years) and quadroscopy with or without random biopsies, were performed in the majority of patients. If no primary cancer was found, and no other disease demonstrated outside of the neck, the patients were divided into the two groups: those with cervical node involvement and those with supraclavicular node involvement. All patients had as their first symptom a lump in the neck.

Among 144 patients seen between 1971 and 1982 and classified as having lymph node metastases in the neck from an unknown primary tumor, 99 patients (69%) had no other demonstrable disease (Fig. 2). There were 52 and 47 patients with tumor limited to

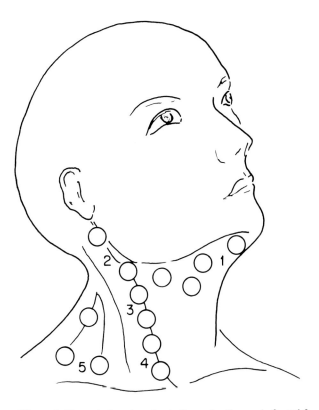

Figure 1 The main lymph nodes in the neck. Groups 1, 2, and 3 in the upper and mid neck are called cervical nodes, and groups 4 and 5 in the lower jugular chain and supraclavicular fossa are called supraclavicular nodes.

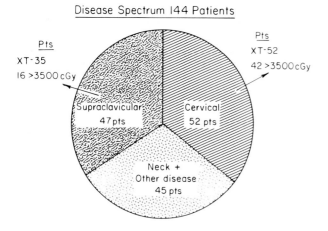

Disease Spectrum 144 Patients

Pts
XT-35
16 >3500 cGy

Pts
XT-52
42 >3500 cGy

Supraclavicular
47 pts

Cervical
52 pts

Neck +
Other disease
45 pts

Figure 2 in 99 (69%) of 144 patients whose first symptom was a lump in the neck, cancer was apparently limited to the cervical or supraclavicular nodes.

the cervical and supraclavicular groups respectively. Males predominated over females, 2.5:1, with 71 male and 28 female patients (Table 1). The median ages for men and women were 57 and 60 years respectively, with a range from 20 to 88 years. There were equal numbers of tumors on the left and right sides, and in nine patients metastases were bilateral. The main symptom was a painless lump in the neck with a median duration of 3 months.

It was not possible to have all the histologic sections reviewed. There was, however, a written pathologic report on every patient, and because of the variety of terms used, the histologic sections were categorized into anaplastic or metastatic carcinoma when the primary cell of origin could not be recognized, into squamous cell carcinoma and adenocarcinoma of all degrees of differentiation, and into a miscellaneous group (Table 2). The diagnosis was made

by incisional or excisional biopsy, with only four patients undergoing radical neck dissection.

RADIOTHERAPY

Radiation therapy aimed at cure or long-term control requires radiation doses of 5000 to 6500 cGy delivered in 4 to 6 weeks. These doses produce a sequence of changes in lymph nodes with progressive shrinkage in lymph node follicles culminating in fibrosis and hyalinization. Radiationtherapy is also used for palliation, usually at lower doses for shorter periods. Occasionally single doses of 1000 cGy are used to retard tumor growth in patients too ill to tolerate multiple daily treatments.

There is a relationship between the size of the primary tumor and the involvement of lymph nodes either at the time of diagnosis or subsequently. The likelihood of control of involved lymph nodes with radiation is dependent not only on clinical features such as size, number, and fixation, but also on the dose of radiation. Metastatic squamous cell carcinoma is not less radiosensitive than the primary tumor from which it is derived.

The optimal arrangement of radiation fields for the treatment of secondary carcinoma in the neck with an unknown primary is not known. A wide range of treatment volumes and techniques have been used. The choices in this regard represent a balance between the need to include the known areas of disease and the likely occult primary site and the knowledge that increasing the treatment volume increases the morbidity of radiation therapy. In regard to the latter a desire to avoid xerostomia predominates.

For most patients, if the nodes are anterior, this means irradiating the lymph nodes from the base of the skull to the clavicle, from the midline anteriorly to the line of the transverse cervical processes pos-

TABLE 1   Distribution of Metastatic Neck Cancer*

	Male	Female	Left	Right	Bilateral	Total Pts.
Cervical	40	12	21	26	5	52
Supraclavicular	31	16	25	18	4	47
Total	71	18	46	44	9	99
	Male : Female 2.5 : 1		57 (20–88) yrs.			

*Males predominated over females 2.5:1. The median age for both sexes was 57 years and there were equal numbers of tumors on both sides.

TABLE 2   Histopathology of 99 Patients with a Secondary Carcinoma in the Neck but no Known Primary Tumor

Neck	Carcinoma				Total
	Anaplastic Metastatic	Squamous	Adeno	Other	
Cervical	29	21	2		52
Supraclavicular	21	11	13	2	47
Total	50	32	15	2	99

teriorly and including a block of tissue in continuity as deep as the midline. This volume will encompass the most likely primary tumor sites in the upper aerodigestive tracts: in particular, the nasopharynx, tonsil, pyriform fossa, and base of tongue. The tissues of the neck must be adequately irradiated to a depth of 3 cm. In general, an ipsilateral wedge pair technique or direct electron beam is preferred. This will reduce the morbidity from radiation including the degree of xe-

rostomia and loss of taste. However, if the nodes are posterior or the primary tumor is presumed to be in the midline, then most of the pharynx, oral cavity and both sides of the neck must be irradiated with parallel opposing lateral beams. Frequently the field size is reduced after 3500 cGy, with the main tumor volume raised to 5000 to 6000 cGy. Persistent nodes are given boost doses of 500 to 1000 cGy using high-energy electrons. Typical treatment techniques and distributions are shown in Figures 3, 4, 5, and 6. The radiotolerance of vital structures must not be exceeded, the most critical organs being the brain, spinal cord, and eye. Usually, the eyes and brain stem can be excluded from the irradiated volume, and the dose to the spinal cord is reduced after 3500 cGy whenever possible. Radiation to the larynx and lungs is lowered with the use of suitable shields.

RESULTS OF TREATMENT AND SURVIVAL

Overall the treatment was well tolerated. The expected usual minor transient radiation symptoms were

A

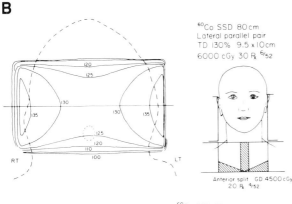

B

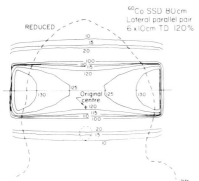

Figure 3 A and B, Set-up and distribution for a patient with undifferentiated carcinoma in the upper neck. A possible primary site in the nasopharynx was postulated. The upper aerodigestive tract together with the upper cervical nodes are irradiated with cobalt-60 using compensated lateral parallel opposed fields. A dose of 5000 cGy in 20 fractions was prescribed and the spinal cord was shielded from 3500 cGy. The lower neck, with no palpable nodes, was treated with an anterior split field to a given dose of 4500 cGy in 20 fractions.

A

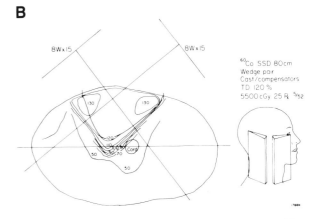

B

Figure 4 A and B, Set-up and distribution for a patient with a moderately well-differentiated squamous cell carcinoma in the upper and midcervical nodes. A primary tumor in the left base of tongue was suspected. The left side of the pharynx together with all of the lymph nodes on that side are irradiated in continuity using cobalt-60 with ipsilateral wedge pair fields. A tumor dose of 5500 cGy in 30 fractions was prescribed.

A

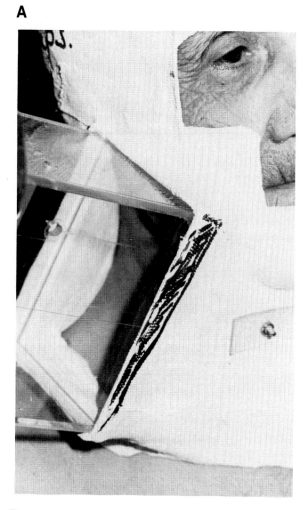

B

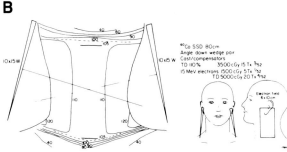

Figure 5 A and B, Set-up and distribution for a patient with a poorly differentiated squamous cell carcinoma in the left mid cervical nodes. A primary tumor in the base of tongue was suspected. The oropharynx and hypopharynx together with the lymph nodes on both sides of the neck are irradiated in continuity using cobalt-60 with an angled-down wedge pair technique. A tumor dose of 3500 cGy in 15 daily fractions is prescribed to be followed with 1500 cGy using a direct 15 Mev electron beam for a total tumor dose of 5000 cGy in 20 fractions.

observed. No serious late complications were recorded.

Survival is determined by the inherent biology of the tumor which can be modified by treatment (Fig. 7). This survival curve has been constructed by the actuarial method and shows a steady mortality with

A

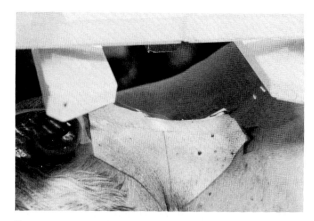

B

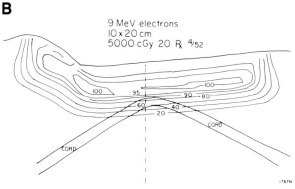

Figure 6 A and B, Set-up and distribution for a patient with metastatic adenocarcinoma in the upper neck. A dose of 5000 cGy in 20 daily fractions was prescribed using 9 Mev electrons.

time and a 5-year survival rate of 22 percent. When cervical metastases are studied alone, the 5-year survival rate is 32 percent but increases to 37 percent and 41 percent for those treated to 3500 cGy and 5000 cGy; their median survival periods are 3 and 4.5 years (Fig. 8, Table 3). Patients with supraclavicular disease fared poorly, with only 19 percent surviving 5 years. The median survival for the 16 patients with supraclavicular disease treated to 3500 cGy or more was only one year.

In some cases it was difficult retrospectively to assess the status of the neck following radiotherapy. However, for 35/52 (67%) patients with cervical disease it was considered controlled (see Table 3). Among a select group irradiated to 5000 cGy or more, re-

**TABLE 3 Treatment of
Neck Metastases: Survival**

	Pts.	cGy.	Median Survival Years
Cervical	52		1.5
	42	> 3500	3
	29	> 5000	4.5
Supraclavicular	47		0.5
	16	> 3500	1
Local control cervical 35/52 67%			

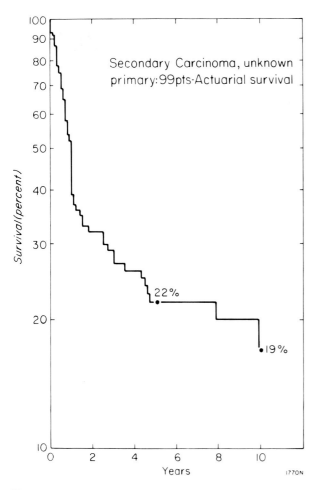

Figure 7 The actuarial survival rate for 99 patients with secondary carcinoma in neck nodes but no known primary tumor. At 5 years, 22 percent of patients are alive.

gional control was achieved in 25/29 (86%).

The study period was concluded in December 1982. At present, although 79 (80%) of the 99 patients with no cancer originally detectable outside of the neck are dead, only 17 (21.5%) have come to autopsy (Table 4). Most patients died elsewhere either in another hospital or at home, but all but two had tumor-related deaths. The primary tumor was only discovered in five autopsies, although these patients had widespread carcinomatosis. To date, a primary

TABLE 4 Mortality from Secondary Carcinoma Primary Unknown*

Patients dead		79/99 (80%)
	Cervical	9/52 17%
Autopsies 17 (21.5%)		
	Supraclavicular	8/47 17%
Diagnosis	Cervical	17/52 33%
Confirmed or 30 (30%) Probable		
	Supraclavicular	13/47 28%

*Although 79 of 99 patients had died, the primary tumor site was confirmed in only 30 (30%).

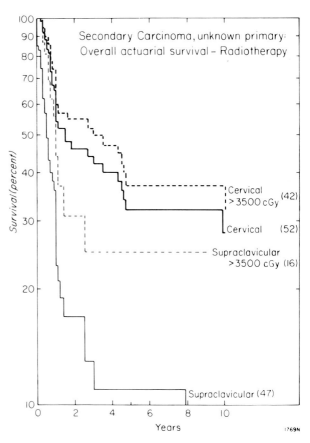

Figure 8 Patients with cervical metastases fare better than those with supraclavicular disease. There appears to be a slight advantage for those treated radically with 3500 cGy or more. The presence of some heterogeneous tumors influences the curves.

tumor has been detected in 30 (30%) of the 99 patients (Table 5).

DISCUSSION AND CONCLUSIONS

The first objective of the study was to research our recent experience of patients with metastatic cancer in the neck and no known primary tumor in order to determine the place of megavoltage radiation in

TABLE 5 Primary Tumor Discovered in 30/99 Patients (30%)

	Neck	Supraclavicular
Nasopharynx	3	
Larynx	1	
Hypopharynx	2	
Histiocytic Lymphoma		1
Hodgkins Disease		1
Lung	2	6
Stomach	3	
Pancreas	1	
Kidneys	1	1
Bladder	1	1
Breast	2	
Melanoma	1	1
Malignant fibrous histiocytoma		1
Choriocarcinoma		1
Total	17/52 33%	13/47 28%

treatment. The second was to compare it with our previously reported experience for the period from 1958 to 1970.[1] In retrospective studies, clinical reviews are handicapped equivalent to the shortcomings of the clinical records, and these limitations must be kept in mind when the results are considered. The first clinical record is the most important and should include a carefully completed staging sheet with the consensus of two experienced observers. A narrative record alone is insufficient. The difficulties we encountered in this retrospective analysis confirm the importance of carefully controlled prospective clinical trials. Although there was a description of the canceorus nodes and a pathologic diagnosis in all patients, it was not possible to have a single pathologist review all of the material. It was also impossible to accurately determine the size and number of nodes in all cases. This missing information would have been valuable in the assessment of results.

Despite the increasing volume of literature on head and neck cancer, papers dealing with the "cervical metastases–unknown primary" syndrome are few and far between.[2-12] This reflects the difficulty in analyzing the material and making meaningful conclusions. Published results from some major cancer institutes are shown in Tables 6 and 7. The principal treatment modality is listed, although all centers used a combination of methods in treating their patients. Although there is some variance in their philosophies of treatment, and despite different techniques and ways of reporting results, most series have similar survival rates. Where there is a difference, it probably represents patient selection.

The results of this review are similar to that of our 1958–1970 study (Table 8).[1] The overall 5-year actuarial survival rate was 18 percent for the first study and 22 percent for the second. The tail on the survival curves is partly accounted for by the presence of a few heterogeneous tumors with a different natural history to squamous cell carcinoma. These include malignant lymphoma, melanoma, malignant fibrous histiocytoma, and choriocarcinoma. The ground rules for the study dictated that, at the time of treatment, disease was limited to metastatic cancer in the neck and no primary cancer was detected. Altogether 87 patients were irradiated, with 58 receiving more than 3500 cGy, the dose that we used as the division between palliative and radical treatment (see Fig. 2). These patients were treated by several physicians who used different techniques and dose-time relationships. Patients with cervical metastases fared better than those with supraclavicular metastases with improved me-

TABLE 6   Reported Survival Rates From Major Institutions With Principal Treatment Modality Used

Clinic	Yr	Pts	Main Treatment	Yrs	% Survival
Cancer Institute, Beijing	1983	69	Radiation	3	45
		60	Radiation	5	37
		46	> 5000 cGy	5	48
		28	Chemotherapy	3	14
		20	Chemotherapy	5	5
Mt. Vernon, London		139	Radiation	2	17
				5	5
M.D. Anderson, Houston	1980	104	Surgery	3	57
		28	Radiation + Surgery	3	47
		52	Radiation	3	48
University, Florence	1981	49	Radiation	2	31
				5	32
University, Wisconsin	1979	54	Radiation	3	38
				5	29
Memorial, New York	1980	132	Surgery	5	50

*If allowance is made for patient selection and different numbers, the results are very similar.

TABLE 7   Reported Cumulative Local Control Rates for Lymph Node Metastases in the Neck*

Clinic	Pts	Main Treatment	% 5 Yrs/Cumulative
PMH, Toronto	52	Radiation	67
University, Wisconsin	54	Radiation	70
M.D. Anderson, Houston	37	Surgery + Radiation	86
Cancer Institute, Beijing	80	Radiation	72
	33	Chemotherapy	39
Memorial, New York	79	Surgery	50

Some selections in all series

*Although the main treatment is listed, many patients had combined therapy.

TABLE 8   Results of PMH Toronto Radiotherapy Studies†

Yr	Pts	cGy	Yrs	% Survival	Local Control Pts	Local Control %
1972	233		3	25		
			5	18		
	68*	> 4500	5	43	50	74
1984	99		3	28		
	52*		5	22	35	67
	29*	> 5000	5	41	25	86

*Cervical nodes only
†Both reports show similar results. A group of patients with disease in the upper and mid neck and treated radically can be identified. They had better survival and local control rates.

dian survivals at all stages. For those receiving more than 3500 cGy the 5-year actuarial survival rate was 37 percent and median survival 4.5 years (Fig. 7, see Table 3). For both study periods it was possible to identify a select group of patients with metastases limited to the upper and middle cervical nodes and radically irradiated (see Tables 3 and 8). The local control rates were 74 percent and 86 percent, and the 5-year actuarial survival rates 43 percent and 41 percent. These results are similar to our reported experience for patients with squamous cell carcinoma of the oral cavity.[13] It is therefore reasonable to assume that a hidden primary tumor in the upper aerodigestive tract was destroyed by irradiation. We have the impression that no one radiation technique had any significant advantage. However, it is recommended that large fields be used in all cases and the technique selected according to the clinical presentation (see Figs. 3, 4, 5, and 6).

For both time periods there was a similar ratio between anaplastic or metastatic tumors when the primary tissue could not be recognized when compared to squamous cell carcinomas of all degrees of differentiation. Adenocarcinomas remained more common in the supraclavicular nodes. In the second study the ratio of cervical to supraclavicular nodes was approximately equal, whereas in the first it was 3:1. This difference is explained by a reduction in the number of anaplastic tumors in the upper and mid neck as a result of a more vigorous assessment with the identification of the primary tumor.

There is good evidence that radiation is a curative agent and that moderate doses will selectively destroy neoplastic cells while in most instances sparing damage to the normal structures.[2-12] Our standard 4-week course for radical treatment using 250 cGy daily fractions to 5000 cGy is of necessity because of limited resources and the large number of patients to be treated. Most radiotherapy centers, however, prefer to use daily fractions of 180 to 200 cGy to a final dose of 6000 to 7000 cGy, using reduced-field techniques and boost radiation. We concur with this approach. Smaller daily fractions may reduce the intensity of the acute mucosal reactions associated with large-volume irradiation. It can also be reduced with ipsilateral radiation techniques.

Survival is determined by the inherent biology of the tumor, which can be modified by treatment. Radiation is equally effective in controlling the primary cancer and regional metastases, and so there is little reason to divide the initial treatment between radiotherapy and surgery. Treatment should always be individualized according to the variables of host, tumor, and best available treatment. From this material we were unable to determine the optimal volume for irradiation. It is important to select patients with a favorable prognosis and give them radical therapy. The regional metastases and probable site of the primary tumor are irradiated in continuity and receive the same dose. If the metastases are fixed, or larger than 3 cm in diameter, boost radiation or surgical dissection is necessary to achieve control. The regional control of a cancer is necessary for improved survival, and so it is good practice to irradiate all of the lymph nodes draining the probable primary tumor site. The known disease should receive the full tumor dose of 5000 to 6000 cGy, whereas the occult metastases can be controlled with 4500 to 5000 cGy.

Our philosophy for treatment is to use irradiation first and to reserve surgery for persistent or recurrent tumor.[14] This delayed combined approach optimizes both treatment modalities. Radiotherapy as the first planned treatment has certain advantages over post-operative radiotherapy or its use in the treatment of recurrence. First, it can destroy an occult cancer. Second, intact lymph node metastases have a better blood supply, thus reducing the risk of radioresistance due to hypoxia, which may be the case for scattered tumor cells. Third, when a large mass is not completely destroyed, the peripheral oxygenated cells are probably sterilized, and so the risk of recurrence following resection is reduced. Following treatment, patients must be examined by competent observers at monthly intervals for at least 2 years and then at increasing periods thereafter. The detection of recurrence in the neck requires immediate surgical intervention.

The place of chemotherapy in the management of these patients still has to be determined. It has been used sporadically, but only anecdotal cases were available for review. A report from Beijing using combination chemotherapy noted 12/33 (36%) patients surviving one year, but only 1/20 (5%) for 5 years (see Table 6).[4] Again, patient selection obscures the result and makes meaningful comparisons difficult. At present there is no reliable information on immunotherapy.

Overall, the results of treating metastatic cervical lymph nodes remain disappointing. Fortunately, owing to a better understanding of the behavior of tumors of the head and neck and more sophisticated assessment of the cervical metastases, unknown primary tumor syndrome is now uncommon. The results are worse when the first planned treatment fails, either in the regional lymph nodes or at the primary site. Optimum care is best defined by a multidisciplinary team that assesses, treats, and follows patients in a single clinic. Many patients require combined treatment.

REFERENCES

1. Fitzpatrick PJ, Kotalik JF. Cervical metastases from an unknown primary tumor. Radiology 1974; 110:659–663.
2. Jose B, Bosch A, Caldwell WL, Frias Z. Metastases to neck from an unknown primary tumor. Acta Radiol Oncol 1979; 18:161–170.
3. Schwarz D, Hamberger AD, Jesse RH. The management of squamous cell carcinoma in cervical lymph nodes in the clinical absence of a primary lesion by combined surgery and irradiation. Cancer 1981; 48:1746–1748.
4. Yang ZY, Hu YH, Yan JH, Cai WM, Qin DX, Xu GZ, Wu XL. Lymph node metastases in the neck from an unknown primary. Report on 113 patients. Acta Radiol Oncol 1983; 22:17–22.
5. Spiro RH, DeRose G, Strong EW. Cervical node metastases of occult origin. Am J Surg 1983; 164:441–446.
6. Fermont DC. Malignant cervical lymphadenopathy due to an unknown primary. Clin Radiol 1980; 31:355–358.
7. Fletcher GH. Textbook of Radiotherapy. Philadelphia: Lea & Febiger. 1980; pp 400–407.
8. Pacini P, Olmi P, Cellai E, Chiavacci A. Cervical lymph node metastases from an unknown primary tumor. Acta Radiol Oncol 1981; 20:311–317.
9. Simpson GT. The evaluation and management of neck masses of unknown etiology. Otolaryngol Clin North Am 1980; 13:489–498.
10. Fried MP, Diehl WH, Brownson RJ, Sessions DG, Oguar JH. Cervical metastases from an unknown primary. Ann Otol 1975; 84:152–157.
11. Dissing I. Metastases from an unknown tumor. Acta Radiol Ther Phys Biol 1976; 15:117–128.
12. Wang CC. Radiation therapy for head and neck neoplasms. Boston: John Wright, 1983; 249–245.
13. Fitzpatrick PJ, Tepperman BS. Carcinoma of the floor of the mouth. Canad J Radiol 1981; 33:148–153.
14. Rider WD, Harwood AR. The Toronto philosophy of management in head and neck cancer. J Otolaryngol 1982; 11:14–16.

THE UNKNOWN PRIMARY: PROGNOSIS AND FOLLOW-UP

JAMES E. M. YOUNG, B.Sc., M.D.
F.R.C.S.(C), F.A.C.S.

PROGNOSIS

The prognosis of an individual patient presenting with a lump in the neck from an unknown primary depends on the site of the node, the likely (or subsequently detected) site of the primary, the size of the node or nodes, and the pathology involved. Well-differentiated thyroid cancer presenting as an unknown primary in the neck with a microscopic or subsequently palpable primary has a very high cure rate. In marked contrast, patients with poorly differentiated adenocarcinoma almost invariably have a primary arising from below the clavicle (with the occasional exception of salivary gland or thyroid gland tumors) and have an exceedingly poor prognosis. Most of these patients are dead within a year. In Spiro's series, 28 of 29 patients were dead within 29 months.[1]

In squamous cell carcinoma, the overall survival rate varies between 15 and 85 percent (with an overall cure rate of about 50%), depending on the size and number of nodes. In Fried's series, no patient survived if the nodal mass at the time of presentation was greater than 4 cm.[2] Coker reported a total 5-year survival of 48 percent for squamous cell or anaplastic carcinoma with an N1 survival of 84 percent, N2 of 60 percent, and N3 of 14 percent.[3] Spiro showed a 5-year cumulative survival for epidermoid carcinoma of 74 percent for patients with N1 disease, and 41 percent for N2 and N3 disease taken together.[1]

Spiro recently emphasized that there has been no increase in survival for patients with an unknown primary over the past 25 years.[1] He also demonstrated a decrease in the incidence of squamous cell carcinoma from 84 to 60 percent, with an increase in adenocarcinoma from 9 to 22 percent during the same period.

The prognosis for patients with an unknown primary is not worse than that for patients with a known primary and similar nodal disease. Several authors have shown that if the primary does subsequently become apparent, the survival rate is poorer than if it never appears. Jesse showed that the 3-year survival for patients in whom the primary was not detected was 58 percent as opposed to 31 percent for those in whom the primary was subsequently detected.[4] Jose showed a similar phenomenon, with an undetected primary 3-year survival rate of 39 percent and a detected primary survival rate of only 25 percent.[5]

It has been suggested that the lower incidence of subsequently detected primary lesions in some series may be related to the use of radiotherapy. However, comparison between series in which patients were treated primarily by surgery, such as that of Spiro (in which 15% of the tumors were subsequently detected),[1] and series in which radiotherapy was the primary modality of treatment, such as those of Pacini (in which 14% of the tumors were subsequently detected)[6] and Jose (in which 17% of the tumors were subsequently detected)[5] show that there is no difference in the incidence of subsequently detected primary. This suggests that radiotherapy does not necessarily prevent the appearance of originally undetected primary tumor. The site of detected primary in these three series was evenly distributed between lesions below the clavicle and those in the head and neck area, further suggesting that radiotherapy does not necessarily sterilize the head and neck primary sites.

It is important to stress that comparison between various series is not only difficult but inappropriate, given the variations of pathology, nodal size, site of lesion, and treatment modalities employed. The cure rate for patients with an unknown primary mass in the neck depends on a cooperative approach among medical, radiation, and surgical oncologists since all have something to contribute to the management of this difficult group of patients.

FOLLOW-UP

The careful follow-up of the patient who has had treated metastatic cancer of the neck from an unknown primary is similar to the evaluation of any patient with a previously treated malignant tumor of the head and neck, and includes a search for recurrence at the original nodal site, evaluation for appearance of primary disease, and an assessment for the development of a new upper aerodigestive tract malignancy.

Efforts to detect the original primary disease require a frequent complete examination of the upper aerodigestive tract with the likely sites of primary receiving the most attention. In most patients, this examination can be carried out by means of palpation and indirect laryngopharyngoscopy and nasopharyngoscopy. When an awake examination is unsatisfactory, complete multiple endoscopy (laryngopharyngoscopy, fiber-optic bronchoscopy, esophagogastroscopy, and palpation of nasopharynx, base of tongue and oropharynx) under general anesthesia is indicated. In patients who originally presented with posterior triangle nodes, the nasopharynx, tonsil, and posterior pharyngeal wall require particularly careful assessment. Patients who had jugulodigastric or middle jugular nodes merit frequent reassessment of the base of the tongue, tonsil, piriform fossa, and supraglottic area. Supraclavicular nodes almost invariably originate from a primary below the clavicle (with the exception of thyroid tumors and very occasionally a laryngopharyngeal or oropharyngeal cancer), and a search for a primary in follow-up should concentrate on those sites where the primary is treatable—thyroid, breast, ovary, and prostate.

When supraclavicular nodes were excluded, it was originally thought that nasopharynx was the most likely site for an unknown primary. However, reevaluation by many authors has shown a predominance for hypopharyngeal area primaries (supraglottic, base of tongue, piriform fossa) as demonstrated in Table 1.[1,4,7] In most series, detection of a primary tumor following completion of treatment varies between 15 and 30 percent (Table 2). Spiro noted that in the original Memorial series reported by Barrie, 29 percent of the primary neoplasms were subsequently found on follow-up,[7] whereas in his own more recent series, only 15 percent of the tumors were subsequently detected.[1] He hypothesized that this might be due to an increasing skill in the ability to detect small inaccessible primaries at the time the patient first presented for treatment. This suggested increased skill may in part be due to the better endoscopic equipment available, particularly to evaluate the tracheobronchial tree, the esophagus, and the stomach. Since 33 of 51 detected subclavicular primaries were discovered in the lung, esophagus, and stomach (64.7%, Table 3), it is obvious that maximum effort should be taken to evaluate these areas both at the time of initial presentation and at the time of follow-up.

TABLE 1 Identified Primary Sites in Head and Neck: 103/879 (11.7%)

Nasopharynx	26
Hypopharynx	17
Supraglottic	13
Base of tongue	13
Tonsil	13
Oral cavity	8
Soft palate	2
Larynx	2
Antrum	2
Nasal cavity	2
Thyroid	2
Skin (squamous cell carcinoma)	1
Skin (melanoma)	1
Ear canal	1

TABLE 2 Primary Identification Following Treatment for Unknown Primary: Total No. of patients in combined series: 879[1-9]

Primary subsequently detected	168	(19%)
Head and neck	103	(61%)
Below clavicle	60	(36%)
Lymphoma	5	(3%)

TABLE 3 Identified Primary Sites Below Clavicle: 60/879 (6.8%)

Lung	19
Esophagus	8
Stomach	6
Pancreas	8
Colon	1
Appendix	1
Ovary	4
Bladder	1
Prostate	1
Breast	2
Unspecified	9

There is a high incidence of multiple primaries in patients with upper aerodigestive tract malignancy. In patients who originally presented as an unknown primary and in whom a primary tumor does subsequently appear, it is impossible to be certain whether the newly found primary is in fact the one that originally metastasized or a new primary appearing following successful treatment of the original one. Accordingly, while a clinician may only expect to find a small percentage of primary tumors following successful treatment of metastatic unknown primary nodal neck disease (Table 2), his frequent assessment of the patient must include the original nodal site, other adjacent nodal areas, and the whole of the upper aerodigestive tract, both for the original malignant tumor and for a second primary lesion.

REFERENCES

1. Spiro RH, DeRose G, Strong EW. Cervical node metastasis of occult origin. Am J Surg 1983; 146:441–445.

2. Fried MP, Diehl WH Jr, Brownson RJ, Sessions DG, Ogura JH. Cervical metastasis from an unknown primary. Ann Otol 1975; 84:152–157

3. Coker DD, Casterline PF, Chambers RG, Jaques DA. Metastases to lymph nodes of the head and neck from an unknown primary site. Am J Surg 1977; 134:517–522.

4. Jesse RH, Perez CA, Fletcher GH. Cervical lymph node metastasis: unknown primary cancer. Cancer 1973; 31:4:854–859.

5. Jose B, Bosch A, Caldwell WL, Frias Z. Metastasis to neck from unknown primary tumor. Acta Radiol Oncol 1979; 18:3:161–170.

6. Pacini P, Olmi P, Cellai E, Chiavacci A. Cervical lymph node metastases from an unknown primary tumor. Acta Radio Oncol 1981; 20:5:311–314.

7. Barrie JR, Knapper WH, Strong EW. Cervical nodal metastases of unknown origin. Am J Surg 1970; 120:466–470.

8. Yan ZY, Hu YH, Yan JH, Cai WM, Qin DX, Xu GZ, Wu XL. Lymph node metastases in the neck from an unknown primary. Acta Radiol Oncol 1982; 22:1:17–22.

9. Comess MS, Beahrs OH, Dockerty MB. Cervical metastasis from occult carcinoma. Surg Gyn Obs 1957; 607–617.

10. Weaver A, Fleming SM, Knechtges TC, et al. Triple endoscopy: A neglected essential in head and neck cancer. Surgery 1979; 86:493–496.

SECTION FOUR / RADIATION THERAPY

22. New Aspects of Radiation Therapy

INTRODUCTION

LESTER J. PETERS, M.D.

This chapter would more properly be entitled "*Some New Aspects of Radiation Therapy*" since it does not address such important new strategies as altered dose fractionation, combined radiation and cytotoxic chemotherapy, and combinations of radiation and hyperthermia. These subjects are discussed elsewhere in this volume. The subjects discussed in this part are fast neutron radiotherapy, radiosensitizers, and radioprotectors. Clinical data relating to radioprotectors are limited to a phase I-II trial sponsored by the RTOG. However, in the case of fast-neutron radiotherapy and radiosensitizers, some data from phase III randomized studies are available.

FAST-NEUTRON RADIOTHERAPY

In his chapter, Duncan reports the results of a randomized trial (of which he was principal investigator) conducted as a collaborative study in Edinburgh, Amsterdam, and Essen. This randomized study failed to show any advantage for fast-neutron radiotherapy in the treatment of head and neck cancer, in contrast to the dramatic advantage previously reported in the trial conducted at the Hammersmith Hospital.[1] Many explanations have been advanced to explain the discrepant results between these two trials: that favored by Professor Duncan is that the biologic dose delivered to the patients in the neutron therapy arm of the Hammersmith trial was greater than that in the photon control arm, as manifested by the higher complication rate in the neutron-treated patients. Using the data for tumor control rates and complications at the mean dose levels used for neutron and photon treatments in the two trials, he constructs dose-response curves which support this interpretation. However, other considerations, such as the tumor stage distribution (higher in the Hammersmith trial), the volume irradiated (larger in the Hammersmith trial), and the number of neutron dose fractions (fewer in the Hammersmith trial), may also have influenced the results.

The results of the Edinburgh trial are generally consistent with the data from the randomized trial of fast-neutron therapy carried out in the United States using a mixed schedule of neutron and photon beam therapy. This trial also failed to demonstrate an overall advantage for patients receiving a component of neutron-beam therapy, although the rate of control of large neck nodes was improved in a subset analysis.[2] Professor Duncan states that in his series neck nodes were controlled in the neutron therapy arm of the study in 63 percent (22/35) of the patients compared with 53 percent (17/32) in the photon therapy arm. However, this difference is not statistically significant.

Whatever the reasons for the discrepant results noted above, the inevitable conclusion one must reach is that fast-neutron therapy has no *across the board* advantage in the treatment of head and neck cancer. This implies that either (1) the radiobiologic rationale for fast-neutron therapy is unsound, or (2) a real benefit for a subset of patients can be masked in random clinical studies by inclusion of other patients who derive no benefit from fast-neutron therapy. From radiobiologic first principles, one can predict that certain tumor characteristics will result in either a positive or a negative therapeutic ratio when fast-neutron therapy is used (Table 1), and thus it is almost certain that in any large series of patients some will benefit from fast-neutron therapy, some will be disadvantaged, and in some the choice of treatment modality will not make any difference. Given this fact, it is not fair to conclude that there is no place for fast-neutron radiotherapy in head and neck cancer based on negative results from randomized trials using unselected patients. The challenge for the future is predictive identification of those patients whose tumors have the

TABLE 1 Radiobiological Parameters Predictive of a Positive or Negative Therapeutic Ratio with Neutrons

Positive	
High intracellular repair capacity	Based on improved
Poor cell cycle redistribution	tumor cell kill
Poor reoxygenation during treatment	with high LET
Rapid regenerative potential	Based on short treatment duration
Negative	
Low intracellular repair capacity	Based on unnecessary
Good cell cycle redistribution	loss of late normal tissue
Good Reoxygenation	tolerance with high LET

radiobiologic features pointing toward an improved therapeutic ratio with fast-neutron radiotherapy. Preliminary data from assays designed to permit this preselection of patients have recently been reported.[3]

HYPOXIC CELL RADIOSENSITIZERS

In his chapter, Phillips presents a comprehensive review of the results of clinical studies of radiation sensitizers in head and neck cancer. With the exception of one small study of halogenated pyrimidines, all the sensitizer strategies have been aimed at hypoxic tumor cells, either by treatment in hyperbaric oxygen or by the use of chemical hypoxic cell radiosensitizers. Relatively few randomized clinical trials of hyperbaric oxygen therapy in the treatment of head and neck cancer have been undertaken. However, the second MRC trial reported by Henk et al[4] did show a significant benefit in terms of both local control and survival for patients treated in hyperbaric oxygen compared with those receiving conventionally fractionated treatment in air (see Table 2 in Phillips' chapter for updated information). Unfortunately, as with the Hammersmith fast-neutron therapy trial, these results have not been reproduced, and hyperbaric oxygen therapy has been abandoned in most modern radiotherapy centers.

Randomized head and neck studies with chemical hypoxic cell sensitizers are more numerous than those with hyperbaric oxygen, but the results are equally inconclusive. Only one trial to date has shown a benefit for patients receiving a sensitizer (misonidazole), and this was limited to one tumor site (see Table 5 in Phillips' chapter).

The same general comments apply to the results of trials of hypoxic cell radiosensitizers as to fast-neutron radiotherapy. However, the rationale for hypoxic sensitizers is more specific than that for fast neutrons: the only patients who could be benefited by their use are those in whom deficient reoxygenation is the limitation to radiocurability, and the proportion of such patients in an unselected series is uncertain.[5] On the other hand, the risk of adversely affecting the therapeutic ratio with hypoxic cell radiosensitizers is small, although some normal tissues may be marginally hypoxic.[6]

Because of the specificity of the rationale for hypoxic cell sensitizers, it is perhaps even more important than with neutron radiotherapy to develop assays capable of quantitating and monitoring tumor cell hypoxia. Another point that should be made with regard to hypoxic cell radiosensitizers is that these agents are dose-modifying, i.e., the effect of a given dose of irradiation with the sensitizer is exactly the same as a higher dose of radiation without the sensitizer. Thus, use of these agents should be limited to categories of tumor where a clear dose-response relationship exists and where the radiation dose in the control arm of the trial is pushed to the limit of normal tissue tolerance.[7]

RADIOPROTECTORS

The concept of using radioprotectors to improve the therapeutic ratio by selectively protecting critical normal tissues from radiation injury is an attractive one. However, the search for effective and sufficiently nontoxic drugs to achieve this goal has been elusive. As Kligerman points out in his chapter, the drug WR-2721 effectively protects against radiation injury in experimental systems and is at least partially specific to normal tissues. As has been pointed out by Milas et al,[8] however, under certain circumstances WR-2721 also protects tumors, and this might be a limiting factor in any clinical application, especially with regard to the treatment of subclinical disease.

Of greater immediate concern, however, is the unexpected nonspecific toxicity that has been observed in clinical trials of WR-2721 given in multiple doses before fractionated x-ray therapy. This toxicity would appear to preclude the use of the drug in any phase III random study, and further evaluation of the role of chemical radioprotectors must await the identification of less toxic compounds.

CONCLUSION

These chapters present a discussion of just three of many possible new strategies available to improve the value of radiation therapy in the treatment of head and neck cancer, and they illustrate different aspects of the difficulties associated with demonstrating a clinical benefit from strategies that have sound laboratory backgrounds. In the case of chemical radiosensitizers and protectors, the toxicity of the available compounds is a severe limitation to their use. Hyperbaric oxygen was (perhaps prematurely) abandoned because of the logistic problems associated with its use. Rigorous testing of fast-neutron therapy has been compromised by the lack of availability of adequate equipment.

However, the greater problem bedeviling clinical application of new treatment strategies is the heterogeneity of human tumors. Heterogeneity is reflected in a wide variety of possible causes of failure to achieve tumor control in a given patient.[5] With so many possible causes of treatment failure, it is not surprising that strategies aimed at one or a few possible causes of failure will have the potential to benefit only a subset of patients, and broadly based random studies may well be inappropriate in elucidating their role in the overall management of head and neck cancer. The dilemma facing the clinical investigator is this: if in a randomized trial the experimental treatment gives approximately the same overall tumor control rates as conventional therapy, can one conclude that there is no place for the new approach? The answer hinges on whether the same subpopulation of patients fails both forms of therapy. If this is true, the experimental therapy can be abandoned. If this is not the case, how-

TABLE 2   Possible Predictive Assays

Estimates of Tumor Cell Survival and Repair Capability

Direct	In vitro clonogenic assays
	Xenograft assays
Indirect	DNA strand breaks and repair
	Micronucleus assay
	Chromosome aberrations
	Suppression of DNA synthesis
	Histologic assessment

Measurement of Parameters Affecting Radiosensitivity

Cellular	Tumor cell kinetics/ploidy
	Nuclear sulfhydryls
Extracellular	Intratumoral PO_2
	Vascularity index
	Sensitizer adducts
	PET imaging of tumor metabolism
	NMR spectroscopy

From Peters et al in press.[3]

ever, there could be an important role for the new treatment, provided the patients in whom it would be beneficial were predictively identified. Along similar lines, predictive identification of specific causes of radioresistance to conventional therapy would permit rational allocation of patients to various experimental studies, thus avoiding dilution of trials of patients who could not hope to benefit from the given experimental approach. These are the goals of research into predicting radiocurability which, although in its infancy, is attracting a great deal of attention at the present time. Possible methods of predicting radiocurability are listed in Table 2 and were reviewed recently.[9] Predictive assays offer the prospect of refining the application of new treatment regimens so that only those patients most likely to benefit will receive the treat-

ment. Until such time as this approach has been tested, it would be premature to conclude on the basis of the studies reported so far that there is no place for fast-neutron therapy or hypoxic cell radiosensitizers in the treatment of head and neck cancer. There is probably little benefit in repeating large-scale nonselective clinical trials, but focused studies on specific subsets of patients should be vigorously pursued.

REFERENCES

1. Catterall M, Bewley DK, Sutherland I. Second report on results of a randomized trial of fast neutrons compared to X and gamma rays in treatment of advanced tumors of the head and neck. Br Med J 1977; 1:1642.
2. Hussey DH, Maor MH, Fletcher GH. A detailed analysis of the MDAH-TAMVEC neutron therapy trials for head and neck cancer. In: Proceedings of the 13th International Cancer Congress, Part D, Research and Treatment. New York: Alan R. Liss, Inc. 1982:267–277.
3. Peters LJ, Brock W, Johnson T. Predicting radiocurability. Cancer 1985, in press.
4. Henk JM, Kunkler PB, Smith CW. Radiotherapy and hyperbaric oxygen in head and neck cancer. The Lancet 1977; ii:101–103.
5. Peters LJ, Fletcher GH. Causes of failure of radiotherapy in head and neck cancer. Radiat Oncol 1983; 1:53–63.
6. Hendry JH. Quantitation of the radiotherapeutic importance of naturally hypoxic normal tissues from collated experiments with rodents using single doses. Int J Radiat Oncol Biol Phys 1979; 5:971.
7. Maor MH, Peters LJ. Selection of appropriate studies for phase III trials of radiosensitizers. Int J Rad Oncol Biol Phys 1983; 9:271 (Letter to Editor).
8. Milas L, Hunter N, Ito H, Peters LJ. Effect of tumor type, size, and endpoint on tumor radioprotection by WR-2721. Int J Radiat Oncol Biol Phys 1984; 10:41–48.
9. Peters LJ, Hopwood LE, Withers HR, Suit HD. Predictive assays of tumor radiocurability. Cancer Treat Symp 1984; 1:67–74.

FAST-NEUTRON THERAPY

WILLIAM DUNCAN, M.D., F.R.C.S.E., F.R.C.P.E., F.R.C.R., F.A.C.R.

Fast neutrons, when attenuated in tissues, produce much more densely ionizing radiations than megavoltage x-rays. The density of ionization is of fundamental importance in determining the biologic effects of these radiations. Fast neutrons are considered to be of special therapeutic interest for two main reasons. First, their biologic effectiveness is much less influenced by hypoxia (and many tumors are thought to be hypoxic) than that of x-rays or photons. The radioresistance of hypoxic cells to photons is greatly reduced when neutrons are used—an effect known as the "oxygen gain factor". Second, the lethal effects

of neutrons are much less dependent on cell age (or position in the cell cycle) than are lethal effects of photons. Some tumors (with a relatively large proportion of cells in S phase) may be more responsive to neutrons than to photons, and this is called the "kinetic gain factor". Other biologic differences, for example, in the capacity to repair radiation-induced damage, may also be important in contributing toward the greater biologic effectiveness of neutron radiation.

The first randomly controlled trial of neutrons in the management of head and neck cancer was reported by Catterall et al in 1975.[1] This trial included patients with very advanced disease, and the majority (76%) had secondary nodes in the neck. The patients randomized to receive neutron therapy were all treated at the MRC Cyclotron Unit, Hammersmith Hospital, London. A mean target-absorbed dose of 15.95 gray in 12 fractions was used over 4 weeks. The photon-treated patients were managed at various radiotherapy centers by whatever dose and fractionation schedule was thought to be appropriate. About one-third of these patients had a relatively low photon dose, and this is confirmed by the fact that the severe radiation-related morbidity was significantly less in the photon-treated group (3%) than in the neutron-treated group (16%). This marked difference in the aggressive approach to radical treatment in the two groups has to be borne in mind when the results of tumor control are compared (Table 1). The local tumor control was only 19 percent in the photon-treated group compared with 76 percent in the neutron-treated group, a highly significant difference. Another remarkable observation in the Hammersmith trial was the very low recurrence rate of only 1.0 percent in the neutron-treated group compared with 24 percent in those treated by photons. This difference has not been explained, but the low recurrence rate after neutrons may simply be another effect of the relatively high absorbed doses delivered. Therefore it has to be acknowledged that the difference observed in total tumor control in the Hammersmith trial may be a quantitative rather than a qualitative effect of neutron therapy. Cohen (1982) has reported his experience at Fermilab with nonrandomized studies treating patients with advanced head and neck cancer, in which he found no evidence of therapeutic gain from neutrons compared with photons.[3] The relative biological effectiveness (RBE) for normal tissue tolerance was similar to that for local tumor control, and so the therapeutic ratio was similar for neutrons and photons in the treatment of head and neck cancer.

Most centers in Europe, unlike those in the United States, have been prepared to compare the effects of neutrons alone with those of megavoltage photon therapy. Centers in Edinburgh, Essen, and Amsterdam have collaborated in a randomly controlled trial of neutrons and photons in patients with head and neck cancer.[3] The disease was on average much less advanced than had been treated in the Hammersmith trial. For example, only 49 percent of patients had involved cervical nodes. The target-absorbed doses were chosen so that the late morbidity would be similar following neutron and photon therapy. That objective was achieved, except that the skin reactions were signif-

icantly more severe after neutron therapy. However, this observation is a reflection of the lack of skin sparing with these energies of neutrons and should not be regarded as a particular disadvantage of neutrons (Table 2). The local tumor control rates in this trial were similar in both treatment groups (68%) (Table 3). After apparently complete regression of tumor, the recurrence rates were also similar (38%) after neutrons and photons. No qualitative advantage was evident when the results of neutron and photon therapy were compared. The overall survival rates were similar in both groups, but there was a statistically significant poorer survival of patients with cancer of the larynx treated by neutrons. It was previously suggested that it may be disadvantageous to treat patients with laryngeal cancer by neutrons,[4] and this trial has confirmed this opinion.

The control rates for metastatic cervical nodes in patients included in the Edinburgh randomly controlled groups have also been compared (Table 4). There is a higher control rate in patients treated by neutrons (63%) than in those treated by photons (53%). However, with such small numbers of patients, this difference is not statistically significant. The magnitude of the difference is similar to that observed in the RTOG trial.[5]

The acute and late normal tissue reactions have also been carefully recorded in the Edinburgh trial.

TABLE 1 Hammersmith Head & Neck Trial: Local Control by Site

	Neutrons		Photons	
Site	No.	Local Control	No.	Local Control
Oral cavity	19	15	19	3
Oropharynx	15	13	16	5
Laryngopharynx	16	9	15	3
Antrum & nasopharynx	8	6	5	1
Neck nodes	9	7	5	0
Salivary tumors	4	4	3	0
Total (p = 0.001)	71	54 (76%)	63	12 (19%)

From Catterall and Bewley, 1974.[4]

TABLE 2 European Head & Neck Trial: Late Radiation Morbidity

	Neutrons	Photons
Skin		
Grade 3	11	1
Grade 4	0	0
Grade 5	0	0
	11 (p < 0.01)	1
Subcutaneous		
Grade 3	10	5
Grade 4	0	0
Grade 5	1	1
Mucosa		
Grade 3	5	14
Grade 4	12	9
Grade 5	5	1
	22	24

From Duncan et al, 1984.[2]

TABLE 3 European Head & Neck Trial: Local Tumor Control

	Neutrons	Photons
Patients assessed	100	95
Complete regression	70 (70%)	63 (66%)
Later recurrence	26 (37%)	25 (39%)
Local control	44 (44%)	38 (40%)

From Duncan et al, 1984.[2]

On analysis of these data, the acute reactions of the mucosa, within the target volume, were found to be significantly more severe in patients treated by photons (Table 5). The late reactions were the same for neutrons and photons. However, had the early reactions to neutrons and photons been similar, the late radiation-related morbidity associated with neutrons would have been disproportionately more severe.

In the United States it has been considered advantageous, in maintaining acceptable levels of late radiation morbidity, to mix neutrons and photons in treatment schedules while attempting to improve local tumor control rates. The RTOG High LET Therapy Group have recently reported an analysis of their randomly controlled trial of head and neck cancer treatment. Photons only were compared with a mixed schedule of neutrons (2/5) and photons (3/5). In their first report,[5] the response of secondary neck nodes in 199 patients has been documented from the total group of 312 patients recruited to this study. Table 6 gives the response rates, which show a statistically significant advantage to the mixed beam group. No data are given in this report of the response of the primary cancers, but there is no significant difference in the overall survival in the two groups. Some insight into the overall control of these tumors is given by the report of Maor et al,[6] which presents the results of the patients in the RTOG trial who were randomized and treated at the MD Anderson Hospital, Houston, Texas. Their analysis has shown similar tumor-control rates in both groups (Table 7) and no significant difference in overall survival. The late radiation morbidity was also similar in both groups (4%), and so no improvement in therapeutic ratio has been demonstrated by the addition of neutrons. It may be that there is a marginal improvement in the control of metastatic cervical nodes following neutron therapy. However, no difference is seen in the response of the primary cancers, and so there is no overall benefit in tumor control or in survival.

TABLE 4 Edinburgh Head & Neck Trial: Response of Neck Nodes

	Neutrons	Photons
No. assessed	35	32
Complete regression	29 (83%)	25 (78%)
Later recurrence	7	8
Local Control	22 (63%)	17 (53%)

TABLE 5 Edinburgh Head & Neck Trial: Assessment of Mucosal Reactions

		Neutrons	Photons
Early	Minor	31	6
	Major	28 (p < 0.001)	56
Late	Minor	36	37
	Major	16	15

TABLE 6 RTOG Head & Neck Trial: Response of Neck Nodes

	Mixed Beam	Photons
No. assessed	111	88
Complete regression (p = 0.025)	77 (69%)	49 (55%)
Later recurrence	16 (21%)	15 (31%)
Local Control (p = 0.03)	61 (46%)	34 (33%)

From Griffin et al, 1983.[5]

TABLE 7 RTOG Head & Neck Trial: Local Tumor Control Follow-up of M D Anderson patients

	Mixed Beam	Photons
Patients assessed	54	41
Complete regression	43 (80%)	28 (68%)
Later recurrence	19 (44%)	11 (39%)
Local control	24 (44%)	17 (41%)

From Maor et al, 1983.[5]

It has to be acknowledged that the neutron therapy facilities available for these trials were suboptimal when compared with modern megavoltage photon machines. The inferior physical characteristics of the neutron beams and other technical limitations may have prejudiced these results to some extent. A new generation of high-energy cyclotrons has been installed in hospitals to provide neutron beams with qualities of penetration and technical refinements similar to those of megavoltage photons. The further evaluation of fast-neutron therapy will have to await randomly controlled trials conducted at these centers, but it is unlikely that the spectacular improvement in tumor control rates originally reported following neutron therapy will be confirmed by future studies.

REFERENCES

1. Catterall M, Sutherland I, Bewley DK. First results of a randomized clinical trial of fast neutrons compared with X or gamma rays in treatment of advanced tumors of the head and neck. Br Med J 1975; 2:653–656.
2. Duncan W, Arnott SJ, Batterman J, Kerr GR, Orr JA, Schmitt G. Fast neutrons in the treatment of head and neck cancers: The results of a multi-center randomly controlled trial. Radiother Oncol 1984 (In press).
3. Cohen L. The absence of a demonstrable gain factor for neutron beam therapy of epidermoid carcinoma of the head and neck. Int J Radiat Oncol Biol Phys 1982; 8:2173–2176.
4. Catterall M, Bewley DK. Tumors of the oral cavity, oropharynx, larynx and hypopharynx. In: Fast Neutrons in the Treatment of Cancer. London: Academic Press, 1979; pp 197–202; p 245.
5. Griffin TW, Davis R, Laramore GE, Hendrickson FR, Rodríguez-Antunez A. Fast neutron irradiation of cervical adenopathy: The results of a randomized RTOG study. Int J Radiat Oncol Biol Phys 1983; 9:1267–1270.
6. Maor MH, Hussey DH, Barkley HT, Peters LJ. Neutron therapy for head and neck cancer. II. Further follow-up on the MD Anderson TAMVEC randomized clinical trial. Int J Radiat Oncol Biol Phys 1983; 9:1261–1265.

USE OF RADIATION SENSITIZERS IN THE TREATMENT OF HEAD AND NECK CANCER

THEODORE L. PHILLIPS, M.D.

Since the recognition of hypoxic cells within tumors in the early 1950s and the discovery of halogenated pyrimidines in the late 1950s, attempts have been made to utilize these approaches in the treatment of head and neck cancer.

Local control and survival in advanced stage III and particularly stage IV squamous cancer of the head and neck are poor, generally below 50 percent and often much lower. Surgery combined with radiation has improved results, but the search for methods to improve the results of radiotherapy alone has continued. Any successful technique must not simply enhance the effect of the radiation on all tissues, but must exhibit a rationale for a differential effect, i.e., greater effect on tumor than on normal tissues.

The majority of studies have concentrated on the presence of hypoxic cells in large numbers in tumors. These cells are generally up to three times more resistant than aerated cells and could be the reason for failure of radiotherapy in some tumors. It is known that in some tumors the cells gain access to oxygen during the course of radiotherapy (reoxygenation). Since hypoxia occurs because of the utilization of oxygen by cells near the capillary, thus depriving the cells more distant, it seemed logical to increase the pressure of oxygen in the blood and get more to the cells. This is the rationale for hyperbaric oxygen treatment (HBO).

Because hyperbaric chambers are cumbersome and not tolerated by some patients, drugs that mimic oxygen in their ability to sensitize hypoxic cells were sought and developed. The electron affinic nitroimidazoles have been the most successful to date. Although less potent than oxygen, they have the advantage of not being metabolized quickly by tumor cells on their way to the tumor center.

Since many tumors proliferate and synthesize DNA more rapidly than surrounding normal tissues, it was obvious that a drug incorporated into DNA which would make it more radiosensitive could sensitize tumor more than normal tissue if a difference in proliferation existed. Uridine analogs containing bromine, iodine, and chlorine were found to mimic thymidine and to be incorporated in large quantities in DNA. High levels can cause up to three times more sensitivity.

Details on the development of sensitizers and their method of action can be found in a recent review.[1]

This presentation will concentrate on the results of sensitizer clinical trials.

METHODS

In order to be as up-to-date as possible in our discussion of sensitizers in head and neck cancer, a complete review of the literature was done using the Cancerline service of the National Library of Medicine. In addition, a number of leading radiation oncologists were contacted who are active in the field and who were kind enough to provide recent data. Because of space limitations, it is not possible to review all the studies or quote all of the references. Key or original references are quoted, updated information is sometimes used in the tables from more recent abstracts or personal communications, and generally only the larger studies are cited. Where possible, the complete response rate, local control, and survival were determined and are presented in the tables.

RESULTS

Halogenated Pyrimidines

After initial work with bacteria and cells by the Stanford group and by others, a clinical trial employing bromodeoxyuridine (BUdR) was started for head and neck patients.[2] Because of detoxification in the liver, the drug was given intra-arterially, using three different drug schedules and a split-course radiation schedule, to 19 patients. The maximum dose was 1 gram per day and maximum replacement of thymidine in tumor DNA was 4.9 percent, most patients achieving much less. Significant increases in radiation mucositis were seen, but no increase in tumor response. In comparison to a randomized control group, the local control and survival was 4/19 for BUdR and 6/18 for controls (Table 1).

A small series of patients was also presented by Nomura and colleagues, who claimed improved results with BUdR, but no control group or specific control or survival rates were quoted.[3]

Hyperbaric Oxygen

Although a large number of phase I and II trials of hyperbaric oxygen were carried out around the world for head and neck cancer, only a small number of randomized phase III trials of any size were completed.[4-7] These are summarized in Table 2. The larg-

TABLE 1 Summary of BUdR Head and Neck Trials

Study Name	Number of Patients	Type Study	CR Rate	NED Survival
Bagshaw	19 BUdR 18 Cont	Rand Ph II	Not given	4/19 BUdR 6/18 Cont
Nomura	20	Phase II	Not given	Not given

CR = complete response; NED = no evidence of disease.

TABLE 2   Summary of Hyperbaric Oxygen Phase III Head and Neck Trials

| | | | | 2 Year | | | |
| | | | | Local Control | | Survival | |
Study Name	Number of Patients	Fractionation Cont	HBO	Cont	HBO	Cont	HBO
MRC UK #1	294	4.5Gy × 10 both		34%	57%	50%	50%
MRC UK #2	127	2.0Gy	4.5Gy	44%	72%	50%	74%
Sause	44	2.5Gy	4.0Gy	57%	62%	52%	57%
Sealy (+ Miso)	114	2.1Gy	6Gy	NA	NA	14%	27%

Cont = control group; HBO = hyperbaric oxygen; Miso = misonidazole.

est and most important were the two trials carried out by Henk for the MRC in the United Kingdom. The first started in 1964, and the final report was given in 1977.[4] The local control or recurrence-free rate at 5 years was 53 percent for the HBO group and 30 percent for the controls. There was identical overall survival in the two groups, probably because of more salvage surgery in the air control group. Both groups were given 10 radiation treatments of 4.5 Gy each.

The second trial, again by the MRC and carried out at Cardiff by Henk, used conventional fractionation for the controls and slightly lower radiation doses for HBO larynx cases. This trial was started in 1971 and closed after 127 patients. Both the 2- and 5-year survival and local control rates were significantly better in the HBO group. A small trial reported by Sause showed a marginal improvement with HBO, but the numbers were too small for significance. An ongoing trial by Sealy combines HBO and misonidazole and is showing better results in the HBO arm.

TABLE 3   Summary of Metronidazole Head and Neck Trials

Study Name	Number of Patients	Type Study	CR Rate	Survival > 1 Yr
Orr	23	Implant Phase II 18 g/m²	16/23	Not given
Lee	9	Phase I/II 4Gy × 11fx 70g/m²	Not given	5/9
Hliniak	18	Phase II 4g/m² Daily	Not given	Not given
Karim	36	Phase II 6.5 Gy 94 g/m²	47%	Not given

Nitroimidazoles

A long search for hypoxic cell sensitizers which would be active in mammals resulted in the identification of two active classes in 1974, the 5-nitro and 2-nitroimidazoles. These drugs had been developed as antitrichomonals, and the first to enter trial as a radiosensitizer was metronidazole, a 5-nitro compound. It has as its limiting toxicity nausea and vomiting and, with cumulative doses near 100 g/m², CNS effects of lethargy and convulsions. A small number of trials totaling less than 100 patients were done without any positive conclusions (Table 3).[8-11] The drug was abandoned because it appeared that the 2-nitro compound misonidazole was more potent and could achieve higher enhancement ratios.

Misonidazole was used in close to a dozen phase II head and neck trials, and five of the largest are shown in Table 4.[12-16] Because of the limit on total dose of misonidazole at 12 g/m² owing to peripheral neuropathy, various fractionation schemes were used to maximize the number of treatments which could be given with misonidazole as well as the size of the drug dose. Higher drug doses were desired in order to maximize sensitization. Radiation fractions ranged from 1.5 Gy tid to 6 Gy bid with misonidazole doses of 1 to 2.5 g/m². The authors concluded that the response and NED (no evidence of disease) survival were better than expected and that phase III trials were indicated.

The five largest randomized phase III trials are summarized in Table 5.[17-21] They were generally based on the phase II schemas and employed multiple daily fractions, conventional fractions, and large 4.1- to 6 Gy fractions of radiation with 0.55 to 2 g/m² of misonidazole. The MRC trial was stopped early because of toxicity and the lack of difference in results be-

TABLE 4   Summary of Misonidazole Phase II Head and Neck Trials

Study Name	Number of Patients	Fractionation	CR Rate	1 year NED survival
RTOG	50	2.5, 2.0, 1.8Gy	50%	NA
Awaad	21	1.5 Gy tid	NA	43%
EORTC	53	1.6Gy tid	83%	50%
Sealy	20	6.0Gy × 6	40%	NA
Paterson	29	4–4.5Gy	83%	66%

TABLE 5 Summary of Misonidazole Phase III Head and Neck Trials

Study Name	Number of Patients	Fractionation		CR Rate		NED survival*	
		Cont	Miso	Cont	Miso	Cont	Miso
RTOG	306	2.0Gy	2.5, 2.1Gy	56%	50%	37%	33%
Sealy	97	6.0Gy	6.0Gy	49%	56%	23%	22%
EORTC	488	1.6Gy	1.6Gy	NA	NA	NA	NA
DAHANCA	554	2/4.1Gy both		53%	77%	26%*	46%†
MRC UK	164	4.1/2.7Gy both		NA	NA	NA	NA

*Generally one year
†Pharynx cases

tween the arms. The RTOG, Sealy, and MRC trials were negative. The EORTC trial has not been analyzed yet, and the Danish (DAHANCA) trial is positive for a benefit with misonidazole. It employed two fraction sizes in both the control and misonidazole arms with or without 0.55 or 1.4 g/m^2 of drug. Stage II cases were included, and the improvement was seen primarily in pharynx patients where the overall disease-free rate was 46 percent vs 26 percent and the 3-year crude survival 53 percent vs 37 percent.

The Danish study is still in interim analysis and the EORTC yet to be analyzed. At this time it can be concluded that misonidazole is of marginal benefit with some radiation schedules and some head and neck sites. Clearly the dose of this drug which could be given was not enough for more than a marginal gain.

CONCLUSIONS

The evaluation of radiation sensitizers in head and neck cancer has been a long process. One can conclude that halogenated pyrimidines are probably not going to change the therapeutic ratio. On the other hand hypoxic cells do appear important in squamous cancer of the head and neck, as shown by the positive trials with HBO and some of the misonidazole trials. Clearly, less toxic and more potent drugs are needed as well as a modern look at hyperbaric oxygen alone or with sensitizers. Several hypoxic sensitizing methods may be combined in the future.

REFERENCES

1. Phillips TL, Wasserman TH. Promise of radiosensitizers and radioprotectors in the treatment of human cancer. Cancer Treat Rep 1984; 68:319–330.
2. Bagshaw MA, Doggett RLS, Smith KC, Kaplan HS, Nelsen TS. Intra-arterial 5-bromodeoxyuridine and x-ray therapy. Am J Roentgenol 1967; 99:886–894.
3. Nomura Y, Matsumura Y, Eguchi S, Yanagida T, Takayama K, Terashima H. BUdR continuous intra-arterial infusion–radiation therapy for cancer of the head and neck. Jibi To Rinsho 1978; 24(Suppl 12):741–750.
4. Henk JM, Kunkler PB, Smith CW. Radiotherapy and hyperbaric oxygen in head and neck cancer. Lancet 1977; 8029:101–103.
5. Henk JM, Smith CW. Radiotherapy and hyperbaric oxygen in head and neck cancer. Lancet 1977; 8029:104–105.
6. Sause WT, Plenk HP. Radiation therapy of head and neck tumors: A randomized study of treatment in air vs treatment in hyperbaric oxygen. Int J Radiat Oncol Biol Phys 1979; 5:1833–1836.
7. Sealy R, Cridland S. The treatment of locally advanced head and neck cancer with misonidazole, hyperbaric oxygen and irradiation. Int J Radiat Oncol Biol Phys 1984; 19:1721–1723.
8. Orr LE, Syed AM, Puthawala A, George FW, McKernan JF, Halikis DN. Radiosensitizers in head and neck cancer. Front Radiat Ther Oncol 1979; 13:215–225.
9. Lee DJ, Wharam MD, Kashima H, Order SE. Short course high fractional dose irradiation in advanced and recurrent head and neck cancer. Int J Radiat Oncol Biol Phys 1979; 5:1829–1832.
10. Hliniak A, Watras J, Maciejewski B, Wojcieszek Z, Widel M. Preliminary clinical investigations on the use of metronidazole as an agent increasing sensitivity to radiation. Nowotwory 1980; 30:127–130.
11. Karim AB. Prolonged metronidazole administration with protracted radiotherapy: a pilot study on response of advanced tumours. Br J Cancer 1978; 37(Suppl III):299–301.
12. Fazekas JT, Goodman RL, McLean CJ. The value of adjuvant misonidazole in the definitive irradiation of advanced head and neck squamous cancer: an RTOG pilot study. Int J Radiat Oncol Biol Phys 1981; 7:1703–1708.
13. Awwad HK, Barsoum M, El Merzabani M, Omar S, El Badawy S, Ezzat S, El Baki HA, Zaki A. The use of misonidazole in association with a three-fractions per day regimen in advanced head and neck epidermoid cancer: a pilot study. Am J Clin Oncol 1983; 6:91–97.
14. Van den Bogaert W, Van der Schueren E, Horiot JC, Chaplain G, Arcangeli G, Gonzalez D, Svoboda V. The feasibility of high dose multiple daily fractionation and its combination with anoxic cell sensitizers in the treatment of head and neck cancer. Int J Radiat Oncol Biol Phys 1982; 8:1649–1655.
15. Sealy R. A preliminary clinical study in the use of misonidazole in cancer of the head and neck. Br J Cancer 1978; 37(Suppl III):314–317.
16. Paterson IC, Dawes PJ, Henk JM, Moore JL. Pilot study of radiotherapy with misonidazole in head and neck cancer. Clin Radiol 1981; 32:225–229.
17. Fazekas JT, Pajak TF, Marcial VA, Davis LW. The RTOG randomized trial–79-15: Misonidazole adjuvant to radiotherapy in advanced head and neck squamous cancers. Proc ASCO 1984; C-719:185.
18. Sealy R, Williams A, Cridland S, Stratford M, Minchinton A, Hallet C. A report on misonidazole in a randomized trial in locally advanced head and neck cancer. Int J Radiat Oncol Biol Phys 1982; 8:339–342.
19. Horiot JC, Van den Bogaert W, Ang KK, Chaplain G, Van der Schueren E, Nabid A, Vessiere M. EORTC experience with misonidazole combined with a multiple daily fractionated radiotherapy. Proc Eur Soc Ther Radiol Oncol (ESTRO) 1982; London, England. 132 pp
20. Overgaard J, Andersen AP, Jensen RH, Hjelm-Hansen M, Jorgensen K, Petersen M, Sandberg E, Sand Hansen H. Misonidazole combined with split course radiotherapy in the treatment of invasive carcinoma of the larynx and pharynx. Acta Otolaryngol (Suppl) 1982; 386:215–220.
21. Henk JM. Misonidazole: MRC trials–head and neck. Proc Eur Soc Ther Radiol and Oncol (ESTRO) 1982; London, England. 132 pp

RADIATION PROTECTION: INCLUDING A REPORT ON THE PHASE I-II STUDY OF SINGLE AND MULTIPLE DOSES OF WR-2721

MORTON M. KLIGERMAN, M.D., M.Sc., M.A.

The most common strategy for increasing the effectiveness of radiation therapy by chemical means is to administer drugs that enhance the sensitivity of tumor cells without significantly changing the radiation resistance of the normal tissue. Such an accomplishment would represent a therapeutic gain. An alternate approach is the use of drugs that would protect the normal tissues, but not significantly raise the radiation resistance of the tumor. To be potentially effective clinically, the radioprotector must be selectively absorbed in normal tissues. It should be a relatively stable, relatively nontoxic compound which could be used by oral administration and/or intravenously. There are several classes of radioprotector drugs such as the sulfur-containing compounds, certain alcohols, and other agents such as 5-hydroxytryptamine (serotonin) and the bacterial endotoxin Pyrexal. However, the most promising class of compounds for radiation protection are the aminothiols. Numerous analogs of the aminothiol cysteamine (mercaptoethylamine) have been synthesized by the United States Army Medical Research and Development Command at Walter Reed Medical Center. Of these, the drug designated WR-2721 appears to be most promising. This presentation will briefly discuss the physical-chemical changes which occur within cells when they are exposed to ionizing radiation and the mechanism of protection by some of the aforementioned compounds with emphasis on the aminothiols. In addition, the present development in the use of WR-2721 clinically will be presented.

The principal mode of action of these compounds utilizes one or more of the following:

1. Produce hypoxia.
2. Scavenge free radicals produced by ionizing radiation.
3. Repair direct and indirect damage to critical molecules including strategic enzymes used to repair radiation-damaged cells.
4. Enzymatically remove slow-reacting products of water radiolysis.

DIRECT AND INDIRECT EFFECT OF IONIZING RADIATION

The excitation and ionization of cellular macromolecules and water occur as the initial event of the interaction of radiation with biologic materials and take place within a time frame of 10^{-17} and 10^{-10} seconds. It is estimated that 30 percent of cell inactivation is due to the direct effect (equation 1) on critical molecules such as DNA and enzymes.[1]

$$RH \rightarrow R^{\cdot} + H^{\cdot} \qquad (1)$$

The free radical $R^{\cdot}$ is inactivated by oxidation, an action that takes place in 10^{-9} to 10^{-8} seconds.

Cellular inactivation by indirect effect results from the products of the initial interaction of ionizing radiation and cellular water (equation 2) reacting with critical macromolecules.

$$H_2O + radiation \rightarrow H^{\cdot}, OH^{\cdot},$$
$$e^-_{aq}, H_2, H_2O_2, H_3O^+, OH^- \qquad (2)$$

Chapman points out that 60 percent of the indirect effect is caused by the interaction of the free radical $OH^{\cdot}$ and critical molecules (targets). This is seen in equations 3, 4, and 5.

$$OH^{\cdot} + T \rightarrow T - OH^{\cdot} \qquad (3)$$

$$OH^{\cdot} + T \rightarrow H_2O + T^{\cdot}. \qquad (4)$$

$$e^-_{aq} + T \rightarrow T^{\cdot-}. \qquad (5)$$

These three free radicals are inactivated by oxidation by the dissolved molecular oxygen, the so-called "radical oxidation".

MECHANISM OF RADIATION PROTECTION BY SULFHYDRYL COMPOUNDS

Sulfhydryl compounds are radioprotectors by virtue of their ability to (1) donate a hydrogen atom to free radicals, thereby reconstituting critical molecules to their active form, and (2) scavenge the products of water radiolysis. The naturally occurring intracellular protector is glutathione (GSH) and the repair reaction is found in equation 6

$$R^{\cdot} + GSH \rightarrow RH + GS^{\cdot} \qquad (6)$$

where RH represents the reconstituted active critical molecule. The scavenging of free radicals by GSH is illustrated in equation 7.

$$^{\cdot}OH + GSH \rightarrow H_2O + GS^{\cdot} \qquad (7)$$

The competition between GSH and oxygen for combining with the free radical of critical molecules overwhelmingly favors oxygen. Ward believes that 10 μM

Supported in part by National Cancer Institute Grants CA-30100, CA-16520 and CA-07153 from the Department of Health and Human Services.

309

of oxygen is reactively equal to 1 mM of GSH;[2] the latter is the intracellular concentration of GSH. Ward points out that the intracellular concentration of oxygen under normal atmospheric conditions is equal to 200 μM. This indicates that to have complete protection, sulfhydryl donors must be present in considerable excess of the intracellular oxygen concentration.

In defining the optimum structure of aminothiols for radiation protection, Doherty and co-workers suggested that the most effective structure was one in which the functional amino group was separated from the available sulfhydryl moiety by a 3-carbon chain. Since then, however, it has been found that in a particular compound, a 2-carbon chain may be ideal.[4]

OTHER RADIATION PROTECTORS

The action of 5-hydroxytryptamine (5-HT) is believed to be mediated through two physiologic changes.[5,6] This drug, which is metabolized very rapidly, acts directly on the central nervous system in the hypothalamic region, affecting the pituitary adrenalcortical system with inhibition of cortical steroid production. This inhibition, Flemming believes, exercizes a beneficial effect on radiation protectors.

Furthermore, 5-HT causes a reduction of intracellular oxygen as measured by a marked increase in hepatic lactate content within 5 minutes after injection. Sulfur-containing compounds other than aminothiols, such as dithiocarbamate, thiourea, and dimethysulfoxide, and certain alcohols, such as isobutinol and ethylene glycol, react with OH and as such are radioprotective agents.

Within the cell itself, enzymatic removal of the more slowly reacting radiation products of water takes place.[1] Superoxide dismutase catalyzes the combination of negatively charged oxygen free radicals and hydrogen to form hydrogen peroxide and oxygen. The hydrogen peroxide so generated is reduced to water by the enzyme catalase or by intracellular peroxidases.

WR-2721 AS A RADIOPROTECTOR

In 1949, Patt demonstrated that rats would experience reduced fatality when exposed to 800 rads of whole-body irradiation when they were pretreated with cysteine.[7] The death rate was reduced from over 90 percent to 20 percent. Further evidence of cysteine protection included reduction in splenic atrophy and a reduction in the degree of leukopenia. In his later review of protective mechanisms, Patt, in commenting on the advisability of using aminothiols in cancer patients, warned that "unless selective protection can be accomplished, the purpose of therapy may be defeated and the area to be treated may also show an increased radioresistance."[8]

Of the numerous analogs of mercaptoethylamine (cysteamine) which have been prepared by the US Army Drug Research and Development Command, S-2-(3-aminopropylamino)-ethylphosphorothioic acid

(WR-2721) was found by Yuhas and Storer to protect mice against fatality with a dose-reduction factor (DRF) of 2.6 to 2.72.[9] They also found that mammary tumors in mice irradiated 15 minutes after the intraperitoneal injection of WR-2721 were only slightly more resistant to irradiation, whereas the skin reaction of the mouse was reduced. This was clearly a therapeutic gain in these experimental animals, since differential protection was achieved. Except for the brain and spinal cord, all normal tissues concentrated this relatively well-tolerated radiation protector. Utley et al[10] and Washburn et al[11] confirmed the localization of WR-2721 in high concentration in normal tissues relative to experimental tumors. In the latter reference, only two experimental tumors tested concentrated WR-2721.

The first clinical experiment with WR-2721 was carried out by Tanaka and Sugahara with daily doses of WR-2721 which corresponded to 60 mg/m^2.[12] Nausea and vomiting were observed in approximately 15 percent of patients. Radiation was given 30 minutes after the intravenous administration. Using the time of onset of first- and second-degree mucosal reactions as criteria, a DRF of 1.7 and 1.3 respectively was observed.

Phase I clinical studies in the United States utilizing WR-2721 were initiated at the Cancer Research and Treatment Center at the University of New Mexico.[13] This effort has been transferred to the University of Pennsylvania. Study of the maximum tolerated dose (MTD) of single doses of WR-2721 before therapeutic doses of radiotherapy and chemotherapy has been completed.[14] The multiple-dose study before fractionated radiotherapy is still in progress and is being carried out in cooperation with the University of Alberta (Dr. R. Urtasun), the University of California (Dr. Theodore Phillips), the University of Rochester (Dr. Philip Rubin), and the M.D. Anderson Hospital (Dr. Lester Peters).

Two hundred and seventy-two patients have been entered in phase I/II studies of WR-2721.[15,16] Patients with advanced malignant disease received WR-2721 before single or multiple doses of radiotherapy or before single doses of cyclophosphamide, cisplatin, or nitrogen mustard. Single doses between 25 mg/m^2 and 1330 mg/m^2 were escalated according to a modified Fibonacci schedule. The work-up for patients receiving palliative therapy consisted of history and physical examination, ECG, SMA12, CBC, platelet count, and fasting blood sugar. These studies, except the ECG, were repeated at appropriate intervals up to 6 months and beyond. Blood pressure was monitored for an hour before the first injection to establish baseline readings. This monitoring was continued during the injection and for an appropriate time after the infusion. WR-2721 is designated NSC296,961 by the National Cancer Institute, who supplied the material in 500-mg vials containing an equal amount of mannitol. To prevent dephosphorylation, the drug is reconstituted in 5% dextrose-lactated Ringer's solution and buffered with sodium bicarbonate to a pH of 7.20. It is infused 15 to 30 minutes before x-ray therapy or chemotherapy. With doses of 450 mg/m^2 and higher, the infusion rate has been between 14 and 20 mg/m^2 per minute, designated as the "long infusion time". The drug was given in 5 minutes when the doses were 25 mg/m^2 to 300 mg/m^2 and in 7 minutes in those patients receiving 340 mg/m^2. More recently, patients have received the larger doses of drug in 15 minutes.

The toxicities observed in the single dose study included hypotension, emesis, somnolence, sneezing, and hypocalcemia. A metallic taste was experienced by some patients. The two major toxicities are emesis and hypotension. Hypotension, somnolence, and sneezing were not dose-related. However, the differences in incidence of these three toxicities when patients were treated over the long infusion time as compared with 15-minute infusion time are set forth in Table 1. A higher percentage of patients were hypotensive when the infusion was given at the rate of 14 and 20 mg/m^2. However, this difference is not statistically significant. Sixteen of the 214 patients receiving single doses became hypotensive to such a degree and persistence that the infusion was not completed. This represents only 7.5 percent of all patients.

The dose-limiting toxicity was emesis. The incidence of emesis increased with dose (Table 2). In the patients who received the long infusion time, 42 percent of 31 patients vomited after the administration of 450 mg/m^2. At 740 mg/m^2, 90 percent of 20 patients were so affected. This difference is significant, p = < .001. However, when patients were infused in 15 minutes, only 35 percent of patients receiving 740 mg/m^2 vomited. This difference, at 740 mg/m^2, 35 percent vs 90 percent, is statistically significant, p = 0.05. At the rate of 910 mg/m^2 delivered in 15 minutes, 12 patients were treated, 9 of whom experienced significant emesis. In addition, these patients complained of a high degree of malaise and indicated that they would not be willing to repeat the treatment.

Of the 214 patients who received single doses, in addition to those who failed to complete treatment because of hypotension, two failed to complete because of emesis. In one instance, this was due to the patient's request, although the amount of vomiting was not considered severe by the attending medical group.

One patient who received WR-2721 before chemotherapy was observed with carpopedal spasm and distal paresthesia, which disappeared spontaneously. The clinical diagnosis of hypocalcemia was confirmed by serum calcium determination.[17] Measurement of the serum calcium before and after infusion of the protective agent revealed a fall in the level from 2.33 to 1.90 mM per liter. This drop was statistically significant, p = < .001. In all of the 8 patients who had serum calcium levels measured at 24 hours, the level remained depressed. Concomitantly, parathyroid hormone levels fell in all patients. It was concluded that WR-2721 inhibits the secretion of parathyroid hormone and increases urinary excretion of calcium, which leads to hypocalcemia.

No other changes in the chemical or enzymatic studies were observed immediately after or at any time subsequent to the administration of WR-2721 with observations made 3 months, 6 months, 9 months, and 12 months after administration of the protector. From these data it was concluded that the dose-limiting toxicity for single doses of WR-2721 was emesis, and 740 mg/m^2 delivered in 15 minutes represented the maximum tolerated dose.

Multiple Doses of WR-2721 Before Fractionated X-Ray Therapy

Fifty-eight patients have been entered into the multiple-dose trial. Doses were escalated from 100 mg/m^2 one to five times a week to 340 mg/m^2 four times a week for 3 weeks and 250 mg/m^2 four times a week for 6 weeks. Tables 3 and 4 reveal the incidence of hypotension and emesis at each dose level. All other dose levels were given over a 3-week period. Seven of the 35 patients at doses of 170 mg/m^2 and above developed symptoms designated as "malaise", which was characterized by a feeling of generalized discomfort, uneasiness, and asthenia. Five of the 58 patients developed symptoms designated as "idiosyncratic",

TABLE 1   Toxicity to WR-2721
Single-Dose: Nondose-Related

	Infusion	
	Long	15-Minute
Number of patients at risk	121	69
Hypotension	14%	7%
Somnolence	22%	13%
Sneezing	19%	38%

TABLE 2   Toxicity to WR-2721, Single-Dose: Emesis

mg/m^2	Long (%)	15-Minute (%)
450	13/31 (42)*	2/8 (25)
740	18/20 (90)*†	14/40 (35)†

*Difference significant, p = < .001
†Difference significant, p = .05

TABLE 3 Hypotension from Multiple-Dose WR-2721
Before Radiation Therapy

(mg/m^2)	Toxic Patients/Total
100	0/14
150	5/9
170	6/16
250*	3/4
250†	3/6
300	2/8
340	0/1

*4 × 3 weeks
†4 × 6 weeks

TABLE 4   Emesis from Multiple-Dose WR-2721 Before Radiation Therapy

(mg/m²)	Toxic Patients/ Total
100	2/14
150	2/9
170	6/16
250*	2/4
250†	2/6
300	5/8
340	1/1

*4 × 3 weeks
†4 × 6 weeks

which included symptoms and signs of fever, chills, rash, and hypotension. All of these symptoms were present in only one patient. Twenty-four of 58 patients failed to complete treatment. Withdrawal of patients from the protocol was either physician-related or patient-related. Physicians withdrew patients because of hypotension, one; idiosyncratic response, five; malaise, five; cancellation of radiotherapy, four; and intractable vomiting, one. In eight instances, patients withdrew themselves from the program. Four of the patients withdrew because of intolerance to nausea and vomiting; four patients withdrew because they feared injury due to the drug.

Bone Marrow Protection Against Cyclophosphamide Toxicity

In animals, WR-2721 was found to protect selected normal tissues against the cytotoxicity of cyclophosphamide and cisplatin.[18] In a phase I trial of WR-2721 pretreatment in patients receiving cyclophosphamide, Glick and co-workers treated 15 patients with 450 mg/m² to 1100 mg/m² of WR-2721 30 minutes prior to cyclophosphamide therapy (1200 to 1800 mg/m²).[16] Four weeks later, these same patients were retreated with the same cyclophosphamide dose without WR-2721. With WR-2721 pretreatment, 11 of 15 patients had improved WBC nadir counts. This was 2700 cells/mm³ with WR-2721 pretreatment compared to 1800 cells/mm³ with the same dose of cyclophosphamide alone (p = 0.008). Seven of the 11 patients showed significant improvement of the nadir granulocyte counts. The mean with pretreatment was 1274 cells/mm³ compared to a mean of 765 cells/mm³ with cyclophosphamide alone (p = 0.05). In a second trial, 25 patients were treated with a reverse sequence. Cyclophosphamide was given alone on the first injection, followed 4 weeks later by WR-2721 pretreatment. The same range of doses of cyclophosphamide and WR-2721 were used as in the first series. With WR-2721 pretreatment, 12 of 25 patients had white counts with a higher nadir. The white count was increased from a mean of 1550 cells/mm³ on cyclophosphamide alone to 1850 cells/mm³ with WR-2721 followed by cyclophosphamide (p = 0.02).

However, when the mean nadir granulocyte count was examined, this had increased from a mean of 449 cells/mm³ to 844 granulocytes/mm³ when patients received WR-2721 before cyclophosphamide, (p = 0.001).

DISCUSSION

There have been no deaths in this phase I trial of WR-2721 involving 272 patients. Patients are able to tolerate nausea and vomiting on the single-dose schedules either before radiation therapy or chemotherapy. Eleven percent of patients exhibit mild transient hypotension, which is quickly reversible. Hypotension and emesis are the two major toxicities of the single-dose schedule, but emesis is the dose-limiting toxicity. The maximum tolerated single dose has been established at 740 mg/m² infused in 15 minutes and is in use in phase II trials.

In the multiple-dose studies, difficulties have been encountered in completing treatment. The major reason for this at the higher dose levels (250 mg/m² and above four times a week for 3 and 6 weeks) has been intolerance of patients to daily nausea and vomiting and the symptoms of generalized discomfort, uneasiness, and asthenia ("malaise") which occur in the second, third, and fourth week of treatment. This problem has been addressed and is currently treated by prescribing single morning doses of dexamethasone in the amount of 4 mg. The experience of bone marrow protection by WR-2721 in patients receiving cyclophosphamide is the first correlation in our group of animal data and clinical experience. Additional patients are showing the same protection of the white count and the granulocyte fraction.

To date, observations are:

1. No evidence of tumor protection.
2. The compound can be given safely; there have been no deaths.
3. Nausea and vomiting are dose-dependent, while hypotension is independent of dose.
4. Patient compliance and maintenance of a feeling of well-being in the multiple-dose study before radiotherapy needs to be investigated.
5. The MTD for single doses of WR-2721 is 740 mg/m² infused in 15 minutes.

REFERENCES

1. Chapman JD, Reuvers AP. The time-scale of radioprotection in mammalian cells. In: Locker A, Flemming K, eds. Radioprotection. Basel and Stuttgart: Birkhauser Verlag, 1977: pp 9–18.
2. Ward JF. Chemical aspects of DNA radioprotection. In: Nygaard OF, Simic MG, eds. Radioprotectors and anticarcinogens. New York: Academic Press, 1983: pp 73–85.
3. Doherty DG, Burnett WT Jr, Shapira R. Chemical protection against ionizing radiation. II. Mercaptoalkylamines and related compounds with protective activity. Radiat Res 1957; 7:13–21.

4. Brown DQ, Pittock JW, Rubinstein JS. Early results of the screening program for radioprotectors. Int J Radiat Oncol Biol Phys 1982; 8:565–570.
5. Streffer C. Studies on the mechanism of 5-hydroxytryptamine in radioprotection of mammals. In: Locker A, Flemming K, eds. Radioprotection. Basel and Stuttgart: Birkhauser Verlag, 1977: pp 71–77.
6. Flemming K. Some ideas concerning the mode of action of radioprotective agents. In: Locker A, Flemming K, eds. Radioprotection. Basel and Stuttgart: Birkhauser Verlag, 1977: pp 79–86.
7. Patt HN, Tyree B, Straube RL, Smith DE. Cysteine protection against X irradiation. Science 1949; 110:213–214.
8. Patt HN. Protective mechanisms in ionizing radiation injury. Physiol Rev 1953; 33:335–376.
9. Yuhas JM, Storer JB. Differential chemoprotection of normal and malignant tissues. J Nat Cancer Inst 1969; 42:331–335.
10. Utley JF, Marlowe C, Waddell WJ. Distribution of 35 S-labelled WR-2721 in normal and malignant tissues of the mouse. Radiat Res 1976; 68–284.
11. Washburn LC, Carlton JE, Hayes RI, Yuhas JM. Distribution of WR-2721 in normal and malignant tissues of rats and mice: Dependence on tumor type drug dose, species. Radiat Res 1974; 59:475–483.
12. Tanaka Y, Sugahara T. Clinical experiences of chemical radiation protection in tumor radiotherapy in Japan. In: Brady LW, ed. Radiation sensitizers. New York: Masson Publishing 1980: pp 421–425.
13. Kligerman MM, Shaw MT, Slavic M, Yuhas JM. Phase I clinical studies with WR-2721. Cancer Clin Trials 1980; 3:217–221.
14. Turrisi AT, Glick JH, Yuhas JM, Glover D, Kligerman MM. Final report: Phase I trial of single doses of WR-2721 before radiotherapy and chemotherapy. In manuscript.
15. Kligerman MM, Glover DJ, Turrisi AT, Norfleet AS, Yuhas JM, Coia LR, Simone C, Glick JH, Goodman RL. Toxicity of WR-2721 administered in single and multiple doses. Int J Radiat Oncol Biol Phys 1984; 10:1773–1776.
16. Glick JH, Glover D, Weiler C, Norfleet L, Yuhas J, Kligerman MM. Phase I controlled trials of WR-2721 and cyclophosphamide. Int J Radiat Oncol Biol Phys 1984; 10:1777–1780.
17. Glover D, et al. Hypocalcemia and inhibition of parathyroid hormone secretion after administration of WR-2721 (a radioprotective and chemoprotective agent). N Engl J Med 1983; 309:1137–1141.
18. Yuhas JM, Spellman JM, Jordon SW. Treatment of tumors with the combination of WR-2721 and cis-Dichlorodiammine platinum or cyclophosphamide, Br J Cancer 1980; 42:574–585.

23. Definitive Radiation Therapy

INTRODUCTION

RODNEY R. MILLION, M.D.

The ensuing chapters on definitive radiotherapy are limited to discussion of lesions arising in the glottic and supraglottic larynx and the pyriform sinus. These common presenting sites represent clinical situations in which there are alternatives of treatment that may affect not only survival, but also the quality of life.

Early glottic, supraglottic, and pyriform sinus carcinomas, when carefully selected for anatomic extent and safe medical condition, may be managed by operation with glottic preservation, or they may be managed by radiation therapy with little regard for anatomic extent or general medical status.

Based on reports from the surgical and radiotherapy literature, it would be difficult to select a treatment for the early lesions based only on the cure rate, and so most decisions are based on local tradition, patient preference, the functional result, the potential for complications, and the like.

These three sites also represent a considerable variation in the risk for spread to the regional lymphatics; glottic carcinomas have a low risk, supraglottic carcinomas an intermediate risk, and pyriform sinus carcinomas a high risk for neck disease. Certainly the risk for subclinical disease, as well as the presence of clinically obvious neck disease, often changes the philosophy in the management of the primary site.

In the chapters that follow, the authors represent two differing philosophies in the approach to definitive radiation therapy of the larynx and pyriform sinus. One hesitates to generalize or characterize a treatment philosophy, as we all individualize our treatment plan to a certain degree. However, it is fair to say that Drs. Harwood and Constable represent what I would call a "moderate-dose" philosophy. Their philosophy is to use a dose that will produce a substantial rate of cure, a minor risk for a complication, and low morbidity for surgical rescue procedures. Their prescribed doses do not usually increase with increasing T stage or tumor volume. The "high-dose" philosophy is represented by Dr. Bataini and me. Adherents to the "high-dose" philosophy believe that slightly higher doses increase the local and regional control rates with minor increase in the complication rate and without significant increase in the morbidity of surgical rescue procedures. The doses are adjusted according to the T or N stage or tumor volume, and the concept of progressively reducing the size of the treatment portal is an essential part of the plan. Although the doses are numerically higher in the "high-dose" approach, there may not be that much difference because of the overall time factor and, in some instances, the way in which the dose is specified. Dr. Goepfert, who presents the viewpoint of the head and neck surgeon, has experience primarily with the "high-dose" school of radiotherapy.

GLOTTIC CARCINOMA

Generally, there is not much controversy about the management of T1 and T2 squamous cell carcinoma of the vocal cord. The local control rates with radiotherapy are fairly uniform, about 90 percent for T1 lesions and approximately 70 percent for T2 lesions. However, one must avoid comparing the results of radiotherapy with those produced by hemilaryngectomy series, as the local control rates for radiotherapy differ, depending on the amount of disease and distribution of disease within T1 and T2 stages.[1] The University of Florida radiation therapy results are analyzed in Tables 1 through 3, according to whether the lesion was initially suitable for cordectomy, hemilaryngectomy, or total laryngectomy.[1]

In my own practice, we choose to use radiation therapy as the initial treatment for nearly all T1 and T2 lesions, with hemilaryngectomy or total laryngectomy reserved for radiation therapy failure. The advantages of radiation therapy are simply that one avoids a major operation and that the quality of the voice is expected to be better with radiotherapy than hemilaryngectomy.

The major controversy that exists today is in the management of T3 and T4 carcinomas of the vocal cord. Dr. Harwood has presented ample evidence to show that the local control rate for T3 and T4 N0 cases is at least 50 percent, and with close observation and surgical salvage there is probably little if anything lost in the overall cure rate. Other studies confirm his findings. Harwood also shows that women have an especially good local control rate compared with men who have similar-stage lesions (see Table 4 in Harwood's chapter). Most surgeons question whether the final survival is as good as if one had proceeded immediately to total laryngectomy, with or without pre-

operative or postoperative irradiation. That is a difficult question to answer, since the reported results tend to come either from surgical centers, where almost all the patients are treated with total laryngectomy with only a few treated with radiotherapy, or from radiotherapy centers, where a large percentage of the patients are treated initially with radiotherapy (see Table 7 in Harwood's chapter). The dichotomy in therapeutic philosophy makes interinstitutional comparisons difficult, but there seems to be little or no difference in 5-year survival. It is our current practice at the University of Florida to individualize the recommendations for T3 and T4 lesions of the glottis.

TABLE 1 Local Control and Voice Retention in Patients Managed by Irradiation and Surgical Salvage: 70 Patients Suitable for Cordectomy (Stage T1)

Results	No. Controlled/ No. Treated	Comments
Control with irradiation alone	68/70 (97.1%)	
Surgical salvage		
Hemilaryngectomy	1/1	Alive and well over 5 years
Total laryngectomy	1/1	Died of intercurrent disease at 8 years
Ultimate control of disease	70/70 (100%)	
Disease control with voice retained	69/70 (98.6%)	

From Dickens WJ, Cassisi NJ, Million RR, Bova FJ. Treatment of early vocal cord carcinoma: A comparison of apples and apples. Laryngoscope 1983; 93:216–219.

TABLE 2 Local Control and Voice Retention in Patients Managed by Irradiation and Surgical Salvage: 84 Patients Suitable for Hemilaryngectomy (Stages T1–T2)

Results	No. Controlled/ No. Treated	Comments
Control with irradiation alone	79/84 (94.0%)	
Surgical salvage		
Hemilaryngectomy	1/1	Alive and well over 5 years
Total laryngectomy	4/4*	Two alive and well over 8 years; two died of intercurrent disease at 3 and 8 years
Ultimate control of disease	84/84 (100%)	
Disease control with voice retained	80/84 (95.2%)	

*Hemilaryngectomy was not considered a treatment option at the University of Florida prior to 1973.

From Dickens WJ, Cassisi NJ, Million RR, Bova FJ: Treatment of early vocal cord carcinoma: A comparison of apples and apples. Laryngoscope 1983; 93:216–219.

TABLE 3 Local Control and Voice Retention in Patients Managed by Irradiation and Surgical Salvage: 55 Patients Not Suitable for Hemilaryngectomy (Stages T1–T2)

Result	No. Controlled/ No. Treated
Control with irradiation alone	36/55 (65.5%)
Surgical salvage	
Hemilaryngectomy	2/3*
Total laryngectomy	11/13†
Refused total laryngectomy: 2‡	
Total laryngectomy for treatment complication: 1§	
Ultimate control of disease	50/55 (90.9%)
Disease control with voice retained	38/55 (69.1%)

*Patient with recurrence after hemilaryngectomy who had total laryngectomy for salvage died of neck node and distant metastases.
†One died of neck node metastases only; one died of distant metastases only.
‡Both died of disease; counted as uncontrolled.
§Necrosis; no tumor found.

From Dickens WJ, Cassisi NJ, Million RR, Bova FJ. Treatment of early vocal cord carcinoma: A comparison of apples and apples. Laryngoscope 1983; 93:216–219.

Our own results in both unselected and selected T3 lesions show a 61 percent local control rate when radiotherapy is used as the initial management.[2] Careful follow-up almost always picks up the recurrences so that salvage surgery can be done. It is our current practice to tell patients that the simplest approach is to have a total laryngectomy and, if needed, postoperative irradiation. However, we tell suitable candidates that radiotherapy is also a reasonable approach, that they have 5 or 6 chances out of 10 of preserving a useful larynx and useful voice. However, they must be willing to come for regular check-ups and have a desire to preserve their larynx. We tell them that they may give reduce survival at 5 years by 5 to 10 percent. Few patients select laryngectomy when presented the facts in this way by the surgeon and radiation therapist.

SUPRAGLOTTIC LARYNX

Early carcinomas of the supraglottic larynx can be treated either with radiotherapy or, in selected cases, with supraglottic laryngectomy. Radiotherapy can be used for all T1 and T2 (and many T3) lesions, but supraglottic laryngectomy is limited by medical conditions as well as the anatomic extent of the lesion. The local/regional control and survival are approximately the same for both surgery and radiation therapy.

There are, however, differences in both acute and late problems. Certainly a patient having a supraglottic laryngectomy must undergo a major operation and a period of retraining to swallow. However, once through the high-risk period, most patients do quite well, have a normal voice, and learn to swallow. Patients treated with radiation therapy have no immediate threat from an operation, but must suffer through 6 to 7 weeks of treatment plus a month for healing. They are at risk for persistent edema, and a very small number develop an incompetent larynx or necrosis. At the University of Florida, when a patient is suitable for either supraglottic laryngectomy or radiation therapy, we have no simple way of selecting the best treatment for the patient, and frequently it is the patient's preference that decides the final management. When a patient presents with major neck disease and an early supraglottic lesion, however, it is our preference to use radiotherapy to the primary site and both sides of the neck with one (or two) neck dissections added, depending on the size and response of the neck nodes. It is our observation that the end result is better in this case, since the larynx is treated only with radiotherapy rather than with surgery and radiotherapy. We strongly dislike performing a supraglottic laryngectomy with one or two neck dissections and then adding postoperative radiation primarily to ensure neck control. In this situation the larynx is incidentally irradiated, which produces significant edema and perhaps the need for a tracheostomy.

For the T3 and T4 supraglottic lesions, the treatment is individualized, depending on location of the lesion, whether it is exophytic or mostly infiltrative, and the degree of involvement of the neck. Although laryngectomy, neck dissection, and preoperative or postoperative radiotherapy are often advised, a proportion of T3 and T4 lesions are favorable for treatment with radiotherapy alone, with surgery reserved for salvage.

PYRIFORM SINUS

Although early primary tumors arising from the pyriform sinus are relatively uncommon, they do occur, and often in combination with major neck disease. Radiotherapy and partial laryngopharyngectomy (PLP) are alternative treatments for the T1 lesions. Dr. Bataini reports a 16 percent local failure rate for T1 lesions, 32 percent for T2 and T3 lesions, and 51 percent for T4 lesions. The University of Florida experience is similar for the T1–T3 lesions, but our success rate with T4 lesions is poor. It has been our usual practice at the University of Florida to recommend radiotherapy for all T1 lesions and for selected T2 and T3 lesions, with surgery reserved for radiation failure. Although PLP is an alternative for T1 lesions, we believe that the PLP may result in permanent difficulty in swallowing and aspiration. Radiation therapy has the added advantage of comprehensive treatment of the entire neck. We frequently combine radiation therapy with a neck dissection 4 to 6 weeks after radiotherapy in the case of N2a or greater neck disease.

TABLE 4 Carcinoma of the Pyriform Sinus: Survival Free of Disease in Patients Treated by Radiation Therapy ± Neck Dissection

AJCC Stage	Absolute Survival		Determinate Survival	
	2 Years	5 Years	2 Years	5 Years
I, II	6/8	5/6	6/8	5/6
III	9/17 (53%)	3/12 (25%)	9/15 (60%)	3/8
IVA*	10/14 (71%)	4/10 (40%)	10/12 (83%)	4/6 (67%)
IVB	4/19 (21%)	1/13 (7%)	4/18 (22%)	1/13 (7%)
Total	29/58 (50%)	13/41 (32%)	29/53 (55%)	13/33 (39%)

*IVA – any combination of T1 or T2 and N2a, N2b, or N3a.
Note: University of Florida data; patients treated 10/64 to 12/80 (to 12/77 for 5-year figures); analysis 2/83 by J. W. Devine, M.D.[5] From Million RR, Cassisi NJ. *Management of Head and Neck Cancer: A Multidisciplinary Approach*. Philadelphia: JB Lippincott, 1984, p 386.

A significant number of patients have a small primary lesion that may be cured with radiotherapy, but also have advanced neck disease; we have had a bit of success with irradiation followed by immediate neck dissection in this group (stage IVa) (Table 4).[3-5] It is important to avoid laryngeal lymphedema in order to detect a recurrence and offer salvage surgery. There are a number of technical tricks that may be used to avoid major laryngeal lymphedema.[4]

Salvage operations for pyriform sinus treatment failures have only been moderately successful and are almost always associated with a fair amount of morbidity. The patient who selects radiation therapy as the initial treatment must be made aware of the risks associated with salvage operations.

For the more advanced lesions, we favor total laryngopharyngectomy and postoperative irradiation; preoperative irradiation is selected for cases in which the neck metastases are considered fixed or borderline operable. We have not had the success with radical irradiation for the advanced lesions reported by Dr. Bataini.

RESCUE OPERATIONS

Surgeons attempting salvage in cases of recurrent disease at the primary site and/or in the neck are always faced with problems in healing, and this is particularly true for recurrent carcinomas of the pyriform sinus. However, with modern surgical technology it is possible to restore the patient to a functional state even after radical resections. It is often possible to do either hemilaryngectomy or supraglottic laryngectomy following radiation therapy failure for early lesions, with complete laryngectomy reserved for recurrence following the conservation procedure. Partial laryngopharyngectomy is rarely a possibility after failure of an early pyriform sinus lesion.

Should more radiotherapists adopt the philosophy of Harwood and Constable and use a slightly more moderate dose of radiation, so that when failures occur, surgery can be done with less morbidity than after high-dose irradiation? Assuming that failure is slightly more common with the "moderate dose" philosophy,

more patients are going to require a rescue procedure. The "high dose" philosophy has the advantage of producing a few more cures, but the probability of a surgical disaster increases. However, when we review our own data and the data of others, it is difficult to see a linear increase in surgical complications related to total dose. Those who adopt the "high dose" philosophy must use every technical trick available (i.e., reducing fields, maximum shielding of normal tissues, treatment beams that spare skin and subcutaneous tissues) to ensure the fewest surgical problems possible. There are advantages and disadvantages to both philosophies, and the selection of irradiation dose is largely governed by the philosophies and abilities of the referring surgeons.

At the University of Florida we have adopted a fractionation scheme that gives 120 rads twice daily. The use of a smaller dose per treatment session should produce a reduction in late effects (for example, fibrosis and chronic lymphedema) and, we hope, help to reduce the problems with rescue surgery. In our 6-year experience we believe that our local control rate is improved and that the late effects are reduced, but we have limited experience so far with salvage treatment and cannot make a statement one way or another about a change in morbidity for rescue procedures.[6]

REFERENCES

1. Dickens WJ, Cassisi NJ, Million RR, Bova FJ. Treatment of early vocal cord carcinoma: A comparison of apples and apples. Laryngoscope 1983; 93:216–219.
2. Mendenhall WM, Million RR, Sharkey DE, Cassisi NJ. Stage T3 squamous cell carcinoma of the glottic larynx treated with surgery and/or radiation therapy. Int J Radiat Oncol Biol Phys 1984; 10:357–363.
3. Million RR, Cassisi NJ. Radical irradiation for carcinoma of the pyriform sinus. Laryngoscope 1981; 91:439–450.
4. Million RR, Cassisi NJ (eds). Hypopharynx: Pharyngeal walls, pyriform sinus, and postcricoid pharynx. In: *Management of Head and Neck Cancer: A Multidisciplinary Approach*. Philadelphia: JB Lippincott, 1984, pp 373–391.
5. Devine JW, Million RR, Cassisi NJ. Squamous cell carcinoma of the pyriform sinus 1984; in preparation.
6. Parsons JT, Cassisi NJ, Million RR. Preliminary report on the results of twice-a-day irradiation of squamous cell carcinomas of the head and neck at the University of Florida. Int J Radiat Oncol Biol Phys 1984; in press.

DEFINITIVE RADIOTHERAPY FOR GLOTTIC CARCINOMA

ANDREW R. HARWOOD, M.B., Ch.B., F.R.C.P.(C)

MANAGEMENT POLICY AND PHILOSOPHY

The treatment of squamous cell carcinoma of the glottic larynx in our hospital is primary moderate-dose radiotherapy for all stages of disease, reserving surgery for biopsy-proved residual or recurrent tumor 3 months or more after completion of irradiation (RRSS).[1] The goal of this management is to combine cure of the tumor with the best quality of life.[1] Since the human larynx is the best method of producing speech, our management policy emphasizes laryngeal preservation when possible.

Moderate-dose radiotherapy is employed with careful attention to radiotherapy technique, and doses used are in the range of 1650 to 1750 rets (i.e., 5000 rads in 4 weeks in 20 fractions, 5500 rads in 5 weeks in 24 fractions, and 6000 rads in 6 weeks in 30 fractions).

The advantages of moderate dose radiotherapy are four-fold:

1. Major radiotherapy complications (such as laryngeal necrosis) are minimized.
2. Complication rate associated with surgery in those failing irradiation is kept within an acceptable range and permits conservative voice-preserving procedures to be carried out in suitable cases.
3. It minimizes postirradiation edema, facilitating early diagnosis of residual or recurrent disease and therefore allowing high control rates to be obtained with salvage.
4. It optimizes voice quality.

These advantages are accomplished without significantly affecting the local and regional control rate of the tumor.[2] In order for the management policy of RRSS to be successful, it is essential that the failures of irradiation be recognized early to permit successful surgical retrieval of the irradiation failures. Since most recurrences, particularly in advanced disease, occur in the first year after irradiation, close follow-up is essential, and the patient is followed monthly in multidisciplinary ENT clinics. Routine direct laryngoscopy and biopsy are performed 3 months after completion of irradiation in all T3 and T4 tumors and anytime thereafter in the patient whose larynx is causing concern. If histologic findings are positive, surgery is carried out. Occasionally, if the laryngeal appearance is deteriorating (e.g., the development of fixity of the larynx), surgery is recommended in the absence of positive histologic findings. Routine follow-up laryngeal tomography is also employed routinely 3 months, 6 months, and 1 year after completion of irradiation. Tomography is particularly useful in the diagnosis of persistent disease in the laryngeal ventricle and subglottic region.[3]

SELECTION OF PATIENTS FOR TREATMENT

Virtually all patients with laryngeal glottic cancer are treated with RRSS. We do not regard the presence of subglottic extension,[4] anterior commissural involvement,[2] a fixed vocal cord or larynx cartilage involvement,[2] presence of nodal disease,[2] or an obstructed larynx necessitating tracheostomy as a contraindication to the use of this management policy.[2] Similarly, verrucous carcinoma is primarily irradiated and the results of irradiation are satisfactory; we have seen only one possible case of anaplastic transformation in more than 40 cases irradiated.[2] We see more than 90 percent of all laryngeal cancers in our draining population of 5 million people, and more than 95 percent of cases seen are treated with RRSS. This experience is unique in North America.

TECHNIQUES OF TREATMENT

These have been described in detail elsewhere.[5] Strict and careful attention to radiotherapy technique is mandatory in the use of definitive radiotherapy in glottic carcinoma. All patients are immobilized with a plastic mask or plaster cast. Patients are treated generally with cobalt-60 with individually made tissue compensators to minimize "hot spots" where necrosis may occur and "cold spots" where recurrence may occur. Technique is particularly important in T1 glottic cancer, in which the local recurrence rate of tumor was reduced from 18 percent to 9 percent with the increase in radiation field size from 5 × 5 cm to 6 × 6 cm.[2] Similarly, in T1 glottic cancer it is vital to make sure that the anterior commissure region receives a full dose of radiotherapy.[2] Since this region is close to the skin surface, bolus or plastic is placed over this region so that full-dose build-up occurs. In our experience, when careful attention is given to radiotherapy technique, involvement of the anterior commissure has no effect on our ability to locally control the tumor.

For patients with subglottic disease, a technique called the angled-down technique has been developed and used for the past 15 years.[5] This technique gives homogeneous irradiation down to the level of the carina (if necessary) from two lateral fields. By means of laryngeal tomography, which precisely delineates the presence or absence of subglottic disease and its extent, we have found that subglottic extension does not affect our ability to cure T2 and T3 glottic cancer with the angled-down technique.

TABLE 1 Results of Definitive Radiotherapy for Carcinoma In Situ (T1sN0)

Series	No. of Patients	Local Control by RT (%)	% Dead from Larynx Cancer
Harwood[2]	92	94	0
Fletcher[6]	86	89	0
Wang[8]	67	83	?

TREATMENT RESULTS

Carcinoma In Situ

The results of definitive radiotherapy of carcinoma in situ of the larynx is shown in Table 1. The incidence of local control by radiotherapy varies between 83 and 94 percent, and virtually all of the recurrences have been controlled with subsequent surgery. In our own experience, plus that of Fletcher,[6] there have been no deaths from tumor.

Invasive Carcinoma Stages T1NO and T2NO

The results of radiotherapy in T1 glottic carcinoma are shown in Table 2, with three large series being documented. It can be seen that the control rate by radiotherapy is approximately 90 percent, with one-half to two-thirds of the recurrences being saved by subsequent surgery. A significant fraction of the failures (one-third to one-half) can be salvaged with partial laryngectomy and preservation of laryngeal speech. In a recent detailed analysis of all our failures with T1 glottic cancer, few (one-third) of the failures died from uncontrolled local tumor alone and the majority (two-thirds) had distant metastases.

In a number of reports it has been shown that the dose-response curve for T1 glottic cancer is flat over the range of 5000 rads in 4 weeks to 7000 rads in 7 weeks.[7] Therefore, our recommendations for the optimal radiotherapeutic treatment of T1 glottic cancer is a dose of 5000 rads in 4 weeks in 20 fractions or equivalent (6000 rads in 6 weeks in 30 fractions) via a compensated or wedged parallel pair technique using a minimum field size of 6 × 6 cm. This will optimize both the control of the tumor and the functional quality of the voice.

The results of radiotherapy of T2 glottic cancer are shown in Table 3. It can be seen that the local control rate by irradiation in more than 600 patients

TABLE 3 Results of Definitive Radiotherapy for T2 Glottic Cancer

Series	No. of Patients	Local Control by RT (%)	% Dead from Larynx Cancer
Harwood[7]	316	68	16
Wang[8]	173	69	14
Fletcher[6]	175	74	6

is approximately 70 percent, with approximately one-half of the postirradiation failures being cured by salvage surgery for a death rate from laryngeal cancer of 6 to 16 percent.[2,6,8] The most important factor determining success of irradiation in T2 glottic cancer is the presence or absence of impairment of mobility of the vocal cord. T2 tumors with normal vocal cord mobility have a local control rate by radiotherapy of 77 to 78 percent, and those with impaired cord mobility, 54 to 58 percent.[4,8] We have not found the presence or absence of subglottic extension to be a significant factor in the success or failure of definitive radiotherapy for T2 glottic cancer, and we do not regard subglottic extension as a contraindication to irradiation. We recommend a minimum field size of 6 × 8 cm for the treatment of patients with T2NO glottic cancer, and we use our standard dose of 5000 rads in 4 weeks in 20 fractions.

One factor of major importance in determining the efficacy of definitive radiotherapy of glottic cancer is sex. The influence of sex on the ability of irradiation to cure glottic cancer is shown in Table 4. In every stage grouping, females have a better control rate than males. The reason for this is unclear, but it is our strongly held belief that it is mandatory that all women with glottic cancer, irrespective of the size of the tumor, should be treated primarily with irradiation, a belief expounded by Lederman 15 years ago.[9]

Advanced Glottic Cancer T3, T4NO, N+

The use of definitive radiotherapy in advanced glottic cancer is extremely controversial. In Toronto and in other centers, RRSS has been the preferred treatment because of the potential to save the larynx and natural voice in a significant proportion of the survivors. The results of definitive radiotherapy in T3 glottic cancer in centers where primary radiotherapy is the preferred modality of treatment are shown in Table 5. With the exception of those reported by

TABLE 2 Results of Definitive Radiotherapy for T1 Glottic Cancer

Series	No. of Patients	Local Control by RT (%)	% Dead from Larynx Cancer
Harwood[2]	571	87	6
Wang[8]	723	90	3
Fletcher[6]	332	89	2

TABLE 4 Influence of Sex on Local Control by Definitive Radiotherapy for Glottic Cancer

Stage	% Local Control	
	Male	Female
T1N0	87	97
T2N0	68	87
T3N0	46	75

TABLE 5 Results of Definitive Radiotherapy for
T3 Glottic Cancer: "Radiotherapy Centers"

Series	No. of Patients	% Control by RT	% Cases Treated by RT
Harwood*	150	51	77
Stewart[13]	67	57	80+
Wang[8]	65	32	65
Trott[14]	300+	50	NA
Lederman[9]	289	47	80+

*Update May, 1984.
NA = not available.

TABLE 6 Results of Definitive Radiotherapy for
T3 Glottic Cancer: "Surgical Centers"

Series	No. of Patients	% Control by RT	% Cases Treated by RT
Skolnick[15]	8	25	6
Kirchner[16]	4	25	13
Martensson[17]	16	19	23

Wang,[8] approximately 50 percent of cases are locally controlled by irradiation. By contrast, in the surgical literature, much poorer results of radiotherapy have been documented and are shown in Table 6. These poor results are almost certainly due to the fact that small numbers of patients were treated by irradiation and that, since surgery was the preferred treatment modality in these centers, only selected unfavorable cases not suitable for surgery were treated by irradiation.

Table 7 summarizes the data from large surgical and radiotherapy series on T3 glottic cancer in terms of survival and proportion of survivors possessing their larynx and natural voice. It can be seen that no difference in survival exists between the surgical and radiotherapeutic series. However, less than 10 percent of the patients in the surgical series possess even a portion of their larynx. In comparison, one-half to two-thirds of the radiotherapy patients possess their larynx

TABLE 7 Survival and Voice Preservation in
T3 Glottic Cancer

	% Alive	% Survivors with Larynx
Surgery (500+ patients)		
Kirchner[16]	60	6
Skolnick[15]	48	3.5
Vermund[18]	61	NA
Ogura[19]	60	NA
RRSS (700+ Patients)		
Harwood[2]	55	66
Lederman[9]	45	63
Wang[8]	57	57
Stewart[13]	57	NA
Vermund[18]	50	66

NA = not available.

and natural voice. Therefore, in view of its potential for laryngeal preservation and better quality of life, we believe that radiation with surgery in reserve is the preferred treatment for T3 glottic cancer.

Our experience in T4 glottic cancer is more limited, with only 68 patients being treated with RRSS.[2] Forty-nine percent of these patients were alive and well at 5 years following treatment. It was found that cartilage invasion per se had no effect on our ability to control T4 glottic cancer.[2] However, the presence or absence of involvement of the hypopharynx had a significant effect on the ability of irradiation to control the disease. For glottic carcinoma involving the hypopharynx, the control rate by irradiation was similar to tht for primary hypopharyngeal carcinoma.

Primary glottic carcinoma presenting with nodal disease is an uncommon problem.[2] Between 1965 and 1979, only 48 patients with advanced glottic cancer combined with nodal disease were seen at the Princess Margaret Hospital and treated with radical radiotherapy with surgery in reserve. Thirty-eight percent were alive and well at 5 years, with 47 percent dying of their laryngeal carcinoma. The majority of these patients had advanced primary disease combined with advanced nodal disease.

COMPLICATIONS OF TREATMENT

The major complications resulting directly from irradiation in the treatment of cancer of the larynx are laryngeal necrosis, laryngeal stenosis, and severe edema requiring tracheostomy or producing aspiration pneumonia. In our experience with more than 1000 patients treated with moderate-dose irradiation for early glottic cancer (T1, T2NO), we have not seen a single case of clinically identifiable cartilage necrosis of the larynx attributable to the irradiation.[2] Similarly, a histopathologic study of larynges removed following failed irradiation in Toronto revealed no histopathologic case of radionecrosis in our early glottic cases, confirming the clinical findings already noted.[10] In a series of patients treated with higher doses of irradiation in Amsterdam, a 7 percent necrosis rate was seen in T1 glottic cancer when a dose of 6200 rads in 4 weeks in 20 fractions was used.[7] We believe strongly, therefore, that moderate doses of irradiation are the optimal treatment for early glottic cancer, optimizing both cure and functional result and minimizing major complications from the irradiation.

In patients with advanced glottic cancer, we have clinically noted laryngeal necrosis in approximately 1 to 2 percent of those radically irradiated. None of the patients who developed laryngeal necrosis from such treatment died as a result of this complication. In a parallel histopathologic study of larynges removed from patients with advanced glottic carcinoma, pathologic radionecrosis of the cartilage was seen in 7 patients.[10] It must be remembered that a significant fraction of these advanced glottic cancer patients who were irradiated had prior invasion of the cartilage. This information therefore demonstrates that it is possible to safely irradiate larynx cancer involving the cartilage with moderate doses of irradiation without running a significant risk of subsequent cartilage necrosis.

The other complication with which one must be concerned when using a deliberate policy of delayed surgery only for persistent disease is the complication rate associated with the surgery. There are a number of reports in the literature which show the high morbidity of operating in previously irradiated tissues.[2] These problems mainly occur in patients who have been heavily irradiated. In our own experience, we have not found an increase in the major complication rate associated with subsequent surgery in patients who have been irradiated with moderate doses of irradiation. Therefore, I see no reason why surgery cannot be delayed for persistent or recurrent disease following moderate doses of irradiation.

FUNCTIONAL RESULTS—QUALITY OF LIFE

The quality of life after treatment for laryngeal cancer is of crucial importance both to the physicians treating laryngeal cancer and to the patients. This can be illustrated by a recent study in which patients were given the option of having primary surgery for laryngeal cancer with no possibility of laryngeal preservation versus an option of radiation with surgery in reserve with a poorer survival, but preservation of the larynx in a significant proportion of patients.[11] A significant proportion of the people interviewed in this study chose to have a poorer survival but better quality of life. According to our own experience, as already noted, we believe that we can produce equivalent survival in advanced glottic cancer using RRSS versus primary surgery. We have carried out some limited studies on the quality of life of patients treated for laryngeal cancer, and we have interviewed patients who had been cured of laryngeal cancer by radical radiation with preservation of the larynx and some who had persistent disease following irradiation, requiring partial or total laryngectomy.[12] In all the parameters tested, the patient with laryngeal preservation had superior quality of life and voice to those who had required total laryngectomy. The majority of the successfully irradiated patients, even with advanced disease, were working, able to use the telephone, and living a normal social life. By contrast, a significant number of the patients who required a laryngectomy were unable to work, were not able to use a telephone, and could not live a normal social life.

In conclusion, therefore, we believe that definitive radiotherapy with surgery in reserve is the optimal treatment for virtually all stages of laryngeal cancer.

REFERENCES

1. Rider WD, Harwood AR. The Toronto philosophy of management in head and neck cancer. J Otolaryngol 1982; 11:14–16.
2. Harwood AR. Cancer of the larynx. The Toronto experience. J Otolaryngol 1982; 11(Suppl 11):
3. Rideout DF, Poon PY. Radiologic studies of the larynx after radiotherapy for carcinoma. Can J Radiol 1977; 28:182–186.
4. Harwood AR, DeBoer G. Prognostic factors in T2 glottic cancer. Cancer 1980; 45:991–995.
5. Harwood AR, Keane TJ. General principles of irradiation therapy as applied to head and neck cancer. J Otolaryngol 1982; 11:69–76.
6. Fletcher GH. Textbook of Radiotherapy. 3rd ed. Philadelphia: Lea & Febiger, 1980, pp 330–363.
7. Harwood AR, Tierie A. Radiotherapy of early glottic cancer. Int J Radiat Oncol Biol Phys 1979; 5:477–482.
8. Wang CC. Radiation Therapy for Head and Neck Neoplasms. Boston: John Wright, PSG Ltd., 1983, pp 165–199.
9. Lederman M. Radiotherapy of cancer of the larynx. J Laryngol Otol 1970; 84:867–896.
10. Keene M, Harwood AR, Bryce DP, Van Nostrand AWP. A histopathological study of radionecrosis in laryngeal carcinoma. Laryngoscope 1982; 92:173–180.
11. McNeil BJ, Weichselbaum R, Parker SG. Speech and survival. Tradeoffs between quality and quantity of life in laryngeal cancer. N Engl J Med 1981; 305:982–987.
12. Harwood AR, Rawlinson E. The quality of life of patients following treatment for laryngeal cancer. Int J Radiat Oncol Biol Phys 1983; 9:335–338.
13. Stewart JG, Brown JR, Palmer MK, Cooper A. The management of glottic carcinoma by primary irradiation with surgery in reserve. Laryngoscope 1975; 85:1477–1484.
14. Macieyewski B, Preuss-Bayer G, Trott KR. The influence of the number of fractions and of the overall treatment time on local control and late complication rate in squamous cell carcinoma of the larynx. Int J Radiat Oncol Biol Phys 1983; 9:321–328.
15. Skolnick EM, Yee KF, Wheatley MA. Carcinoma of the laryngeal glottis; therapy and end results. Laryngoscope 1975; 85:1452–1466.
16. Kirchner JA, Owen JR. Five hundred cancers of the larynx and pyriform sinus. Results of treatment by radiation and surgery. Laryngoscope 1977; 87:1288–1303.
17. Martensson B, Fluer E, Jacobsson F. Aspects of treatment of cancer of the larynx. Ann Otol 1967; 76:313–329.
18. Vermund H. Role of radiotherapy in cancer of the larynx as related to the TNM system of staging. Cancer 1970; 25:485–504.
19. Ogura JH, Sessions DG, Spector GJ. Analysis of surgical therapy for epidermoid carcinoma of the laryngeal glottis. Laryngoscope 1975; 85:1522–1530.

CANCER OF THE SUPRAGLOTTIC LARYNX

WILLIAM C. CONSTABLE, M.B., Ch.B., D.M.R.T.

TABLE 1 Stage At Presentation of Supraglottic and Glottic Cancer (%)

Stage	I	II	III	IV
Supraglottic cancer (present series)	6	27	27	40
Glottic cancer[1]	63	13	21	3

The otolaryngologist, spoiled by the excellent results obtained in glottic cancer, is often pessimistic about the results in supraglottic malignant disease. Despite the dramatic differences in stage at presentation, modern results in cancer of the supraglottic larynx stand comparison with malignant tumors at many other head and neck sites (Table 1).

The present series represents recent experience and spans the period in which surgeons have experimented with conservative surgery and preoperative and postoperative radiotherapy and the radiotherapists have introduced higher energy equipment and have experimented with higher total dose, hyperfractionation, and radiosensitizers. At the University of Virginia most of the radiotherapeutic fads have been avoided and the cobalt-60 unit has retained its role in the treatment of laryngeal malignant tumors.

ANATOMY AND LYMPHATIC DRAINAGE

For radiotherapy to be correctly administered, an understanding of certain key features concerning the mode of spread in supraglottic cancer is vital. First, there is no barrier to spread within the supraglottic region itself, and extensive but still localized lesions occur (no apparent nodal involvement). For example, 50 percent in the present series were T2, T3, T4 NO. Second, spread to the pre-epiglottic space occurs and is usually unsuspected as, in certain instances, involvement of cartilage is only discovered at operation. Third, the lymphatic drainage is abundant and bilateral spread can occur and, except in the *earliest* T1 lesions, must be a paramount consideration in management. Fourth, the entire chain of nodes from mastoid to clavicular head must be considered as the target volume. On the other hand, in the majority of instances the posterior triangle can be omitted.

Cartilage necrosis following radiotherapy has proved an evanescent issue, and treatment of even localized lesions has serendipitously resulted in treatment of the first echelon of nodes.

STAGING

We have employed the TNM staging as recommended by the American Joint Committee (Table 2).[2]

As already indicated, spread to the pre-epiglottic region or cartilage involvement may not be appreciated. Difficulty is also experienced in ascertaining the site of origin within the supraglottic larynx of any but the earliest lesions. A defect in the staging is the lack of emphasis on fixation with its attendant poor prognosis whether the lesion is a T3 or T4, vis à vis the other lesions lumped together in their category. Finally, it is impossible to define whether an advanced lesion has arisen in the glottis or the supraglottic larynx; it has been our practice to guess at the epicenter and, if this is above the vocal cords, to classify the lesion as supraglottic.

Over half the tumors in this series were classified T3 and T4, and 44 percent had nodes detected on presentation.

HISTOLOGY

All cancers in the present series were squamous cell carcinomas, 39 percent poorly differentiated and 42 percent moderately well differentiated. The only other histologies were a carcinoid tumor and an adenocarcinoma. Given the anatomic and lymphatic considerations, it can be appreciated that supraglottic malignant tumors are potentially highly aggressive.

SITE OF ORIGIN

The most common site of origin within the supraglottic larynx was the false cord (48%), the next being the epiglottis (37%). The former figure represents the advanced nature of many tumors and the impracticality of precise localization.

TREATMENT PHILOSOPHY AND POLICIES AT THE UNIVERSITY OF VIRGINIA

Radiotherapy

Unquestionably, the overriding philosophy has been conservation: spare the larynx whenever possi-

TABLE 2 T Staging (abbreviated) of Supraglottic Cancer

T1	Confined to site of origin, normal mobility.
T2	Involves adjacent supraglottic site(s) or glottis, without fixation.
T3	Limited to larynx with fixation and/or extension to postcricoid, medial wall of pyriform sinus, or pre-epiglottic space.
T4	Massive tumor involving oropharynx, soft tissues, or cartilage.

ble, use moderate doses for cure and accept, possibly, a higher surgical salvage rate but lower radiotherapy morbidity. At the same time it must be appreciated that a *relatively* small number of tumors are amenable to conservative management in view of the preponderance of advanced tumors necessitating aggressive combined therapy to attain cure and consequent sacrifice of the larynx.

The standard radiotherapy approach for the exceptional early lesion has been 6000 rads in 5 weeks encompassing the primary and first-echelon nodes. For more advanced tumors, the standard approach has been 5000 rads in 5 weeks to the primary and nodes, with 1000 rads/week as a supplement to the primary. In rare instances, the supplement has been 1250 rads or greater. The philosophy has been that the additional gain (a few percent) in local control is bought at the expense of a substantial increase in morbidity, particularly postoperatively. Our results would seem to support this view.

Preoperative or Postoperative Radiotherapy

Although subscribing to the view that moderate-dose (5000 rads) preoperative radiotherapy has substantial advantages over postoperative radiotherapy,[3] our policy has been modified to encompass advances in surgical technique and evaluation. Preoperative radiation is still the optimal approach when the lesion is demonstrably inoperable or doubtfully operable; certain of these lesions may be rendered operable, nutrition improved, and recurrence reduced. When lesions are operable, surgery as an initial approach with postoperative radiation has been employed and is perhaps appropriate where a large number of surgeons operate on a small number of cases and are not comfortable with preoperative radiation. We believe, however, that if radiotherapy is delayed longer than 2 or 3 weeks, the effectiveness of this approach is decreased.

With the introduction of partial laryngectomy techniques and preservation of voice, this approach has been employed in selected cases with postoperative irradiation to a modest dose (5000 rads) as a vital part of the treatment. This policy, then, has been restricted to those well-defined lesions, usually T2, with considerable success.

TABLE 3   Nodal Management in Supraglottic Cancer: T1, T2, T3 (mobile)

Nodal Staging	Nodal Mobility	Treatment Policy
N0		Radiotherapy for control
N1, N2, N3	Mobile or fixed	Preoperative radiotherapy & surgery whenever possible
N1, N2, N3	Fixed & remaining inoperable	Radiotherapy & supplemental electron therapy or brachytherapy

Chemotherapy Regimen

Methotrexate has been used on occasion for the primary treatment and for recurrences, but without enthusiasm. More recently, as reported elsewhere in this book, 5-FU and mitomycin have currently been in vogue in combination with radiotherapy and surgery.

Treatment of Neck Nodes

The policy at the University of Virginia has been to operate on all *palpable* lymph nodes. Although the place of radiotherapy in the treatment of undetected lymph node metastases is undisputed, it has been felt that the additional dose of radiation to eliminate palpable disease carries an unnecessary morbidity rate compared with a radical neck dissection. The surgery is usually preceded by preoperative radiation (5000 rads) and discouraged as an initial procedure. Obviously, for unresectable lymph nodes and for the less involved neck when bilateral nodes are present, radiotherapy is employed as the definitive treatment (Table 3).

The Epiglottis

Cartilage involvement, either of the epiglottis or elsewhere, has not proved a deterrent to radiotherapy either alone or in combination.

PRESENT SERIES: MATERIAL AND METHODS

All cases of supraglottic cancer seen at the University of Virginia from 1968 through 1980 have been reviewed. A minimum follow-up of 3 years is available in all cases. A total of 156 patients were seen with supraglottic cancer, a ratio of 1:1.5 when compared with glottic cancer. The average age was 60.6 years for males and 55.7 years for females, the ratio of males to females being 2.9:1. Caucasians exceeded blacks 6.4:1. Smoking and alcohol were concomitant vices in a high percentage of cases—smokers, 100 percent; drinkers, 74 percent.

Crude survival rates were estimated after excluding (1) patients treated elsewhere, (2) patients with distant metastases at presentation, (3) patients who declined treatment, and (4) patients who received planned palliative treatment. The remaining 139 patients were considered eligible for curative attempts at treatment.

Determinate survival rates were calculated after excluding (1) patients who did not complete treatment, (2) patients who died of a second primary before the year of evaluation, and (3) patients who died of intercurrent disease before the year of evaluation. This resulted in 119 patients for analysis at 3 years and gave a conservative estimate of treatment effectiveness since, in the majority of patients with a second primary or dying of intercurrent disease, the larynx was free of disease.

RESULTS

The results by stage are suprisingly good for the advanced tumors, with figures in the same range as for other head and neck tumors in the early stages. Overall, the crude 3-year survival was 61 percent and the determinate 5-year survival 65 percent for patients among whom 67 percent were stage III and IV. Considering nodal involvement, a similar encouraging picture emerges, although less so for the more advanced nodes (Tables 4 and 5).

As expected, T stage was related to prognosis. More interesting was the importance of fixation in comparably staged tumors (Table 6). Undoubtedly the suprisingly good survival in stage IV (T4 lesions) relates to the relative lower incidence of fixation compared to T3 lesions.

The distribution of treatment policy by stage and 3-year determinate survival rates are given in Tables 7 and 8.

The results demonstrate that radiotherapy is a competitive treatment through stage III for selected cases, but a combined approach is appropriate for advanced disease. The selection of patients for partial laryngectomy and postoperative radiotherapy has been gratifying.

Radiotherapy has as one of its main attractions the fact that the larynx can be conserved (Table 9).

TABLE 4 Crude and Determinate Survival Rates in Supraglottic Cancer

Stage		Crude 3-year	Determinate	3-	5-	7-year
I	(8)	62.5		86	80	75
II	(37)	73		90	92	57
III	(37)	65		75	57	43
IV	(57)	50		56	50	31
All	(139)			71	65	43

Figures in parentheses represent number of patients.

TABLE 5 Three-year Determinate Survival by Nodal Stage (%)

Nodal Stage	Survival Rate	
N0	66	69
N1	79	
N2	50	45
N3	41	

TABLE 6 Three-year Determinate Survival Considering Fixation

T3 mobile	6/9	(67%)
T3 fixed	15/26	(58%)
T4 mobile	13/19	(68%)
T4 fixed	5/9	(56%)

TABLE 7 Distribution by Stage and Treatment Policy (%)

Treatment		Stage			
		I	II	III	IV
Radiation alone	(50)	86	63	31	30
Preoperative irradiation	(43)	0	10	50	48
Postoperative irradiation	(26)	14	27	19	22

Figures in parentheses represent number of patients.

TABLE 8 3-year Determinate Survival by Treatment Policy (%)

Treatment		Stage				
		I	II	III	IV	All
Radiation alone	(50)	5/6 83	17/19 89	8/10 80	3/15 20	66
Preoperative irradiation	(43)	—	3/3	11/16 69	17/24 71	72
Postoperative irradiation (total Laryngectomy)	(18)	1/1	3/4	3/4	6/9 67	72
Postoperative irradiation (partial Laryngectomy)	(8)	—	4/4	2/2	2/2	100

Figures in parentheses are number of patients.
Patients salvaged following recurrence are included.

TABLE 9 Results of Treatment by Initial Radiotherapy

Radiation Control		Salvage	Overall Survival	Larynges Saved	
T1	5/7	1/2*	6/7	6/7	(86%)
T2	13/25	8/11**	21/25	15/25	(60%)
T3	5/11	0/1	5/11	5/11	(46%)
All	23/43 53%	9/14 64%	32/43 74%	26/43	60%

*3 cases had partial laryngectomy.

RECURRENCES

All except two recurrences in the larynx or neck occurred within 36 months, for a 77 percent local control rate. The two exceptions recurred at 40 months. The 3-year survival rates are therefore reasonable reflections of long-term control. In the entire series of radically treated patients, there were five stomal recurrences (4%). None of these was controlled. As stressed by other authors, the best treatment is prevention of recurrence with pre- or postoperative radiation in all advanced cases.

INTERCURRENT DISEASE, METASTASES, AND SECOND PRIMARIES

An insidious influence in assessing survival and effectiveness of treatment is the frequency of death from intercurrent disease, distant metastases, and second primaries in this age group. By eliminating the patients dying of intercurrent disease and second primaries, we are depressing our control and survival rates because frequently these patients are well as far as their larynx is concerned. By recording those with distant metastases as "dead of cancer", we often overlook the fact that the primary site is controlled. In the present series 36/156 patients developed second primaries, with the lung (35%) and head and neck (30%) being the most common sites. Six patients who died from their second cancer appeared to have their primary lesion controlled; 17/156 were recorded as dead of intercurrent disease, and most of these patients were well as far as their larynx was concerned. Patients dying with metastases (26/156) represented 17 percent of the series—not excessively high considering the advanced nature of supraglottic cancers in general, ther high malignancy (histologic grade), and good survival. Many of these metastases developed late, with the lung and thorax being the most frequent sites (65%) and liver and axilla being other common sites (each 12%). In five patients recorded as dying of metastases, the primary area appeared to be free of disease.

COMPLICATIONS

In general, the rate of complications has been low, subcutaneous edema and xerostomia being the major

TABLE 10   Present Policy for Treatment of Supraglottic Cancer—University of Virginia, 1984

Stage I (T1N0)		Radiotherapy with surgery for salvage
Stage II (T2N0)	Early	Radiotherapy with surgery for salvage
	Others	Partial laryngectomy and postoperative radiotherapy
Stage III (T3N0 and T1, T2, T3, N1)	Mobile	Radiotherapy with surgery for salvage*
	Fixed	Preoperative radiotherapy and total laryngectomy*
Stage IV (All T4s and T1, T2, T3, N2, N3)	Mobile	Preoperative radiotherapy and total laryngectomy*
	Fixed	Preoperative radiotherapy and total laryngectomy

*Total laryngectomy and postoperative radiotherapy may be preferred

TABLE 11   3-year survival rates using the AJC recommendations[2]

Stage	Observed	Adjusted	
		Reflecting death from cancer of the larynx*	Reflecting survival without local recurrence
I	62.5%	83.3	83.3
II	73.0	88.2	88.2
III	64.1	69.4	74.5
IV	50.0	58.9	68.8

* Includes those dying of distant metastases alone.

side effects of radiation. The complications from combined treatment failed to show a preponderance for the preoperative over the postoperative cases, although they represent the more advanced cases subjected to combined therapy.

COMMENTS

In spite of the frequently advanced and high-grade malignancy of supraglottic cancers, control and survival are good beyond 5 years. Radiotherapy can save a large number of larynges with T1, T2, and T3 lesions, either alone or in combination with partial laryngectomy. Combined therapy forms the basis for cure in the advanced cases at the sacrifice of laryngeal speech (Table 10).

The future control of supraglottic malignant tumors lies in preventing or detecting cancers at an early stage. Why do patients frequently present with T3 and T4 lesions? This probably relates to the high incidence of smoking and drinking alcohol, the patient dismissing minor throat problems as a consequence of his habits. Education is necessary to improve results because we have the means to cure early and even locally advanced cancers (Table 11).

REFERENCES

1. Constable WC et al. Radiotherapeutic management of cancer of the glottis, University of Virginia, 1956–1971. The Laryngoscope 1975; 9:1494–1503.
2. American Joint Committee (AJC) on Cancer. Manual for Staging of Cancer. 2nd ed, Chicago, IL, 1983.
3. Constable WC et al. Intermediate dose preoperative radiotherapy for cancer of the larynx–end results. Canad J Otolaryngol 1975; 4:246–250.

DEFINITIVE RADIATION THERAPY OF CANCER OF THE PYRIFORM SINUS

JEAN P. BATAINI, M.D.
JACQUES M. BRUGERE, M.D.

In France, cancer of the pyriform sinus (CaPS) constitues 85 to 90 percent of the carcinomas of the hypopharynx and is rare in females (2 to 3%). In a prospective study of 300 patients with CaPS treated at the Institute Curie (IC), a higher percentage were heavy smokers and alcohol drinkers, had chronic ailments and poor nutritional status, and were unskilled laborers, than 1700 patients with cancer of other sites of the upper aerodigestive tract. Moreover, the majority presented with advanced stages of tumor, which accounts for the fact that only one-third to one-half of the patients in a specialized French center were eligible for surgical treatment[1] or could be entered into prospective studies assessing chemotherapy or radiosensitizers.[2] The purpose of this report is to evaluate the results of radiation therapy (RT) as the primary therapeutic approach for this lethal disease.

PATIENTS AND METHODS

We have previously described the entire population of 619 patients with hypopharyngeal cancer registered at the IC from 1958 through 1974 and the analyzed series of 434 patients with M0 tumors who were treated with megavoltagle RT for squamous CaPS and who did not have prior or simultaneous malignant tumors or distant metastases.[3] All of these patients were treated by megavoltage RT regardless of their general condition and locoregional extent of disease; during this period no alternatives were offered as primary treatment. For this presentation, an analysis of the current status of the series has been performed using the 1978 UICC classification with four T classes and, for certain end points, the 1976 AJC classification. Fourteen patients have been added: 7 females previously excluded and 7 patients treated in early 1975. The series thus comprises 448 consecutive patients followed for at least 5 years. The mean age was 57;

56 patients were above 70 years of age. During the same period, 13 patients presented with distant metastases. The distribution of the patients according to TN classifications is shown in Table 1.

Surprisingly, despite the fact that the classifications of nodal status are different, the TN stages of the tumors according to UICC and AJC systems were almost similar, stages I and II accounting for about 8 percent, stage III for 16 percent, and stage IV for 76 percent of tumors.

The RT techniques have been described.[3] Treatments were individualized, using the shrinking field technique with total tumor doses (TD) of 65 to 75 Gy to the primary in 30 to 40 fractions over 40 to 50 days and booster doses to residual nodes, for a total of 80 to 85 Gy. In this series, the mean basic dose was 47 Gy and mean TD 65 Gy in 34 fractions over 46 days. Sixty-two patients received TD less than 55 Gy (in terms of 6 weeks' equivalent dose).

RESULTS

Tumor Regression. Complete regression of the *primary* occurred in 58 percent of the patients. Two months after RT, the tumors had regressed completely in 314 patients (70%) and incompletely in 69 (15%), but regression could not be assessed in 65 patients. Complete *nodal* regression occurred in only 30 percent of patients at the end of RT, but increased to 62 percent 2 months afterward, and the status of nodes could not be assessed in 15 percent. Regression of large nodes continued for as long as 4 months after RT.

Survival. The absolute survival for the entire series was 35 percent, 26 percent, and 18 percent at 2, 3, and 5 years respectively. At 10 years, 28 of 411 patients (7.5%) were alive. The causes of death at 3 years are reported in Table 2.

Survival according to UICC staging is shown in Figure 1, and the determinate survival according to stage for patients who received TD greater than 55 GY is shown in Figure 2. In this report, patients who died of indeterminate causes during the first 2 years after RT or who were lost to follow-up were considered as having died from the tumor, although there was no suspicion of relapse at their last regular check-up. Survival according to AJC staging was similar. Direct correlation between the two systems has been reported.[4] The determinate survival (see Fig. 2) was

TABLE 1   Stage of Cancer of the Pyriform Sinus in 448 MO Patients

	UICC		AJC	Stages :
T1+T2 : 20%	N0	29%	29%	I + II : 8%
T3 : 19%	N1	28%	26%	III : 16%
T4 : 61%	N2	2%	23%	IV : 76%
	N3	41%	22%	

TABLE 2   CaPS: Causes of Death at 3 Years in 448 patients

Loco-regional failure*	68%
Distant metastases alone	8%
Second primary	4%
Intercurrent disease	5%
Unknown disease	13%
Lost to follow-up	1%

* Alone or associated with other causes of failure and treatment complication

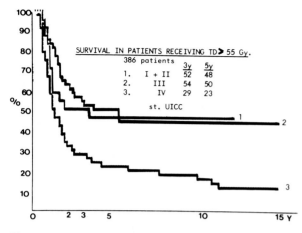

Figure 1 Absolute survival according to UICC stage (448 M0 patients).

TABLE 3 Radiotherapy of CaPS: 3 Year Absolute Survival (Institut Curie UICC T N staging)

St. I + II	T1 + T2 N0	42%
	T1 − T2 N1	43%
St. III	T3 N0	50%
	T3 N1	46%
	T4 N0	29%
St. IV	T4 N1	28%
	T1 T2 N2N3	22%
	T3 T4 N2N3	13%

significantly better than absolute survival (see Fig. 1), indicating that a significant number of patients died of unrelated causes. The absolute 3-year survival rates according to stage of disease are shown in Table 3.

Time of Appearance of Failures. Ninety-five percent of all treatment failures in both primary and neck sites occurred within 2 years after RT. Table 4 shows the sites of loco-regional failure at 2 years. Almost all nodal failures in T1 and T2 tumors occurred with major nodal metastases. Distant metastases were diagnosed in 74 patients and, in 73 percent of these, within 2 years.

Solitary Distant Metastases and Second Primary Tumors. Solitary distant metastases were responsible for the death of 41 patients. Second primary tumors were diagnosed in 8 patients at 2 years, in 13 at 3 years, in 20 at 5 years, and in 28 at 10 years among the survivors.

Control of the Primary. In the determinate group (386 patients), the 2-year control of the primary pharyngeal tumor was 54 percent for all stages. The

total number of local failures (with unlimited follow-up) was 16 percent for T1 tumors, 32 percent for T2 and T3 tumors, and 51 percent for T4 tumors.

Control of neck nodal metastases. In the determinate group, 86 percent of patients with controlled primaries had controlled neck nodal metastases (334 patients) at 2 years. Total isolated treatment failures for neck nodal metastases are 4 percent in N0, 13 percent in N1, 0 percent in N2, and 17 percent in N3 patients. Using AJC staging, the failure rate was the same in N0, 11 percent in N1, 16 percent in N2, and 19 percent in N3 patients.

PROGNOSTIC FACTORS

Site of Origin. Local control decreased with site of origin in the following order: lateral wall, medial wall, anterior angle. The differences are significant, but site had no effect on survival.

Gross Pathology. With predominantly exophytic tumors (36% of patients), the 2-year control rate was 69 percent; with predominantly ulcerated or infiltrating tumors (64% of patients), the 2-year control rate was 46 percent. These differences are statistically significant (p <0.03).

Histologic Differentiation. Among the 66 percent of patients with well-differentiated tumors, the 2-year control rate was 51 percent, whereas in poorly differentiated tumors, it was increased to 72 percent (p <0.002), but there was no correlation with survival.

Extent of Tumor. In the determinate group, extent of tumor influenced the 2-year control rates. The control rates were 77 percent in the absence of extension beyond the hypopharynx (31 patients); 62 percent with laryngeal involvement (215 patients); 41 percent with oropharyngeal extensions (90 patients); 38 percent with esophageal extension (10 patients),

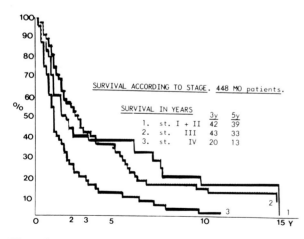

Figure 2 Determinate survival according to UICC stage in patients recieving TD ≥55 Gy (386 patients).

TABLE 4 CaPS: Sites of Loco-regional Failure 2 Years After RT in 434 M0 patients (M)

	T1 T2 (90)		T3 T4 (344)	
P	26%		28%	
P + N	7%	32%	19%	46.5%
N	12%		8%	

and 28 percent with invasion of the cartilage and neck soft tissues (40 patients).

Cord Mobility. Fixation of the vocal cords is usually due to tumor growth. In the determinate group, control was approximately 75 percent with normal or impaired mobility versus 47 percent with fixation of the cords (p = 0.0001). However, local control was the same in T2 and T3 patients.

Dose-control Correlations for primary and neck metastases have been discussed.[2] Local control for early stages (T1–T2) reached 65 percent with doses of 65 Gy or higher vs 36 percent with lower doses. For T3 and T4 tumors, there was no significant improvement with increasing doses, but nodal control was improved by increasing radiation doses.

Regression of the primary had prognostic significance at the end of the RT in the determinate group. With complete regression, the 3-year survival was 32 percent vs 16 percent with incomplete regression. The same relations were observed with 2-year control rates, being 69 percent and 34 percent respectively. These differences in control rates were greater at 2 months after completion of RT.

Regression of lymph nodes. Correlation of nodal regression with control of the nodes was significant at the end of therapy (p = 0.02) and even more significant after 2 months (p = 0.0001) in patients who received more than 55 Gy and in whom the primary was controlled. There also appeared to be a relation between nodal regression and survival.

COMPLICATIONS AND FUNCTIONAL RESULTS

In most patients, fatal complications were related to progression of disease; however, 11 patients (2.5%) died of complications without evidence of loco-regional recurrence: one of laryngeal edema, one of aspiration pneumonia, two of cachexia, and seven of hemorrhage.

Of the 154 patients surviving 2 years, complications were reported in 17 (11%). They were severe in six, with three requiring tracheostomy and three requiring tracheostomy and gastrostomy. Two additional patients had temporary tracheostomy; nine others developed moderately severe complications, including four instances of pharyngeal necrosis, which were treated conservatively. Among the 79 5-year survivors, five have tracheostomies and 1 a gastrostomy.

Fatal hemorrhage occurred only in patients receiving TD higher than 65 Gy. The complication rate in survivors was dose-dependent: 3 percent with doses less than 70 Gy versus 22 percent with doses higher than 70 Gy.[3] The occurrence of complications was also related to local tumor extent, occurring more frequently in patients with advanced tumors and especially in patients with tumor extension to the oropharynx, or to the cartilage and soft tissues of the neck.

Surgical Salvage. In the present series, attempts at surgical salvage were undertaken in 28 patients after failure of RT. Six of the patients were alive at 2 years (1 out of 15 in the previous report).

DISCUSSION

The almost exponential shape of the survival curve (see Fig. 1) is typical of all head and neck cancers except cancer of the glottis, but its slope is definitely steeper in CaPS. These survival figures are exactly the same as those of the 619 patients with hypopharyngeal cancer registered at the IC, which also included cancers of other sites and histologies and patients with prior, concomitant, or secondary malignant disease.

These absolute survival figures are the only reliable ones for evaluating the impact of treatment, whether single or combined modality, or alternative approaches on the entire population presenting with a given cancer over an appreciable time, preferably in a single institution with at least a 3-year follow-up. Other characteristics of the cancer and the host, e.g., distant metastases, second primaries, and intercurrent diseases, are appreciated by 5-year survival data. Mutilation and complications due to a given therapy should be honestly weighed against the real benefits of treatment and the expense.

Comparison of the results of the systematic radiotherapeutic approach to treatment of CaPS with those of surgical or combined radiotherapy-surgical management is extremely difficult because of (1) the differences in "patient population" (socioeconomic status, life style, age, sex, stage distribution, nutritional status), (2) inclusion of epilaryngeal tumors with better prognosis, (3) differences in the tumor classification systems utilized and, for some, special staging, and (4) differences in presentation of results, as with the ambiguities inherent in "corrected" or "determinate" results. In addition, retrospective analysis of data within institutions that simultaneously offer other approaches must be cautiously interpreted, for example, the type of treatment offered, whether "curative" or "palliative".

Voice-preserving surgery is performed by few surgeons in the management of CaPS and condemned by many others. Its indications are limited by the highly malignant nature of the disease, with its tendency to submucosal spread, the frequent paraglottic and oropharyngeal extensions, and by the age and the general condition of the patients. The percentage of patients subjected to partial surgery evidently reflects a definitive selection in certain centers. Ogura et al reported 85 partial procedures vs 57 radical ones,[5] whereas André reported 105 vs 400 total procedures.[6] Moreover, the value of partial surgery could not be accurately assessed because of the inclusion of epilaryngeal cancers[6] and because of individualized staging.[5] Combined treatment with RT is indispensable because of the very high incidence of neck node involvement verified at surgery,[1] which increases complication rates. Reported results for these selected patients with minimal or moderate disease in the primary and the neck are not superior to results reported herein for stages I, II, and III tumors. Ogura et al reported a 59 percent 3-year actuarial rate with partial laryngopharyngectomy and 36 percent with total laryngopharyngectomy.

The necessity of combining RT with ablative surgery is obvious from many reports.[1,7,8] El Badawi et al claimed 50 percent and 40 percent 2-year and 5-year survival rates respectively in a series of 125 patients who received planned postoperative RT.[8] Serious local complications were reported. In Shah's series, a minority of patients had advanced malignant tumors, 24 percent at the primary site, and only 11 percent fixed nodes.[9] The experience and successively reported results obtained from the Institut Gustave Roussy in Villejuif are exemplary regarding patient selection and extent of follow-up.[1,7] The patterns of failure with combined modalities are different, but the 5-year survival rate, if not the 3-year survival rate, is not superior to those obtained by radical and individualized RT, even if the local control rate is higher. The determinate 5-year survival in patients receiving TD exceeding 55 Gy approaches 50 percent for stages I, II, and III tumors and is 23 percent for stage IV tumors.

Results of primary RT are favorable, with a substantial surgical salvage rate in the small series reported by Million.[10] Results of the largest series, from the Princess Margaret Hospital, treated by RT were: 15 percent 5-year actuarial survival for all patients,[11] which is similar to the survival experience reported by larger cancer registries in the United States over a comparable period for patients treated with salvage surgery for a large percentage of loco-regional failures. A recent evaluation of 496 patients with CaPS treated from 1976 through 1980 in a major tumor center in Northern France (Dr. Lefeurt, Centre Oscar Lambret in Lille) yielded 22 percent and 14 percent actuarial 3- and 5-year survival rates. In this series, 49 percent of patients were treated by RT, 42.5 percent by surgery and RT, and 8.5 percent were treated palliatively. Recent figures from the M.D. Anderson Hospital for patients managed by combined modality or RT differ somewhat from those previously published.[8]

A randomized trial at the IC assessing the radiation therapy sensitizer misonidazole in head and neck cancer, with two schedules of administration of the drug from 1980 to 1982, did not show improvement in tumor control.[2] A randomized prospective trial assessing the value of two cycles of chemotherapy prior to radiotherapy is under way.

The use of new constructive procedures with fewer and less serious complications argues for more frequent attempts at salvage surgery after failure of RT. In a new series of 32 salvage pharyngolaryngectomies, 11 of 24 and 5 of 20 are alive at one and 5 years respectively. Moreover, planned postradiation neck surgery after 60 to 65 Gy is often considered in some patients with multilevel or bulky unilateral nodes.

CONCLUSIONS

The survival and functional results obtained in this large, homogeneous, and unselected series seems to justify the primary radiotherapeutic approach utilized in the management of CaPS. Better control and survival rates can be reasonably achieved with more adequate management in T1 and T2 tumors. The possibility of improving the results with a short course of chemotherapy given prior to definitive RT is being explored for more extensive tumors. Closer follow-up in the first few months after therapy, especially if regression is not complete by the end of RT, now allows more frequent salvage procedures with fewer complications if neck disease is not extensive. Moreover, surgery should be considered at 60 Gy (i.e., by the end of the sixth week of treatment) if tumor regression is unsatisfactory, since the local status at the end of RT is the best prediction of the final result with RT. New surgical procedures permit wide excisions with greatly reduced morbidity, thus rehabilitating high-dose preoperative irradiation, especially since the larynx is preserved in a fair number of patients. Tumor doses greater than 70 Gy must be given only exceptionally and through small portals to avoid complications.

Neck nodal treatment failures with control of the primary were rare in this series, but neck surgery should be performed in patients with residual nodes 2 to 3 months after RT if the primary is controlled, and planned postradiation neck surgery may be considered in certain AJC N2 and N3 tumors.

Improvement can reasonably be expected in stages I, II, and III, and perhaps in certain stage IV tumors, in terms of loco-regional control and survival, but prognosis remains poor for the majority of stage IV tumors, which constitute about one-third to one-half of the tumors at presentation. For this very lethal malignancy, prevention and early diagnosis remain most important approaches for tumor control.

REFERENCES

1. Vandenbrook C, Luboinsky B, Marandas P, et al. Association radio-chirurgicale et résultats obtenus par une chirurgie première suivie d'irradiation post-opératoire. In: Veronesi U, Bocca E, Molinari R, Emmanuelli H (eds). *I Tumori della Testa e del Collo*. Milano: Casa Editrice Ambrosiana 1979: 413–420.
2. Brunin F, Bataini JP, Asselain B, et al. Résultats préliminaires d'un essai thérapeutique sur l'effet radiosensibilisant du misonidazole dans les cancers de la tête et du cou. J Eur Radiothér 1983; 4:181–188.
3. Bataini P, Brugere J, Bernier J, et al. Results of radical radiotherapeutic treatment of carcinoma of the pyriform sinus: Experience of the Institut Curie. Int J Radiat Oncolo Biol Phys 1982; 8:1277–1286.
4. Black RS, Gluckman JL. Staging systems for cancer of head and neck region. Comparison between AJC and UICC. Clin Otolaryngol 1983; 8:305–312.
5. Ogura J, Marks JE, Freeman RB. Results of conservative surgery for cancers of the supraglottis and pyriform sinus. Laryngoscope 1980; 90:591–600.
6. André P. Chirurgie conservatrice du cancer du sinus piri-

forme. Indications, techniques et résultats. In: Veronesi U, Bocca E, Molinari R, Emmanuelli H (eds). *I Tumori della Testa e del Collo*. Milano: Casa Editrice Ambrosiana 1979: 391–394.

7. Vandenbrook C, Sancho H, Lefur R, et al. Results of a randomized clinical trial of preoperative irradiation versus postoperative in treatment of tumors of the hypopharynx. Cancer 1977; 39:1445–1449.

8. El Badawi SA, Goepfert H, Fletcher GH, et al. Squamous cell carcinoma of the pyriform sinus. Laryngoscope 1982; 92:357–364.

9. Shah J, Shaha A, Spiro R, Strong EW. Carcinoma of hypopharynx. Ann J Surg 1976; 132:439–443.

10. Million RR, Cassisi NJ. Radical irradiation for carcinoma of the pyriform sinus. Laryngoscope 1981; 91:439–50.

11. Keane TJ, Hawkins NV, Beale FA, et al. Carcinoma of the hypopharynx. Results of primary radical therapy. Int J Radiat Oncol Biol Phys 1983; 9:659–664.

CANCER OF THE LARYNX AND PYRIFORM SINUS: THE SURGEON'S VIEWPOINT

HELMUTH GOEPFERT, M.D.

The two principal goals of the treatment of cancer in or about the larynx are to eradicate the cancer and to do so by preserving or rehabilitating the best possible phonatory function. In this chapter, I will attempt to define the way we perceive the role of radiotherapy in the management of cancer in these areas. The choices of treatment include (1) surgical resection either by partial or total laryngectomy, (2) radiation therapy, and (3) depending upon the clinical situation, a sequential use of both methods for the treatment of either the primary tumor or metastases in the cervical lymph nodes.

Both surgery and radiation therapy have made substantial advances in the last four decades, and specialists in each field have presented arguments concerning their respective discipline's abilities to meet the end points of tummor eradication and preservation of function. Unfortunately for our patients, these two disciplines have seldom presented their statements in an ecumenical fashion above and beyond the limitations imposed by disputes over "specialty turfs".

The two forms of treatment are often presented as mutually exclusive, rather than as integrated or complementary disciplines. Narrow-minded polarization often results in one institution treating everyone by radiation therapy regardless of the stage of disease, while the medical center next door treats every patient by surgery.

Whether or not radiation therapy is the best modality for treating primary cancer, we must be sure it eliminates disease in a high percentage of patients and preserves laryngeal function. When cancer recurs following radiation therapy, it can be successfully managed only by some form of surgical resection.

Adequate evaluation of patients and proper staging of tumors are mandatory. The cancer itself should be evaluated through indirect and direct examination by trained observers and appropriate radiographic studies.

Review of the literature and analysis of our own material at the University of Texas M.D. Anderson Hospital has allowed us to define a policy of treatment that, although far from ideal and certainly not inflexible, attempts to give every patient the best possible result. Each patient should be considered individually, because not only must the characteristics of the cancer be taken into account, but the patient's own characteristics and idiosyncrasies must be respected as well. To dwell on every possibility of tumor presentation would take up more space than this chapter permits, and thus some generalizations will be necessary.

There is little argument that both radiotherapy and surgery are effective treatments for early glottic cancer, and T1 and T2 lesions can be controlled at the primary site by either modality with preservation of phonation. Even bulky exophytic tumors of the vocal cord can be treated by radiation therapy alone with a high rate of success. Under optimal circumstances, the larynx recovers a far better voice quality following treatment than most conservation surgical procedures can provide. Local control of T1 lesions by radiation therapy only is close to 90 percent, and for T2 lesions it is about 75 percent. However, when a T2 lesion combines all three descriptive features (i.e., reduced mobility, extension beyond the cord, and subglottic extension), the local failure rate reaches 40 percent. In these circumstances we believe conservation surgery and, if necessary, surgery followed by radiation therapy have distinct advantages. Obviously, patient selection factors such as age and pulmonary status have a strong influence on this decision. One alternative that works well on occasion is to start a patient on radiation therapy; if by the fifth week of treatment (1000 rads per week) the cord has become mobile and there is marked tumor reduction, we proceed with this treatment to completion. Conversely, should these results not be evident by the fifth week, we stop radiation therapy and perform a conservative operation, if possible. I must admit that occasionally a total laryngectomy becomes necessary with this course.

Edema of the larynx following radiation therapy for glottic cancer is seldom a problem, and on followup the organ appears relatively undisturbed.

T1, T2, and certain early T3 lesions of the supraglottic larynx, especially exophytic and superficially infiltrating cancers of the suprahyoid epiglottis and of the aryepiglottic fold, even if bulky, are well suited to radiation therapy as the only treatment for the primary tumor. The portal size necessarily varies with the anatomic site of the tumor, and because surface landmarks cannot be sharply defined for the supraglottic larynx, as they can for vocal cord tumors, the immediately surrounding structures must be included in the treatment field. It is important that the head and neck surgeon be familiar with the different radiotherapy portals and participate in the evaluation of these patients during planning and treatment to avoid geographic misses. The control rate of the tumor at the primary site is approximately 90 percent for T1 and T2 cancers and between 75 percent and 80 percent for T3 cancers. There is no question that with proper selection the same local control can be achieved by conservation surgery.

A complicating factor in treating cancers of the supraglottic larynx is the presence of lymph node metastases, which are present in 50 to 60 percent of patients and influence the treatment selection process. The management of primary tumors and neck disease under these circumstances is integrated. The lymphatic supply of the epilarynx (suprahyoid epiglottis and aryepiglottic fold) is abundant, and tumors originating within these areas have a marked propensity for nodal metastases. The lymphatic supply of the vestibulum (infrahyoid epiglottis and false cord) is less abundant than that of the epilarynx, and cancers of the vestibulum have less tendency to metastasize to lymph nodes. Subclinical or microscopic cancer in regional lymphatics (whatever the definition of this term might imply) is amenable to radiation therapy, and for this reason we include the upper and midjugular nodes in the initial treatment field for every patient who receives radiation therapy to the primary tumor when the neck is free of palpable metastases. After 5000 rads in 5 weeks, the fields are reduced to encompass the primary tumor only. In the event of large clinically positive nodes, combined treatment is used for the treatment of regional lymphatics. If in these circumstances the primary cancer is amenable to radiation therapy, up to 5000 rads in 5 weeks, to the appropriate neck fields (bilateral opposed superor fields and anterior inferior fields). The treatment fields are then reduced to carry the treatment of the primary tumor to the required therapeutic level (6500 to 7000 rads in 7 weeks). Four to 6 weeks after completion of radiation therapy, the appropriate planned neck dissection is performed, either regional or modified as the circumstances dictate.

If cancer of the supraglottic larynx is deeply infiltrating, with invasion of the pre-epiglottic space or the full thickness of the laryngotracheal wall, the tumor is growing in poorly vascularized tissues and has varying degrees of hypoxia. Such cancers are more suited to surgical treatment. Partial laryngeal surgery often can be performed with preservation of phonation. Furthermore, if radiation therapy is used to treat a deeply infiltrating lesion of the supraglottic larynx, in many cases the structures and motility do not return to normal, and follow-up examinations are more difficult because the observer cannot distinguish between residual tumor or active disease and posttherapy changes (e.g., edema, dryness, hyperkeratosis).

Total laryngectomy is not necessary for all patients who have deeply infiltrating lesions of the supraglottic larynx, nor is it necessary for some patients with pyriform sinus cancer. In the past two decades, better perioperative care has allowed proper selection of patients for partial laryngectomy with preservation of laryngeal function. Not all patients need radiation therapy after partial laryngectomy, and the criteria for such combined treatments are still under evaluation.

Mention should be made of the so-called "borderline histology lesions". These include atypical hyperplasia, dysplasia, carcinoma in situ, and atypia with hyperkeratosis. Often these differential diagnoses are a matter of interpretation, and can vary between pathologists and between multiple biopsies. At times in bulky lesions, a biopsy yields only the diagnosis of carcinoma in situ or noninvasive squamous carcinoma despite repeated biopsies. It may be debated whether some of these lesions are verrucous carcinomas.

Microsurgical stripping and laser vaporization of superficial and small lesions often are sufficient to control preinvasive cancer, and such techniques are fast, efficient ways of dealing with these problems. When "borderline histology" lesions are multicentric and margins cannot be obtained, it has been the policy at the University of Texas M.D. Anderson Hospital to give the same treatment as for invasive carcinoma. The percentage of local failure is the same as for invasive squamous carcinoma, that is, around 10 percent for T1 lesions and about 25 percent for T2 lesions.

When there are contraindications to laryngectomy (usually medical), indications for radiation therapy are extended to more advanced cancers. The portals are determined by the extension of tumor above and below the glottic area. Patients with unresectable cancer (either massive primary or unresectable neck disease) may be irradiated radically. The final dose to primary tumors in these circumstances is usually about 7500 to 8000 rads, which can be delivered at a weekly rate of 900 rads because of the large volume of tissue. Hyperfractionation with twice-daily treatment may have a place under these circumstances. Because no surgery can be contemplated for these patients, a higher risk of local complications must be accepted to achieve tumor control.

In general, treatment similar to that for cancer of the supraglottic larynx can be used for pyriform sinus cancer whenever the primary tumor is suitable for curative radiation therapy, as when (1) primary disease is considered favorable for primary radiation therapy (T1 and some T2 lesions, especially of the vestibulum), (2) the patient is a prohibitively high surgical risk, and (3) the patient has unresectable neck node metastases fixed to either the carotid vessels or the deep cervical fascia.

Unfortunately, few patients with pyriform sinus cancer are eligible for either radiation or surgical lar-yngeal conservation therapy. The local regional and distal failure rates are higher than in supraglottic cancers, and therapy of subclinical or obvious regional or nodal metstases is always part of the integral treatment plan.

24. Fractionation

INTRODUCTION

SIMON KRAMER, M.D., F.A.C.R.

As J. Robert Andrews has pointed out,[11] ever since the introduction of radiation therapy as a means of managing cancer some 80 years ago, we have had two avenues only for optimizing differential cancericidal effects. One is the optimization of the macroscopic distribution of the radiation dose, and the other is the manipulation of the time/dose/fraction aspect of radiation therapy. More recently, combined management by surgery, radiation therapy, and chemotherapy have come into prominence as well as the adjuvant use of sensitizers, protectors, and hyperthermia, all of which are discussed in this book. But if one looks at the radiotherapeutic portion specifically, we are still confined to those two avenues, and in the chapters of this Part, we shall discuss the time/dose/fraction aspect.

In the first two decades of radiation therapy, there were essentially two methods of using it. One was to use rather massive doses given in one or two treatments, as advocated by Holzknecht in Vienna and Wintz in Erlangen; the other was to give fractionated doses, as advocated by L. Freund in Vienna and others, wherein doses were so discontinuous and sometimes widely spaced that it earned itself the term "Verzettelte Dosen" (frittered-away doses). It was really through the work of Regaud in basic research[2] and Coutard in the clinic[3] that modern fractionated radiation therapy came into being. Most of the methods employed since that time rested largely on empiric clinical findings, and it is only fairly recently that an explanation is forthcoming of the biologic basis underlying fractionated therapy. Even so, the basic methodology of one fraction per day of about 180 to 200 rads remains essentially the standard of a course of radiation therapy. Most of us are comfortable with this, we know that the normal tissues can tolerate it, that an effective therapeutic ratio can be obtained with this, and that in the majority of epithelial tumors the effect on the tumor is relatively predictable and satisfactory. Still, many questions remain:

Is it really reasonable to assume that all the different tumors that we are called upon to treat will respond to the same fraction size in the same way?

Is it not possible that a more cost-effective, that is to say, shorter course of treatment, might do equally well without causing excessive damage to normal tissues?

If adjuvant therapy is used, such as hypoxic cell sensitizers or other sensitizers, or hyperthermia, may not the interaction of these agents with radiation therapy be more effective if the standard fractionation is changed?

Finally, is it possible to get the same or better effect, i.e., to increase the therapeutic ratio, by using more than one fraction of radiation therapy per day, as suggested by Zuppinger 40 odd years ago?

Weichselbaum and Ervin, in their chapter, briefly review the biologic factors that affect the delivery of ionizing radiation alone or in conjunction with chemotherapeutic agents. This work emphasizes the importance of potential lethal damage repair (PLDR), a phenomenon that exists in tumors when cells enter a crowded density inhibited state of growth, when there may exist a large number of nondividing, but potentially clonogenic cells. By using explants from biopsies obtained from patients with head and neck cancer, they were able to study radiobiologic parameters from cells in which radiocurability was known. The potential of measuring PLDR is somewhat diminished by the known heterogeneity of tumor cells in human tumors, but nonetheless, PLDR may be of great importance in attempting to alter fractionation schemas in clinical management. Other biologic factors are discussed as they may have impact on different fractionation programs.

In his chapter, Cox gives an excellent overview on fractionation dose and time considerations. After defining terms for various fractionation schemes, he makes a rather convincing case for the disadvantage of few large fractions rather than the classic five fractions per week, as far as both tumor control and late normal tissue changes are concerned. These late effects would not have been predicted from the various iso effect formulas used in recent years. Late normal tissue damage appears to be related to fraction size more than expected from the immediate early radiation effects on these tissues. An interesting observation concerns the relatively rapid course of therapy often employed in the United Kingdom and Canada (3 to 4 weeks) compared with the more extended course usually employed in the United States (6 to 7 weeks). Equally good results are claimed by protagonists of both methods, and further studies are needed for the evaluation of these two methods. His conclusions stress the need for further clinical studies with hyperfractionation rather than few or large fractions.

Leeper, in his chapter, summarizes the biologic basis of localized hyperthermia as an adjunct to radiation therapy. He points out that at large fractions of radiation, there is an interaction with heat, and that the higher the radiation dose and the higher the temperature and time of heating, the greater the combined effect. At the level of radiation dose commonly employed in clinical radiation therapy, there is an additive effect of heat and radiation, but the action is probably independent rather than synergistic. Nevertheless, since the clinical indications favor the lower radiation dose fractions, it would seem more advantageous to explore the effect of hyperthermia using conventional fractionation as the baseline. The difficulties of both generating heat in deep tissues and measuring the heat dose are pointed out. Another area of concern is the development of heat tolerance so that at present there remains a question whether once weekly or twice weekly heating is the more advantageous method. Further studies are under way to determine these issues before this promising adjuvant therapy can be taken to clinical practice.

In the chapter by Arcangeli, he reports on several studies of the Radiation Therapy Group of the European Organization for Research on Treatment of Cancer.

In the first study, a pilot study of accelerated fractionation, patients received radiation therapy three times daily. In some of these patients misonidazole, a hypoxic cell sensitizer, was given before the first daily fraction. Since this was a pilot study, no data on control patients are available for comparison. But the feasibility of such a study was established. The results of the pilot study have prompted the group to undertake a randomized prospective trial as of February, 1981. This trial compares the standard single fraction per day with a three-fraction-per-day schema, with and without misonidazole, in advanced head and neck cancer.

The final contribution, mine, reports on the studies in hyperfractionation performed by the Radiation Therapy Oncology Group. The first, a pilot study, established the feasibility of two fractions per day for advanced head and neck cancer. The second, a randomized prospective study, documented that twice-daily fractions to a dose of 60 Gy in 5 weeks provided the same local control as standard therapy to a dose of 66 to 73.8 Gy. The third study now under way is a randomized prospective dose-seeking study to establish the highest tolerated dose in a two-fraction-per-day regimen.

REFERENCES

1. Andrews JR. The radiobiology of human cancer radiotherapy. 2nd Ed. Baltimore: University Park Press, 1978.
2. Regaud CL, Ferroux R. Influence du "facteur temps" sur la sterilisation des lignees cellulaires normales et neoplasiques par la radiotherapie. Acta Radiol 1929; (Suppl. III):107–123.
3. Coutard H. Roentgentherapy of epitheliomas of the tonsillar region, hypopharynx, and larynx from 1920-1926. Am J Roentgenol 1932; 28:313.

RADIOBIOLOGIC FACTORS INFLUENCING FRACTIONATION IN HEAD AND NECK CANCER THERAPY

RALPH R. WEICHSELBAUM, M.D.
THOMAS J. ERVIN, M.D.

Advanced head and neck cancer is a major oncologic challenge with unique therapeutic limitations imposed by vital structures in this region. Therefore, a multidisciplinary approach, including surgery, radiotherapy, and chemotherapy, has evolved in many centers. Radiation therapy has the potential to occupy a central role in the management of these patients since this group of tumors has a predominantly local mode of failure. Enhancement in the radiotherapeutic ratio, therefore, may yield an increase in the number of surviving patients with potential for decreased morbidity. We will briefly review the biologic factors that effect the delivery of ionizing radiation alone and/or in combination with chemotherapeutic agents.

INHERENT RADIATION SURVIVAL CURVE PARAMETERS AND REPAIR OF SUBLETHAL AND POTENTIALLY LETHAL DAMAGE

The term radiosensitive refers to the D_0 which is the inverse of the slope of the straight line portion of the radiation survival curve when data are plotted in a semilogarithmic fraction. This is the dose necessary to reduce the surviving fraction in the straight line portion of curve by 0.63 to a level of 0.37. The radiobiologic definition of death is the inability to reproduce.[1]

It has been demonstrated that when a single dose of x-rays is divided into two fractions separated by an interval of several hours, an enhancement in survival occurs. This split-dose recovery phenomenon has been interpreted as reflecting the repair of sublethal damage induced by the first dose in cells that survive this dose. The magnitude of this effect can be expressed by the extrapolation number $\bar{n}$ of the single-dose survival curve, which is the back extrapolation of the slope to the ordinate (the shoulder of the survival curve).[2]

When monolayer cultures of mammalian cells are maintained under conditions of constant media renewal without subculture, they enter a crowded density inhibited state of growth in which the fraction of dividing cells is reduced and a large population of nonproliferating cells accumulates. This is an experimental condition which may resemble the physiologic state of tumor cell populations in vivo since these may contain a large population of nondividing but potentially clonogenic cells. When such plateau-phase cultures are treated with x-rays or chemical agents and subcultures of cells is delayed, an enhancement in survival occurs. This phenomenon is described as reflecting recovery from potentially lethal damage and as analogous to liquid-holding recovery in bacteria and yeast.[3] PLDR has been described in animal solid and ascites tumors as well as in established human tumor cell line.[3,4]

Experimental evidence indicates that many established human tumor cell lines in culture are not intrinsically more sensitive or resistant to the lethal effects of x-rays than are cells obtained from normal tissues. Exceptions have been reported, however. Weichselbaum et al described an inherently radioresistant melanoma line and Gerweck et al and Nillson et al have described several radioresistant glioblastoma lines.[4-6] Unusual repair parameters have been reported in some human tumor cell lines as well. For example, Barranco et al reported a melanoma line with a large shoulder,[7] and Carney et al investigated two large cell lung cancer lines with relatively large extrapolation numbers, although smaller than those reported by Barranco et al.[8] Selby and Courtenay reported a large shoulder for two human melanoma xenografts grown in agar diffusion chambers.[9] Courtenay et al found a xenografted pancreatic carcinoma proficient in the repair of potentially lethal damage (PLDR),[10] and Weichselbaum and Little studied two human melanoma lines and an osteosarcoma line especially proficient in PLDR.[4] Both groups suggested that one factor in the failure of x-ray to sterilize malignant tumor could be the ability of noncycling cells to recover from potentially lethal damage.

Weichselbaum et al studied the possible contribution of cellular radiosensitivity and of sublethal and potentially lethal damage repair in head and neck cancer treatment.[11] They studied 10 early-passage tumor-cell populations derived from patients with head and neck squamous carcinoma. Five biopsies were obtained from patients before the institution of therapy, and five from patients who suffered radiation failures. Their study is unique in that cell populations from each tumor were serially cultivated under identical conditions and were studied between 10 and 15 passages after initial explant. It is the first study to examine radiobiologic parameters from cells where radiocurability is known. This investigation found that D_0s ranged from 107 to 193 rads. Extrapolation numbers ranged from 1.17 to 2.14 and PLD recovery at 24 hours from 1.4 to 20.3. Despite significant differences in parameters among cell lines, a firm correlation between radiocurability and individual radiobiologic parameter could not be etablished. The data suggested that the mechanism associated with radioresistance was complex and that any single radiobiologic parameter would not predict clinical success or failure. It is interesting that inherent radioresistance was associated with failure in four of eight cases, and significant repair of potentially lethal damage was associated with failure in one case. These results point out that large-fraction radiotherapy proposed for some human tumors may not be optimal since any noncycling cells in a condition analogous to stationery phase tumor cells may be efficient in the repair of PLD. Thus large fractions may induce initial damage analogous to 0 hours survival, much of which may be repaired in 6 to 24 hours. Therefore, large-fraction treatment regimens should be employed with caution if PLDR is shown to be a significant factor in head and neck cancer radiotherapy.

HYPOXIA

Since the radiation acts through free radical-mediated DNA damage, hypoxic or anoxic cells are more radioresistant than well-oxygenated cells. There is evidence from hyperbaric oxygen trials that hypoxic cells may be important in head and neck cancer. Therefore, low dose rate radiation and hyperfractionation have been suggested as alternatives to hyperbaric oxygen and hypoxic cell sensitizers to partially circumvent the problem hypoxia.[1] The reasons for this, based on laboratory investigations, are as follows: In hypoxic cells the repair of sublethal damage may be slow to absent, so that the killing of hypoxic cells from accumulated damage may be possible. Another advantage of hyperfractionation is that the redistribution of tumor cells to a more radiosensitive portion of the cell cycle may occur and/or allow reoxygenation of hypoxic tumor cells. This has been demonstrated in experimental animal tumors exposed to low dose rate continuous radiation.

CELL CYCLE EFFECT

The lethal effects of radiation are cell cycle-specific, and the effects of radiation at different stages in the cell cycle can be studied using synchronizing populations of cells. This may vary from cell line to cell line, although there are some generalizations: (1) cells are generally more sensitive near or at mitosis, (2) if G1 is an appreciable length, a resistant period is evidenced followed by a decline in survival toward S, (3) in most cell lines resistance rises during S to a maximum in the latter part of the S phase (4) in most cells G2 is as sensitive as M. Thus protracted fractionation or hyperfractionation may allow the advantage of cells passing through a more sensitive portion of the cell cycle more frequently.

NORMAL TISSUE EFFECTS

It has been demonstrated from many normal tissues that large fraction sizes increase the frequency of normal tissue damage when the same total dose is delivered. Withers and Peters have elegantly investigated aspects of fractionation with regard to normal tissue damage.[1]

REFERENCES

1. Withers HR, Peters LJ. Basic principles of radiotherapy. In: Fletcher G (ed). Textbook of radiotherapy. Philadelphia: Lea & Febiger, 1983:3:103.
2. Elkind MM, Sutton A. X-ray damage and recovery of mammalian cells in culture. Nature 1969; 184:1293–1295.
3. Little JB, Hahn GM, Frindel E, Tubiana M. Repair of potentially lethal radiation damage in vitro and in vivo. Radiology 1973; 106:689–694.
4. Weichselbaum RR, Schmidt A, Little JB. Cellular factors influencing radiocurability of human malignant tumors. Br J Cancer 1982; 45:10–16.
5. Gerweck LE, Kornblith PL, Burlett EP, Wang J, Seiger S. Radiation sensitivity of cultured human glioblastoma cells. Radiology 1977; 125:231–234.
6. Nilsson S, Carlson J, Larsson E, Ponten J. Survival of irradiated glia and glioma cells studied with a new cloning technique. Int J Radiat Biol 1980; 37:267–279.
7. Barranco SC, Romsdahl MM, Humphrey RM. The radiation response of human malignant melanoma cells grown it vitro. Cancer Res 1971; 31:830–833.
8. Carney DN, Mitchell JB, Kinsella T. In vitro radiotherapy and chemotherapy sensitivity of established cell lines in human small cell lung cancer and large cell morphological variance. Cancer Res 1983; 43:2806–2811.
9. Selby PJ, Courtenay D. In vitro cellular radiosensitivity of human malignant melanoma. Int J Radiat Biol Oncol Phys 1982; 8:12–35.
10. Courtenay D, Smith IE, Peckam MJ, Steel GG. In vitro and in vivo radiosensitivity of human tumor cells obtained from a pancreatic carcinoma xenograft. Nature 1976; 263:771–772.
11. Weichselbaum RR, Dahlberg W, Little JB, Ervin TJ, Miller D, Hellman S, Rheinwald JG. Cellular x-ray parameters of early passage squamous cell carcinoma lines derived from patients with known responses to radiotherapy. Br J Cancer 1984 (In Press).

FRACTIONATION: DOSE-TIME CONSIDERATIONS IN THE MANAGEMENT OF CARCINOMA OF THE UPPER AERODIGESTIVE TRACT

JAMES D. COX, M.D.

Fractionation, the combination of individual dose, total dose, and interval from the first treatment to the last, is the oldest "modality" in the radiotherapeutic armamentarium. From the earliest work at the Fondation Curie by Regaud and Coutard, it was apparent that manipulations of fractionation had important differential effects on malignant tumors and normal tissues. In spite of this long history, much has been learned in the past 15 years that permits a more sound scientific basis for altering fractionation with the hope of increasing the probability of tumor control, decreasing effects on normal tissues, or providing a fractionation regimen optimal for combinations with other modalities such as radiosensitizers, biologic response modifiers, and hyperthermia.

In the middle 1960s, most radiation therapy in the United States, Canada, the United Kingdom, and France was administered 5 or 6 days per week without interruption for 4 to 8 weeks.[1] Since that time, many variations were introduced, some to attempt to increase tumor control or decrease normal tissue effects, but many were selected for the convenience of the patients and the radiation therapists. Since the possible combinations of individual and total doses and the overall period of treatment are infinite, it was reasonable to attempt to reduce the combinations to single numbers if they could be shown to be isoeffective by some measure. By far, the most frequently used expression was the nominal standard dose (NSD) of Ellis.[2] Variations on this approach have been introduced by others, but the basic concept of a "biologic dose", isoeffective in regard to normal tissues, was widely accepted. Some of the variations that have been explored are defined in Table 1. The following brief review will evaluate results in the treatment of carcinomas of the upper aerodigestive tract, tumors that require total doses near the tolerance of the surrounding normal tissues.

HYPOFRACTIONATION: TUMOR CONTROL

Three Fractions Per Week. The minimal departure from common fractionation for which there are clinical data of interest is thrice-weekly fractionation. Such treatment has been considered "classic" in some departments.[3] Total doses were usually re-

TABLE 1   Fractionation Definitions*

Schedule	d	N/Wk	Ti (hrs.)	N	T (Wks)	D
Common	1.0–2.5	5–6	24	25–40	5–8	55–75
Hypo	> 3.0	1–4	48–168†	↓	NC	↓
Hyper	.7–1.3	10–25	2–12	↑	(↓) NC	NC (↑)
Rapid	> 2.5	5	24	↓	↓	↓
Accelerated	1.5–2.5	10–15	4–12	↓	↓↓	↓

*= assumes dose-rate of 0.5 to 3.0 gy/min; d = dose per fraction (Gy); N/wk = number of fractions per week; Ti = interval between fractions; † = intervals > 168 hrs. constitute "split-course"; N = total number of fractions; T = duration of treatment course; D = total dose (Gy)

duced to compensate for effects that were anticipated in normal tissues. Based on the NSD formula of Ellis,[2] approximately 600 patients were treated with fewer than five fractions per week at the Medical College of Wisconsin between 1971 and 1975:[4] the most frequent fraction size was 3 gray (Gy), and the total doses were usually 54 to 57 Gy in approximately 6 weeks. Byhardt et al retrospectively analyzed the results for carcinomas of the oral cavity and oropharynx comparing three fractions per week with five fractions per week during the period 1965 to 1975;[5] all of the patients treated with hypofractionation came from the more recent 4-year period. Table 2 shows that local control was achieved in 60 percent (38 of 63) of patients treated with five fractions per week compared with 13 percent (4 of 31) for those treated with three fractions a week. Indeed, it was not possible to find a single patient with a T3 or T4 primary lesion which was controlled with three fractions per week.

The British Institute of Radiology conducted a cooperative trial comparing three versus five fractions per week for carcinomas of the larynx and hypopharynx. The most recently published analysis of the data showed a consistent difference for all sites combined and all subsets in favor of five fractions per week, but in no case were the differences considered statistically significant. The laryngectomy-free survival curves favored five fractions per week with a p value of 0.035. However, the fraction sizes in the five-times-per-week arm of this study exceeded that which was defined as "common" in Table 1. Therefore, this trial can more appropriately be considered a comparison of hypofractionation with rapid fractionation.

Another randomized trial comparing three versus five fractions per week was reported by Henk and James.[7] A wide variety of tumors in the upper aerodigestive tract of different sites of origin and extent were studied, with patients allocated to a regimen of 39 to 46.5 Gy in ten fractions in 22 days or 55 to 65 Gy in 30 fractions in 42 days. No differences in survival, local tumor control rates, or late effects on normal tissues were apparent.

Two Fractions Per Week. A prospective randomized trial was conducted by Handa et al;[8] patients with carcinomas of the oral cavity were treated with "radical" cobalt 60 teletherapy if the primary tumor was 5 cm or less and there was no regional adenopathy or a single mobile node was present. The patients were assigned to receive 60 to 65 Gy in 6 to 6½ weeks, 5 fractions per week, or a two-fraction-per-week regimen which was equivalent by the NSD formula. The results are shown in Table 3. The authors concluded that the two-fraction-per-week regimen was disadvantageous in regard to both tumor control and radiation sequelae.

Rapid Fractionation. In many radiotherapy centers in the United Kingdom and Canada, rapid fractionation is considered the norm. Thus, most patients treated with curative intent undergo a course of radiotherapy that is accomplished in 3 to 4 weeks. As with common fractionation in the United States, decades of experience of countless clinicians have resulted generally in satisfactory therapeutic ratios, i.e.,

TABLE 2   Squamous Cell Carcinomas of the Oral Cavity and Oropharynx: Local Control by Fractionation Regimen

Biologic Dose (NSD)₂	Tumor Size	Fractions per Week	
		Three	Five
< 1850	T1–2	1/3	10/12
	T3–4	0/2	2/6
1850–1950	T1–2	2/3	11/12
	T3–4	0/16	6/14
> 1950	T1–2	1/5	2/2
	T3–4	0/2	7/17
		4/31	38/63
		(13%)	(60%)

Data from Byhardt et al.[5]

TABLE 3   Comparison of Fractionation Regimens for Carcinomas of the Oral Cavity

	2 fractions/wk		5 fractions/wk	
Number of patients	23		21	
Alive free of cancer (12 months)	13	(57%)	15	(71%)
Number evaluable at 12 months for sequelae	17		18	
Fibrosis	3		2	
Radionecrosis	2	47%	1	28%
Other morbidity	3		2	

Data from Handa et al.[8]

the best control rates within the limitations of acceptable effects of normal tissues. However, it is worth noting experiences that have attempted to compress the course of irradiation further.

Lee et al reported 23 previously untreated patients with stage III and IV carcinomas of the "head and neck" who received 44 to 52 Gy in 11 to 13 fractions of 4.0 Gy, five fractions per week.[9] Three patients also had interstitial implants, two had resection for recurrence, and nine received the nitrofuran "radiosensitizer" metronidazole. The actuarial survival rate at 2 years was 45 percent, and the actuarial local control rate was 59 percent. However, only four patients had been followed 2 years or longer. They summarized 89 patients from the literature or from previous protocols and concluded the results were satisfactory in regard to local control and complications. Direct comparisons were not made with concurrent or historical control groups. Weissberg et al reported a randomized clinical study comparing similar fractionation (4.0 Gy, 5 fractions per week, to 40 to 48 Gy compared with 2.0 Gy, 5 fractions per week, to 60 to 70 Gy).[10] Thirty-one patients received common fractionation and 33 had rapid fractionation. The results were similar in regard to local control and disease-free survival. They also concluded that acute and late effects of radiations were the same; however, only eight patients (4 in each group) were alive at the time of the report, too few to provide adequate assessment of late effects.

Rapid Split-Course Regimens. The interposition of a period without treatment during a course of radiotherapy for carcinomas of the upper aerodigestive tract developed naturally in response to the initial wave of mucosal reactions at the end of the second week and during the third week of treatment. Thus, this "rest" period permitted the patients' symptoms to subside more completely, if not more rapidly, to the satisfaction of both the patient and the physician. Parsons et al allowed such a rest period in the middle of a course of common fractionation in the management of patients with carcinomas of the upper aerodigestive tract.[11] In a retrospective evaluation of local control compared with an immediately prior series of patients who received identical common fractionation without the rest, they found that the control rates with tumors of all sizes were lower with the split-course regimen. They concluded that the recovery of normal tissues in the 2-week interval was accompanied by recovery, presumably repopulation, of the tumor. Others have not found such split-course regimens with common fractionation to be disadvantageous,[12] but comparisons with control groups without the split-course have not been attempted.

Most split-course regimens have combined rapid fractionation with the interruption, based on a recognition of the potential for tumor recovery during the rest period and therefore the necessity of achieving a greater degree of reduction of the population of tumor cells prior to the rest. The Radiation Therapy Oncology Group (RTOG) has conducted several studies in which a rapid-fractionation split-course regimen has been compared with common fractionation. The experimental arm used 30 Gy in 10 fractions in 2 weeks, a rest period of 3 weeks, and another course of 30 Gy in 10 fractions for a total dose of 60 Gy in 7 weeks; this was compared with common fractionation with 2.0 Gy or 2.2 Gy per fraction, five fractions per week, continuously for thirty fractions and a total dose of 60 to 66 Gy in 6 weeks. Analysis of 109 evaluable patients with carcinoma of the nasopharynx (54 in continuous arm; 55 in "split" arm) showed no significant differences in acute reactions, late effects, proportions of patients whose primary tumors or cervical adenopathy disappeared, or disease-free survival.[13] A recent report of the results in 141 patients with carcinoma of the base of the tongue (73 in continuous arm; 68 in "split" arm) indicated that the two regimens were similar in regard to control of the primary tumor and cervical lymph nodes, time to failure, and survival; however, there was a suggestion that late effects, especially necrosis, were more frequent in the "split" regimen.[14] Similar results had been presented for 131 patients with carcinoma of the tonsillar fossa.[15] Future reports of these studies will contribute important information about late effects as a function of the size of the individual fraction.

NORMAL TISSUE EFFECTS

Considerable information is available on tumor control probability and late effects of irradiation with common fractionation.[16] However, there is a paucity of data concerning late effects on normal tissues in patients treated for carcinomas of the upper aerodigestive tract with reduced fractionation. Since the survival rate is low for patients irradiated for advanced carcinomas of the upper aerodigestive tract, the numbers of patients followed for sufficient periods of time to assess late effects are few. The experience from the Medical College of Wisconsin did not permit assessment of late effects on normal tissue since nearly every patient treated with three fractions per week had progression of the primary tumor and short survival.[5] A review of the effects of hypofractionation on a variety of normal tissues led to the following conclusions:[17] (1) there was a significantly greater late effect on the normal tissues (skin, bowel, spinal cord) than was predicted by the NSD equation; (2) acute reactions did not predict the differences observed in late effects comparing hypofractionation and common fractionation; (3) although "late" effects were seen within the first 12 months, they continued to progress between 12 and 60 months.

Few data are available pertaining to late effects from rapid fractionation with or without the interruption ("split"). A suggestion of increased late effects with larger-sized fractions has been reported by Horiot et al from the experiences at M.D. Anderson Hospital of Houston in the treatment of carcinoma of the vocal cord; they found late edema or necrosis in six of 68 (9%) of patients who were treated with 2.75 Gy per fraction compared with three of 236 (1%) of patients who received 2.0 or 2.2 Gy per day.[18] Stewart and Jackson reported similar results (4% to 10% of patients with "prolonged reaction" and 5% with necrosis) following irradiation with 3.7 to 3.87 Gy per fraction, with 15 fractions over a 3-week period for carcinoma of the larynx.[19]

DISCUSSION

Since "fractionation" has been important in radiotherapy for at least three-quarters of a century, it is impossible to review and categorize all the literature available. In addition, there are several confounding factors which prevent meaningful conclusions being drawn from the data in the literature. Clinical trials, even prospective and randomized, in which both arms involve an inadequate total dose, contribute little to our understanding; conclusions from these studies usually have been that there were no differences, but both study arms were unsatisfactory. Studies that have used survival as the only end point have limited value since survival may be a very indirect measure of control of the tumor within the irradiated volume, and may be determined more by patient characteristics than by treatment approaches. Tumors that can grow very slowly are poor indicators of tumor control since very long periods of follow-up are necessary to assess success or failure; an obvious example is well-differentiated carcinoma of the thyroid, but carcinomas of the prostate and breast present similar difficulties. The addition of either brachytherapy or surgery to any regimen of fractionated external irradiation complicates evaluation of local control.

A summary of studies of reduced fractionation is presented in Table 4. The data for this table are derived from the studies reviewed above and those included in a broader review of the literature, which included malignant epithelial tumors of other sites in addition to those arising in the upper aerodigestive tract.[17] The evidence available to date suggests that larger doses delivered in fewer fractions are disadvantageous in regard both to control of the tumor within

TABLE 4 Summary of Studies of Reduced Numbers of Large Fractions

Regimen	Tumor control	Late effects*
3 × per week	NC or ↓	NC
2 × per week	↓	↑
1 × per week	NC or ↓	↑↑
Rapid	NC	NC or ↑
Rapid-split	NC or ↓↓	NC or ↑

*Relative to common fractionation
NC = no change

the field of irradiation and to late sequelae from treatment. The former might not have been anticipated from isoeffect formulas based on effects of radiations on normal tissues. However, there was a clear underestimation of the magnitude of late effects on normal tissues resulting from large fraction sizes. Thames et al have reviewed a large body of data from irradiation of normal tissues in laboratory studies.[20] They have also concluded that late effects are more sensitive to increasing fraction size than acute effects.

SUMMARY

Fractionation in radiation therapy has been manipulated to attempt to improve control of malignant tumors, to decrease effects on normal tissues, or to provide more convenient schedules for the patient and radiation therapist. In addition, some fractionation regimen must be selected as the basis for addition of such potential modifiers of radiation effects as radiosensitizers, biologic response modifiers, and hyperthermia. A considerable literature derived from clinical experiences with reduced numbers of large fractions has become available in the last fifteen years. A review of this literature focused upon tumor control and effects on normal tissues resulting from hypofractionation (fewer than five fractions per week), rapid fractionation (large daily fractions treated five times per week), and rapid split-course regimens which included a rest interval in the course of treatment. The evidence available indicated that a decrease in tumor control was associated with each of these large-dose fractionation approaches. At the same time, late effects on normal tissues were increased as the result of the large-sized fractions.

The overall reduction in therapeutic ratio suggests that reduced numbers of large-sized fractions should no longer be pursued in clinical research, and such regimens should be adopted with great caution in clinical investigations combining radiosensitizers or hyperthermia. The data now available strongly suggest that any decision to choose altered fractionation in clinical practice, even if justified on the basis of a formula of alleged isoeffectiveness, must be undertaken with great caution. Conversely, it is natural to pursue clinical investigations with increased numbers of smaller fractions than employed with common fractionation with the hope of diminishing late effects on normal tissues for a given probability of tumor control. If this were realized, total doses might be increased, still with an acceptable level of late effects on normal tissues, with improved radiotherapeutic control of carcinomas of the upper aerodigestive tract.

REFERENCES

1. Marcial VA. Time-dose-fractionation relationships in radiation therapy. Natl Cancer Inst Monogr 1967; 24:187–203.
2. Ellis F. The relationship of biological effect to dose-time-frac-

tionation factors in radiotherapy. In: Ebert M, Howard A (eds). Current Topics in Radiation Research. Amsterdam: North Holland Publishing Co, 1968:357–397.

3. Dutreix J, Hayem M, Pierquin B, Zummer K, Hesse C, Wambersie A. Epitheliomas de la region amygdalienne. Comparaison entre fractionnement classique et irradiation en deux series (split-course). Acta Radiol Ther Phys Biol 1974; 13:167–184.

4. Greenberg M, Eisert DR, Cox JD. Initial evaluation of reduced fractionation in the irradiation of malignant epithelial tumors. Am J Roentgenol Rad Ther Nucl Med 1976; 126:268–278.

5. Byhardt RW, Greenberg M, Cox JD. Local control of squamous carcinoma of oral cavity and oropharynx with 3 vs 5 treatment fractions per week. Int J Radiat Oncol Biol Phys 1977; 2:415–420.

6. Wiernik G, Bates TD, Berry RJ, Brindle J, Bullimore J, Dalby JE, Flatman GE, Fowler JF, Hadden RCM, Haybittle JL, Henk JM, Howard N, Ledda J, Lindup R, Phillips DL, Pointon RS, Sambrook DK, Skeggs D. Seventh interim progress report of the British Institute of Radiology fractionation study of 3F/week versus 5F/week in radiotherapy of the laryngo-pharynx. Br J Radiol 1982; 55:505–510.

7. Henk JM, James KW. Comparative trial of large and small fractions in the radiotherapy of head and neck cancer. Clin Radiol 1978; 29:611–616.

8. Handa K, Edoliya TN, Pandey RP, Agarwal YC, Sinha N. A radiotherapeutic clinical trial of twice per week vs five times per week in oral cancer. Strahlentherapie 1980; 156:626–631.

9. Lee D, Wharam MD, Kashima H, Order SE. Short-course high fractional dose irradiation in advanced and recurrent head and neck cancer. Int J Radiat Oncol Biol Phys 1979; 5:1829–1832.

10. Weissberg JB, Son YH, Percarpio B, Fischer JJ. Randomized trial of conventional versus high fractional dose radiation therapy in the treatment of advanced head and neck cancer. Int J Radiat Oncol Biol Phys 1982; 8:179–185.

11. Parsons JT, Bova FJ, Million RR. A re-evaluation of split-course technique for squamous cell carcinoma of the head and neck. Int J Radiat Oncol Biol Phys 1979; 6:1645–1652.

12. Scanlon PW, Soule EH, Devine KD, McBean JB. Cancer of the base of the tongue. 116 Patients treated radiotherapeutically in the 11 year period 1952 through 1962. Am J Roentgenol Rad Ther Nucl Med 1969; 55:26–36.

13. Marcial VA, Hanley JA, Chang C, Davis LW, Moscol JA. Split-course radiation therapy of carcinoma of the nasopharynx: results of a national collaborative clinical trial of the Radiation Therapy Oncology Group. Int J Radiat Oncol Biol Phys 1980; 6:409–414.

14. Marcial VA, Hanley JA, Hendrickson F, Ortiz, H. Split-course radiation therapy of carcinoma of the base of the tongue: results of a prospective national collaborative clinical trial conducted by the Radiation Therapy Oncology Group. Int J Radiat Oncol Biol Phys 1983; 9:437–443.

15. Marcial VA, Hanley J, Rotman M. Split-course radiation therapy of carcinoma of the tonsillar fossa: results of a prospective national collaborative clinical trial of the Radiation Therapy Oncology Group. Int J Radiat Oncol Biol Phys 1978; 4(Suppl 1):17–18. (Abstract)

16. Fletcher GH, Shukovsky LJ. The interplay of radiocurability and tolerance in the irradiation of human cancers. J Radiol Electrol 1975; 56:383–400.

17. Cox JD. Large dose fractionation (Hypofractionation). Cancer (Suppl). In Press.

18. Horiot JC, Fletcher GH, Ballantyne AJ, Lindberg RD. Analysis of failures in early vocal-cord cancer. Radiology 1972; 103:663–665.

19. Stewart JG, Jackson AW. The steepness of the dose response curve both for tumor cure and normal tissue injury. Laryngoscope 1975; 85:1107–1111.

20. Thames Jr HD, Withers HR, Peters LJ, Fletcher GH. Changes in early and late radiation responses with altered dose fractionation: implications for dose-survival relationships. Int J Radiat Oncol Biol Phys 1982; 8:219::226.

ADJUVANT HYPERTHERMIA IN RADIATION THERAPY

DENNIS B. LEEPER, Ph.D.

Although we still do not understand the exact mechanisms involved in hyperthermia cytotoxicity or thermal radiosensitization, much data now exist, and human tumors are being treated with combinations of hyperthermia and radiation. Two excellent reviews have been recently published, and the reader is referred to these.[1,2] Briefly, the G_1 phase is the most resistant to hyperthermia, and cells die from membrane-related damage before entering mitosis, whereas S-phase cells are quite sensitive to hyperthermia and die of chromosome-related damage after passing through mitosis. Hyperthermia damage is enhanced by membrane active agents and cells are sensitized to hyperthermia by low pH and nutritional deprivation, but the cell response to hyperthermia damage is not affected by acute hypoxia. Hyperthermia does not appear to cause in vitro cell transformation to malignancy. Hyperthermia sensitizes cells to low LET radiation damage (decreased D_0), it inhibits repair of sublethal and potentially lethal radiation damage, and cell-cycle sensitivity to the combined modalities is complementary. G_2 arrest and G_1 S delay are much longer after hyperthermia than after radiation.

In spite of the biologic rationale for combining hyperthermia with radiation, great technical difficulties still exist in thermometry and uniform heating of tumors. In spite of these technical limitations, and limitations in the understanding of the nature of hyperthermia damage and thermal radiosensitization, many clinical investigations have sought to combine hyperthermia with radiation therapy for superficial malignant tumors, and attempts are being made to heat deep-seated tumors by interstitial applicators, regional hyperthermia, and systemic hyperthermia. It is the purpose of this paper to review the experimental and clinical data relevant to developing a rational concept for applying hyperthermia to radiation therapy.

Supported by Grant CA11602 from the National Cancer Institute, NIH, USA.

RESULTS

Thermal Dose

A unit of thermal exposure or thermal dose is critical to comparing results from different clinics. Two similar approaches to establishing a unit of thermal dose have recently been described based on the in-activation energy for cell killing from the Arrhenius plot.[3,4] Sapareto and Dewey have defined equivalent minutes at 43° by the formula

$$Eq43° = tR^{(43-T)} \text{ where } t = \text{time, } T =$$

temperature, and R = 0.5 for T >43 and R = 0.25 for T <43°.

They have established a nomogram relating any time and temperature combination to Eq43° (Fig. 1), and they have published a computer program to calculate Eq43°.[4]

Thermotolerance

Thermotolerance is a nonheritable resistance to hyperthermia that is induced by heat and several other cytotoxic agents.[5] Maximal thermotolerance develops during 3 to 4 hours of exposure of cells to temperatures below 42.5° and by 8 to 10 hours after exposure of cells to >43° and their return to 37°.[6] Thermotolerance then decays over 80 to 120 hours depending on the amount of thermotolerance that was induced.

Thermotolerance increases the resistance of sur-

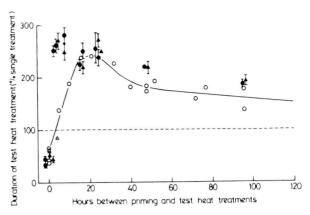

Figure 2 Thermotolerance in the mouse ear induced by 1, 2, or 5 daily treatments of 43.5° for 20 minutes. The duration of a test treatment to cause necrosis in 50 percent of the ears, expressed as a percent of that required in a single treatment, is plotted against the time between the last priming treatment and the test dose. ○ Priming treatment of 1 × (43.5°, 20 min); ● 2 × (43.5°, 20 min); ▲ 5 × (43.5°, 20 min). (From Law et al.[7])

viving cells by several orders of magnitude and is a factor to be reckoned with in fractionated hyperthermia. Thermotolerance develops in normal tissues after single or multiple hyperthermia fractions[7] (see Fig. 2 for example of mouse skin). Since maximal thermotolerance occurs by 24 hours, daily fractionation completely wastes heating subsequent to the first fraction. All experimental normal tissues studied to date develop thermotolerance. Tumors are no exception, and it has recently been shown that mouse C3H mammary tumors are quite adept at developing thermotolerance, with the development time and decay time being quite similar to those for skin and other normal tissues;[8](Fig. 3). As with skin, if heat fractions are given

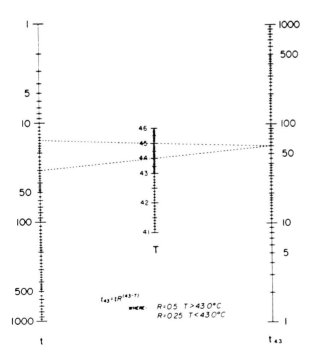

Figure 1 A nomogram relating time at any temperature to an equivalent time at 43° (Eq43°). Two examples of use are shown by dashed lines: a 30-minute treatment at 44° is equivalent to 60 minutes at 43°, which is also equivalent to 15 minutes at 45°. (From Sapareto and Dewey.[4])

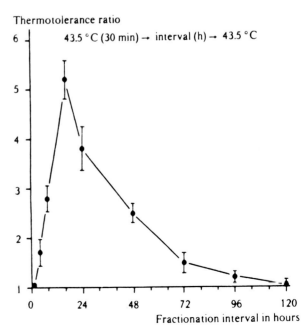

Figure 3 The kinetics of thermotolerance development and decay in the C3H mammary carcinoma after preheating at 43.5° for 30 minutes. (From Kamura, Nielsen, et al.[9])

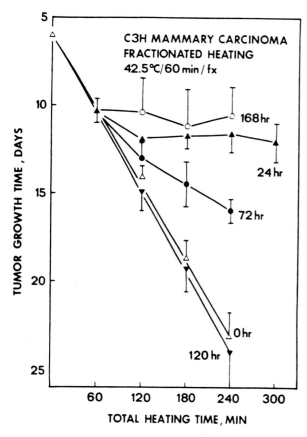

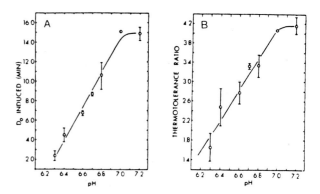

Figure 5 Impact of pH on 45° hyperthermia sensitivity and thermotolerance development in CHO cells. *Panel A*, D$_0$ of 45° hyperthermia survival curve as a function of pH. *Panel B*, Thermotolerance ratio at 8 hours post-heating (maximum thermotolerance development) as a function of pH. (From Goldin and Leeper.[11])

Figure 4 Tumor growth time as a function of fractionated hyperthermia treatment given with fractionation intervals ranging from 0 hours (single treatment) to 7 days. Note the effect of fractionation at 24-hour intervals indicating the impact of thermotolerance development in tumor cells. (From Overgaard and Nielsen.[9])

lead to selective tumor heating.[14] Figure 6 shows a compilation of a number of observations on rat tumors, muscle, and skin by Song et al[14] and shows that muscle and skin have a greatly enhanced blood flow at temperatures above 42° relative to transplantable tumors[14]. Waterman et al have shown that human tumors exposed to temperatures of 43.5 to 45° have a slightly increased blood flow during heating for 60 minutes (rather than a decreased blood flow), but

every 24 hours, all fractions subsequent to the first are wasted, whereas if the fractionation interval is 120 hours, the effect of fractionation is similar to that of a single treatment[9] (Fig. 4). There is no reason to suspect that human normal tissues and well-perfused tumor cells are not perfectly capable of developing thermotolerance just the same as murine tissues.

pH

Cells are sensitized to hyperthermia damage by low pH[10] and thermotolerance development is reduced by low pH[11] (Fig. 5). Since much of a tumor population is at low pH, and these cells are very likely to be hypoxic and radioresistant,[12] this offers one of the strongest reasons for combining hyperthermia with radiation therapy in the treatment of human tumors. Reduced pH also enhances thermal radiosensitization.[13]

Blood Flow

The neovasculature of tumors does not respond to increased temperatures as do blood vessels in normal tissues, and thus differences in blood flow may

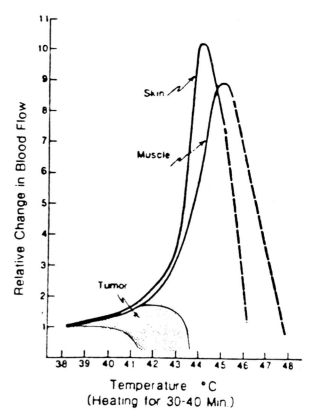

Figure 6 Relative changes in blood flow in skin and muscle of the rat and in various animal tumors during 30- to 45-minute exposure to different temperatures. (From Song et al.[14])

nonetheless do not respond with the greatly increased flow as do normal tissues[15] (Fig. 7). Interestingly, Kang et al have shown that in transplantable mouse tumors, vascular volume decreases to a minimum between 4 and 6 hours post-heating at 43.5° (Fig. 8), and as might be expected, pH and Po^2 also fall.[16] Recovery occurs between 24 and 48 hours. Such studies have not been conducted in human tumors.

Radiosensitization

The mechanism of heat cytotoxicity is quite independent of that from ionizing radiation, and heat cytotoxicity is influenced by thermotolerance, pH, and nutritional deprivation. Also, blood flow influences the heating characteristics of a tumor relative to normal tissues, and vascular collapse may occur after heating. While these factors alone are independent of radiation damage, thermal radiosensitization can also affect the response of human tumors to the combined modalities.[1,2] While different cell lines respond differently to heat followed by radiation or radiation followed by heat, invariably the greatest interaction results when irradiation occurs in the middle of the

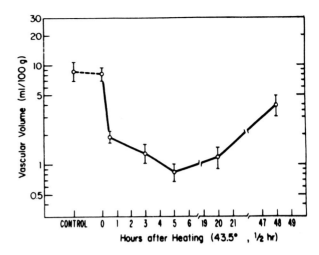

Figure 8 Changes in blood volume in SCK tumors of the A/J mouse as a function of time after heating at 43.5° for 30 minutes. Each point is the average of 10 to 15 tumors. (From Kang et al.[16])

heating interval.[17] Hyperthermia reduces the shoulder of the radiation survival curve in addition to reducing the D_O,[18] but at modest heat doses the primary effect is on the shoulder (inhibition of repair of DNA damage).

One would not be surprised, then, if modest hyperthermia had little sensitizing effect on low-dose fractions where much of the damage consists of single-hit lesions.[19] Gerner et al have shown a decreasing thermal radiosensitizing effect of 43° for 30 minutes with decreasing dose rate down to 6.25 cGy/minute, although they did find increased sensitization at 0.57 cGy/minute by this heat dose.[20] Their data with CHO cells demonstrated that a clinically relevant heat dose enhances very low dose rate as well as very high dose rate ionizing radiation, but suggest that little benefit is to be gained by using dose rates intermediate between conventional radiotherapeutic high dose rates or dose rates representative of interstitial implants. Gerner and Leith also demonstrated that 43° for 60 minutes does not sensitize CHO cells to high LET radiation (34 KeV/μ).[21] Therefore, clinically, one would expect to see the greatest effect of thermal radiosensitization the higher the heat dose, the higher the radiation dose, and the closer the two are together.

Denekamp and Stewart,[22] and Overgaard[23] examined the effect of sequence and interval between radiation and heat on mouse tumors and skin. As shown in Figure 9, the response was much less predictable for heat followed by radiation than vice versa. For the sequence radiation followed by heat, the repair of radiation damage in skin occurred by 2 to 4 hours, and the TER (thermal enhancement ratio) fell to 1, whereas between 4 and 8 hours, the TER for tumor remained at 1.5. Thus, the therapeutic gain factor comparing the response of tumor to that of skin was enhanced by separating radiation and hyperthermia by a 4-hour interval compared to simultaneous treatment.[23] The question is, do these findings have any impact on the

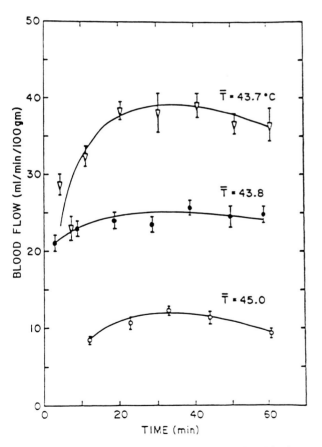

Figure 7 Blood flow (determined by thermal washout) in three human tumors during local hyperthermia. The upper curve is from a malignant melanoma in the groin, the center curve from a squamous cell carcinoma in the neck, and the lower curve a squamous cell carcinoma in the groin. (From Waterman et al.[15])

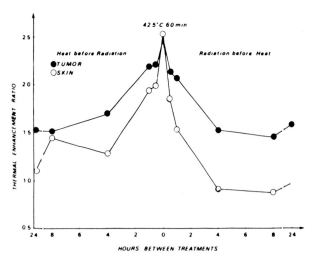

Figure 9 Thermal enhancement ratio (TER) as a function of time interval and sequence between hyperthermia (42.5° for 1 hour) and radiation treatments of a mouse mammary carcinoma and its surrounding skin. Maximal TER values were observed after simultaneous treatment, and any interval reduces the thermal effect. Note that in the tumor for the sequence radiation followed by heat there was persistent thermal enhancement with intervals of >4 hours, whereas in the skin the TER was markedly reduced within 1 hour and after 4 hours no thermal enhancement of the skin was retained. (From Overgaard.[23])

response of human tumors to combinations of hyperthermia and radiation?

Clinical Findings

Large Fractions Vs Small Fractions. Both Overgaard and Overgaard,[24] studying human melanomas (Fig. 10), and Arcangeli et al,[25] studying miscellaneous surface lesions (Fig. 11) using various protocols, but all in paired lesions, have shown enhancement of the therapeutic gain factor for tumor control vs skin damage when large radiation fractions were separated from hyperthermia by an interval of 4 hours. When large radiation fractions and hyperthermia were given simultaneously, the TER for tumor

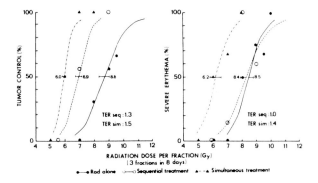

Figure 10 Dose-response relationship for radiation alone, or radiation and hyperthermia combined given either simultaneously or sequentially (4 hours) to human malignant melanomas (*left*) and the surrounding skin (*right*). (From Overgaard and Overgaard.[24])

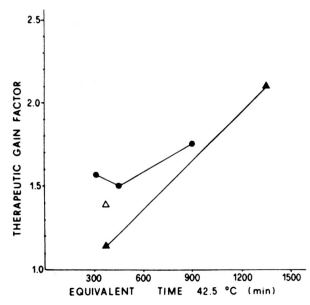

Figure 11 Therapeutic gain factor (ratio of tumor TER to skin TER) as a function of equivalent heating time (Eq42.5°). ▲ large RT fractions (5 to 6 Gy) and simultaneous heat; △ large RT fractions and sequential heat; ● small RT fractions (1.5 to 2.0 Gy) and simultaneous or sequential heat. (From Arcangeli et al.[26])

control was enhanced, but so was the skin reaction. However, when 2-Gy fractions were used, Arcangeli et al found no difference between simultaneous and sequential heating.[26] In fact, there was no difference in the TER or therapeutic gain factor between 2-Gy fractions combined with heat and large radiation fractions and sequential heat, indicating that for both situations there was independent interaction between radiation and hyperthermia effects, and the primary effect of heat was probably direct cytotoxicity (Fig. 12).

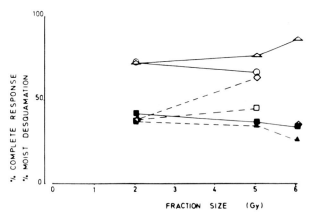

Figure 12 Percent complete tumor response (paired lesions) and moist desquamation as a function of radiation fraction size for radiation therapy only (RT) or radiation therapy plus hyperthermia (HT). △ Simultaneous treatment (tumors); ○ sequential treatment (tumors); ■ RT alone (tumors); ◇ simultaneous treatment (skin); □ sequential treatment (skin); ▲ RT alone (skin). *Note*: No difference in simultaneous or sequential treatment for a fraction size of 2 Gy. (From Arcangeli et al.[25])

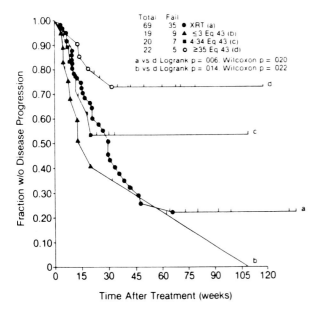

Figure 13 Response duration as a function of minimum temperature obtained during the first heat treatment in spontaneous pet tumors. The response duration increased significantly when >35 Eq43° (*d*) was obtained compared with no heat (RT alone, *a*) or <3 Eq43° (*b*). Tumors with intermediate heat doses (4–34 Eq43°, *c*) fell between the two extremes. (From Dewhirst et al.[27])

Furthermore, there was no increased skin damage for heat combined with 2-Gy fractions compared to 2-Gy fractions only[25,26] (Fig. 12).

Uniformity of Heating. Dewhirst et al,[27] in an elegant study of the effects of hyperthermia and radiation in spontaneous pet tumors, have shown that the minimum tumor temperature is the best predictor of local control. In fact, they have shown that the minimum temperature during the first heat treatment is a good predictor of response (Fig. 13). Oleson et al have verified these results in human tumors.[28] These results indicate that not only is temperature uniformity critical, but it is the first heat treatment that exerts the greatest hyperthermia effect on tumor control.

Thermotolerance. Most clinical studies on hyperthermia and radiation have employed two heat sessions per week with a 72- to 96-hour interval between heat fractions. Perez has recently tabulated several clinical studies showing the response of matched superficial lesions to radiation or radiation plus hyperthermia.[29] The complete response rate after heat plus radiation varied between 67 and 86 percent, whereas after radiation therapy only it was 7 to 46 percent (Table 1). Table 2 shows the complete response rate of human tumors treated with interstitial radiation plus hyperthermia using either resistive or microwave heating techniques prior to implanting [192]Ir. In some

TABLE 1 Efficacy of Combining External Hyperthermia and Radiation: Responses of Matched Superficial Lesions to Irradiation or Irradiation Plus Heat

Author	Tumor Histologies	Patients	Irradiation Alone	Hyperthermia Irradiation
Kim et al (1979)[30]	Various	54	26% CR	78% CR
Kim et al (1982)[31]	Malignant melanoma	38	46% CR	70% CR
Marmor et al (1980)[32]	Various	15	7% CR	47% superior
U et al (1980)[33]	Various	7	14% CR	86% CR
Arcangeli (1980)[34]	Neck node metastases from head and neck primary sites	15	46% CR	85% CR
Arcangeli (1983)[25]	Various	52*	42% CR	73% CR
Arcangeli (1983)[25]	Various	28†	37% CR	67% sequential heat 77% simultaneous heat

CR = complete response; superior = complete response vs. partial response, or more than 6 weeks' difference in time to regrowth.
*Randomized study = conventional radiotherapy fractionation, 42.5° for 45 minutes.
†Randomized study = high dose fractions (600 rads × 5), 45° for 30 minutes.

TABLE 2 Efficacy of Combining Interstitial Hyperthermia and Radiation

Author	Tumor Histologies	Lesions	Radiation Dose (rads)	No. of Heat Fractions	% CR
Manning et al (1982)[35] Aristizabal & Oleson (1984)[36]	Various	64	2,850	1*	38
Cosset et al (1982)[37]	H & N	17	3,000	1	88
Vora et al (1982)[38]	Various	15	< 6,000 > 6,000	1 1	36 90
Emmami et al (1984)[39]	Various	26	4,000–6,000	2†	69

*Heat administered prior to radiation.
†Heat before and after radiation.

cases a second heat treatment was applied after re-moving the [192]Ir.[39] The best responses were also in the range of 69 to 90 percent complete response. The similarity of the complete response rate for one frac-tion of heat, two fractions of heat, or eight fractions of heat given twice a week imply that either ther-motolerance is diminishing the response to subse-quent heat fractions or the first heat fraction has killed most of the heat-sensitive cells. The fact that the min-imum tumor temperature during the first heat session correlates with response also supports this conclusion. Nevertheless, there is currently no direct evidence for thermotolerance in human tumors or normal tissues.

DISCUSSION

A unit of thermal dose has been described[4] and is available for clinicians to use to facilitate compar-ison of results. Although this unit of thermal dose is not a good predictor of thermotolerance or sensitiza-tion to heat cytotoxicity,[4] it is at least one way to be-gin quantitation of thermic damage. Thermotolerance has the potential for influencing clinical results, and probably does. Likewise, low pH and nutritional dep-rivation sensitizing to hyperthermia cytotoxicity prob-ably have a large role to play in the therapeutic gain from heat on human tumors. It is also likely that the differential response of blood flow in tumors com-pared to normal tissues results in differential heating of human tumors, thus leading to a therapeutic gain based on physical parameters. However, well-per-fused tumor cells probably have the same heat sen-sitivity as normal cells, and hyperthermia alone yields only limited local control;[25,26] therefore, hyperthermia must be combined with radiation therapy or chemo-therapy. The nonproliferative, hypoxic cells at low pH that are thought to be "resistant" to radiation are "sensitive" to hyperthermia, and the well-perfused tumor cells that are "resistant" to hyperthermia are "sensitive" to radiation and cytotoxic chemotherapy.

Regarding radiosensitization affecting human tu-mor response to combined heat and radiation: for small radiation fractions (1.5 to 2 Gy), heat and radiation probably interact independently since there is no dif-ference between simultaneous and sequential combi-nation of heat and 2-Gy fractions and there is no in-creased skin damage when conventional fraction sizes of radiation are combined with moderate heat[25] (see Fig. 12). For large radiation fractions (5 to 6 Gy), when heat is applied simultaneously one sees heat ra-diosensitization for both tumor and skin (see Figs. 10 through 12). This is probably due primarily to the in-hibition of repair of radiation damage. A therapeutic gain is observed when large radiation fractions and heat are separated by 4 hours or more since, although the TER of tumor response is reduced, in skin it is reduced even further.

The first heat treatment of multiple heat fractions given less than 5 days apart is the most effective, and the minimum tumor temperature of the first heat ses-

sion is a good predictor of response.[27,28] It is not known yet whether this is because of thermotolerance. Also, a similar response is seen whether interstitial radiation is combined with one or two treatments, and the re-sponse is similar to that of external radiation com-bined with 3 to 8 heat treatments at two fractions a week (see Tables 1 and 2). This indicates that ther-motolerance may have an impact on human tumor re-sponse.

RECOMMENDATIONS

Because of the current technical difficulties of obtaining uniform thermal distributions throughout the tumor, and because tumor cells adjacent to normal tissue vasculature at normal pH probably exhibit the same hyperthermia sensitivity as normal cells, a full-dose efficacious radiation protocol for a given site is indicated. In that way, the radiation oncologist is se-cure in predicting normal tissue morbidity and tumor response. A standard radiation protocol would prob-ably include daily fractions of 1.5 to 2 Gy; this is the dose-fraction that the radiation oncologist finds most comfortable since it is the least likely to lead to late tissue damage.

It is the peripheral proliferative cells that are most responsive to ionizing radiation and the least respon-sive to hyperthermia; and it is the nutritionally de-prived cells at low pH and hypoxic that are the most sensitive to heat and the most resistent to radiation.

It is recommended that hyperthermia be added to a conventional low-dose-per-fraction protocol in the form of one heat treatment per week to avoid ther-motolerance. Heating should begin early in the ther-apy before reoxygenation occurs. The sequence should be radiation followed soon by heat to avoid hypoxia induced by vascular collapse as well as for conven-ience and consistency. One should try to achieve a minimum temperature of >35 Eq43° per hyperther-mia session, and it is highly recommended that one use some form of thermal dose calculation to facilitate comparison with other investigators. Surface cooling should be employed since it only makes sense to uti-lize any method possible to increase the therapeutic gain.

The question of using large dose fractions com-bined with heat to take advantage of radiosensitization to reduce the total radiation dose, and the use of other intriguing fractionation sequences to take advantage of reduced blood flow and pH following heating, or to take advantage of differential thermotolerance be-tween normal and tumor tissues, probably should wait until more clinical experience can be gained.

REFERENCES

1. Hahn GM. Hyperthermia and cancer. New York: Plenham, 1982.
2. Storm FK, ed. Hyperthermia in cancer therapy. Boston: GK Hall, 1983.
3. Field SB, Morris CC. The relationship between heating time

and temperature: Its relevance to clinical hyperthermia. Radiother Oncol 1983; 1:179–186.

4. Sapareto SA, Dewey WC. Thermal dose determination in cancer therapy. Int J Radiat Oncol Biol Phys 1984; 10:787–800.

5. Henle KJ, Dethlefsen LA. Heat fractionation and thermotolerance: A review. Cancer Res 1978; 38:1843–1851.

6. Li GC, Hahn GM. A proposed operational model of thermotolerance based on effects of nutrients and the initial treatment temperature. Cancer Res 1980; 40:4501–4508.

7. Law MP, Ahier RG, Somaia S, Field SB. The induction of thermotolerance in the ear of the mouse by fractionated hyperthermia. Int J Radiat Oncol Biol Phys 1984; 10:865–873.

8. Kamura T, Nielsen OS, Overgaard J, Andersen AH. Development of thermotolerance during fractionated hyperthermia in a solid tumor in vivo. Cancer Res 1982; 42:1744–1748.

9. Overgaard J, Nielson OS. The importance of thermotolerance for the clinical treatment with hyperthermia. Radiother Oncol 1983; 1:167–178.

10. Gerweck LE. Modification of cell lethality at elevated temperatures. The pH effect. Radiat Res 1977; 70:224–235.

11. Goldin EM, Leeper DB. The effect of low pH on thermotolerance: induction using fractionated 45°C-hyperthermia. Radiat Res 1981; 85:472–479.

12. Wike-Hooley JL, Haveman J, Reinhold HS. The relevance of tumor pH to the treatment of malignant disease—A review. Radiother Oncol 1984; 2:343–366.

13. Holahan EV, Highfield DP, Holahan PK, Dewey WC. Hyperthermic killing and hyperthermic radiosensitization in Chinese hamster ovary cells: Effects of pH and thermal tolerance. Radiat Res 1984; 97:108–131.

14. Song CW, Lokshina A, Rhee JG, Patten M, Levitt SH. Implications of blood flow in hyperthermia treatment of tumor. IEEE BME 1984; 31:9–16.

15. Waterman FM, Nerlinger RE, Moylan DM III, Leeper DB. Blood flow in human tumors during local hyperthermia. Int J Radiat Oncol Biol Phys 1984; submitted.

16. Kang MS, Song CW, Levitt SH. Role of vascular function in response of tumors in vivo to hyperthermia. Cancer Res 1980; 40:1130–1135.

17. Meyer KR, Hopwood LE, Gillette EL. The response of mouse adenocarcinoma cells to hyperthermia and irradiation. Radiat Res 1979; 78:98–107.

18. Gerner EW, Oval JH, Manning MR, Sim DA, Bowden GT, Hevezi JM. Dose rate dependence of heat radiosensitization. Int J Radiat Oncol Biol Phys 1983; 9:1401–1404.

19. Keller AM, Rossi HH. The theory of dual radiation action. Curr Top Radiat Res Q 1971; 8:85–158.

20. Chadwick KH and Leenhouts HP. The molecular theory of radiation biology. New York: Springer-Verlag 1981:377.

21. Gerner EW, Leith JT. Interaction of hyperthermia with radiations of different linear energy transfer. Int J Radiat Biol 1977; 31:283–288.

22. Denekamp J, Stewart F. Evidence for repair capacity in mouse tumors relative to skin. Int J Radiat Oncol Biol Phys 1979; 5:2003–2010.

23. Overgaard J. Simultaneous and sequential hyperthermia in radiation treatment of an experimental tumor and its surrounding tissue in vivo. Int J Radiat Oncol Biol Phys 1980; 6:1507–1517.

24. Overgaard J, Overgaard M. A clinical trial evaluating the effect of simultaneous or sequential radiation and hyperthermia in the treatment of malignant melanoma. In: Overgaard J, ed. Hyperthermic Oncol 1984. Vol. I. London and Philadelphia: Taylor & Francis 1984:383.

25. Arcangeli G, Cividalli A, Nervi C, Creteon G. Tumor control and therapeutic gain with different schedules of combined radiotherapy and local external hyperthermia in human cancer. Int J Radiat Oncol Biol Phys 1983; 9:1125–1134.

26. Arcangeli G, Nervi C, Stefano VS, Cividalli A, Lovosilo GA, Mauro F. The clinical use of experimental parameters to evaluate the response to combined heat and radiation. In: Overgaard J, ed. Hyperthermic Oncol 1984. Vol. I. London and Philadelphia: Taylor & Francis 1984:329.

27. Dewhirst MW, Sim DA, Sapareto S, Connor WG. Importance of minimum tumor temperature in determining early and long-term responses of spontaneous canine and feline tumors to heat and radiation. Cancer Res 1984; 44:43–50.

28. Sim DA, Oleson JR, Grochowski KJ. An update of the University of Arizona human clinical hyperthermia experience including estimates of therapeutic advantage. In: Overgaard J, ed. Hyperthermic Oncol 1984. Vol. I. London and Philadelphia: Taylor & Francis 1984:367.

29. Perez CA. Clinical hyperthermia: Mirage or reality. Int J Radiat Oncol Biol Phys 1984; 10:935–937.

30. Kim JH, Hahn EW. Clinical and biological studies of localized hyperthermia. Cancer Res 1979; 39:2258–2261.

31. Kim JH, Hahn EW, Antich PP. Radiofrequency hyperthermia for clinical cancer therapy. J Natl Cancer Monogr 1982; 61:339–342.

32. Marmor JB, Hahn GM. Combined radiation and hyperthermia in superficial human tumors. Cancer 1980; 47:1986–1991.

33. U R, Noell KT, Woodward KT, Word BT, Fishburn RI, Miller LS. Microwave-induced local hyperthermia in combination with radiotherapy of human malignant tumors. Cancer 1980; 45:638–646.

34. Arcangeli G, Barni E, Cividalli A, Morrow F, Morelli D, Nervi C, Spanno M, Tabocchini A. Effectiveness of microwave hyperthermia combined with ionizing radiation: Clinical results on neck node metastases. Int J Radiat Oncol Biol Phys 1980; 6:143–148.

35. Manning MR, Cetas TC, Miller RC, Oleson JR, Connor WG, Gerner EW. Clinical hyperthermia: Results of a phase I trial employing hyperthermia alone or in combination with external beam or interstitial radiotherapy. Cancer 1982; 49:205–216.

36. Aristizabal SA, Oleson JR. Combined interstitial irradiation and localized current field hyperthermia: Results and conclusions from clinical studies. Cancer Res 1984; 44:4457s–4760s.

37. Cossett JM, Dutreix A, Gerbaulet A, Damia E. Combined interstitial hyperthermia and brachytherapy: The Institute Gustave Russy experience. In: Overgaard J, ed. Hyperthermic Oncol 1984. Vol. I. London and Philadelphia: Taylor & Francis 1984:587.

38. Vora N, Forell B, Joseph C, Lipsett J, Archambaau J. Interstitial implant with interstitial hyperthermia. Cancer 1982, 50:2518–2523.

39. Emami B, Marks J, Perez C, Nussbaum G, Laybovich L. Treatment of human tumors with interstitial irradiation and hyperthermia. In: Overgaard J, ed. Hyperthermic Oncol 1984. Vol. I. London & Philadelphia: Taylor & Francis 1984:583.

MULTIPLE FRACTIONS PER DAY IN THE RADIOTHERAPY OF HEAD AND NECK CANCER: AN UPDATED STUDY OF THE EORTC RADIOTHERAPY GROUP

GIORGIO ARCANGELI, M.D.
CARLO NERVI, M.D.
ANTONIO GUERRA, Ph.D.
WALTER VAN DEN BOGAERT, M.D.
EMMANUEL VAN DER SCHUEREN, M.D.
JAN CLAUDE HORIOT, M.D.
DIONISIO GONZALES, M.D.
VLADIMIR SVOBODA, M.D.

TABLE 1   Distribution of Patients, according to Subsite

Larynx	15	} 53
Hypopharynx	30	
Pharynx (extensive)	8	
Neck nodes	6	
Oropharynx	56	
Tongue	24	} 50
Flour of mouth	6	
Oral cavity (other)	20	
Paranasal sinuses	12	
Nasopharynx	1	
Salivary glands	1	
	179	

TABLE 2   TNM Distribution

	All	N0	N1	N2	N3
T1	5	1	2		2
T2	20	11	1	1	7
T3	89	33	20	6	30
T4	45	15	5	4	21
No Prim.	4				4
No T Staging	16	6	2	0	8
	179	66	30	11	72

Recent advances in radiobiology indicate that a therapeutic advantage may be accomplished by treating tumors with several sessions of irradiation per day. In comparison with standard treatment, this implies a modification of one or more treatment parameters which may be combined in several varieties of treatment schedules, summarized as follows: (1) accelerated fractionation: conventional fraction size in a reduced overall treatment time; (2) hyperfractionation: reduced fraction size in a conventional overall time; and (3) combined rationales: reduced fraction size with increased fraction number in a reduced overall time. All these schedules have been tested in recent studies.[1]

In view of the encouraging results, a pilot study was started in the Radiotherapy Group of the EORTC on patients with advanced cancer of the head and neck. The aim of the study was twofold: (1) to investigate the feasibility of three fraction per day radiotherapy using 1.6 Gy per fraction (4 hours between fractions); and (2) to perform the same scheme combined with the hypoxic cell sensitizer misonidazole. The early results of this study were published in 1982.[2] In this paper an updated analysis of the result (April 1983) is presented.

TREATMENT REGIMENS

From the end of 1978 to December 1980, 179 patients with advanced head and neck tumors were entered in the study. The patient's characteristics and the treatment techniques, previously described in detail[2] will be presented briefly here.

Patients were irradiated three times daily, with intervals of 3 to 4 hours, using 1.6 Gy per fraction. Patients were usually treated for 2 weeks (10 irradiation days) to a dose of 48 Gy; 3 to 4 weeks later a boost was added to a total dose of 67 to 72 Gy in 6 to 7 weeks.

In 55 patients, misonidazole was given 2 hours before the first irradiation fraction of each treatment day in a dose of 1 g/m^2.

Tumor localization and TNM distribution are shown in Tables 1 and 2, respectively. Survival and local control were calculated by the Kaplan and Meier product limit method.[3] The statistical significance was tested by the Mantel Haenszel test.[4]

RESULTS

At the time of analysis, the minimum period of follow-up for all patients was 2 years. Forty-five patients were still alive, five with local failure, three with a second tumor, and one with distant metastases. One hundred and thirty-four patients were dead: four died of a second tumor, but with the first disease locally controlled; in 64 patients a local recurrence was seen, in 14 combined with distant metastases and in four with a second primary; distant metastases alone occurred in 13 cases (1 combined with a second tumor). In the 28 patients with distant metastases, the site of spread was lung in 21 cases, bone in five, liver in four, and brain in three. Causes of death were complications in 17 patients (eight necrosis, five pharyn-

TABLE 3   Status of Patients Treated, April 1983

NED local	43	24%
Local failure	87	49%
Metastases	28	16%
Second tumor	12	7%
Complications	17	9%

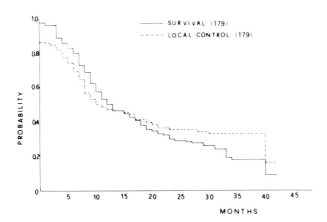

Figure 1 Estimated overall survival and local control distribution according to the product limit method of Kaplan and Meier. Median length of life = 11.9 ± 1 months. Median length of local control time = 10 ± 1.4 months.

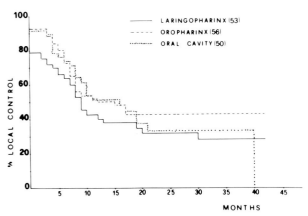

Figure 3 Estimated local control distribution in patients with tumor of oral cavity, oropharynx, and laryngopharynx. Median length of local control time = 12.7 ± 0.9, 11.8 ± 2.6, and 8.4 ± 0.7 months, respectively. The differences are not statistically significant (see text).

geal hemorrhage, three postoperative complications, and one severe neuropathy) and intercurrent disease in 14; the cause was unknown in three cases. One patient was lost to follow-up. The general outcome of disease is summarized in Table 3.

A general idea of survival and local control can be obtained from Figure 1, which shows an actuarial analysis of survival and local control. The median length of life and of local control time is 11.9 and 10 months, respectively; at 36 months, survival is 17.5 percent and local control is 32.5 percent.

More detailed information on local control is given in Figures 2 and 3. In patients treated with misonidazole, the median length of local control time is 9.9 months, but compared to the patients not given the drug (10 months), the difference is not significant (Fig. 2).

No statistically significant differences in local control are observed when the different subregions are compared (Fig. 3): the median length of local control

time is 12.7, 11.8, and 8.4 months for cancer of the oral cavity, oropharynx, and laryngopharynx, respectively. However, when we compare local control in the laryngopharynx, which is the worst, to that in the oral cavity and oropharynx, the differences become close to the 0.05 percent level of significance (p = 0.14 and 0.09, respectively).

More detailed information on survival is reported in Figures 4 and 5. In patients treated with misonidazole, the median length of life is 19.9 months (Fig. 4); in comparison to that observed in patients not given the drug (10.3 months), the difference is highly significant (p < 0.01).

The survival for cancers in the different subregions is shown in Figure 5; the median length of life is 16.8, 12.8, and 8.6 months for disease of the oral cavity, oropharynx, and laryngopharynx, respectively. No significant difference in survival is observed when statistics for oral cavity cancer are com-

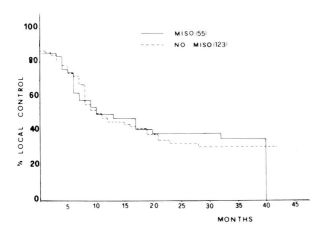

Figure 2 Estimated local control distribution in patients treated or not treated with misonidazole. Median length of local control time = 9.9 ± 1.5 and 10 ± 2 months, respectively. The difference is not statistically significant.

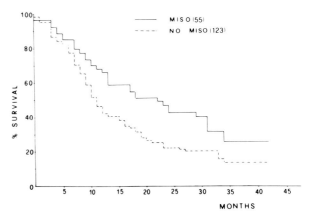

Figure 4 Estimated survival distribution in patients treated or not treated with misonidazole. Median length of life = 19.9 ± 9.5 and 10.3 ± 0.7 months, respectively. The difference is statistically highly significant (p < 0.01).

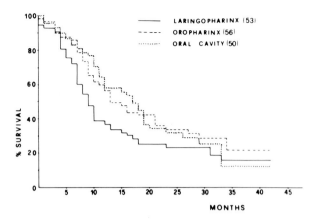

Figure 5 Estimated survival distribution in patients with tumors of oral cavity, oropharynx, and laryngopharynx. Median length of life = 16.8 ± 1.4, 12.8 ± 1.5, and 8.6 ± 0.7 months, respectively. Statistical significance: oral cavity vs oropharynx p = 0.46; oropharynx vs laryngopharynx p = 0.06; oral cavity vs laryngopharynx p < 0.05.

pared to those for oropharynx disease. The difference is at a borderline level of significance when the survival in laryngopharynx cancer is compared to that in oropharynx cancer (p = 0.06), and is statistically significant (p < 0.05) when the comparison is made between laryngopharynx and oral cavity cancer survival rates.

Acute tolerance has already been reported.[2] Briefly, skin reaction is moderate and is not affected by the addition of misonidazole. Mucosal reaction starts at the end of the first week and reaches the maximum (confluent mucosity) between the tenth and the fifteenth days. Reaction lasts for about 10 days and subsides rapidly thereafter. The addition of misonidazole does not seem to affect the intensity or the duration of mucosal reaction. A peripheral neuropathy was observed in 11 patients receiving misonidazole; in nine patients this neuropathy was slight and in two it was serious. Three patients developed a rash, and in one patient hepatitis was seen, possibly caused by misonidazole. One fatal complication was seen (coma ending in death), possibly caused by the drug. In two patients, the drug was discontinued because of gastrointestinal intolerance. Late reactions in 45 long-term survivors are shown in Table 4. Severe reactions were seldom observed. The most common reactions were skin fibrosis and xerostomia, the latter being severe in four cases. In general, it does not seem that late

TABLE 4   Late Reactions in Survivors (45 Patients)

	Mild	Moderate	Severe
Fibrosis	11	9	1
Xerostomia		16	4
Edema	14	2	—
Radiation myelitis			1
Interstitial pneumonitis			1

reactions are heavier than those expected after a conventional fractionation schedule.

DISCUSSION

There is some experimental evidence that irradiation given in multiple fractions per day is more efficient than the standard treatment in killing fast-growing tissues because of the self-sensitization induced by the redistribution of cells through the cycle. For actively proliferating normal tissues, this self-sensitization is probably the cause of increased acute reactions that would be even more exaggerated if the opportunity for cell proliferation is reduced by shortening the overall treatment time, as in accelerated fractionation regimens.[5] In many situations (i.e., when considerable mucosa is included in the treatment field), it is possible for acute reactions to be dose-limiting. However no change in the response of the slowly cycling target cells, which are much less sensitized by redistribution and which are responsible for late damage, would be expected with accelerated fractionation.

The present study confirms the radiobiologic predictions that a short course with high daily dose rates is feasible. Giving three fractions per day for a period of 2 weeks allows delivery of about the same total dose as that delivered in 5 weeks by means of a standard fractionation regimen. The time course of acute reaction is drastically changed, resulting in an earlier appearance and a shorter plateau of the radiation mucositis. The boost dose, after 3 to 5 weeks of rest, carries the total dose to about 72 Gy. The overall time of 7 weeks is not changed in comparison to the single-fraction-per-day regimen; however, the number of treatment days is reduced from about 40 to 15. This allows misonidazole to be given during all treatment sessions in doses within the range of drug tolerance. Overall survival and local control do not seem to be high, but most patients had very large lesions that were treated mainly with palliation as the goal. From this point of view, it can be considered a success to have 45/179 patients surviving more than 2 years.

Local control does not seem to differ significantly between the various subregions, although a complete and persistent tumor response is clearly more difficult to achieve in the laryngopharynx than in the oral cavity and oropharynx. This is confirmed by the significantly better survival observed in patients with intraoral and oropharyngeal lesions than in patients with laryngopharyngeal lesions.

The addition of misonidazole does not seem to affect local control rate, but in patients treated with the radiosensitizer, survival appears to be significantly higher than in patients treated without the radiosensitizer. This peculiarity may be the consequence of a different number and a biased selection of patients in the two series, since there was no randomization for the administration of the drug.

In conclusion, these results indicate that it is possible to shorten the treatment time while administering total doses equal to those used with standard fractionation regimens. Whether an accelerated treatment like that employed in this study could achieve better results remains to be proved, although the present results indicate a possible improvement in local control and survival, and misonidazole could have a further beneficial effect.

To test these findings, a randomized clinical trial has been activated in the EORTC Radiotherapy Group since February 1981. It compares the standard single-fraction-per-day regimen to a three-fractions-per-day scheme, with and without misonidazole, in advanced head and neck cancer.

REFERENCES

1. Kotalik JF. Multiple daily fractions in radiotherapy. Cancer Treat Rev 1981; 8:127–146.
2. Van den Bogaert W, van der Schueren E, Horiot JC, Chaplain G, Arcangeli G, Gonzales D, Svoboda V. The feasibility of high-dose multiple daily fractionation and its combination with anoxic cell sensitizer in the treatment of head and neck cancer. Int J Radiat Oncol Biol Phys 1982; 8:1649–1655.
3. Kaplan EL, Meier P. Non-parametric estimation from incomplete observations. J Am Stat Assoc 1958; 53:457–481.
4. Mantel N. Evaluation of survival data and two new rank order statistics arising in its consideration. Cancer Chemother Rep 1966; 50:163–170.
5. Arcangeli G, Nervi C, Mauro F. Experimental multiple daily fractionation. Cancer Bull 1982; 34:234–238.

HYPERFRACTIONATION STUDIES OF THE RADIATION THERAPY ONCOLOGY GROUP IN PATIENTS WITH ADVANCED SQUAMOUS CELL CARCINOMA OF THE HEAD AND NECK

SIMON KRAMER, M.D., F.A.C.R.

In the Radiation Therapy Oncology Group there are three studies dealing with hyperfractionation.

The first was a pilot study (77–03) initiated in 1977 (Fig. 1). All patients with advanced head and neck cancer not previously treated were included in this pilot study in which the primary site and stage were recorded. Treatment consisted of 1.5 Gy twice daily at a 4-hour interval to a total dose of 60 Gy in 4 weeks initially. Roughly the first half of these patients were treated with the schema as indicated. At this point it was observed that the acute mucosal reactions were unacceptably severe, and the schema was changed to 1.25 Gy twice daily at a 4-hour interval

to a total dose of 60 Gy in just over 5 weeks. There were 69 patients that could be evaluated. The study chairmen were Richard Marks and Victor Marcial. The results of that study indicated that at 1.25 Gy twice daily, skin and mucosal reactions were less when compared with conventional treatment, but still remained the limiting factor. Late changes such as necrosis, fibrosis, and loss of salivary function seemed less than expected with the 1.25 Gy twice daily fractions. Tumor control and local control seemed to be equal to those of conventional treatment by comparing with historical controls.

On the basis of these findings, a randomized clinical trial was undertaken in 1979 with V. Marcial as study chairman and T. Pajak as the statistician (Fig. 2). Some 210 patients were randomized into either conventional radiation therapy at 1.80 to 2.00 Gy/fraction to 66 to 73.8 Gy at five fractions per week or hyperfractionation using two fractions of 1.20 Gy per day with a 3- to 6-hour interval to a total of 6 Gy at ten fractions per week over 5 weeks.

In brief, major treatment symptoms and reactions

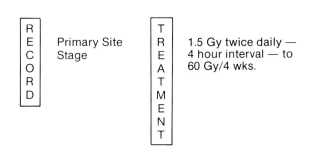

Figure 1   RTOG 77-03 schema. Study chairmen: R. Marks, M.D., V. Marcial, M.D.

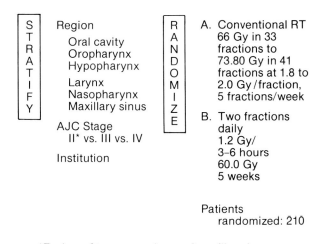

*For base of tongue, nasopharynx, & maxillary sinus.

Figure 2   RTOG 79-13 schema. Study chairman: Victor A. Marcial, M.D.; statistician: Thomas Pajak, Ph.D.

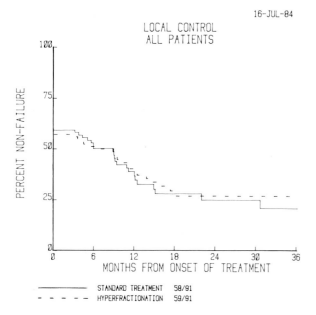

16-JUL-84

LOCAL CONTROL
ALL PATIENTS

PERCENT NON-FAILURE

MONTHS FROM ONSET OF TREATMENT

——————— STANDARD TREATMENT   58/91
– – – – – HYPERFRACTIONATION   59/91

Figure 3 Local control rates for patients treated with one fraction per day versus hyperfractionation.

Stratify
1. Site within URDT oval cavity, oropharynx (except base of tongue), larynx vs other sites

2. Nodal metastases N0 vs. N+

3. Karnofsky performance status 80–100 vs. 50–70

R
A
N
D
O
M
I
Z
E

Treatment
1. 20 Gy twice daily × 4 wks. (50.40 Gy in 42 fractions) to primary and regional nodes
       plus
Boost to reduced field to primary of:

A. 16.80 Gy in 14 fractions in 1.5 wks. Total dose: 67.20 Gy in 56 Fx/28 Rx days/5.5 wks.

B. 21.60 Gy in 18 fractions in 2 wks. Total dose: 72.00 Gy in 60 Fx/32 Rx days/6 wks.

C. 26.40 Gy in 22 fractions in 2 wks. Total dose: 76.80 Gy in 64 Fx/32 Rx days/6.5 wks.

Escalations

D. 31.20 Gy in 26 fractions in 2.5 wks. Total dose: 81.60 Gy in 68 Fx/34 Rx days/7 wks.

E. 36.00 Gy in 30 fractions in 3 wks. Total dose: 86.40 Gy in 72 Fx/36 Rx days/7.5 wks.

Figure 4 RTOG 83-13 URDT schema. Study chairman: James Cox, M.D.; statistician: Marie Diener, Ph.D.; data manager: JoAnn Stetz, R.N.

appear to be the same for the two arms of the study, and local control, as shown in Figure 3, is the same. It is noteworthy that a dose of 60 Gy in 5 weeks was being compared with a dose of 66 Gy to 73.8 Gy in 1.80 to 2.00 Gy fractions with essentially the same outcome and the same reactions, thus indicating that hyperfractionation, even with a compressed overall time and at somewhat lower dose than conventional fraction size, can obtain at least equally good results.

The third study now undertaken by the Radiation Therapy Oncology Group is a dose-seeking study (Fig. 4). The schema indicates the stratification and a number of arms into which patients are randomized. This type of study is also being done at other sites. The dose-seeking feature of this study consists of randomly allocating patients to the first three arms in the first place and comparing a total dose of 67 Gy in 56 fractions over 5.5 weeks with 72 Gy in 60 fractions over 6 weeks and 76 Gy in 64 fractions over 6.5 weeks. When, in comparison of these three arms, no exces-

sive morbidity is found, the first arm is dropped and replaced with the next higher dose arm, which is 81.6 Gy in 68 fractions, 34 treatment days over 7 weeks; if possible, proceed in the same fashion, dropping arm B and replacing it with arm E for a total dose of 86.4 Gy in 72 fractions over 36 days in 7.5 weeks. By progressing in this stepwise fashion we hope to be able to find the highest tolerable dose delivered by two fractions a day, not changing each fraction size, but rather the total dose. This study has now been active for approximately one year, and data so far have not indicated excessive morbidity, but the projected completion date of that study does not occur until July, 1988.

25. Brachytherapy in Head and Neck Cancer

INTRODUCTION

C. C. WANG, M.D.

The method of radiation therapy for head and neck cancer may be external beam or interstitial (including intracavitary) implant or a combination of the two. The external beams include x-ray with energies of 4 to 10 mv from a linear accelerator, cobalt-60 machine, or electron beams with energies ranging from 4 to 18 Mev. Particle radiations consisting of protons and neutrons are still in the experimental stage and are used primarily as research tools.

Implant or brachytherapy is used with various isotopes which are placed within the tumor or adjacent to the tumor. The former is called interstitial implant and the latter is intracavitary implant. The radioisotopes for removable implants include radium-226, cesium-137, cobalt-60, iridium-192, gold-198, and iodine-125, among others.

External-beam irradiation is suitable for most lesions of the head and neck, and in most instances, it is the procedure of choice. It is commonly used as the major portion of the radiation to include the primary as well as the regional nodes. External-beam therapy may traverse the jaw, teeth, TM joint, or salivary gland resulting in radiation sequelae. For most external-beam therapy, the irradiated volume is generally large and the tumor dose is limited to 70 Gy in 7 weeks.

In contrast to external-beam therapy, interstitial implant is most suited to lesions of the lip, floor of the mouth, tongue, buccal mucosa, nasal vestibule, or skin. The irradiated volume generally is small, and therefore the total dose delivered is intense. The implant procedure requires skill, experience, and judgment. It is often used as a boost to the primary lesions. Unfortunately, inhomogeneity of dose distribution often unavoidably results in "hot" and "cold" spots. Interstitial implantation is not suitable for any lesions invading or adjacent to the mandible because of the risk of osteoradionecrosis. For most implants, the dose rate is low, ranging from 50 to 60 cGy per hour. From the radiobiologic standpoint, low-dose irradiation is more effective in local tumor control and there is a decrease in late radiation changes.

With a combination of external beam and interstitial implant, a dose of 70 to 80 Gy may be given without risk of complications. With the modern afterloading techniques, unnecessary exposure of the professional staff to radiation hazards is very much reduced.

It is to be noted that any treatment for cancer of the head and neck for local control should always be the prime objective. Cosmetic and functional results should also be taken into serious consideration. In highly selected instances, these two objectives can be better achieved by brachytherapy with or without external beam therapy than by external beam therapy alone.

The following chapters describe the experience of each author in the field of brachytherapy.

BRACHYTHERAPY OF CARCINOMA OF THE TONGUE (MOBILE PORTION) AND FLOOR OF THE MOUTH

FRANÇOIS ESCHWEGE, M.D.
CHRISTINE HAIE, M.D.
ALAIN GERBAULET, M.D.
JEAN-MARIE RICHARD, M.D.
GÉRARD MAMELLE, M.D.
PIERRE WIBAULT, M.D.
DANIEL CHASSAGNE, M.D.

Head and neck carcinomas represent 12 percent of tumors reported in France, approximately 30 percent of these being carcinomas of the mobile portion of the tongue and of the floor of the mouth.

Brachytherapy by iridium-192 (^{192}Ir) wires and pins was introduced at the Institut Gustave-Roussy by B. Pierquin and D. Chassagne in 1960 and has been practiced at this institution since that time. Currently, treatment by brachytherapy alone or combined with external radiotherapy is the standard treatment for T1, T2, and some T3 tumors of the oral cavity.

TECHNIQUES AND INDICATIONS

Wires of ^{192}Ir (half-life: 74 days; average energy of gamma rays: 0.31 Mev; HVL: 2 mm of lead) are used which consist of an alloy of 25 percent iridium and 75 percent platinum. The wires are coated with a 0.1-mm layer of platinum. Two sizes of wire are used, 0.1-mm diameter (total: 0.3 mm) and 0.3-mm diameter (total: 0.5 mm). Because the wires are not sufficiently rigid to be introduced directly into the tissues, implantation requires use of rigid guide material, either guide gutters or plastic tubes. Implantation is done under radiographic control with nonradioactive material to permit corrections and adjustments before introduction of the radioactive wires.

For the more frequent T1 and T2 tumors of the borders of the mobile part of the tongue with infiltration that does not exceed 12 mm, the guide gutter technique of the implantation is used. Twin guide gutters consisting of parallel tubes of stainless steel (external diameter: 1.8 mm) are used. The internal diameter of the tubes is sufficient to allow passage of the radioactive wires. The radioactive wire pairs are 40 mm in length and shaped like the letter M in cross section, with the parallel bars connected by a connecting bar 12 mm long.

Implantation is done under local anesthesia, with the patient in the sitting position. Two or three guide gutters are placed in a row from front to back. Their exact position is verified under fluoroscopy and corrected if necessary to obtain parallelism between the guide gutters.

If the lesion is greatly infiltrating, a sagittally oriented guide gutter is added at the points of maximum infiltration. Nylon sutures are placed under the heads of the twin guides, and the radioactive wires are then placed and rapidly inserted in the gutters. Next the guides are removed, and the sutures are gently tied over the wires. Dosimetry is then performed.

For minimally infiltrating tumors of the floor of the mouth, the guide gutter technique is used. Under local anesthesia, twin guide gutters are inserted vertically into each half of the tumor in a plane perpendicular to the long axis of the floor of the mouth. With some tumors it is possible to complete this implantation with a simple guide.

For infiltrating tumors of the mobile part of the tongue and floor of the mouth, the plastic techniques first described by Henscke is used. This technique utilizes plastic tubes containing the radioactive wires that are inserted through the skin. Under general anesthesia and with the patient supine, a projection of the tumor is drawn on the skin of the submental and submaxillary regions, and the points of entry of hollow guide needles are indicated.

It is usually necessary to implant 3 to 6 radioactive wires into the tumors. The wires (0.3 mm in diameter) are inserted into plastic tubes that have an internal diameter of 0.5 mm. The tubes containing the wires are placed in outer plastic tubes after the outer tubes have been inserted into the tumor.

Since it is not possible to insert the large plastic tubes directly into the tumor, the following pulling technique is used: (1) a hollow stainless steel guide needle is inserted into the tumor in a posterior to anterior direction by inserting the needle through the skin and soft tissues in the submaxillary region, then along the inner surface of the mandible to the tongue, and finally through the tongue to exit at the tip; (2) a nylon cord is passed through the guide needle, after which the needle is extracted; (3) the outer plastic tube is passed over the nylon cord in a posterior to anterior direction; and (4) the nylon cord is removed. A second guide needle is inserted and, like the first one, traverses through skin, muscle, and finally mucosa at the tip of the tongue. The anterior end of the nylon cord inserted through the first needle is passed through the guide needle in an anterior to posterior direction. The end of the plastic tube at the tip of the tongue, previously placed, is then passed along the nylon cord through mucosa and muscle to exit in the submaxillary region and the nylon cord is removed. A median loop of plastic tubing is thus formed for insertion of the radioactive wires.

With the same technique, right and left lateral loops of plastic tubing are placed. These extend from the skin in the submaxillary region, through the musculature, and finally through the mucosa of the tongue. Next, parallel tubes, spaced 1.5 to 2.5 cm from each other, are inserted posteriorly into the tumor. Depending on the results of the dosimetry calculations, a transverse loop of outer plastic tubing is added if the space between the anterior and posterior tubes is excessive. The tubes are immobilized with metallic buttons, and heparin solution is injected to clean blood clots from the tubes. The radioactive wires are inserted, but not necessarily into all of the tubes, after dosimetry is completed.

In all patients, dosimetry calculations are derived from both transverse tomographic studies and computer-generated dosimetry data. The dosimetry is based on the Paris System and the fundamental concept of the flexible relationship between the length of the radioactive wires and their spacing. According to the Paris System, when brachytherapy is used alone, the delivered dose is generally 70 Gy; when associated with external radiotherapy, the dose is approximately 25 to 30 Gy.

RESULTS

Tumors of the Mobile Portion of the Tongue

From 1970 to 1978, 155 patients were treated by brachytherapy for tumors of the mobile portion of the tongue at the Institut Gustave-Roussy. The protocol consisted of brachytherapy alone for T1 tumors and T2 tumors ≤3 cm, and for selected T3 tumors, and external radiotherapy combined with brachytherapy for T2 tumors >3 cm and for selected T3 tumors. In this series, 119 patients were treated exclusively by brachytherapy and 36 were treated by a combination of external radiotherapy and curietherapy. The 1979 UICC classification was used for all patients. The TNM classification of the tumors treated by curietherapy is shown in Table 1 and those treated by combined therapy in Table 2.

All patients were treated with iridium wires: the guide gutter technique was used in 104 patients (T1, 22%; T2, 60%; T3, 18%) and the plastic tube technique was used in five patients (T1, 2%; T2, 29%; T3, 68%). The mean dose used for curietherapy was 72 Gy. In patients treated with combined therapy, the external radiation dose was 50 Gy and was followed after a 3- to 5-week rest by curietherapy of 25 Gy.

TABLE 1   TNM Classification of Cases Treated by Brachytherapy Alone

	T1	T2	T3	Total
N0	21	53	19	93
N1	1	6	5	12
N2	0	0	3	3
N3	1	3	7	11
Total	23	62	34	119

TABLE 2   TNM Classification of Cases Given Combined Treatment

	T1	T2	T3	Total
N0	1	12	16	29
N1	—	1	2	3
N2	—	—	—	—
N3	—	2	2	4
Total	1	15	20	36

Figure 1 shows the 5-year survival (Kaplan-Meier) for patients treated by brachytherapy alone (50%) and by brachytherapy combined with external radiotherapy (31%). Table 3 shows the 5-year actuarial survival correlated with the classification of the tumors. Survival appeared to be better with brachytherapy alone than with combined treatment, but the difference may be due to patient selection. The local control rate was excellent (83%) and was related to the size of the tumor (Table 4). These results show that brachytherapy is a satisfactory treatment for tumors of the mobile tongue, and 75 percent of our patients with these tumors are treated with this modality alone or in combination with radiotherapy.

Complications consisted of mucosal necrosis (MN) and bone necrosis (BN). BN was infrequent with curietherapy alone (7%) and was more frequent with T3 tumors (15%). In patients treated by combined therapy, BN occurred in 19 percent and did not correlate with the size of the tumors (5 of 15 T2 and 2 of 20 T3 tumors).

Tumors of the Floor of the Mouth

From 1972 to 1978, 61 patients with tumors of the floor of the mouth were treated at the Institut Gustave-Roussy by curietherapy alone (55 patients) or by combined treatment (6 patients). The 1979 UICC TNM classification was used. Table 5 shows the TNM classification of the tumors. In patients with poor general health or with extensive tumors, curietherapy was combined with external radiotherapy. Combined ther-

TABLE 3   Five-Year Crude Survival Rate and Size of Tumor

	T1	T2	T3	Total
Brachytherapy	62% (23)	50% (62)	35% (34)	50% (119)
Combined treatment	— (1)	40% (15)	25% (20)	35% (36)

TABLE 4   Local Recurrence Rate and Size of Tumor

	T1	T2	T3
Brachytherapy	4%	6,5%	14%
Combined treatment	—	20%	50%

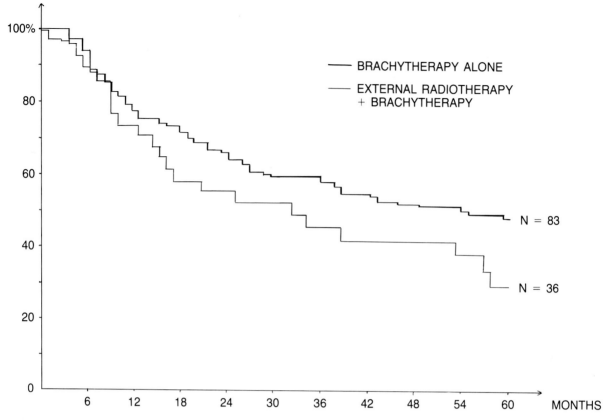

Figure 1 Survival rate for tumors of the mobile part of the tongue (Kaplan-Meier method).

TABLE 5 TNM Classification of Tumors of Floor of Mouth

	T1	T2	T3	T4	Total
N0	19	22	2	1	44
N1	2	7	3	—	12
N2	1	1	—	—	2
N3	—	2	1	—	3
Total	22	32	6	6	61

apy was used for one T1 and five T2 tumors. No T3 or T4 tumors were treated with combined therapy.

At 5 years, the survival (Kaplan-Meier) was 77 percent for patients treated with curietherapy alone and 18 percent for patients treated with combined therapy (Fig. 2). There were no local recurrences with T1 and T3 tumors, but six occurred in 32 (18%) T2 tumors. Two of the five T2 tumors treated with combined therapy developed local recurrences. Three patients died of a second primary cancer. The most frequent cause of death was distant metastases, which developed in 8 of 61 (13%) of patients. Two of these latter patients also had regional lymph nodal recurrences.

The most common complication was necrosis. Among the 61 patients, 19 (31%) had mucosa necrosis and 17 (28%) had bone necrosis, which was severe in 14 patients. Size of tumor and technique were not clearly correlated with bone necrosis; however, proximity of tumor to mandible and dental extractions appeared to be important factors. The onset of bone necrosis usually occurred within 2 years (median 19 months), and the necrosis persisted for approximately 3 years. Bone or mucosal necrosis was not related to prognosis, since the percentage NED at 3 years was the same with or without necrosis. Thus, the local control (90% of tumors) achieved in this series recommend brachytherapy for treatment of tumors of the floor of the mouth, with bone necrosis and distant metastases being the major problems associated with this treatment.

CONCLUSIONS

Brachytherapy with ^{192}Ir implants is an excellent treatment for carcinomas of the mobile tongue and the floor of the mouth. Excellent control of T1, T2, and some T3 tumors was achieved in this series. Complications were infrequent after treatment of the tongue cancers; however, with floor of mouth cancers, necrosis of bone adjacent to the tumors occurred in a significant number of patients.

The results with the treatment of limited tumors was the same as that achieved with surgery in terms of local control and survival. The advantage of treat-

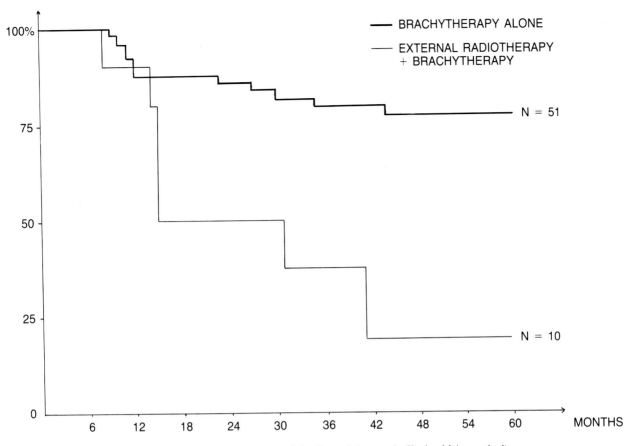

Figure 2 Survival rate for tumors of the floor of the mouth (Kaplan-Meier method).

ment with brachytherapy is the preservation of the functional status and quality of life that is achieved with the technique.

REFERENCES

1. Haie C, Gerbaulet A, Wibault P, Chassagne D, Marandas P. Résultats de la curiethérapie et de l'association radiothérapie transcutanée curiethérapie dans 155 cas de cancers de la langue mobile. Expérience de l'Institut Gustave-Roussy de 1970 à 1970. Actualités de Carcinologie Cervico-faciale. No 9, Paris: Masson et Cie, 1983.
2. Henscke U, Hilaris BS, Mahan GD. Afterloading in interstitial and intracavitary radiation therapy. Am J Roentgenol 1963; 90:386–395.
3. Pierquin B, Chassagne D, Chahbazian CM, Wilson JF. Brachytherapy. St. Louis: Warren H. Green Inc, 1978.
4. Pierquin B, Chassagne D, Perez R. Précis de curiethérapie. Paris: Masson et Cie, 1964.
5. Pierquin B, Chassagne D. La préparation non radioactive en curiethérapie interstitielle de contact. J Radiol 1972; 43:65–72.
6. Pierquin B, Chassagne D, Baillet F, Castro JR. The place of implantation in tongue and floor of mouth cancer. JAMA 19791; 215:961–963.
7. Pierquin B, Chassagne D, Cachin Y, Baillet F, Fournelle Le Buis F. Carcinomes épidermoides de la langue mobile et du plancher buccal. Acta Radiol 1970; 9:465–480.
8. Raynal M, Chassagne D, Pierquin B. Utilisation d'un mandrin plastique dans la technique d'endocuriethérapie par tubes plastiques. Ann de Radiol 1965; 8:393–396.

ROLE OF INTERSTITIAL IRRADIATION IN THE TREATMENT OF PRIMARY AND RECURRENT TUMORS OF TONSILLAR REGION AND SOFT PALATE

A. M. NISAR SYED, M.D., F.R.C.S.(Lond)
F.R.C.S.(Edin), D.M.R.T.(Eng)
AJMEL A. PUTHAWALA, M.D.

External irradiation alone has been proved efficacious in the treatment of many early-stage head and neck cancers. Several recent studies have reported long-term local tumor control as high as 70 to 80 percent for T1 and T2 carcinoma of the tonsillar region treated by external irradiation alone. However, in contrast, irradiation alone in the treatment of locally advanced (T3 and T4) lesions has shown poor local control, i.e., 20 to 35 percent.[1-3] This is apparently due to the large tumor volume that is frequently associated with hypoxic radioresistant cell populations. Much higher doses of radiation are required to sterilize these tumors. Several investigators have recommended radiation doses of 6000 to 6500 rads in 6 to 7 weeks for T1 and T2 lesions and 7000 to 8000 rads over 8 to 9 weeks for T3 and T4 lesions.[1-4] In spite of higher doses of external irradiation, which are often associated with high morbidity, results obtained so far for locally advanced cancer of the tonsillar region are unsatisfactory. The surgical salvage rate for these patients also remains poor. Adjuvant systemic chemotherapy with irradiation and/or surgery also has failed to show appreciable improvement in overall survival of patients with advanced or recurrent head and neck cancers.

In 1974, we began to use interstitial irradiation in the treatment of recurrent head and neck cancers with gratifying results.[5,6] Subsequently, we started the treatment protocol for various primary head and neck cancers to be treated with definitive radiation therapy. All patients have been treated with a combination of limited external irradiation to the primary site and the neck, followed by interstitial iridium-192 implant boost. This regimen allows safe delivery of relatively higher tumor doses and considerable sparing of the surrounding normal tissues, which results in higher local tumor control and less acute and late radiation sequelae. We will discuss here our clinical experience in the treatment of primary and recurrent or persistent cancer of the tonsillar region and soft palate utilizing a combination of external and interstitial irradiation for primary tumors and interstitial implant alone for recurrent cancers.

MATERIALS AND METHODS (Table 1)

Between February of 1974 and March of 1982, a total of 127 patients with a histologically proved diagnosis of carcinoma of the tonsillar region and soft palate were analyzed with a minimum follow-up period of 2 years. In the primary treatment group there were 80 patients, and in the retreatment group, 47 patients. In the former group there were 54 males and 26 females ranging in age from 38 to 82 years (median 62); in the latter group there were 32 males and 15 females ranging in age from 36 to 78 years (median 60). Sixty-five of the 80 (81%) patients in the primary treatment group presented with locally advanced (stage III and IV) tumors. Thirty-five of the 80 (44%) patients presented with clinically palpable ipsilateral neck disease. Only one had contralateral disease, and three additional patients had bilateral disease. Greater than 60 percent of the patients had extension of their tumor to the base of the tongue, and 70 percent had extension of the tumors to the soft palate. Twenty patients who were classified as having primary tumor of the soft palate are included in this study because the tumor extended clearly to involve either the anterior tonsillar pillar or the tonsillar bed. All patients with recurrent disease had received external irradiation to a minimum tumor dose of 5000 rads to the oropharynx 4 to 36 months prior to re-irradiation. Twenty-six of these 47 (56%) patients also had recurrent neck disease besides recurrent tumor at the primary site. Twelve patients had previous composite resection of the primary with radical neck dissection, three patients had only local excision, 15 additional patients had radical neck dissection as part of the initial treatment. Seventeen of the 47 (36%) were treated with external irradiation alone with doses of 7000 to 8000 rads. Ten of these 47 patients had also received systemic chemotherapy.

TREATMENT TECHNIQUE (Primary Group)

All the patients underwent a course of megavoltage external irradiation to the primary site and the upper neck nodes through bilateral parallel opposing ports (except three patients who were treated with ipsilateral ports) to a tumor dose of 4500 to 5000 rads over $4^1/_2$ to $5^1/_2$ weeks. The lower neck was also treated through a single anterior port to include the lower cer-

TABLE 1   Primary Carcinoma of the Tonsillar Region and Soft Palate: Distribution of Patients according to TNM Classification

	N0	N1	N2	N3	Total
T1	3	—	—	—	3
T2	12	1	2	—	15
T3	19	6	13	5	43
T4	7	—	4	8	19
Total	41 (51%)	7 (9%)	19 (24%)	13 (16%)	80

vical nodes as well as supra- and infraclavicular lymph nodes to a similar dose. The interstitial iridium-192 implant was performed under general anesthesia 2 to 3 weeks after completion of external irradiation. Various techniques of interstitial implants were utilized to encompass the original extent of the tumor with adequate margins. The ipsilateral side of the soft palate and base of the tongue were implanted routinely in all patients. The residual palpable neck disease was also implanted using flexible plastic tube and button technique.[7,8] Computerized dosimetry was obtained in all cases (Figs. 1 and 2). Interstitial irradiation boost doses ranged between 2000 to 2500 rads over 50 to 60 hours for T1 and T2 tumors and 3000 to 4000 rads over 75 to 100 hours for T3 and T4 tumors. Similar radiation doses were given to the persistent neck masses, depending on the initial N staging.

All patients with recurrent disease were treated with interstitial iridium-192 implant alone. Similar techniques were utilized to encompass the visible and palpable extent of the disease with adequate margins. Palpable neck disease was always separately implanted, using a minimum of 2 planes to a maximum of 4 planes. A minimum tumor dose of 5000 to 6000 rads over 100 to 134 hours was delivered. The radioactive iridium-192 seed ribbons were afterloaded into

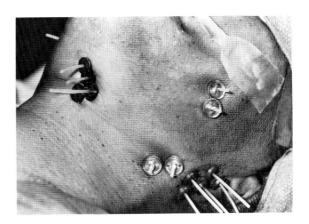

Figure 2   Patient with implanted afterloading plastic tubes for squamous cell carcinoma (T3 N0 M0) of left tonsillar region.

the implanted plastic tubes with due radiation precautions in the patient's room. The empty implant tubes were again removed under general anesthesia with orotracheal intubation. Elective tracheostomy was performed in a few patients with extensive tumor involving the vallecula and laryngopharynx.

RESULTS (Table 2)

The loco-regional control is defined as complete resolution of visible and palpable disease. Patients who expired within 6 months after treatment in the recurrent group and 12 months in the primary group were automatically counted as treatment failure. The overall local control of the disease was achieved in 67 of the 80 (84%) patients, with a minimum follow-up period of 24 months to a maximum of 84 months. Seven patients failed in the neck only, and two patients failed at the primary site as well as in the neck. Both of these patients had T4 N3 lesions. Of the 30 patients who underwent iridium-192 implant for residual palpable neck disease at the time of interstitial implant to the primary site, none developed recurrent metastatic neck disease. Seven of the nine patients (78%) who initially failed in the neck were subsequently salvaged by radical neck dissection (three patients) and

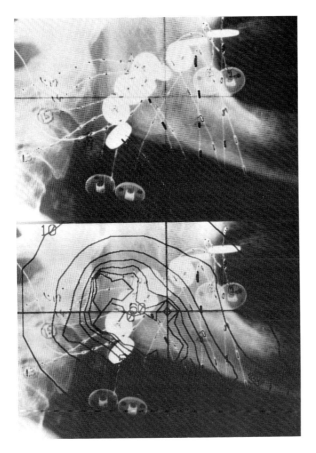

Figure 1   AP (top) and lateral (bottom) roentgenograms of left tonsillar region implant for stage T3 N0 M0 carcinoma, with overlying computerized dosimetry plot.

TABLE 2   Primary Carcinoma of Tonsillar Region and Soft Palate: Tumor Control according to TNM Distribution*

	N0	N1	N2	N3	Total
T1	3/3	—	—	—	3/3
T2	12/12	1/1	1/2	—	14/15
T3	16/19	5/6	8/13	3/5	32/34
T4	5/7	—	3/4	3/8	11/19
Total	36/41 (88%)	6/7 (86%)	12/19 (63%)	6/13 (46%)	60/80 (75%)†

*Minimum follow-up period of 24 months to maximum of 84 months (median, 40 months).

†7 patients failed in neck only. Therefore, primary was controlled in 67/80 (84%) of patients.

interstitial re-irradiation (four patients). Five of 13 patients (38%) who failed at the primary site were ultimately salvaged, three with surgery and two with interstitial re-irradiation. Thus an ultimate loco-regional control was possible in 81 percent of patients; 3-year absolute survival for the entire group was 81 percent while 5-year actuarial survival was 72 percent. Thirty-five of 47 (75%) patients with recurrent disease achieved loco-regional tumor control with re-irradiation. Ninety percent of the patients with uncontrolled disease were dead within 6 to 8 months. Two-year absolute survival for these patients was 42 percent. The most frequent cause of death in this group of patients was poor nutrition and inability to thrive despite local tumor control. Six patients developed distant metastases and four additional patients died of new primary tumor in the upper aerodigestive tract.

COMPLICATIONS

The expected mucosal reactions were mild-to-moderate in most patients; loss of taste was transient and loss of saliva was moderate since the dose of external irradiation was limited to 4500 to 5000 rads. Transient mucosal ulceration at the implanted site, noted in 30 percent of the patients, usually healed on conservative management within 8 to 12 weeks. Late sequalae such as soft tissue necrosis or osteoradionecrosis of the mandible occurred in five patients (6%). Eleven of the 47 (23%) patients in the retreatment group developed severe complications such as soft tissue necrosis (four patients) and soft tissue necrosis plus osteoradionecrosis (seven patients). Two of these seven patients also developed pharyngocutaneous fistulization. Six of these 11 patients with such complications had evidence of uncontrolled disease and died within 12 to 18 months after re-irradiation.

DISCUSSION

It has become clear over the past two decades that small T1 and T2 tumors of the tonsillar region can be successfully treated with external irradiation alone. However, locally advanced tumors require much more aggressive treatment. Several investigators now recommend preoperative external irradiation of 5000 to 6000 rads followed by surgical resection of the primary tumor with radical neck dissection for patients with T3 and T4 tumors of the oropharynx.

A 3-year disease-free survival of 41 to 65 percent has been cited.[9] On the other hand, Perez et al and Kaplan et al found no significant improvement in the ultimate results by addition of surgery.[1,2] Furthermore, the incidence of complications was considerably higher in the patients treated with combined therapy than in those treated with irradiation alone. Gelinas and Fletcher reported a 32 percent surgical salvage rate in 106 patients who failed after definitive irradiation for carcinoma of the faucial arch, the tonsillar fossa, and the base of the tongue.[10] Williams reported

a 16 percent surgical salvage rate in 144 patients treated for head and neck cancer initially by surgery alone.[11]

In the past decade systemic chemotherapy, either with a single agent or with multiple agents, has been utilized by several investigators as an adjuvant to surgery and/or irradiation in the treatment of locally advanced head and neck cancers. A complete remission rate of 30 to 60 percent was reported.[12] However, chemotherapy has not proved successful in the retreatment of recurrent head and neck tumors.

We have previously reported 64 patients with persistent or recurrent head and neck tumors after definitive irradiation with or without surgery; 49 percent of these 64 patients achieved complete local tumor control with good palliation for 18 to 36 months following re-irradiation with interstitial iridium-192 implant.[5,6] We have also reported similar results in the retreatment of recurrent carcinoma of the anterior mobile tongue and the base of the tongue.[8] In the present series we report excellent local tumor control in relatively advanced stages of carcinoma of the tonsillar region with absolute 3-year disease-free survival of 81 percent and 5-year actuarial survival of 72 percent. The ultimate salvage of the patients either failing at the primary site or in the neck, using either surgery or interstitial iridium-192 implant alone, was feasible and has yielded a 54 percent salvage rate. The late severe radiation sequelae such as soft tissue necrosis and osteoradionecrosis are minimal in our series (6%). These late side effects of radiation could be as high as 50 percent in patients who are cured of their disease after high-dose megavoltage external irradiation.[13]

The use of interstitial irradiation alone in the present study for the patients with recurrent tumors of the tonsillar region has also proved quite effective, with 42 percent of the patients surviving two or more years with no evidence of disease after re-irradiation with interstitial iridium-192 implant. These results are encouraging. In the retreatment group, as expected, the severe complication rate of 23 percent is relatively high and is most likely related to the radiation dose employed. We are now studying the effects of some chemotherapeutic agents such as 5-fluorouracil or hydroxyurea, given concurrently with interstitial irradiation. We are also investigating the use of localized interstitial hyperthermia with interstitial irradiation as radiosensitizing agent, which may allow reduction of radiation dose and thus reduce radiation sequelae and improve tumor control.

REFERENCES

1. Kaplan R, Million RR, Cassisi NJ. Carcinoma of the tonsil: Results of radical irradiation with surgery reserved for radiation failure. Laryngoscope 1977; 87:600–607.
2. Perez CA, Purdy JA, Breaux BA, Ogura JH, von Essen S. Carcinoma of the tonsillar fossa. Cancer 1982; 50:2314–2322.
3. Fayos JV, Morales P. Radiation therapy of carcinoma of the tonsillar region. Int J Radiat Oncol biol Phys 1983; 9:139–144.

4. Shukovsky LJ, Fletcher GH. Time-dose and tumor volume relationships in the irradiation of squamous cell carcinoma of the tonsillar fossa. Radiology 1973; 107:621–626.
5. Syed AMN, Feder BH, George FW, Neblett D. Iridium-192 afterloaded implant in the treatment of head and neck cancers. Br J Radiol 1978; 51:814–820.
6. Syed AMN, Puthawala AA, Fleming P, Burton RH, George FW. Afterloading interstitial implant in head and neck cancer. Arch Otolaryngol 1980; 106:541–546.
7. Syed AMN, Feder BH. Techniques of afterloading interstitial implants. Radiol Clin 1977; 46:458–475.
8. Puthawala AA, Syed AMN, Neblett D, McNamara C. The role of afterloading iridium (IR-192) implant in the management of carcinoma of the tongue. Int J Radiat Oncol Biol Phys 1981; 7:407–412.
9. Rabuzzi DD, Mickler AS, Chung AT, Chatter DJ, Sagerman RH. Treatment results of combined high-dose preoperative radiotherapy and surgery for oropharyngeal cancer. Laryngoscope 1982; 92:989–992.
10. Gelinas M, Fletcher GH. Incidence and causes of local failure of irradiation in squamous cell carcinoma of faucial arch, tonsillar fossa and base of tongue. Radiology 1973; 108:393–398.
11. Williams RC. Recurrent head and neck cancer: The results of treatment. Br J Surg 1974; 61:691–697.
12. O'Connor D, Clifford P, Edwards WG, Dailey VM, Durden-Smith J, Hollis BA, Calman RM. Long-term results of VDM and radiotherapy in advanced head and neck cancer. Int J Radiat Oncol Biol Phys 1982; 8:1525–1531.
13. Larson DL, Lindberg RD, Lane E, Goepfert H. Major complications of radiotherapy in cancer of the oral cavity and oropharynx. Am J Surg 1983; 1146:531–536.

HEAD AND NECK BRACHYTHERAPY EMPHASIZING AFTERLOADING REMOVABLE OROPHARYNGEAL IMPLANTS

DON R. GOFFINET, M.D.

There are many implant techniques available for the treatment of head and neck cancers. At present, both removable afterloading and permanent implant techniques are performed, primarily involving the use of iridium-192 seeds for the former and iodine-125 seeds for the latter (Table 1). Permanent implants are useful for irradiating involved surgical margins at the primary site or neck and for neoplastic extension to the ptergyopalatine area and the base of the skull.[1-4] [125]I seeds may be implanted by the use of such devices as the Mick or Scott applicators, or may be inserted into the central core of a resterilizable, absorbable suture and sewn into the tissues intraoperatively with preplanned spacing and symmetry.[5-8] A variety of surface applicators, molds, moulages, and afterloading catheter techniques utilizing either high-intensity ^{125}I seeds, ^{192}Ir line sources, or cesium-137 sources are also useful for delivering intracavitary booster radiation doses to such sites as the nasopharynx and nasal cavity, and may also be applied postoperatively for neoplasms of the sinuses and orbits.

Since the use of [125]I Vicryl sutures is discussed elsewhere in this book, I will describe here the results of afterloading iridium-192 implants in the oropharynx, one of the more technically difficult head and neck areas to implant successfully, but one that, once the techniques are mastered, is amenable to high local control rates through the use of interstitial radiation boosts.

Cancers of the oral cavity have long been treated either with interstitial radioisotope implantation alone or by combinations of external beam irradiation and implantation.[9,10] However, since oropharyngeal neoplasms are less accessible than those in the oral cavity, fewer interstitial implants have been performed in these sites, although excellent results in limited numbers of patients have been obtained by various authors.[1,10-14] Resection of tonsillopalatine neoplasms is often the treatment of choice and may be followed by the use of a prosthetic obturator to restore speech, with excellent results.[11,15-18] Operative procedures on the base of the tongue have been accompanied by aspi-

TABLE 1 Brachytherapy: Head and Neck Cancer

[125]I Permanent Implant
  Suture carrier
    Surgical margins
    Neck (and carotid)
  Applicator or suture
    Pterygoid
    Base of skull

Removable Implant
  Oral cavity
    Floor of mouth
    Tongue
    Other sites
  Oropharynx
    Base of tongue
    Tonsillopalatine
    Oropharyngeal walls
  Laryngopharynx
  Lymph nodes (vs. [125]I)
  Facial skin, nose, etc.
  Intracavitary — molds, plaques, catheters
    Nasopharynx
    Nose
    Sinuses
    Ear canal
    Postresection

A portion of this chapter is reprinted from Proceedings of 5th Annual Brachytherapy Oncology Update, Memorial Sloan-Kettering Hospital, New York, March 1984. Permission of Basil Hilaris, M.D.

ration and garbled speech; total laryngectomy is frequently required, either at the time of base tongue resection or as a secondary procedure for chronic aspiration.[19-24] A radiotherapeutic alternative to surgery has therefore been developed which utilizes combined external beam and interstitial irradiation, taking into account the patterns of spread of these tumors and including the surrounding tissues such as the tonsilloglossal groove, lateral pharyngeal walls, epiglottis when necessary, and most importantly, the pharyngoepiglottic folds in the implant volume when appropriate.[12]

In this chapter, the results of a 7-year experience with oropharyngeal neoplasms involving the tonsil, tonsillar pillars, soft palate, and base tongue, all implanted by removable ^{192}Ir techniques, will be presented.

MATERIALS AND METHODS

All newly referred patients with head and neck cancer are seen by a multimodality tumor board in which head and neck surgeons, radiation therapists, medical oncologists, dentists, speech therapists, social workers, and dietitians are all involved in the initial evaluation. Fifty-four previously untreated patients with oropharyngeal squamous carcinomas were evaluated by the combined Head and Neck Tumor Board between 1975 and 1983.

Tonsillopalatine Implants

Twenty-four patients with neoplasms in these locations were treated between 1975 and 1983 by removable ^{192}Ir implants. American Joint Committee on Cancer (AJC) staging and TNM distribution are shown in Tables 2 and 3. External beam irradiation consisting of 5000 to 5500 rads in 5 weeks was given to the primary lesion and lower cervical lymph nodes at a rate of 200 rads per day, five fractions per week, with

TABLE 2 Tonsillopalatine Swage Implants: Stanford 1975–83 (24 Patients)

Stage (AJC)	No. of Patients
I	4
II	3
III	9
IV	8

TABLE 3 TNM Staging of Patients with Tonsillopalatine Swage Implants: Stanford 1975–83 (24 Patients)

Tumor	No. of Patients	Nodes	No. of Patients
T1	7	N0	11
T2	10	N1	7
T3	6	N2	4
T4	1	N3	2

a 6 Mev linear accelerator. The spinal cord dose was limited to 4000 rads or less. The primary sites were generally treated by opposed lateral portals, while the cervical lymph nodes were irradiated by an anterior port with a midline bar at a depth of 3 cm. If multiple lymph nodes were clinically involved or if massive adenopathy was present, the midline bar was omitted, and a mediastinal T field was irradiated instead.

Instead of inserting trocars percutaneously to implant these oropharyngeal sites (tonsil, soft palate, and tonsillar pillars), a method of crimping or swaging needles onto the ends of ^{192}Ir seed-containing nylon ribbons was developed which allows the implant to be performed intraorally by sewing the ^{192}Ir seed-containing ribbons into position.[25] The implant was preplanned as previously described.[6] Once all of the ribbons were positioned, the seed-containing ends (which were kept in a shielded, sterile container until that time) were drawn into the implant volume. The ribbons were then stabilized by applying hemostatic clips, to which 3–0 silk traction sutures were tied to both ends so as to facilitate the removal of the implant. If the neoplasm extended to the level of the tonsillopharyngeal junction, lateral percutaneously inserted loops which cross the pharyngoepiglottic fold (to be described) were added. After the implant was completed, orthogonal localizing radiographs were obtained, and a General Electric treatment planning computer was used to obtain isodose distributions and radiation dose rates to tissue volumes.[26]

Base of Tongue Carcinoma

Between 1975 and 1983, 30 patients with base of tongue carcinomas have been treated by either (1) resection of the primary neoplasm and simultaneous radical or modified neck dissections if indicated, combined with postoperative irradiation, or (2) external beam irradiation followed by removable ^{192}Ir implantation approximately 2 weeks after completion of the course of external beam irradiation. Sixteen patients were treated by interstitial and external beam irradiation, while 14 were treated by surgery and postoperative irradiation by surgeon preference. These 30 patients all had squamous cell carcinomas, were previously untreated, and were evaluated by the combined Head and Neck Tumor Board. All underwent direct laryngoscopy and examination under anesthesia prior to the initiation of treatment. The AJC staging of the patient groups is shown in Table 4. The patients in the two treatment categories were equally distributed with regard to the various stages.

The surgical group, in general, was managed by composite resection and radical neck dissection, with or without supraglottic or total laryngectomy. In the surgical group, postoperative irradiation was delivered with a 6-Mev linear accelerator through opposed lateral portals to the primary site, which received at least 5000 rads in 5 weeks (spinal cord dose limited to 4000 rads) with booster doses of 6000 to 6600 rads

TABLE 4 Staging (AJC) of Base of Tongue Carcinoma:
Stanford 1975–83 (30 Patients)

Surgery and Radiation Therapy (14)		Radiation Therapy and ^{192}Ir (16)	
Stage	No. of Patients	Stage	No. of Patients
II	2	II	3
III	9	III	5
IV	3	IV	8

in 6 to 6^{1}/$_{2}$ weeks if the surgical margins were close or involved. Elective supplemental bilateral low cervical nodal irradiation was also given, utilizing an anterior portal for a total dose of 5000 rads in 5 weeks to a depth of 3 cm with a midline bar, unless massive adenopathy was present, in which case a mediastinal T field was used.

Patients managed by radiation therapy alone received 5000 to 5500 rads to the primary site at a similar rate, with the spinal cord dose limited to 3800 rads, while 5000 rads in 5 weeks were delivered to the low cervical lymph nodes, as already described, using a midline bar in most cases. Approximately 2 to 3 weeks after the completion of external beam irradiation, the ^{192}Ir base of tongue and pharyngoepiglottic fold implant was carried out.

Our initial implants consisted of multiple percutaneously placed trocar pairs, the first of which entered the submental skin and emerged in the vallecula; the other pairs extended in an anterior direction to the level of the circumvallate papillae. The trocar pairs were inserted into the submental skin close to each other and diverged as they approached the base of the tongue, so as to effectively "cross" the deep or free ends of the loop that is ultimately formed when a hollow nylon ribbon is inserted as the trocars are removed; in addition, inferior trocar approximation submentally helps to spare the lingual arteries, which are more laterally placed.

After the first eight implants, which were limited to the tongue, two patients suffered relapses at the base of tongue-pharyngoepiglottic fold junction independently of implant radiation doses. Therefore, a technique was developed in which a lateral cervical trocar pair was placed superior to the hyoid bone, with the posterior trocar passing anterior to the carotid artery to emerge at the posterolateral oropharyngeal wall junction, while the second anterior trocar emerged in front of the tonsillar pillars. In this way, a loop was formed which traversed the oropharyngeal wall, pharyngoepiglottic fold, and base of the tonsil. If necessary, a second, more inferiorly placed lateral loop can also be positioned inferior to the hyoid bone if the oropharyngeal wall at this level is involved by inferolateral extension of the base of tongue neoplasm. Therefore, a simple three- to four-loop submentally placed ^{192}Ir implant was transformed into a complex, multiloop procedure extending from the vallecula an-

teriorly into the oral tongue. Additional loops may be placed at right angles in the base of the tongue if the anterior-posterior row of loops, which are usually 2 cm across at the tongue surface and separated from each other by 1 cm, do not adequately cover the entire oropharyngeal tongue surface. In addition, lateral ipsilateral or bilateral pharyngoepiglottic fold and tonsilloglossal groove loops are also inserted, depending on the location of the neoplasm in the base of the tongue and its anatomic extent.

The spacing and symmetry of all implants were preplanned, as previously described. A tracheostomy was performed either when the base of tongue was implanted or when the pharyngoepiglottic fold region was included in the procedure. Prophylactic antibiotics were begun preoperatively, and corticosteroids were administered intravenously for the first 48 to 72 hours after implantation. Again, computerized dosimetry utilizing orthogonal radiographs was used to determine radiation doses to tissue volumes, as well as isodose distributions.

RESULTS

Tonsillopalatine Implants

Table 5 gives details of the implant parameters used, whereby a mean dose of 2800 rads was delivered to an 18.5-cc volume, utilizing an average seed strength of 0.46 mg Ra eq; the total mean milligram radium equivalents implanted was 10.8 for these 24 implants. Twenty of these 24 patients have remained without evidence of local or distant failure (83%) after a mean follow-up of 33 months (Table 6). Of the four failures, two occurred in the implant volume, either in a low-dose area or in an inadequately implanted site, while the third occurred in the cervical region. A single patient who died with distant metastases did so without a local recurrence.

TABLE 5 Mean Implant Parameters of Tonsillopalatine
Swage Implants: Stanford 1975–83 (24 Patients)

Dose (rads)	2800
Mg Ra equiv	
Total	10.8
Per seed	0.46
Volume	18.5 cc

TABLE 6 Results of Tonsillopalatine Swage Implants:
Stanford 1975–83 (24 Patients)

NED	20/24 (83%)
Failures	4/24
Implant volume	2
Neck	1
Metastases	1
Mean F/U	33 mos. 6–73

Table 7 lists the NED (no evidence of disease) percentages for the various anatomic sites of the primary neoplasms. No patient has relapsed with a tonsil cancer, but one of the eight patients with soft palate cancers had a local relapse and another failed in a cervical lymph node. In the four patients whose cancers involved the adjacent anterior tonsillar pillars, one had base of tongue extension and a second developed distant metastases. The base of tongue was *not* implanted in the single patient who relapsed at that site.

Finally, survival for these 24 patients is presented in Table 8: 13 patients are alive, while four have succumbed to their neoplasms, five died with second primary malignant disease, and two expired from intercurrent causes. Eight patients had second primary neoplasms, including three involving the esophagus and two in head and neck sites.

Only two postimplant complications were noted in these 24 patients, both self-limited and mild. A single patient developed acute bilateral parotitis immediately following implantation, but this cleared spontaneously in a few days; the second patient developed a soft tissue palatal ulcer, which ultimately healed with antibiotic therapy and superficial debridement.

Base of Tongue Carcinoma

Table 9 presents the results of treatment for the 30 patients with base of tongue carcinomas. The 14 patients who underwent resection and postoperative irradiation have been followed for a mean of 40 months, and five are without evidence of disease. There have been relapses in nine of these 14 patients, including five failures in the tongue, seven in cervical lymph

TABLE 7 Results of Tonsillopalatine Swage Implants Based on Primary Site: Stanford 1975–83 (24 Patients)

Primary Sites	NED
Tonsil 12	12 (100%)
Soft palate 8	6 (75%)
Tonsil pillar 4	2 (50%)

TABLE 8 Results of Tonsillopalatine Swage Implants and Occurence of Second Primaries: Stanford 1975–83 (24 patients)

Result	No. of Patients
Alive	13
Dead	11
Died of cancer	4
2nd 1°	5
Intercurrent	2
Second Primaries	8
Esophagus	3
Head & neck	2 (FOM, FVC)
Lung	1
Ovary	1
Breast	1

TABLE 9 Results of Treatment for Base of Tongue Carcinoma: Stanford 1975–83 (30 patients)

	Surgery and Radiation Therapy (14)	Radiation Therapy ^{192}Ir (16)
Mean F/U	40 mos.	34 mo.
NED	5 (36%)	11 (69%)
Relapse		
Tongue	*5 (36%)	2 (12%)
Neck	*7 (50%)	1 (6%)
Metastases	*4 (29%)	2 (12%)
	*9 Pateints	

nodes, and four instances of distant metastases. Two total and three partial laryngectomies were performed in this group, along with 12 radical and two partial neck dissections.

Eleven of the 16 patients treated with external beam irradiation and ^{192}Ir implantation remain without evidence of disease, while only two have failed in the tongue (prior to the implantation of the pharyngoepiglottic fold). A single patient suffered relapse in a cervical lymph node, while distant metastases have occurred in two patients. The single patient in this group who failed in the neck received external beam irradiation in another institution, but elective cervical lymph node irradiation was not given. Four of the 12 irradiated patients had radical neck dissections at the time of implantation and none have relapsed in the neck. (The ^{192}Ir radiation doses to tissue volumes are shown in Table 10.) Seven of the 14 surgical patients are alive, four without evidence of disease; 13 of the 16 irradiated patients are alive, 11 remaining NED.

Complications occurred in almost 70 percent of the surgical patients, including fistulas, wound infections, dysphagia, and aspiration. A variety of mainly self-limited complications occurred in seven of the 14 irradiated patients, including tongue ulcers and temporary dysphagia, each in two patients; miscellaneous complications took place in three other patients. Local control appears to be improved in the irradiated patients compared to the 14 patients treated by resection and postoperative irradiation.

DISCUSSION

Extensive base of tongue resections which sacrifice hypoglossal nerve function, performed without a laryngectomy, frequently result in aspiration, poor speech, and a difficult existence for the patient. Combined total glossectomy and laryngectomy, while po-

TABLE 10 Implant Doses for Base of Tongue Carcinoma: Stanford 1975–83 (16 Patients)

Implant Dose (rads)	Volume (Mean)
1,500	150 cc
2,500	74 cc

tentially curative in some patients with advanced base of tongue cancers, produces grave functional deficits. Composite resection of tonsillar and/or palatine cancers interferes less with function, and with proper postoperative rehabilitation and obturation of palate lesions, satisfactory results may be obtained. We were dissatisfied with the poor local control rates resulting from external beam irradiation alone for soft palate carcinomas, even when booster radiation doses totaling 7000 rads or more were given to the primary site.[11,27] We therefore utilized interstitial ^{192}Ir boosts after external beam radiation doses of 5000 to 5500 rads to the primary and cervical lymph nodes, with apparently improved local control. When necessary, radical neck dissection is carried out at the time of implantation for persistent adenopathy; complications are not increased when these procedures are performed simultaneously.

A tracheostomy is mandatory for patients receiving base of tongue implants; corticosteroids (dexamethasone) and prophylactic antibiotics are also used. When a tonsillopalatine neoplasm involves the base of the tongue or tonsilloglossal groove, a tracheostomy is performed prior to the addition of base of tongue implantation and/or pharyngoepiglottic fold looping to the standard swage implant at the primary site.

High local control rates have been obtained in all oropharyngeal sites implanted, and no base of tongue relapses have occurred since the high-dose implant volume was extended laterally by the pharyngoepiglottic fold brachytherapy technique. To obtain optimal results with minimal morbidity, we believe that careful preimplantation planning to obtain proper source placement and dose distribution is vital. Postimplant dosimetry calculates not only isodose distributions, but also dose rates to tissue volumes, which helps to eliminate overdosages. Complications from these techniques of oropharyngeal implantation are ordinarily self-limited and not severe. We believe that the intraoral implantation approach to the tonsillopalatine region and the complex, technically difficult percutaneous loop technique for the base of the tongue, tonsilloglossal groove, and pharyngoepiglottic fold are very effective in reducing the risk of local recurrence, compared to external beam irradiation alone. The epiglottis may also be implanted through the submental approach should the lingual surface of this structure be involved by direct extension from a carcinoma of the base of the tongue or vallecula.

SUMMARY

Between 1975 and 1983, 40 patients were treated with removable ^{192}Ir implants to either the base of tongue-pharyngoepiglottic fold region (16) or the tonsillopalatine area (24) combined with preimplantation external beam irradiation. Another 14 patients with base of tongue carcinomas underwent resection and postoperative external beam irradiation.

Twenty of the 24 patients with tonsillopalatine cancers (83%) are without evidence of disease; only two of the 24 patients experienced local recurrences. The 16 patients who underwent external beam radiation therapy and interstitial implantation of their base of tongue neoplasms had fewer local relapses (12% vs 36%), cervical lymph node failures (6% vs 50%), and distant metastases (12% vs 29%) than a group of 14 similarly staged patients with base of tongue cancers who were treated by resection and postoperative irradiation. We believe that implantation of the pharyngoepiglottic fold and lateral oropharyngeal wall regions appears to be the important radiotherapeutic variable in obtaining high local control rates in cancers of the base of the tongue.

REFERENCES

1. Goffinet DR, Martinez A, Fee WE. [125]I Vicryl suture implants as a surgical adjuvant in cancer of the head and neck. Int J Radiat Oncol Biol Phys In press.
2. Goffinet DR, Martinez A, Fee WE et al. Intraoperative pterygo-palatine ^{125}I seed implants. Int J Radiat Oncol Biol Phys 1983; 9:103–106.
3. Kim JH, Hilaris B. Iodine-125 source in interstitial tumor therapy. Am J Radiol 1974; 123:163–169.
4. Vikram B, Hilaris BS, Anderson L et al. Permanent iodine-125 implants in head and neck cancer. Cancer 1983; 51:1310–1314.
5. Martinez A, Goffinet DR, Palos B et al. Sterilization of ^{125}I seeds encased in Vicryl sutures for permanent interstitial implantation. Int J Radiat Oncol Biol Phys 1979; 5:411–413.
6. Palos B, Pooler D, Goffinet DR et al. A method for inserting ^{125}I seeds into Vicryl absorbable sutures in preparation for permanent implantation into tissues. Int J Radiat Oncol Biol Phys 1980; 6:381–385.
7. Sandor J, Palos B, Goffinet DR et al. Dose calculations for planar arrays of ^{192}Ir and ^{125}I seeds for brachytherapy. Applied Radiol 1979; 8:41–44.
8. Fee WE, Goffinet DR, Paryani S et al. Intraoperative iodine-125 implants: Their use in large tumors in the neck attached to the carotid artery. Arch otolaryngol 1983; 109:727–730.
9. Puthawala AA, Syed AMN, Neblett D et al. The role of afterloading iridium (^{192}Ir) implant in the management of carcinoma of the tongue. Int J Radiat Oncol Biol Phys 1981; 7:407–412.
10. Gilbert EH, Goffinet DR, Bagshaw MA. Carcinoma of the tongue and floor of the mouth: Fifteen years' experience with linear accelerator therapy. Cancer 1975; 35:1515–1525.
11. Fee WE, Schoeppel SL, Rubenstein R et al. Squamous cell carcinoma of the soft palate. Arch Otolaryngol 1979; 105:710–718.
12. Goffinet DR, Fee WE, Wells J et al. [192]Ir pharyngoepiglottic fold interstitial implants: The key to successful treatment of base of tongue carcinoma by radiation therapy. Cancer. In press.
13. Martin CL, Martin JA. Treatment of epithelioma of the lateral oropharynx with low intensity radium needle implants. Am J Roentgenol 1965; 93:7–18.
14. Syed AMN, Puthawala A, Fleming P et al. Afterloading interstitial implant in head and neck cancer. Arch Otolaryngol 1980; 106:541–546.
15. Healy GB, Strong MS, Uchmakli A et al. Carcinoma of the palatine arch. Am J Surg 1976; 132:498–503.
16. Kaplan R, Million RR, Cassisi NJ. Carcinoma of the tonsil: Results of radical irradiation with surgery reserved for radiation failure. Laryngoscope 1977; 87:600–607.
17. Mickler AS, Chung CT, Clutter DJ et al. Treatment results of combined high-dose preoperative radiotherapy and surgery

for oropharyngeal cancer. Laryngoscope 1982; 92:989–992.

18. Perez CA, Purdy JA, Breaux SR et al. Carcinoma of the tonsillar fossa. Cancer 1982; 50:2314–2322.

19. Dupont JB, Guillamondegui OM, Jesse RH. Surgical treatment of advanced carcinomas of the base of the tongue. Am J Surg 1978; 136:501–503.

20. Harrold CC. Surgical treatment of cancer of the base of the tongue. Am J Surg 1976; 42:670–674.

21. Jesse RH, Lindberg RD. The efficacy of combining radiation therapy with a surgical procedure in patients with cervical metastasis from squamous cancer of the oropharynx and hypopharynx. Cancer 1975; 35:1163–1166.

22. Novack AJ. Treatment of carcinoma of the base of the tongue and larynx. Laryngoscope 1975; 85:1332–1343.

23. Rabuzzi DD, Mickler AS, Chung CT et al. Treatment results of combined high dose preoperative radiotherapy and surgery for oropharyngeal cancer. Laryngoscope 1982; 92:989–992.

24. Weisberger EC, Lingeman RE. Modified supraglottic laryngectomy and resection of lesions of the base of tongue. Laryngoscope 1983; 93:20–25.

25. Goffinet DR, Martinez A, Palos B et al. A method of interstitial tonsillo-palatine implants. Int J Radiat Oncol Biol Phys 1977; 2:155–162.

26. Goffinet DR, Martinez A, Pooler D et al. Brachytherapy renaissance. Front Radiat Ther Oncol 1981; 15:43–57.

27. Weller SA, Goffinet DR, Goode RL et al. Carcinoma of the oropharynx: Results of radiation therapy in 305 patients. Am J Roentgenol 1976; 126:236–247.

BRACHYTHERAPY FOR SELECTED CANCERS OF THE HEAD AND NECK

C. C. WANG, M.D.

Appropriate application of brachytherapy is a highly effective means of delivering intensive radiations to a limited volume of tissue in which the tumors lie. It is commonly used as a dose-boosting procedure. The combination of implant and external-beam radiation therapy can deliver uniform radiations to the tumors while sparing the adjacent radiosensitive organ from a full dose of radiation therapy.

In this chapter I will describe the experience of our institution in the treatment of some superficial lesions of the head and neck, such as cancer of the skin, parotid lymph node metastases, lip, buccal mucosa, nasal vestibule, and nasopharyngeal carcinoma. The technique will be briefly outlined for each lesion and individual cases so treated will be described.

For the interstitial work, the technique consists of the use of Angiocaths and iridium-192 seeds.[1] The applicators and the irradiation sources are commercially available and have been found to be highly applicable for daily clinical operation.

DOSE CONSIDERATION

In general, the dose for external-beam therapy, which may or may not include the regional nodes, is approximately 30 to 40 Gy in 3 to 4 weeks; to be followed by 30 to 40 Gy interstitial implant in 3 to 4 days. The total dose and fraction size for external-beam therapy is determined by the extent of the primary lesion, the necessity of inclusion of regional nodal disease, and, consequently, the volume of tissue to be encompassed.

TUMOR SITES

Cancer of the Skin of the Head and Neck

The most common sites suitable for brachytherapy for skin lesions include cancer of the nasolabial fold or nasal ala and lesions overlying the temporomandibular joint and mastoid tip. By using combined external-beam radiation therapy and brachytherapy, permanent damage of the temporomandibular joint in the form of ankylosis and osteoradionecrosis of the temporal bone can be prevented. In general, the cartilages of the nose and auricle tolerate interstitial implant well, and no increase in radiochondritis or necrosis is encountered after a therapeutic dose of radiation therapy.

Parotid Lymph Node Metastases

Parotid lymph nodes may be the site of metastases from carcinoma of the skin or other sources. The inoperable lesions can be effectively treated by combined external beam and brachytherapy with good local control. Since the effective range of high-dose brachytherapy is no more than 1 cm from the implant, the use of brachytherapy allows the adjacent mandible and temporomandibular joint to be spared a full dose of radiation therapy and yet the superficial parotid nodes can be fully irradiated. Experience at the Massachusetts General Hospital with such a combined approach shows that the local control rate for early parotid lymph node metastases was 89 percent at 24 months, without significant bone, joint, and soft tissue complications[2] (Table 1).

Lip and Buccal Mucosa Carcinomas

If small-to-moderate-sized, these lesions are eminently suited for treatment by combined external beam and brachytherapy. They are treated by interstitial implant by the cutaneous route. Frequently, a single-plane implant is used. The adjacent mandible is excluded from the high-dose zone, while the tumors are irra-

TABLE 1 Parotid Lymph Node Metastases:
Results of Radiation Therapy ≥ 24 months (1964–1980)

	No. NED/ No. Risk	Local Control	
N1	7/9 (78%)	8/9 (89%)	} 16*/18 (89%)
N2a	7/9 (78%)	8*/9 (89%)	
N2b	3/8 (38%)	5/8 (63%)	} 8/12 (67%)
N3c	1/4 (25%)	3/4 (75%)	
Total	18/30 (60%)	24/30 (80%)	

*One patient living with disease in the neck; in parotid area locally, NED. Analyzed 1982.

diated by a full course of radiation therapy without complications.[3] Table 2 shows the results of treatment of lower lip cancer by radiation therapy. For most T2 lesions, the combination of x-rays and brachytherapy was used with a resultant 3-year NED (no evidence of disease) rate of 88 percent, including a surgical salvage rate of 91 percent.

Nasal Vestibule Carcinomas

Lesions of the nasal vestibule are frequently irradiated by combined external beam and brachytherapy with good local control and cosmesis. The ipsilateral nasal vestibule and the nasal septum are irradiated to high-dose radiations and yet the contralateral nasal vestibule is spared from the high-dose zone; thus excessive dryness of the entire nasal cavity can be avoided. Table 3 shows that local control rate of early carcinomas (T1) of the nasal vestibule was 89 percent at 3 years. For the T2 and T3 lesions, the rates were 72 percent and 43 percent respectively.[4]

TABLE 2 Carcinoma of Lower Lip

	NED after RT	Overall NED Inc. Salv. Surg.	
T1	14/14 (100%)	14/14 (100%)	N0 75/79 (95%)
T2	50/57 (88%)	52/57 (91%)	N1 —
T3	12/14 (86%)	12/14 (86%)	N2 1/5
			N3 0/1
Total	75/85 (89%)	78/85 (92%)	

TABLE 3 Nasal Vestibule: 3-year NED Rates
Following Radiation Therapy (1960–1978)

	NED after RT
T1	27/27 (89%)
T2	13/18 (72%)
T3	3/7 (43%)
Total	40/52 (77%)

TABLE 4 Carcinoma of Nasopharynx: Comparison of Local
Control Rates of Primary Lesions by "Boost" Techniques

	Implant Boost		External Beam Boost	
T1	10/15 67%		23/35 66%	
T2	12/15 80%	} 15/18 (83%)	23/41 56%	} 24/47 (51%)
T3	3/3 100%		1/5 17%	
Total	25/33 76%		47/82 57%	

Analyzed 1981.

Carcinomas of the Nasopharynx

Brachytherapy of this site is in the form of intracavitary implant. Frequently, the primary lesions are treated by external-beam therapy to approximately 64 Gy, to be followed by intracavitary implant for a boost dose of 7 Gy. A special technique employing pediatric endotracheal tubes and cesium-137 sources is used for this procedure.[5] Table 4 shows the local control rates of the primary lesions following implant oost as compared to external-beam boost alone. For the T1 lesions, no significant difference was noted. For the combined T2 and T3 lesions, the rates were 83 percent after implant and 51 percent after external beam alone. Brachytherapy boost is used mostly for the T1 and T2, and some T3, lesions of the nasopharynx.[6]

CONCLUSION

Brachytherapy is highly effective in delivering localized curative doses of radiation to the desired tumor volume and yet sparing the adjacent normal tissues a full dose of radiation therapy. In highly selected cases, the procedure is worthwhile to achieve maximum local control and minimum complications.

REFERENCES

1. Wang CC, Boyer AL, Mendiondo O. Afterloading interstitial radiation therapy. Int J Radiat Oncol Biol Phys 1976; 1:365–368.
2. Wang CC. The management of parotid lymph node metastases by irradiation. Cancer 1982; 50:223–225.
3. Wang CC. In: Radiation therapy for head and neck neoplasms—indications, techniques and results. Littleton, MA: Wright-PSG, 1983, pp 61–62, 113.
4. Wang CC. Treatment of carcinoma of the nasal vestibule by irradiation. Cancer 1976; 38:100–106.
5. Wang CC, Busse J, Gitterman M. A simple afterloading applicator for intracavitary irradiation for carcinoma of the nasopharynx. Radiology 1975; 115:737–738.
6. Wang CC. In: Radiation therapy for head and neck neoplasms—indications, techniques and results. Littleton, MA: Wright-PSG 1983, pp 203–210.

26. Hyperthermia

INTRODUCTION

CARLOS A. PEREZ, M.D.

In the past ten years there has been a growing interest in the use of hyperthermia for the treatment of malignant tumors, thus reviving previous efforts that had been hampered by the lack of adequate equipment for heat delivery and thermometry. This modality certainly represents a new approach to overcome some of the deficiencies observed at this conference in the management of patients with head and neck cancer by current classic modalities (surgery, irradiation, chemotherapy).

As Hahn indicates in his chapter, in vitro and in vivo experiments have shown that heat selectively kills cells that are deprived of oxygen or nutrients, have a low pH, or are in the S phase of the cell generation cycle. Furthermore, blood flow measurements have demonstrated that tumors have abnormal microcirculation with slow blood flow, resulting in less dissipation of heat in comparison with the surrounding normal tissues. Therefore, higher temperatures can be reached in tumors without injury to normal structures. In addition, as also discussed by Hahn, heat has been noted to enhance the cellular effects of irradiation, cytotoxic drugs, and even hypoxic cell sensitizers.[1-3]

Heat can be delivered by electromagnetic or ultrasound methods. Unfortunately, present microwave equipment utilizes frequencies in the range of 915 to 433 mHz, with limited penetration (3 to 4 cm). Ultrasound, with a greater penetrability, cannot be utilized in areas where there is interface with bone or air cavities. Thus, there is a relative limitation to our ability to deliver adequate hyperthermia to a number of head and neck tumors, although superficial lesions, particularly cervical lymph nodes, can be adequately treated with current techniques. Interstitial hyperthermia (microwaves or radiofrequency) is increasingly used in accessible lesions because of its ability to deliver heat adequately to a limited volume. Its main limitation resides in the accessibility of the lesion to the implantation of the catheters or electrodes for the introduction of the microwave antennas or the placement of the RF electrodes. However, significant advances have been made recently in the commercial development of effective equipment for localized hyperthermia.

It is extremely important to measure the temperature delivered to the tumor and the normal tissues throughout every treatment session. Unfortunately, techniques available at this time are invasive and allow only the temperature determination in selected points in the tumor. Usually, Teflon catheters are inserted in the tumor and the normal tissues, through which the thermometry probes are later introduced. As indicated by Perez et al, there are several types of probes available, the most desirable being nonconducting optical probes, such as the gallium arsenide system developed by Christensen.[4] It is anticipated that in the near future clinical thermometry systems will combine computer based mathematical models of the bioheat equation with empiric direct measurements of temperature, blood flow, and other parameters at selected points in the patient, permitting a reliable prediction of three-dimensional representation of thermal distribution in the tumor volume and in the normal tissues. In his chapter, Stewart demonstrates a method described by Gibbs et al which utilized multiple catheters and a sophisticated system to obtain temperature measurements in multiple points along the tract of a probe (thermal mapping).[5] Thermal distribution is critically affected by the choice of hyperthermia modality, frequency, size, and design of the external applicators and coupling devices, as well as the size and characteristics of the interstitial heating sources.

Since there are temperature variations throughout a treatment, Sapareto et al and others have attempted to develop thermal dose models that allow the expression of equivalent temperatures based on a reference point (43°C).[6]

It is extremely important to develop the appropriate systems to measure the temperatures and represent the thermal doses adequately in the tumor and normal tissues. Dewhirst et al, treating spontaneous tumors of dogs and cats with irradiation and hyperthermia, reported a correlation between the minimal temperature and the tumor volume and the tumor response and subsequent tumor control.[7] There has also been a good correlation noted between the maximum temperature and the incidence of complications from heat therapy.

Heat alone has been shown to be relatively ineffective in animal tumors and in the treatment of patients. Approximately 15 percent of the tumors treated with temperatures in the range of 42.5° to 43°C for 45 to 60 minutes have shown a complete response, usually of short duration. Because of this, most clinical trials have included the combination of irradiation and heat. Perez et al and Arcangeli, in their chapters that follow, as well as others, have reported 50 to 60 percent complete responses in patients with recurrent or metastatic head and neck tumors treated with irradiation and hyperthermia. Arcangeli, in elegant experiments which he reports here, has described a tumor response of 35 to 40 percent with irradiation alone in contrast to 67 to 87 percent with irradiation and heat. He has noted increasing tumor control and skin reactions with higher doses of irradiation (400 to 600 cGy TD, 2 to 3 times weekly) and increasing thermal doses. However, with conventional fractionation (200 cGy TD), the reaction of normal tissues is less, resulting in a greater therapeutic gain. Furthermore, the delay of 4 hours between irradiation and heat delivery, as opposed to the immediate administration, or the selective cooling of the skin also yields a greater therapeutic gain.

Regional hyperthermia is more complex in its delivery and thermometry. At present, equipment is not available to adequately heat any major portion of the head and neck, particularly deeper-seated tumors or those near the base of the skull or the cervical spine. In his chapter, Stewart reviews the physical principles of regional hyperthermia and associated thermometry problems, offering possible solutions to prevent limitations to the use of this modality in the head and neck.

Similar observations have been reported by Overgaard et al.[8]

Hahn has carried out extensive studies analyzing the interaction of heat and cytotoxic agents, many of which are not only interactive but synergistic. The potential for the combination of irradiation, hyperthermia, and cytotoxic drugs in the treatment of head and neck tumors, in addition to surgery when feasible, should be explored in the future.

There are several unknown factors that may affect the interaction of these various modalities, and well-designed prospective clinical trials should be fostered to determine the optimal way in which hyperthermia can be integrated into the armamentarium for the treatment of head and neck malignant disease.

Certainly, hyperthermia is in the early developmental stages; yet, over 4000 patients have been treated with this method, and it appears that it has a definite role in the palliative management of patients with recurrent or metastatic carcinomas of the head and neck, particularly in patients failing after definitive radiotherapy. With moderate doses of irradiation (4000 cGy) and hyperthermia, which can be tolerated by normal tissues, noteworthy tumor regression and control have been noted in 50 percent of the patients treated.

At present, hyperthermia should be practiced only in institutions that have adequate staff and resources including physicians, physicists, engineers, technologists, and nurses, so that the theoretic and practical intricacies of this new modality can be studied under controlled conditions.

REFERENCES

1. Dewey WC, Hopwood LE, Sapareto SA, Gerweck LE. Cellular response to combinations of hyperthermia and radiation. Radiology 1977; 123:463–474.
2. Field SB, Bleehen NM. Hyperthermia in the treatment of cancer. Cancer Treat Rev 1979; 6:63–94.
3. Hahn GM. Potential for therapy of drugs and hyperthermia. Cancer Res 1979; 39:2264–2268.
4. Christensen DA. Current techniques for non-invasive thermometry. In: Nussbaum GH, ed. Physical aspects of hyperthermia. New York: American Institute of Physics, 1982:266–279.
5. Gibbs FA Jr. "Thermal mapping" in experimental cancer treatment with hyperthermia: Description and use of a semi-automatic system. Int J Radiat Oncol Biol Phys 1983; 9:1057–1063.
6. Sapareto SA, Dewey WC. Thermal dose determination in cancer therapy. Int J Radiat Oncol Biol Phys 1984; 10:787–800.
7. Dewhirst MW, Sim DA, Sapareto SA, Connor WG. The importance of minimum tumor temperature in determining early and long term responses of spontaneous pet animal tumors to heat and radiation. Cancer Res 1984; 4:43–50.
8. Overgaard J, Overgaard M. A clinical trial evaluating the effect of simultaneous or sequential radiation and hyperthermia in the treatment of malignant melanoma. In: Overgaard J, ed. Proceedings of 4th International Symposium on Hyperthermia Oncology. Vol 1. London: Taylor & Francis, 1984:383.

POTENTIAL EFFICACY OF HYPERTHERMIA IN TREATMENT OF HEAD AND NECK TUMORS

CARLOS A. PEREZ, M.D.
BAHMAN N. EMAMI, M.D.
RONALD S. SCOTT, PhD., M.D.

Although some forms of hyperthermia have been used for over 100 years in the treatment of malignant tumors, interest in this modality has only recently been rekindled, in the light of technical advances in heat delivery and thermometry systems. Biologic phenomena indicate that tumors may be more sensitive to heat because they are oxygen-deprived, nutritionally deficient, and have a low pH. Moreover, cells in the S phase of the proliferative cycle, usually radioresistant, are known to be sensitive to hyperthermia. Tumors are less vascularized than normal tissues and do not dissipate heat as easily; these differences in microcirculation and blood flow accentuate the sensitivity of the tumors to heat. Temperature elevation within the tumor destroys existing blood vessels, further contributing to decreased vascularity, oxygen tension, and nutrition and creating a low pH environment. Selective killing of tumor cells occurs at about 42 to 45°C, whereas at higher temperatures, normal and tumor tissues may have the same response to heat.

MODALITIES OF HEATING

At the present time, the physical agents used for power deposition in local and regional clinical hyperthermia are (1) microwaves (MW), (2) radiofrequencies (RF), and (3) ultrasound (US). These modalities, which deposit thermal energy in tissues primarily by generating electromagnetic field or mechanical ultrasonic motion, have different physical properties influencing the power deposition. For instance, microwaves have limited penetration in soft tissues, with greater propagation in fat; ultrasound will not propagate in media with different density than water, such as bone or air. External contour and tissue composition of the anatomic area to be treated, as well as the size and depth of the tumor, determine the appropriate method of heating to be used.

Depending on the anatomic area to be treated and modality used, *external hyperthermia* can be delivered by surface applicators for microwaves or external electrodes, coils, plates, or crystal transducers for ultrasound.

Interstitial hyperthermia employs conducting electrodes or antennas implanted directly in the tissues for RF or microwaves, respectively. Intracavitary antennas (MW) or large electrodes (RF) encased in special applicators can be introduced into natural cavities such as the oropharynx and larynx.

THERMOMETRY

Direct and continuous monitoring of temperature in clinical applications of hyperthermia is necessary for thermal treatment verification. Subsurface thermometry is carried out with invasive probes in 20- to 29-gauge hypodermic needles or in 16-gauge plastic tubes. The most frequently used instruments are (1) *conducting probes*—standard thermistors and thermocouples, (2) *minimally conducting probes*—high resistivity thermistors with high resistivity leads (Bowman), and (3) *nonconducting optical probes*—smaller gallium arsenide (Christensen). Field-induced artifacts often occur with the conducting probes in electromagnetic fields, making high resistivity and optical probes preferable.

For satisfactory clinical thermometry, appropriate standard thermistors and probes must be used, and the temperature must be measured in at least two or three locations at the greatest possible depth of the tumor to permit adequate description of the thermal state of the tissue. A probe is placed on the skin to measure surface temperature.

Noninvasive thermometry is the subject of current research. Techniques under development, not available for clinical applications today, include infrared and microwave thermography and ultrasound reconstruction.

CLINICAL MATERIALS AND METHODS

Three different groups of patients will be described.

Group A: Superficial Metastatic or Recurrent Head and Neck Tumors Treated with External Microwaves.

A total of 82 superficial metastatic or recurrent tumors were treated with combinations of irradiation (9 to 15 Mev electrons) and hyperthermia (915 MHz external microwaves) between March 1978 and June 1983 (minimum 3-month follow-up). Seventy-two percent of the patients had received previous irradiation (from 5000 to 6500 cGy (rads)). Doses of irradiation ranged between 2000 and 4000 cGy in fractions of 400 cGy delivered every 72 hours (twice weekly) followed by hyperthermia (41 to 43°C, 60 minutes). The desired temperature was reached in the majority of patients in about 10 minutes. Fractionation every 72 hours was chosen to avoid the thermotolerance reported in some in vitro biologic experiments.[1] Commercial microwave generators at 915 MHz (MCL 15222), specially interfaced for clinical use, and dielectric filled waveguide applicators were utilized. A plastic bag containing deionized water was used after $1^{1}/_{2}$ years, to improve coupling of the applicators to irregular surfaces of the patient. A minimum of two thermistor probes (YSI, 524) encased in 24-gauge needles were inserted at the depth of the tumor (one at central axis, one peripheral when possible), and one thermistor embedded in a 22-gauge plastic tube was placed at the skin surface during each treatment session. The temperature at these sites was continuously recorded on a dual-channel strip chart recorder. Temperatures were measured every 15 minutes with the power off. Variations of temperature of 0.5 to 2°C were noted with the RF generator power on or off, and appropriate corrections were made to obtain the actual tissue temperature. Since 1981 high resistivity (Bowman) thermistors or gallium arsenide (Christensen) probes were used.

Group B: Patients with Recurrent or Metastatic Head and Neck Carcinoma Treated with Interstitial Thermoradiotherapy.

From October 1981 to November 1983, a total of 22 recurrent and/or persistent tumors (21 patients) were treated with interstitial thermoradiotherapy in the Division of Radiation Oncology, Mallinckrodt Institute of Radiology (MIR). The average dimensions of the tumors were calculated by the formula $\frac{A+B+C}{3}$. There were 8 lesions less than 4 cm, and 14 lesions of 4 to 10 cm in average diameter. These patients had all undergone extensive previous treatment by surgery and/or radiation therapy. In all patients, a life expectancy of at least 3 months was anticipated; the investigational nature of the therapy was explained in detail, and an informed consent form was signed by every patient.

All patients were treated with interstitial thermoradiotherapy following an institutional Phase I-II protocol:

Radiation Therapy. Interstitial irradiation was administered with [192]I after loading interstitial implant. The total dose was dependent on the initial radiotherapy dose and was generally 4000 to 6000 cGy delivered in 4 to 7 days. The implantation was performed according to standard interstitial brachytherapy techniques[2] following the Quimby system implantation technique.[3]

Hyperthermia. In the majority of the patients interstitial hyperthermia was administered with coaxial microwave antennas (915 MHz) placed in Teflon catheters (Angiocaths) which had been previously implanted in the tumor tissue. The space between one Teflon tube and the other was 10 to 12 mm. The inner diameter of the Teflon tubes was adequate for placement of both radioactive sources (ribbons) and microwave coaxial antennas. In our patients, we utilized 16-gauge Angiocaths (Deseret Medical Inc., Sandy, Utah). The implantation was done in the operating room. After the patient was transferred from the recovery room to the isolated floor room, [192]I was loaded on the same day. The following day, the [192]I wires were temporarily removed and the patient was transferred (with Teflon catheters secured in place) to the radiotherapy department for a dosimetry procedure and then to the hyperthermia suite. The basic goal in the heating applications was the achievement of minimal tumor temperatures of 43°C for 60 minutes. This often required accepting temperatures, e.g., necrotic centers, well above the protocol-specified temperature of 43°C. In virtually all cases, the maximum measured tumor temperature was less than 50°C. After completion of the hyperthermia, the patient was taken back to his room and the [192]I wires were reinserted. This procedure was repeated 72 to 96 hours later for the second course of hyperthermia.

Heat was produced in a few patients through resistive heating induced by radiofrequency electric currents (frequency range was 0.1 to 1.0 MHz) driven between pairs of electrically connected arrays of hollow stainless steel stylets. The slabs of tissue between respective pairs of adjacent arrays were all heated simultaneously by connecting alternative arrays together to form a circuit with two "multiplane" electrodes. In all but one of the patients, the heating was performed in one session in the operating room, with patients under general anesthesia. After completion of the hyperthermia session, the metallic guides were replaced with Teflon tubes for routine afterloading [192]I implant. Hyperthermia was performed an average of 4 to 8 hours before loading the radioactive [192]I wires.

For most of the patients, steady-state temperatures were mapped along at least one of the catheter tracks during each treatment. In carrying out thermometry with RF interstitial hyperthermia, standard thermistor probes were employed. For interstitial hyperthermia produced with microwave antennas, both high-resistivity thermistors with carbon-impregnated plastic leads and gallium arsenide "optical" thermometers were employed.

Group C: Patients with Advanced Head and Neck Malignant Tumors Treated with Definitive Doses of Radiotherapy and External Microwaves.

A total of 9 patients with squamous cell carcinoma of the head and neck were treated with definitive radiotherapy, to a total dose of 6000 cGy delivered in 200 cGy TD daily fractions, five times weekly. A smaller group of patients, who could not be treated daily, received a total of 4800 cGy TD in fractions of 400 cGy TD per day, twice weekly. The two-dose schedules are claimed to be equivalent.[4] Hyperthermia was delivered with 950 MHz external applicators twice weekly, within 30 minutes following radiotherapy. When the central tumor temperature was 42 to 43°C, 45-minute exposures were used. When the central tumor temperature reached 43 to 44°C, 30-minute exposures were used. All patients have been followed for at least 6 months after therapy and many for one year. Therefore, they are better suited for long-term analysis of tumor control and late effects of radiotherapy and hyperthermia in normal tissues.

RESULTS

Group A: Superficial Metastatic or Recurrent Tumors Treated with External Microwaves.

Of 64 measurable epidermoid lesions in the head and neck, 29 (45.3%) exhibited a complete response (CR) and 23 (35.9%) a partial response (PR), defined as more than 50 percent regression in all diameters. In 12 patients with recurrent or metastatic epidermoid carcinoma infiltrating the neck that could not be measured, 10 (83%) showed tumor control (no evidence of recurrence) lasting several months after therapy or until the patient's death (Table 1).

Approximately 80 percent of the tumors less than 2 cm in thickness achieved satisfactory temperatures (over 42.5°C) in contrast to only 55 percent of those 2 to 4 cm in depth and 15 percent of the tumors with diameter greater than 4 cm.

A greater proportion of complete regressions was noted in tumors measuring less than 2 cm in diameter (70%) or 2 to 4 cm in diameter (60%), whereas only 20 percent of lesions larger than 4 cm in diameter showed complete regression (Table 2). This correlation must be analyzed in the light of the few temperature points taken and the variation in temperature throughout the tumor and during the daily hyperthermia sessions.

A correlation was made of the tumor regression with doses of irradiation. With doses over 3200 cGy, a higher incidence of complete tumor regression was noted in comparison with lower doses (Table 3).

Side Effects of Therapy. Of the 82 sites treated, 18 (22%) developed tumor necrosis or ulceration which did not heal spontaneously. One additional patient (1.2%) showed a thermal burn which involved the skin and/or subcutaneous tissues. In most instances these

TABLE 1 Head and Neck Cancer Group A, Irradiation and Hyperthermia: Summary of Tumor Response and Control

	No. of Lesions Treated	Tumor Regression		Tumor Control in CR*
		Complete	Partial (≥ 50%)	
Epidermoid ca (measurable)	64	29 (45.3%)	23 (35.9%)	22/29 (75.9%)
Epidermoid ca (nonmeasurable)	12	NA	NA	10/12 (83.3%)
Melanoma	3	3 (100%)	—	3/3 (100%)
Sarcoma	3	3 (100%)	—	3/3 (100%)

*No evidence of tumor recurrence.

TABLE 2 Head and Neck Cancer Group A, Irradiation and Hyperthermia: Correlation of Average Temperature and Complete Tumor Response as a Function of Depth of Tumor

Depth of Tumor	≤ 2 cm			2.1–4 cm			≥ 4 cm		
Average Temperature °C	≤ 41	41–42	≥ 42.5	≤ 41	41–42	≥ 42.5	≤ 41	41–42	≥ 42.5
Measurable	1/3 (33.3%)	2/3 (66.7%)	12/17 (70.6%)	2/4 (50%)	6/10 (60%)	10/18 (55.6%)	0/3	0/1	2/11 (18.2%)
Nonmeasurable	2*/2 (100%)	1*/1 (100%)	7*/9 (77.8%)						

*Denotes nonmeasurable patients with tumor control.

TABLE 3 Head and Neck Cancer Group A, Irradiation and Hyperthermia: Correlation of Doses of Irradiation with Tumor Control

Dose of Irradiation (cGy)	Epidermoid (measurable)	Epidermoid (nonmeasurable)	Sarcoma	Melanoma
1000–2000	—	1/1 (100%)	—	—
2001–3199	2/8 (25%)	—	—	—
3200–4000	19/54 (35.2%)	9/11 (81.8%)	1/1 (100%)	3/3 (100%)
> 4000	1/2 (50%)	—	2/2 (100%)	—

burns healed with conservative management in 8 to 12 weeks. Other reactions of the skin and subcutaneous tissues, such as erythema, dry or moist desquamation, and fibrosis, were observed in a proportion similar to those noted with irradiation alone and indicated no significant enhanced normal tissue effects because of the hyperthermia.

Group B: Recurrent or Metastatic Carcinoma Treated with Interstitial Thermoradiotherapy.

A total of 22 recurrent or metastatic lesions were treated in 21 patients (Fig. 1). All but one were squamous cellcarcinoma, the other being a mucoepidermoid carcinoma of the salivary gland. Eight of the tumors were less than 4 cm, whereas the remaining 14 lesions were 4 to 10 cm in average diameter.

Fifteen of the lesions were heated with microwave antennas while seven received hyperthermia with RF interstitial electrodes. There was no significant difference in the overall response depending on the type of heating (7/15 complete responses with microwaves and 4/7 with RF; 4/15 partial responses with microwaves in contrast to 2/7 with interstitial RF).

Of the patients receiving satisfactory heating over (42.5°C for at least 30 minutes in both sessions), 11/17 exhibited a complete response and five a partial response. Only one showed no regression after therapy. In contrast, there were no complete responses in five lesions with inadequate heating and only one had a partial response (Table 4). As in the patients treated with external hyperthermia, there was a significant correlation between the size of the tumor and the response to therapy. Six of eight lesions with diameters less than 4 cm showed a complete response and one partial response. Of nine tumors with average diameters of 4 to 10 cm, five had a complete response and four a partial response.

In seven of the patients, rapid tumor necrosis was observed. In such patients, after debridement of necrotic tissue, no gross tumor could be identified. In

A

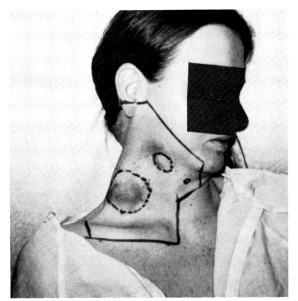

B

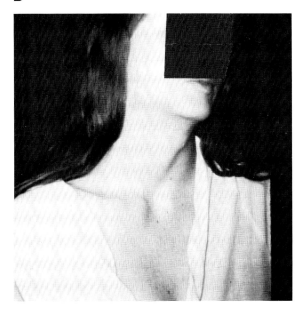

Figure 1 *A*, Patient with recurrent malignant melanoma in the right neck 2 years after wide local excision and radical neck dissection. Patient was treated with 4000 cGy in 10 fractions, delivered twice weekly followed by hyperthermia (915 MHz microwaves, 43°C, 60 minutes). *B*, Photograph of patient 3 months after completion of radiotherapy, showing complete regression of tumor. No significant effect of treatment in normal tissues.

two patients in whom skin overlying the tumor was involved, the aforementioned phenomenon resulted in an open wound which, despite weekly debridement and conservative management, took several weeks to heal.

Tumor necrosis resulted in a cutaneous sinus in two of those patients. In two of the seven patients in whom a massive floor of mouth recurrence was reach-

TABLE 4 Head and Neck Tumors Group B, Interstitial Thermoradiotherapy: Tumor Response versus Quality of Heating

Quality	CR	PR	NR	Not Evaluable	Total
Satisfactory	11/17	5/17	1/17	—	17
Unsatisfactory	0/5	1/5	2/5	2/5	5
Total					22

From Emami et al, Unpublished data.

ing the mandible, complete and massive tumor necrosis resulted in a large cavity in the floor of the mouth with marked mandibular pain for several weeks. It is planned for one of these patients to have surgical reconstruction with resection of a portion of the mandible. Finally, in another patient with a massive floor of mouth tumor invading the skin of the submental region, the rapid tumor necrosis resulted in an orocutaneous fistula (Fig. 2). The long delay in healing of the foregoing process was most likely due to poor blood supply resulting from extensive prior treatments such as surgery and/or radiation.

Group C: Advanced Tumors Treated with Definitive Radiotherapy and External Microwaves.

Of the 9 patients with squamous cell carcinoma of the head and neck treated, with a minimum of 6-month follow-up, approximately 70 percent have shown a complete response, and most of them have no evidence of recurrence. The one-year survival rate is 59 percent. At 6 months, seven patients treated with irradiation and heat exhibited a complete response and two a partial response, in contrast to only two complete responses and seven partial responses in a comparable group treated with similar doses of irradiation alone (Table 5).

Except for a few thermal burns, combined therapy has been well tolerated, and the late effects observed are similar to those from the surrounding radiotherapy fields.

TABLE 5 Head and Neck Tumors Group C: Nine Patients with Paired Lesions

	Hyperthermia and Radiation Therapy			Radiation Therapy Alone		
	CR	PR	NR	CR	PR	NR
End of therapy	3	6	0	1	5	3
6 months following therapy	7	2	0	2	7	0
1 year following therapy	5	0		2	3	
2 years following therapy	1			1		

From Scott, et al.[4]

A

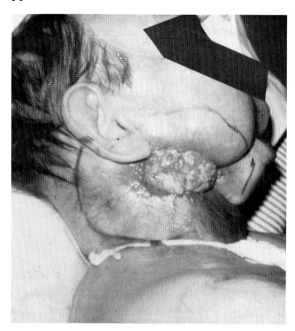

B

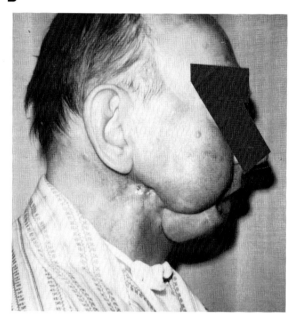

Figure 2 *A*, Patient with recurrent epidermoid carcinoma of the floor of the mouth in the right upper neck following surgical resection and postoperative radiotherapy (6000 cGy TD). Additional resection and reconstruction was done for recurrence. Subsequent recurrence (shown in photograph) was treated with irradiation (4000 cGy, 10 fractions delivered twice weekly) combined with interstitial and external hyperthermia. *B*, Photograph 6 months after completion of therapy, showing complete regression of tumor. A small ulceration and subcutaneous fibrosis are noted.

DISCUSSIONS AND CONCLUSIONS

From preliminary data reported by us,[5] Arcangeli et al,[6] and others,[7–10] it appears that a combination of irradiation and hyperthermia will produce more complete responses and better tumor control than comparable doses of irradiation alone. Further improvements are needed in patient selection, equipment, and techniques for heat delivery and temperature monitoring. The need to develop a reliable thermal dose expression to accommodate variations in temperatures throughout the treatment sessions has been emphasized.[11] Dewhirst et al, in 130 tumors in pet animals, reported a significant correlation between the minimal temperature achieved during treatment and tumor response and control.[12]

Arcangeli et al have noted increasing tumor control with higher doses of irradiation and increasing number of hyperthermia treatments.[13] Although these preliminary data are encouraging and certainly should support continued efforts in clinical evaluation of hyperthermia, it is obviously imperative to develop stringent quality assurance programs to ensure the reliability of the treatments given and the data generated. Furthermore, preliminary results must be confirmed by clinical trials which randomly allocate patients with comparable lesions to be treated with irradiation alone or with irradiation and hyperthermia. The Radiation Therapy Oncology Group (RTOG) is conducting a large multi-institutional cooperative trial randomizing measurable recurrent superficial lesions (less than 4 cm in diameter) to be treated with irradiation alone (3200 cGy in eight fractions, twice weekly) or irradiation and hyperthermia (same dose of irradiation plus hyperthermia consisting of 42.5° to 43°C for 60 minutes after each irradiation exposure). In addition, a protocol to assess the late effects of definitive doses of irradiation and hyperthermia, similar to that reported here, has registered over 65 patients and should be analyzed in the near future. Furthermore, a protocol to evaluate efficacy of interstitial thermoradiotherapy compared with brachytherapy alone is in the final stages of implementation, and preliminary results should be available within the next 2 years.

It is known that patients with large epidermoid carcinomas of the larynx, pyriform sinus, and pharynx with palpable neck nodes have a high incidence of local and neck failures following combined therapy with surgery and irradiation.[14,15] At Washington University a protocol has been developed, based on preliminary results presented in this report, to deliver a combination of irradiation and hyperthermia after surgical resection of the primary tumor and radical neck dissection on patients with advanced tumors of the larynx and pharynx.

In summary, hyperthermia has the potential to contribute significantly to the management of patients with primary or recurrent head and neck tumors who have high local or regional failure rate following treatment with existing modalities.

It will be extremely important to develop well-structured programs to adequately train physicians, physicists, technologists, and nurses who will be knowledgeable in the basic concepts and clinical administration of hyperthermia.

REFERENCES

1. Henle KJ, Bitner AF, Dethlefsen LA. Induction of thermo-tolerance by multiple heat fractions in Chinese hamster ovary cells. Cancer Res 1979; 39:2486–2491.
2. Hilaris BS, Henschke UK. General principles and techniques of interstitial brachytherapy. In: BS Hilaris, ed. Handbook of Interstitial Brachytherapy. Acton, Massachusetts Sciences Group Inc., 1975:61.
3. Emami B, Marks JE. Retreatment of recurrent carcinoma of the head and neck by afterloading interstitial Iridium 192 implant. Laryngoscope 1983; 93:1345–1347.
4. Scott RS, Johnson RJR, Story KV, Clay L. Local hyperthermia in combination with definitive radiotherapy: Increased tumor clearance, reduced recurrence rate in extended followup. Int J Radiat Oncol Biol Phys 1984; 10:2119–2123.
5. Perez CA, Nussbaum G, Emami B, Von Gerichten D. Clinical results of irradiation combined with local hyperthermia. Cancer 1983; 52:1597–1603.
6. Arcangeli G, Cividalli A, Nervi C, Creton G, Lovisolo G, Mauro F. Tumor control and therapeutic gain with different schedules of combined radiotherapy and local external hyperthermia in human cancer. Int J Radiat Oncol Biol Phys 1983; 9:1125–1134.
7. Fazekas JT, Nerlinger RE. Localized hyperthermia adjuvant to irradiation in superficial recurrent carcinomas: A preliminary report on 46 patients. Int J Radiat Oncol Biol Phys 1981; 7:1457–1463.
8. Hornback NB, Shype RE, Shidnia H, Joe BT, Sayoic E, Marshall E. Preliminary clinical results of combined 433 megahertz microwave therapy and radiation therapy on patients with advanced cancer. Cancer 1977; 40:2854–2863.
9. Kim SH, Hahn GM. Clinical and biological studies of localized hyperthermia. Cancer Res 1979; 39:2258–2261.
10. Marmor JB, Pounds D, Postic TB, Hahn GM. Treatment of superficial human neoplasms by local hyperthermia induced by ultrasound. Cancer 1979; 43:188–197.
11. Sapareto SA, Dewey WC. Thermal dose determination in cancer therapy. Int J Radiat Oncol Biol Phys 1984; 10:787–800.
12. Dewhirst MW, Sim DA, Sapareto S, Connor WG. The importance of minimum tumor temperature in determining early and long term responses of spontaneous pet animal tumors to heat and irradiation. Cancer Res 1984; 44:43–50.
13. Arcangeli G, Nervi C, Cividalli A, Lovisolo GA. The problem of the sequence and fractionation in the clinical application of combined heat and radiation. Cancer Res (SUPPL) 1984; 44:48575–48635.
14. Marks JE, Kurnik B, Powers WE, Ogura JH. Carcinoma of the pyriform sinus. An analysis of treatment results and patterns of failure. Cancer 1978; 41:1008–1015.
15. Mittal B, Marks JE, Ogura J. Transglottic carcinoma. Cancer 1984; 53:151–161.
16. Emami B, Marks JE, Perez CA. Nussbaum GH, Leybovich L, Von Gerichten D. Interstitial thermoradiotherapy in the treatment of recurrent/residual malignant tumors. Am J Clin Oncol, in press.

EXPERIENCE WITH LOCAL HYPERTHEMIA AND RADIATION

GIORGIO ARCANGELI, M.D.

The combination of heat and radiation is a treatment modality that has been widely studied in recent years. However, the interaction between heat and radiation is complex and not yet completely understood. Furthermore, unlike most experimental studies, which are related to a single administration of heat and radiation, the clinical combination of the two modalities is more likely to be applied as fractionated regimens.[1] In this situation, the influence of some treatment parameters, such as the time-temperature relationship, the sequence of the two modalities, the fractionation interval, and the size of radiation fractions, and that of some physiologic factors, such as blood flow, pH, and thermotolerance, strongly increase the complexity of delivering optimal treatment and make it difficult to know whether the addition of heat to radiation can increase the therapeutic effect.

In our series of studies we have tested in patients several combination schedules of fractionated heat and radiation in search of the optimal approach to cancer therapy and the influence of the various biologic phenomena.

TREATMENT REGIMENS

The study reported here is based on the treatment of 77 patients with a total of 163 multiple superficial lesions. This multiplicity of lesions allowed us to compare, in the same patient, the response to both radiotherapy alone and combined treatment.

The lesions were metastases from primaries of several sites and histologies; however, almost one-third were neck node metastases (N2 or N3) from squamous cell carcinomas of head and neck.

The treatment techniques have been extensively described elsewhere.[1] Briefly, radiation was given with a 6 Mev photon beam or with electrons of appropriate energy by linear accelerators. Heat was applied by means of various microwave or radiofrequency external applicators; the time-temperature relationships varied according to the several treatment regimens, which are summarized in Table 1.

In the first regimen, radiation was delivered as three fractions per day of 1.5 to 2 Gy at 4-hour intervals, up to a total of 60 Gy, and heat, at 42.5° for 45 minutes, was applied every other day, immediately after the second daily fraction of radiation, for a total of seven hyperthermic treatments.

In the second regimen, radiation was given as daily fractions of 2 Gy up to a total of 50 Gy, and heat, at 43.5 for 45 minutes, was applied once or twice a week immediately after the last or the second and the last radiation fraction of each week, for a total of five or 10 hyperthermic treatments.

The third regimen was designed to give radiation as biweekly fractions of 5 Gy up to a total of 40 Gy

TABLE 1 Treatment Regimens for Local Hyperthermia and Radiation

Treatment Regimens	Heat Treatment		Radiation Treatment		
	°C/min	Tot (N°/Week)	Fract.	Size (Gy)	Dose (Gy)
1. Simult./Sequent.	42.5/45	7 (3/w)	3/d	1.5–2.0	60
2. a. Simultaneous	43.5/45	5 (1/w)	1/d	2.0	50
b. Simultaneous	43.5/45	10 (2/w)	1/d	2.0	50
3. a. Simultaneous	42.5/45	8 (2/w)	2/w	5.0	40
b. Sequential	42.5/45	8 (2/w)	2/w	5.0	40
4. Simultaneous	45/30	5 (2/w)	2/w	6.0	30

and to apply heat, at 42.5° for 45 minutes, either immediately (immediate treatment) or 4 hours after (delayed treatment) each radiation fraction for a total of eight hyperthermic treatments.

In the fourth regimen, radiation fractions of 6 Gy were delivered twice per week up to a total of 30 Gy, and heat, at 45° for 30 minutes, was applied immediately after each radiation fraction for a total of five hyperthermic treatments; in this case, the skin around the lesions was cooled by means of circulating cold water.

RESULTS

Table 2 shows that the addition of heat resulted in a remarkable improvement in the percentage of complete tumor response over that to radiation alone, whichever treatment schedule was employed. The difference was statistically significant for the lesions treated with regimens 1, 2b, and 4. The highest improvement rate was obtained with the regimen that utilized large radiation fractions and intense heating: 87 percent (13/15) versus 33 percent (5/15) complete tumor responses were observed after combined modality and radiation alone, respectively.

However, by employing large radiation fractions, the immediate addition of heat resulted in an increased percentage of skin reaction: 64 percent (9/14) versus 36 percent (5/14) moist desquamation was observed after combined and single modality, respectively. The introduction of an interval of 4 hours between the two modalities or the use of a skin cooling system produced less skin reaction, approaching, with regimen 4, the intensity of that observed after radia-

tion alone. No increased skin reaction was seen when small radiation fractions were employed.

These observations stimulated us to calculate the thermal enhancement ratio (TER), which, unlike experimental studies in which it represents a dose modifying factor,[2] in our clinical study is defined as the ratio of percent response (complete tumor response or moist desquamation) after combined modality to percent response after radiation alone. Consequently, the therapeutic gain factor (TGF: tumor to skin TER ratio) also could be evaluated.

From Table 2 it can be observed that, by using large radiation fractions, the immediate addition of moderate heat induced an enhancement in the skin (TER = 1.8), almost as high as in the tumor (TER = 2.05), resulting in a poor therapeutic effect (TGF = 1.16).

By introducing an interval of 4 hours between the two modalities or by cooling the skin around the lesion, the enhancement in the skin was low, resulting in better therapeutic effects (TGF = 1.38 and 2.08, respectively). In addition, with the use of small radiation fractions the skin TERs were low, resulting in therapeutic gain factors ranging from 1.50 to 1.75.

The thermal enhancement in the tumor is related to both the magnitude of the applied heat and the size of radiation fraction. Figure 1 shows the tumor and skin TER as a function of the equivalent heating time at 42.5°, calculated following the rule of thumb that an increase of 1° in temperature was equivalent to increasing the time by a factor of 2, a value that has been reported in vivo and in vitro in large series of experimental studies.[3]

TABLE 2 Tumor and Skin Response to Combined and Single-modality Treatment

Treatment Regimens	Tumor Response		Skin Reaction		TER		
	RT + HT	RT Alone	RT + HT	Rt Alone	Tumor	Skin	TGF
1.	19/26 (.73)*	11/26 (.42)*	11/26 (.42)	10/26 (.38)	1.72	1.10	1.57
2. a.	9/14 (.64)	6/17 (.35)†	6/14 (.43)	6/17 (.35)	1.82	1.21	1.50
b.	7/9 (.78)†		4/9 (.44)		2.20	1.26	1.75
3. a.	10/13 (.77)	6/16 (.37)	9/14 (.64)	5/14 (.36)	2.05	1.80	1.14
b.	8/12 (.67)		6/13 (.46)		1.78	1.29	1.38
4.	13/15 (.87)‡	5/15 (.33)‡	5/15 (.33)	4/15 (.27)	2.60	1.25	2.08

Statistical difference: *†$p < 0.05$;   ‡$p = 0.01$

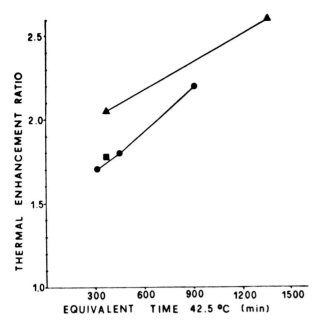

Figure 1 Thermal enhancement ratio of tumor as a function of the equivalent heating time at 42.5°. Triangles-large radiation fractions (immediate treatment); square-large radiation fractions (delayed treatment); circles-small radiation fractions.

In general, tumor TER increased as the equivalent heating time increased; the enhancement was higher after large than after small radiation fractions, probably a consequence of the radiosensitization induced by heat applied immediately after radiation. When an interval of 4 hours between the two modalities was introduced, the tumor TER decreased to a value close to those observed after small radiation fraction, probably a consequence of the direct hyperthermic cytotoxicity which is selective against acidic and chronically hypoxic tumor cells.[4,5]

The use of an equal number of small radiation fractions (i.e., 25 fractions of 2 Gy) caused tumor TER to increase from 1.83 to 2.2 when the equivalent heating time was increased from 450 to 900 minutes (i.e., when the number of equal hyperthermic treatments was doubled from 5 to 10), indicating that no thermotolerance was induced with this treatment regimen.

In Figure 2A, tumor and skin TER is shown as a function of the radiation fraction number. When the magnitude of hyperthermic treatment was similar (i.e., equivalent heating time between 300 and 450 minutes), tumor TER decreased by increasing the number of radiation fractions, probably a consequence of both lower number of radiation fractions sensitized by heat and/or less hyperthermic impairment of sublethal damage repair at small radiation fractions, since the mechanism of cell killing, at low doses, is predominantly by "single-hit" lethal events. In this case, the enhancement in the tumor could be the result of the selective hyperthermic cytotoxicity against acidic and chronically hypoxic tumor cells. This mechanism of

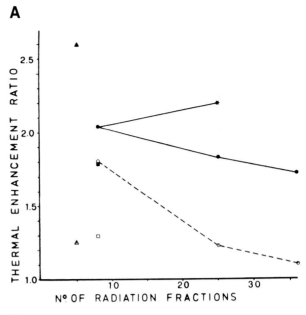

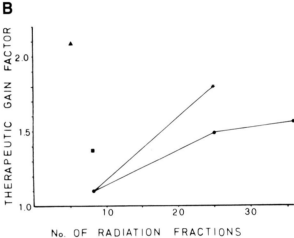

Figure 2 *A*, Thermal enhancement ratio for tumor and skin as a function of the number of radiation fractions. *Immediate treatment*: ● tumor (300 to 450 minutes equivalent heating time); ☆ tumor (900 minutes equivalent heating time); ▲ tumor (1350 minutes equivalent heating time); ○ skin; △ cooled skin. *Delayed treatment* (360 minutes equivalent heating time): ■ Tumor; □ Skin. *B*, Therapeutic gain factor as a function of the number of radiation fractions. *Immediate treatment*: ● 300 to 450 minutes equivalent heating time; ★ 900 minutes equivalent heating time; ▲ 1350 minutes equivalent heating time. ■ *Delayed treatment* (360 minutes equivalent heating time).

cell killing is probably utilized also by the delayed treatment which resulted, in fact, in a tumor TER lower than that observed after immediate treatment.

When the magnitude of hyperthermic treatment was higher (900 minutes equivalent heating time), tumor TER increased by increasing the number of radiation fractions. Again, as in Figure 1, employing equal radiation schedules (i.e., 25 daily fractions of 2 Gy), tumor TER increased from 1.83 to 2.2 when the number of equal hyperthermic treatments (i.e., 43.5° for 45 minutes) was doubled from 5 to 10.

Although the number of radiation fractions associated with hyperthermia was different in the two schedules, as were the interval and the total magnitude of the applied heat, our data do not seem to demonstrate any thermotolerance induction in human tumors, at least by using clinical treatment schedules like those employed in this study.

Finally, by using large radiation fractions, the immediate addition of the largest magnitude of hyperthermic treatment (i.e., 5 treatments at 45° for 30 minutes, or 1350 minutes equivalent heating time) resulted in the highest thermal enhancement ratio in the tumor, probably a consequence of radiosensitization induced by heat applied immediately after each radiation fraction.

The skin TER, in general, appeared to decrease by increasing the number of radiation fractions. However, when few fractions were employed, the enhancement in the skin was lower if an interval of 4 hours was introduced between the two modalities, or if skin was actively cooled. Consequently, the therapeutic effect increased, in general, by increasing the number of radiation fractions and/or the magnitude of hyperthermic treatment (Fig. 2B). However, by using large radiation fractions, the therapeutic gain was higher with delayed than with immediate treatment, and because of the preferential tumor heating, the highest therapeutic gain was accomplished when the largest magnitude of hyperthermic treatment was combined with radiation.

In conclusion, when heating tumor and normal tissue to the same temperature, the best therapeutic advantage was obtained by using small radiation fractions or by introducing an interval between the two modalities. When the tumor could be preferentially heated in respect to the surrounding normal tissue, the immediate combination of the highest hyperthermic treatment and the largest radiation fractions resulted in a high therapeutic effect. This practically suggests that in patients in whom radiotherapy has never been delivered, an optimal treatment should result by simply adding, once or twice a week, a simultaneous session of moderate heat to a full conventional fractionation radiotherapy course. In heavily irradiated tissues or when fast treatments of multiple lesions are required for palliation, an optimal treatment should result from delivery of five to seven biweekly fractions of 5 to 6 Gy in combination with hyperthemia. If the tumor can be selectively or preferentially heated in respect to normal tissue, a simultaneous application of intense heating can be safely administered with a significant probability of tumor control. On the contrary, the sequential administration of moderate heat should provide an effective treatment with a lower incidence of normal tissue damage.

A further development of better heating techniques is now necessary to employ heat in all clinical situations as adjuvant to radiotherapy.

REFERENCES

1. Arcangeli G, Cividalli A, Lovisolo G, Mauro F, Nervi C. Tumor control and therapeutic gain with different schedules of combined radiotherapy and local hyperthermia in human cancer. Int J Radiat Oncol Biol Phys 1983; 9:1125–1134.
2. Robinson JE, Wizenberg MJ, McCready WA. Radiation and hyperthermal response of normal tissues in situ. Radiology 1974; 113:155–198.
3. Field SB, Morris CC. The relationship between heating time and temperature: its relevance to clinical hyperthemia. Radiother Oncol 1983; 1:179–186.
4. Dewey WC, Freeman ML, Raaphorst GP, Clark EP, Wong RS, Highfield DP, Spiro IJ, Tomasovic SP, Denman DL, Coss RA. Cell biology of hyperthemia and radiation. In: *Radiation Biology in Cancer Research*. Meyn RE, Withers HR (eds) New York: Raven Press, 1980:589–621.
5. Overgaard J, Nielsen OS. The importance of thermotolerance for the clinical treatment with hyperthermia. Radiother Oncol 1983; 1:167–178.

DEEP REGIONAL HYPERTHERMIA: OVERVIEW OF METHODS AND POTENTIAL APPLICATION IN THE TREATMENT OF HEAD AND NECK CANCERS

J. ROBERT STEWART, M.D.

The use of hyperthermia in the treatment of cancer, especially as an adjunct to radiation therapy, rests on a strong and convincing rationale. In his chapter, Hahn reviews in detail the biologic rationale for its use. At temperatures above 42°C, heat is cytotoxic, and the cytotoxicity is quantitatively related to the temperature and to the duration of exposure to that temperature. Lowering the pH of the medium or causing nutritional exhaustion increases the cells' sensitivity. Hypoxic cells are not heat-resistant, and in tumors, hypoxic cells are apt to be more heat-sensitive owing to the nutritional deprivation and low pH that one would expect in poorly vascularized regions containing hypoxic tumor cells. Relatively radioresistant S-phase cells show an increased sensitivity to hyperthermia. In addition to these cytotoxic effects, hyperthermia is also a potent radiation sensitizer. Thus, the rationale for incorporating hyperthermia into multimodality cancer treatment rests on both *complementary* and *synergistic* properties. Clinical experience so far has suggested that complications of hyperthermia are rare; however, one must continue to be cautious since effective heating of deep, radiation dose-limiting organs has infrequently been achieved. In their chapters, Perez and Arcangeli review results of hyperthermia plus radiation versus radiation alone in superficial lesions. Other authors have reviewed the reports of superficial hyperthermia used with ionizing irradiation.[1-3] Both the complete response rates and duration of response are better in the group receiving hyperthermia than in those treated only with radiation. It can now be stated with confidence that hyperthermia has efficacy in man in superficial tumor sites. This important finding adds to the rationale for further study of hyperthermia in an attempt to define its role in primary multimodality therapy of cancer, and particularly to develop and refine methods applicable to deep tumor sites, including primary cancers

in the head and neck, which are inaccessible to currently available techniques.

METHODS OF PRODUCING DEEP HYPERTHERMIA

In some instances the tumor might be implanted with catheters to carry electrodes for RF interstitial heating or microwave antennae. The same catheters can be used for thermometry and for interstitial radiotherapy. When this is feasible, one can achieve good heating patterns by these methods; however, the tumor must either be in an accessible site or be approachable through surgical exposure. In attempting to induce hyperthermia by external means, either ultrasound energy or electromagnetic energy can be used. For ultrasound to be useful for deep-lying lesions, some method of scanning[4] or the use of multiple transducers[5] becomes essential. Since ultrasonic waves are not conducted in air, tumors lying beyond air-containing structures cannot be heated by ultrasound, and there is also a problem at bone–soft tissue interfaces which leads to excess deposition of energy and consequently hot spots. Limited available clinical data suggest that ultrasonic devices will be useful in some deep tumor sites. Head and neck primary tumors tend to occur in regions where both air cavities and bone-tissue interfaces would be expected to present severe problems.

Electromagnetic (EM) methods are highly dependent on the frequency of the energy applied. High-frequency (915 to 2450 MHz) propagated waves give effective local heating, but the depth of penetration is limited to a few centimeters. At lower frequencies, where penetration is greater, the applicators must be large because of the long wave lengths, and heating becomes regional rather than local. EM methods have been applied using (1) magnetic induction, (2) capacitance heating, and (3) combined propagated-wave and near-field heating from coupled electromagnetic-wave applicators. The largest deep heating clinical experience to date has been with magnetic induction by a concentric coil.[6,7] This method has the disadvantage of maximal heating at the surface with rapid drop-off to zero at the center of the heated object.[8] These physical characteristics would predict for inhomogeneous heating with little or no heating centrally, and these characteristics have been confirmed in clinical studies.[9,10] The major disadvantage of capacitance heating is that the maximal heating occurs in tissues of greatest electrical resistance, especially the superficial fat layer. A new device, the Thermotron 8, has recently been introduced[11] and has the added modification of efficient surface cooling. This device has been said to produce good deep heating in the hands of investigators in Japan, and it may have application in head and neck sites. The only propagated-wave device for deep heating that has undergone any systematic clinical evaluation is the annular-phased array operated with the BSD-1000 system. This device relies on the central reinforcement that occurs when electromagnetic-wave applicators are operated in electrical phase

Supported by PHS Grant #1PO1 CA29578 and NCI #NO1 CM17523.

(Fig. 1). Effective deep heating has been documented in the pelvis and abdomen with the device shown in Figure 2.[12,13]

THERMOMETRY

We have learned from previous clinical and laboratory studies that the degree of response to hyperthermia is directly related to the temperatures achieved. Methods that produce inhomogeneous heating patterns with cold spots lead to decrease in tumor response.[14] The work of Dewhirst et al suggests that the response will be related mainly to the minimum temperatures and time at temperature achieved.[15] Multiple temperatures can be measured simultaneously by thermometers with multiple sensors along a single probe. However, there is little experience with such probes, which are not interactive with EM fields. In our own work we have found that mapping by sampling temperatures with a single sensor at multiple sites along a preplaced catheter through the tumor and relevant normal tissues has given an improved assessment of temperature distributions achieved. Gibbs has developed a semi-automated system for achieving this thermal mapping.[16] When multiple thermal maps are

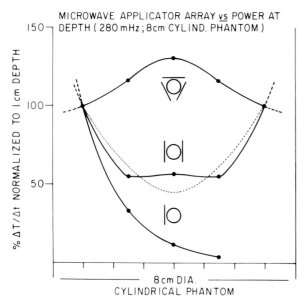

Figure 1 Illustrated here is a simple experiment by Dr. Gibbs at the University of Utah in an 8-cm diameter cylindrical phantom to demonstrate the phenomenon of central reinforcement of power when EM-propagated wave applicators are operated in phase. The lower curve shows the drop-off with depth when a single applicator is used. The middle solid curve shows the result of opposed applicators operated with the electric fields in phase. Note that central heating is more than double that achieved with a single applicator (phase reinforcement). The top curve shows the preferential central heating from reinforcement from three applicators in phase. The dotted curve represents the pattern achieved when the three applicators are turned 90° (out of electric phase), a simple summation rather than reinforcement of the three outputs. This phenomenon of phase reinforcement is the physical basis of the apparatus shown in Figure 2 and the schematic in Figure 4.

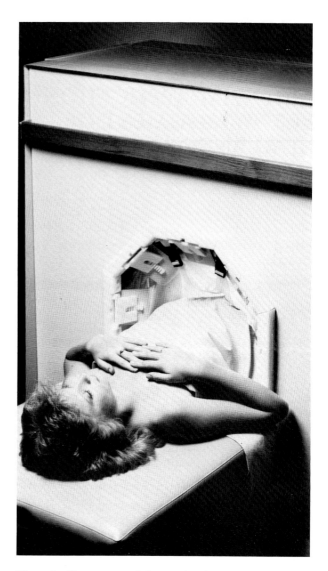

Figure 2 The aperture of the annular-phased array (APA) operated with the BSD-1000 hyperthermia device (BSD Medical Corporation, Salt Lake City, Utah) for deep regional heating of the trunk.[12,13] Note the plastic water-containing bags which encircle the patient to provide coupling of the EM waves to the body of the patient. Within the octagonal aperture are two banks of eight waveguide applicators converging toward the patient. Heating is predominantly from central reinforcement of the applicators operated in electric phase (see Fig. 1).

made from multiple thermometers during multiple courses of therapy, a staggering amount of data is generated which becomes extremely difficult to analyze in terms of the effectiveness of heating of a given tumor. This problem becomes even more complex when one attempts to compare one device with another. Because of this we have developed a system of data analysis using a "thermal dose," which takes into consideration both the temperature achieved and the time that temperature was maintained at multiple sites over time within the tumor and normal tissues. The units of "thermal dose" in this system are equivalent degree minutes at 42°C. With this system it is possible to reduce to a single plot the thermometry results from an entire treatment. Furthermore, one can determine the minimal tumor thermal dose, the mean tumor thermal dose, the mean normal tissue thermal dose, and the fraction of tumor that achieves the stated prescribed dose. The ratio then of the mean tumor thermal dose to the mean normal tissue thermal dose gives a measure of effectiveness of tumor versus normal tissue heating. When applying this concept, it is essential to achieve the desired temperature as rapidly as possible to minimize the effect of thermotolerance. This procedure is described elsewhere in detail.[10,17]

POTENTIAL APPLICATIONS OF DEEP HEATING METHODS TO HEAD AND NECK CANCER

A large number of patients have had metastatic adenopathy treated by hyperthermia with promising results. Certain sites within the head and neck are amenable to interstitial implants which can give satisfactory thermal distributions; however, many primary sites in the head and neck are not accessible to this procedure. The complex anatomy of the head and neck with constantly changing external and internal contours, the presence of large air cavities, and many bone–soft tissue–air interfaces presents some rather severe constraints on what approaches might be used for primary cancers inaccessible to interstitial methods. Ultrasound approaches are not promising because of the bone and air interfaces. Two possible approaches that warrant investigation are capacitance devices and phased arrays of electromagnetic-wave applicators. With more efficient water bolus coupling and surface cooling, capacitance devices may find a role (Fig. 3). Phased arrays of electromagnetic-wave applicators operating at frequencies between 200 and 400 MHz might also be applicable. There has recently been some experimental evaluation of such phased arrays,[18,19] and there is some promise for their being applicable to sites in the head and neck (Fig. 4).

SUMMARY

The biologic and metabolic rationale for the use of hyperthermia is very strong indeed. The methods to achieve deep regional heating are complex, and at this point the technology is a relative impediment to further application; however, there are proved approaches which might well be modified to provide more effective heating for primary head and neck cancers. Whatever techniques are used, extensive thermometry and detailed analysis of thermal patterns are essential to understand responses to hyperthermia. Several thousand patients have been analyzed following treatment of superficial metastases, and we can now state with confidence that hyperthermia, especially when combined with radiation therapy, has efficacy in man. With the encouraging results seen from superficial treatment, more effort is indicated to adapt techniques or develop new techniques to provide adequate hy-

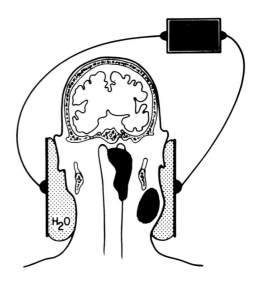

Figure 3 Diagramatic representation of a sagittal section showing tumor extent of an advanced carcinoma of the nasopharynx with ipsilateral node metastases. A possible hyperthermia treatment approach is shown schematically with capacitance plates in place and the RF generator shown as the "black box". Flexible water bolus bags would ensure conformational electrical coupling to the region and could be cooled with circulating water to avoid excessive superficial heating. This approach, tested at other sites,[11] warrants investigation, but there may be hot spots treated along the base of the skull anterior to the spine and along the mandible owing to concentration of electric fields. The diagram is not meant to show realistic features of the actual design of the applicators.

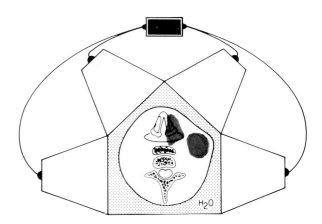

Figure 4 Schematic representation of a possible design of an array of applicators for treatment of tumors of the aerodigestive tract and regional nodes in the neck. The example shown is an advanced carcinoma involving the hypopharynx and supraglottic larynx with ipsilateral node metastasis. The array could be designed so that any or all of the applicators could be operated to achieve the desired regional power deposition with or without phase reinforcement, as described in Figure 1. The concept has been the subject of preliminary testing in phantoms.[18,19]

perthermia for primary sites, such as many in the head and neck, where improved control of local and regional cancer will have a major impact on morbidity and mortality. The major clinical research question with hyperthermia at this point is to define its place in primary multimodality therapy.

REFERENCES

1. Overgaard J. Hyperthermia modification of the radiation response in solid tumors. In: Fletcher G, Nervi C, and Withers H, eds. Biological Bases and Clinical Implications of Tumor Radioresistance. New York: Masson, 1983:337.

2. Meyer JL. The clinical efficacy of localized hyperthermia. Cancer Res 1984, 44:4745s–4751s.

3. Stewart JR, Bagshaw MA, Corry PM, Gerner EW, Gibbs FA Jr, Hahn GM, Lele PP, Oleson JR. Hyperthermia as a treatment of cancer. Interdisciplinary Program for Radiation Oncology Research, Report of the American College of Radiology. Cancer Treat Sym 1984; 1:135–145.

4. Lele PP, Parker K. Temperature distributions in tissues during local hyperthermia by stationary or steered beams of unfocused and focused ultrasound. Br J Cancer 1982; 45(Suppl):108–121.

5. Marmor JB. Cancer therapy by ultrasound. Adv Radiat Biol 1983; 10:105–133.

6. Storm K, Elliott R, Harrison W, et al. Radiofrequency hyperthermia of advanced human sarcomas. J Surg Oncol 1981; 17:91–98.

7. Baker H, Snedecor P, Goss J, et al. Regional hyperthermia for cancer. Am J Surg 1982; 143:586–590.

8. Paliwal B, Gibbs FA, Wiley A. Heating patterns induced by a 13.56 MHz radiofrequency generator in large phantoms and pig abdomen and thorax. Int J Radiat Oncol Biol Phys 1982; 8:857–864.

9. Oleson JR, Heusinkveld R, Manning M. Hyperthermia by magnetic induction: II. Clinical experience with concentric electrodes. Int J Radiat Oncol Biol Phys 1983; 9:549–556.

10. Sapozink MD, Gibbs FA Jr, Thomson JW, Eltringham JR, Stewart JR. A comparison of deep regional hyperthermia from an annular array and a concentric coil in the same patients. Int J Radiat Oncol Biol Phys, in press, Jan. 1985.

11. Morita K, Watanabe M, Niwa K, et al. Local RF-wave hyperthermia (8MHz) combined with radiotherapy: One year's clinical experience. In: Matsuda T, Kikuchi M, eds. Hyperthermic Oncology. Tokyo General Komosome Hospital, Tokyo, Japan, 1984:168.

12. Sapozink MD, Gibbs FA Jr, Gates KS, Stewart JR. Regional hyperthermia in the treatment of clinically advanced, deep seated malignancy: Results of a pilot study employing an annular array applicator. Int J Radiat Oncol Biol Phys 1984; 19(6):775–786.

13. Stewart JR, Gibbs FA Jr, Sapozink MD, Gates KS. Regional hyperthermia using an annular phased array system: Preliminary patient and thermometry data. Front Radiat Ther Oncol 1984; 18:103–107.

14. Gibbs FA Jr, Dethlefsen LA. Temperature uniformity in subcutaneous murine tumors heated by water bath immersion. Radiat Res 1981; 87:187–197.

15. Dewhirst M, Sim D, Sapareto S, et al. The importance of minimum tumor temperature in determining early and longterm responses of spontaneous pet animal tumors to heat and radiation. Cancer Res 1984; 44:43–50.

16. Gibbs FA Jr. "Thermal mapping" in an experimental cancer treatment with hyperthermia: description and use of a semiautomatic system. Int J Radiat Oncol Biol Phys 1983; 9:1057–1063.

17. Sapozink MD, Gibbs FA Jr, Sandhu TS. Practical thermal dosimetry. Int J Radiat Oncol Biol Phys, still in press.

18. Nilsson P, Persson B. Absorbed power distributions from single or multiple electromagnetic direct-contact waveguide applicators. In: Overgaard J, ed. Hyperthermic Oncology 1984, Volume 1, Summary Papers. Proceedings of the 4th Int Symposium on Hyperthermic Oncology, Aarhus, Denmark, 2-6 July, 1984. London and Philadelphia: Taylor and Francis, 1984:643.

19. Johnson RH, James JR, Hand JW. Field penetration of multiple compact applicators in localised deep hyperthermia. In: Overgaard J, ed. Hyperthermia Oncology 1984, Volume 1, Summary Papers. Proceedings of the 4th Int. Symposium on Hyperthermic Oncology, Aarhus, Denmark, 2-6 July, 1984. London and Philadelphia: Taylor and Francis, 1984:667.

BIOLOGIC RESPONSES OF CELLS, NORMAL TISSUES, AND TUMORS TO HEAT

GEORGE M. HAHN, Ph.D.

Inactivation of mammalian cells, whose normal host temperature is around 37°C, starts at 40 to 41°C. (Temperatures discussed herein are centigrade.) When cell survival is plotted against time at temperatures below 43°, it is found that cell inactivation continues for the first few hours. After that time the surviving cells appear to be resistant to heat.[1] Careful studies have shown that this is not a selection of a heat resistant subpopulation nor an effect associated with progression of cells in the cell cycle. It results from a heat-induced resistance to heat. This resistance is transient, decays in 100 to 150 hours, and is usually referred to as thermotolerance. At higher temperatures, above 43°, cell inactivation with time is exponential (except for a shoulder in the survival curve) and thus resembles cell inactivation by ionizing radiations or by many chemotherapeutic agents. During heating at temperatures above 43°, no evidence for the development of thermotolerance is usually detected. However, if the cells are placed at 37° after an initial treatment at these high temperatures, within a few hours the surviving cells become heat-resistant. This heat resistance can be quite dramatic. An exposure of Chinese hamster cells for 45 minutes at 45° kills approximately 99.9 percent of the cells. However, if such heating is preceded 4 hours earlier by an exposure of 20 minutes at 43°, the same 45° 45-minute heat exposure leaves at least 50 percent of the cells as survivors. Clearly, thermotolerance is an important factor in determining heat resistance of cells. Thermotolerance must be taken into account when scheduling fractionated heat treatments of tumors. Thermotolerance has also been demonstrated to occur in normal tissue and, if used carefully, could therefore improve the therapeutic ratio. This would be done by mildly preheating the critical normal tissue and then heating the entire tissue-tumor volume. Thermotolerance can also greatly modify the cells' response to many chemotherapeutic agents (protecting, in most cases, but accentuating in some), but apparently has much less effect on the cells' responses to x-irradiation.

Heat sensitivity can also be modulated by changing the cells' environment. For example, suddenly lowering pH from the "normal" value of 7.4 to below 7.0,[2] reducing available nutrients and/or oxygen, and a variety of other relatively minor modifications of the cellular milieu can all increase the heat sensitivity of cells. The relevance of these observations to the response of tumor cells in vivo has not yet been demonstrated. Lower pH and reduced nutrient availability do characterize the interior of many tumors and therefore may be responsible for the frequently made claim that tumor cells are more heat-sensitive than their normal counterparts.[3]

As has been discussed earlier, it is also possible to demonstrate heterogeneity for heat responses of cells from single tumors. Table 1 lists survival values of cells from a permanent line isolated from surface variants of B16 melanoma cells and exposed to different heat doses.[4] We estimate that only one cell in 10^4 to 10^5 shows this pronounced heat resistance. Nevertheless, if human tumors show a similar heterogeneity, then in order for heat treatments by themselves to be curative, it is necessary to design protocols to eliminate even these resistant cells. Oncologists are familiar with similar problems: one likely reason that multidrug chemotherapy is effective is that drugs are chosen so that a cell resistant to one member of a multidrug regimen is not likely to be resistant to others. Similarly, it might be argued that heat is likely to be most effective when combined with other modalities that do not show cross-resistance with hyperthermia.

HEAT AND X-IRRADIATION

Heat enhances the cytotoxicity of x-rays, in both a synergistic and a complementary fashion. Synergism is shown by comparing survival curves of cells irradiated at various temperatures. Studies have shown that the shoulder of such survival curves is reduced and their slope enhanced when radiation is carried out at temperatures above about 39°.[5] Actually, radiation and heat do not have to be applied simultaneously in order for a synergistic effect to be measurable. As the time between the two treatments is lengthened, however, the interaction is reduced, and it completely disappears once the separation of the two treatments has

reached about 6 hours. In practice, if the synergistic effect is to be used in the clinic, heat and x-irradiation should be spaced closely together. Complementary results from the findings that cells particularly resistant to radiation tend to be heat-sensitive. This seems to hold for those cells in tumors that are hypoxic and therefore highly radiation-resistant. This heat sensitivity does not necessarily result from hypoxia, but from the fact that these cells are away from blood vessels and therefore find themselves at low pH; they also tend to be deprived of adequate nutrients. As I have pointed out earlier, such cells tend to be heat-sensitive. The additional feature of complementarity is related to the response of cells in various parts of the cell cycle. Cells in late S phase tend to be x-ray-resistant; these same cells, however, are particularly sensitized by heat and are also sensitive to killing by heat.[6] These results suggest that heat and x-irradiation together should greatly enhance antitumor responses provided tumors can be heated adequately. Many studies on murine tumors have verified this hypothesis. For example, a one-hour exposure at 43° of mammary carcinomas reduces the dose required to cure 50 percent of these tumors from 5000 to 1700 rads.

HEAT AND DRUGS

The relationship between drug cytotoxicity, temperature, and pH is varied and fascinating. A drug whose mode of action is primarily chemical (e.g., alkylating agents) has increased reaction rates at elevated temperatures. The rate of alkylation, or the chemical conversion of a drug to a cytotoxic intermediate that does not require enzymatic action, can be expected to proceed at higher rates when the temperature is elevated. Indeed, studies have shown that alkylating agents, the nitrosoureas, and cisplatin all show killing rates that vary smoothly with increasing temperatures.[8] In mouse tumors, similar findings are observed: when local heating is performed at times when drug concentration in the lesion is expected to be high, a synergistic effect can readily be demonstrated.[7]

There are, however, other anticancer agents whose cytotoxicity is only little changed by temperatures in the range of 37° to 42°.[7] Above that temperature, however, their activity is greatly enhanced. Drugs showing such thresholds of increased activity include bleomycin and Adriamycin. At clinically usable doses, the polyene antibiotic amphotericin B is relatively noncytotoxic over the temperature range of 37° to 41°. Above 42°, however, it becomes a potent cytotoxic drug. This is also true for agents rich in sulfhydril groups, as well as for some local anesthetics. Thus, it is likely that whole classes of drugs exist that could be useful agents at elevated temperatures, but are useless at 37°. On the other hand, cytotoxicity of various analogs such as methotrexate or FUdR usually is not enhanced at elevated temperatures. Again, findings in animal studies tend to reflect the tissue culture studies.

TABLE 1 Survival of Wild Type and of a Heat-resistant Mutant (B-HR 44) of B16 Melanoma Cells

Time at 43° (min)	Survival	
	B16	B-HR-44
80	10^{-1}	5×10^{-1}
120	5×10^{-3}	2×10^{-1}
160	10^{-5}	8×10^{-2}

The dependence of cytotoxicity on pH for any of the chemotherapeutic agents examined is minimum at 37°. At elevated temperatures, cell killing by drugs can be increased dramatically if the extracellular pH is changed from 7.4 to below 7.0.[9] For agents such as BCNU, the increased cytotoxicity at low pH is most dramatic. For that drug at 43°C, a mere change in proton concentrations of .6 pH unit results in increased cell kill by about a factor of 10^5! If one compares the survival curve of BCNU at 37°C with that obtained at 43° and pH 6.8, a dose-modifying factor as high as 30 is seen (i.e., it would take 30 times the drug concentration to achieve equivalent cell kill at 37° than at 43° and pH 6.8). Because of the low pH found within certain regions of many tumors, the combination of BCNU (and probably other nitrosoureas) and heat should be quite effective against large lesions. Manipulation of blood flow could result in even lower tumor pH, accentuating this effect. This suggests that treatment involving sequential reduction of blood flow and heating during administration of nitrosoureas might be unusually effective against large lesions.

CONCLUSION

The biologic rationale leading to the use of heat in the clinic is well established. The data of studies carried out over the last 10 years have demonstrated precisely and quantitatively the cell killing ability of mildly elevated temperatures and the increased cytotoxic effectiveness of x-irradiation and chemotherapeutic agents when combined with mild heat.

However, treatment of tumors in human beings is a much more complicated problem. Uniform heating of such lesions usually requires invasive techniques; with noninvasive approaches, nonuniform energy deposition as well as nonuniform cooling by blood flow frequently, if not invariably, cause large temperature variations to occur across the tumor. Often it is difficult, if not impossible, to raise the temperature of portions of the tumor to therapeutic levels. Physiologic or local modifications of blood flow could alleviate the problem. Such manipulations have not yet been tried on humans. Combinations of heat treatments with drugs that are not used as anticancer agents, but do accentuate effects of heat, are also possible. Examples are agents like lidocaine; these lower the heat requirements to achieve a given level of cell kill and thereby ease the tumor-heating requirements, but show no cytotoxicity at 37°. The development of the clinical use of hyperthermia has been somewhat unusual when compared to x-ray therapy, for example, in that (at least within the last few years) it has been achieved via a rational transfer to the clinic of information gained in the laboratory. Blood flow manipulations and the clinical use of "heat modifiers" that have been shown in the laboratory to have considerable promise should also lead to improved treatment of patients.

REFERENCES

1. Westra A, Dewey WC. Heat shock during the cell cycle of Chinese hamster cells in vitro. Int J Radiat Biol 1971; 19:467–477.
2. Gerweck LE. Modification of cell lethality at elevated temperatures: the pH effect. Radiat Res 1977; 70:224–235.
3. Rossi-Fanelli A, Cavaliere R, Mondovi B and Moricca G, eds. Selective heat sensitivity of cancer cells. Berlin, Heidelberg and New York: Springer Verlag, 1977:1.
4. Tao TW, Calderwood SK, Hahn GM. Stable heat-resistant clones selected from wild-type and surface variants of B16 melanoma. Int J Cancer 1983; 32:533–535.
5. Sapareto S, Raaphorst G, Dewey WC. Cell killing and the sequencing of hyperthermia and radiation. Int J Radiat Oncol Biol Phys 1979; 5:343–347.
6. Kim SH, Kim JH, Hahn EW. The enhanced killing of irradiated HeLa cells in synchronous culture by hyperthermia. Radiat Res 1976; 66:337–345.
7. Hahn GM, Shiu EC. Effect of pH and elevated temperatures on the cytotoxicity of some chemotherapeutic agents in vitro. Cancer Res 1983; 43:5789–5791.
8. Hahn GM. Hyperthermia and cancer. New York and London: Plenum, 1982.

SECTION SIX / CHEMOTHERAPY

27. Mechanisms of Cancer Cell Resistance

INTRODUCTION

EMIL FREI, III, M.D.

Drug resistance is a ubiquitous problem in biomedicine, particularly in cancer chemotherapy. There are two primary needs in cancer chemotherapy: (1) the development of qualitatively different and more specific chemotherapeutic agents, and (2) improved understanding of the nature of drug resistance. The latter should provide insights and opportunities into the prevention or circumvention of drug resistance. There is ample evidence, for example, in microbiology, to the effect that once resistance to an antibiotic is understood at a biochemical level, the antibiotic can be appropriately altered, so as to circumvent the resistance mechanism. Although the complexity of mammalian cells is substantially greater than that of microorganisms, there is no a priori reason that comparable approaches should not prove successful in cancer chemotherapy. Indeed, developing knowledge of the mechanisms of drug resistance on the part of chemotherapeutic agents is already providing fundamental insights into drug resistance on the part of the cancer cell as well as therapeutic intervention.

As regards head and neck cancer, the agent methotrexate is effective in producing tumor regression in some 50 percent of patients with squamous cell carcinoma of the head and neck. However, in such patients tumor progression, that is, relapse, occurs at a median time of 3 to 4 months, at which time the tumor is no longer responsive to methotrexate. Thus, 50 percent of patients are naturally resistant to methotrexate, and in 50 percent, such resistance presumably occurs as a result of selection pressure. Using the technique of Rheinwald, we have cultured squamous cell carcinoma from 12 patients with head and neck cancer. The cells from one patient were exposed to increasing concentrations of methotrexate (selection pressure) for a 12-month period, during which time resistance progressively increased until 10,000-fold resistance was achieved. In this cell line, early resistance was characterized by a marked decrease in the capacity of the cell to actively transport methotrexate. At slightly higher levels of resistance, the cell lost the capacity to polyglutamate methotrexate, a mechanism that increases retention of methotrexate within the cell and also increases the affinity of meth-

otrexate for thymidylate synthetase. Finally, above 100-fold resistance, gene amplification occurred with a substantial increase in the target enzyme, dihydrofolate reductase, and a lesser but definite increase in the gene coding for the target enzyme, as determined by southern blots. The earliest mechanism for resistance (that is, impaired active transport) could be circumvented by a methotrexate ester, tertiary butyl methotrexate, a lipid-soluble compound which enters cells by passive diffusion and is at least as active against transport-resistant lines as it is against the parent line. In his chapter, Colvin presents evidence concerning resistance to cyclophosphamide that relates to intracellular catabolism. Inhibition of aldehyde oxidase, a catalytic enzyme, represents a potential approach to preventing or circumventing drug resistance. Vistica and Ozols have demonstrated experimentally that ovarian cancer resistance to phenylalanine mustard contains increased concentrations of glutathione, a material that can complex with reactive compounds such as alkylating agents, inactivating them before they reach the presumed target site DNA. Glutathione within cells can be reduced by DSO, an inhibitor of glutathione synthetase, and at least in the test tube, this has been shown to be capable of rendering such resistant cells sensitive to phenylalanine mustard. Ling makes the important observation that there may be cross-resistance among seemingly unrelated agents. Although it is generally appreciated clinically that second-line chemotherapy is less effective than earlier, first-line, treatment, there are numerous clinical variables that have precluded interpretation of this phenomenon. Pleiotropic drug resistance, as described by Ling, is a possible explanation. More important, it is subject to experimental study, since the mechanism of such resistance relates, at least in part, to the presence of the cell surface glycoprotein, which is thought to modify uptake or egress of structurally unrelated compounds. Finally, Goldie addresses the genetics of drug resistance, with emphasis on quantitative models. These mathematical models have been confirmed in part by in vivo biologic studies by Skipper. Among the many important clinical implications of these observations is the fact that large tumors invariably have relatively large numbers of resistant cells to a given antitumor agent. This supports the approach involving combination chemotherapy. Furthermore, Goldie's modeling supports the position that microscopic tumor (present often in the adjuvent situation) might transit from drug sensitivity to drug resistance as a result of mutations in a relatively short period of time (weeks). This has major implications for such therapeutic strategies as adjuvant and neoadjuvant chemotherapy.

In summary, the revolution in molecular biology will provide increasingly precise insight into the nature of drug resistance. The biggest problem, I suspect, will relate to tumor cell heterogeneity; that is, we may learn that, even within a given tumor and with selection pressure with a given drug, multiple mechanisms of resistance might exist. In any event, such insight, coupled with advances in biochemical pharmacology and drug synthesis, will undoubtedly have positive impact on the effectiveness of cancer chemotherapy in the future.

MECHANISMS OF RESISTANCE TO ALKYLATING AGENTS

MICHAEL COLVIN, M.D.

The alkylating agents have activity against many tumors and are important components of most effective combination drug regimens. Their important role in such combinations may derive from the fact that alkylating agents can be cytotoxic to cells at all stages of the cell cycle and therefore may serve to eradicate noncycling cells which have survived other components of the combination regimen. Furthermore, since the mechanism of action of the alkylating agents is distinct from those of other classes of antitumor agents, cells that are resistant to other agents may still be sensitive to alkylating agents.

At one time the alkylating agents as a group were thought to be so similar in their activity that a cell resistant to one alkylating agent would be resistant to other alkylating agents. However, the work of the late Frank Schabel and other investigators demonstrated lack of cross-resistance between alkylating agents in animal tumor models[1,2] (Table 1). A great deal of work has demonstrated that the effects of different alkylating agents on nucleic acids and the biologic consequences of these effects are very similar. However, the chemical nature, mechanisms of alkylation, mode of transport into the cell, and susceptibility to metabolic inactivation are different among the alkylating agents and provide the molecular basis for different mechanisms of resistance to different alkylating agents. On the other hand, the chemical requirements for alkylation and similarity of nucleic acid damage provide the potential for mechanisms of broad cross-resistance between alkylating agents which can and does occur. The purpose of this discussion is to describe and discuss mechanisms of resistance to alkylating agents which have been described.

The alkylating agents fall into one of two categories, bifunctional and monofunctional agents. Most alkylating agents fall into the first category and have two reactive sites on the drug molecule, thus allowing the cross-linking, or bonding together, of biologic molecules. A great deal of evidence has now been accumulated to strongly support the concept that the bifunctional alkylating agents exert their cytotoxic activity by cross-linking complementary strands of DNA (interstrand cross-linking), thus preventing the proper functioning of this cross-linked DNA in macromolecular synthesis. Certain of the clinically effective alkylating agents, such as procarbazine and DTIC, are clearly monofunctional and do not cross-link DNA. These compounds appear to mediate their cellular toxicity through the production of DNA strand breaks.

Figure 1 shows three aspects of the cellular interaction of an alkylating agent which are likely targets for resistance mechanisms. These aspects are entry into the cell, traverse through the cell to the target, and damage to the DNA. Potential mechanisms of resistance would be decreased uptake of drug into the cell (or increased exit of the drug from the cell), more rapid inactivation of the drug inside the cell, and enhanced repair of the macromolecular damage produced by the agent. Variations of all of these mechanisms have now been described.

DECREASED UPTAKE OR INCREASED EFFLUX OF DRUG

In order to react with DNA, the alkylating agent must penetrate the cell membrane to gain access to the cytoplasm and, ultimately, to the nucleus of the

TABLE 1 LOG_{10} Reduction in Viable Tumor Cells by Optimal Single-dose, I.P., Treatment ($\leq LD_{10}$) of 10^5–10^6 Tumor Cell Implants

Alkylating Agent	L1210/0	L1210/CPA	L1210/BCNU	L1210/L-PAM
CPA	6	0	6	4
BCNU	>6	>6	2	6
CCNU	>6	>6	1	>6
MECCNU	>6	>6	3	>6
Chlorozotocin	6	6	4	4
BIC	>6	*	0	6
L-PAM	6	4	6	2
Dianhydrogalactitol	5	5	5	4
Piperazinedione	5	3	4	5
Thiotepa	3–4	2	NA	2
Cis-DDPT (QD 1–5)	5	5	NA	0

NA = not available; *similar to L1210/L-PAM; unconfirmed exp. IP = intraperitoneal

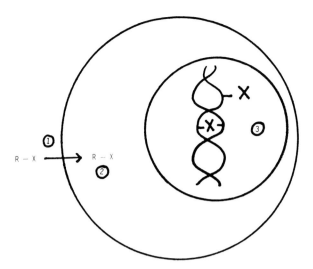

Figure 1 Mechanisms of resistance. *1*, Decreased cell entry. *2*, Metabolic interaction with active species. *3*, Repair of damage.

cell. Some alkylating agents have been shown to enter the cell by active carrier systems which usually serve to transport cellular nutrients. Other alkylating agents, such as the nitrosoureas, appear to enter the cell by simple diffusion. Obviously, one mechanism of resistance would be for the cell to reduce the uptake of an agent. It would seem more feasible for such a reduction of uptake to occur in the situation in which the agent is actively transported into the cell, by modulation of aspects of the active transport system.

In 1970 Goldenberg and colleagues found that nitrogen mustard was actively transported in mouse L5178Y lymphoblasts and established that the carrier by which nitrogen mustard was being transported was the carrier for the natural substrate choline.[3,4] As can be seen in Figure 2, choline and nitrogen mustard bear a close structural resemblance. In nitrogen mustard-resistant L5178Y lymphoblasts, both the rate of accumulation and total cellular accumulation of nitrogen mustard were decreased. These results were similar to those of Wolpert and Ruddon, who had found decreased drug uptake in nitrogen mustard-resistant mouse Ehrlich ascites cells.[5]

Work by Vistica and colleagues[6] and by Goldenberg and co-workers[7] has shown that melphalan is transported into murine L1210 lymphoblasts, Chinese hamster ovarian cells, and human tumor cells and lymphocytes by two amino acid transport systems, which had previously been described by Christen-

sen.[8,9] One of these systems, the ASC system is a high-affinity, low-velocity system, and is the carrier for the amino acids alanine, serine, and cysteine. The other system, the L system, serves as the transport carrier for leucine and is a lower-affinity, higher-velocity system.

Redwood and Colvin found that L1210 cells resistant to melphalan had a less rapid uptake of melphalan and only accumulated about one-half the intracellular concentration of melphalan, as compared to the wild type cells[10] (Fig. 3). Further investigation suggested that a mutation had occurred in the L carrier system, resulting in a lower affinity of the carrier for melphalan in the resistant cell line. Subsequent work by Goldenberg and colleagues[11] found no difference in the initial rate of uptake of melphalan by drug-resistant Chinese hamster ovarian cells (CHO), but found that significantly lower intracellular concentrations of melphalan were achieved in the drug-resistant cells, as had been described by Redwood and Colvin. The resistant CHO cells were demonstrated to have an enhanced rate of efflux, which was postulated to account for the lower intracellular content of melphalan. However, the differences in accumulation of melphalan between the resistant and sensitive cells were thought to be insufficient to account for the differences in sensitivity to the drug. The resistant cells were also found to contain higher levels of sulfhydryl groups (to be discussed), and the drug resistance was thought to be multifactorial.

INTRACELLULAR DEGRADATION OF DRUG AND PROTECTION BY NUCLEOPHILES

Several investigators have found cellular resistance to alkylating agents associated with increased cellular levels of sulfhydryl compounds.[12–14] It has been postulated that such nucleophilic compounds might react with alkylating agents to reduce the intracellular levels of the drug or to protect critical targets by re-

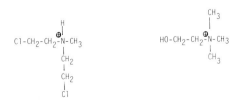

Figure 2 Chemical structures of nitrogen mustard and choline.

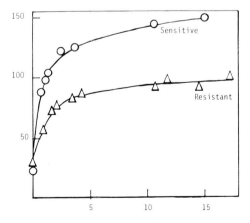

Figure 3 Time course of (^{14}C) melphalan uptake by L1210 cells in vitro measured at 37°. The concentration of (^{14}C) melphalan in the incubation medium was 36 μM. (Reprinted with permission from Redwood and Colvin.[10])

acting with the alkylating agent more readily than the critical target does. In this regard, several aspects of the chemistry of the alkylating agents should be pointed out. A few of the alkylating agents, such as busulfan, appear to react as pure SN_2 reactants (Fig. 4).

In such a reaction the parent compound reacts directly with an electron-rich atom, such as an amino nitrogen, to displace a proton, as shown in Figure 4. Thus the electron-rich sulfhydryl groups can react with the busulfan to deplete the concentrations of the agent and to protect vital targets.

However, the majority of the alkylating agents, such as the nitrogen mustards, are SN_1 in character, as shown in Figure 5. The parent nitrogen mustard is not sufficiently reactive to alkylate thiols in a spontaneous reaction. The aziridine moiety will react rapidly with thiols, but since reaction 1 is irreversible, reaction of the aziridine with a thiol will not reduce the concentrations of the nitrogen mustard more rapidly than if the thiol were not present. The aziridine is very short-lived and does not migrate an appreciable distance during this lifetime. Therefore, a protective compound such as a thiol does not deplete the intracellular concentrations of the alkylating agent and is protective of biologic targets only if the thiol is present in the immediate vicinity of the biologic target and traps the aziridine formed there. However, there are enzymes which are capable of catalyzing the dechlorination of hydrocarbons such as a nitrogen mustard. These enzymes might well utilize sulfhydryl compounds as acceptors for dechlorination products.

In the earlier studies of resistance associated with increased sulfhydryl levels, the products of degradation of the agent have not been identified. Vistica and colleagues have recently reported that in murine L1210 cells resistant to melphalan, there was a more rapid dechlorination of the melphalan to the inactive dihyroxy derivative[15] (Fig. 6). The drug-resistant cells were found to contain elevated levels of intracellular glutathione. Growth in cysteine-free media reversed the melphalan resistance of cells and lowered the intracellular glutathione content. Reversal of melphalan resistance could also be achieved by brief exposure

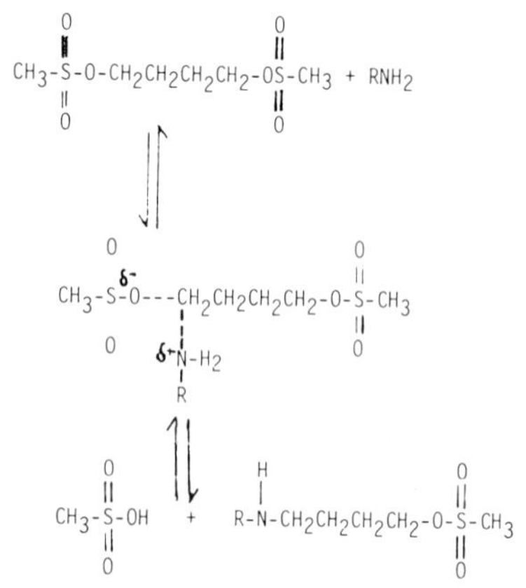

of the drug-resistant cells to the sulfhydryl reagent N-Ethyl Maleimide. The mechanism of the dechlorination has not been established.

Cyclophosphamide is activated to alkylating and cytotoxic activity, as shown in Figure 7. The compound 4-hydroxycylophosphamide enters cells readily and is spontaneously converted to phosphoramide mustard, which can alkylate and cross-link DNA.

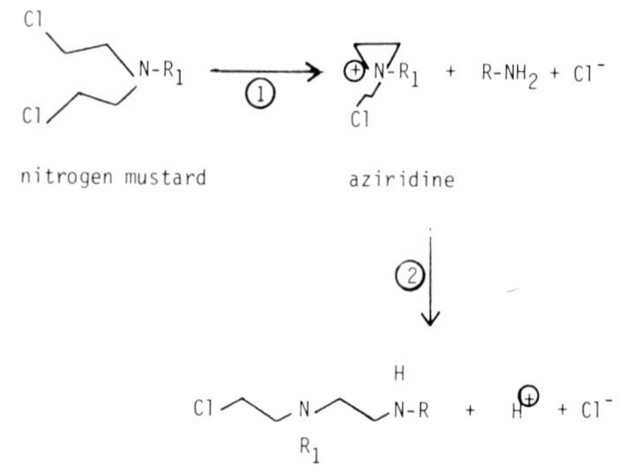

Figure 5   Alkylation by nitrogen mustard.

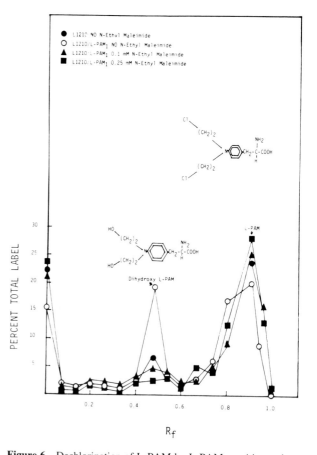

Figure 6   Dechlorination of L-PAM by L-PAM-sensitive and resistant murine L1210 leukemia cells and its inhibition by N-Ethyl Maleimide. L1210 (●) and L1210/L-PAM₁ (○) cells were exposed to (¹⁴C)-L-PAM (1.25 μg/ml) for 3 hours. L-PAM₁ cells were treated for 5 minutes with 0.1 mM (▲) or 0.25 mM (■) Ethyl Maleimide, prior to exposure to L-PAM. (Reprinted with permission from Suzukake et al.[15])

Figure 4   Alkylation by busulfan.

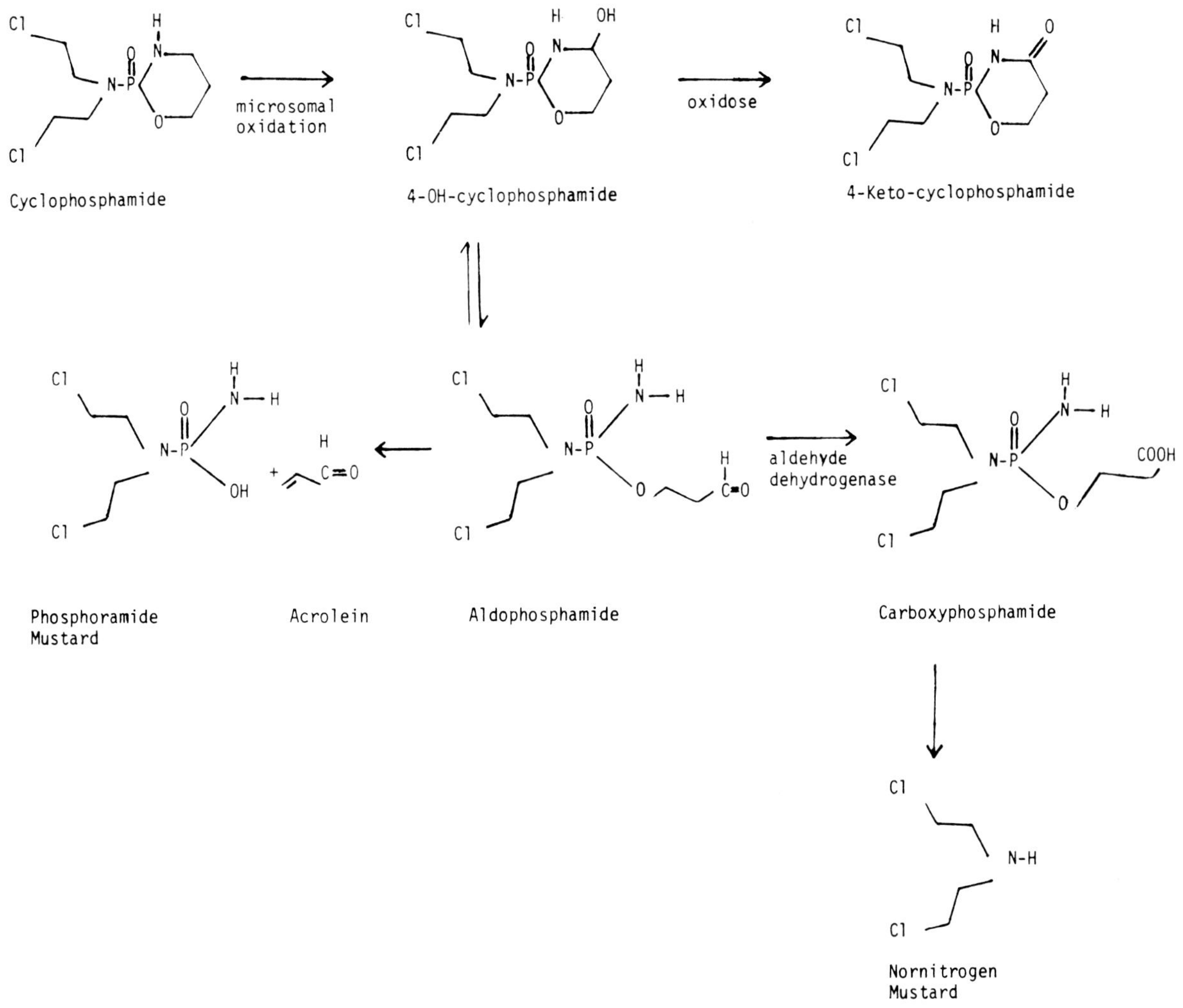

Figure 7 Metabolism of cyclophosphamide.

Further oxidation of aldophosphamide by aldehyde dehydrogenase in the liver produces the inactive compound carboxyphosphamide, the major metabolite of cyclophosphamide, which is excreted in the urine and accounts for approximately 70 percent of an administered dose of cyclophosphamide. Recent work by Hilton has demonstrated that the presence of elevated intracellular aldehyde dehydrogenase is responsible for the in vitro cellular resistance to 4-hydroxycyclophosphamide and the in vivo resistance to cyclophosphamide of resistant murine L1210 cells.[16] Figure 8 illustrates an experiment in which either wild type or cyclophosphamide resistant L1210 cells are exposed in vitro to radioactive 4-hydroxycyclophosphamide. After 5 minutes the cells are washed and lysed, and the intracellular contents examined for the various cyclophosphamide metabolites by high pressure liquid chromatography. As can be seen in the lower panels, after 5 minutes there is a substantial quantity of carboxyphosphamide in the resistant cells, but not in the sensitive cells. As shown in Figure 9, the addition of disulfiram, an inhibitor of aldehyde dehydrogenase,

renders the resistant cells sensitive to the active metabolite.

One of the clinical characteristics of cyclophosphamide is the relative sparing of the hematopoietic stem cells, as reflected in the rapid recovery of hematopoiesis, lack of cumulative bone marrow damage, and platelet sparing. We have recently accumulated evidence that the resistance of the bone marrow stem cells is due to elevated aldehyde dehydrogenase levels (Hilton and Colvin, unpublished data).

RESISTANCE BY REPAIR OF DNA DAMAGE

Another mechanism by which generation of cellular resistance to an alkylating agent could occur is by an increase in activity of enzymes to repair the macromolecular damage which the alkylating agent has produced. There is extensive evidence for enzymes which repair and remodel DNA, and the repair of light-induced and carcinogen damage has been described. Furthermore, studies have established that in sensitive cells, many of the interstrand cross-links

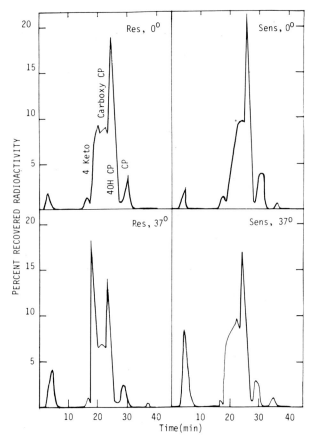

Figure 8 Chromatography of extracts from L1210 cells exposed to (^{14}C) ring hydroxycyclophosphamide.

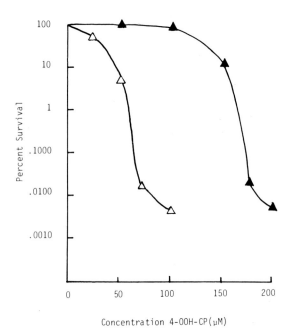

Figure 9 Survival of cyclophosphamide-resistant L1210 cells following exposure to 4-hydroperoxycyclophosphamide (▲) for 30 minutes. One portion of the culture was pretreated with 10 μM disulfiram in dimethyl sulfoxide (DMSO) for 60 minutes before 4-hydroperoxycyclophosphamide treatment (△). The remaining half received an equal amount of DMSO.

produced in DNA by alkylating agents are removed with time.[17,18] Therefore, it has long been postulated that the enhanced enzymatic repair of DNA would also be a mechanism of resistance to alkylating agents. Also, it might be anticipated that such a mechanism of resistance would produce cross-resistance to a number of alkylating agents. However, definitive evidence for the enzymatic repair of alkylating agent damage as a mechanism of resistance has only been recently described.

The mechanism of DNA alkylation of nitrosoureas has been shown to proceed through the initial regeneration of a chloroethyldiazonium entity, as shown in Figure 10.[19] Kohn and colleagues have shown that cells with an enzyme which repairs 0–6 methylguanine lesions by demethylation (Mer+ phenotype) are resistant to the cytotoxicity of the chloroethyl nitrosoureas[20] (Fig. 11). On the basis of these observations, the investigators postulated that the initial lesion of the nitrosoureas is chloroethylation of the 0–6 position of a guanylic acid residue (Fig. 12), fol-

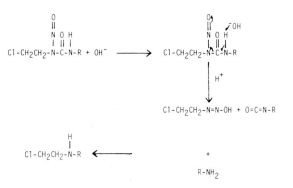

Figure 10 Mechanism of decomposition and alkylation of chloroethylnitrosoureas.

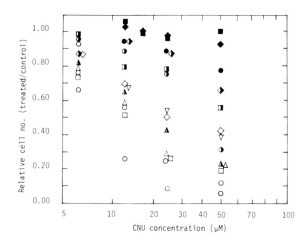

Figure 11 Effect of CNU treatment on proliferation of various cell strains. Cells were treated with CNU for 1 hour. After drug removal, the cells were allowed to proliferate in fresh medium for 3 days (three to five doubling times for control cells). Open symbols—Mer⁻ strains; closed and half-closed symbols—Mer⁺ strains. (Reprinted with permission from Erickson et al[20])

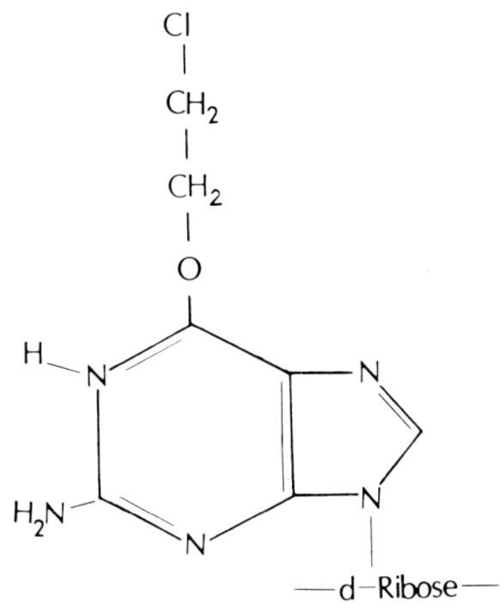

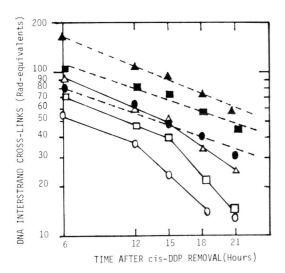

Figure 12 0–6 Chloroethylation product of guanylic acid residue.

lowed by a slow reaction of the bound chloroethyl group with a nucleophilic site on the complementary strand of DNA to produce an interstrand cross-link. The protective effect of the Mer+ phenotype is postulated to be the removal of the chloroethyl monoadduct at the 6 position of guanylic acid, preventing the formation of the cross-link.

In a recent study, Kohn and co-workers have shown that melphalan-resistant (L1210/L-PAM) cells are resistant to cisplatin.[21] An increased rate of disappearance of DNA interstrand cross-links (Fig. 13) seen in the resistant cells initially suggested that the resistance was due to enhanced cross-link repair. However, further studies have indicated that the decreased net number of interstrand cross-links in the resistant cells is due to the repair or neutralization of

Figure 13 Decline of net DNA interstrand cross-linking between 6 and 21 hours after treatment of parent [L1210/NCI (●, ■, ▲)] or resistant [L1210/PAM (○, □, △)] cells treated with 20, 20, or 40 μM cis-DDP for 1 hour. (Reprinted with permission from Micetich et al[21])

monofunctional adducts, analogous to the nitrosourea resistance already described. The mechanisms of the monoadduct repair must be different from that described for nitrosoureas, since the melphalan-resistant and cisplatin-resistant cells remain fully sensitive to the chloroethylnitrosoureas (see Table 1).

As already described, removal of DNA interstrand cross-links, probably by an excision repair process, appears to occur in cells treated with alkylating agents. However, enhanced repair of cross-links as a general mechanism of resistance to alkylating agents has not yet been definitely demonstrated.

CONCLUSIONS

As discussed in this presentation, a number of specific mechanisms of cellular resistance to alkylating agents have now been described. Most of these mechanisms are relatively specific to particular alkylating agents. However, at least two of the mechanisms, increased degradation of the agents associated with increased sulfhydryl compounds and excision repair of DNA cross-links, provide potential mechanisms for general cross-resistance, but such a mechanism for general cross-resistance has not yet been described.

Many of the cell lines studied appear to have multiple mechanisms responsible for the resistance observed. An important question is whether each cell has several mechanisms of resistance, or whether the cells being studied consist of several populations of resistant cells, each with a single mechanism of resistance. To answer this question, approaches that allow the study of single cells, such as flow cytometry, must be used.

The advances in cellular and pharmacologic techniques which have enabled the studies described herein to be carried out should allow the further elucidation of mechanisms of resistance, descriptions of patterns of cross-resistance, better testing of human tumor cells for drug resistance, and evolution of successful strategies to minimize and overcome drug resistance.

REFERENCES

1. Schabel FM, Trader MW, Laster WR, Wheeler GP, Witt MH. Patterns of resistance and therapeutic synergism among alkylating agents. Antibiot Chemother 1978; 23:200–215.
2. Schmid FA, Otter GM, Stock CC. Resistance patterns of Walker carcinosarcoma 256 and other rodent tumors to cyclophosphamide and L-phenylalanine mustard. Cancer Res 1980; 40:830–833.
3. Goldenberg GJ, Vanstone CL, Israels LG, Ilse D, Bihler I. Evidence for a transport carrier of nitrogen mustard in nitrogen mustard-sensitive and resistant L5178Y lymphoblasts. Cancer Res 1970; 30:2285–2291.
4. Goldenberg GJ, Vanstone CL, Bihler I. Transport of nitrogen mustard on the transport-carrier for choline in L5178Y lymphoblasts. Science 1971; 172:1148–1149.
5. Wolpert MK, Ruddon RW. A study on the mechanism of resistance to nitrogen mustard (HN21) in Ehrlich ascites tumor cells: comparison of uptake of HN2-14-C into sensitive and resistant cells. Cancer Res 1969; 24(49):873–879.

6. Vistica Ct. Cytotoxicity as an indicator for transport mechanism: evidence that melphalan is transported by two leucine-preferring carrier systems in the L1210 murine leukemia cell. Biochim Biophys Acta 1979; 550:307–317.

7. Begleiter A, Lam H-Y, Grover J, Froese E, Goldenberg GJ. Evidence for active transport of melphalan by two amino acid carriers in L5178Y lymphoblasts in vitro. Cancer Res 1979; 39:353–359.

8. Oxender CL, Christensen HN. Distinct mediating systems for the transport of neutral amino acids by the Ehrlich cell. J Biol Chem 1963; 238:3686.

9. Christensen HN, Handlogten ME, Lam I, Tager HS, Zand R. A bicyclic amino acid to improve discriminations among transport systems. J Biol Chem 1969; 244:1510–1520.

10. Redwood WR, Colvin M. Transport of melphalan by sensitive and resistant L1210 cells. Cancer Res 1980; 40:1144–1149.

11. Begleiter A, Grover J, Froese E, Goldenberg GJ. Membrane transport, sulfhydryl levels and DNA cross-linking in Chinese hamster ovary cell mutants sensitive and resistant to melphalan. Biochem Pharmcol 1983; 32:293–300.

12. Calcutt G, Connors TA. Tumor sulphydryl levels and sensitivity to the nitrogen mustard merophan. Biochem Pharmacol 1983; 12:839.

13. Goldenberg GJ. Properties of L5178Y lymphoblasts highly resistant to nitrogen mustard. Ann NY Acad Sci 1969; 163:936–953.

14. Hirono I. Non-protein sulphydryl group in the original strain and sub-line of the ascites tumor resistant to alkylating reagents. Nature 1960; 186:1059.

15. Suzukake K, Vistica BP, Vistica DT. Dechlorination of L-phenylalanine mustard by sensitive and resistant tumor cells and its relationship to intracellular glutathione content. Biochem Pharmacol 1983; 32:165–167.

16. Hilton J. Deoxyribonucleic acid crosslinking by 4-hydroperoxycyclophosphamide in cyclophosphamide-sensitive and resistant L1210 cells. Biochem Pharmcol 1984; 33:1867–1872.

17. Zwelling LA, Michaels S, Schwartz H, Dobson PP, Kohn KW. DNA cross-linking as an indicator of sensitivity and resistance of mouse L1210 leukemia to cis-diamminedichloroplatinum (II) and L-phenylalanine mustard. Cancer Res 1981; 41:640–649.

18. Pera MF Jr, Rawlings CJ, Shackleton J, Roberts JJ. Quantitative aspects of the formation and loss of DNA interstrand crosslinks in Chinese hamster cells following treatment with cisdiamminedichloroplatinum (II) (cisplatin). II. Comparison of results from alkaline elution, DNA renaturation and DNA sedimentation studies. Biochim Biophys Acta 1981; 655:152–166.

19. Colvin M, Brundrett RB, Cowens W, Jardine I, Ludlum DB. A chemical basis for the antitumor activity of chloroethylnitrosoureas. Biochem Pharmacol 1976; 25:695–699.

20. Erickson LC, Laurent G, Sharkey NA, Kohn KW. DNA cross-linking and monoadduct repair in nitrosourea-treated human tumor cells. Nature 1980; 288:727–729.

21. Micetich K, Zwelling LA, Kohn KW. Quenching of DNA: platinum (II) monoadducts as a possible mechanism of resistance to cis-diamminedichloroplatinum (II) in L1210 cells. Cancer Res 1983; 43:3609–3613.

INFLUENCE OF TUMOR GROWTH RATE AND MUTATIONS ON DRUG RESISTANCE

JAMES H. GOLDIE, M.D., F.R.C.P.(C)

A large amount of currently available data indicates that the development of drug-resistant cells within tumors is a critical factor in determining curability by chemotherapeutic agents. Evidence strongly implies a genetic origin for most of these drug-resistant phenotypes and that such drug-resistant cells are arising continuously within neoplastic cell populations.[1]

This capacity to generate a large number of drug-resistant variants is one property that distinguishes most neoplastic cell lines from those of normal cell populations. For reasons that have not been clearly elucidated, tumor cells readily generate a great range of phenotypic variability, including resistance to all types of cancer chemotherapeutic agents, whereas normal cell systems have little or no capacity to produce this variability. This tendency to generate a great range of altered cell types due to genetic changes has been referred to as genetic instability, and is probably intimately related to the fundamental process of neoplastic transformation itself.[2] Whatever the precise basis of this genetic instability, it has the effect of permitting the neoplastic cell population to spontaneously generate a huge range of variant cell types, at least some of which will by chance have the biochemical properties that will render them resistant to therapeutic doses of anticancer drugs.

There are no known methods whereby this capacity of tumor cells to produce drug-resistant variants can be prevented or diminished, and in fact, it is likely that many therapeutic modalities employed in the treatment of cancer, such as radiation and many antineoplastic agents themselves, may actually increase the overall mutation rate to resistance in cells that survive the killing effect of these modalities. However, analysis of the phenomenon of spontaneous mutations to resistance does permit us to examine how different chemotherapeutic strategies might be expected to exert their effect and to evaluate which ones may be superior to others. I will describe briefly in this review how certain well-characterized processes in tumors may lead to diminished curability and, from this, develop inferences as to how chemotherapeutic strategy may be better directed to circumvent the development of resistance and to increase cure rates in neoplasms.

James H. Goldie acknowledges the support of the British Columbia Health Care Research Foundation and the Cancer Control Agency of British Columbia.

RELATIONSHIP BETWEEN TUMOR BURDEN AND CURABILITY

It has been long appreciated in the chemotherapeutic treatment of experimental tumors that there is a strong inverse relationship between tumor burden and curability.[3] That is, small tumor populations are likely to be far more easily cured by tolerable doses of drug than larger tumors. The same general relationship has been observed in a significant number of human neoplasms in which it is possible to produce at least a proportion of drug-induced cures.[4] In every clinical neoplasm in which it is possible to generate cures, one can usually define an approximate relationship between extent of tumor burden at the time of treatment and the overall likelihood of cure. Although tumor burden cannot be estimated with the same accuracy in patients that it can in experimental animals, the various clinical, biochemical, and radiographic markers that correlate with extent of disease clearly demonstrate that it is in those patients in whom lower tumor burdens can be inferred that greater percentage cures are achieved.

The logical extension of this observation is to employ chemotherapy at a time when tumor burden is microscopic and not to wait until the disease has become clinically overt. Under these conditions it may be possible to produce cures directed against microscopic disease when drug-induced cure would not be achievable if treatment were delayed until the tumor was clinically apparent.

Study of the phenomenon of spontaneous mutations to resistance provides a strong rationale and a useful conceptual basis for the utility of adjuvant chemotherapy. If we imagine a tumor population increasing in size over time and we further postulate that at each cell division there is a certain probability (which may be quite low, i.e., in the order of 1 in a million) that that cell and its progeny will display resistance to a particular chemotherapeutic agent or combination of such agents, then it is apparent that the larger the neoplastic cell population becomes, the greater the likelihood that at least one resistant cell will have emerged.

As this process is random and is not directed or caused by the chemotherapeutic agents themselves, there is an inherent unpredictability about the point in time when the first drug-resistant mutant will appear in any given tumor or discrete tumor colony. For a given value of the mutation rate, there is an overall average time at which the first resistant mutant appears, but there is substantial variation in individual cases, with some mutations occurring well before the average time and others occurring much later.

Translated into biologic terms, this would mean that one could have a series of tumor cell populations of the same size and with the same average mutation rate to drug resistance and yet each individual tumor population might contain significantly different numbers of drug-resistant cells. If a mutation occurs early, by chance, in the growth of the tumor, there will be considerable time for that resistant mutant to generate a large number of progeny with the consequent development of a high fraction of resistant cells.

The converse of this situation would be the instance in which the first mutation appears quite late and therefore has little time to produce large numbers of descendents; in this case the ratio of drug-sensitive to drug-resistant cells will be very high. In these two extreme examples, though the tumor is biologically and histologically identical, there will be a marked difference in terms of response to a given chemotherapeutic treatment. When the proportion of resistant cells is high, such a tumor responds for only a short time to treatment and, in fact, may not regress sufficiently to produce even partial remission. In contrast, if the proportion of resistant cells is very low, there may be substantial or even complete regression of clinically detectable tumor, which may persist for a considerable period of time. The duration of the remission is dictated essentially by the growth rate of the resistant subpopulation and its absolute size. If this is small and the growth rate is slow, the patient may display a sustained remission following discontinuance of therapy. However, eventually the tumor recurs and in the great majority of instances, it is composed largely of drug-resistant cells and therefore shows little or no response to reapplication of therapy.

It is also possible that no resistant cells will be present in the tumor at the time treatment is commenced, but this possibility is clearly related to the size of the tumor and the frequency with which resistant cells appear in that particular tumor line (i.e., the mutation rate). If the tumor size is relatively small and if the mutation rate is relatively low, there is a significant probability that no resistant cells will be present within the tumor at the time therapy is started. Under these conditions, if sufficient courses of therapy are given to eliminate the sensitive tumor cells, such a tumor is potentially curable by means of chemotherapy.

The majority of types of clinical solid tumors are not curable with existing drug or drug combinations if treatment is initiated when the tumor is far advanced or clinically overt. This strongly argues for the utilization of chemotherapy in an adjuvant setting when this is feasible.

RELATIONSHIP BETWEEN TUMOR GROWTH RATE AND CURABILITY

In addition to the aforementioned well-documented relationship between tumor mass and drug curability, there also exists a relationship between overall tumor growth rate and the sensitivity to antineoplastic drugs.[5] In general, tumors that exhibit the fastest growth rates in terms of clinical doubling time are most likely to be curable at an advanced stage and display the highest cure rates when treatment is directed at them in adjuvant circumstances.

There are exceptions to this general correlation between tumor growth rate and curability, and these are sufficiently frequent to suggest that growth rate on its own appears unlikely to be the principal factor in dictating the basis for this relationship. Some slow-growing neoplasms (e.g., adenoid-cystic carcinoma) are relatively sensitive to chemotherapeutic effect, and some rapidly growing neoplasms (e.g., blast cell crisis of chronic myelogenous leukemia, bronchiolar cell carcinoma) are poorly responsive to existing chemotherapy protocols.

We have recently examined the question of the relationship between tumor growth rate and curability by studying the effects of certain time-dependent processes, which are thought to occur in tumors, on the overall probability of drug-resistant cells emerging.[6]

Although the data are still far from conclusive, a considerable amount of evidence suggests that the intermitotic time of cells within tumors is relatively short, with estimated values ranging between 24 and 48 hours.[7] Further evidence clearly suggests that within spontaneous clinical tumors, only a small fraction (probably considerably less than 1%) of the cells within the tumor have the capacity for indefinite sustained growth.[8] These cells with indefinite growth capacity, i.e., tumor stem cells or clongenic cells, dictate the overall growth rate of the entire neoplastic cell population itself. If few or none of the clonogenic cells within the tumor lose the capacity for indefinite proliferation, the entire cell population of the tumor will in effect be composed of clonogenic cells. Such a cell system then grows at the same rate as the generation time of the clonogenic cells. These conditions are closely approximated by some experimental tumors, but this does not appear to be the case for most clinical malignant tumors. In clinical solid tumors, the evidence favors a cellular model of the tumor in which only a small subpopulation of clonogenic cells sustains the indefinite growth of the neoplasm as a whole. For most clinical solid tumors, nearly half the progeny of each clonogenic cell division results in the production of a differentiated or nonclonogenic cell which will have only a limited capacity for proliferation. These cells divide a variable number of times, cease division, then ultimately become senescent and die.

It can be shown, by the appropriate mathematical and computer modeling techniques, that it is the frequency with which the clonogenic cells produce either two new clonogenic cells or produce differentiated cells that will dictate the overall growth rate of the tumor.

If the proportion of differentiated cells produced is close to 50 percent, the overall growth rate or doubling time of the system is very slow. Moreover, it requires many more divisions occurring within the clonogenic cell compartment to produce a tumor of any given size.

In other words, the slow growing system is, in effect, equivalent to a much larger rapidly growing tumor from the point of view of the number of divisions that have occurred within the stem cell compartment. If the mutation rate is constant, the increased number of divisions that occur within the clonogenic cell fraction in a slow-growing tumor results in an enhanced probability that mutations will appear.

Thus the slowing up of growth due to this mechanism has the effect of magnifying the mutation rate to resistance. One would predict accordingly that relatively slow-growing tumors are going to exhibit significantly higher orders of resistance than an equivalent cell system which is characterized by more rapid growth, even if the mutation rates to resistance are identical in both cases.

With specific reference to the problem of carcinomas of the upper aerodigestive tract, we can see that these tumors as a group tend to be relatively slow-growing, especially compared with the rapidly growing pediatric tumors, many lymphomas, and germ cell neoplasms. One might anticipate that on its own this would tend to render such cancers less likely to be curable by chemotherapy, and if this is combined with a tendency toward higher mutation rates to resistance, the resulting neoplasms would be very unlikely to be cured by drugs alone when the advanced disease is treated.

The behavior of clinically apparent squamous carcinomas of the head and neck area is consistent with this general model of tumor dynamics. Typically, these tumors respond to a variety of antineoplastic agents, but the duration of response is generally short, and most studies of the chemotherapy of advanced head and neck carcinoma have demonstrated little in the way of significant increase in survival, despite the relatively frequent occurrence of at least partial regression of disease.

CONCLUSIONS

The clinical behavior of most head and neck carcinomas suggests a significantly high fraction of drug resistant cells present in the tumor by the time the disease is clinically overt. The fact that measurable responses to treatment occur with significant frequency does suggest that in most instances the proportion of sensitive tumor cells is greater than that of the resistant fraction. The frequency of measurable responses seen in this disease is perhaps deceptive as the generally short duration of such responses argues for a relatively low sensitive-to-resistant cell ratio in most cases.

The fact that not all adjuvant chemotherapy trials in this disease have yielded positive results suggests that the subclinical burden of disease in many patients is probably greater than is appreciated. If, as appears to be the case, many patients with squamous cell head and neck carcinomas are presenting with subclinical but still noncurable burdens of metastatic disease, this argues for the following strategic approaches. First, adjuvant programs may have to be targeted at better selected subgroups of patients who are more likely to benefit from the adjuvant intervention, i.e., patients in whom it can be inferred that their average tumor burden is less and whose tumor type is known to display greater responsiveness to chemotherapy. In addition, more attention will have to be paid the design of effective chemotherapy protocols involving the use of noncross-resistant agents which are delivered at an effective dose rate and intensity.

REFERENCES

1. Ling V. Genetic basis of drug resistance in mammalian cells. In: Bruchovsky N, Goldie JH (eds). Drug and hormone resistance in neoplasia. Vol. 1. Boca Raton: CRC Press, 1982.
2. Nowell PC. Tumor progression and clonal evolution: The role of genetic instability. In: German J (ed). *Chromosome Mutation and Neoplasia*. New York: Alan R. Liss, 1983, pp 413–432.
3. Skipper HE, Schabel FM Jr., Wilcox WS. Experimental evolution of potential anticancer agents. XII, On the criteria and kinetics associated with "curability" of experimental leukemia. Cancer Chemother Rep 1964; 35:1–111.
4. De Vita VT Jr. The relationship between tumor mass and resistance to chemotherapy. Cancer 1983; 51:1209–1220.
5. Schachney SE, McCormack GW, Cuchural GJ Jr. Growth rate patterns of solid tumors and their relation to responsiveness to therapy: An analytical review. Ann Intern Med 1978; 89:107–121.
6. Goldie JR, Coldman AJ. Quantitative model for multiple levels of drug resistance in clinical tumors. Cancer Treat Rep 1983; 67:923–931.
7. Hill BT. Biochemical and cell kinetic aspects to drug resistance. In: Bruchovsky N, Goldie JH (eds). Drug and Hormone Resistance in Neoplasia. Vol 1. Boca Raton: CRC Press, 1982; 21–53.
8. Bush RS, De Boer G, Hill RP. Long-term survival with gynecological cancer. In: Stoll BA (ed). Prolonged Arrest of Cancer. New York and London: John Wiley and Sones, 1982; 27–58.

MULTIDRUG RESISTANCE AND CHEMOTHERAPY

VICTOR LING, Ph.D.

Nonresponse to chemotherapeutic treatment in advanced cancers often extends to drugs or combinations of drugs with which the patient had not been treated previously. In many instances, an initially responsive disease is followed subsequently by a nonresponsive one. Many factors may contribute to this nonresponsive state. One possibility is the development of variant tumor cells resistant to the anticancer drugs applied.[1–3] Such malignant cells could ultimately play a dominant role in limiting successful chemotherapy.

In tumor cell populations used for experimental studies, drug-resistant variants are normally observed in low frequencies (10^{-5} or lower); however, clonal lines resistant to the major anticancer agents have now been isolated for investigation, and mechanisms of resistance have been elucidated.[1,4] Studies of such lines have resulted in the development of probes and approaches for the detection of drug-resistant cells in heterogeneous populations of tumor cells. Recently, drug-resistant tumor cells have been identified directly in patient biopsy samples.[5,6] Such findings are consistent with the hypothesis that in these patients, drug-resistant tumor cells are generated during tumor progression, and that during chemotherapeutic treatments, such variant cells enjoy a growth advantage

and are selectively propagated, thus occupying a significant proportion of the tumor cell population.

The discovery that lines selected for resistance with a single agent frequently display an unanticipated *multidrug resistance* phenotype further supports the hypothesis that drug-resistant tumor cells could limit successful chemotherapy. This is a highly complex phenotype involving resistance to a plethora of functionally and structurally unrelated drugs. Features of this phenotype will be described in greater detail below; however, it is worth noting that acquisition of such a phenotype could render tumor cells refractile to a combination of apparently unrelated "non-crossreacting" drugs. This could very well provide a rational explanation for the nonresponse to a variety of drug combinations observed in many cases of advanced cancers.

MULTIDRUG RESISTANCE PHENOTYPE

The multidrug resistance phenotype has been observed in a wide variety of animal and human cell lines.[1,4,7–9] The major characteristic of cells acquiring this phenotype is their response to a variety of unrelated cytotoxic compounds. This is illustrated in the mutant line CH^{R}C5 isolated in Chinese hamster ovary tissue culture cells for resistance to the antimitotic compound colchicine (Table 1). Both cross-resistance and collateral sensitivity are observed. The phenotype is complex in that the pattern of response to various drugs displayed by a particular resistant line appears not to be readily predicted a priori. Similar results have been observed in human and animal cell lines isolated for resistance to compounds such as Adriamycin, actinomycin D, daunorubicin, emetine, podophyllotoxin, puromycin, taxol, vinblastine, and vincristine.

The basis of the resistant phenotype appears to result from a reduced accumulation of the drugs in-

This work was supported by grants from the National Cancer Institute of Canada, Medical Research Council of Canada, and National Institutes of Health, U.S.A.

TABLE 1 Multidrug Resistance in CH^R C5

Drug	Relative Resistance*
Colchicine	180
Puromycin	~100
Daunomycin	76
Adriamycin	90
Vinblastine	30
Emetine	29
Taxol	~20
Melphalan	15
Chlorambucil	2
Nitrogen mustard	3
Deoxycorticosterone	0.1
1-Dehydrotestosterone	0.1
Acronycine	< 0.06
Triton X-100	0.3

* Relative resistance was determined by the concentration of drug required to inhibit growth or colony formation in the drug-resistant line compared with that required for the parent drug-sensitive line. A value greater than 1 denotes cross-resistance and one less than 1 denotes collateral sensitivity. The CH^R C5 line was derived from a Chinese hamster ovary cell line by selection in three steps for colchicine resistance. Data presented in this table are compiled from previous studies from this laboratory.

volved. The mechanism by which this is mediated is not well understood. Data to support a mechanism involving reduced drug influx or increased drug efflux have been obtained with different labeled drugs in different systems. This altered drug accumulation can be modulated by inhibitors of energy metabolism, calcium antagonists, nonionic detergents, steroids, or local anesthetics. The basis for collateral sensitivity is not known. However, all these findings are consistent with the basis of the multidrug resistance phenotype involving an altered cell surface membrane. Mutations in such an organelle could result in a wide-ranging pleiotropy.[10]

P-GLYCOPROTEIN AND MULTIDRUG RESISTANCE

Increased expression of a cell surface glycoprotein of approximately 170,000 daltons is closely associated with the expression of multidrug resistance in cell lines from different species isolated with different drugs.[9] This has been called the P-glycoprotein because of its association with the pleiotropic phenotype of multidrug resistance. The amount of P-glycoprotein found in resistant cells appears to correlate with the degree of resistance. The carbohydrate portion of P-glycoprotein, which accounts for approximately 30,000 daltons, appears not to be directly involved in the pleiotropic phenotype.[8] Nevertheless, this cell surface moiety appears to be conserved both with respect to molecular size and to maintaining immunologic identity among the ''P-glycoproteins'' found in the multidrug resistance lines from different species.[9] Monoclonal antibodies have been raised which react with P-glycoproteins from human and rodent cells.

The actual role played by P-glycoproteins in the multidrug resistance phenotype is not known, nor is it known whether its overexpression in the resistant cells is alone sufficient for expression of the multidrug resistance phenotype. It is possible that P-glycoprotein interacts with different membrane and cytoplasmic components to mediate this complex phenotype. Other molecular changes have been identified in a number of multidrug-resistant lines; however, those changes are not consistently seen in different isolates. To date, overexpression of P-glycoprotein appears to be the best molecular marker that is quantitatively correlated with expression of the multidrug resistance phenotype.

GENETICS OF MULTIDRUG RESISTANCE

Cell:cell hybrid studies indicate that the multidrug resistance phenotype is expressed in a dominant manner. This implies that this phenotype can be readily expressed in fully diploid or in polyploid tumor cells. Analyses of independent clonal isolates, revertants, and DNA-mediated transfectants indicate that the different features of the multidrug resistance phenotype (e.g., cross-resistance, collateral sensitivity, increased expression of P-glycoprotein) are probably coded for by a single gene or by a group of very closely linked genes.

Karyotypic changes have also been identified in mutant cell lines expressing the multidrug resistance phenotype. Most notable are homogeneous staining regions (HSRs) and double minute (DM) chromosomes. These are features generally associated with gene amplification. Recently, amplified DNA sequences associated with multidrug resistance in hamster cells have been identified and cloned.[11] These findings indicate that multidrug resistance probably arises from gene amplification and that P-glycoprotein is one of the amplified genes.

CONCLUSIONS AND FUTURE PROSPECTS

The question of whether multidrug resistant malignant cells do in fact occur in human neoplasms deserves continued attention. The availability of immunologic probes for P-glycoprotein expression and application of recombinant DNA technology should greatly facilitate investigation in this area. As already noted, a preliminary study clearly indicated that tumor cells containing greatly increased amounts of P-glycoprotein are found in some cases of advanced ovarian cancer nonresponsive to chemotherapy.[5] This finding is consistent with the notion that in these cases, multidrug-resistant tumor cells are resistant to the chemotherapeutic treatment applied and are selectively propagated to the detriment of the patient. More detailed studies will be required to confirm this hypothesis.

The finding that multidrug resistance probably involves gene amplification provides a basis for speculation on the origin of malignant disease innately resistant to chemotherapy even prior to treatment. In such an instance, a mechanism involving a selective outgrowth of a resistant subpopulation in the presence of drugs could not be invoked. One possibility is that genes involved in multidrug resistance (e.g., P-gly-coprotein gene) are coincidentally amplified in such malignant tumors. The involvement of gene amplification in malignant development has gained support from studies of tumor cells at the cytologic level (e.g., presence of DMs and HSRs) and at the DNA level (e.g., amplification of oncogenes). Because gene amplification can often be accompanied by translocation, it seems possible that malignancy genes may in some cases become closely linked to genes involved in drug resistance and that during malignant progression, the drug resistances genes are co-amplified. Such speculations can be tested directly and may provide new insights to the process of malignant progression.

The fact that the multidrug resistance phenotype is a complex one, involving resistance to a wide variety of apparently unrelated anticancer agents, raises the practical issue of how "non-cross-reacting" drugs can be identified. Information of this nature will probably be required to design appropriate alternating drug combinations for therapy. Screening of the current anticancer agents to determine their effect on model multidrug resistance lines would constitute a first approach toward this objective. The prospect of identifying collaterally sensitive compounds is an exciting one.

The intimate association of increased P-glycoprotein expression with expression of multidrug resistance in a variety of tumor cell lines raises the possibility that this cell surface antigen may potentially be exploited for diagnostic and therapeutic purposes. For example, hitherto unresponsive tumor cells may become amenable to treatment with P-glycoprotein-targeted antibodies conjugated with cytotoxic agents.

REFERENCES

1. Ling V. Genetic basis of drug resistance in mammalian cells. In: Bruchovsky N, Goldie JH (eds). Drug and Hormone Resistance in Neoplasia. Vol 1. Boca Raton: CRC Press, 1982; 1–19.
2. Goldie JH, Coldman AJ. Clinical implication of the phenomenon of drug resistance. In: Bruchkovsky N, Goldie JH (eds). Drug and Hormone resistance in neoplasia. Vol II. Boca Raton: CRC Press 1982; 111–127.
3. DeVita VJ Jr. The relationship between tumor mass and resistance to chemotherapy. Cancer 1983; 51:1209–1220.
4. Curt GA, Clendeninn NJ, Chabner BA. Drug resistance in cancer. Cancer Treat Rep 1984; 68:87–99.
5. Bell RD, Gerlach JH, Kartner N, Buick RN, Ling V. Detection of P-glycoprotein in ovarian cancer: a molecular marker associated with multidrug resistance. J Clin Oncol (in press).
6. Carman MD, Schornagel JH, Rivest RS, Srimatkandada S, Portlock CS, Duffy T, Bertino JR. Resistance to methotrexate due to gene amplification in a patient with acute leukemia. J Clin Oncol 1984; 2:16–20.
7. Biedler JL, Chang T, Meyers MB, Peterson RHF, Spengler BA. Drug resistance in Chinese hamster lung and mouse tumor cells. Cancer Treat Rep 1983; 67:859–867.
8. Ling V, Kartner N, Sudo T, Siminovitch L, Riordan JR. The multidrug resistance phenotype in Chinese hamster ovary cells. Cancer Treat Rep 1983; 67:869–874.
9. Kartner N, Riordan JR, Ling V. Cell surface P-glycoprotein associated with multidrug resistance in mammalian cell lines. Science 1983; 221:1285–1288.
10. Baker RM, Ling V. Membrane mutants of mammalian cells in culture. In: Korn E (ed). Methods in Membrane Biology. Vol 9. New York and London: Plenum Press, 1978; 337–384.
11. Roninson IB, Abelson HT, Housman DE, Howell N, Varshavsky A. Amplification of specific DNA sequences correlate with multidrug resistance in Chinese hamster cells. Nature 1984; 309:626–628.

28. Tumor Response to Chemotherapy and Its Measurement

INTRODUCTION

STEPHEN K. CARTER, M.D.

The measurement of objective response is a critical component of evaluating the results of cancer chemotherapy. Objective response means measurable shrinkage of clinically evident tumor. In head and neck cancer, as in other types of malignant tumor, responses break down into several varieties (Table 1). Complete response means complete disappearance of all evidence of neoplastic disease. The patient, after complete response, should be completely free of any clinical and/or pathologic residue of the disease. A clinical complete remission means that the evaluation of the measurable tumor disappearance has been limited to physical examination, radiologic or isotopic

TABLE 1   Responses in Head and Neck Cancer

Complete
Clinical
Pathologic
Partial
> 50% Shrinkage
< 50% Shrinkage

examination,and laboratory studies. Pathologic complete remission means that tissue has been examined for evidence of malignant cells. In head and neck cancer, this can involve biopsy of primary and nodal sites or examination of operative specimens when drugs are given in a preoperative or neoadjuvant (induction) mode. In general, pathologic complete response rates are lower than clinical complete response rates. Therefore, in the comparative evaluation of different regimens from different studies, it is essential that the type of complete response reported be clearly elucidated. Along with this elucidation should come details as to what examinations were performed to search for residual cancer. Unfortunately, the methods section of most papers do not go into great detail concerning response criteria and the aspects just discussed.

Partial response means that tumor shrinkage has occurred to a degree less than 100 percent. The most common definition of partial response is a greater than 50 percent shrinkage of the products of the measurement of a lesion in its two perpendicular diameters. This shrinkage should last some minimal period of time; 4 weeks is the most commonly used duration, although there is no absolute consistency in this aspect. The clinically evident disease in head and neck cancer is not always bidimensionally measurable. Some are only unidimensionally measurable and some are not measurable at all but can be deemed "evaluable".

A further problem in the determination of a partial response in head and neck cancer is that multiple lesions exist in many cases. With multiple lesions, there are at least four approaches to the definition of a partial response within the framework of a 50 percent shrinkage concept (Table 2). The most stringent criterion would be that all lesions have to shrink by at least 50 percent. The most liberal criterion would be to demand that only one shrink, while all the others do not progress in size. All of the four approaches listed in Table 2 are valid as defined, and it is up to the reader to decide what biologic meaning to give the results. The major problem is that there is no comparability of criteria across clinical trial groups and centers so that making cross comparisons between studies is a complicated process.

Yet another problem in evaluating partial response is the question whether a shrinkage in the range of 25 to 50 percent is acceptable. This type of shrink-

age is usually described as a "minor response" or "stable disease". If this is allowed, the response rate rises, but it is questionable whether these responses are biologically important, given the difficulty of measuring lumps and bumps in patients in a reproducible fashion.

Duration of response is an important consideration, and a variable in reporting this is the zero point chosen. Some groups choose the zero point as the date of initiation of treatment. Other groups use the zero point of when response was first observed or determined to actually exist by the utilized criteria. If the initiation of treatment is used, this can add 3 to 12 weeks, or even longer, to the response duration in comparison to the other approach. Again, both approaches are valid as defined, but the issue is biologic importance and across-study comparisons.

An often neglected (and possibly important) measurement is the time to treatment failure in all patients treated, independent of response, using initiation of therapy as the zero point. This is a determination which relates to potential benefit for all patients regardless of whether they have fully measurable disease and whether it shrinks.

Survival is the bottom-line determination in any study, but it can be a heterogeneous determination and not easy to evaluate in specific relation to the therapy in question. With survival, the end point is finite and easily measured. The zero point, hopever, is less clearcut. Survival can be measured from diagnosis, first treatment, diagnosis of recurrent disease, or from initiation of the chemotherapy being evaluated. The latter is the most common zero point utilized. The heterogeneity within this zero point relates to where, in the sequential flow of therapies, chemotherapy has been used. The first use of chemotherapy can be the third treatment after surgery, failure, radiation therapy, and a second failure. It can be the second treatment after either surgery or radiation therapy and failure. It can also be the first treatment in a patient presenting with metastatic disease or with disease not amenable to local control approaches.

Another heterogeneity that exists with survival is the impact of therapy given after progressive disease has been discovered after chemotherapy. This secondary therapy can have an impact on survival by either lengthening it, if it is effective, or shortening it, if it is excessively toxic. Nevertheless, impact on survival must be demonstrated if an objective response is to be considered meaningful. The demonstration of this is difficult and has eluded most of the chemotherapy studies in head and neck cancer published to date. It is easy to fall into a trap by showing that the objective responders live longer than the nonresponders and using this fact to claim proof of chemotherapy's benefit. This type of analysis ignores several biases which are described in detail by Vogl in his chapter. In addition, it ignores the bias that responders tend to have a more favorable mix of prognostic variables for survival than do nonresponders, independent of response. The proof

TABLE 2 Possible Approaches to Defining a Partial Response, Utilizing a > 50% Shrinkage Criterion, when Faced with Multiple Lesions in Head and Neck Cancer

All lesions must shrink by ≥ 50%.

≥ 50% of the lesions must shrink by ≥ 50%.

One lesion must shrink by ≥ 50% with all other lesions remaining stable.

The sum of the product of all lesions must shrink by ≥ 50%.

that response is an independent variable for survival prolongation requires a multiple regression analysis utilizing all known and available prognostic variables. Even so, there is still the possibility that an imbalance of unknown, or not measured, prognostic variables may be the reason for the observation.

The clearest determination that chemotherapy improves survival in advanced head and neck cancer would be a randomized study comparing chemotherapy with best supportive care. This trial would be difficult, if not impossible, to perform in the United States today.

The importance of objective response in head and neck cancer can be viewed from both a patient care and research perspective. From a patient care perspective, objective response is important only if it is associated with palliation and survival gains which are achieved with reasonable toxicity. This involves an evaluation of the impact of therapy on quality of life, which is often ignored in the research-oriented literature reports on chemotherapy. The research perspective views objective response as an indication of tumor cell kill and the drug(s) in question as a potential building block for further research studies.

In the chapters that follow, there is general agreement that partial responses are probably not meaningful in a patient care sense, but that they might be meaningful in a research sense. Although cisplatin alone and 5-FU alone give mainly partial responses, the combination of the two appears to be giving higher complete response rates and may be highly important in a combined-modality setting.

ISSUES IN DEFINING PARTIAL RESPONSE

MARCEL ROZENCWEIG, M.D.

The outcome of clinical trials is affected by a number of well-recognized and somewhat interrelated factors including patient selection, response criteria, and method of data analysis. These variables may account for conflicting results such as those concerning the single-agent activity of bleomycin in head and neck cancer (Table 1). Even carefully designed randomized trials do not fully preclude misleading reports as interpretation of the data may also be obscured by inadequate sample sizes or by a subtle effect of the very nature of the hypothesis under investigation.[7]

The selection of useful end-points for assessing a therapeutic option is limited, practically, by the stage of the disease and the developmental status of available therapy. Despite disputable definitions, partial responses play an important role in chemotherapeutic strategies for advanced disease. Active drugs must first be identified with activity commonly defined as a 20 percent or greater overall response rate. These active agents are then incorporated into various combination chemotherapy regimens, resulting eventually in improved effectiveness. As further progress is made, evaluation of new chemotherapeutic programs may become increasingly based on complete response and survival, which are more reliable indicators of drug efficacy than partial response.

In head and neck cancer, a superiority of combination chemotherapy over single-agent treatment has not yet been firmly established. In recurrent and metastatic disease, complete responses remain generally infrequent and, consequently, partial responses are still largely used to evaluate the respective value of currently available regimens.[8] Response duration is short with no or minimal impact on survival.

Much effort has been devoted to standardizing response criteria.[9,10] The following discussion focuses on the difficulties of defining partial response in head and neck cancer, and particular attention is given to recurrent and metastatic disease.

MEASURABILITY OF THE DISEASE

Detection of partial tumor shrinkage implies the presence of measurable or evaluable malignant disease. The reliability of this observation varies greatly with the degree of measurability of the tumor deposits. Well-circumscribed lesions in which the surface area may be estimated by the product of the two largest perpendicular diameters measured by ruler or calipers are most appropriate to identify objective tumor regression (e.g., isolated metastatic lung nodules, neck lymph nodes). Measures in one dimension may also be useful when the cross-sectional tumor area cannot be determined. Thus, liver enlargement due to tumor involvement is evaluated clinically by the distances of the inferior liver edge from the costal margins and the tip of the xiphoid. A minimum distance of 5 cm is required according to ECOG criteria.

TABLE 1 Single-Agent Activity of Bleomycin in Head and Neck Cancer

| No of Patients | Response Rate (%) | | Investigator |
	Complete	Overall	
53	6	45	Halnan[1]
48	4	38	Bonadonna[2]
64	0	19	Haas[3]
54	2	17	EORTC[4]
46	—	13	Yagoda[5]
81	1	6	Durkin[6]

Extreme interpretations are possible with poorly measurable malignant disease, as is frequently the case with primaries from the head and neck region. The line between clearly and poorly evaluable lesions is a matter of individual judgment. Poorly evaluable lesions leave ample room for subjective assessment. They cannot be simply ignored since the meaning of a partial response would become highly questionable. If they represent the bulk of disease, this could make a patient ineligible for clinical trials, which in turn could have serious impact on available accrual. Biases could also be introduced in the selection of patients by excluding those with poor prognostic characteristics such as previously irradiated lesions.

DEFINITION OF PARTIAL RESPONSE FOR INDIVIDUAL LESIONS

Partial response is commonly defined as a ≥ 50 percent decrease in tumor area for at least 4 weeks without increase in size by >25 percent in any area of known malignant disease or appearance of new areas of malignant disease. For unidimensionally measurable lesions, the cut-off point is lowered to 30 percent according to ECOG criteria (Table 2). For nonmeasurable, evaluable lesions, an estimated improvement by at least 75 percent is required by a number of investigators whereas ECOG and WHO requirements are less stringent. Following the ECOG system, however, this estimated improvement should be agreed upon by two independent investigators and documented serial evaluations are recommended.

Whatever the criteria, the weight given to a partial regression is the same regardless of the initial tumor volume. One might advocate the need for taking this variable into consideration despite its speculative biologic significance. However, adding this information could seriously confuse response definitions and make a widely accepted consensus even more remote.

Striking limitations of measurement accuracy have been demonstrated by Moertel and Hanley with simulated bidimensionally measurable tumor masses.[11] The experimental conditions mimicked ideal clinical situations which minimized discrepancies that could be expected with real tumors in patients. A true difference in surface area by 50 percent was detected in 88 percent of the cases when measurements were repeated by the same investigators and 73 percent of the cases when these measurements were obtained by two different investigators. When two masses of the

TABLE 2 Partial Response

Lesion	Required Reduction (%)
Measurable, bidimensional	50
Measurable, unidimensional	30–50
Nonmeasurable, evaluable	50–75

TABLE 3 Repeated Measurements of the Same Simulated Tumor Masses

	% Erroneous Observations			
	Decrease		Increase	
	$\geq 25\%$	$\geq 50\%$	$\geq 25\%$	$\geq 50\%$
Same investigators	19	8	19	19
Different investigators	25	7	32	18

Adapted from Moertel and Hanley[11]

same diameter were measured, a reduction by 50 percent in cross-sectional area was found in nearly 10 percent of the cases (Table 3). The data also indicated that lesser degrees of clinical response (>25 to 49% decrease in cross-sectional tumor area) would be subject to considerable measurement errors. Although often reported as minor and less than partial responses, these should not be considered objective tumor regression.

The time element incorporated into the definition of partial response is another source of variability in data reporting. Response duration might be considered to last from the initiation of therapy until the eventual verification of disease progression. At least the former event is fixed, and it is reasonable to assume that an antitumor response begins with the onset of treatment, when indeed it occurs. On the other hand, using the date when partial response is fully demonstrated as a starting point could identify more meaningful responses. Very transient therapeutic effects classified as responses by the previous approach would be excluded and, by definition, confirmatory findings would become necessary, often at a time when further tumor growth would be expected.[11]

A key definition is that of treatment failure. Appearance of a new tumor is a reliable indication of tumor progression, although occasionally it may occur concomitantly with regression elsewhere. Such mixed responses may be worth noting, but must still be classified as progressions. In many instances, progressive disease is established with difficulty, and one must rely on increases in tumor size or less definable changes (Table 4). Relapse after regression may pose additional difficulties since its recognition is based on the maximum regression that has been observed. In

TABLE 4 Common Criteria for Treatment Failure

Appearance of new lesions
Progressive growth ($> 25\%$ increase in area)
Symptomatic deterioration, stable objective measurements*
Symptomatic deterioration, after partial response*
Death from disease, with or without toxicity†
Severe toxicity with cumulative, irreversible, or unpredictable manifestations

*Must document decline in performance status or weight loss, or increase in specific symptoms, and exclude drug toxicity or other complications (not applicable until patient has received minimum prescribed course of therapy).
†"Early death" should be defined if excluded from analysis.

addition, minimal changes in very small tumors may easily show increases greater than 25 percent. To require increases in excess of 50 percent would not necessarily safeguard against prematurely interpreting termination of a response. In the study of Moertel and Hanley,[11] repeated measurements of simulated tumor masses which had remained the same size indicated an increase in cross-sectional area by 50 percent in about one-fifth of the cases (see Table 3).

DETERMINATION OF TOTAL RESPONSE

Total response is an assessment of response when many indicator lesions are present and many organ systems are affected. For ECOG and WHO, this total response is based on organ site evaluation. Accordingly, insufficient consideration may be given to tumor burden and number of tumor deposits. Partial response in an organ site denotes a greater than 50 percent decrease in the sum of the measurements of all measurable lesions. The absence of change in unmeasurable disease does not detract from a partial response by organ site. Total partial response indicates that the number of organ sites with complete or partial response is equal to or greater than that of organ sites designated as "no change".

Various theoretic examples illustrate the problems associated with this method of assessment. Partial regression of a small measurable lesion might qualify for an overall partial response even with concomitant unchanged bulky disease that is evaluable but not measurable. In the presence of two lesions, with partial response in one and no change in the other, total response would be partial if these lesions were in different sites, although there could be unchanged disease if they were in the same site.

Practically, many investigators evaluate total response based on the sum of the measurements of all measurable lesions regardless of organ site involvement. Improvement or defined estimated regression of nonmeasurable, evaluable disease may or may not be required. In the vast majority of publications on clinical trials, the broad description of response criteria does not lend itself to detailed analysis and may conceal wide variations in the individual understanding of the commonly used 50 percent tumor reduction definition.

INITIAL WORK-UP AND FOLLOW-UP

Initial work-up should consist of detailed history, thorough physical examination with skilled evaluation of the head and neck region, complete blood counts and chemistries, chest roentgenogram, lung tomograms if routine chest films are unremarkable, radionuclear bone scan, as well as CT scans of the head and neck and of the liver. Additional diagnostic tests might be necessary to ascertain and document the extent of local or distant dissemination.

Clear documentation of head and neck lesions is not always possible. Minute descriptions are often more useful than photographs. CT scans are of definite value for diagnostic purposes, but their actual contribution in assessing tumor response remains to be determined.

Extensive baseline studies might prove difficult in patients with limited therapeutic expectations. On the other hand, distant metastases occur in 10 to 30 percent of the patients with advanced head and neck cancer,[12] and missing a single site of metastatic dissemination might modify a partial response to a "no change" status or vice versa. Moreover, concomitant disease such as alcoholic cirrhosis or multiple primaries are common features in these patients, and their blurring effect on the total assessment should not be neglected, particularly with incomplete pathologic investigations. Thus, in a recently reported study on 36 patients with head and neck cancer and a suggestion of malignant pulmonary invasion on chest roentgenogram,[13] biopsy or postmortem examination revealed a second malignant tumor in 19 (53%), benign lesions, mostly of chronic organizing pneumonia, in 10 (28%), and metastatic head and neck cancer in seven (19%).

Repeated measurements confer confidence to response data, especially when a continuous trend toward tumor regression is found prior and after the occurrence of partial response. Frequent evaluaations may be needed as time to tumor shrinkage by 50 percent may be very brief, duration of this shrinkage may be borderline, and no consistent relationship has been noted between these variables. Whichever starting date of response duration is selected, widely spaced follow-up (e.g., 4-week intervals) could miss a true partial response or falsely identify a response while undetected regrowth is ongoing. Such errors could barely be avoided when special tests are needed for tumor evaluation, e.g., endoscopic examination of the primary, lung tomograms, or CT scans. These considerations should be kept in mind when analyzing partial response rates by organ sites.

DISCUSSION

Establishing the relative efficacy of chemotherapeutic agents in a wide range of malignant diseases has been a difficult and complex endeavor. Initially, the lack of statistical sophistication in clinical trials led to many inconclusive results of drug evaluation. While interest in chemotherapy was expanding, major efforts were made to identify active single agents, setting the stage for the development of combination chemotherapy. The methodology of clinical trials improved with better knowledge of prognostic factors influencing response and with greater emphasis on fulfillment of statistical requirements. The need for standardized response criteria was also recognized as an essential ingredient of a systematic, rigorous, and successful search for increased chemotherapeutic activity.

Despite several attempts at standardization, common criteria are not yet uniformly utilized. Major discrepancies in assessment may result from variable definitions of indicator lesions and total response. Moreover, clinical measurements lack reproducibility, particularly in poorly measurable lesions, which frequently represent the bulk of disease in previously operated and irradiated patients. An added complication is short response duration, which gives great weight to the definition of its starting point as well as the extent and frequency of follow-up.

Some flexibility in response criteria might be allowed for phase II trials with new anticancer agents. These trials are primarily designed to rapidly reject ineffective drugs. Any hints of antitumor activity might be important and would justify additional drug testing. The consequences of false-negative evaluations are difficult to estimate, whereas those generated by false-positive evaluations are more predictable. Generally, these reports constitute no major problem in diseases wherein even preliminary borderline activity demands further exploration, and a more thorough experience is worthwhile and achievable. However, labeling an agent as active may continue to bring about trials based on inadequate rationale. Thus, cyclophosphamide, which has been extensively used in combination against carcinomas of head and neck origin, was deemed active based essentially on data from one study using inadequate definitions of response.[14]

Detailed criteria such as those of ECOG or WHO do not preclude substantial background noise in partial response data. The resulting effect can hardly be determined, but conceivably this could totally obscure the outcome of the most carefully designed randomized studies. Significant differences in overall response rates that are not supported by significant differences in complete response rates should be interpreted with the greatest caution. Adding accuracy to current criteria might prove to be an academic exercise because increasing their complexity would probably prevent wide acceptance. Restricting accrual to patients with no prior radiotherapy would solve only part of the problem. Another option for phase III trials would be merely to ignore partial responses and to base treatment evaluations on complete responses only. The possible impact of such an option on chemotherapeutic straegies is uncertain, but it deserves at least critical consideration.

REFERENCES

1. Halnan KE, Bleehen NM, Brewin TB, et al. Early clinical experience with bleomycin in the United Kingdom in a series of 105 patients. Br Med J 1972; 4:635–638.
2. Bonadonna G, De Lena M, Monfardini S, et al. Clinical trials with bleomycin in lymphomas and in solid tumors. Eur J Cancer 1972; 8:205–215.
3. Haas CD, Coltman CA Jr, Gottlieb JA, et al. Phase II evaluation of bleomycin. A Southwest Oncology Group study. Cancer 1976; 38:8–12.
4. Clinical Screening Cooperative Group of the European Organization for Research on Treatment of Cancer: Study of the clinical efficiency of bleomycin in human cancer. Br Med J 1970; 2:643–645.
5. Yagoda A, Mukherji B, Young C, et al. Bleomycin, an antitumor antibiotic. Clinical experience in 274 patients. Ann Intern Med 1972; 77:861–870.
6. Durkin WJ, Pugh RP, Jacobs E, et al. Bleomycin (NSC-125066) therapy of responsive solid tumors. Oncology 1976; 33:260–264.
7. Staquet MJ, Rozencweig M, Von Hoff DD, et al. The delta and epsilon errors in the assessment of cancer clinical trials. Cancer Treat Rep 1979; 63:1917–1921.
8. Rozencweig M, Decoster G. Chemotherapy in squamous cell carcinoma of the head and neck. In: Bonadonna G, Veronesi U, eds. Clinical trials in cancer medicine. New York: Academic Press (in press).
9. Oken MM, Creech RH, Tormey DC, et al. Toxicity and response criteria of the Eastern Cooperative Oncology Group. Am J Clin Oncol 1982; 5:649–655.
10. World Health Organization: WHO handbook for reporting results of cancer treatment. WHO Offset Publication No. 48, Geneva, 1979.
11. Moertel CG, Hanley JA. The effect of measuring error on the results of therapeutic trials in advanced cancer. Cancer 1976; 38:388–394.
12. Papac RJ. Distant metastases from head and neck cancer. Cancer 1984; 53:342–345.
13. Malefatto JP, Kasimis BS, Moran EM, et al. The clinical significance of radiographically detected pulmonary neoplastic lesions in patients with head and neck cancer. J Clin Oncol 1984; 2:625–630.
14. Harrison D, Espiner H, Glazebrook G. Cyclophosphamide in head and neck cancer. In: Fairley G, Simister J, eds. Cyclophosphamide. Baltimore: Williams & Wilkins, 1965, pp 48–55.

TUMOR RESPONSE TO CHEMOTHERAPY AND ITS MEASUREMENT: RESPONSE DETERMINATION IN COMBINED-MODALITY SETTINGS

JAMES Y. SUEN, M.D.

TABLE 1 Chemotherapy As Neoadjuvant: Results of Three Studies

Spaulding, Loré et al[3]	
Cis-platinum	46 pts. Stages III & IV
Bleomycin	86% response
Vincristine	10 CR
Posner et al[5]	
Cis-platinum	93 pts. Stages III & IV
Bleomycin	88% response
Methotrexate with L.R.	24% CR
Al-Sarraf, Weaver et al[4]	
Cis-platinum	85 pts. Stages III & IV
5-FU	93% response
	54% CR

It is well known that the cure rates for advanced (stages III and IV) cancer of the head and neck are poor. The standard acceptable treatment for years has been surgery and radiation therapy. In an effort to improve the poor prognosis, chemotherapy has been added to the treatment modalities.

The methods of combined modality treatment using chemotherapy have been numerous, but basically can be categorized into three methods: neoadjuvant, concurrent, and maintenance. These methods will be discussed in this chapter.

The measurement of response to chemotherapy is obviously important. When responses are given for various studies, we seldom question how the responses were measured. There are some problems with measuring response and these must be addressed.

CHEMOTHERAPY AS NEOADJUVANT (INDUCTION CHEMOTHERAPY)

The primary indication for chemotherapy as a neoadjuvant is the patient with an advanced (stage III or IV) resectable, potentially curable head and neck cancer. This can include previously untreated as well as recurrent cancers. These patients must also be in good enough health to tolerate this prolonged treatment.

It is generally accepted that previous radiation therapy significantly decreases the chances of response to chemotherapy, whereas chemotherapy administered as the first treatment modality can give impressive responses.

Most oncologists believe that advanced cancer of the head and neck is a systemic disease on initial presentation. Therefore, it seems appropriate to treat these patients with chemotherapy initially, especially if it is more effective at that time. It is hoped that the chemotherapy, if effective, will destroy micrometastases as well as reduce the local tumor bulk.

Several studies which have reported high rates of partial and complete responses when chemotherapy was used as a neoadjuvant.[1-3] These are summarized in Table 1. These responses with combination chemotherapy, using cis-platinum as the primary base drug, are significantly better than with single-drug chemotherapy.

As a neoadjuvant, the chemotherapy could be administered in several ways. These methods are outlined in Table 2. At present most studies are using chemotherapy as an induction therapy followed by surgery and radiation therapy.

The measurement of response to chemotherapy as a neoadjuvant should not be difficult since it is the only treatment being administered at that time. The accepted responses are (1) no response with progression, (2) no response with stable or less than 50 percent regression, (3) partial response (50% or greater regression), and (4) complete response (no clinical evidence of residual cancer).

Since patients with distant metastases are rarely cured, they would not normally be treated with chemotherapy as a neoadjuvant. Therefore, discussion of the response determination can be confined to the primary cancer and regional cervical lymph node metastases.

There are two major issues of defining and measuring response which must be addressed. One is the difficulty in measuring the primary upper aerodigestive cancer and its cervical metastases in an objective manner. The other is deciding how many courses of chemotherapy should be administered to obtain the optimal response.

One must be careful in assessing some of the advanced cancers in which there is erythema, induration and pain from ulceration, necrosis, and secondary infection. These conditions can regress somewhat with antibiotic treatment only, and when antibiotics and chemotherapy are given simultaneously it may be dif-

TABLE 2 Methods of Administering Neoadjuvant Chemotherapy

1. CT ⟶ S
2. CT ⟶ S ⟶ XRT
3. CT ⟶ S ⟶ XRT ⟶ CT
4. CT ⟶ S ⟶ CT
5. CT ⟶ XRT

CT = chemotherapy; S = surgery; XRT = radiation therapy.

ficult to assess whether the regression is due to the chemotherapy.

Measurement of a primary cancer in the upper aerodigestive tract during the physical examination is usually an estimate and frequently differs with different examiners. This difference can be considerable at times. I have treated over 500 head and neck cancer patients with chemotherapy, and my assessment of tumor response in most upper aerodigestive tract cancers has been more subjective than objective. I feel that I can safely state that most other examiners also use subjective measurements. If complete clinical regression of the primary is noted while the patient is on chemotherapy, the assessment is more likely to be correct. On the other hand, assessment of regressions between 25 and 75 percent can be difficult. Since a 40 percent regression is considered a "no response" and a 50 percent regression is considered a partial response, one can easily see that this type of assessment may be very inaccurate, especially when there is no satisfactory objective way of measuring the tumor directly.

These measurements of response should be performed by an experienced examiner with as much objective measurement as possible. Computerized tomography (CT scan) is valuable in delineating the extent of disease and can be used as a method of objective measurement. It can sometimes be difficult to define the exact limits of the tumor because the tumor density may be very close to the density of adjacent normal structures. A combination of an experienced examiner's physical assessment and a CT scan assessment should give the best measurement of response at this time.

The same problems exist with the measurement of cervical node metastases. The intervening tissue of the neck skin, subcutaneous tissue, and neck muscles must be taken into account, and a measuring tape should definitely be used. I believe that there is a significant amount of subjective measuring of the lymph nodes and that the response determination may frequently be erroneous. The CT scan can be helpful in measurement of the lymph node responses.

The other major issue which must be addressed is how many courses of chemotherapy should be administered during this induction chemotherapy. The goal of this type of therapy is to reduce the local tumor burden (we hope completely) and to destroy micrometastases which are certain to exist in at least 20 percent of the patients.

Although the data are not yet conclusive, there is growing evidence that a patient who has a complete clinical regression during induction chemotherapy has a greater chance for cure. Patients who have a partial response do not seem to have an improved cure rate, but may experience longer disease-free intervals following surgery and/or irradiation than do nonresponders.

There have been no studies to indicate how many courses of induction chemotherapy are required to give the maximum number of complete responders. A study by the Wayne State group using cis-platinum and 5-FU as induction chemotherapy reported that after one course of induction chemotherapy, 11 percent had complete regression (CR).[4] After two courses of chemotherapy, 29 percent had CR, and after three courses, the percentage of CR was 67 percent. It is difficult to know whether further courses of chemotherapy would have increased the number of patients with CR.

One would think that if all local and regional disease regressed with the induction chemotherapy, all of the micrometastases would be destroyed. There is no known method of measuring whether the micrometastases have been destroyed, and so one can only assume it. The proof would be in long-term followup to see whether those who had a complete response to the induction chemotherapy remain free of distant metastases.

CONCURRENT CHEMOTHERAPY

Most concurrent chemotherapy has been with a combination of a single drug and radiation therapy (RT). Many studies have shown that most chemotherapy-RT treatment regimens effect dramatic regressions during treatment, but the side effects are significantly greater, and the cure rate is not significantly improved over that of irradiation alone. The primary problem is severe mucositis, which in many cases necessitates interruption of RT. Mucositis has not proved to be a major problem when cisplatin is combined with RT.

The patient population selected for concurrent chemotherapy-RT are those with advanced squamous cell carcinomas, which would normally be treated with RT alone for one reason or another. The chemotherapy is usually administered as a sensitizer for the RT.

It is not known whether the chemotherapeutic agent destroys part of the tumor cells and the RT destroys another group or whether the drug sensitizes the cells to RT so that the RT destroys more cells. It may be immaterial which is the case, as long as more cancer cells are killed. Since most randomized studies have shown that survival is not improved with concurrent therapy, it would appear that these single drug regimens are not destroying the micrometastases.

When two different treatment modalities are being administered concurrently, it is difficult to measure the response from the chemotherapy except by prospective randomized studies comparing concurrent therapy to RT alone to assess the local control rate, disease-free intervals, and survival.

CHEMOTHERAPY AS MAINTENANCE OR PROPHYLACTIC THERAPY

In the adjuvant breast studies, prophylactic chemotherapy was given postoperatively. The data seem to indicate that the cure rate is improved. In advanced resectable carcinomas of the head and neck, there was interest in treating these patients with chemotherapy prophylactically after surgery and RT. Ten years ago a study was initiated by Jesse, Goepfert, and me in which we treated approximately 25 patients in this manner. The study was discontinued because it was our impression that the additional chemotherapy had no significant effect.

In our experience, after previous RT the best expected response rate with chemotherapy was only about 25 to 30 percent. This meant that 70 to 75 percent of the patients were receiving prolonged chemotherapy without any benefit. Since there was no measurable disease during this treatment, the end-point was recurrent or metastatic disease or no evidence of disease after 5 years. Another problem, besides that of having no measurable disease to follow for response determination, was the increased incidence of major complications such as brain necrosis, bilateral blindness, and severe fibrosis. To my knowledge, no reported controlled studies have been conducted randomizing patients with head and neck cancer to either adjuvant (prophylactic) treatment or "no treatment" following surgery and/or RT.

DISCUSSION

Of the different combined-modality approaches discussed, the method that seems most appealing is the "induction chemotherapy" or neoadjuvant method. Chemotherapy is definitely more effective when given prior to irradiation and surgery. When chemotherapy is administered initially, the responses are easier to measure, although there are the problems with objective measurements, which have been discussed. Even though we define the measurement of a tumor as the product of the largest perpendicular diameters of all measurable tumor, I would seriously doubt that this measurement is commonly used when assessing tumors. The subjective measurements used surely have a significant error rate.

The issue of how many courses of induction chemotherapy should be administered is still unresolved. The primary goal is to improve the cure rate, and it appears that the cure rate is improved only if a complete clinical regression is obtained. It would seem logical that a patient should proceed with surgery and radiation therapy as soon as a complete regression is obtained, even if it only takes one course of chemotherapy. If a patient has not had a complete regression after three courses of chemotherapy, but has shown significant regression after each course, then a fourth course should be considered in the hope of obtaining

a complete response before proceeding with surgery and RT.

If there has been little or no response after two courses of chemotherapy a complete regression is highly unlikely no matter how many courses are administered. In this group of patients, treatment with surgery and RT should proceed.

Another issue is the significance of finding no tumor in the surgical specimen after induction chemotherapy. We are all aware that it would be extremely difficult to examine the entire specimen histologically, and it certainly is not practical to do so. It would be easy to miss small microscopic foci of tumor cells that might persist, and these would be capable of growing if no further treatment were administered. It is common knowledge that these last few cancer cells are difficult to destroy with chemotherapy alone. Therefore, additional therapy, such as surgery/ and or RT, is still essential.

Any subsequent surgery should encompass the original extent of disease. Prospective, randomized studies will need to be performed to determine whether surgery or irradiation can be deleted if a complete regression is obtained with induction chemotherapy.

In an effort to improve our methods of measuring response to chemotherapy, we should develop a uniform method of objective measurements of the local and regional cancers and use it for reporting purposes. This should include more exact methods of measuring lesions on physical examination and utilizing the CT scan.

Since the primary response to be measured with chemotherapy as an adjuvant is an improved cure rate, the most accurate method of assessment would be large, prospective, randomized studies.

REFERENCES

1. Decker DA, Drelichman A, Jacobs J, et al. Adjuvant chemotherapy with cis-diamminodichloroplatinum II and 120-hour infusion 5-fluorouracil in stage III and IV squamous cell carcinoma of the head and neck. Cancer 1983; 51:1353–1355.
2. Ervin TJ, Weichselbaum RR, Fabian RL, et al. Advanced squamous carcinoma of the head and neck. Arch Otolaryngol 1984; 110:241–245.
3. Spaulding MB, Kahn A, Santos RDL, Klotch D, Loré JM. Adjuvant chemotherapy in advanced head and neck cancer. Am J Surg 1982; 144:432–436.
4. Weaver A, Fleming S, Vandenberg H, et al. Cis-platinum and 5-fluorouracil as initial therapy in advanced epidermoid cancers of the head and neck. Head Neck Surg 1982; 4:370–373.
5. Posner MR, Ervin TJ, Weichselbaum RR, et al. The role of chemotherapy in treatment of advanced squamous cell cancer of the head and neck. Laryngoscope 1984; 94:481–482.

IS PARTIAL RESPONSE OF VALUE IN THE CHEMOTHERAPY OF ADVANCED HEAD AND NECK CANCER?

STEVEN E. VOGL, M.D.
DAVID A. SCHOENFELD, Ph.D.

Partial response to chemotherapy of head and neck cancer has generally been found to be of little value. In our group's initial experience with combination chemotherapy based on cisplatin (diamminedichloroplatinum(II) or DDP),[23] median duration of partial remission was 5 months (a respectable figure when compared to the 6-month median duration of remission to combination chemotherapy of metastatic breast cancer with cyclophosphamide, methotrexate, and 5-fluorouracil), but the median survival of partial responders was only 6 months, not much longer than the median survival of nonresponders (4 months). Complete responses, on the other hand, lasted much longer (median 11 months) and were associated with a median survival of 22 months. Unfortunately, only 17 percent of patients achieved complete remission in this pilot study.

One of the reasons partial response may fail to predict for prolonged survival relates to the high risk of intercurrent illnesses in this population. The tumors often interfere with nutrition because of their position, and the patients are particularly susceptible to aspiration pneumonia. Catastrophic events involving the larynx, the trachea, or the carotid artery are common and have been observed in our series even in situations in which the tumor was responding (e.g., an ischemic stroke occurred as the carotid artery seemed to collapse with the tumor mass). Furthermore, the epidemiologic correlates of head and neck cancer in this country, abuse of alcohol and tobacco, produce major illnesses which in themselves limit the survival of head and neck cancer patients, even if the tumor is completely controlled. Be that as it may, it seems reasonable to assume that such catastrophic events and intercurrent illnesses are more likely to occur when the tumor is growing than when it is shrinking.

We set out to search for a definition of partial remission, which is indeed correlated with prolonged survival. We fortunately had at our disposal intimate knowledge of a large cooperative group trial of chemotherapy of head and neck cancer with distant metastases or recurrence after radiation therapy which were not amenable to complete surgical excision. This Eastern Cooperative Oncology Group trial (EST 1377) accrued patients between 1978 and 1980, and so essentially complete follow-up is available.[1] Eligibility was restricted to squamous cancer and lymphoepithelioma in patients who were out of bed at least once a day, who had no other primary cancer, and who had adequate bone marrow, liver, and renal function to allow safe administration of chemotherapy. Details of the results of this trial are being reported elsewhere in this book (in the chapter on single-agent versus combination chemotherapy). Therefore only a few points related to response will be emphasized here.

The study randomized patients to methotrexate (MTX) alone, MTX with weekly subcutaneous *Corynebacterium parvum*, or MTX with concurrent bleomycin and cisplatin (a program given the acronym MBD). After 37 evaluable patients had entered the MTX + C. parvum arm, it was closed to patient entry because of poor overall accrual on the study and experience elsewhere suggesting lack of efficacy for this immune modulator. Indeed, in this trial, *C. parvum* did little but make skin sores and fevers. It had no effect at all on the rate, quality, or duration of response, on the severity or incidence of toxicity from methotrexate, or on survival. After randomization to the C. parvum arm was stopped, the response rate to single-agent methotrexate rose, so that by the end of the trial the overall response rate was 35 percent versus 48 percent for MBD. Complete responses were observed in 16 percent of MBD patients and 8 percent of MTX patients. These differences were not significant when other prognostic factors for response were taken into account, even if it was assumed that MBD could not be less active than MTX. For the purpose of this analysis, all three groups on the study will be combined.

Survival on the two arms of the study was identical, with a median of 5.6 months from entry, and with only 20 percent of the patients living longer than one year. Median time to disease progression for all patients was 3 months, with only 10 percent of patients free of progression at one year. Taking only responding patients, median time to progression was similar between the arms, 5 months for TMX and 5.8 months for MBD, with 20 percent on each arm free of progression at 10 months. Time to treatment failure for responding patients is a measure of duration of treatment benefit that ignores date of onset of response. This is not always precisely known, since tumors are not always measured weekly, and onset of response therefore cannot always be precisely determined. The median time from entry to coding of remission was 6 weeks on MBD and 5 weeks on MTX. Responses were noted as early as 1 week on both treatments, and as late as 34 weeks for MBD and 23 weeks for MTX. Median duration of therapy for nonresponders was 7 weeks on each arm.

Response was strongly correlated with survival

This study was conducted by the Eastern Cooperative Oncology Group, Paul P. Carbone, Chairman, and Barry H. Kaplan, Chairman of the Head and Neck Committee.

404

TABLE 1 Median Survival in Months

	From:	
Response	Entry	Response
None	4.8	4.8
Partial	8.1	6.0
Complete	11.3	8.9

in this study, especially complete response. Complete responders had a median survival of 11.3 months, compared to 8.1 months for partial responders and 4.8 months for nonresponders. This analysis, however, does not take into account a major bias related to survival until an event occurred. For instance, there is little doubt that patients who survive until their next birthday will live longer than those who do not, only because we require them to survive until an event occurs, whether or not that event relates independently to their disease or the cause of death. Although there is no perfect way to correct for this, subtracting the time until remission was first noted is a reasonable approximation. This carries with it the problems mentioned earlier of imprecise determination of date of response, but is the best estimate we can make of the extent of bias. This approach really is most appropriate if survival follows an exponential pattern.

Fully one-third of the patients did not achieve their responses before the end of 2 months of treatment. Correcting for the time to remission, median survival of complete responders from complete remission was 8.9 months; partial responders from partial remission 6.0 months; and nonresponders, 4.8 months from entry (Table 1). The benefit for partial responders is small indeed if one corrects for the bias of required survival time to enter the group of partial or complete responders.

Given this minor benefit from partial remission, defined as it was in this trial as a 50 percent decrease in the product of the largest diameter of a lesion and its largest perpendicular diameter, or in the sum of which products if more than one measurable lesion is present, we wondered whether more restrictive definitions of partial response would give better results for the partial responders. We reviewed tumor measurement forms on all the cases, and coded the percent reduction in the sum of the products of tumor diameters by decades, as shown in Table 2. In this table mean survivals are given, since with such small groups this is a better estimate of true results than the median, and since this appropriately weights longer responses as being of greater value. The analysis of data included all points for statistical purposes, however. Excluding two very long survivors with regressions of 70 to 80 percent, there is no correlation at all between percent partial regression and survival.

We next wondered whether within some of the categories of higher tumor regression we were not missing benefits because patients in response were dying early of intercurrent illnesses or catastrophes relating to the tumor or its shrinkage. We therefore looked at survival from maximum tumor regression, excluding patients who received less than 2, 4, or 6 weeks of chemotherapy. It was fair to do this, since the original study protocol had stipulated that all patients should receive at least 6 weeks of chemotherapy to ensure an adequate trial. As shown in Table 2, restricting analysis to those who received defined periods of treatment had the effect only of making those nonresponders left in the analysis appear to survive longer. Obviously, most of those receiving less than 6 weeks of therapy did so because of early death, tumor progression, general deterioration, or drug-related mortality (there were three treatment-related deaths on each arm), and these events occurred far more often in nonresponders than in those with objective regression of tumor.

Having found no more useful definition of partial response in extent of regression, whether or not corrected for adequate duration of therapy, we now turned to a requirement that partial remission last a minimum of a fixed period of time. The traditional period in the Eastern Cooperative Oncology Group has been 4 weeks. Median survival from entry of 16 partial responders whose response lasted <4 weeks was 4.3 months, less than that of nonresponders (4.8 months), and much less than that of responders whose partial response lasted τ4 weeks (9.0 months), p = 0.0035. While the 9-month median sounds impressive, it is

TABLE 2 Mean Survival In Months By Extent Of Regression

	Treatment			From Maximum Tumor Regression: Duration of Protocol Chemotherapy			
Extent Regress.	MTX #119	MBD #80	From Entry	Any	> 2 weeks	> 4 weeks	> 6 weeks
None	69%	54%	6.4	6.4 (#125)	7.3 (#108)	8.0 (#92)	9.3 (#69)
50–59%	5%	5%	8.3	6.4 (#10)	*	*	6.7 (#9)
60–69%	3%	3%	10.4	5.7 (#6)	*	*	7.0 (#4)
70–79%	2%	8%	6.1†	4 5† (#8)	*	*	*
80–89%	6%	8%	8.5	5.7 (#13)	*	*	*
90–99%	7%	8%	9.4	6.8 (#14)	*	*	*
Complete	8%	16%	12.5	10.5 (#23)	*	10.8 (#22)	*

*No change from leftward column
†excludes two long survivals (mean survival 19.1 months from entry and 17.4 months from maximum response with them included)

uncorrected for the bias in waiting for response to occur. When this is done, median survival from onset of response is 7.2 months, versus 3.6 months for those whose response lasted < 4 weeks.

However, the median survival of 7.2 months is uncorrected for the bias of having to wait an additional month of survival before being eligible to enter this group. If one takes survival of partial responders with remissions lasting τ4 weeks from date of partial response, and subtracts the one month of subsequent survival guaranteed by the definition, the median survival is 6.2 months, versus 4.8 months survival from entry for those without response or shorter partial responses. Survival for both groups is 20 percent at 12 months. This difference is not statistically significant (p = 0.06). In clinical terms, this 6-week prolongation of median survival without any effect on long-term survival is of little consequence.

It is possible that correcting for the influence of known significant prognostic factors for survival in this trial (ambulatory performance status, absence of distant metastases, absence of heavy smoking history, absence of adjacent organ invasion from primary site, absence of major weight loss, absence of tumor in the neck, and absence of history of heavy alcohol ingestion) will make partial response defined as lasting >4 weeks seem more important. However, the major prognostic factors for response (ambulatory performance status, absence of fixed neck nodes, and absence of distant metastases) are not very different from those for survival, and so are likely to diminish the apparent effect of partial response in prolonging survival. A formal covariate analysis of the effect of partial response on survival is now under way.

We therefore conclude that partial response defined in any way we could design is of little consequence in terms of survival of patients with advanced head and neck cancer. Complete remissions seem to be of some value, and these should be used to compare different therapeutic approaches rather than overall remission rate. There is little to be said, in the development of new therapeutic programs, for improving the rate of partial remission unless more complete remissions are also produced. It is disappointing to note that in the ECOG trial we have been discussing, complete remission on MBD lasted no longer than those on MTX, though there was a higher rate of developing them on MBD. Obviously, in terms of recurrent and metastatic disease, not only *more* complete remissions are needed, but better ones that last longer.

Finally, it is of interest to look at the influence of partial remission on survival after induction chemotherapy of regional, previously untreated head and neck cancer. In the largest series reported to date, that of Al-Sarraf and co-workers at Wayne State University in Detroit, the median survival of partial responders to induction chemotherapy (13 months) is not significantly longer than that of nonresponders (8 months), even though the nonresponders almost uni-

formly failed to benefit with even a "partial" response to subsequent radiation therapy.[5] Complete responders survived longer than either of the other groups, a median of 24 months after entry. This confirms earlier data from Einstein,[4] Memorial, and Walter Reed suggesting that partial response to induction chemotherapy leads to no obvious improvement in survival for patients with far advanced, inoperable lesions. Al-Sarraf's series is important because earlier lesions were included, and many patients received surgical resection as part of their treatment program after induction chemotherapy, although patients undergoing subsequent resection and irradiation did not survive significantly longer than those receiving radiation only.

Thus it appears that the goal of clinical research in the area of head and neck cancer chemotherapy should be enhancement of the rate of complete remission, and that this should be the goal of therapy for the individual patient as well. The number of patients so far achieving complete remission of recurrent and metastatic disease remains small, and even the duration of *these* remissions leaves a lot to be desired for most of the patients. Similarly, the quality of complete remission for induction chemotherapy patients is inadequate, since fully 60 percent of Al-Sarraf's responders have died by 36 months by actuarial analysis.

The lack of value of partial remission has important implications for patient treatment. If a patient has reached a stable partial response, with no further shrinkage of tumor on continued treatment, it may well be that treatment can be stopped with no loss to the patient, since statistical methods can detect no benefit in survival after this point even if therapy is continued. If alternate effective chemotherapy is available, the point of maximum regression might be a reasonable point in time to introduce it, since the prognosis for prolonged survival is poor in the presence of only partial remission, and complete remission should be the goal.

REFERENCES

1. Vogl SE, Schoenfeld DA, Kaplan BH, Lerner HJ, Engstrom PF, Horton HJ. A randomized prospective comparison of methotrexate with a combination of methotrexate, bleomycin and cisplatin in head and neck cancer. Cancer (in press).
2. Chiuten D, Vogl SE, Kaplan BH, Greenwald E. Effective outpatient combination chemotherapy for advanced cancer of the head and neck. Surg Gynecol Obstet 1980; 151:659–662.
3. Vogl SE, Lerner H, Kaplan BH, Coughlin C, McCormick B, Camacho F, Cinberg J. Failure of effective initial chemotherapy to modify the course of stage IV(MO) squamous cancer of the head and neck. Cancer 1982; 50:840–844.
4. Vogl SE, Schoenfeld DA, Kaplan BH, Lerner HJ, Horton J, Paul AR, Barnes LE. Methotrexate alone or with regional subcutaneous corynebacterium parvum in the treatment of recurrent or metastatic squamous cancer of the head and neck. Cancer 1983; 50:2295–2302.
5. Rooney M, Kish J, Jacobs J, Kinzie J, Weaver A, Crissman J, Al-Sarraf M. Improved complete response rate and survival in advanced head and neck cancer after 3 course induction therapy with 120 hour 5-FU infusion and cisplatin. Cancer, in press.

WHICH RESPONSES ARE MEANINGFUL IN HEAD AND NECK CANCER?

ROBERT E. WITTES, M.D.

When a physician gives medicine to sick people, his therapeutic objective is invariably to make life better in quality, or longer in duration, or both. The goal of treatment with anticancer agents does not differ from that with cardiotonics, antibiotics, anti-inflammatory agents, or psychotropics. Therefore, the only meaningful response to chemotherapy in head and neck cancer is an increase in the quantity or quality of life.

In the examining rooms, however, oncologists can usually be found puttering around with rulers or calipers in an attempt to see whether the "measurable disease" is shrinking on treatment. If questioned about this curious practice, the oncologist would probably respond with one or more of the following statements:

1. Shrinkage of tumor is an objective sign of treatment effect; malignant masses should be followed on therapy just as the cardiologist monitors râles at the lung bases, cardiac gallops, or irregular rhythms.
2. Patients whose tumors shrink commonly feel better as a result.
3. Responders generally live longer than nonresponders; if the treatment results in a response, therefore, it produces improved survival, which is admittedly what we really care about.

SHRINKAGE OF TUMOR AS AN OBJECTIVE MEASURE OF DRUG EFFECT

The primacy of the ruler and caliper comes from the reasonable assumption that if cytotoxic agents are to exert beneficial effects on a patient's clinical course, they will do so by causing tumor shrinkage or at least slowing the rate of tumor progression. There are theoretically two separate issues here (measurement of response and the significance of tumor shrinkage), but they cannot be disentangled.

Obviously it is possible to assign measurements to many malignant lesions and to document changes in these measurements as treatment is given. Often however, because of the location or character of a lesion, measurement is patently impossible, and the estimation of what is happening with a cancer which is only "evaluable" is necessarily quite subjective. Ill-defined masses in the hypopharynx or ulcerated lesions with serpiginous borders plastered onto the posterior pharyngeal wall bedevil all rigorous attempts at assessment. Evaluation by multiple observations may be more reliable than the observations of a single physician, but even in clinics where several physicians see the patient at each visit, the examiners often vary considerably in skill and the assessments may not really be independent observations.

Even when measurements may be meaningfully assigned to apparent lesions, the bulk of tumor may be largely inapparent, and using the "tip of the iceberg" as an indicator of what is happening with the patient's disease is at best an unverified extrapolation. This problem may reach ludicrous proportions when, as often happens, one or two discrete skin nodules or palpable neck nodes are employed as indicator lesions for a very extensive tumor invading fascial planes and muscles in the neck, the upper mediastinum, and other anatomic compartments inaccessible to the examiner.

It also seems certain that even in the case of discrete lesions, substantial measurement error contributes to confusion about treatment effects. Measurement error obviously becomes a greater problem as one encounters smaller lesions or when less tumor shrinkage is required to qualify as a "response". One could significantly increase the reliability of response assessment by redefining response as > 75 percent reduction in estimated tumor bulk instead of the current 50 percent and by requiring that lesions exceed a certain size before they can be used as markers of treatment effect. Stiffening the response criteria is likely to deal with another potential problem in evaluation: the nonspecific nature of some apparent responses. The late Dr. Richard Jesse was fond of pointing out that he could get dirty, infected lesions, and presumably their regional draining nodes, to regress 25 to 50 percent just by adequate local treatment of the infection.

For all these reasons, objective response is surely a lot less objective than we would like to think. Much of the annoying variation in response rates from study to study may no doubt be laid at this particular doorstep.

For all the ink that has been spilled on the subject of response evaluation, however, one important fact remains very clear: the reason that responses are hard to measure in head and neck cancer is that the agents currently available are not strikingly active. In the hematologic malignant diseases, testis cancer, and several pediatric cancers, for which truly effective chemotherapy exists, clinicians do not spend valuable time at symposia deliberating the "meaning of response" or refinements in response criteria. Complete response rate and serious acute toxicities are the early end points of significance; survival and late side effects are the ultimate measures of a treatment's value. One can refine response criteria ad infinitum; the outcome of the effort will only be better definition of various categories of incomplete response. Insofar as complete response is the only worthy objective of treatment, the exercise has limited value. The real problem in the developmental therapy of epithelial tumors is the discovery of truly active agents. When these are at hand, the problem of response assessment recedes into the background.

CORRELATION OF OBJECTIVE RESPONSE WITH SUBJECTIVE STATUS

Objective response may certainly result in an improved quality of life. Decrease in the extent of local infection or pain, a decrease in trismus, and shrinkage in the bulk of disease at certain sites can all translate into greater patient comfort and lessened need for ancillary palliative measures.

Tumor shrinkage and increased well-being, however, do not necessarily go hand in hand. Rapid tumor necrosis sometimes results in increased bleeding or the creation of fistulas that can be difficult to deal with. In addition, side effects from the treatment itself may override any subjective benefits that might otherwise have been derived from the oncolytic effect.

The point here is simply that measuring tumor regression in no way replaces an adequate accounting for the impact of treatment on the comfort and day-to-day functioning of the patient. Effects of therapy on quality of life are not easy to document with precision. Performance status scores, which make a crude attempt to do this, are not precisely defined, and probably for this reason their use is characterized by high interobserver variability. Better instruments for measuring quality of life in cancer patients on therapeutic trials are badly needed; some promising ones are currently in development.

CORRELATION OF RESPONSE WITH INCREASED SURVIVAL

Comparison of the survivorship of responders and nonresponders has been very common practice. The rationale of the comparison rests on the assumption that patients who do not respond will have survival similar to untreated cases. If this is so, the nonresponders constitute a kind of control group against which the effect of response can be measured; if responders live longer than nonresponders, the argument continues, the treatment has a favorable impact on survival.

As has been pointed out in the recent literature, this kind of comparison is fallacious. In the first place, there is no reason to assume a priori that the survival of nonresponders is equivalent to that of an untreated control. Deleterious effects of various kinds of treatment on survival have been documented enough to make the assumption of no effect in nonresponders untenable. Furthermore, since patients have to live a certain length of time to exhibit a response, whereas no such requirement is imposed on nonresponders, a time bias is built into the very definition of a responder. This bias can be eliminated by somewhat more sophisticated kinds of survival analyses than are usually performed (see chapter by Vogl and Schoenfeld, this volume).

A far more serious problem, however, and one that cannot be overcome by analytical tricks, relates to the impossibility of establishing a cause and effect relationship between treatment and the prolonged survival that one may see in the responders. There is no way to know whether response itself produced the long survival or whether the patients who did indeed respond to treatment were destined for long survival anyway because of a favorable combination of (unknown) prognostic factors.

For these reasons, survival comparisons of this type are best avoided. One cannot deduce simply from the superior survival of complete responders (CRs) compared to partial responders (PRs), for example, that CR should be the goal of all therapy. Most of us do, in fact, believe that CR should be the goal of therapy, but the real reason for this belief is that in other clinical settings the attainment of CR is associated with long survival or cure that is *unprecedented* in patients not attaining CR. In these settings, the benefit of treatment is easily seen when the survivorship of the entire treated population, and not just the responders, is compared with that of patients treated in some other way, and it is this type of comparison that really provides conclusive evidence of benefit. It is therefore impossible to use calipers or rulers to measure the impact of treatment on survival.

CONCLUSION

The clinical assessment of objective response is full of uncertainty. In early clinical trials tumor shrinkage is about the only parameter available for judging an agent's potential. In the phase I and II study, therefore, response assessment should be done with attention to the various details already mentioned. It is certainly desirable for the many investigators in clinical trials to employ similar methodology in assessing response. How could any reasonable person argue otherwise? If we all were to do so, the phase II literature would be much more meaningful, and decisions about which drugs were worth a phase III evaluation would be easier than they often are.

It is likely that impending advances in diagnostic imaging may yield quantum improvements in the non-invasive assessment of cancers with regard not only to their anatomic extent, but also to their viability and metabolic characteristics. Such improvements, however, will be significant additions to our ability to assess response only if the therapeutic agents of the future are much better antitumor treatments than the ones we have now. The situation is analogous to the use of circulating chorionic gonadotropin in following the response of gestational choriocarcinoma to treatment: if the treatment itself were not so effective, the value of the very sensitive marker would be much less than it is.

Phases I and II, however, are a small part of the total clinical trials effort and a miniscule part of the total treatment effort. It is really the phase III trial that ought to tell the practitioner what he needs to know for intelligent clinical decision-making. Here, instead of agonizing about response criteria and assessment, oncologists should move to the direct comparative trial much earlier in a drug's development than they currently do. And in doing so, they should move the vital end points of therapeutic trials—survival duration and quality of life—back to center stage where they belong.

29. Chemosensitivity Assays

INTRODUCTION

MICHAEL E. JOHNS, M.D.

Tissue culture and other techniques have been utilized in attempts to study the effects of chemotherapeutic agents on human neoplasms. Some of these techniques have included: (1) morphologic assessment of cellular damage in monolayer or in organ cultures,[1-3] (2) parametric measurements of inhibition of cellular metabolism,[4,5] and (3) in vitro measured inhibition of radioactive nucleotide or amino acid precursor incorporation into cellular protein or DNA.[6,7] Unfortunately, the in vitro effects of the cytotoxic agents correlated poorly with the clinical actions.

Because these methods are technically cumbersome, subjective in interpretation, and only moderately successful in predicting in vivo effects, and/or because they become so time-consuming that they are not clinically feasible, interest in them as useful methods was not maintained.

In 1977 Hamburger and Salmon described a soft agar colony assay to measure in vitro the number of clonogenic cells in a given tumor cell population and to measure the in vitro effects of cytotoxic agents on tumor colony formation.[8] Their early reports and reports from other investigators generated enthusiasm for this assay and a resurgence of interest in developing other assays to measure chemotherapeutic sensitivity. Analogies were made to in vitro antibiotic sensitivity testing.

In the case of squamous cell carcinomas of the head and neck, time has not borne out the projections for this assay. In squamous cell carcinomas, only about 35 percent of tumors will grow in the assay.[9,10] Of those tumors that grow, a very small percentage have sufficient cloning efficiencies to allow in vitro manipulations that are meaningful. Furthermore, squamous cell carcinomas of the head and neck do not usually provide large enough cell yields or allow easy preparation of single cell suspension, a requirement for a clonogenic assay.

The chapters in this Part are written by four leaders in the area of chemosensitivity testing in squamous cancers of the head and neck. Hill discusses the pitfalls in the soft agar clonogenic assays and compares the Hamburger and Salmon assay to that of Courtenay and Mills. Mattox presents a variation of the clonogenic assay technique using capillary tubes that overcome several of the problems of the Hamburger and Salmon assay. McCormick addresses the use of the mouse subrenal capsule assay and Braakhuis and Snow describe the nude mouse model as predictive assays for head and neck cancer.

It is important to realize that there are limitations in all of these model systems. The four authors have been good enough to point out the limitations that exist in these different systems. In order to have a clonogenic assay, a viable single-cell tumor population is a requirement. It is clear that preparation of this suspension is the single most difficult problem in these assays. In addition, once single cells are obtained, they must maintain the ability to grow in the culture system. It is the consensus among all who have worked with squamous cell carcinomas that it is impossible to obtain a pure single-cell preparation. There has also been some concern that for squamous carcinoma the preparation of the single-cell suspension might cause significant damage to the cells, thus precluding growth.

My laboratory has used the Hamburger and Salmon Assay to culture head and neck tumors for more than $2\frac{1}{2}$ years. Particular problems that we have encountered have been: (1) high contamination rate, (2) low cell yields from small specimens, (3) low growth rates, (4) low cloning efficiencies, (5) extreme difficulty in obtaining single-cell suspensions, and (6) in vitro growth rate inversely proportional to the purity of the single-cell suspension (Table 1).

In summary, the chemotherapeutic sensitivity assays all leave something to be desired in terms of predicting a drug response for the head and neck cancer patient. However, the clonogenic assay, subrenal capsule assay, and nude mice model assay are important tools for the study of head and neck tumor cell growth and head and neck tumor biology. Diagnostic and therapeutic advances in squamous carcinoma are dependent on a better understanding of the cellular behavior of these tumors, and these assays provide valuable avenues for such efforts.

TABLE 1   Squamous Cancer Cell Colony Formation in Soft Agar

Sample Identification	No. of Cells plated/dish	Viability (%)	No. of colonies 30 cells or greater on day 1	No. of clumps in 4-mm circle on day 1	Colonies on day 13	Cloning efficiencies
H212 A	5.0×10	95%	6	0	7	0.0002
B	5.0×10^5	95%	5	2	6	0.0002
C	5.0×10^5	95%	4	0	3	0.0002
H215	1.0×10^5	90%	5	2	7	0.0019
H216 A	5.0×10^5	93%	17	13	60	0.0086
B	5.0×10^5	93%	10	19	34 (day 7)	0.0048
H217 A	2.5×10^5	90%	3	2	3	—
B	2.5×10^5	90%	5	4	3	—
H219	5.0×10^5	95%	12	9	29	0.0034
H218 (Parotid)	4.8×10^5	92	27	32	61	0.0071

REFERENCES

1. Wright JC, Plummer-Cobb J, Gumport S, et al. Investigation of the relation between clinical and tissue culture response to chemotherapeutic agents on human cancer. N Engl J Med 1957; 257:1207–1211.
2. Wright JC, Plummer-Cobb J, Gumport SL, et al. Further investigation of the relation between the clinical and tissue culture response to chemotherapeutic agents on human cancer. Cancer 1962; 15:284–293.
3. Ambrose EJ, Andrews RD, Easty DM, et al. Drug assays on cultures of human tumor biopsies. Lancet 1962; 1:24–25.
4. Black MM, Speer FD. Further observations on the effects of cancer chemotherapeutic agents on the in vitro dehydrogenase activity of cancer tissue. J Natl Cancer Inst 1954; 14:1147–1158.
5. Knock FE. Qualitative and quantitative in vitro sensitivity tests for cancer chemotherapy. Natl Cancer Inst Monogr 1971; 34:247–249.
6. Freshney RI. Some observations on assay of ant culture. In: Dendy PP, ed. New York: Academic Press 1976, pp 150–155.
7. Volm M, Wayss K, Kaufmann M, et al. Pretherapeutic detection of tumor resistance and the results of tumor chemotherapy. Eur J Cancer 1979; 15:983–993.
8. Hamburger AW, Salmon SE. Primary bioassay of human tumor stem cells. Science 1977; 197:461–463.
9. Johns ME. The clonal assay of head and neck tumor cells: results and clinical correlations. Laryngoscope 1982; 92(Suppl 28):1–26.
10. Mattox DE, Von Hoff DD, Clark GM, Aufdemorte TB. Factors that influence growth of head and neck squamous carcinoma in the soft agar cloning assay. Cancer 1984; 52:1736–1740.

CAPILLARY CLONING ASSAY IN HEAD AND NECK CANCER

DOUGLAS E. MATTOX, M.D.
DANIEL D. VON HOFF, M.D.
IBRAHIM RAMZY, M.D.
H. DANIEL SCHANTZ, CMIAC
JOY BUCHOK, B.A.

Chemotherapy response rates in head and neck cancer are poor and of short duration, especially in heavily pretreated patients. The sensitivity of an individual tumor to a drug or combination of drugs is unpredictable based on the histologic characteristics, clinical behavior, site of primary, or previous response to other drugs. In this chapter we will discuss the results of a pilot study of a modification of the soft agar cloning assay using capillary tubes as the culture vessel. An attempt was also made to correlate culture results with the cytologic appearance of the single cell suspension used for the cultures.

The soft agar cloning assay was developed as a means of determining chemosensitivity of individual tumors, and in clinical trials it has correctly predicted in vivo chemosensitivity in 65 percent of patients and resistance in 97 percent.[1] Unfortunately, the experience in head and neck cancer has been disappointing. Successful cultures were obtained in only 36 percent of specimens and contamination rates were high.[2] The number of specimens in which there were enough cells to permit testing of multiple drugs ranged from 11 to 13 percent.[2,3]

The capillary cloning system uses techniques and media similar to the Petri dish method, except that 0.1-ml capillary tubes are used as the culture vessel.[4] This modification in technique offers a number of practical and theoretic advantages. Whereas the Petri dish method uses 500,000 cells per dish, each capillary tube needs only 50,000 to 100,000 cells, giving

Supported by NIH Grants CA 27733 and CA 30195.

a five- to tenfold increase in the number of drugs that could be tested. The ends of the capillary tube are permanently sealed and the surface area during preparation is greatly reduced, decreasing the chances of contamination. In other tumor types cultured with this technique, the cloning efficiencies were increased by a factor of 3.[5] This increase in growth may be the result of improved local conditioning of the small volume of media by tumor cells or by hypoxic conditions in the center of the tube. In practical terms, the capillary tubes are easier to handle and require less storage and incubator space than 15-mm Petri dishes. Finally, automated scanning equipment for counting colonies in a capillary tube is simpler and less expensive than similar equipment for counting plates.

The results of in vitro cloning are generally expressed as a cloning efficiency, i.e., the number of colonies divided by the number of initial cells plated expressed as a percent. The appropriate dilution of the cell suspension is determined by measuring the concentration of nucleated viable cells on a hemocytometer. Although erythrocytes and polymorphonuclear cells can be excluded during this count, clonogenic tumor cells are indistinguishable from nonclonogenic tumor cells and benign cells including fibroblasts and histiocytes. Therefore, the cloning efficiency may not accurately reflect the clonogenic potential of the actively growing tumor. Theoretically, a more accurate assessment of the potentially clonogenic fraction of the single cell suspension could be made with cytologic techniques. The cloning efficiency could then be calculated based on the fraction of cells that appear clonogenic, i.e., parabasal cells.

METHODS

One cubic centimeter tumor samples were harvested directly from patients or from surgical specimens and immediately transported to the laboratory in enriched McCoys 5A medium with penicillin and streptomycin. A single-cell suspension was made mechanically by mincing and teasing the tissue with needles, and passing it through a 100-mesh screen and 25- and 27-gauge needles. Red cells were lysed with $0.15M$ NH_4Cl in phosphate buffer. The cells were centrifuged at $1000 \times g$ for 7 minutes and the pellet resuspended in 5 to 10 ml McCoys 5A. The total nucleated cell count was determined in aliquot of the suspension in 3 percent glacial acetic acid. The culture medium contained CRML 1066, asparagine, dextran, 2-mercaptoethanol, and 0.3 percent agar. Serial concentrations of cells were adjusted to 20K, 40K, 60K, 80K, and 100K/0.1 ml tube, and at least six capillary tubes were filled at each concentration. An air space was maintained on each side of the culture medium to avoid contamination, and the tube was sealed with hematocrit clay. Control tubes with 50K cells/tube treated with 100 μg/ml Chromomycin were used to assess the number of clumps of cells remaining in the suspension at the time of plating. For ad-

equate quality control, the clusters in Chromomycin-treated tubes should be ≤30 percent of the untreated control tubes. The capillary tubes were incubated at 37°C in a 7 percent CO_2 humidified atmosphere and counted at 14 days.

A separate aliquot of the cell suspension was taken for cytologic analysis and immediately mixed with an equal volume of a 50 percent ethyl alcohol and 2 percent Carbowax mixture. Two to four slides were prepared using a cytocentrifuge, postfixed in 95 percent ethyl alcohol, and stained with a modified Papanicolaou method. A differential count of the cells in the single-cell suspension was performed. The squamous cells present were identified and classified according to their degree of maturation into (1) anucleated squamous cells (keratinized), (2) superficial and intermediate squamous cells, (3) isolated parabasal squamous cells, (4) parabasal cells in clusters of 3 to 10 cells, and (5) parabasal cells in clusters of 11 or more cells. An additional category, (6) fibroblasts and histiocytes, was included in the differential.

Anucleated squamous cells are polygonal cells with eosinophilic cytoplasm, 40 to 60 μm in diameter and without a discernible nucleus. Superficial squamous cells are also polygonal, eosinophilic cells, 40 to 60 μm in diameter, and have small pyknotic nuclei. Intermediate squamous cells, 30 to 50 μm, are polygonal, cyanophilic cells with centrally placed vesicular nuclei. Parabasal cells are generally smaller, 20 to 40 μm, and are round to oval with a dense cyanophilic cytoplasm. The nuclei of the parabasal cells are centrally located and vesicular, and have varying degrees of chromatin clumping and nucleoli.

Cell clusters, large and small, have nuclear and cytoplasmic features similar to those of parabasal cells. No attempt was made to count the individual cells in clusters because the three-dimensional nature of the clusters prevented an accurate count.

Histiocytes and fibroblasts are both small cells, 10 to 15 μm, with oval to reniform vesicular nuclei. These were grouped together in one category, and no attempt was made to cytologically separate them.

Preparation and plating of specimens occurred within 3 hours of biopsy, and cytospin preparations were done within 2 hours of completion of the single-cell suspension. Informed consent was obtained in accordance with local Institutional Review Board guidelines.

RESULTS

In this pilot study, capillary cloning was attempted on 13 tumor specimens. Nine of the 13 (70%) grew and had a median cloning efficiency (calculated on the basis of total nucleated cells plated) of 0.014 percent (range 0.009 to 0.15%). Three tumors failed to grow, and one was contaminated by fungus.

Serial concentrations of cells in suspension were used to determine the optimum concentration for plating. In six cases, enough cells were present to perform a series from 20K to 100K/tube. Figure 1 shows the results. For a given tumor the number of colonies at each concentration is expressed as a percent of the maximal number of colonies for that tumor. In five of the six cases, the optimum plating concentration was between 80K and 100K. The "colonies" in the Chromomycin-treated tubes represent clumps of cells present at the time of plating, but these clumps were never more than 40 percent of the colonies at the optimum concentration.

Twelve specimens were examined by the cytopathologist. The cells were divided into the following categories: (1) anuclear (keratinized) cells, (2) superficial and intermediate cells, (3) parabasal cells, (4) small clusters of parabasal cells (3 to 11 cells), (5) large clusters of parabasal cells (11 or more), and (6) fibroblasts. The median and range for each category is shown in Table 1. One specimen was very degenerated and a differential could not be done; this specimen did grow in the assay. The number of fibroblasts and histiocytes was small. Superficial and intermediate cells were the most common kinds of isolated cells. Parabasal cells, presumably the clonogenic fraction of the culture, had a median of 14 percent and a range of 1 to 48 percent for isolated cells. Clus-

TABLE 1 Cytopathology: Squamous Carcinoma Single-Cell Suspensions

	Median (%)	Range (%)
Parabasal	14	1–48
Superficial and intermediate	50	5–92
Anuclear (keratinized)	7	2–35
Cluster (3–10)	3	0–31
Cluster (11 or more)	0.6	0–14
Histiocytes and fibroblasts	2	1–12

ters of parabasal cells had medians of 3 percent and 0.6 percent for small and large clusters respectively.

The three specimens that did not grow at all had less than 10 percent isolated parabasal cells. Otherwise a trend could not be demonstrated between the cloning efficiency and the fraction of single parabasal cells (Fig. 2). However, there did appear to be a relationship between the cloning efficiency and the number of parabasal cell clusters. Figure 3 shows the cloning efficiency plotted against the sum of the large and small clusters.

DISCUSSION

This pilot study substantiates the feasibility of using the capillary cloning assay for head and neck squamous carcinoma. However, the numbers are too

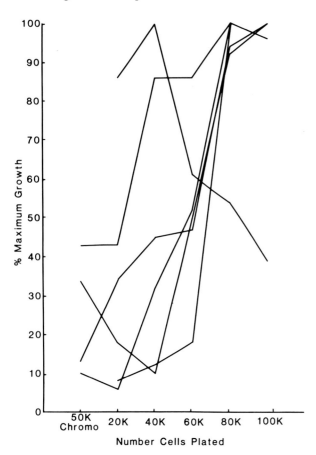

Figure 1 Optimum plating concentration for capillary cloning. For each tumor the number of colonies at each concentration is expressed as a percent of the maximum number of colonies. The optimum plating concentration was 80K to 100K/tube.

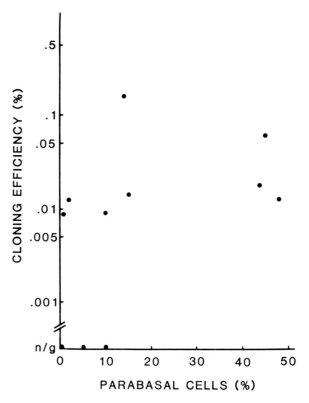

Figure 2 Cloning efficiency vs single parabasal cells. The cloning efficiency (log scale) is plotted against the percent of single parabasal cells in the cytology. There is no trend for increased cloning with increased number of cells. (n/g = no growth)

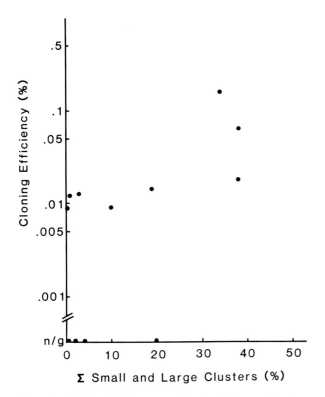

Figure 3 Cloning efficiency vs parabasal cell clusters. The cloning efficiency (log scale) is plotted against the sum of small and large clusters seen in the cytology. There is a trend toward higher cloning efficiency with a greater percentage of clusters. (n/g = no growth)

small to predict its usefulness in a clinical setting. In its favor is the fact that successful growth was obtained in 9 of 13 trials with 100,000 cells or less per capillary tube, as opposed to 500,000 per Petri dish in the traditional method. The median cloning efficiency in this trial was 0.014 percent, whereas it was 0.001 percent in a series of 57 tumors grown in Petri dishes. Thus the previously reported trend toward higher cloning efficiencies with the capillary system was also seen for head and neck cancer.[5]

Our original objective was to recalculate the cloning efficiency according to the percent of isolated parabasal cells in the suspension. However, the trend for increasing cloning efficiency with clusters rather than with isolated parabasal cells made it unlikely that this was a useful calculation. The low numbers of "colonies" in the Chromomycin controls indicated that these clusters were not large enough at the time of plating to be counted as colonies. These data may suggest that small clumps of cells are more able to cope with the trauma of tissue preparation and the in vitro environment. Finally, the clusters may be an artifact produced by reaggregation of cells in suspension occurring during the time of transport and preparation for cytology.

There is a continued need for a rapid, reliable method of evaluation chemosensitivity of individual tumors. This pilot study suggests that the capillary tube modification of the soft agar clonogenic assay deserves further investigation and development.

REFERENCES

1. Salmon SE, Alberts DS, Durie BGM, et al. Clinical correlations of drug sensitivity in the human tumor stem cell assay. In: Mathe G, Muggia FM, eds. Recent results in cancer research. Vol 74. Berlin: Springer-Verlag, 1980:300.
2. Mattox DE, Von Hoff DD, Clark GM, Aufdemorte TB. Factors that influence growth of head and neck squamous carcinoma in the soft agar cloning assay. Cancer 1984; 52:1736–1740.
3. Johns ME. The clonal assay of head and neck tumor cells: Results and clinical correlations. Laryngoscope 1982; 92:1–26.
4. Von Hoff DD, Hoang M. A new perfused capillary cloning system (PCCS) to improve cloning of human tumors. Proc Am Assoc Cancer Res 1983; 24:310.
5. Von Hoff DD. Plating efficiency of human tumor in capillary versus petri dishes. In: Salmon SE, Trent JB, eds. Human tumor cloning. New York: Grune and Stratton, 1984:(In press).

PITFALLS IN THE SOFT AGAR CLONOGENIC ASSAYS; RECOMMENDATIONS FOR IMPROVING COLONY-FORMING EFFICIENCIES AND THE POTENTIAL VALUE CELL LINES DERIVED FROM HEAD AND NECK TUMORS

BRIDGET T. HILL, Ph.D., F.R.C.S., F.I.Biol.
RICHARD D. H. WHELAN, M.I.Biol.
ANGELA S. BELLAMY, Ph.D.
H. THOMAS RUPNIAK, Ph.D.

The publication of Salmon and his colleagues in 1978,[1] describing the quantitation of differential sensitivity of human tumor stem cells to antitumor agents using an in vitro agar assay, fired our enthusiasm to adapt this procedure to investigate two tumor types in which our group had a major clinical interest, namely, head and neck squamous cell carcinomas and colorectal carcinomas. In our initial attempts we employed not only the Hamburger and Salmon assay,[2] but also the procedure described by Courtenay and Mills.[3] Our complete lack of success in obtaining colony formation in soft agar from biopsies taken from 17 primary squamous cell carcinomas of the head and neck and from 11 primary colorectal carcinomas was reported in 1980.[4] This contrasted with our relatively high success rate working with ascitic ovarian carcinomas, neuroblastoma-infiltrated bone marrows, and tumor cells from pleural effusions. In these preliminary studies, however, we found consistently that both colony-forming efficiencies (CFEs) and colony size were significantly superior when the Courtenay and Mills methodology was used.

These preliminary studies served to highlight various problems associated with these clonogenic assays,

1. Certain tumor types are more amenable to these procedures, so that there is a need to select carefully the tumor material for study.
2. Many "solid" tumors cannot be adequately dissociated to provide the mandatory "single cell suspension."
3. Colony-forming efficiencies are frequently very low and inadequate for attempting in vitro drug sensitivity testing, so that conditions for optimizing colony formation need to be established.

We have concentrated our attention on this latter problem, attempting to enhance CFEs by varying the assay conditions. We elected to use tumor cells derived from continuous lines for these comparative studies rather than being restricted by the limited supply of tumor cells frequently available from biopsies of head and neck tumors; in this way have also circumvented problems of "solid" tumor disaggregation.

We have used the HN-1 human tumor cell line derived from a squamous cell carcinoma of the tongue, originally established by Easty et al.[5] Using the Courtenay assay we have consistently obtained CFEs of approximately 15 percent (Table 1). In contrast, CFEs using the Hamburger and Salmon assay were 10-fold lower. We have reported similar discrepancies in a range of other human tumor cell lines.[6] To attempt to improve the results of the Hamburger and Salmon procedure, we modified their methodology. We omitted certain "extra factors," including DEAE dextran and tryptic soy broth, which were toxic to cells under our experimental conditions, and substituted components of the Courtenay assay such as "lethally irradiated" feeder cells, August rat red blood cells (rbc), conditions of low oxygen tension (i.e., 5% O_2, 5% CO_2, 90% N_2), and 95 percent humidity. These modifications resulted in significantly enhanced CFEs with these HN-1 cells (see Table 1), a finding also confirmed in other human tumor lines.[6] Unfortunately, with these higher CFEs obtained when this modified Hamburger and Salmon assay was used, we noticed a further problem, with the formation of a variable yet significant number of colonies on the lower plastic dish surface. This was not encountered in the Courtenay assay carried out in Falcon plastic tubes. We therefore recommend wider use of the Courtenay and Mills clonogenic assay.

If these assays are to be used for drug sensitivity evaluations, it is important to establish whether the CFE obtained or the assay procedure adopted influences the drug sensitivity pattern. Using the HN-1 cell line, we have established the effect of a 1-hour exposure to a range of Adriamycin (ADR) concentrations on cell survival using each of the three assay

TABLE 1   Comparison of CFE Values Obtained and IC_{50} and IC_{10} Values for Adriamycin from In Vitro Dose-Response Curves Using Various Clonogenic Assay Procedures*

Assay Procedure	% CFE	1 hr. exposure to ADR	
		IC_{50} ($\mu g/ml$)	IC_{10} ($\mu g/ml$)
Courtenay and Mills	14.8 ± 0.8	0.14	0.48
Hamburger and Salmon	1.50 ± 0.17	0.16	0.42
Modified Hamburger and Salmon†	12.9 ± 1.5	0.15	0.46

IC_{50} = concentration required to reduce survival to 50%
IC_{10} = concentration required to reduce survival to 10%
* In part after Hill & Whelan[6].
† + rbc + low O_2 tension + 95% humidity.

methods. Our results show that irrespective of the assay used and the CFE obtained, the survival curves were essentially similar and yielded comparable IC_{50} (drug concentration reducing cell survival to 50%) or IC_{10} values (see Table 1). Similar data have been reported using a series of other human tumor lines and other drugs including cisplatin and VP-16-213.[7]

Our earlier studies employing either tumor cell lines[7] or tumor cells obtained directly from ovarian ascites[8] have also served to emphasize that a critical factor in drug sensitivity testing is the duration of in vitro drug exposure. This observation also holds for the HN-1 cells (Fig. 1). We have therefore concluded that employing a single standard set of conditions, irrespective of the drug under evaluation, is inadequate because for certain drugs, for example, vincristine or VP-16-213, negligible cell kill occurs during a 1-hour exposure, but by prolonging the exposure duration,

significant drug-induced cytotoxicity results.

In *summary*, therefore, in these experimental studies with a human tumor line derived from a squamous cell carcinoma of the tongue we have:

1. Obtained significantly higher CFEs using the clonogenic assay procedure described by Courtenay and Mills as opposed to that of Hamburger and Salmon,
2. Shown that the addition of red blood cells under conditions of 95 percent humidity ± low oxygen tension to the Hamburger and Salmon assay significantly enhanced the CFEs obtained,
3. Demonstrated that in vitro drug sensitivity evaluations were not markedly influenced either by the assay procedure adopted or by the resultant CFE,
4. Provided evidence that duration of drug exposure in vitro is a critical determinant of drug-induced cytotoxicity.

In view of our initial lack of success in soft agar cloning of head and neck tumor cells directly from biopsy material, we have been investigating the potential of human tumor continuous cell lines for in vitro drug sensitivity testing. We were encouraged by the report by Carney et al that such lines derived from small cell lung cancers may be as useful a screening system for clinical correlations as the original tumor biopsy material.[9] From 20 biopsy specimens taken from the head and neck region we have successfully established four new tumor cell lines, all derived from tumors from previously irradiated patients. Two of the lines were established from laryngeal tumors, one from a tumor of the tongue, and the fourth from a neck node taken from a patient with a buccal cavity lesion. The population doubling times of in vitro culture were not markedly different, ranging from 21 to 34 hours. Of particular interest, however, was the fact that while all four lines readily formed colonies on a plastic substratum with CFEs of 6 to 46 percent, all were virtually incapable of forming colonies in soft agar with CFEs of <0.0001 to 0.013 percent, even using the Courtenay assay. The proliferation of this group of tumor-derived cell lines therefore appears highly anchorage-dependent. Other groups working with tumor cell lines derived from squamous cell carcinomas of the head and neck have also reported that only a minority of lines appear capable of "genuine" colony formation in a semisolid medium.[5,10]

However, there are now a few reports of some success in directly cloning cells from head and neck tumors in soft agar or agarose, although only with CFEs of 0.002 to 0.15 percent.[11] Thus it would appear that, depending on the culture conditions employed, different tumor cell populations can be cultivated. It now becomes important to establish whether the drug sensitivity patterns of these tumor cell subpopulations are comparable, an aspect we are currently considering.

In addition, we have shown that cell lines derived from head and neck tumors can be used suc-

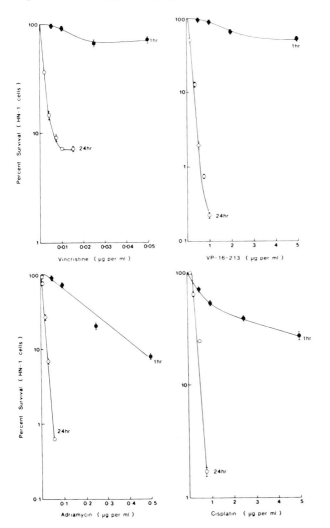

Figure 1 Influence of duration of exposure to a range of drug concentrations on the survival of logarithmically growing HN-1 cells. A significant reduction in cell survival occurred following a 1- or 24-hour exposure to Adriamycin or cisplatin. However, a 1-hr exposure to VP-16-213 or vincristine proved inadequate since significant cytotoxicity resulted only from the longer drug exposure.

cessfully to (1) evaluate new analogs, and (2) investigate drug-radiation interactions.

A number of anthracycline analogs have been developed recently, and we have used a series of human tumor cell lines as an initial preclinical screen. Figure 2 depicts the effects of 24-hour drug exposures on the survival of HN-1 cells, as judged by clonogenic assays. Although 4'-epi-Adriamycin (EPI-ADR) exhibits comparable activity to Adriamycin (ADR), the other three agents have significantly enhanced cytotoxic effects, with IC_{50} values being reduced by factors of 16, 7.3, or 2.4 compared with Adriamycin, mitoxanotrone (DHAD), 4'-0-methyladriamycin (40-ADR), and 4'-deoxyadriamycin (4'-ADR) respectively. A similar pattern of response has also been noted using two tumor lines derived from colon carcinomas.

Prior radiotherapy adversely influences subsequent clinical response rates and durations of response to chemotherapy in squamous cell carcinomas of the head and neck. To determine whether any cellular events mediate these effects, we exposed HN-1 cells

TABLE 2 Summary of Patterns of In Vitro Drug Responses following Fractionated Radiation Exposure of HN-1 cells

Increased Sensitivity	Unchanged Response	Marked Resistance
Cisplatin	Adriamycin	Vincristine
5-Fluorouracil	4'-Deoxyadriamycin	VM 26
Hydroxyurea	Bleomycin	VP-16–213
	Methotrexate	

to fractionated irradiation in vitro. ID_{10} values (dose required to reduce survival to 10%) for radiation were derived from dose-response curves, and cells were exposed to 11 fractions, allowing the cell population to recover between each fraction, to a total dose of 60 Gray. For a number of antitumor drugs already used to treat head and neck cancer and certain newer agents, dose-response curves were constructed for these radiation-treated cells and the parent line, assessing survival following a 24-hour drug exposure. Three distinct patterns of response were noted with the radiation-pretreated cells showing resistance, or an unaltered response, or enhanced sensitivity, depending on the drug tested (Table 2).[12] If confirmed, these results could have major biologic and clinical significance. They provide some preliminary evidence that three of the drugs (namely, cisplatin, 5-fluorouracil, and hydroxyurea) may be particularly beneficial in patients who have received prior radiotherapy. Therefore, in this group of patients with recurrent disease and such a poor prognosis, we have set up a feasibility study at the Royal Marsden Hospital in London, based on these findings, to evaluate a combination of "high-dose" 5-fluorouracil and hydroxyurea.

SUMMARY

Therefore a cell line derived from a human squamous cell carcinoma of the head and neck has been used as a preclinical screening system for new drug evaluation and has provided a useful model for further investigating mechanisms associated with drug-radiation interactions which is particularly relevant in this tumor type.

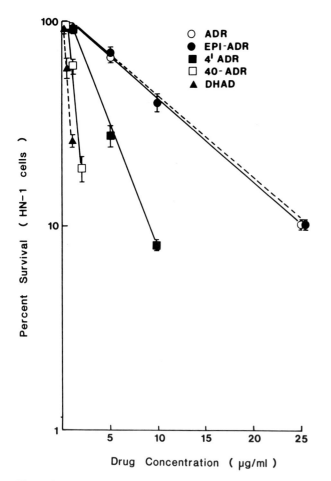

Figure 2 In vitro evaluation of anthracyclines: comparative lethal effects of anthracycline derivatives, as determined by colony-forming assays following a 24-hour drug exposure of logarithmically growing HN-1 cells. Each point represents the mean of 4 determinations ± s.e.m.

REFERENCES

1. Salmon SE, Hamburger AW, Soehnlen BJ, et al. Quantitation of differential sensitivities of human tumor stem cells to anticancer drugs. N Engl J Med 1978; 298:1321–1327.
2. Hamburger AW, Salmon SE. Primary bioassay of human tumor stem cells. Science 1977; 197:461–463.
3. Courtenay VD, Mills J. An in vitro colony assay for human tumours grown in immune-suppressed mice and treated in vivo with cytotoxic agents. Br J Cancer 1978; 37:261–268.
4. Rupniak HT, Hill BT. The poor cloning ability in agar of human tumour cells from biopsies of primary tumors. Cell Biol Int Rep 1980; 4:479–486.
5. Easty DM, Easty GC, Carter RL et al. Ten human carcinoma cell lines derived from squamous cell carcinomas of the head and neck. Br J Cancer 1981; 43:772–785.

6. Hill BT, Whelan RDH. Attempts to optimise colony-forming efficiencies using three different survival assays and a range of human tumor continuous cell lines. Cell Biol Int Rep 1983; 7:617–624.
7. Hill BT, Whelan RDH, Hoskin LK, et al. The value of human tumor continuous cell lines for investigating aspects of the methodologies used for *in vitro* drug sensitivity testing. In: Salmon SE, Trent JM (eds). *Human Tumor Cloning*. Orlando, Florida: Grune and Stratton, 1984; 487–496.
8. Rupniak HT, Whelan RDH, Hill BT. Concentration and time-dependent interrelationships for antitumour drug cytotoxicities against tumor cells *in vitro*. Int J Cancer 1983; 32:7–12.
9. Carney DN, Gazdar AF, Minna JD. *In vitro* chemosensitivity of clinical specimens and established cell lines of small cell lung cancer. Stem Cells 1982; 1:296.
10. Rheinwald JG, Beckett MA. Tumorigenic keratinocyte lines requiring anchorage and fibroblast support cultured from human squamous cell carcinomas. Cancer Res 1981; 41:1657–1663.
11. Schiff LJ, Shugar MA. Growth of human head and neck squamous cell carcinoma stem cells in agarose. Cancer 1984; 53:286–290.
12. Hill BT, Bellamy AS. Establishment of an etoposide-resistant human epithelial tumor cell line *in vitro*: characterization of patterns of cross-resistance and drug sensitivities. Int J Cancer 1984; 33:599–608.

MURINE SUBRENAL CAPSULE (SRC) ASSAY IN HEAD AND NECK CANCER

KENNETH J. McCORMICK, Ph.D.
WILLIAM R. PANJE, M.D., F.A.C.S.
ROGER H. MERRICK, B.S.M.T.

The development of in vitro assays for the assessment of the chemosensitivities of a patient's autochthonous tumor may become an important tool in attempts to individualize a particular patient's chemotherapeutic regimen. The human tumor stem cell assay[1] and the treatment of nude mice bearing subcutaneous xenografts of human tumors[2] have been investigated for their applicability to the clinical situation. However, the difficulties encountered in utilizing tissue culture techniques[3] or the nude mouse model[4] with squamous cell carcinomas of the head and neck prompted us to assess the chemosensitivities of these tumors in the in vivo murine subrenal capsule (SRC) assay developed by Bogden et al.[5]

The SRC assay is performed by surgically positioning a 1 cu mm fragment of tumor tissue under the renal capsule of normal immunocompetent mice. The fragment is measured in situ prior to closure of each animal. One day following surgery, single-agent chemotherapy is initiated and is continued through day 5 in groups of mice bearing the human tumor implants. On day 6, the animals are sacrificed, and the in situ measurements of the xenografts are repeated. Cytotoxic activity is demonstrated by shrinkage (oncolytic activity) of implants in drug-treated groups. The SRC assay has been used by the Division of Cancer Treatment, National Cancer Institute in evaluating the response of transplantable human tumor xenografts to new drugs.[6] Its potential usefulness in assays to predict clinical responses in individual patients has been reported.[7] In this chapter, the results of our studies with the SRC assay for head and neck tumors will be presented, and some of the problems inherent in the assay will be discussed.

MATERIALS AND METHODS

Tumor Tissue. Tumor tissue was obtained at the time of biopsy or surgical resection and processed with sterile techniques. Frozen sections were used to guide both the selection of neoplastic tissue and the removal of stroma and normal epithelium. In general, tumors were prepared for the SRC assay immediately after excision.

MURINE SRC ASSAY

The assay, described in detail by Bogden et al,[8] was adapted for use in our laboratory.[9]

In situ tumor size (TS) was estimated microscopically in ocular micrometer units: TS = (length + width)/2.[5] The change in tumor size (ΔTS) following treatment was calculated by the formula:

$$\Delta TS = TS_{(final)} - TS_{(initial)}.$$

The ΔTS values from individual animals within one treatment group were pooled. A negative mean ΔTS value (shrinkage of tumor) indicated oncolytic activity within that treatment group if the control mean ΔTS was positive (enlargement of implant). The percent reduction in tumor weight (% reduction TW) was calculated by the formula:

$$\% \text{ reduction TW} = [(\text{length (mm)} \times \text{width}^2 {}_{(mm)}/2)_{(final)} - /(\text{length (mm)} \times \text{width}^2 {}_{(mm)}/2)_{(initial)} - 1] \times (-100).$$ [5]

STATISTICAL ANALYSIS

Only drug-treated groups that produced mean ΔTS values with a negative sign (oncolytic activity) were

This study was partially supported by American Cancer Society Institutional Grant No. IN-122 and by NIH grant CA-28848. Drugs were kindly supplied by Bristol-Myers Company, Syracuse, NY.

analyzed. Initial results (Fig. 1) were assessed by comparing $\triangle TS_{(control)}$ to $\triangle TS_{(treated)}$ by Student's t test after proving the homogeneity of variances.

Statistical significance of oncolytic activity in current experiments was determined by a paired t test comparing initial and final TS within a treatment group (to be discussed).

RESULTS

Initial Evaluation of SRC Assay

We have reported the sensitivities of 20 squamous cell carcinomas (SCC) from 17 patients to several cytotoxic drugs using the SRC assay.[9] Figure 1 summarizes these results. Approximately 60 percent of the tumors responded to methotrexate or cyclophosphamide; however, all tumors were not sensitive to both drugs. Sensitivities to cisplatin or bleomycin occurred in 20 percent and 11 percent of tumors, respectively.

Examples of other head and neck tumors tested in the SRC assay are presented in Table 1. Although no drugs tested resulted in regression of the adenoid cystic or mucoepidermoid carcinomas, cyclophosphamide was effective against the anaplastic carcinoma, and doxorubicin produced strong oncolytic activity against the osteosarcoma and two of the three melanomas. The latter finding is especially interesting since doxorubicin, a drug with little clinical activity against malignant melanoma, has induced partial regression in a melanoma patient treated with doxorubicin which was selected on the basis of the SRC assay.[7]

Mechanisms of the Assay

The in situ microscopic measurement of tumor size provides a sensitive method with which to evaluate drug sensitivity. Correlations between SRC assays and clinical results in a prospective clinical trial will aid in determining the degree of oncolytic activity needed in order to select a clinically active drug. However, studies on the basic mechanisms of the assay are also needed. In a histologic study of our SRC series,[10] Seltzer et al found that tumor cells, both in interphase and mitotic, could be found in implanted tumor in control animals 6 days after surgery; however, the host inflammatory response was usually marked at that time. This histologic feature suggested that the increase in tumor size in saline-treated controls may reflect the inflammatory activity of the host rather than the kinetics of tumor cell growth. Initial experiments in mice implanted with SCC and immunosuppressed with hydrocortisone suggested that the increase in ΔTS values of saline-treated animals resulted from host reaction to the implanted tissue (Table 2). The mean ΔTS in control animals was +2.0; in hydrocortisone-treated mice, the mean ΔTS was −0.5.

Statistical Analysis of Drug Sensitivities

In our initial report,[9] sensitivity of implanted tumor to cytotoxic agents was determined statistically by comparing mean ΔTS values of treated groups to the mean ΔTS value of animals treated with saline. This analysis does not compare the size of the implants at day 6 to the size of control implants at day

TABLE 1   Other Head and Neck Tumors (Non-Squamous Cell) Tested in the SRC Assay

Tumor Type	Drug of Choice*	ΔTS	% Reduction in Tumor Weight
Adenoid cystic carcinoma	none	---	---
Mucoepidermoid carcinoma	none	---	---
Anaplastic carcinoma	cyclophosphamide	-2.2	51
Osteosarcoma	doxorubicin	-4.8	83
Melanoma #1	doxorubicin	-1.1	35
#2	doxorubicin	-3.4	72
#3	doxorubicin	-3.6	71

* Drug producing the greatest oncolytic effect.

TABLE 2   Effect of Hydrocortisone* on Increase in Tumor Size

Experiment Number	Change in Tumor Size (mean ΔTS)	
	Control	Hydrocortisone
1	+ 0.9	- 0.6
2	+ 0.6	- 0.4
3	+ 5.6	+ 0.4
4	+ 0.9	- 0.9
5	+ 1.9	- 1.0
Mean ± SE	+2.0 ± 1.0	-0.5 ± 0.3[+]

* 100 mg/kg on days 1, 3, and 5.
[+]p < 0.05

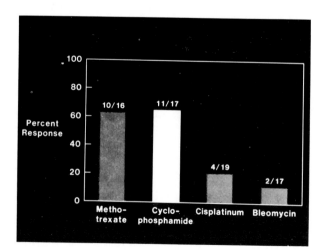

Figure 1 Distribution of chemosensitivities of 20 squamous cell carcinomas to single-agent chemotherapy in the SRC assay.

6; it compares the *change* in size of the treated implants to the *change* in size of control implants. However, if the increase in size of the controls is predominantly due to an active host response, such comparisons are meaningless. As described by Bogden et al,[5] control groups are used to identify an unevaluable assay (i.e., an assay in which control implants shrink spontaneously as a result of the poor quality of the tumor tissue). In our studies of approximately 60 tumor samples, only three assays have been unevaluable.

In an attempt to eliminate statistical comparisons of $\triangle TS_{(treated)}$ to $\triangle TS_{(control)}$, we have used the paired t test to compare the initial size of each implant in a group to the final size of the same implant in the group. The more powerful paired t test thus eliminates comparisons of size changes in treated groups to those in control groups in which implants have enlarged as a result of host response.

Chemosensitivities of SCC

Using the paired t test ($p < 0.05$) as the criterion of significant oncolytic activity, we have assessed the chemosensitivities of 31 SCC (Table 3) to single-agent chemotherapy with four standard cytotoxic drugs: methotrexate, cisplatin, bleomycin sulfate, and cyclophosphamide. The mean ΔTS values ($\pm$ SEM) for control animals was $+2.7 \pm 0.4$. Of the 31 SCC tested, approximately one-third (10/31) were resistant to all four drugs (Fig. 2). Forty two percent of tumors (13/31) were sensitive to only one cytotoxic agent; 22 percent of tumors (7/31) responded to three or more drugs. Previous surgery or radiotherapy did not influence sensitivity or resistance to drugs in the assay (data not shown). The general order of decreasing drug activities was: cyclophosphamide, 45 percent (14/31); methotrexate, 32 percent (10/31); cisplatin or bleomycin, 23 percent (7/31).

Table 4 presents the drug of choice selected by the SRC assay for the 21 drug-responsive SCC. Cyclophosphamide and methotrexate were selected with equal frequency (9 tumors versus 7 tumors, respectively). Cisplatin and bleomycin sulfate were selected with equal frequency (4 tumors each), but less often than were cyclophosphamide or methotrexate. No

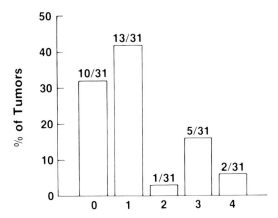

No. of Drugs Producing Significant Regression

Figure 2 Distribution of multiple chemosensitivities or resistance of 31 squamous cell carcinomas to single-agent chemotherapy in the SRC assay.

evidence of a consistent linkage between multiple drug sensitivities was found with this small number of tumors (data not shown).

From these data, the SRC assay appears to provide a selective test for differentiation of chemosensitivities for SCC of the head and neck. The cytotoxic drugs used fall into two groups: highest activity is obtained with cyclophosphamide or methotrexate; lower activity is found with cisplatin or bleomycin sulfate. The data suggest that combination chemotherapy may be appropriate only for a subset of head and neck tumors.

Changes in Drug Sensitivity Following Chemotherapy

SCC from three patients have been tested before and after chemotherapy with methotrexate. Table 5 demonstrates that tumors which were sensitive to methotrexate before treatment (patients 2 and 3) lost

TABLE 3 Distribution of Squamous Cell Carcinomas Tested In The Murine SRC Assay

Primary Site	No.	Type Primary	Type Recurrent	Type Metastasis
Oral cavity	12	7	4	1
Oropharynx	12	3	7	2
Larynx	3	2	---	1
Salivary gland	1	---	1	---
Cervical esophagus	1	1	---	---
Scalp	1	1	---	---
Unknown	1	---	1	---
Total	31	14	13	4

TABLE 4 Drug of Choice for Squamous Cell Carcinomas In The Murine SRC Assay

Drug*	No. of Tumors	ΔTS ($\bar{x} \pm SEM$)	% Reduction in Tumor Weight ($\bar{x} \pm SEM$)
Cyclophosphamide	7	-2.3 ± 0.4	49 ± 6
Methotrexate	5	-2.1 ± 0.3	47 ± 4
Cisplatin	3	-1.6 ± 0.3	40 ± 7
Bleomycin sulfate	3	-1.3 ± 0.4	33 ± 11
Methotrexate or cyclophosphamide	1	-2.2	50
Methotrexate or cisplatin	1	-2.2	50
Cyclophosphamide or bleomycin sulfate	1	-2.0	44

* Ranked first in oncolytic activity by ΔTS value and statistically significant by paired t test.

TABLE 5   Ranking of Drug Sensitivities in SCC Obtained Before and After Clinical Chemotherapy with Methotrexate

Patient. No.	Sensitivity Before Treatment	Sensitivity After Treatment
1	none	none
2	Bleomycin sulfate, methotrexate, cyclophosphamide	none
3	Methotrexate, cyclophosphamide, bleomycin sulfate	Cisplatin, cyclophosphamide, methotrexate

sensitivity to this drug (completely or by changing the ranking order of drug sensitivity). One tumor (patient 1) was not sensitive at the time of either test.

LIMITATIONS OF THE ASSAY

Although the rate of evaluability for the SRC assay is high, there are limitations to the use of the test. The first problem is the quality of the tumor specimen. In our laboratory, frozen sections are performed to evaluate the character of the tissue. When a nonnecrotic, tumor-rich area is obtained, the fragments are prepared from the cut surface adjacent to that used to prepare the section. The section also serves to guide the removal of normal tissue and stroma. Necrotic specimens produce a negative ΔTS in the assay, and tests therefore become unevaluable.[11]

Since tumor fragments, even from a tumor-rich specimen, may lack tumor cells, some form of quality control is necessary to validate each experiment. Using a 4-day SRC assay, Levi et al have suggested that frozen sections of 10 randomly selected tumor fragments can be used to assess the quality of each assay.[12] If 70 percent of fragments contained tumor, good correlation with microscopic responses to drug were observed.

The primary tumor cell population itself may be composed of subsets of cells with differing sensitivity to a given antitumor agent. Therefore, the portion of tumor sampled may not reflect the entire tumor or its metastases. In our series of SCC, the majority of responding tumors (13/21) were sensitive to only one agent; however, this may reflect only the tumor cell population in that particular area of the tumor chosen to prepare the fragments. In primary and metastatic tumors we have tested,[9] a metastasis could be shown to lose a sensitivity that was present in the primary tumor mass, suggesting that the original tumor contained subsets of cells with differing metastatic potentials and drug sensitivities.

Another problem associated with the assay involves the method of determining the degree of oncolytic activity necessary to consider the test positive. Bogden et al state that "effective chemotherapeutic agents act either by inhibiting cell division or by accelerating cell death, with either mode of action re-sulting in a reduction in tumor size."[13] Nevertheless, as a result of the host response to the implant, Edelstein et al have suggested that macroscopic changes in tumor size do not agree with the microscopic evaluation of drug efficacy.[14] For similar reasons, Levi et al suggest a microscopically evaluated assay which is terminated at day 4, prior to the time of infiltration.[12] However, these variations in technique significantly increase the cost of the assay and perhaps the time for final analysis of the data. We have chosen to define a positive response as one that is statistically significant by the paired t test (already discussed). This eliminates comparison of treated ΔTS values to the control ΔTS value which can be influenced by the inflammatory response.

We suggest that (1) frozen sections be used to guide tissue selection and trimming, (2) the quality of the tumor fragments be tested randomly by frozen section prior to implantation,[12] (3) the number of animals per group be increased to seven to enhance the sensitivity of differences observed in drug susceptibility, and (4) statistical analysis should not compare changes in tumor size of treated groups to those of control groups.

CONCLUSIONS

The relevance of the murine SRC assay to clinical oncology can only be determined through well-designed prospective clinical studies, which involve close cooperation between the head and neck surgeon, medical oncologist, surgical pathologist, and the basic science laboratory. The initial reports utilizing the SRC in small retrospective studies are encouraging.[7,15] Nevertheless, the limitations of the assay must be considered in order to ensure the validity of such studies. Clinical studies with various types of tumors will provide data on the degree of oncolytic activity needed to herald a potential clinical response and will enable us to determine the most suitable methods with which to analyze the laboratory results.

REFERENCES

1. Von Hoff DD, Clark GM, Stogdill BJ, et al. Prospective clinical trial of a human tumor cloning system. Cancer Res 1983; 43:1926–1931.
2. Fujita M, Taguchi T. Comparison between the chemotherapy of human cancer xenografts in nude mice and the clinical responses observed in the donor patients. In: Reed ND, ed. Proceedings of the Third International Workshop on Nude Mice. New York: Gustave Fischer, 1982:621–630.
3. Johns ME. The clonal assay of head and neck tumor cells: results and clinical correlations. Laryngoscope 1982; 28(Suppl 92):1–25.
4. Braakhuis BJM, Sneeuwloper G, Snow GB. The potential of the nude mouse xenograft model for the study of head and neck cancer. Arch Otorhinolaryngol 1984; 239:69–79.
5. Bogden AE, Cobb WR, LePage DJ, et al. Chemotherapy responsiveness of human tumors as first generation xenografts in the normal mouse: six-day subrenal capsule assay. Cancer 1981; 48:10–20.

6. Venditti JM. The model's dilemma. In: Fidler IJ, White RJ, eds. Design of models for testing cancer therapeutic agents. New York: Van Nostrand Reinhold, 1982:80–94.
7. Griffin TW, Bogden AE, Reich SD, et al. Initial clinical trials of the subrenal capsule assay as a predictor of tumor response to chemotherapy. Cancer 1983; 52:2185–2192.
8. Bogden AE, Kelton DE, Cobb WR, Esber HJ. A rapid screening method for testing chemotherapeutic agents against human xenografts. In: Houchens DP, Ovejera AA, eds. Proceeding of the Symposium on the Use of Athymic (Nude) Mice in Cancer Research. New York: Gustave Fischer, 1978:231–250.
9. McCormick KJ, Panje WR, Seltzer S, Merrick RH. Single agent chemotherapy for head and neck cancers. Arch Otolaryngol 1983; 109:715–718.
10. Seltzer S, McCormick KJ, Panje WR, Platz CE, Merrick RH. Assessment of the subrenal capsule (SRC) assay in the determination of chemotherapeutic sensitivities of head and neck cancers. Proc AACR 1983; 24:319.
11. Bogden AE, Griffin W, Reich SD, Costanza ME, Cobb WR.

12. Levi F, Blum J-P, Lemaigre G, et al. A 4-day (d) subrenal capsule (SRC) assay for evaluating the responsiveness of human tumors to anticancer drugs: a macroscopic and histologic investigation. Proc AACR 1983; 24:308.
13. Bogden AE, Houchens DP, Ovejera AA, Cobb WR. Advances in chemotherapy studies with the nude mouse. In: Fogh J, Giovanella BC, eds. The nude mouse in experimental and clinical research. Vol. 2. New York: Academic Press, 1982:367–400.
14. Edelstein MB, Fiebig HH, Smink T, Van Putten LM, Schuchhardt C. Comparison between macroscopic and microscopic evaluation of tumor responsiveness using the subrenal capsule assay. Eur J Cancer Clin Oncol 1983; 19:995–1009.
15. Favre R, Verrier C, Marotia L, Carcassonne Y. Chemosensitivity testing of advanced human tumors by the 6-day subrenal capsule mice implant assay. In: Proceedings of the International conference on predictive drug testing on human tumor cells. University Hospital of Zurich: 1983; 85:22.

Predictive testing with the subrenal capsule assay. Cancer Treat Rev 1984;11 (Suppl A):1–12.

NUDE MICE MODEL AS A PREDICTIVE ASSAY IN HEAD AND NECK CANCER

BOUDEWIJN B.J.M. BRAAKHUIS, M.Sc.,
GORDON B. SNOW, M.D., Ph.D.

In general xenografts, that is, grafts exchanged between different species, are rejected by the recipient. Some success in xenografting human tumors has been achieved with newborn rats and mice, with immunosuppressed animals, or on privileged sites such as the brain, the anterior chamber of the eye, or the cheek pouch of the hamster. Since the congenitally athymic nude mouse became available,[1] a large number of reports appeared during the last 15 years, which concerned the use of this host for human tumors. The nude mouse has a T-cell immunodeficiency which allows xenografting, but makes the animal susceptible to viral, bacterial and parasitic infections.

Special care is required in handling these animals, and special housing systems have been developed for maintaining them.[2] The nude mice must be kept in plastic cages with a sealed air filter or in a laminar flow hood, located in a temperature- and humidity-controlled environment. Moreover, it is necessary that food, cages, bedding, and water be sterilized before use. These conditions make this type of research expensive and laborious.

FUNDAMENTALS AND APPLICATIONS OF THE NUDE MICE MODEL

The rate of tumor take varies with the tumor type. For instance, melanomas and adenocarcinomas of the colon take well, whereas leukemias and prostatic carcinomas take poorly. The reasons for these differences are unknown. That the remaining immune system can indeed play a role has been shown by Habu et al,[3] who effected an increase in tumor take by blocking natural killer cells with an antiserum. The establishment of a first transplant generation does not always lead to a serially transplantable tumor line, but depends on the tumor type.

The human origin of tumor cells in the xenografts is preserved according to the results of chromosome analyses and lactate dehydrogenase isoenzyme patterns. However, some reports describe a transformation into a murine tumor. To what extent the characteristics of the original tumor are maintained is still undetermined. The transplanted tumors can grow faster when the number of passages increases,[4] and an increase in the rate of DNA synthesis was found during the first serial passages.[5] Most xenografted tumors are well circumscribed and surrounded by a connective tissue capsule. Metastasis and invasion, characteristics of malignant tumor growth, are rarely found.[6] The immune system of the nude mouse can play an inhibiting role in the development of metastasis. In 3-week-old mice, which have low levels of natural killer cells, the incidence of metastasis is elevated.[7]

The nude mice model can be used for the study of tumor pathology. In the testing of tumor-specific antisera, it has been shown to be of value. This model is also suited for the study of metastasis and tumor growth kinetics. Another application is experimental therapy. Radiotherapy and hyperthermia studies have

The experimental work was supported by the Netherlands Cancer Foundation (KWF) with grant AUKC 82-11.

been reported, but much more attention is focused on chemotherapy. Xenografted tumors generally respond to agents that are active in the clinic. For a few tumors it could be demonstrated that xenografts reproduced the patterns of response of the source tumors. (reviewed by Steel et al[8]).

If a tumor starts to grow in the mice, it takes 3 to 5 months before the response to a limited number of drugs can be evaluated. Therefore, this model is not suitable for selecting chemotherapeutic agents for individual patients, but may be of use if the tumor recurs. The model seems very suitable for the selection of new chemotherapeutic agents, as this model might well be more predictive with respect to human tumors than those using transplanted animal tumors.

GROWTH CHARACTERISTICS OF HUMAN HEAD AND NECK CANCER XENOGRAFTS IN NUDE MICE

In our laboratory, 26.9 percent of 130 transplanted head and neck tumors started to grow in the first passage[9] (Table 1). These transplants consisted of small biopsies taken under local anesthesia as well as tumor pieces obtained from surgical specimens in the operating room. Tumor material, preserved in ice-cold Hanks' buffered salt solution with streptomycin and pencillin, was immediately transported to the laboratory. Slices measuring 3 × 3 × 1 mm were dissected and implanted within 2 hours subcutaneously in the lateral thoracic region on both sides of the animal. The take rate we observed is somewhat less than that reported by Wennerberg et al,[5] who xenotransplanted a total of 54 head and neck tumors. Thus far we have been able to obtain nine tumor lines with at least 10 passages. Poorly differentiated squamous cell carcinomas tend to take better than moderately and well-differentiated ones. These results may reflect the more malignant character of poorly differentiated squamous cell carcinomas. Tumor material from lymph node metastases tended to show initial growth more often than material from primary tumors. An explanation for this tendency might be that the proliferation rate of metastasized tumor cells is higher than that of cells of primary tumors. Absence of contamination might also be important in this regard.

TABLE 2 Growth Characteristics of Tumor Lines that could be Transplanted in More than Nine Passages (May 1984)

Line	Maximum passage number	Mean take rate* (%) (± SD)	Mean tumor-doubling time† (days ± SD)
HNX-DU	15	70.7 ± 21.4	4.4 ± 1.4
HNX-G	16	96.7 ± 6.0	6.0 ± 2.4
HNX-KE	10	68.6 ± 15.9	6.6 ± 0.7
HNX-LA	10	52.2 ± 18.8	7.5 ± 2.8
HNX-OV	11	55.1 ± 15.5	9.2 ± 1.8
HNX-P	10	71.5 ± 21.2	7.2 ± 1.6
HNX-PV	11	84.8 ± 18.5	8.2 ± 5.8
HNX-TI	10	48.8 ± 25.7	5.6 ± 0.9
HNX-W	15	86.8 ± 13.9	7.1 ± 1.9

*Take rate is defined as the number of tumors that have reached a volume of 100 mm³ as a percentage of the number of tumors transplanted.

†Tumor doubling time is defined as the number of days needed by the tumor to grow from 100 to 200 mm³.

These mean values are calculated from the individual passages starting with the third passage.

Considering the nine lines that have reached more than nine passages, it was found that in three of these lines the take rate per passage was at a mean level of over 80 percent (Table 2). Furthermore, in most lines the take rate varies considerably with passage number, without a tendency toward a higher take rate with increasing passage number. In general the xenotransplanted tumors grow with a tumor volume-doubling time (TD) between 5 and 9 days. In four of the nine lines, the TD decreased after a few passages to a level of 4 to 6 days. This characteristic is perhaps a less general phenomenon than could be expected from earlier results.[9] In two lines the TD is at a constant level; in three lines the TD varies with the passage number.

The histologic characteristics of the original tumor are maintained well in the xenografts. The tumors are well circumscribed and surrounded by a connective tissue capsule originating from the mouse. No microscopic signs of metastasis to other organs could be found in ± 500 tumor-bearing animals. Mouse-grown tumors of all lines showed necrosis. The extent varied between tumor lines and increased according to tumor volume.

TABLE 1 Take of Various Types of Head and Neck Tumors obtained from Untreated Patients

Tumor type	No. tumor takes/ No. transplanted (%)		No. of lines with at least 10 passages/ No. attempted (%)	
Squamous cell carcinoma				
Poorly differentiated	7/13	(53.8%)	3/6	(50.0%)
Moderately differentiated	13/45	(28.8%)	2/9	(22.2%)
Well differentiated	11/59	(18.6%)	3/10	(30.0%)
Salivary gland	2/9	(22.2%)	1/2	
Chondrosarcoma	0/1		0/0	
Non-Hodgkin's lymphoma	0/1		0/0	
Mucosal melanoma	2/2		0/2	
Total	35/130	(26.9%)	9/29	(31.0%)

Owing to a temporary lack of animals, tumor lines were frozen in liquid nitrogen. Pieces of tumor tissue were incubated in McCoy's medium with 20 percent fetal calf serum and 10 percent dimethylsulfoxide. With a standard program used for preservation of lymphocytes, the liquid nitrogen temperature was attained. With five of seven lines (71.4 percent), it was possible to continue passaging after storage at low temperatures.

THE SCREENING POTENTIAL OF THE NUDE MICE MODEL FOR ANTICANCER DRUGS IN HEAD AND NECK CANCER

A total of 19 lines were found to be suitable for chemotherapy studies. Some of these results were published previously.[10] Chemotherapy studies could not be done in each passage because of a varying pattern of tumor take. Drug activity was expressed as growth delay,[8] defined as the difference between the mean values of the time required by the tumors of treated and control mice to double their volume, divided by the mean value of the time required by the tumors of control mice to double their volume. Growth delay was thus expressed in terms of the fold increase in volume doubling time gained by the treatment. To get an idea of the screening potential of this model, five drugs with known clinical activity were tested (Table 3). Maximum tolerated dose levels were used. Cis-platinum and bleomycin appeared to be the most effective drugs, causing a growth delay of more than two in 45.5 and 40 percent of the lines respectively. Methotrexate (MTX), at a daily dose schedule for 5 to 7 days, caused in only one line a growth delay of more than one. In the remaining 11 lines it was inactive or minimally active. Using a schedule of high doses on days 1 and 8 in only one line, a moderate response was observed (growth delay 1.0). For two

tumors, the reaction of the xenografts to MTX did not correlate with the source tumors. The patients' tumors showed a 90 percent and 50 percent remission after monochemotherapy with MTX; the xenografts did not respond, regardless of the schedule used. 5-Fluorouracil caused a growth delay of about one in three lines and was minimally active in four others. Cyclophosphamide was moderately active in four lines and minimally active in one line.

In Table 3 the chemotherapy results in the tumor lines are compared with overall patient response rates, known from the literature.[11] Cis-platinum and bleomycin tend to be more effective in this model than would be expected from the clinical data. It is possible that in our model, by chance, more sensitive tumors were tested than could be expected. It is interesting to note that MTX elicited only a minimal response. This observed lack of activity of MTX in this model might be attributed to a difference in pharmacokinetics between man and mouse. However, this is unlikely since a MTX-sensitive rat rhabdomyosarcoma was very sensitive to MTX in this model using both aforementioned schedules. Known resistance mechanisms can play a role in this model. The intracellular pool of dihydrofolate reductase, the target enzyme to which MTX binds reversibly, may be increased, or the rate of MTX uptake into the tumor cells may be decreased. Another possibility is a reversal of MTX toxicity by purine and pyrimidine nucleotide precursors released by a population of dying tumor cells.

CONCLUSIONS

Owing to a low take rate, the use of the nude mice model to test drugs for head and neck cancer is expensive and laborious. The tumor take rates vary per passage, and this complicates the planning of ex-

TABLE 3   Xenograft Response Compared with Clinical Findings, Obtained from the Literature[11]

Drug	Xenograft response				Patient response[11]
	Sensitive (%)	Moderatley sensitive (%)	Inactive or minimally sensitive (%)	Total no. of lines	Percentage partial or complete remissions (no. of patients)
Cis-platinum	5 (45.5%)	2 (18.2%)	4 (36.4%)	11 (100%)	33% (108)
Bleomycin	4 (40.0%)	2 (20.0%)	4 (40.0%)	10 (100%)	18% (298)
Methotrexate (I)	0	1 (8.3%)	11 (91.7%)	12 (100%)	50% (100)
Methotrexate (II)	0	1 (11.1%)	8 (88.9%)	9 (100%)	50% (100)
Cyclophosphamide	0	4 (80.0%)	1 (20.0%)	5 (100%)	36% (77)
5-Fluorouracil	0	3 (42.8%)	4 (57.2%)	7 (100%)	15% (118)

Sensitive = growth delay > 2; moderately sensitive = growth delay between 1 and 2; insensitive of minimally sensitive = growth delay < 1.
Cis-platinum dose = 3 mg/kg daily for 3–5 days (intraperitoneally); bleomycin dose = 15 mg/kg daily for 4–7 days (subcutaneously); methotrexate (1) dose = 5 mg/kg daily for 5–7 days (intraperitoneally); methotrexate (11) dose = 250 mg/kg on day 1 and 8 (intraperitoneally); cyclophosphamide dose = 100 mg/kg on day 1 and 8 (intraperitoneally); 5-fluorouracil dose = 25 mg/kg daily for 4–5 days (intraperitoneally).

periments. Good cooperation between investigators and clinicians is essential.

Our results show that with the nude mice model methotrexate would not have been selected as a promising drug against head and neck cancer. Since methotrexate is the drug most widely used against this type of cancer, our results indicate that this model has certain limitations as a screening model. Further investigation of the ineffectiveness of MTX in this model is needed. Preliminary results indicate that this model can be suitable for the testing of analogs of a drug that has been found to be active in this model, such as cis-platinum.

REFERENCES

1. Rygaard J, Povlsen, CO. Heterotransplantation of a human malignant tumor to "nude" mice. Acta Pathol Microbiol Scand 1969; 77:758–760.
2. Ediger R, Giovanella BC. Current knowledge of breeding and mass production of the nude mouse. In: Foqh J, Giovanella BC (eds). The nude mouse in experimental and clinical research. New York: Academic Press, 1978, pp 16–28.
3. Habu S, Fukui H, Shimamura K, Kasai M, Nagai Y, Okumura K, Tamaoki N. In vivo effects of anti-asialo GM. I. Reduction of NK activity and enhancement of transplanted tumor growth in nude mice. J Immunol 1981; 127:34–38.
4. Mattern J, Haag D, Wayss K, Volm M. Growth kinetics of human lung tumours in nude mice. Exp Cell Biol 1981; 49:34–40.
5. Wennerberg J, Tropé C, Biörklund A. Heterotransplantation of human head and neck tumors into nude mice. Acta Otolaryngol. 1983; 95:183–190.
6. Sharkey FE, Fogh J. Metastasis of human tumors in athymic nude mice. Int J Cancer 1979; 24:733–738.
7. Hanna N, Fidler IJ. Expression of metastatic potential of allogeneic and xenogeneic neoplasms in young nude mice. Cancer Res 1981; 41:438–444.
8. Steel GG, Courtenay VD, Peckham MJ. The response to chemotherapy of a variety of human tumour xenografts. Br J Cancer 1983; 47:1–13.
9. Braakhuis BJM, Sneeuwloper G, Snow GB. The potential of the nude mouse xenograft model for the study of head and neck cancer. Arch Otorhinolaryngol 1984; 239:69–79.
10. Braakhuis BJM, Schoevers EJ, Heinerman ECM, Sneeuwloper G, Snow GB. Chemotherapy of human head and neck cancer xenografts with three clinically active drugs: cis-platinum, bleomycin and methotrexate. Br J Cancer 1983; 48:711–716.
11. Hong WK, Bromer R. Chemotherapy in head and neck cancer. N Engl J Med 1983; 308:75–79.

30. Single Agent Versus Combination Chemotherapy

INTRODUCTION

ROBERT E. WITTES, M.D.

Is combination chemotherapy superior to single-agent treatment for squamous head and neck cancer? The question is obviously an important one. Single-agent treatment is of very limited value for most patients; with any of the so-called active drugs, significant tumor shrinkage occurs in a minority of patients, lasts for 2 to 4 months, and has minimal impact on survival. In the absence of more effective drugs, therefore, drug combinations represent the best hope for developing regimens of real value.

The question is also important for day-to-day decision making in clinical care. The patient who has failed attempts at cure with radiation and surgery deserves at least that the therapy chosen by his oncologist be selected on the basis of the best evidence available. If two regimens do not differ significantly concerning major therapeutic end points, then side effects, convenience, and cost become particularly important in selecting treatment.

As with every other neoplasm for which multiple active agents exist, the promise of combination chemotherapy has been explored intensively in squamous head and neck cancer. Reviews of this literature have been published elsewhere.[1,2] The heterogeneity and relative rarity of the head and neck cancers, the heavily pretreated nature of most of the patients entered on exploratory trials, and the high incidence of major medical co-morbidity have until recently been major obstacles to the conduct of meaningful therapeutic trials. The literature is cluttered with small pilot studies of empirically derived drug combinations, most of which do not explicitly address questions of comparative efficacy. Before even beginning to decide whether drug combinations have been superior to single agents, therefore, one must acknowledge that prevailing patterns of clinical trial methodology do not permit an answer to the question in most cases. The absence of control groups and the small size of most trials obscure any but the most extreme results.

It has certainly become clear, though, that however brilliantly the promise of combination chemotherapy has been realized in other diseases, the construction of regimens which can yield appreciable complete response rates in head and neck cancer has been very difficult indeed. No less disturbing has been the failure of drug combinations to improve the very short durations of response seen with single drugs; indeed, the rapidity with which clinical drug resistance develops in head and neck cancer is one of its most striking features.

Even a cursory look at the literature reveals an obvious part of the problem: many combinations have been put together without adequate attention to selection of agents or details of dose and schedule. Particularly in the precisplatin era, agents were incorporated into regimens with little regard for their activity; the use of the nitrosoureas, bifunctional alkylating agents, vincristine, hydroxyurea, and doxorubicin is very difficult to defend if established single-agent activity is a valid criterion for use in combination. In addition, since the toxicities of many of these drug classes are at least partially overlapping, the individual constituents of a combination cannot be given at or even near full single-agent doses. It follows that additive toxicity is more likely than an additive (or synergistic) therapeutic effect.

Since the mid 1970s, most combination regimens have been based on methotrexate and/or cisplatin, with or without bleomycin. In his interesting chapter, Vogl discusses various possible reasons why the MBD regimen developed at the Albert Einstein Medical Center and further tested by the ECOG failed to surpass weekly methotrexate alone in therapeutic effect. After considering the issues of optimal dose and schedule of the three constituent agents and reported results with similar combinations, he includes that "there is no consistent evidence that other ways of giving the drugs are superior"; the implication is clearly that the results with MBD very likely represent the state of the art for combinations of these particular agents.

Perhaps so. The absence of "consistent evidence" for better ways of giving these drugs, however, is based on evidence of largely unsatisfactory quality. The fact is that very few studies provide direct evidence for or against dose or schedule dependency of response. Can one expect methotrexate at 40 mg/m^2 every other week (as in MBD) to be equivalent therapeutically to the same dose weekly which ECOG used as its control? Can one expect the relatively small bolus dose of bleomycin weekly in MBD to have any therapeutic effect at all?

Vogl's main conclusion, however, is certainly valid. In patients who have failed local therapy, there is no ethical imperative to treat with conventional agents, singly or in combination, before moving on to trials with experimental drugs. The totality of experience with head and neck cancer strongly suggests that empirically derived combinations of existing agents have very limited utility. The most pressing need remains the discovery of drugs with significantly greater efficacy than those available today.

REFERENCES

1. Wittes RE. Combination chemotherapy of head and neck cancer in the United States. In: Carter SK, Sakurai Y, Umezawa H (eds). Recent Results in Cancer Research. Vol. 76, Berlin, Heidelberg: Springer Verlag, 1981: 276–289.
2. Million R, Cassizzi N, Wittes RE. Cancer in the head and neck. In: DeVita V, Hellman S, Rosenberg S (eds). Principles and Practice of Oncology. Philadelphia: J.B. Lippincott Company, 1982: 301–386.

SINGLE AGENT VERSUS COMBINATION CHEMOTHERAPY IN HEAD AND NECK CANCER

JOSEPH R. BERTINO, M.D.
ENRICO MINI, M.D.

The rationale for combination chemotherapy, and its firm basis in the treatment of experimental tumors, is now well established. The major reasons for use of combination chemotherapy are (1) enhanced cytotoxicity when drugs with different mechanisms of action are employed, and (2) prevention or delay of drug resistance. Although not always observed, general principles for using drugs in combination have evolved over recent years based on experimental data, and are worth reemphasizing.

First, some evidence for biochemical or pharmacologic synergy should be present. This might derive from in vitro or in vivo animal studies. For example, methotrexate (MTX) and asparaginase are synergistic when the sequence is MTX followed by asparaginase 24 hours later, but have less than additive antitumor effects versus lymphoblasts when given together.[1] Similarly there is experimental rational for the sequence MTX followed by 5-fluorouracil (5-FU) rather than the reverse sequence.

Second, drugs used in combination may be used in maximum dosage when the limiting toxicities are different, e.g., vincristine and cyclophosphamide. If limiting toxicities are not different, e.g., both drugs are marrow suppressants, then two-thirds of the maximum dose of each agent may be safely employed. Often in combination therapy regimens, one-half the dose of drug A and one-half the dose of drug B are utilized. Assuming the activity of A>B or B>A, in both circumstances the net effect will be less than expected with full dose A or B. At best, if A=B in potency, the result will be the same for A+B versus full-dose A or B alone. Therefore, it follows that not all drug combinations are necessarily better than or even equal to single-agent therapy.

Third, drugs used in combination lessen the chance of drug resistance. This is true if multidrug resistance does not occur. This recently discovered phenomenon may be very important and limit the value of combination chemotherapy. Drugs sharing in this multi-drug-resistant phenotype are the anthracyclines, the vinca alkaloids, actinomycin D, and perhaps certain alkylating agents (e.g., melphalan).[2] Finally, since almost all agents that react with DNA are mutagens, the use of these agents in combination may actually enhance the number of drug-resistant mutants emerging after treatment. Recent reports from the laboratories of Schimke[3] and Varshavsky[4] also demonstrate that exposure of tumor cells in early S phase to antimetabolites as well as agents that effect DNA synthesis may also increase the drug-resistant mutant frequency via gene amplification. Thus, timing of drugs, as well as dose, may be important in the clinic in regard to generation of drug resistance.

HEAD AND NECK CANCER AND COMBINATION CHEMOTHERAPY

The number of effective drugs available (defined as giving at least a partial remission (PR) rate of $>20\%$) is limited in the treatment of patients with head and neck cancer. These drugs are cisplatin, MTX, and perhaps bleomycin. Infusion therapy with 5-FU, as used in the cisplatin-FU combination,[5] has not been tested as a single agent, although it has been used together with radiation therapy.[6] Determination that a given drug combination is clearly superior to single-agent therapy in head and neck cancer is difficult, and requires a sufficient number of patients properly stratified for stage, location, performance status, and degree of differentiation. In addition, pretreatment variables such as previous treatment are known to hae a significant effect on chemotherapy outcome.[7]

Two combinations have been tested that appear to give greater than single-agent activity: MTX and 5-FU, and cisplatin and 5-FU by infusion. While the sequence MTX followed by 5-FU may not be better than simultaneous or the reverse sequence (with a one-hour interval), all studies save one have reported a 50 to 70 percent response rate (Table 1). Although this combination has not been compared to single-agent MTX, the groups reporting these results (including a study by ECOG that has not been reported yet) have not had this high a response rate to MTX as a single agent. Nevertheless, unless a larger randomized trial is performed, the superiority of MTX/FU over MTX alone may not be considered established.

The second combination that has produced exciting results is cisplatin-FU. The need for the infusion of 5-FU rather than a rapid injection was recently established, and thus presumably the superiority of the combination over cisplatin therapy alone. This combination is now being tested as part of multimodality approaches to treatment of epidermoid cancer of the head and neck, and these results will be awaited with interest.

TABLE 1 MTX and 5-Fluorouracil in Head and Neck Cancer

Author	Schedule	No. Pts*	% CR+PR
Pitman et al[8]	MTX —> FU	35	71
Ringborg et al[9]	MTX —> FU†	36	64
Jacobs[10]	MTX —> FU‡	14	21
Bowman et all[11]	MTX —> FU§	42	62
	MTX + FU#	37	38
Coates et al[22]	MTX —> FU**	26	65
	FU —> MTX††	23	39

*Patients not previously treated with chemotherapy.
‡One-hour interval: Dose — MTX, 125 to 250 mg/m²; FU, 600 mg/m². LV, 10 mg/m² q6h × 6, 24 h after MTX. Treatments were weekly.
†Two-hour interval: Dose — MTX, 200 mg/m²; FU, 600 mg/m². LV, 10 mg/m² q6h×5, 24 h after MTX. Treatments were weekly.
§One-hour interval, MTX and FU doses as in footnote (†). Treatments were given days 1 and 8 of a 21-day cycle.
#FU given immediately after MTX. Same doses as in footnote (†).
**One-hour interval: Dose — MTX, 250 mg/m²; FU, 600 mg/m². LV at 24 h, 8 doses q6h, 15 mg each. Treatment was weekly.
††FU preceded MTX by one hour. Doses as in footnote (**).

CONCLUSIONS AND PROSPECTS

Chemotherapy for head and neck cancer has now entered a new phase of combination therapy. The superiority of combination regimens over single-agent programs has not been established, but results with two combinations suggest that there now may be combinations available that are better than single-agent treatment.

Future work should build on this information once it has been established that these combination are more effective than cisplatin or MTX alone. New combinations should be developed on the basis of pharmacologic and biochemical leads rather than by complete empiricism.

REFERENCES

1. Capizzi RL. Schedule-dependent synergism and antagonism between methotrexate and asparaginase. Biochem Pharmacol 1974; 23:151–161.
2. Ling V. Genetic basis of drug resistance in mammalian cells. In: Bruchovskky W, Goldie JH (eds). Drug and Hormone Resistance in Neoplasia. Vol. 1. Florida: CRC Press, 1982: 1–19.
3. Schimke RT. Gene amplification in cultured animal cells. Cell 1984; 37:705–713.
4. Varshavsky A. Phorbol ester dramatically increases incidence of methotrexate-resistant mouse cells: Possible mechanisms and relevance of tumor promotion. Cell 1981; 25:561–572.
5. Decker DA, Drelichman A, Jacobs J, Hoscher J, Kinzre J, Lik JJ, Weaver A, Al-Saraf M. Adjuvant chemotherapy with high dose bolus cis-diamminedichloroplatinum II and 120 hour infusion 5-fluorouracil in stage III and IV carcinoma of the head and neck. Proc Am Soc Clin Oncol 1982; 1:195.
6. Byfield JE, Sharp TR, Frankel SS, Tang SG, Callipari FB. Phase I and II trial of five-day infused 5-fluorouracil and radiation in cancer of head and neck. J Clin Oncol 1984; 2:406–413.

7. Mead GM, Jacobs C. The changing role of chemotherapy in the treatment of head and neck cancer. Am J Med 1982; 73:582–599.
8. Pitman SW, Kowal CD, Bertino JR. Methotrexate and 5-fluorouracil in sequence in squamous head and neck cancer. Semin Oncol 1983; 10:15–19.
9. Ringborg U, Evert G, Kinnman J, Landquist PG, Strander H. Sequential methotrexate-5-fluorouracil treatment of squamous cell carcinoma of the head and neck. Cancer, in press.
10. Jacobs C. Use of methotrexate and 5FU for recurrent head and neck cancer. Cancer Treat Rep 1982; 66:1925–1928.
11. Browman GP, Archibald SD, Young JEM, et al. Prospective randomized trial of one-hour sequential versus simultaneous methotrexate plus 5-fluorouracil in advanced and recurrent squamous cell head and neck cancer. J Clin Oncol 1983; 1:787–792.
12. Coates AS, Tattersall MHN, Swanson C, Hedley D, Fox RM, Raghavan D. Combination therapy with methotrexate and 5-fluorouracil: A prospective randomized clinical trial of order of administration. J Clin Oncol 1984; 2:756–761.

RATIONALE FOR COMBINATION CHEMOTHERAPY AS TREATMENT OF ADVANCED HEAD AND NECK CANCER

THOMAS J. ERVIN, M.D.
RALPH R. WEICHSELBAUM, M.D.
JOHN R. CLARK, M.D.
KLAUS BOEHEIM, M.D.

The usefulness of any chemotherapeutic program must be assessed in relationship to the desired treatment goals. Chemotherapy as the only treatment for solid malignant tumors is restricted to a few pediatric or germ cell tumors. Advanced adult solid tumors remain a major treatment dilemma requiring the skills of the surgeon, radiotherapists, and oncologist for optimal management. Within this multidisciplinary framework, the role of the oncologist (and chemotherapy) may differ depending on the clinical goals. An evaluation of single agent vs combination chemotherapy programs must be viewed with these issues in focus.

CLINICAL PROBLEM

Squamous carcinoma of the head and neck (SCCHN) is a malignant tumor that presents with loco-regional disease. Even in its advanced stages, SCCHN does not present with distantly metastatic disease.[1] Radiation therapy and/or surgery may be effective in eradicating all disease, even for patients with stage III and IV disease. An analysis of failure of such patients indicates that persistence of local tumor cells is the major problem.[2] Conversely, fewer patients fail with distant metastasis, only suggesting that the distantly metastatic tumor burden is low. These principles outline the goals for the addition of chemotherapy to standard local treatment. These goals are (1) to improve local control via loco-regional cytoreduction, and (2) to eradicate a small but finite number of distantly metastatic cells. In addition to the curative goals of chemotherapy, palliation of symptoms caused by recurrent disease is also an issue.

When stage III or IV SCCHN presents clinically, it is likely that the tumor burden approximates 10^{10} cells.[3] Within these cellular compartments, tumor cells may be sensitive or resistant to available chemotherapeutic agents. Even if the initial malignant clonal event produces a drug-sensitive tumor cell line, naturally occurring resistance may occur. It has been estimated that such mutational resistance may occur at a frequency approximating 10^{-6}.[4] Given a presenting cellular burden of 10^{10} or more cells, it is highly probable that clonogenic SCCHN cells resistant to any one chemotherapeutic agent exists. Current in vitro evidence suggests that drug resistance mechanisms may affect more than single drugs so that any mutation affecting SCCHN drug sensitivity may produce resistance to other drugs as well.[5] These resistant tumor cells would be expected to be randomly distributed throughout the loco-regional and distantly metastatic drug compartments.

In addition to cellular compartments, there appear to be environmental compartments within tumors as well. These micro and macro environments may produce conditions resulting in a decreased sensitivity to chemotherapy. Oxygen delivery to tumors appears to be disorganized and incomplete.[6] Resulting tumor tissue hypoxia will decrease drug as well as irradiation sensitivity.[7] Tumor cells may respond to hypoxia by expansion of G0 or by initiation of anaerobic glycolysis. These changes in cellular functioning may be circumvented by utilizing selective chemotherapies which are active under these conditions. For instance, mitomycin may be more active under conditions favoring anaerobic glycolysis.[8] Additionally, inhibition of repair of potentially lethal DNA damage by drug combinations may improve cellular killing of G0 phase cells.[9]

CHEMOTHERAPY TARGETS

Head and neck cancer presents with macroscopic disease. For patients presenting for induction chemotherapy, the goal of chemotherapy is maximum tumor cytoreduction. In surgical terms, this cytoreduction can increase the potential for resectability of resistant or persistent cancer cells at the primary site. Radiation therapy may be more effective as the treatment volume is lower and the number of cells to be killed are fewer. Tumor cells may become re-oxygenated and more radiosensitive by the disappearance of tumor cells killed by chemotherapy. For the reasons just mentioned, such cytoreduction via chemotherapy is achieved to a greater degree by combination chemotherapy.

Microscopic disease is present in a finite but limited number of patients with advanced squamous carcinoma of the head and neck. Given that many of the patients will present with a limited number of distant micrometastases, this group of patients should benefit from combination chemotherapy. A 2- to 3-logarithm cell kill is possible with multiple drug regimens such as cisplatin, bleomycin, and methotrexate or cisplatin and fluorouracil.[10,11]

TREATMENT RESULTS

Single-agent chemotherapy for advanced head and neck cancer can, under certain conditions, produce a high partial response rate. Such response rates in the range of 20 to 50 percent have been reported for methotrexate, bleomycin and cisplatin.[12] Despite these high response rates, tumor recurrence is universal. Early recurrences following single-agent chemotherapies suggest that the log-kill produced by single agents is limited. Studies of in vitro squamous cell carcinoma, treated with bleomycin have demonstrated that for exponentially growing cells, the agent is highly effective. This phenomenon has been reported for methotrexate and ArA-C, a drug which has no known efficacy in squamous carcinoma of the head and neck. For plateau phase cells, however, the effectiveness of bleomycin is limited, possibly due to repair of bleomycin-induced DNA damage. The combination of other drugs such as Adriamycin and cisplatin, which inhibit DNA repair in addition to their direct DNA damaging effects, may produce a potential advantage therapeutically. The combination of cisplatin and 5-fluorouracil has gained favor as induction treatment for advanced head and neck cancer. Responses are in the range of 80 to 90 percent, and for the first time clinical complete responses are documented in 30 to 50 percent of patients following chemotherapy alone. This magnitude of response suggests an increased cytotoxic effect. This degree of cytotoxic antitumor effect is necessary for translation into curative chemotherapy treatment program.

SUMMARY

Overall, several lines of evidence suggest that combination chemotherapy is appropriate for squamous carcinoma of the head and neck. Clinical data now accumulating from Wayne State, Dana-Farber Cancer Institute, and Roswell Park Memorial Institute all suggest that antitumor effect with multiple drugs exceeds that seen with single-agent chemotherapies. Additionally, survival advantages have been reported by Spaulding[13] and by Ervin[14] with the use of chemotherapy as initial treatment of advanced, previously untreated squamous carcinoma of the head and neck.

Chemotherapy as palliative treatment for previously treated squamous carcinoma of the head and neck is still experimental. Performance status problems, mechanical debilities, and mucosal intolerance from previous treatment limit the use of effective combination chemotherapies. Response rates in such patients can exceed 50 percent with a duration of response of approximately 6 months.[15] Further research in the use of non-cross-resistant combinations of chemotherapies are needed for these patients.

REFERENCES

1. Cancer, Facts and Figures. American Cancer Society, 1980:8–19.
2. Suit HD. Potential for improving survival rates for the cancer patient by increasing the efficacy of treatment of the primary lesion. Cancer 1982; 50:1227–1234.
3. Ervin TJ, Karp DD, Weichselbaum RR, Posner MR, Fabrois RL, Miller D. The role of chemotherapy in the multidisciplinary approach to advanced head and neck cancer: potentials and problems. Ann Otol Rhinol Laryngol 1981; 90:506–511.
4. Goldie JH, Coldman AJ, Gadaushes GA. Rationale for the use of alternating non-cross-resistant chemotherapy. Cancer Treat Rep 1982; 439:449.
5. Frei E III. Personal communication, 1984.
6. Weichselbaum RR, Ervin TJ. Chemical nodulation of the hypoxic fraction in the treatment of advanced head and neck cancer. Arch Otolaryngol 1981; 107:237–240.
7. Withers HR, Peters LJ. Basic principles of radiotherapy. In: Fletcher G, ed. Textbook of radiotherapy. Philadelphia: Lea & Febiger, 1983:103.
8. Teicher BA, Lazo JS, Sartorelli AC. Classification of antineoplastic agents by their selective toxicities toward oxygenated and hypoxic tumor cells. Cancer Res 1981; 41:73–81.
9. Bocheim K, Weichselbaum RR. Personal communication, 1984.
10. Ervin TJ, Weichselbaum RR, Miller D. Treatment of advanced carcinoma of the head and neck with cis-platinum, bleomycin, and methotrexate (PBM). Cancer Treat Rep 1981; 65:787–791.
11. Weaver A, Fleming S, Kish J, Vanderbery H, Jacob J, Gussman J, Al-Sarral M. Cis-platinum and 5-fluorouracil as induction therapy for advanced head and neck cancer. Am J Surg 1982; 144:445–448.
12. Glick JH, Taylor SG IV. Integration of chemotherapy into a combined modality treatment plan for head and neck cancer: A review. Int J Radiat Oncol Biol Phys 1981; 7:229–242.
13. Spaulding MB, Kahn A, Delos Santos R, Klotch D, Love J. Adjuvant chemotherapy in advanced head and neck cancer. Am J Surg 1982; 144:432–436.
14. Ervin TJ, Weichselbaum RR, et al. Neoadjuvant cis-platinum, bleomycin, and methotrexate chemotherapy for advanced squamous carcinoma of the head and neck. Preliminary report. Arch Otolaryngol 1984, in press.
15. Carter SK. The chemotherapy of head and neck cancer. Semin Oncol 1977; 4:413–424.

IS COMBINATION CHEMOTHERAPY OF DEMONSTRATED VALUE FOR ADVANCED HEAD AND NECK CANCER?

STEVEN E. VOGL, M.D.

Considerable excitement occurred in the early and mid 1970s when new and effective agents became available for the chemotherapy of advanced head and neck cancer. The excitement was fueled by extraordinary response rates (over 70 percent) reported from Memorial Hospital for a combination of a bleomycin infusion and a high dose of cisplatin (DDP) as initial therapy before radiation for regionally confined but far-advanced lesions. Multiple programs combining these agents, with or without the most active known agent from the past, methotrexate (MTX), were developed. In keeping with our philosophy of keeping patients out of the hospital as much as possible, and with limited resources, we at the Albert Einstein College of Medicine designed for the Eastern Cooperative Oncology Group (ECOG) an outpatient program combininng these three agents, given the acronym MBD:

	Day				
	1	4	8	15	22
Methotrexate 40 mg/m² IM	X			X	Repeat cycle
Bleomycin 10 units IM	X		X	X	
Cisplatin (DDT) 50 mg/m² IV		X			

Details of the program have been published, including the pharmacologic rationale for the unusual scheduling of cisplatin apart from methotrexate in order to keep the former from impairing the excretion of the latter, leading to enhanced toxicity.[1] The initial response rates were encouraging; the overall response rate was 63 percent among patients who had an "adequate" 3-week trial of therapy, with 17 percent complete remissions. Partial remissions lasted a "respectable" median of 5 months, measured from date of entry to relapse, though median survival for partial

responders was only 6 months, and only 2 months longer than that of nonresponders. Median duration of complete remission was 11 months, and median survival for complete responders was 22 months. These results were far better than we had previously observed for methotrexate alone in the Eastern Cooperative Oncology Group: 25 percent rate of largely partial remissions. This response rate was not improved by administration of high doses of methotrexate with citrovorum rescue alone or combined with cyclophosphamide and cytosine arabinoside.

We therefore proceeded to design a randomized trial to prove that a combination of these drugs was indeed superior to methotrexate alone in terms of rates of overall and complete remission, remission duration, and survival. Eligibility was restricted to patients with histologically proved squamous cancer or lymphoepithelioma of the upper aerodigestive tract with either recurrence after radiation therapy or distant metastases, without second primary tumors, out of bed at least once a day, and with adequate bone marrow, liver, and renal function to tolerate chemotherapy. No patient eligible for the trial was excluded from analysis for any event occurring after entry. Of 168 patients entered on these two treatments (a third immuno-chemotherapy arm was dropped early), three were never treated and two were excluded as ineligible. Methotrexate (MTX) was given in the standard ECOG regimen of 40 mg/m² intravenously weekly, with an escalation to 60 mg/m² on the eighth day of treatment and thereafter in the absence of toxicity during the first week.

The ultimate results proved disappointing! The overall response rate was 48 percent for MBD and 35 percent for methotrexate, with 16 percent and 8 percent complete response rates, respectively. This difference is of borderline statistical significance, and becomes significant only if one performs a statistical test which weights complete responses as being better than partial responses, and if one further assumes that the combination could not possibly be less active than MTX alone. The difference in rate of response is not significant if one takes into account the major prognostic factors for response: ambulatory performance status, absence of fixed nodes in the neck, and absence of distant metastases. Neither complete nor partial remissions were longer for MBD than for methotrexate, with approximate median durations (measured from date of entry to relapse) of 5 and 8 months, respectively.

There was no difference in survival between the two arms: the median was 5.6 months on each, with only 20 percent of patients alive one year after entry. Responders, especially complete responders, lived considerably longer than nonresponders. Significant prognostic factors for prolonged survival include ambulatory performance status, absence of distant metastases, lack of a heavy smoking history, absence of adjacent organ invasion from the primary site, absence of major weight loss, absence of tumor in the

The study whose results are reported extensively in this chapter was performed by the Eastern Cooperative Oncology Group, Paul Carbone, chairman, and Barry H. Kaplan, chairman of the head and neck committee.

neck, and lack of a history of heavy alcohol ingestion. There was no significant difference in response rate according to primary site. A complete discussion of the limited value of partial response in this trial is presented elsewhere in this volume. Hmatologic toxicity with the combination was only slightly worse than with MTX, and mucosal toxicity was identical. Renal toxicity was trivial, and pulmonary toxicity occurred in 3 percent of patients on MBD.

We were profoundly disappointed by the failure of MBD to prove itself superior to MTX. We went back to the data to see if we had introduced any major biases along the way. No major imbalances in pretreatment characteristics existed between the groups. We then examined whether requiring a minimum 2, 4, or 6 weeks of therapy would change the response rates. It did, but did not make the difference between MBD and MTX any more impressive: requiring 6 weeks of therapy left 61 patients evaluable on MBD, with 20 percent complete remissions and 38 percent partial remissions; for MTX the results were 13 percent complete remissions and 36 percent partial remissions. Probably as a result of a chance variation, MTX produced a 44 percent response rate in the second half of the study versus 25 percent in the first half; no such variation was found for MBD.

Given the finding of no major difference between the two treatments, we used our data on 163 patients to determine whether we missed major differences (a process statisticians call posterior probabilities). The chance that there really is a ≥25 percent increase in response rate from 35 percent for methotrexate to ≥60 percent for MBD is only 6 percent. The chance of a true increase ≥15 percent in complete response rate from 7 percent for MTX to ≥22 percent for MBD is only 8 percent. The chance that MBD really prolongs median survival ≥2 months from 5.5 months for MTX to ≥7.5 months for MBD is only 10 percent. We can be quite convinced then (and quite depressed) that we did not miss major differences for these end points in our large study.

It seems that the combination program we chose is not much better than single-agent methotrexate, the most obvious reason being that the drugs are not as effective as expected on the basis of early data. Initial results with methotrexate alone suggested response rates as high as 60 percent for standard doses and 75 percent for high doses with citrovorum rescue. In a prior study in the Eastern Group, however, this drug produced a 26 percent response, only 7.5 percent of them complete, and only a 15-week median duration of response from onset to relapse. Cisplatin (DDP) initially was reported to produce a 35 percent response rate in patients with tumor resistant to MTX, but in previously untreated patients in randomized studies, response rates of 18 percent (10% complete remission [CR]) have been reported among 40 patients from the Northern California Oncology Group (NCOG), 8 percent (no CR) among 46 from the Southwest Group, 29 percent (5% CR) among 13 at the Boston VA, and

13 percent (3% CR) among 30 in New Jersey.

No prospective well-designed study of the activity of bleomycin as a single agent in head and neck cancer with modern response criteria is available, and certainly not one with a randomized control group receiving some other therapy.

It is worthwhile to examine the reasons why single-agent data from randomized trials just cited so often seem inferior to those reported in early trials from single institutions. For instance, the response rate for single-agent cisplatin (DDP) treatment reported by NCOG after failure of MTX was 39 percent in their initial series, and fell to 18 percent in a randomized trial using the same dose and schedule of DDP. The first and most obvious explanation is that patient selection is less rigorous and certainly less personalized in a large trial, so that patients with lower likelihoods of response are entered. This effect can be looked for and corrected in analysis. Probably more important are factors of "trial selection" that tend to operate in a competitive and public clinical research environment. First, trials of new drugs which show early promise tend to be completed, whereas some of those with no initial effect are abandoned for lack of interest to complete them. Thus, initial chance positive findings will go into the literature, but chance negative results may be lost. Furthermore, early and final positive results tend to be reported more quickly, finished sooner because of investigator enthusiasm, submitted for presentation at meetings more often, accepted for presentation and publication more readily (in more complete form and in journals with wider circulation than are negative results), given wider media coverage, cited more often, repeated more often, rewarded by funding agencies and rewarded by academic promotion committees. All this works in the converse for negative trials. All these influences are at work in the reporting of combination results, with the added incentive that the combination design is more likely a personal product of the investigator than a single agent, so that he has a personal and understandable bias in its favor.

These biases tend to be minimized in fully funded large randomized trials because of the tremendous inertia of these studies; once they get going they are hard to stop because of the presence of statisticians dedicated to avoiding beta error (missing a significant difference) and because of the penalties imposed by the funding agencies for failure to complete a planned randomized trial. In doing a critical analysis of the value of combination chemotherapy, it is therefore worthwhile to weight data from such trials as being less likely to be influenced by "trial selection" than that those from single institutions.

Returning to the ECOG negative trial, perhaps it was negative because we used the wrong drugs. This does not appear to be the case. There is already a huge body of literature on combination chemotherapy without any evidence of substantial activity as single agents from trials with modern response criteria for

Adriamycin, vincristine, cyclophosphamide, CCNU, vinblastine, mitomycin, mechlorethamine, hydroxyurea, procarbazine, and methyl-CCNU, with no evidence that any of these agents enhances the response rates reported with MTX or DDP. It is possible that bolus injection of 5-fluorouracil fits into this category, although there is one retrospective study from Wayne State University suggesting single-agent activity. Most of these drugs add little to combination chemotherapy except toxicity, with the possible exception of hydroxyurea, which in a retrospective comparison seemed to significantly reduce the toxicity of the MBD program for reasons that are yet unclear.

Perhaps the MBD program did not make optimal use of the "big three": MTX, BLM, and DDP. Unfortunately, there is no consistent evidence that other ways of giving the drugs are superior. Certainly higher doses of all the agents can be given, with concomitant increases in toxicity, expense, and difficulties and complexities of administration.

There are four randomized studies comparing high doses of methotrexate with citrovorum rescue, one of them using doses in grams, that show no enhanced activity when compared to standard doses without rescue. A nonrandomized comparison at the Dana-Farber Center of standard doses given semi-weekly with rescue compared to high doses (in grams) with rescue showed no obvious advantages to the high doses, with response rates of 60 percent for low-dose and 50 percent for high-dose MTX in patients who had no prior MTX. Responses on both programs were all partial, with a median duration of 11 or 12 weeks from onset of response to relapse.

Three studies used high doses of methotrexate with rescue in combination with DDP. The best of these was the Northern Oncology Group Trial in which the MTX dose was 250 mg/m^2 weekly and the DDP dose 80 mg/m^2 every 21 days. The overall remission rate was 33 percent (15% CR) and not significantly better than that of DDP alone with 40 patients per arm. We suspect that the response rate in this trial was reported to be lower than that of MBD because 4 weeks of response were required to code remission, and tumor was only measured every 3 weeks. Elias gave a single high dose of methotrexate (1550 mg/m^2) followed by a bleomycin infusion and a high dose of DDP and found only a 62 percent response rate (0 complete) in eight cases. Ervin gave 200 mg/m^2 MTX with rescue on days 7 and 14 of a 4-week cycle containing a bleomycin infusion and 100 mg/m^2 DDP over 5 days and observed a 100 percent response rate, but only three CRs among 11 patients. These response rates, especially the CR rate, are not significantly better than those of MBD, especially considering "trial selection".

Perhaps MBD should have used higher doses of DDP. In patients refractory to MTX, published response rates cluster around 35 percent regardless of dose, including doses of 50 mg/m^2 in an uncontrolled Southwest Oncology Group study. A single random-

ized trial has just been reported from Italy in which single-agent cisplatin was given to patients without prior chemotherapy, with response rates of 18 percent (0 CR) for 50 mg/m^2 and 16 percent (3% CR) for 120 mg/m^2 every 3 weeks with 30 patients per arm.

As part of combination chemotherapy, higher doses also did not improve response rate or duration in a randomized study from Australia (50 vs 100 mg/m^2) in combination with 40 mg/m^2 MTX with rescue weekly and 15 mg/m^2 weekly of BLM. With 90 patients per arm, about two-thirds of them "induction" patients being treated before planned radiation and/or surgery, overall response rates were 75 percent. There was no difference between the arms, with 26 percent CR for the high dose and 16 percent for the standard dose. The difference was not statistically significant.

The Northern California trial suggests that MTX + DDP at 80 mg/m^2, produces response rates no higher than those of MBD with 50 mg/m^2. Although Ervin, in his small series of 11 cases receiving 20 mg/m^2 DDP daily X5, achieved a 100 percent response rate, only 3/11 had CR, and the series is small and subject to trial selection. Caradonna, in Albany, gave 120 mg/m^2 DDP every 10 weeks with standard dose MTX and weekly BLM, but results were not much better than with MBD (74% response with 19% CR), considering trial selection in a study of 19 patients, and toxicity was severe. Responses in the NCOG and Albany trial lasted no longer than those with MBD. It appears that higher doses of DDP offer little or no advantage over 50 mg/m^2, alone or in combination.

Higher doses of bleomycin have generally been given by continuous infusion, largely based on historical comparisons of efficacy in testis cancer and a single pharmacologic trial at Memorial Hospital in New York. In patients with recurrent or metastatic disease, bleomycin infusions with cisplatin, alone or with vincristine, gave response rates of 33 percent (0 CR), 41 percent (11% CR), and 50 percent (0 CR) in three trials from Memorial and Wayne State, no better than those reported with MBD, and perhaps no better than results of single institution trials with DDP alone. The small Ervin and Elias trials included BLM infusions and were not obviously superior to MBD in the treatment of refractory disease.

It is reasonable at present to question whether bleomycin adds any efficacy at all to combination chemotherapy of head and neck cancer. A randomized study of 51 patients at Wayne State showed no advantage for a BLM infusion at 30 mg/day for 4 days with high-dose DDP and vincristine (41% response with 11% CR) over standard-dose single-agent MTX (33% response with 8% CR). A large Southeast Oncology Group trial of 167 patients showed no advantage of BLM at 15 mg every 7 days with vinblastine and cisplatin over standard dose MTX alone (23% vs 17% responses). A study of 57 patients from New Jersey showed twice-weekly doses of 15 mg/m^2 with high-dose DDP and biweekly standard dose MTX to have responses in 11 percent (0 CR), compared to 13 percent (3% CR) for 3 mg/kg DDP alone.

All this does not leave those of us who "build" combination chemotherapy programs much to work with in terms of MTX, BLM, and DDP. There was an exciting presentation in 1980 from Yale suggesting that giving 5-fluorouracil (5-FU) one hour after 250 mg/m^2 of methotrexate produced a very high response rate, presumably because MTX inhibition of purine biosynthesis led to increased phosphoribosyl-pyrophosphate concentration in the tumor cells, enhancing 5-FU entry by rapid combination to form FUMP, which is then incorporated into messenger RNA, leading to "nonsense" message and cell death. Specificity of this effect for tumor cells over normal cells has never been shown. Although the initial report from Yale was immediately confirmed in Stockholm, response rates with the same combination were only 50 percent in a subsequent ECOG study managed from Yale, and 23 percent at Stanford. Furthermore, a randomized study from Hamilton, Ontario, suggested (p<.03) that simultaneous administration of the two drugs is superior to sequential administration. Including 43 cases given "induction" therapy among 71 in the trial, simultaneous administration gave a 62 percent response rate (13% CR) and sequential administration gave 32 percent (3% CR). Two trials gave sequential MTX then 5-FU with DDP, one from ECOG using standard dose MTX in the MBD schedule and the other from M.D. Anderson using 250 mg/m^2 MTX and 100 mg/m^2 DDP over 2 days every 4 weeks. The response rate in patients with recurrent or metastatic disease in each trial was 41 percent, and response duration was singularly unimpressive. The utility of sequential MTX-FU in head and neck cancer remains to be conclusively demonstrated.

The only promising lead in the combination chemotherapy of head and neck cancer is a program developed at Wayne State using DDP, 100 mg/m^2, in combination with infusion 5-FU, 1000 mg/m^2/day for 4 days for patients with recurrent or metastatic disease, and 5 days as "induction" chemotherapy. Allopurinol was given with 5-FU, ameliorating the toxicity. The initial trial at Wayne State on 30 patients with recurrent or metastatic disease showed a response rate of 70 percent with 27 percent CR (mean duration 11.3 months). The same group then conducted a randomized trial in patients with recurrent or metastic disease, using the same dose of DDP and with 5-FU given either as a bolus (600 mg/m^2 on days 1 and 8) or as an infusion (1000 mg/m^2 daily for 4 days) every four weeks. The overall response rate for the infusion was 72 percent (22% CR) versus 20 percent for the bolus (10% CR). The partial remissions were all short (median 10 weeks), and the complete remissions were mostly ongoing at the time of last analysis. If one assumes that the bolus 5-FU plus DDP is no better than DDP alone, then the infusion program may be the first combination program found to be superior to single agents in the treatment of recurrent or metastatic disease. Ob-

viously, these results need to be repeated and confirmed. Such studies are under way at many centers.

Finally, this paper has not addressed the role of single agents or combination chemotherapy as "induction" programs before radiation and/or surgical resection. This literature is difficult to interpret. Studies from the 1960s and 1970s failed to show benefit from single agent MTX in this setting. More recent experience with DDP-based programs suggests response rates of 70 to 90 percent, but complete remission rates with induction chemotherapy have generally been about 20 percent. Multiple studies have shown that the achievement of partial remission before radiation for far advanced (T4 or N3) regional disease has little impact on the dismal prognosis of these patients. A recent national trial of chemotherapy given before surgery and irradiation, which produced only a 50 percent response rate, almost all partial, showed no benefit in operable stage III and IV patients. In this setting the infusion 5-FU + DDP programs offer the hope of improved CR rates of 40 percent and 54 percent in two studies (one at Wayne State and one in the Radiation Therapy Oncology Group). However, the value of induction chemotherapy in ultimate tumor control has never been conclusively demonstrated. In Al-Sarraf's series of 164 patients given induction chemotherapy with one of three cisplatin-based programs, complete responders did indeed live longer (median 24 months) than partial responders (median 13 months) or nonresponders (median 8 months), but 62 percent of complete responders by actuarial analysis are *dead* within 3 years of diagnosis. Of those complete responders with poorly differentiated tumors, 82 percent are projected to be dead by 3 years, despite consolidation therapy with radiation and/or surgical resection. Dr. Al-Sarraf tells us that most of the complete responders are dying with disease above the clavicles. We must conclude that complete response to currently available chemotherapy is of questionable value in enhancing the rate of regional control, presumably because it is unable to control microscopic disease beyond the surgical margin, even with the help of subsequent radiation therapy.

The point of this review is not to say that single-agent chemotherapy should be given either for recurrent or metastatic disease or as part of induction therapy. Rather, it is to give an honest appraisal of the relatively small amount of progress we have made in the chemotherapy of this terrible group of diseases, and to unencumber the research community from programs of marginal value so that new approaches and new active agents, such as methylglyoxal bis-guanylhydrazone, may be investigated more quickly and thoroughly.

REFERENCES

1. Vogl SE, Schoenfeld DA, Kaplan BH, Lerner HJ, Engstrom PF, Horton HJ. A randomized prospective comparison of methotrexate with a combination of methotrexate, bleomycin

and cis-platinum in head and neck cancer. Cancer; In press.

2. Chiuten D, Vogl SE, Kaplan BH, Greenwald E. Effective outpatient combination chemotherapy for advanced cancer of the head and neck. Surg Gynecol Obstet 1980; 151:659–662.

3. Vogl SE, Lerner H, Kaplan BH, Coughlin C, McCormick B, Camacho F, Cinberg J. Failure of effective initial chemotherapy to modify the course of stage IV (MO) squamous cancer of the head and neck. Cancer 1982; 50:840–844.

4. Vogl SE, Schoenfeld DA, Kaplan BH, Lerner HJ, Horton J, Paul AR, Barnes LE. Methotrexate alone or with regional subcutaneous Corynebacterium parvum in the treatment of recurrent or metastatic squamous cancer of the head and neck. Cancer 1983; 50:2295–2302.

5. Rooney M, Kish J, Jacobs J, Kinzie J, Weaver A, Crissman J, Al-Sarraf M. Improved complete response rate and survival in advanced head and neck cancer after 3 course induction therapy with 120 hour 5fu infusion and cis-platinum. Cancer; In press.

6. DeConti RC, Schoenfeld D. A randomized prospective comparison of intermittent methotrexate, methotrexate with leu-

covorin, and a methotrexate combination in head and neck cancer. Cancer 1981; 48:1061–1072.

7. Randolph VL, Vallejo A, Spiro RH, Shah J, Strong EW, Huvos AG, Wittes RG. Combination chemotherapy of advanced head and neck cancer: induction of remissions with diamminedichloroplatinum (II), bleomycin and radiation therapy. Cancer, 1978; 41:460–467.

8. Williams SD, Einhorn LH, Velez-Garcia E, Essessee I, Ratkin G, Birch R, Garrard J. Chemotherapy of head and neck cancer: comparison of cis-platinum plus vinblastine plus bleomycin versus methotrexate. Cancer; In press.

9. Woods RL, Gill PG, Levi JA. Chemotherapy for advanced squamous cell carcinomas of the head and neck: a randomized comparison of high dose versus low dose cis-platinum in combination with bleomycin and methotrexate. Proc Am Assoc Cancer Res 1984; 25:193.

10. Jacobs C, Meyers F, Hendrickson C, Kohler M, Carter S. A randomized phase III study of cis-platinum with or without methotrexate for recurrent squamous cell carcinoma of the head and neck. Cancer 1983; 52:1563–1569.

31. Combination Radiation and Chemotherapy for Stage IV Tumors

INTRODUCTION

JOHN M. LORÉ, Jr., B.S., M.D.

Since the survival rate of patients with advanced cancers of the head and neck is so poor, utilizing the time honored combination of surgery and radiation therapy, regardless of sequence, it is appropriate to review and attempt to evaluate the effectiveness of combining these modalities, either alone or in combination with chemotherapy. Whether surgery and radiation should be utilized each alone or together with either induction chemotherapy or chemotherapy after surgery and/or radiation is a question that must be addressed.

This charge is a big task for a number of reasons. Even without chemotherapy, the effectiveness of combined surgery and radiation treatment is not entirely clear. Another problem is the paucity of large randomized series of patients with long-term follow-up from any one institution. Variations of the "fine specifics" of protocols are bound to occur in multi-institutional series and even in a single institution. These variations have clouded the issue of combined chemotherapy and, unfortunately, appear to have cast a poor light on the use of combined chemotherapy and advanced head and neck cancer. The haphazard use

of these combined modalities must be avoided; strict protocols must be followed. Very accurate pretreatment and post-treatment data must be kept for ongoing and future analysis. Staging is a sine qua non, and the staging system to be used must be specified.

It must be emphasized that the combined modalities in the management of advanced head and neck cancer are not intended to facilitate a lesser surgical procedure, but rather to improve the survival and lengthen the disease-free period.

Our own pilot program of 46 patients treated by combined induction chemotherapy (Fig. 1) followed by surgery emphasizes the absolute requirement of precise prechemotherapy evaluation of the extent of

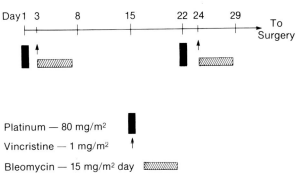

Figure 1 Protocol of induction chemotherapy followed by surgery (Spaulding and Loré)

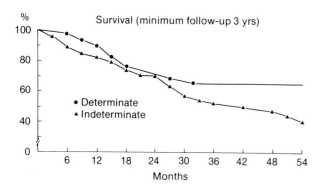

Figure 2 Survival of patients treated with induction chemotherapy (Spaulding and Loré)
▲ Survival of all patients
● Survival of patients dying of head and neck cancer only

ROLE OF CHEMOTHERAPY FOR STAGE IV TUMORS

MUHYI AL-SARRAF, M.D., F.R.C.P.(C), F.A.C.P.

In patients with stage IV epidermoid cancer of the head and neck, the standard treatment is surgery and/or radiotherapy. Unfortunately, the overall 3- and 5-year survival of these patients continues to be poor, and further clinical trials are needed to improve the length and the incidence of cure. A recent and significant development in the treatment of these patients has been the introduction of chemotherapy. In an attempt to achieve better results, systemic chemotherapy has been added as part of the multimodality therapy for patients with stage IV previously untreated cancer[1] (Table 1).

It is well accepted that the best cure rate can be obtained in patients with advanced head and neck cancer by the first most successful therapy attempted.

TABLE 1   Chemotherapy as Part of Multimodality Treatment in Head and Neck Cancer

Combination of Chemotherapy and Radiation
  Combined chemotherapy agents and radiotherapy
  Hydroxyurea and radiotherapy
  Methotrexate and radiotherapy
  5-Fluorouracil and radiotherapy
  Bleomycin and radiotherapy
  Cis-platinum and radiotherapy
Initial Induction Chemotherapy
  High-dose methotrexate
  Cis-platinum and bleomycin combination
  Cis-platinum and 5-FU combination
  Non-cis-platinum combination
Adjuvant chemoimmunotherapy
Chemotherapy postradiotherapy
Chemotherapy between surgery and radiotherapy

the disease. Regardless of the clinically favorable results of the chemotherapy, the surgery must encompass the original extent of the disease. Results in our pilot, nonrandomized program for stage III (6 patients) and stage IV (40 patients) cancers is shown in Figure 2.

In the evaluation of patients' statistics, there is a difference of opinion among the authors of the ensuing chapters regarding the distinction between operability and resectability. Operability refers to whether the patient can safely undergo a major surgical procedure, whereas resectability refers to whether a neoplasm can in fact be removed by the surgeon. Nonresectability distinctly implies advanced disease, and actually further implies a stage beyond stage IV, almost a "stage V".

At the time of first recurrence, the chance of salvage is very low. For this reason and for the investigation of the antitumor effect in previously untreated patients as well as the side effects of chemotherapy and the feasibility of the combined modality approach, chemotherapy was given before surgery and radiotherapy.

At present, clinical trials of chemotherapy in patients with previously untreated advanced head and neck cancer are focused primarily in three directions: (1) to continue optimizing the effectiveness and the safety of induction chemotherapy; (2) combining cisplatin and radiotherapy; and (3) investigating the timing of chemotherapy in relationship to surgery and radiotherapy.

Since most of the investigations reported have dealt with chemotherapy before surgery and radiotherapy, the rest of this chapter will focus on this area.

If chemotherapy is used as initial, induction therapy before surgery and/or radiotherapy, many factors may affect the response rate (Table 2).

With the introduction of cisplatin as an effective agent in patients with recurrent cancers of the head and neck, many trials were initiated with cisplatin combinations.[1]

In most of the studies, the combination of cisplatin and bleomycin was used or was used in combination with other agents (Table 3). Cisplatin combinations have proved effective in producing objective

TABLE 2   Factors Affecting Response Rate to Induction Chemotherapy in Previously Untreated Head and Neck Cancer

Stage (T and N)
Performance status
Tumor differentiation
Site of primary cancer
Type of chemotherapy
Number of courses of chemotherapy
Single institution vs. cooperative group
Other

TABLE 3   Response to Induction Chemotherapy with Cis-Platinum and Bleomycin
in Previously Untreated Head and Neck Cancer

Author	Year	No. Eval. Patients	No. of Courses	Agents	CR	PR	%
Al-Sarraf[2,3]	1979, 81	77	2	COB	22	39	80
Amrein[4]	1983	37	2	COB	2	23	67
Brown[5]	1980	23	3	CVB	5	12	74
Elias[6]	1979	22	1	CMB	4	12	73
Ervin[7]	1981	29	2	CMB	7	22	100
Glick[8]	1980	29	2	CB	—	14	48
Hong[9,10]	1979,82	41	2	CB	7	22	73
Kloss[11]	1981	16	3	CB	1	12	81
Kuten[12]	1983	10	3	CMB	2	5	70
Randolph[13]	1978	21	2	CB	4	11	71
Schuller[14]	1983	58	1–3	CMOB	15	20	66
Spaulding[15]	1982	50	2	COB	11	33	88
Tannock[16]	1982	33	2	CMB	3	17	60
Vogl[17]	1982	22	2	CMB ± MC	2	15	77
Wittes[18]	1979	21	1	CMVB	—	10	48

C = cis-platinum; O = oncovin; B = bleomycin; V = Velban; M = methotrexate; MC = Mitomycin-C.

tumor response in patients with locally advanced and previously untreated cancers.

CYTOTOXIC AGENTS AND RESPONSE RATE

Cisplatin alone, in doses of 120 mg/m^2 intravenously every 3 weeks for no more than three courses, was given to 22 patients with previously untreated head and neck cancers.[18] Most of these patients (19/22) had stage IV disease. Six patients had no clinical node involvement. The overall response rate was 40 percent with 1 (4%) CR and 8 (36%) PR.

The combination of cisplatin and bleomycin, given in two to three courses, produced a response rate of 48 percent to 81 percent (average 72/105, 69%). Complete response rates ranged from 0 percent to 21 percent.

The addition of methotrexate and/or vinca alkaloid agents (vincristine or vinblastine), given for one to three courses every 3 weeks, did not improve the overall response rate of 78 percent (281/382), with a range of 48 to 100 percent. The complete response rate ranged from 0 percent to 28 percent.

In an attempt to avoid the pulmonary toxicity of bleomycin and to maintain a high tumor response rate, we chose two courses of the combination of cisplatin and 96-hour infusion of 5-FU for patients with previously untreated head and neck cancer.[19,20] Twenty-six patients were treated with this combination, all with epidermoid carcinoma and all clinically stage IV and inoperable. Fifty percent (13 patients) had multiple primaries of the head and neck or esophagus, and many had poor pulmonary functions that excluded them from higher priority protocols containing bleomycin. Twenty-four patients had no previous therapy, and two had had previous radiotherapy and had developed a second primary 2 and 7 years later.

The response rate we observed was 19.2 percent (5/26) complete and 69.3 percent (18/26) partial, for

an overall response of 88.5 percent. Toxicities were acceptable and reversible without any fatalities. No impairment was produced that precluded other therapies; we started utilizing three courses (every 21 days) of cisplatin and 120-hour 5-FU infusion in patients with locally advanced head and neck cancers.[19,21] The complete response rate was 54 percent (33/61), and in 39 percent (24/61), partial response was achieved with an overall response rate of 93 percent. Toxicities again were acceptable and reversible.[21]

Although the overall response rate to three courses of cisplatin and 120-hour 5-FU infusion was no greater than that to two courses of the cisplatin, Oncovin, bleomycin (COB) combination, the increase in complete response rate with the three courses of cisplatin and 5-FU was statistically significant (p = 0.04).

The overall types and severity of drug-produced toxicities were not different between the three studies (Table 4). Fever, alopecia, and pulmonary toxicity were more common with the cisplatin, Oncovin, bleomycin combination. The higher incidence of leukopenia in the last group of patients treated may be related to the three courses of chemotherapy and/or simultaneous

TABLE 4   Drug Toxicity in Three Separate Studies by Wayne State University

Type	COB (77)	CACP + 96-hr. 5-FU (26)	CACP + 120-hr 5-FU (61)
Leukopenia	21 (27%)	7 (27%)	25 (41%)
Thrombocytopenia	3 (4%)	1 (9%)	7 (11%)
Nausea/Vomiting	55 (71%)	19 (70%)	35 (57%)
Diarrhea	—	—	8 (13%)
Stomatitis	5 (7%)	2 (8%)	7 (11%)
Renal	8 (10%)	7 (27%)	26 (43%)
Skin	10 (13%)	—	2 (3%)
Fever	23 (30%)	—	—
Alopecia	40 (52%)	1 (4%)	5 (8%)
Pulmonary	4 (%)	—	—
Phlebitis	—	2 (8%)	6 (10%)

radiotherapy to the second primary cancer of the esophagus in five patients.

In summary, the cisplatin combination produced a high tumor response rate (80 to 90 %) in patients with previously untreated advanced epidermoid cancer of the head and neck. The complete response rate was up to 54 percent, and the drug toxicities were acceptable and reversible.

The one most important question which still needs to be answered is the optimal chemotherapy in reference to the number of courses and the incidence of clinical complete response rate. Also, the placement of combined chemotherapy in the multimodality treatment regimen for patients with resectable advanced head and neck cancer needs to be investigated. We do believe that initial administration of chemotherapy may not be the ideal method in the resectable cases, since the antitumor effect of up to three courses of chemotherapy is directed toward the local and regional disease. Why should there be a significant difference in survival after shrinking a cancer which the surgeon will resect as much as possible as staged before any therapy started? Having confirmed the feasibility of post-surgery chemotherapy at Wayne State University and subsequently at the Radiation Therapy Oncology Group (RTOG), the efficacy of this modality is now being tested at Inter-group.

FACTORS THAT INFLUENCE RESPONSE TO INDUCTION CHEMOTHERAPY

Sex. There was no statistically significant difference between the overall response rate and the incidence of complete response according to the sex of the patients. The response rate in females was 97 percent (28/29), and in males it was 84 percent (113/135). The complete response rates were 42 percent and 36 percent respectively. Our patient population was drawn from two hospitals, Harper-Grace of Detroit and Veterans' Administration Hospital of Allen Park, Michigan. All patients from the VA Hospital were male, but no differences were found between their response rates to induction chemotherapy and those of the males or females of Harper-Grace Hospital, nor were there any differences between response rates of the sexes of Harper-Grace Hospital patients only.

Race. The overall response rate to initial chemotherapy was not different in white patients (88%) as compared to response rates in black patients (84%) with locally advanced head and neck cancer.

The clinically complete response rate in black patients (41%) was higher than complete response to chemotherapy in white patients (33%); however, this difference was not statistically significant.

Site. The overall tumor response ranged from 33 percent in patients with unknown head and neck primaries and N3 neck disease to 90 percent in patients with cancer of the tonsil. No statistical differences were found between the overall response rate

or the complete response rate to systemic chemotherapy and the site of the primary cancer.

Morphology. The overall response rate to initial chemotherapy in patients with well-differentiated cancers of the head and neck was 79 percent (11/14); in patients with moderately differentiated lesions it was 85 percent (82/96), and in poorly differentiated lesions, it was 88 percent. These differences were not significant. The complete clinical response rate to induction chemotherapy ranged from 29 percent in patients with well-differentiated tumor to 46 percent in patients with poorly differentiated cancers. Again, no statistical differences were found between the complete response rate and the tumor morphology.

Stage. No differences were found between the overall response rate and the stage of the head and neck cancer. The majority of the patients included in our studies on induction chemotherapy had stage IV disease. During the last trial of cisplatin and 120-hour 5-FU infusion for three courses, we analyzed the patients in more detail to evaluate the stage of the cancer and the response rate to chemotherapy.[21] Again, no differences were found between the overall response rate and those for stage III or IV tumors of the head and neck. At the same time, no differences were found between the overall response rate and the size of the primary lesion (T) or of the regional node involvement (N). When we analyzed the clinically complete tumor responses, the incidence of CR dropped the higher the T or the N disease, and it seemed clear, as shown in Table 5, that the N disease is the factor that influences the complete response to chemotherapy. In patients with T4 N0 M0 disease, the complete response rate was 89 percent as compared to those patients with T4 N3 M0 disease who had complete responses of only 25 percent.

FACTORS THAT INFLUENCE SURVIVAL OF PATIENTS ON MULTIMODALITY THERAPY

It is very important for any multimodality therapy or adjuvant therapy to prove its effectiveness. This includes not only the response rates to such therapy, but more importantly, whether this response rate can be translated to improvement in disease-free survival, quality of survival, and the overall survival of these patients. In patients treated with multimodality therapy, many factors may influence the disease-free sur-

TABLE 5 Stage IV (T4N0–3 Only) and Complete Response to Induction Chemotherapy with Cis-Platinum and 120-Hour 5-FU Infusion

Response	T4N0	T4N1	T4N2	T4N3
CR	8	1	1	3
PR	—	1	1	9
NR	1	—	—	—
CR/Total	8/9 (89%)	1/2 (50%)	1/2 (50%)	3/12 (25%)

vival and the overall survival results reported: stage, performance status, tumor differentiation, response to initial chemotherapy, type of response to initial chemotherapy, site of primary cancer, and other factors.

RESPONSE TO INITIAL CHEMOTHERAPY AND SURVIVAL

Patients on multimodality therapy had initial chemotherapy of 2 or 3 courses 3 weeks apart. Two weeks after the end of the last chemotherapy, these patients usually underwent surgery and/or radiotherapy. The usual delay for starting the standard and definitive therapy of surgery and/or radiation is 5 to 8 weeks.

In our first trial with two courses of COB in 77 patients with locally advanced head and neck cancer, all patients have had minimum follow-up of 4 years. We found that responders to chemotherapy (CR or PR) had statistically better survival than nonresponders to initial chemotherapy; in spite of that, these patients had the standard therapy subsequent to the completion of chemotherapy. Patients with a complete response to induction chemotherapy had median survival of 80 weeks; patients with partial tumor response had median survival of 79 weeks; those patients who did not respond to chemotherapy had a median survival of 35 weeks (p = 0.004).

STAGE AND SURVIVAL

As expected and already mentioned, the stage of the head and neck cancer statistically influenced the survival of patients on any multimodality therapy they received which included initial chemotherapy, regardless of the other factors (including response to the chemotherapy). Patients with stage III disease had a median survival of 91 weeks compared to a median survival of 67 weeks for patients with stage IV cancer (p = 0.04). We are certain that the different types of the stage IV disease influenced the survival of these patients; patients with stage T4 N0 have better survival than patients with T4 N3 disease.

MORPHOLOGY AND SURVIVAL

Although there were no differences between the overall response or the complete response rate to induction chemotherapy and the tumor morphology, we found and reported statistical differences in survival according to the tumor differentiation.[3] In our first trial with COB, the median survival of 54 patients with moderately differentiated epidermoid head and neck cancers was 85 weeks as compared to the median survival of those patients with poorly differentiated tumors which was 45 weeks. This finding needs further documentation by other institutions; we are evaluating patients treated with two or three courses of 5-FU and cisplatin. Statistical differences in survival and the morphology of cancer are seen in spite of the response

to chemotherapy, the stage, the site, or subsequent treatment with surgery and/or radiation.

SUMMARY

The feasibility and the antitumor effectiveness of cisplatin combinations prior to definitive surgery and/or radiotherapy has been established. The definitive role of such combinations in improving survival and the quality of such survival needs to be proved with good randomized and stratified national studies. The placement of chemotherapy in relationship to surgery and/or radiotherapy in an effort to achieve the best results from the multimodality approach has to be evaluated and studied.

The need for better and safer cytotoxic agents and the need for evaluation of what is considered as adequate therapy with these agents must continue to add to the improved results of multimodality therapy. The possibility of delayed radiotherapy or limiting the extent of ablative surgery for cosmetic or other reasons needs to be evaluated in the future.

REFERENCES

1. Al-Sarraf M. Chemotherapy strategies in squamous cell carcinoma of the head and neck. CRC Crit Rev Oncol Hematol 1984; 1:323–355.
2. Al-Sarraf M, Amer MH, Vaishampayan G, et al. A multidisciplinary therapeutic approach for advanced previously untreated epidermoid cancer of the head and neck. Preliminary report. Int J Radiat Oncol Biol Phys 1979; 5:1421–1423.
3. Al-Sarraf M, Drelichman A, Jacobs J, et al. Adjuvant chemotherapy with cisplatin, Oncovin, and bleomycin followed by surgery and/or radiotherapy in patients with advanced previously untreated head and neck cancer. Final report. In: Jones SE, Salmon SE, eds. Adjuvant therapy of cancer III. New York: Grune and Stratton, 1981; 145–152.
4. Amrein PC, Fingert H, Weitzman SA. Cisplatin-vincristine-bleomycin therapy in squamous cell carcinoma of the head and neck. J Clin Oncol 1983; 1:421–427.
5. Brown AW, Blom J, Butler WM, et al. Combination chemotherapy with vinblastine, bleomycin, and cis-diamminedichloroplatinum (II) in squamous cell carcinoma of the head and neck. Cancer 1980; 45:2830–2835.
6. Elias EG, Chretien PB, Monnard E, et al. Chemotherapy prior to local therapy in advanced squamous cell cancer of the head and neck: Preliminary assessment of an intensive drug regimen. Cancer 1979; 43:1025–1031.
7. Ervin TJ, Weichselbaum R, Miller D, Mashad M, Posner M, Fabian R. Treatment of advanced squamous cell carcinoma of the head and neck with cisplatin, bleomycin, and methotrexate (PBM). Cancer Treat Rep 1981; 65:787–791.
8. Glick JH, Marcial V, Richter M, et al. The adjuvant treatment of inoperable stage III and IV epidermoid carcinoma of the head and neck with platinum and bleomycin infusions prior to definitive radiotherapy. An RTOG Pilot Study. Cancer 1980; 46:1919–1924.
9. Hong WK, Shapshay SM, Bhutani R, et al. Induction chemotherapy in advanced squamous head and neck carcinoma with high-dose cisplatin and bleomycin infusion. Cancer 1979; 44:19–25.
10. Pennacchio JL, Hong WK, Shapshay S, et al. Combination of cisplatin and bleomycin prior to surgery and/or radiotherapy compared with radiotherapy alone for the treatment of advanced squamous cell carcinoma of the head and neck. Cancer 1982; 50:2795–2801.

11. Kloss R, Oster M, Blitzer A, et al. Cisplatin (P) and bleomycin (B) for previously untreated locally advanced squamous cell carcinoma of the head and neck. Proc Am Soc Clin Oncol 1981; 22:535.

12. Kuten A, Zidan J, Cohen Y, Robinson E. Multi-drug chemotherapy using bleomycin, methotrexate and cisplatin alone or combined with radiotherapy in advanced head and neck cancer. Cancer Treat Rep 1983; 67:573–574.

13. Randolph VL, Villajo A, Spiro RH, et al. Combination therapy of advanced head and neck cancer. Induction of remissions with diamminedichloroplatinum (II), bleomycin, and radiation therapy. Cancer 1978; 41:460–467.

14. Schuller DE, Wilson HE, Smith RE, Batley F, James AD. Preoperative reductive chemotherapy for locally advanced carcinoma of the oral cavity, oropharynx, and hypopharynx. Cancer 1983; 51:15–19.

15. Spaulding MB, Kahn A, De Los Santos R, Klotch D, Lore JH Jr. Adjuvant chemotherapy in advanced head and neck cancer. An update. Am J Surg 1982; 144:432–436.

16. Tannock I, Cummings B, Sorrenti V, and the ENT Group. Combination chemotherapy and prior to radiation therapy for locally advanced squamous cell carcinoma of the head and neck. Cancer Treat Rep 1982; 66:1421–1424.

17. Vogl SB, Lerner H, Kaplan BH, Caughlin C, McCormick B, Camacho E, Ginsberg J. Failure of effective initial chemotherapy to modify the course of stage IV (M0) squamous cancer of the head and neck. Cancer 1982; 50:840–847.

18. Wittes R, Heller K, Randolph V, et al. Cis-dichlorodiammineplatinum (II) based chemotherapy as initial treatment of advanced head and neck cancer. Cancer Treat Rep 1979; 63:1533–1538.

19. Al-Sarraf M, Drelichman A, Peppard S, et al. Adjuvant cisplatin and 5-fluorouracil 96 hour infusion in previously untreated epidermoid cancers of the head and neck. Proc Am Soc Clin Oncol 1981; 22:428.

20. Kish J, Drelichman A, Jacobs J, et al. Clinical trial of cisplatin and 5-fluorouracil as initial treatment for advanced squamous cell carcinoma of the head and neck. Cancer Treat Rep 1982; 66:471–474.

21. Weaver A, Fleming S, Kish J, et al. Cisplatin and 5-fluorouracil as induction therapy for advanced head and neck cancer. Am J Surg 1982; 144:445–448.

MULTIMODALITY THERAPY FOR ADVANCED EPIDERMOID CARCINOMA OF THE HEAD AND NECK

WILLIAM A. MADDOX, M.D., F.A.C.S.
MARSHALL M. URIST, M.D., F.A.C.S.

In 1978, data had accumulated showing that chemotherapy administered to previously untreated patients with advanced epidermoid carcinoma of the upper aerodigestive tract produced substantial responses. The agents used included methotrexate, with and without leucovorin rescue,[1,2] bleomycin and cisplatin,[3] cisplatin alone,[4,5] and bleomycin, methotrexate, Leucovorin (L), vincristine, 5-FU, and hydrocortisone.[5] Results appeared to be best when no prior radiation therapy was given and when the agent was methorexate with rescue. Cisplatin toxicity appeared to be dose-dependent and was reduced by mannitol diuresis. Because of these and other considerations, protocol 79 HN 357 used the schedule of methotrexate, cisplatin and bleomycin to a tolerable, easily administered combination for previously untreated late stage IV (T4 and/or N3) patients. In addition, the same combination was used for another study of operable stage III and early stage IV patients as follows: (1) methotrexate, 70 mg/m² IV push every 6 hours × 4, days 0 and 21 with IV leucovorin rescue; (2) bleomycin, 30 mg IV push every 7 days × 6; and (3) cisplatin, 2 mg/kg IV drip in 200 cc normal saline over one hour, days 3 and 24 with mannitol diuresis.

OBJECTIVES

Objectives of this study are to determine the response rate of previously untreated patients with inoperable stage IV epidermoid carcinoma of the oral cavity, oropharynx, hypopharynx, and larynx to a combination chemotherapy regimen of cisplatin, bleomycin, and methotrexate with folinic acid rescue, followed by radiation therapy, and to compare the disease-free survival of the patients rendered operable with historical controls and with that of those not rendered operable.

BACKGROUND AND RATIONALE

Many studies have demonstrated very gratifying partial or complete responses to chemotherapy regimens in the 65 to 85 percent range. Generally, the responses are inversely proportional to the tumor volume. In this study, 55 patients were evaluable for chemotherapy, with complete or partial responses of 67 percent. The CT regimen was well tolerated, with 17 percent grade 3 and 11 percent grade 4 granulocyte toxicity, and active, with 5 percent complete responses (CR) and 62 percent partial responses (PR). Because of early death or poor compliance, only 75 percent of patients received radiation therapy (RT) after completion of chemotherapy (CT). Forty-four patients were evaluable for radiation therapy, with 48 percent PR and 16 percent CR rate; 11 percent of the patients had progression of disease.

It is too early to report results of this study. This review is intended to point out problems with clinical trials in this patient population. Seventeen of 24 institutions entered 173 patients into the protocol (Table 1). It is too early to evaluate 24 of these patients. There were a total of 39 patients who did not complete the study because of unpreventable errors (Table

2). There were a total of 45 preventable errors (Table 3) and 18 protocol violations (Table 4), making a total of 64 inevaluable patients. The total number of evaluable patients was 46 or 31 percent. The preventable errors combined with the protocol violations comprise 42 percent of this review (Table 5).

I personally reviewed the records submitted to the Statistical Office. The preventable errors are, for the most part, inherent to multimodality protocols for these patients with advanced cancer in this anatomic area. I do think that preventable errors can be reduced. However, we were unable to identify the discipline or individual responsible for these errors. In spite of this negative report I believe there are lessons to be learned from this.

Suggestions are:

1. Institutions participating must be able to enter enough patients to establish and maintain familiarity with the protocol.
2. All patients must be staged by a competent head and neck oncologic surgeon.
3. A nurse oncologist must follow all patients through

TABLE 1   SECSG 79 HN 357: Institutions Ranked by Induction Registrations

Institutions	Registrations	Percent
New Jersey	38	22.0
Case Western Res. — CLEV VA	25	14.5
Univ. of Alabama in Birmingham	17	9.8
Louisville KY	17	9.8
Lexington KY	16	9.2
Indiana	11	6.4
Miami	9	5.2
Emory	8	4.6
Tampa	8	4.6
Temple	6	3.5
Tennessee — Knoxville	5	2.9
Tennessee — Memphis	4	2.3
Cincinnati	4	2.3
St. Louis	2	1.2
Puerto Rico	1	0.6
Rush Presbyterian — St. Luke	1	0.6
Georgetown	1	0.6

TABLE 2   Unpreventable Errors: SCSG – 79 HN 357 (N = 149)

Lost to follow-up	1
Intercurrent disease	2
Refused treatment	10
Early removal	7
Early death	16
Insufficient recovery	1
Drug toxicity	2
Total	39

TABLE 3   SCSG – 79 HN 357: Preventable Errors (N = 149

Incorrect dose	2
Inadequate data	23
Schedule not followed	16
Inappropriate dose chemo	3
Wrong surgical procedure	1
Total	45

TABLE 4   SCSG – 79 HN 357: Ineligible Patients; Protocol Violations (N = 149)

Incorrect stage	2
Ineligible site	12
Another uncontrolled primary	2
Total	18

TABLE 5   SCSG – 79 HN 357 (N = 173)

Total entered	173	
Too early to evaluate	24	
Total evaluated	149	
Unpreventable errors	39	(27%)
Total potentially evaluable	110	(74%)
Preventable errors	45	(30%)
Protocol violations	18	(12%)
Evaluable	46	(31%)

all phases of the protocol to ensure patient and staff compliance.
4. Good statistical office review and follow-up are necessary.

Based on this experience with the Southeastern Cancer Study Group, it is probably not possible to implement phase III randomized clinical trials in a single study group. An intergroup study is being planned. It is essential that we develop more effective treatment in an accurate and timely fashion for advanced cancer of head and neck origin.

REFERENCES

1. Bertino JR, Mosher MB, DeConti RC. Chemotherapy of cancer of the head and neck. Cancer 1973; 31:1141–1149.
2. Livingston RB, Carter SK. Single Agents in Cancer Chemotherapy. New York: Plenum, 1970; pp 137–172.
3. Randolph VL, Vallejo A, Strong EW, Wittez RE. Combination treatment with chemotherapy and radiation therapy in head and neck cancer. Proc Am Assoc Can Res and Am Soc Clin Oncol 1977; 18:336.
4. Wittes RE, Cuitkovie E, Strong E. DDP in epidermoid carcinoma of head and neck. Wadley Med Bulletin 1976; 6:85.
5. Price LA, Hill BT, Calvert AH, Dalley V, Shaw JH. Improved results in combination chemotherapy of head and neck cancer. Proc Am Assoc Can Res and Am Soc Clin Oncol 1977; 18:271.

EVALUATION OF PATIENTS WITH ADVANCED HEAD AND NECK CANCER: SELECTION OF PATIENTS FOR COMBINATION THERAPY

M. STUART STRONG, M.D.

The survival of patients with advanced head and neck cancer has not been enhanced by the introduction of supra-radical surgical procedures or radiotherapy techniques; the combination of surgery and radiotherapy has resulted in disappointing outcomes at 3 years, although the tumor-free survival has been modestly increased.

The value of adjuvant chemotherapy has not yet been defined; initial experience is often encouraging, but further experience leads to disappointment. Nonetheless, not all combinations of chemotherapy with surgery or radiotherapy have been explored, and the surgeon must strive to identify more effective methods of palliation and cure.

The issues are compounded by the fact that not all patients can tolerate chemotherapy and that the expense and toxicity of chemotherapy may outweigh the potential benefits. Furthermore, the circumstances of the disease vary so much from patient to patient that not all can be treated similarly, and a selection must be made in treatment planning.

The solution to the problem is to carry out a comprehensive evaluation of the local disease and the patient's general condition, to discuss the findings in an interdisciplinary conference, and to make an informed selection of the most suitable treatment for each patient.

CLINICAL APPROACH

Virtually all patients suspected of having advanced head and neck cancer will benefit from an in-depth evaluation of the disease as well as the general status; the only patients who would not benefit are those so debilitated by the disease or other conditions that the use of general anesthesia for endoscopy would be precluded. Most often supportive care is all that is available for this group of patients. All patients require a careful history, a thorough review of systems, and a search for evidence of distant metastases; a chest film, liver scan, and bone scan are mandatory examinations.

Following the history and physical examination, a *barium swallow* examination using air contrast should be performed; although it cannot be depended on to identify all early lesions of the food passages, it often provides useful information regarding areas of suspicion requiring special attention, limitation and/or incoordination of motion of the swallowing muscles, and early signs of aspiration.

An unhurried *endoscopy* should be carried out on all patients under general anaesthesia. The airway should be secured by passage of an endotracheal tube; if a laryngeal tumor is suspected, a 6-mm or smaller tube should be selected to facilitate the laryngeal examination. If it is thought to be unsafe to attempt intubation after induction because of the bulk of the tumor, an awake intubation under local anaesthesia should be carried out. Occasionally the airways are compromised to such a degree that a preliminary tracheotomy must be carried out under local anaesthesia before general anaesthesia can be induced safely.

The lesion should be carefully *inspected* and *palated*, and its margins *tattooed* with carbon particles. *Measurements* in two dimensions should be made as accurately as possible, and an estimation should be made of the third dimension. Measurements and tattooing will be very important when it comes time to reevaluate the lesion after initial treatment (for example, after induction chemotherapy) or prior to surgical resection following radiotherapy or chemotherapy. A generous biopsy should always be taken.

Laryngoscopy and esophagoscopy should be carried out on all patients because of the known instances of occult simultaneous second primaries; examination in the esophagus should be confined to the upper two-thirds if the size of vertebral osteophytes constitutes a threat to the safe passage of the esophagus into the lower esophagus and stomach. In the presence of an abnormal chest film, bronchoscopy should be carried out with bronchial washing; if the roentgenogram is clear, the chances of uncovering an occult neoplasm of the tracheobronchial tree is very low and may be omitted.

At the conclusion of the endoscopic examination, the neck should be carefully examined for nodes and the size of the nodes measured; evidence of extracapsular spread (fixation to surrounding structures) should be sought and noted. Equivocal nodes should undergo *fine-needle aspiration biopsy* in order to clarify the nodal status. Occasionally, a CT scan will clarify the nature and location of extensive primary tumors and large metastases.

At this time, the details of the tumor should be committed to a *"tumor map"*, and the disease staged according to the American Joint Committee on Staging; measurements of lesions depicted on the tumor should be entered (Fig. 1). Observations regarding fixation of nodes to surrounding tissues, immobility of vocal cords, extension of tumor across natural barriers, etc. should be recorded. A decision must be made regarding *resectability* of the tumor and the nodal disease: a determination must be made as to whether an operation could be carried out that would circumvent the disease and provide the patient with at least a small chance of cure along with a tolerable degree of moribidity and/or deformity. It is this important information that will allow an informed, intelligent discussion of the patient's problem at the interdisciplinary conference so that the most ideal treatment plan can be developed and a decision made regarding combined treatment.

Before the plan can be developed, it must be determined whether the patient is *operable* if it has al-

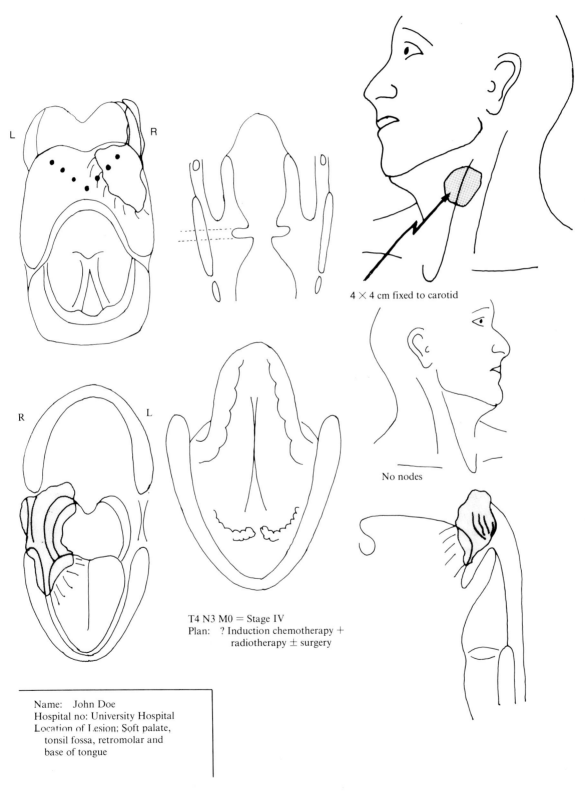

4 × 4 cm fixed to carotid

No nodes

T4 N3 M0 = Stage IV
Plan: ? Induction chemotherapy +
        radiotherapy ± surgery

Name: John Doe
Hospital no: University Hospital
Location of Lesion: Soft palate,
    tonsil fossa, retromolar and
    base of tongue

Figure 1 Tumor map.

ready been determined that the *lesion is resectable*. Operability is dependent on a variety of factors, including the following:

The *Karnofsky performance status* of the patient will often make it clear than an operation is a reasonable or unreasonable possibility; rarely is a major resection in the best interest of the patient if his Karnofsky performance status is less than 70 percent.

The *mental capacity* of the patient and his ability to understand and to cooperate are of the utmost importance in treatment planning; the patient must understand the nature of his disease and the rationale of the various treaments that are eventually selected and advised. It is this understanding that will make it possible for him to cooperate in the postoperative period.

The *cardiac status*, particularly the history of a recent myocardial infarction, will influence the decision regarding an operation as part of the treatment plan; if an operation is carried out within 3 months of a myocardial infarction, it carries a high risk of further myocardial damage so that the patient may not be operable.

The *acceptability* of an operation to the patient and the patient's *motivation* to proceed in spite of anticipated morbidity and risk of mortality are critical aspects of operability; without the commitment to an operation, some other form of treatment probably should be selected.

The *quality of life* that can be anticipated postoperatively is an appropriate consideration in deciding operability; if the patient cannot be returned to his family and friends and be free from major equipment and appliances, the wisdom of the operation remains in question. An operation that will leave a patient embarrassed by deformity or unacceptable to his family and friends is almost always ill-advised.

Tumor characteristics have an influence on operability. The cell type is important and may dictate that an operation is not indicated (for example, lymphoma). The growth pattern of the tumor, whether it grows diffusely or discretely, whether it grows slowly or explosively, should influence the decision whether to operate. Rarely can a rational operation be designed to control a rapidly growing tumor which expands and infiltrates in all directions.

The *site of the tumor* often indicates the wisdom or folly of an operation. Tumors occurring at the thoracic inlet rarely lend themselves to an operation carried out from above or below or even by a combination of approaches. The lack of natural tissue barriers to tumor expansion dooms an operation to failure. The finding of distant metastases or extensive multiple synchronous primaries usually constitute a contraindication to operation.

The *skill and bias of the surgeon* have a lot to do with operability; whether or not he is surrounded by skilled surgeons in other fields (for example, vascular, thoracic, or neurologic) and is supported by expertise in medical oncology and radiotherapy should profoundly influence the decision whether to advise an operation. Operability is intimately dependent on the circumstances surrounding the surgeon.

The *availability of alternate treatments* should have impact on operability; if the patient has had previous radiotherapy in the head and neck, precluding further radiotherapy, or if he has renal, pulmonary, or auditory problems that preclude use of radical chemotherapy, he may be deemed operable even though under other circumstances he might be deemed inoperable.

TREATMENT PLANNING AND SELECTION OF PATIENTS FOR COMBINED THERAPY

The patient's interests are best served by a thorough discussion of his problems by an *interdisciplinary tumor conference*; the conference is not a tumor board where binding decisions are made and handed down to the team responsible for the patient, but a conference where ideas are aired and alternatives are discussed so that a rational decision can be made by the physicians in charge.

The tumor conference should be attended by the surgeons who have been responsible for the work-up, evaluation, and biopsy of the patient's lesion. It is extremely important that the endoscopist be present and be able to describe the clinical features of the lesion in detail. The tumor map should be available to all of those attending the conference so that everyone has a visible image of the patient's problem. The patient's general medical status, his Karnofsky performance data, details of portals and dosages of any previous radiotherapy, or contraindications to chemotherapy should all be made available to the conference. A firm decision must have been made by the surgical team regarding the resectability of the tumor and operability of the patient; this must be presented to the conference.

In addition to the surgical team, the conference should be attended by representatives from medical oncology, oral surgery, maxillofacial prosthodontics, speech pathology, and nursing. Only by interaction of these groups can all facets of the patient's problems be properly addressed and the best treatment option selected.

The goals of treatment must be clearly defined. Is there a realistic hope of cure, and if not, what symptoms require palliation at this time? On occasion, it may be necessary to arrive at the decision to withhold all active treatment because there is no hope of cure and no symptoms that demand relief at this time. In cases of advanced tumors in head and neck cancer, this is often the wisest and most compassionate form of management; under these circumstances, social service may be needed to help in the placement of the patient if he is already too ill to be cared for by the family at home.

If there is a hope for cure, discussion of the problem and the available options will allow the selection of the particular combination of treatments to be made and contingency plans to be developed. For example, induction chemotherapy followed by endoscopic reevaluation might be advised; in the event of a limited clinical response, surgery might be carried out followed by radiotherapy. If a complete response to chemotherapy is obtained, it may be deemed wise to omit the surgery and to proceed to radical radiotherapy.

Decisions made in the milieu described above are likely to be wise and to be followed by the fewest regrets on the part of the patient and the physicians in charge.

SUMMARY

Patients with advanced head and neck cancer usually benefit from combination therapy. Selection of the particular combination should be made after a thorough evaluation and discussion of the options at an interdisciplinary tumor conference.

COMBINATION TREATMENT OF HEAD AND NECK CANCER WITH INDUCTION CHEMOTHERAPY

RALPH R. WEICHSELBAUM, M.D.
JOHN R. CLARK, M.D.
DANIEL MILLER, M.D., F.A.C.S.
MARSHALL R. POSNER, M.D.
JOHN T. CHAFFEY, M.D.
RICHARD L. FABIAN, M.D.
CARL M. NORRIS Jr., M.D.
THOMAS J. FITZGERALD, M.D.
CHRISTOPHER M. ROSE, M.D.
THOMAS J. ERVIN, M.D.

Advanced squamous cell carcinoma of the head and neck region (SCCHN) remains a therapeutic challenge in clinical oncology. Chemotherapy regimens employed to treat recurrent disease following surgery and/or radiation have never been shown to be curative, and are only marginally effective in prolonging survival. Although chemotherapy does not provide significant palliation in most patients with SCCHN, the overall response rates reported with newer combination chemotherapies have improved. Several investigations have reported response rates in excess of 50 percent in patients with recurrent SCCHN.[1-8]

A novel approach in the treatment of advanced previously untreated SCCHN employs the use of induction chemotherapy as part of an overall treatment program prior to surgery and/or radiation therapy. Such an approach has been increasingly reported, and response rates exceeding 75 percent are frequently recorded prior to definitive treatment.[9] In this report, we will discuss the results of treatment with induction cisplatin, bleomycin, and methotrexate-leucovorin chemotherapy followed by definitive surgery and/or radiation therapy with respect to the patterns and predictors of response, the toxicity of multidisciplinary

therapy, and the patterns of failure following local treatment.

MATERIALS AND METHODS

From October 1, 1979 to August 1, 1983, 114 patients with advanced stage III and IV, previously untreated squamous cell carcinoma of the head and neck region were entered into a protocol study. All 114 patients had histologically confirmed squamous cell carcinoma and were evaluable for response and/or toxicity. Patients with distant metastasis at the time of presentation were excluded from this study as were patients whose tumor represented a second primary carcinoma. No patient had received specific therapy for carcinoma prior to entry into this study.

The characteristics of the 114 entered patients are noted in Table 2 and the proportion of patients in each T-N combination in Figure 1. All patients entered in this protocol were evaluated at the Multidisciplinary Head and Neck Cancer Clinic at the Dana-Farber Cancer Institute and seen simultaneously by participating physicians from each service. At that time, the patient's pretherapy examination was reviewed and all patients were staged according to the American Joint Committee for Cancer Staging System.[10]

All 114 evaluable patients received their chemotherapy as induction chemotherapy prior to definitive treatment. All patients receiving chemotherapy on this protocol were hospitalized at the Dana-Farber

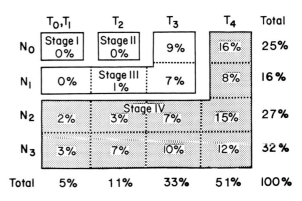

Figure 1 Proportion of Patients by T-stage and N-stage

Cancer Institute, the Children's Hospital Medical Center, or the Beth Israel Hospital (Boston, Massachusetts). The treatment protocol is outlined in Figure 2. Induction chemotherapy consisted of two cycles of a previously described regimen known as PBM.[5,11] In brief, patients received cisplatin, 20 mg/m^2 per day as a 2-hour daily infusion on days 1 through 5; bleomycin, 10 mg/m^2 per day as a continuous infusion on days 3 through 7; and methotrexate, 200 mg/m^2 on days 15 and 22, followed by leucovorin rescue orally, 20 mg every 6 hours for 12 doses beginning 24 hours after each methotrexate infusion. This regimen was then repeated beginning on day 29 for a second treatment cycle. At the end of the second course of PBM chemotherapy, all patients were evaluated for response. A complete response (CR) was defined as the complete disappearance of all clinically detectable disease, and a partial response (PR) was defined as a greater than 50 percent reduction in the product of the largest perpendicular diameters of all measurable tumor. No response (NR) was defined as a less than 50 percent reduction in the product of the largest perpendicular diameters of any measurable tumor.

Patients with surgically resectable lesions, for whom surgery was the appropriate treatment, then underwent standard surgical resection. Surgical resection as part of initial local treatment was undertaken in 63/114 (55%) patients and was based on the initial volume of disease present prior to the initiation of chemotherapy. When performed, surgical resection was carried out within 3 weeks of the last dose of chemotherapy. Radiation therapy was administered postoperatively in patients undergoing surgical resection. A minimum of 6000 rads were administered to the regions of the primary tumor bed and the involved neck disease. A minimum of 4500 rads were delivered bilaterally to clinically uninvolved necks. For unresectable tumors, or when radiation was the preferred method of definitive treatment, radiation therapy was begun within 3 weeks of the last dose of chemotherapy and carried to a minimum of 6800 rads delivered to the primary tumor site and involved nodal areas.

Twenty-six patients received additional, adjuvant chemotherapy with PBM as part of a randomized trial involving 47 patients who had responded to induction chemotherapy and subsequently been rendered free of clinical disease by definitive surgery and/or radiation therapy. Results of this later study will be reported elsewhere.[12]

RESULTS

For all sites of disease, the cumulative response rates to PBM were: CR, 26 percent; PR, 52 percent; and NR, 18 percent; 4 percent of patients were not evaluable for response (Table 1). The response to PBM chemotherapy as a function of primary tumor site is recorded in Table 2. At all major sites of disease, a significant response was noted. No one site of disease was resistant to PBM chemotherapy when used prior to definitive surgery and/or radiation therapy.

Patient Age and Performance Status

In our study, neither patient age nor performance status correlated with response to induction PBM chemotherapy (see Table 2). The finding of a high response rate in patients with a poor performance status at protocol entry is in contrast to results reported from

TABLE 1 Response to PBM Chemotherapy

Response	Number (%)
Complete response	30 (26)
Partial response	59 (52)
No response or progression	20 (18)
Not evaluable*	5 (4)
Total	114

*Includes one patient with unmeasurable middle ear carcinoma and 4 deaths during induction therapy.

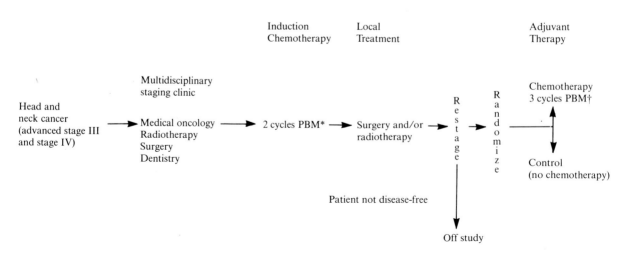

Figure 2   Treatment Protocol

TABLE 2 Patient Characteristics and Response Data (114 patients)

Characteristic	Number (% of 114)		Total Response Rate (%)		CR (%)		PR (%)	
Age								
< 30	6	(5)	6/6	(100)	4	(67)	2	(33)
30–39	1	(1)	1/1	(100)	—	—	1	(100)
40–49	15	(13)	11/15	(73)	1	(7)	10	(67)
50–59	32	(28)	20/32	(63)	6	(19)	14	(44)
60–69	38	(33)	34/38	(90)	2	(32)	22	(58)
70–79	22	(19)	17/22	(77)	7	(32)	10	(45)
Sex								
Male	83	(73)						
Female	31	(27)						
Performance Status (ECOG)								
Asymptomatic (0)	48	(42)	38/48	(79)	7	(15)	31	(65)
Minor symptoms (1)	38	(33)	29/38	(76)	14	(37)	15	(39)
In bed < 50% (2)	20	(18)	16/20	(80)	7	(35)	9	(45)
In bed > 50% (3 + 4)	8	(7)	6/8	(75)	2	(25)	4	(50)
Primary site								
Tongue*	20	(18)	17/20	(85)	10	(50)	17	(85)
Oral cavity†	11	(10)	10/11	(91)	1	(9)	10	(91)
Tonsil	15	(13)	12/15	(80)	—	—	12	(80)
Oropharynx	7	(6)	5/7	(71)	3	(43)	2	(29)
Hypopharynx	28	(25)	22/28	(79)	8	(29)	14	(50)
Larynx‡	12	(11)	7/12	(58)	2	(17)	7	(58)
Nasopharynx	16	(14)	13/16	(81)	6	(38)	13	(81)
Other sites§	3	(3)	1/3	(33)	—	—	1	(33)
Unknown	2	(2)	2/2	(100)	—	—	2	(100)

*Includes 10/20 base of tongue
†Includes cheek, floor of mouth
‡Includes supraglottic larynx
§Includes ear, sinus, nose

TABLE 3 Relationship of Histologic Grade and Response to PBM Chemotherapy (114 evaluable patients)

Histologic Grade*	Total Response Rate (%)		CR (%)		PR (%)	
Well-differentiated	10/14	(71)	2	(14)	8	(57)
Moderately well-differentiated	45/55	(81)	15	(27)	30	(54)
Poorly differentiated	34/45	(76)	13	(29)	21	(47)

*Broders classification
†Includes undifferentiated nasopharynx cancer (lymphoepithelioma)

trials of previously treated patients with advanced SCCHN, where poor performance status at presentation correlated with both response to chemotherapy and survival.[6,13,14]

Histologic Grade

The response rate of poorly differentiated SCCHN was not found to be significantly different from that of other histologic subtypes. Nasopharyngeal carcinomas (lymphoepithelioma, Schminke tumor) respond as well to PBM chemotherapy as other histologic subtypes of SCCHN. These data are shown in Table 3.

Initial Tumor Size

Initial tumor volume was considered a possible predictor for response to subsequent chemotherapy, but an accurate and reproducible determination of tumor volume was considered impossible to obtain. An easily obtained parameter of tumor size is the largest diameter of the largest evaluable tumor mass, considering both primary site and involved neck masses when present. Response to induction PBM chemotherapy was evaluated as a function of greatest initial tumor diameter in Table 4. In this study, tumor size, as eval-

TABLE 4 Relationship of Initial Tumor Size* and Response to PBM Chemotherapy (113 evaluable patients)

Tumor Size	Total Response Rate (%)		CR (%)		PR (%)	
3–6 cm	73/86	(85)	24	(28)	49	(58)
>6 cm	16/27	(59)	6	(22)	10	(37)

*Largest evaluable diameter of largest tumor mass.

uated by largest tumor diameter, did predict for response to subsequent chemotherapy. Tumors with an initial diameter of greater than 6 cm responded less well to PBM chemotherapy than tumors having a smaller initial tumor diameter. Although the response rate for larger tumors remains high, the difference compared with smaller tumors appears significant. This finding is in contrast to a previously published report from our group; in a smaller study of 97 untreated patients with advanced SCCHN treated with induction PBM chemotherapy, an initial tumor diameter greater than 6 cm was not associated with a lessened response to induction chemotherapy.[11]

EFFECT OF LOCAL THERAPY ON RESIDUAL TUMOR FOLLOWING CHEMOTHERAPY

Ninety of the 114 patients entered into this protocol study completed induction chemotherapy and subsequent definitive local treatment with surgery and/or radiation therapy. These 90 patients were followed for local and regional (locoregional) control of disease (Table 5); duration of follow-up was measured from the completion date of local treatment with surgery and/or radiation therapy to the date of locoregional relapse, death related to reasons other than local relapse, or, if alive without locoregional recurrence, until November, 1983 when this study was completed.

When the incidence of locoregional recurrence was stratified according to local treatment and greatest tumor diameter following induction PBM chemotherapy, no difference between standard local treatment with surgery and radiation versus radiation therapy alone was apparent in the control of locoregional disease, regardless of the extent of residual tumor burden following chemotherapy. Patients exhibiting a complete response to PBM, with a residual tumor size of zero prior to local treatment, did well with a low incidence of locoregional recurrence following either standard surgical resection based on the volume of disease at presentation with postoperative radiation (0/9 recurrences), or radiation therapy alone (3/13 recurrences). Patients with extensive residual disease of 3 or more centimeters in greatest diameter following induction chemotherapy did poorly, with early locoregional recurrences developing in 13/14 (93%) patients treated with combined surgery and radiation and in 9/10 (90%) patients treated with radiation alone. The two patients within the latter group of 24 with extensive residual disease following PBM that did not develop a local recurrence following local treatment both died of early distant metastasis. Patients with minimal residual disease up to 3 cm in greatest diameter prior to local treatment did moderately well and also had similar incidences of locoregional recurrence whether treated with standard surgical resection plus radiotherapy (38% recurrences, 10/26 patients) or radiation therapy alone (35% recurrences, 6/17 patients).

Locoregional recurrence following a complete response to induction chemotherapy and subsequent definitive surgery and/or radiotherapy was uncommon, occurring only in three of 22 (14%) evaluable patients. None of these 22 patients have developed distant metastasis. Of the three patients who developed a local or regional recurrence, all received radiation therapy as the sole form of local treatment. Two of these three patients had unresectable disease involving the base of tongue: one with T3N0 disease relapsed 4 months after completion of radiation therapy, and the other with T4N0 disease developed an in-field recurrence during radiation therapy. The third patient refused laryngectomy for a T4N2B lesion of the hypopharynx and relapsed 8 months after completion of radiation therapy.

Postinduction chemotherapy tumor size strongly correlated with locoregional control. Tumor reduction to a greatest diameter of less than 3 cm following induction chemotherapy was associated with early locoregional control. Sixteen of 19 patients with tumors less than 3 cm following PBM have developed a locoregional recurrence after a median of 12 months' observation following the completion of local treatment with surgery and/or radiation therapy. This is contrasted with a 92 percent (22/24) locoregional relapse rate for patients with tumors greater than, or

TABLE 5 Effect of Postinduction Chemotherapy Tumor Size and Local Treatment on Local Recurrence (90 evaluable patients*)

Tumor Size†	Local Treatment	Local Recurrences/ Evaluable Patients	Alive at Risk	Median Follow-up‡	
0	Surgery + RT	0/9	8	19	(7–40)
	Radiation	3/13	10	11	(0–42)
0–2.9 cm	Surgery + RT	10/26	13	10	(5–41)
	Radiation	6/17	10	10	(0–41)
3–6 cm	Surgery + RT	13/14	0	5	(0–9)
	Radiation	9/10	0	0	(0–4)

*Ninety patients who completed induction chemotherapy and definitive local treatment, followed until local recurrence or for a minimum of 6 months following completion of local treatment.

†Largest diameter of tumor mass present upon completion of PBM chemotherapy.

‡In months from completion of local treatment until local relapse, until death for reasons not related to local relapse, or until November 1983 if alive without local relapse.

equal to, 3 cm in greatest diameter after induction chemotherapy.

Another predictor of relapse following local therapy appeared to be a nonresponse to induction chemotherapy. Nineteen of the 20 patients in this study recorded as having no response to induction chemotherapy completed subsequent local treatment and were evaluable for analysis of locoregional failure. All 19 patients were found in the group of patients with residual disease of 3 or more centimeters in greatest diameter following induction chemotherapy and account for 86 percent (19/22) of locoregional relapses in that group of patients. Of the 19 nonresponders to induction chemotherapy, nine received subsequent therapy with both surgery and radiation, nine with radiation alone, and one with surgery alone. Only five of the 19 nonresponders (26%) were considered to have no residual tumor at the end of local treatment, with the remaining 15 relapsing rapidly with symptomatic disease. Of the five nonresponders to induction PBM who were considered without evidence of clinical disease upon the completion of local treatment, all received both surgery and radiation therapy as local treatment and all ultimately recurred locally with a mean time to locoregional relapse of 5 months.

TOXICITY OF MULTIMODALITY THERAPY

Table 6 records the frequency of the more common toxicities experienced during induction chemotherapy with PBM. This regimen was generally well tolerated, with nausea and vomiting being the most common mild toxicity (35%) and thrombocytopenia being the most moderate or severe complication (14 and 14% of patients, respectively) of initial therapy. Leukopenia was less frequently a moderate or severe problem, present in 6 and 5% of patients respectively. Nephrotoxicity was of similar frequency. Myelosuppresion was rare and usually associated with noncompliance in taking oral leucovorin at home, or with mild nephrotoxicity at the time of methotrexate administration. Pulmonary toxicity was uncommon, with 95 percent of patients experiencing no toxicity. Other induction toxicities not included in Table

6 included one case of mild pulmonary edema; two cases, one moderate and one severe, of weight loss; one case of syndrome of inappropriate antidiuretic hormone (SIADH); two cases of severe seizures; one case of moderate penumonitis; one case of moderate hyponatremia; one case of life-threatening neuropathy; one case of reactivated tuberculosis; and one case of lethal aspiration pneumonia.

Four patients died during the induction regimen: a 77-year-old male developed fatal methotrexate or bleomycin lung toxicity characterized by acute-onset shortness of breath and bilateral pulmonary infiltrates one day after receiving his second dose of methotrexate, followed by progressive pulmonary failure; a 70-year-old male died of a pulmonary embolism after one course; a 62-year-old male died of a myocardial infarction after one course; and a 49-year-old female with a performance status of 4 died of aspiration pneumonia after one course of therapy.

In 27 (23%) cases, induction dose modifications were made generally as a result of therapy-induced bone marrow suppression or nephrotoxicity. In five cases, only one course of PBM was administered, and in one case, three courses of PBM were received prior to definitive local treatment. Two patients received no methotrexate at any time, and one patient received no methotrexate in the second cycle of therapy. Twelve patients received reduced methotrexate doses of 50 to 80 percent the standard dose and six patients received reduced doses (60 to 90%) of cisplatin and/or bleomycin, and/or methotrexate. Complications of subsequent local treatment with surgery and/or radiation therapy included seven patients with weight loss greater than 10 pounds, three cases of wound infection, one case of wound breakdown, and two cases of osteoradionecrosis. One patient died of a pulmonary emoblism after surgery, and another patient died from aspiration pneumonia, which was reported to be a radiation therapy complication.

DISCUSSION

Spaulding et al has reported promising results of induction cisplatin, bleomycin, and vincristine (two

TABLE 6   Frequency of Toxicity to Induction PBM

Toxicity	Total	Mild[1]	Moderate[2]	Severe[3]	Lethal
Nausea/Vomiting	46%	35%	10%	1%	—
Thrombocytopenia	45%	18%	13%	14%	—
Leukopenia	30%	19%	6%	5%	—
Nephrotoxcity	20%	7%	6%	7%	—
Mucositis	14%	5%	4%	5%	—
Fever	9%	5%	2%	2%	—
Rash	7%	3%	1%	3%	—
Respiratory[4]	5%	3%	1%	—	1%
Diarrhea	2%	1%	1%	—	—

1–3 Toxicity code criteria: Thrombocytopenia: 0 = >150,000; 1 = 100,001–150,000; 2 = 50,000–1000,000; 3 = <50,000; Leukopenia: 0 = >2000; 1 = 1001–2000; 2 = 501–1000; 3 = 0–500; Nephrotoxicity (creatinine × baseline): 0 = <1.25; 1 = 1.25–1.50; 2 = 1.5–2.0; 3 = >2.0; Respiratory: 1 = asymptomatic CXR infiltrates; 2 = external dyspnea; 3 = dyspnea at rest 4 = Drug-related toxicity cycles) followed by surgery in advanced, but technically resectable stage III and IV SCCHN.[7] Ervin will soon report survival data from the 114 patients considered in this paper and, with a mean follow-up of 24 months, will document an improved tumor-free and absolute survival in patients with advanced SCCHN treated with multimodality therapy including induction PBM as compared with historical controls.[12] In addition, that study will report an improved tumor-free survival in a subgroup of patients treated with continued adjuvant chemotherapy following the completion of definitive local treatment. Previous studies have reported no effect of short-course adjuvant combination chemotherapy following definitive local treatment, or single-agent induction chemotherapy, on survival.[15-18]

In our study, we report the response data from 114 patients with advanced, previously untreated SCCHN treated with PBM chemotherapy. The specifics of this regimen have been reported previously.[5,11] The response rate to PBM chemotherapy is high (78%), with 26 percent of patients achieving a complete response. These response rates are comparable to those reported by Weaver et al[19] and Spaulding et al[7] with alternative cisplatin-containing chemotherapy protocols. While other reports of high response rates are available,[9] it appears that cisplatin-containing drug regimens most consistently produce high response rates in previously untreated patients with SCCHN. In such studies, cisplatin is usually employed at high doses (100 mg/m[2]) and is combined with at least one other active drug (5-fluorouracil, bleomycin, vincristine, or methotrexate), which is also administered at full dosage.

In this study, differences in patient age, performance status, histologic grade, and tumor site did not correlate with response to PBM chemotherapy. These parameters appear not to be true predictors of cellular resistance to effective combinations of antineoplastic drugs. Patient age and performance status correlated more often with toxicity than with antitumor response. In single-agent trials, there appeared to be a site-specific sensitivity pattern for both bleomycin and methotrexate. Although such an analysis has not been performed for cisplatin alone, this study failed to note a site-specific sensitivity to PBM when using these three drugs in combination. It is possible that previous studies reflected a response pattern related to tumor size and dosage of drug delivered rather than to inherent drug resistance by certain SCCHN tumors.

The analysis of local failures in our study suggests that chemotherapy may add to definitive local treatment by reducing tumor size prior to surgery and/or radiation therapy. Patients with residual tumors less than 3 cm in greatest diameter following induction PBM have done well, with local or regional relapses developing in only 10/35 (29%) patients subsequently treated with surgery and radiation therapy, and in 9/30 (30%) patients treated with radiation therapy alone.

Local control in patients with residual tumors of 3 or more centimeters in greatest diameter following PBM was limited, with 22/24 (92%) patients developing an early local or regional recurrence. The remaining two patients died of distant metastasis in the absence of locally recurrent disease, 1 and 5 months following the completion of radiotherapy.

The failure of surgery and radiation therapy to control larger tumor volumes after induction chemotherapy is a new finding. The failure of radiotherapy to locally control larger tumor volumes in trials utilizing induction chemotherapy and radiation alone has been previously reported.[15-17] In some cases, large residual masses following induction chemotherapy are a reflection of the relative ineffectiveness of the chemotherapy.

SUMMARY

In this report, we have presented evidence that high-dose combination chemotherapy can be effective in producing a significant antitumor response in the majority of patients with advanced, untreated SCCHN. Traditional parameters of patient age, performance status, histologic grade, and tumor site did not predict for response to PBM chemotherapy. Initial tumor size was a weak predictor of response. Our analysis of local failures suggests that for tumors proved unresponsive to induction PBM or with a residual size of 3 or more centimeters in greatest diameter following induction chemotherapy, local treatment with either surgery and radiation therapy or radiotherapy alone is ineffective in achieving lasting control of local disease. For tumors less than 3 cm in greatest diameter following induction chemotherapy, radiation therapy appeared as effective as surgery plus radiotherapy in controlling locoregional disease, given that local treatment recommendations were based on standard criteria considering site and volume of disease present prior to the initiation of chemotherapy. The analysis of failure in our study suggests that maximum standard treatment is necessary in addition to induction chemotherapy for increasing locoregional control of advanced squamous cell carcinoma of the head and neck. This final point is emphasized because patients receiving less than standard local treatment relapsed despite excellent responses to induction chemotherapy with PBM.

REFERENCES

1. Al-Sarraf M, Binns P, Vaishampayan G, Loh J, Weaver A. The adjuvant use of cis-platinum, Oncovin, and bleomycin (COB) prior to surgery and/or radiotherapy in untreated epidermoid cancer of the head and neck. In: Salmon and Jones. Adjuvant therapy of cancer II. New York: Grune and Stratton, 1979, 145–152.
2. Cardonna R, Paladine R, Ruchdechel JC, et al. Methotrexate, bleomycin and high-dose dichlorodiammineplatinum (II) in the treatment of advanced epidermoid carcinoma of the head and neck. Cancer Treat Rep 1979; 63:489–491.
3. Chivten D, Vogl S, Kaplan B, et al. Effective out-patient

combination chemotherapy for advanced cancer of the head and neck. Surg Obstet 1980; 151:659-662.

4. Elias EG, Chretien PB, Monnard E, et al. Chemotherapy prior to local therapy in advanced squamous cell carcinoma of the head and neck: Preliminary assessment of an intensive drug regimen. Cancer 1979; 43:1025–1031.

5. Ervin TJ, Weichselbaum RR, Miller D, Meshad M, Posner MR, Fabian RL. Treatment of advanced squamous cell carcinoma of the head and neck with cisplatin, bleomycin and methotrexate (PBM). Cancer Treat Rep 1981; 65:787–791.

6. Kish JA, Weaver A, Jacobs J, et al. Cisplatin and 5-fluorouracil in patients with recurrent and disseminated epidermoid carcinoma of the head and neck. Cancer 1984; 53:1819–1824.

7. Spaulding SE, Kahn A, De Los Santos R, Klotch D, Lore JM. Adjuvant chemotherapy in advanced head and neck cancer. Am J Surg 1982; 144:432–436.

8. Vogl SE, Kaplan BH. Chemotherapy of advanced head and neck cancer with methotrexate, bleomycin, and cis-diamminedichloroplatinum II as an effective outpatient schedule. Cancer 1979; 44:26–31.

9. Glick JH, Taylor SG IV. Integration of chemotherapy into a combined modality treatment plan for head and neck cancer: A review. Int J Rad Oncol Biol Phys 1981; 7:229–242.

10. American Joint Committee for Cancer Staging and End-Results. Reporting Manual for Staging of Cancer. Chicago, IL, 1977.11. Ervin TJ, Weichselbaum RR, Fabian RL, Miller D, Norris CR, Posner MR, Rose C, Tuttle SA, MacIntyre JM, Frei E. Neoadjuvant cis-platinum, bleomycin, methotrexate chemotherapy for advanced squamous cell carcinoma of the head and neck: A preliminary report. Arch Otolaryngol 1984; 110:241–245.

12. Ervin TJ. Personal communication.

13. Amer MH, Al-Sarraf M, Vaitkevicius VK. Factors that effect response to chemotherapy and survival of patients with advanced head and neck cancer. Cancer 1979; 43:2203–2206.

14. Drelichman A, Cummings G, Al-Sarraf M. A randomized trial of the combination of cis-platinum, oncovin, and bleomycin (COB) versus methotrexate in patients with advanced squamous carcinoma of the head and neck. Cancer 1983; 52:399–403.

15. Wittes R, Heller R, Randolph V, Howard J, Vallejo A, Farr H, Harold C, Cvitkovic A, Shah J, Gerald RP, Strong EW. Cis-dichlorodiammineplatinum (II) based chemotherapy as initial treatment of advanced head and neck cancer. Cancer Treat Rep 1979; 63:1533–1538.

16. Fazekas JT, Sommer C, Kramer J. Adjuvant intravenous methotrexate or definitive radiotherapy alone for advanced squamous cancer of the oral cavity, oropharynx, supraglottic larynx or hypopharynx. Int J Rad Oncol Biol Phys 1980; 6:533–541.

17. Vogl SE, Lerner H, Kaplan BH, Coughlin C, McCormick B, Camacho F, Ginberg J. Failure of effective initial chemotherapy to modify the course of stage IV (MO) squamous carcinoma of the head and neck. Cancer 1982; 50:840–844.

18. Pennacchio J, Hong W, Shapsay S, Blutani R, Gillis T, Strong S, Gromer R. A comparison of combined modality therapy vs. radiotherapy alone in the treatment of stage IV unresectable head and neck cancer. Proc Am Soc Clin Oncol 1981; 21:430.

19. Weaver A, Flemming S, Kish J, Vandenberg H, Jacob J, Crissman J, Al-Sarraf M. Cis-platinum and 5-fluorouracil as induction therapy for advanced head and neck cancer. Am J Surg 1982; 144:445–448.

32. Intra-Arterial Chemotherapy

INTRODUCTION

BENJAMIN F. RUSH, Jr., M.D.

History repeats itself and medicine is no exception. We are currently in the midst of an exciting surge of interest in the technique of intra-arterial infusion therapy. This technique was introduced some 34 years ago by Calvin Klopp,[1] who described the introduction of nitrogen mustard into the external carotid artery by means of an intra-arterial catheter. The medication was given as bolus injection. Later in the same year, Berman et al described the same technique in an abstract at the Fifth International Cancer Congress in Paris.[2] We should be mindful that these reports appeared only 6 years after the first patient had been treated with systemic nitrogen mustard and only 4 years after the use of nitrogen mustard for cancer therapy was permitted to escape the shackles of wartime censorship. During the fifties, there were scattered reports of the use of this technique. Sullivan et al reported various modifications of the implantation of the catheter in

1953.[3] Reese et al reported effective use of intra-arterial chemotherapy via the internal carotid artery in the treatment of patients with retinoblastoma.[4] TEM (triethylenemelamine), given in this way, combined with radiation therapy showed promise of sparing the less involved contralateral eye in patients with bilateral retinoblastoma.

The intra-arterial approach did not really grip the imagination of oncologists until the early sixties, when new drugs were introduced, particularly 5-fluorouracil. Regression rates with this drug, administered by continuous infusion into the external carotid, were reported to be quite high. Johnson et al reported 20 partial (more than 50% decrease in size) and 8 complete remissions in 47 patients with head and neck tumors who had not had prior radiation, a 60 percent remission rate.[5] There was a rash of similarly optimistic reports in the early 1960s. By the mid-sixties, a substantial experience with the technique emerged as well as a better understanding of some of the drawbacks.

Perhaps the most disappointing observation was that the great majority of these tumors treated by arterial infusion showed rapid regrowth despite dramatic initial regressions, and on the average, tumors that had appeared to respond would begin to increase in size again by the end of 3 to 6 months. In addition, cerebral emboli and infarction occurred in a number of these patients, devastating complications in a patient when the only gain was a transient period of remission in perhaps 50 to 60 percent of those treated. Hotspots would sometimes emerge in the rheology of the external carotid distribution. Drugs administered slowly into the system would sometimes be swept primarily into single branches, and therefore some areas of the arterial distribution would receive much more drug than others.[6]

Certainly there are a number of theoretic advantages. These include the much higher dose that can be safely deposited in the tumor-bearing area without much in the way of systemic toxicity. Another development that attracted interest to the technique was the development by Watkins of an external portable pump which was spring-driven and which could permit the patient to receive long periods of chemotherapy at home.[7] Management of the catheter always remained a problem, however, and patients being treated on an outpatient basis would often dislodge the catheter with resulting failure of the portal of access. Patients would also occasionally blow out the carotid, especially if the catheter had been implanted in the wall of this vessel rather than through a branch.

Animal models recently developed seemed to confirm that many agents are more effective when given intra-arterially than when given systemically for regional treatment. However, to date there has been no truly successful randomized study of the effectiveness of systemic treatment as compared to intra-arterial treatment.

The factors which have led to the current wave of new enthusiasm for the use of the intra-arterial technique are (1) the availability of an implantable pump, which greatly simplifies the administration of the drug or drugs over a long period of time, (2) the appearance of new drugs, particularly cisplatin, and, to a lesser extent, of new drug combinations, and (3) the final impetus—the concept of "neoadjuvant treatment", whereby the intra-arterial drugs are used to supplement radiation and/or operation in patients not previously treated.

Using this concept, the brief period of dramatic remission seen in many of these patients is thought by many to permit a safer removal of the tumor, with wider margins and a lesser likelihood of local recurrence. Again, these are all hypothetical and await rigorous proof.

The chapters that follow bring together a vast experience. Each of the three authors approaches the problem of intra-arterial therapy in a somewhat different way. Sessions describes a technique whereby the intra-arterial area to be treated was approached very specifically by transfemoral cannulation, with insertion of the tip of the catheter in the arterial area to be treated. This is complemented by the fibrin embolization of vessels that do not supply the tumor area. Thus it is possible to exclude the superifical temporal and the occipital vessels when they do not supply the

tumor area and to avoid alopecia, while at the same time increasing the volume of chemotherapeutic agent carried to the tumor-bearing region. His most exciting report relates to results in the nasopharynx, which is an area that can be isolated very specifically by this technique and in which he has obtained regression rates in excess of 50 percent in 100 percent of his patients. The impact of this neoadjuvant treatment can not be clearly predicted, since all patients received radiation therapy subsequent to chemotherapy. Eleven of the 15 patients are alive without recurrence at the time of this report; however, results of radiation therapy for this lesion are favorable enough so that it is difficult to be sure whether the effects on long-term survival will be significant.

Molinari reports his series from the Milan Cancer Institute. With over 260 patients, this is probably one of the world's largest series. Patients were treated by an intra-arterial catheter passed retrograde by way of the temporal artery. The drugs used were methotrexate, vincristine and bleomycin in various combinations.

Baker of Ann Arbor is the final author and reports his results after using an implantble pump. Unlike those of the other two authors, Baker's patients had all received previous radiation therapy and, in some cases, surgery and chemotherapy as well. Thus he is dealing with the treatment of therapeutic failures. Most of his patients received 5-Fluorouracil deoxyribonuclease (5-FUDR) and cisplatin, and using this protocol, he obtained a partial or complete remission rate of 80 percent of the patients treated. This figure suggests a response rate that rivals the results seen in treatment of untreated patients by the systemic route.

All of the investigators demonstrate results that are highly provocative and suggestive. However, none are able to show data which are definitive, since all of the studies are based on a single mode of therapy, compared to data from other institutions or on historical controls. Certainly the results reported are intriguing enough to illustrate the urgent need for randomized controls to demonstrate whether local regional control achieved by this technique is indeed superior to systemic therapy and, if so, whether it is worth the somewhat increased morbidity that the technique incurs. It is hoped that by the time of another international conference, in 4 years or so, this type of control data will be available.

REFERENCES

1. Klopp CT, Alford TC, Bateman J, Berry GN, Winship T. Fractionated intra-arterial cancer chemotherapy with methyl bis amine hydrochloride, preliminary report. Ann Surg 1950; 132:811.
2. Bierman HR, Shimkin MB, Byron RL, Miller EC. The effects of intra-arterial administration of nitrogen mustard. Fifth International Cancer Congress, Paris, 1950:187–188 (abstract).
3. Sullivan RD, Jones R, Schnobel TG Jr, Sharey JMcC. The treatment of human cancer with intra-arterial nitrogen mustard utilizing a simplified catheter technique. Cancer 1953; 6:121.
4. Reese AB. Treatment of retinoblastoma by radiation and trieth-

ylenemelamine. Trans Am Acad Ophthal Otolaryngol 1957; 61:439.

5. Johnson RO, Kisken WA, Curreri AR. A report upon arterial infusion with 5-fluorouracil in 100 patients. Surg Gynecol Obstet 1965; 120:530.

6. Rush BF, Horie N, Klein NW. Intra-arterial infusion of the head and neck: anatomical and distributional problems. Am J Surg 1965; 110:510.

7. Watkins E. Chronmetric infusor—an apparatus for protracted ambulatory infusion therapy. N Engl J Med 1963; 269:850.

INTRA-ARTERIAL CISPLATIN IN THE TREATMENT OF AERODIGESTIVE SQUAMOUS CARCINOMA AND NASOPHARYNGEAL CARCINOMA

ROY B. SESSIONS, M.D., F.A.C.S.
DANIEL E. LEHANE, M.D.
R. NICK BRYAN, M.D.
BARRY L. HOROWITZ, M.D.

This report concerns a clinical experience gathered during the period between 1978 and 1983, a time during which 68 patients with aerodigestive squamous cell carcinoma (ADSC) and nasopharyngeal carcinoma (NPC) were treated with intra-arterially administered cisplatin. This project was undertaken jointly by the Departments of Otolaryngology, Medicine, and Pharmacology, and Radiology at the Baylor College of Medicine in Houston, Texas. The patient group consisted of a consecutive, but nonrandomized series of stage III and IV patients that included NPC, and squamous cell carcinoma of the nose, paranasal sinuses, oropharynx, hypopharynx, and larynx.[1] This report is, in effect, somewhat anecdotal, and attempts only to report observations and speculation on potential for both methodology and drug. In analyzing such a series of patients, one must impose stern restrictions on the conclusions drawn; one must realize, for example, that in order to attain a high confidence level in a stage-to-stage comparison of the efficacy of intravenous versus intra-arterial methods of drug delivery, nearly 75 evaluable patients in each study arm would be needed to show a 20 percent difference in response rates. To further construct the ideal study, comparison of patients that have been matched for site as well as stage should be undertaken. The numeric demands of such an endeavor, however, render its development by a single institution unlikely.

Regarding our report, it should be pointed out that we consider the natural history of NPC somewhat unique, and we believe that including these patients with the other aerodigestive carcinomas is somewhat inappropriate when analyzing response and survival data. We have treated 20 NPC patients with intra-arterial cisplatin, and observations regarding both their tumor responses and their survival are included in this report, but in a separate listing from the other patients.

With regard to the methodology employed, we treated all of these patients by bolus delivery, employing a transcutaneous, retrograde femoral artery approach, isolating the particular artery in the carotid system most suitable for the tumor to be infused. Gelfoam (Upjohn) embolization was often used to divert flow and thereby enhance the site selectivity of the infusion. The drug was administered over a 1- to 2-hour period, and the catheters were then withdrawn. Cisplatin was prepared as a 1 mg/ml solution, with 0.9% sodium chloride as a diluent. Solutions were prepared immediately before infusion and were passed through a 0.2-micron filter before use. Patients with a creatinine clearance (CCR) of 70 ml/min or greater received a dose of 100 mg/m^2. Those with a CCR of 45 to 70 ml/min recieved a reduced dose. The cisplatin dose was reduced appropriately in the second and third infusions of responding patients whose CCR decreased during treatment. Treatment was repeated at 4-week intervals. Immediately prior to the infusion, metoclopramide (3 mg/kg) was used, and this was repeated 2 hours later; nausea was thus minimized.

In an effort to prevent nephrotoxicity, a simple hydration scheme was instituted. Prehydration was accomplished with 0.2% NaCl, 200 ml/hour, given 3 to 12 hours before infusion; this usually resulted in a water diuresis. After cisplatin administration, hydration was continued intravenously for 24 to 48 hours with 0.2% NaCl, until the patient was able to maintain an oral hydration rate of 3 L/24 hours, which was continued for one week. Nephrotoxins, such as aminoglycoside antibiotics, were avoided whenever possible.

Regarding the preparation of the cisplatin solution, filtration seems to lower the incidence of CNS toxicity. In a group of brain tumor patients who had previously been treated with this method in the same institution, there had been a tendency for them to develop cerebral edema, and for that reason mannitol and dexamethasone had become part of the treatment routine. This has not been the case in the head and neck group, however, despite the "wash" of cisplatin into the internal carotid system in some patients. As a result, mannitol has not been included in the treatment plan. On the other hand, corticosteroids have been administered in a number of these patients.

With reference to the patient series with which

this report is concerned, a total of 68 patients with aerodigestive squamous carcinoma (ADSC) or NPC were treated with this method between 1978 and 1983. We graded responses to chemotherapy as complete (CR), partial (PR), or none (NR). CR was evidenced by no visible tumor remaining following treatment; PR represented at least a 50 percent measurable decrease in tumor mass; NR represent anything less than a 50 percent measurable decrease in tumor mass. In patients with primary and cervical disease, the sum of the two-dimension product of individual tumor sites was used to calculate the responses. In the case of the NPC patients, final response was measured by CT evaluation. Recurrence was established by biopsy. The 68 patients were divided into three groups, depending on stage of their disease and whether or not they had received previous treatment. Group I included patients who had received previous radiation therapy (RT) and had failed this modality either by disease persistence or recrudescence. Group II was made up of previously untreated tumors that were considered inoperable at the time of initial evaluation. Finally, group III included patients with advanced but operable disease that had not been previously treated.

Group I consisted of 21 patients with recurrent ADSC and five recurrent NPC patients who had originally been stage III or IV (Table 1, 2). These patients were given three cycles of intra-arterial cisplatin (IACP), 3 to 4 weeks apart. Of the 21 ADSC patients, 18 responded (86%); 11 showed a PR, and seven a CR. Three patients demonstrated no response to treatment (Table 1). Of the 18 responders, the median survival time is 39 weeks. It is noteworthy that two pa-

TABLE 1 Response to Intra-arterial Cisplatin: Group I, Recurrent ADSC

Site	Response	Survival Weeks (Months)	
Palate	NR	4	(1)
FOM	PR	12	(3)
Hypop	PR	17	(4)
Max	PR	17	(4)
Max	PR	19	(5)
Eth	PR	19	(5)
Tonsil	CR	20	(5)
Max	PR	20	(5)
Hypop	PR	20	(5)
Hypop	PR	30	(8)
Max	PR	39	(9)
Pyriform	PR	39	(9)
Larynx	CR	45	(12)
Larynx	CR	47	(12)
Hypop	CR	48	(12)
BOT	CR	53	(13)*
Max	PR	58	(15)
FOM	CR	67	(17)
OP	NR	69	(17)
Nose	CR	157	(39)*
Hypop	NR	204	(51)
Total responders	18/21 (86%)		

*Still alive

TABLE 2 Response to Intra-arterial Cisplatin: Group I, Recurrent NPC

	Response	Survival	
NPC	PR	35	(8.7)
NPC	CR	100	(25)*
NPC	CR	100	(25)*
NPC	CR	172	(43)*
NPC	CR	192	(48)*
Total responders	5/5		

*Still alive

tients who had CRs are still alive and show no evidence of disease (NED), one at 13 months, and the other at 39 months. It should also be noted that two patients with relatively long survival times, one with an oropharyngeal lesion at 17 months and the other with a hypopharyngeal lesion at 51 months, were NRs. Both ultimately died from their disease. In this group, there was no apparent relationship between site and responsiveness.

There were five NPC patients treated in group I, all of whom had failed by persistence or recurrence following RT. The failures had been at the primary site, and these were treated with the same cycling of IACP as was used for the ADSC patients in this group. All five patients responded; one with a PR and four with CRs (Table 2). The four CRs remain alive and are NED 25 to 48 months after IACP treatment. The patient who had a PR died almost 9 months following treatment.

Group II consisted of previously untreated patients with stage III or IV disease, and these were treated with IACP plus RT. The drug was given in three cycles—prior to, at the midpoint of, and at the completion of radiation. The standard ADSC in this group were advanced and were considered inoperable at the time of initial evaluation; of these, there were 19 patients. Eighteen of the 19 responded (94%). Of the 18 responders, 14 were PRs and four were CRs (Table 3). The median survival time in this group is 36 weeks or 9 months. All of the CRs have had relatively extended survival times. Again, as with group I, these data do not reflect a site and responsivity relationship.

We have treated 15 NPC patients as part of group II (Table 4). They were, as were all patients in this group, previously untreated. All 15 demonstrated tumor response, three in partial fashion (PR) and 12 in complete fashion (CR). Four of those patients (2 PRs and 2 CRs) have died at 10, 15, 16, and 22 months respectively.

In group III, patients with advanced primary disease that was considered surgically resectable were treated with a combined protocol of induction IACP, followed by extirpative surgery 10 days later (Table 5). One month following surgery, radiation therapy was begun and carried to full course. There were eight patients in this group, and all of their tumors re-

TABLE 3 Response to Intra-arterial Cisplatin: Group I, CIS DDP & RT—Untreated ADSC

Site	Response	Survival Wks (Months)	
BOT	PR	20	(5)
Palate	PR	21	(5)
BOT	PR	22	(6)
Eth	PR	24	(6)
OP	PR	24	(6)
FOM	PR	28	(7)
OP	NR	30	(8)
BOT	PR	32	(8)
Hypop	PR	35	(9)
Tonsil	PR	36	(9)
BOT	PR	56	(14)
Epiglottis	PR	56	(14)
BOT	CR	56	(14)
Palate	CR	56	(14)
Max	CR	62	(16)*
FOM	PR	104	(26)*
Hypop	PR	104	(26)*
FOM	PR	128	(32)*
Max	CR	128	(32)*
Total responders	18/19 (94%)		

*Still alive

TABLE 4 Response to Intra-arterial Cisplatin: Group II, NPC—Previously Untreated

	Response	Survival Wks (Months)	
NPC	PR	8	(2)*
NPC	CR	17	(4)*
NPC	CR	21	(5)*
NPC	CR	22	(6)*
NPC	CR	35	(9)*
NPC	PR	40	(10)
NPC	PR	61	(15)
NPC	CR	64	(16)
NPC	CR	82	(21)*
NPC	CR	86	(22)
NPC	CR	100	(26)*
NPC	CR	100	(26)*
NPC	CR	104	(26)*
NPC	CR	108	(27)*
NPC	CR	108	(27)*
Total responders	15/15		

*Still alive

TABLE 5 Response to Intra-arterial Cisplatin: Group III, combined Therapy—Untreated ADSC

Site	Response	Survival Wks (Months)	
BOT	PR	15	(4)
Epiglottis	PR	17	(4)
OP	PR	44	(11)
Max	PR	60	(15)
Ethmoid	CR	65	(16)
Hypop	PR	74	(18)
Hypop	PR	116	(29)*
FOM	PR	156	(39)*
Total responders	8/8		

*Still alive

sponded to the induction drug; there were seven PRs and one CR. Those responses were to one cycle of CP. There were no NPC in this surgical group.

There was noticeable toxicity seen in a moderate percentage of patients; four patients demonstrated complete facial nerve paralysis on the side of the infused lesion; one patient demonstrated a transient cerebral ischemic episode during catheter placement (but prior to embolization); one patient developed a stroke one day following infusion; a small number of patients developed partial alopecia in the distribution of the ipsilateral superifical temporal artery; and 35 percent of the patients developed mild-to-moderate renal impairment resulting in elevation of serum creatinine. Patients with facial nerve paralysis concomitantly developed substantial parotid gland swelling in the ipsilateral side; in each of these patients, the nerve function eventually returned, although it took up to one year to do so in two of these cases. The patient who developed a stroke had only moderate neurologic recovery; the deficits were permanent. Twenty-five percent of the patients (17) had up to a 25 percent elevation of serum creatinine, and 10 percent (6 patients) doubled their serum creatinine. In all cases, the elevations were reversed to some degree. Patients who lost hair all had regrowth following cessation of treatment.

Regional drug administration (RDA) is an alluring methodology that, at least theoretically, offers the opportunity to increase drug concentration at a given tumor site while decreasing systemic drug levels, and creates a more thorough tumor cell exposure to the antineoplastic agent. The most common methods of RDA are intra-arterial (IA), intraperitoneal, and intrathecal delivery. With regard to IA administration, despite the potential advantages, there has not been a substantial number of oncologists who have adopted these methods in anything other than a sporadic manner. In the past, difficulty with a safe and consistent delivery system has been one hinderance. The lack of well-designed clinical or animal experiments showing an enhancement of either responsiveness or survival has been another deterrent. In addition, it might be said that enthusiasm for IA drug methods has been diminished by clinical studies that were poorly designed with respect to pharmacodynamics and pharmacokinetics. Ideally, the selection of a drug for IA use should be based on the need for drugs with high total body clearance and/or body sites with low regional exchange rates.[2] For example, use of a low total body clearance drug such as methotrexate in an area with a high regional exchange rate such as the liver ignores these principles.

Nevertheless, enthusiasm for the potential of IA therapy continues. In theory, head and neck cancer patients are particularly suited to IA chemotherapy because essentially they have loco-regional disease and the anatomy of the part generally provides a readily accessible arterial blood supply from the external carotid arterial system. This system can be entered and manipulated with relative safety, given technical competence and experience, and methodology for delivery continues to improve. In the particular study that is reported herein, femoral artery puncture and standard retrograde angiographic techniques were used for drug delivery, but as implantable pumps and/or reservoirs are perfected,[3] these methods may dominate future studies.

Recent laboratory studies done with a rabbit Vx-2 tumor system have demonstrated a more complete and rapid response in IA administration of Adriamycin as compared to the IV method of administration.[4] Other recent work has suggested an enhancement of survival with IA over IV administration of chemotherapeutic agents.[5] There are other studies that have suggested the superiority of activity of IACP over IVCP.[6]

To date, no clinical study with appropriate stage and site matching has been carried out comparing the efficacy of IA versus IV drug administrtion in ADSC patients. Again, the numbers involved in such a study have probably been the major reason for the failure of the development of such an undertaking.

Regarding the matter of employing IA techniques in body sites with low regional exchange rates, the head and neck is ideal because of the low flow rates of the carotid artery system.[2] Regarding total body clearance of different drugs, cisplatin is theoretically not ideal for intra-arterial use. In theory, FUdR, 5-fluorouracil, CBNU, and others are better suited (Table 6). Despite these theoretic contradictions, the data presented within this study suggest a superiority of response of the IA route of administration of cisplatin over IV methods.[7,8] What is needed is a randomized study comparing stage-matched ADSC patients in sufficient proportions to give numeric credibility to the endeavor. Further substage breakdown into individual "T" and "N" categories would be useful for definitive comparisons. A study is just begining at MSKCC in which we will be treating patients with advanced ADSC who have failed with cisplatin that was administered intravenously. This will be a harsh

TABLE 6   Regional Drug Delivery

Drug	ClTB (ml/min)*
Thymidine	40,000
FUdR	25,000
5-Fluorouracil	4,000
Cytosine arabinoside	3,000
BCNN	1,000
Doxorubicin	900
AZQ (Diaziquone)	400
Cisplatin	400
Methotrexate	200

*ClTB = total body clearance
From Collins[2].

test for IA methods, and if an enhancement of response is seen, it will produce strong data.

Regarding the information derived from the study reported in this paper, some carefully drawn conclusions are appropriate, but because of limited numbers, and also because of a lack of randomized comparisons with other methods, there must be stern restrictions imposed. The median survival of our group I patients is about the same as that reported by others who used systemic CP in a single-drug regimen. It is, however, the responsiveness (86%) of the advanced tumors in this group that is noteworthy. These are a group of patients who have failed radiation and/or surgery, and except for patients who were eliminated because previous surgery had abolished arterial access to the tumor site, they were a consecutive group. It would seem that the patients who had a CR seemed to do better than the PRs in terms of survival. This re-inforces, but in no way legitimizes, the suspicion that a good response may be related to enhancement of survival time; however, any attempt to directly attribute an enhancement of survival time should be made with the consideration that the longest surviver in this group (54 months) had NR to drug.

Regarding the NPC patients in group I, the number is small—only five, but it is worth noting that all responded, and four of those are currently NED 2 to 4 years post-treatment as evidenced by CT scan. Considering the fact that these are persistent or recurrent tumors following radiation, this datum, while extremely limited numerically, is provocative. Overall, of the 26 patients in the recurrent group (group I), 23 responded (89%).

Analysis of group II shows again what seems to be a very high response rate. Analysis of this has to be carefully interpreted because of the fact that 10 days to 2 weeks after these patients received the first dose of CP, radiation was begun. All of the responders in the ADSC group (18/19) had substantial responses prior to the beginning of radiation, but how many of these had CRs vs PRs at that time has not been studied. How many of the CRs would have been CRs with drug alone, or conversely, how many would have been CR with RT alone is unknown. Our general impression throughout most of our series of patients was that if there failed to be an early response, repeated cycles were not likely to produce a difference. From looking at the parties in ADSC group II, there does not seem to be any definitive correlation with responsiveness and survival time. To emphasize the unreliability of ascribing survival time enhancement to response degree, one should consider that three of the four patients who were alive longer than two years after treatment were only PRs and continue to live in relative harmony with residual tumor. We consider it noteworthy to see such a high response in advanced, inoperable, but previously untreated patients.

The 15 NPC patients in group II showed 100 percent responsiveness, but as with the ADSC group, how many of the CRs were due to drug and/or radiation is unknown. They all had substantial responses prior to the first RT treatment, but because no CTs were obtained prior to the commencement of radiation, quantitating this is impossible. Ideally, to measure this, one would have to treat these patients with only drug. In light of the excellent control figures being reported with modern-day radiation methods, one could hardly justify eliminating this modality for anything less than a guaranteed method. Regarding survival times, this group shows 30 percent to be 2 years or better, but considering the disease and the combined treatment plan, no statement can be made. In effect, therefore, as one looks at response rates in these previously untreated patients, 33/34 responded (95%).

Group III is a very limited group of previously untreated patients with advanced disease who were managed with combination therapy. It is virtually impossible to make a meaningful statement about anything other than the responsivity of these tumors. In reality, from the standpoint of initial tumor response to CP, these patients could be grouped with the patients in group II. When these 8/8 responders are pooled with this group, the response rate is 41/42 (97%).

With the exception of the instances of facial nerve paralyses, the complications incurred in this study are fairly representative of what one would expect with these methods and this drug. Regarding the facial paralysis, it is doubtful that parotid swelling would be the direct cause. The salivary engorgement was probably a parenchymal reaction to infusion of CP; that the swelling was adjacent to the nerve is probably only a fact rather than a causal explanation. It is our goal to examine such a parotid gland by biopsy if this circumstance occurs again. Regarding the facial nerve dysfunction in these cases, in the absence of other abnormal neurologic findings, it is also unlikely that this was due to a central phenomenon. We would suggest that these paralyzed nerves are a manifestation of a peripheral neuropathy that was secondary to the known neurotoxic capabilities of CP, which in these cases was delivered to the nerve by the delicate vascularity of the individual nerve sheaths.

The transient ischemic episode seen in one case was not followed by permanent sequelae. Considering the fact that intraluminal catheterization is capable of causing vasospasm, and considering the relatively advanced age group of our patient population, it is surprising that we have not encountered this problem more often. The infrequency of the problem may reflect, at least in part, the technical delicacy of the interventionists who have participated in this study.

The one patient who had a stroke did so the day following IACP infusion. Whether the stroke was secondary to misdirection of Gelfoam embolism is unknown, but its occurrence serves to emphasize the fact that such techniques as employed in this study are fraught with some degree of danger, and with their employment by inexperienced and unsupervised radiologic interventionists, the risks assume unacceptable levels.

Finally, we have learned to selectively embolize the superficial temporal artery during the administration of IACP and, in so doing, have eliminiated the problem of alopecia in these patients.

In summary, it would seem that despite decades of experience with IA chemotherapy, there still is not widespread use of this method. Scientifically, there has been no clear demonstration of a difference in its efficacy over that of systemic therapy; however, there are provocative data to suggest this fact. Although from a pharmacokinetic and pharmacodynamic standpoint, CP should not be the best drug for this method, our feasibility study, as well as the work of others, would suggest a unique responsiveness in head and neck tumors. If in fact this suggestion is borne out, the addition of a maintenance drug added to the treatment plan probably will be the next step in the evolution of our methods. There is, in our opinion, enough encouragement in the suggestive response numbers offered in this paper to warrant a well-designed study of the topic in question.

REFERENCES

1. American Joint Committee on Cancer. Staging of cancer of the head and neck site and melanoma, 1980.
2. Collins JM. Pharmacologic rationale for regional drug delivery. J Clin Oncol 1984; 2:
3. Baker SR. Intra-arterial chemotherapy for head and neck cancer, Part I: Theoretical consideration and drug delivery systems. Head Neck Surg 1983; 6:664–682.
4. Swistel AJ, Bading JR, Roaf JH. Intra-arterial versus intravenous Adriamycin in athe rabbit Ux-2 tumor system. Cancer 1984; 53:1397–1464.
5. Arcangeli G, Nervi C, Righiri R, et al. Combined radiation and drugs: The effect of intra-arterial chemotherapy followed by radiation therapy in head and neck cancer. Radiother Oncol 1983; 1:101–107.
6. Lehane DE, Session SR, Johnson P, et al. Intra-arterial cisplatin administration for advanced squamous cell carcinoma of the head and neck region. Int Head Neck Oncol Res Con 1980; 2:11.
7. Wittes RE, Cuitkovic E, Shah J, et al. Cis-dichlorodiammineplatinum (II) in the treatment of epidermoid carcinoma of the head and neck. Cancer Treat Rep 1977; 61:359–66.
8. Panieltiere FJ, Lehane D, Fletcher WS, et al. Cisplatin therapy of previously treated head and neck cancer: The Southwest Oncology Group's two-dose-per-month outpatient regimen. Med Pediatr Oncol 1980; 8:221–25.

PRELIMINARY INTRA-ARTERIAL CHEMOTHERAPY IN CANCER OF THE ORAL CAVITY: LONG-TERM RESULTS OF COMBINED TREATMENTS WITH SURGERY OR RADIOTHERAPY

ROBERTO MOLINARI, M.D.

From 1971 to 1981, 207 patients with more or less locally advanced, previously untreated epidermoid carcinoma of the oral cavity, anterior oropharynx, and infrastructure of the maxillary sinus were treated with courses of regional intra-arterial chemotherapy (IAC). Except for a small number of cases treated for palliative purposes only, IAC was administered as preliminary treatment prior to surgery or radiotherapy, according to two main indications. In a first group of cases that were inoperable or theoretically only suitable for palliative radiotherapy, IAC was used with the aim of inducing a shrinkage of the tumor mass, to reduce it within the boundaries of feasible surgery or probable curative radiotherapy ("salvage" IAC). In a second group of relatively less extended cancers directly suitable for primary radical surgery or curative radiotherapy, IAC was used as a preliminary adjuvant procedure in order to offer to subsequent major treatments less viable cells, a decreased tumor mass, and safer margins of resection (planned IAC).

TECHNICAL PROCEDURE OF IAC

Arterial cannulation (Table 1) was performed almost always via the superficial temporal artery (superior thyroid artery in 7 cases), pushing the catheter tip into the lumen of the external carotid artery, below the origin of the appropriate branch. This procedure was performed unilaterally in 150 cases and bilaterally in 57 patients in whom the cancer was located astride the midline. In some of the latter cases, cannulation of terminal branches (i.e., lingual artery after radical neck dissection) was combined with contralateral external carotid artery catheterization. The catheter position was controlled by injecting methylene blue or by arteriography in some cases.

In all patients the indwelling polyethylene catheter remained in place for a relatively short period, the maximum duration being 24 days. As a rule in this series, the IAC course lasted 10 to 15 days, according to the chemotherapy schedule.

COMPOSITION OF THE SERIES AND INDICATIONS FOR IAC

Indications for IAC depended basically on size, extent, and location of the primary tumor as well as on size and characteristics of the neck nodes, when present. According to the treatment protocols at the INT of Milan, all epidermoid carcinomas of the oral cavity and oropharynx classified T1 and T2 smaller than 3 cm, or strictly exophytic, were treated with single modalities (interstitial brachytherapy whenever possible, primary surgery, transcutaneous radiotherapy). For T2 tumors 3 to 4 cm in size, the treatment planned was (1) transcutaneous ^{60}Co teletherapy (40 to 45 Gy) followed by a boost with interstitial brachytherapy (fungating, superficial ulcerating tumors), or (2) primary surgery (older patients, tumors adherent to or directly invading bony structures), or (3) IAC followed by surgery or RT (T2 infiltrating). Except for clearly untreatable patients, both T3 and T4 cases were generally treated with IAC as a preliminary procedure, followed by surgery or RT according to the immediate response to IAC. In other cases, regardless of the T value of their primary tumor, patients with palpable nodes greater than 3 cm with reduced mobility or fixed were treated with a combined radiosurgical approach. IAC has little effect on the neck node metastases.

The present series consists of tumors classified as T2 greater than 3 cm, infiltrating or involving bony structures, and T3 with or without bone involvement (Table 2). As a rule, bone involvement dictates a T4 classification, but since bone involvement can take place regardless of the tumor size, with possibly different prognostic implications, we prefer to retain the

TABLE 1   Arteries used for IAC

	Patients	Arteries
IAC indications	233	294
Unsuccessful cannulations	26 (11%)	30 (11%)
Successful cannulations	207	264
Cannulated arteries		
Superf. temporal a., unil.	142	142
Superf. temporal a., bilat.	55	110
Superf. temporal a. + contralat. lingual a.	2	4
Lingual a., unilat.	1	1
Super. thyroid a.	7	7

TABLE 2   Composition of the Series (TNM)

	N0	N1	N2	N3	Total
T2	29	13	—	—	42
T3	33	31	1	—	65
T2–3 bone	24	10	4	2	40
Totals	86	54	5	2	147

older (1974) UICC TNM classification. At the same time, N2 and N3 categories are rare in this series.

CHEMOTHERAPY REGIMENS

Several drugs and combinations of them were used during this time. Single drugs (MTX at various dosages, ADM, BLM) were administered up to 1975-1976; since then multiple drug regimens have been used almost exclusively (VCR + BLM + MTX, and more complex schemes after 1978). All drugs were administered daily by slow intra-arterial infusion lasting 6 to 12 hours (median 8.2 hours), by means of various types of infusion sets. Table 3 lists drugs, doses, and schedules of each regimen.

COMPLICATIONS AND FEASIBILITY OF IAC

Technique-related complications occurred quite frequently; they were generally minor (obstructions,

breakage, displacement) and simply required treatment interruption. In 14 patients, CNS disorders appeared; in 6 cases, they were minor and of short duration, in 8 cases, intensive care was required. One patient died of embolism that resulted from maneuvers to relieve catheter obstruction. In all these cases but one, IAC was interrupted.

Drug-related complications were generally slight (Table 4), except for the first part of our experience with single drugs (low-dose MTX, ADM). Two of these patients died, and one additional death occurred recently during treatment with VCR + BLM + MTX; in all cases bone marrow depression was the determinant cause of death. On the whole (Table 5), the mortality was low (4/207, or 1.9%), and 80 percent of the patients could receive a full course of the planned chemotherapy. In an additional 12 cases, IAC was interrupted after administration of sufficient drug (more than two-thirds of the planned regimen), thus bringing to 86 percent the number of patients receiving helpful treatments.

TABLE 3 Drugs and Schedules used for IAC

Drugs	Daily dose (mg)	Schedule day(s)	Total dose (mg)	No. Treated Patients
ADM	10	1 → 15	120–150	9
MTX	5–10	1 → 12	60–120	8
MTX (+CF)	50	1 → 10	500	10
BLM	15	1 → 13	150–195	36
VCR + BLM	1 / 15	1-5-9 / 1 → 12	3 / 180	77
VCR + BLM + MTX	1 / 15 / 50	1-6-11 / 1 → 4, 6 → 9, 11 → 14 / 5, 10, 15	3 / 180 / 150	52
Miscellaneous		Various	Various	15
				207

TABLE 4 Drug-related Complications

	MTX low-dose (8 cases)	MTX 50 mg (10 cases)	ADM (9 cases)	BLM (36 cases)	VCR BLM (77 cases)	VCR BLM MTX (52 cases)	Miscell. (15 cases)
General complications							
Fever (38°C)	2	2	2	9	9	2	2
Neurologic (CNS excl.)	—	—	—	2	3	—	—
Gastrointestinal	1	1	—	—	1	—	—
Cardiotoxic	—	—	1	1	2	—	—
Dermatologic	—	2	—	2	6	—	—
Bronchopulmonary	1	—	—	5	3	—	—
Hematologic	1†	2	3	1	2	5†	1
Renal	1†	—	—	—	—	—	1
Local complications							
Mucositis	2	3	6	1	2	15	3
Bleeding	—	—	—	1	2	—	—
Alopecia	—	—	1	1	2	1	—

†Death

TABLE 5   General Feasibility of IAC

	No. Treatments	Attempts
Attempted cannulations		233
Successful cannulations	207	
No complications	88 (42.5%)	
Transient minor complications	77 (37.2%)	
Total full-dose treatments	165* (79.7%)	71%
Partial treatments	42	
After sufficient dose ($> \frac{2}{3}$)	12 (5.8%)	
After insufficient dose ($< \frac{2}{3}$)	30† (14.5%)	
Total useful treatments	177 (85.5%)	76.5%
* 2 deaths		
† 2 deaths		
4 deaths total	1.9%	1.7%

TABLE 7   Combined Treatments by Indication

IAC alone	18	
IAC + Radiotherapy	44	
Interstitial brachytherapy		9
Transcutaneous RT		35
IAC + Surgery	112	
Salvage IAC + Surgery		76
Planned IAC + Surgery		36

TABLE 8   Surgical Procedures used after IAC

Surgical Treatment	No. of Cases
Pull-through anterior pelvectomy	29
Transoral hemiglossectomy	12
Transmand. cons. hemiglossectomy (ant.)	11
Transmand. demol. hemiglossectomy (ant.)	28
Transmand. demol. post. hemiglossectomy	11
Hemimandibulectomy (gingiva, retrom. space)	14
Total subglossolaryngectomy	1
Superior maxillary resection	6
Total	112

IMMEDIATE RESPONSE TO IAC

Immediate response was evaluated in the 174 patients who received adequate chemotherapy. Regression was expressed as reduction of the tumor in percent of its initial size (Table 6). Responses depended somewhat on T stage, but were strictly related to the chemotherapy regimen used. Multiple drug regimens induced more frequent and more important regressions than did single drugs, with the sequence VCR + BLM + MTX achieving the highest response rates (74% of regressions greater than 50% and 41% exceeding 75% of the initial size). More complex combinations of drugs have recently been tried, adding CisDDP or ADM to VCR, BLM, and MTX; toxicity is relatively higher, but response rates also have increased.

SUBSEQUENT TREATMENT

Eighteen patients did not receive any further treatment (Table 7). In 112 patients, subsequent treatment consisted of various surgical procedures (Table 8), generally combined with en bloc neck dissection (78 cases). In 12 patients the neck dissection was delayed, whereas in 2 cases it preceded IAC. As a rule, postoperative radiotherapy was also administered when positive nodes with extracapsular spread were found

in the surgical specimen; in some of these cases (18), the site of the primary lesion was also included in the radiotherapy fields. This was the rule in patients with histologically positive margins (7).

In 44 patients radiotherapy was the subsequent treatment; transcutaneous ^{60}Co teletherapy (55 to 72 Gy, median 61 Gy) was used in 35 cases, encompassing both primary tumor and lymphatic areas. In 9 relatively less extended tumors the treatment of choice was interstitial brachytherapy (radium or iridium).

CLINICAL COURSE AFTER COMBINED TREATMENTS

IAC + RT

In this group of cases local complications occurred more frequently and earlier than during RT alone. Mucositis and skin reactions were earlier and more intense, with nearly one-quarter of the treatments more protracted than usual. In spite of this, only 3 cases were not able to receive the planned dose,

TABLE 6   Immediate Response to IAC, by CT Regimen

	Cases	Eval.*	Regression			Total
			< 50%	50–75%	> 75%	> 50%
MTX (5–10)	8	2	2	—	—	0%
MTX 50	10	10	3	7	—	70%
ADM	9	8	5	3	—	38%
BLM	36	33	21	5	7 (21%)	37%
VCR + BLM	77	65	38	16	11 (17%)	42%
VCR + BLM + MTX	52	42	11	14	17 (41%)	74%
Others (various drugs)	15	14	12	1	1	14%
Total	207	174	92	46	36 (21%)	47%

*Excluded: upper jaw; incomplete treatments.

which was reduced to 48, 54, and 55 Gy, respectively. Soft tissue fibrosis occurred later with the same frequency as after RT alone. No major complication was observed.

Radionecrosis did not seem increased in comparison with RT alone or after transcutaneous or interstitial administration.

IAC + Surgery

No postoperative death was observed. In 2 cases serious complications occurred: (1) bronchial pneumonia followed by pleural empyema, which needed adequate treatment and a long stay in the hospital, and (2) necrosis of submandibular soft tissues after a pull-through glossopelvectomy with bilateral neck dissection, which required several operations for plastic repair, but was corrected in 3 months. All the other postoperative courses were completed in 15 to 38 days, with a median of 29 days.

LONG-TERM RESULTS OF COMBINED TREATMENTS

IAC + Brachytherapy

One patient was lost to follow-up; all of the remaining 8 patients are living and well, with one patient salvaged by surgery (hemiglossectomy) after local recurrence. Seven also received delayed neck dissection.

IAC + Transcutaneous Radiotherapy

Of 35 patients receiving this sequence, 9 were good responders to IAC (regression greater than 75%). Five-year actuarial survival in this group was high (60%), whereas in the remaining 26 patients it was remarkably disappointing (9%), with no significant difference among various levels of response to IAC. Overall and disease-free survivals were strictly related to the extent of the primary tumor.

IAC + Surgery

Of 112 patients who underwent surgery, 36 were initially inoperable but became operable after IAC. They represent nearly half of those locally far-advanced cases in which IAC was attempted as a salvage procedure. Overall 5-year survival was only about 7 percent (Fig. 1), with median survival of 16 months, the same observed after IAC + RT.

Planned IAC + surgery in 76 already operable patients achieved 5-year actuarial survival as high as 60 percent. Survival (Fig. 2) was strictly related to the extent of the primary tumor before IAC (T2, 76%; T3, 53%) and dependent on the degree of initial response obtained by IAC (Fig. 3). As for the latter prognostic factor, the difference in disease-free survival was statistically significant only between regres-

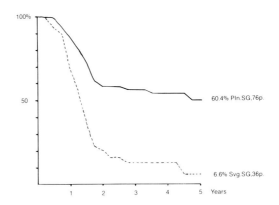

Figure 1 Overall survival after IAC + surgery, by indication for IAC. (Pln = planned IAC; Svg = salvage IAC; SG = surgery; p = patients).

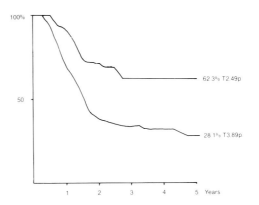

Figure 2 Overall survival after IAC + surgery, by T stage.

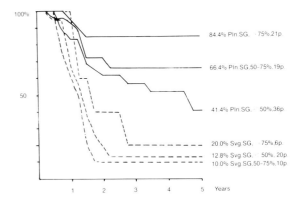

Figure 3 Overall survival after IAC + Surgery, by indication of IAC and degree of regression achieved. (Pln = planned IAC; Svg = salvage IAC; SG = surgery; p = patients).

sions greater or smaller than 75 percent (Fig. 4); no difference was found among the intermediate degrees of response comprising 0 to 75 percent.

Figure 5 compares the impact of the immediate regression after IAC on the whole series, by the type of combination treatment.

As far as the IAC regimen is concerned (Fig. 6), no significant difference in survival was found after

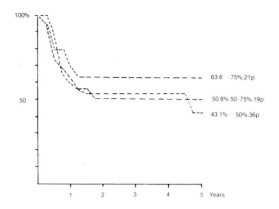

Figure 4 Overall survival after planned IAC + surgery, by degree of regression achieved by IAC.

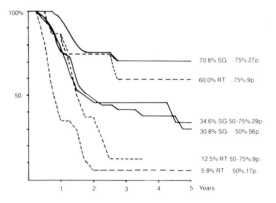

Figure 5 Overall survival in the whole series (IAC + surgery or RT), by type of subsequent treatment and by degree of regression observed after IAC. (SG = surgery; RT = radiotherapy).

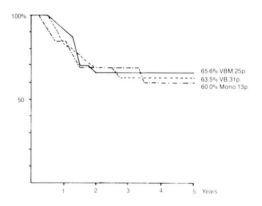

Figure 6 Overall survival after planned IAC + Surgery, by type of chemotherapy regimen. (VBM = VCR + BLM + MTX; VB = VCR + BLM; Mono = single drugs).

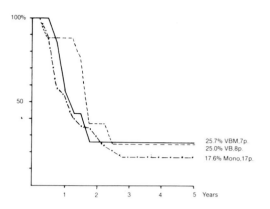

Figure 7 Overall survival after IAC + transcutaneous RT (worse cases), by type of chemotherapy. (VBM = VCR + BLM + MTX; VB = VCR + BLM; Mono = single drugs).

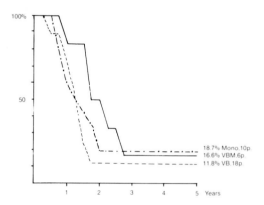

Figure 8 Overall survival after salvage IAC + Surgery, by type of chemotherapy. (Mono = single drugs; VB = VCR + BLM; VBM = VCR + BLM + MTX).

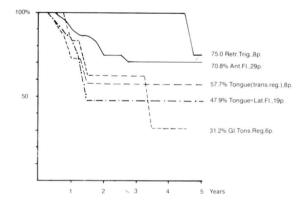

Figure 9 Overall survival after planned IAC + surgery, by site of the primary tumor. (Retr Trig = retromolar triqoue; Ant Fl = Anterior floor; Trans reg = transitional region; Lat Fl = lateral floor; Gl Tons Reg = glossotonsillar region).

IAC + surgery among the three main types used (single drugs, VCR + BLM, VCR + BLM + MTX). Nevertheless, some difference seems to exist in the shape of the curves concerning V-B and V-B-M schedules in far-advanced cases (Figs. 7 and 8). The free interval is longer for V-B when followed by radiotherapy, for V-B-M after IAC + surgery.

The contribution of preliminary IAC seems to vary, depending on the location of the primary tumor (Fig. 9): tumors in the retromolar space, inner gingiva, and hard palate show a better 5-year survival than tumors in the tongue, lateral floor of the mouth, and glossotonsillar region.

CAUSE OF FAILURE OF COMBINED TREATMENTS

Tumor recurred locally in 95 percent of the patients treated with IAC + radiotherapy and in 70 percent of those who received IAC as a salvage procedure before surgery.

In the group treated by planned IAC + surgery, tumor recurred in 19 of 76 patients (25%). The recurrence rate in these patients was not strictly related to the initial response to IAC.

Practically no local recurrence was observed after the third year. The main cause of death after this interval is a second primary tumor.

CONCLUSIONS

Our experience indicates that chemotherapy administered intra-arterially in intensive short courses is a feasible procedure, evidently giving rise to fewer complications than reported in the literature.

Multiple-drug regimens cause more frequent and especially more important regressions than do single drugs, with lower general complication rates.

When used as a preliminary procedure prior to major treatments, IAC does not significantly increase postradiotherapy or postoperative complications. Long-term results of these combined treatments seem to be better than those achieved by radiotherapy or surgery alone, in retrospective comparisons. It is more evident when surgery follows IAC, whereas the contribution of preliminary chemotherapy prior to radiotherapy looks more shaded. Nevertheless, the final outcome seems to be clearly related to the degree of immediate response to chemotherapy.

IAC does not modify prognosis related to the lymphatic spread. Its most significant contribution is in decreasing local primary recurrence rates. Apart from this retrospective evaluation, a controlled randomized trial conducted in the framework of the Head and Neck Cooperative Group of the EORTC, comparing surgery alone with surgery preceded by IAC in some locations of the oral cavity, seems to show a real benefit from the use of preliminary chemotherapy.

At present new combinations of drugs, including CisDDP given either intra-arterially or intravenously, are giving promising results, with an increase in response rates.

CisDDP can also be used as a radiosensitizer by intra-arterial administration of small doses immediately before or concurrently with single or multiple daily sessions of radiotherapy. The feasibility of this combination was excellent in a series of advanced cancers of the maxillary antrum which we have been treating for the last 18 months.

RECENT DEVELOPMENTS IN THE MANAGEMENT OF HEAD AND NECK CANCER WITH INTRA-ARTERIAL CHEMOTHERAPY

SHAN R. BAKER, M.D., F.A.C.S.
RICHARD H. WHEELER, M.D.
ARLENE A. FORASTIERE, M.D.
BARBARA N. MEDVEC, R.N., B.S.N.

One of the main reasons intra-arterial (IA) infusion chemotherapy has not been more widely accepted has been the need for prolonged hospitalization and the many complications accompanying its use. Most of the complications are related to the use of an indwelling catheter. The catheter must remain in place, which requires constant nursing care and a cooperative patient.

To circumvent many of the complications of IA chemotherapy, a percutaneously refillable, totally implantable pump has been developed. It consists of a hollow titanium disk separated into two chambers by a metal bellows (Fig. 1). The inner chamber contains the infusate, the outer a charging liquid in equilibrium with its vapor phase. At 37°C, the vapor pressure is approximately 450 mmHg greater than atmospheric pressure. This vapor pressure provides the power source, exerting pressure on the bellows, and forcing the infusate through a 0.22-micron bacterial filter and a fluid resistance element. The pump is placed beneath the skin and the drug chamber is periodically refilled through percutaneous injections of infusate. The drug chamber is refilled through a self-sealing

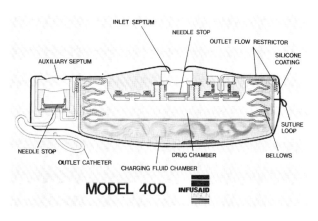

Figure 1 Infusaid pump Model 400, schematic. (Courtesy of the Infusaid Corporation, Sharon, MA).

silicone rubber septum in the top of the pump. The pressure of the refill injection forces the bellows to extend, reducing the volume of the outer chamber and recondensing the volatile-driving vapor. Thus, refilling the drug chamber simultaneously recharges the power source for the next infusion cycle. The fluid resistance element is connected to a silicone rubber delivery catheter, which can be inserted into a vein, artery, or body cavity.

Certain models of the pump feature an auxiliary injection port with a second self-sealing rubber septum (see Fig. 1). This port connects directly with the infusion catheter bypassing the pump, and may be used for injection of fluorescein or radioactive microspheres to confirm the region of infusion. It may also be utilized for bolus injections of the same or a different drug from that being infused by the pump.

IMPLANTATION

Implantation of the pump and delivery catheter may be accomplished under local or general anesthesia. Neoplasms confined to the head and upper neck are perfused through the external carotid artery. A branch of the external carotid artery which does not perfuse a region of the neoplasm is selected to receive the catheter. An arterotomy is performed, and the delivery catheter is threaded into the vessel. The catheter tip is advanced until it is located just at the origin of the vessel from the external carotid artery. The placement of the catheter tip flush with the lumen of the external carotid artery permits delivery of the infusate directly into the blood stream of the external carotid artery without the need of the catheter to occupy any of the vessel's luminal space.

Implantation of the infusion pump requires an incision parallel to and 2 cm below the clavicle. A subcutaneous pocket is made superficial to the fascia of the pectoralis major muscle to receive the pump. The catheter from the pump is connected to the delivery catheter or may be tunneled into the neck and placed directly into the arterotomy already described.

The pump delivers 45 ml of antineoplastic drug solution over a time period of 1 to 5 weeks, dependent on the flow rate. The drug concentration in the pump is determined by the desired dose rate and the flow rate. Patients are able to perform their regular activities without limitation while receiving IA chemotherapy on an outpatient basis.

AMBULATORY PATIENT CARE

During one of the early outpatient visits, the infusion distribution is checked by slowly injecting radioactive-labeled microspheres into the auxiliary port of the pump. The head and neck area is then scanned for localization of the microspheres in the region of the cancer.

During each outpatient visit, patients are assessed for tumor response, pump function, and possible drug toxicity. Tumor response is assessed by physical examination and, when necessary, computerized tomography. The pump is emptied by percutaneous needle entry through the subcutaneous septum. The flow rate is then calculated (by subtracting the residual pump infusate volume from the volume used to recharge the pump at the time of previous refill), and the pump is refilled with antineoplastic drug or sterile heparinized saline.

The recent development of a dual-catheter implantable pump initiates a new frontier in head and neck infusion chemotherapy. The pump permits infusion of both external carotid arteries simultaneously. This has obvious advantages for the treatment of tumors extending across the midline. Likewise, for the first time, unilateral local-regional disease that extends inferiorly beyond the nutrient field of the external carotid artery may be treated with IA chemotherapy by cannulating both the thyrocervical trunk and the external carotid artery.

For the past 4 years we have been employing the Infusaid Pump for outpatient regional therapy of patients with cancer of the head and neck. This report summarizes our experience with the Infusaid implantable Infusion Systems and discusses single agents and combination drug regimens delivered through this system. The Infusaid Pump is a safe, reliable delivery system that permits long-term, continuous intra-arterial infusion in ambulatory head and neck cancer patients.

MATERIALS AND METHODS

Patient Population

The patient and tumor characteristics of the 22 patients who have had the Infusaid Pump implanted between January 1980 and June 1983 are shown in Table 1. The eligibility criteria for patients to receive an infusion pump are as follows: (1) a biopsy-proved primary malignant tumor of the head and neck, (2) the vasculature of the entire neoplasm confined to the distribution of the external carotid artery and/or thyrocervical trunk, (3) performance status ≥ 50 Karnofsky (4) Creatinine clearance ≥ 50 ml/min, WBC 4000/ml, platelet count $\geq 150,000$ ml, $\geq 150,000/\mu l$, bilirubin 1.5 mg/μl, and (5) no prior radical neck dissection on the side of the tumor unless an accessible vascular supply can be demonstrated by angiography. Patients who have received prior methotrexate or cisplatin are not excluded; however, patients who have received systemic bleomycin are not candidates to receive this agent intra-arterially.

Chemotherapeutic Agents

Fluorodeoxyuridine (FUdR), dichloromethotrexate, and bleomycin are the drugs with which we have had the most experience in delivering chemotherapy through the pump by continuous infusion. FUdR and

TABLE 1   Patient Population Treated with the Infusaid Pump

No. Treated	22
Male/female	15/7
Median age	55
	(18–72)
Prior radiation	18
Prior chemotherapy	8
No prior therapy	4
Cell type	
Squamous	14
Basal cell	2
Undifferentiated	2
Salivary gland	2
Sarcoma	1
Sebaceous cell	1
Primary Site	
Tongue/tonsil	9
Palate	2
Ethmoid sinus	2
Parotid	3
Skin	3
Larynx	1
Floor of mouth	1
Maxillary sinus	1

bleomycin are dissolved in normal saline containing 200 units/ml sodium heparin. Dichloromethotrexate (obtained from the National Cancer Institute) is dissolved in 0.5% sodium bicarbonate without heparin.

Cisplatin (1 mg/ml) and mitomycin C (total dose in 30 ml of normal saline) are given by short-term infusion through the auxiliary port of the pump using a Harvard Pump. The Harvard Pump is connected with polyethylene tubing to a bent Huber needle inserted into the auxiliary port. Cisplatin is infused over 90 minutes and mitomycin C over 30 minutes.

RESULTS

Pump Performance

Pump performance is described in detail in Table 2. Twenty-seven pumps have been implanted in 22 patients. Before the dual-catheter pump became available, two patients had two pumps implanted to provide bilateral head infusion. Surgical implantation has been well tolerated. All patients have been discharged within a week of surgery and most within 4 days. Four cases of failure of the infusion system have occurred.

TABLE 2   Pump Performance

No. implanted	27
Single catheter	(19)
Dual catheter	(8)
No. infusion days	7500+
Median duration of therapy	7+ months
	(3+ – 31+)
Infections	2
Bleeding	0
Emboli	2
System failure	4

An abrupt decrease in flow rate occurred in three patients receiving dichloromethotrexate dissolved in normal saline. The pump was replaced in two patients, and dichloromethotrexate crystals were noted in the arterial catheter or resistance element. The pump was not replaced in the third patient. Dichloromethotrexate has subsequently been dissolved in 0.5% sodium bicarbonate to increase drug solubility, and no further infusion malfunctions have occurred utilizing this drug. The fourth case of system failure was due to kinking of the catheter near the site of the arterotomy and subsequent obstruction of the catheter from blood clot. The catheter was removed. However, the pump, which continued to function, was connected to a second catheter placed in the subclavian vein so that the patient could receive intravenous systemic chemotherapy utilizing the infusion pump as the primary vehicle.

Two patients developed an infection of the pump pocket, necessitating removal of the pump. One infection was probably precipitated during the 3 weeks the catheters were external prior to pump implantation; the second occurred after skin breakdown over the catheter in a patient who had undergone a previous radical neck dissection and neck irradiation. Two patients developed a single small area of facial skin necrosis, presumably from small emboli dislodged from the tip of the infusion catheter. These were isolated episodes and occurred several months after pump implantation. Such episodes have not recurred in spite of the fact that the infusion system was not removed. However, both patients received a 24-hour infusion of urokinase through the auxiliary port.

One patient was returned to the operating room for catheter revision. The patient had ligatures, previously placed around the internal maxillary arteries, removed because the postoperative radionuclide infusion scan showed infusion of the brain. Catheters were placed in the superior thyroid arteries, which in this patient arose at the carotid bifurcation. Shunting of blood in the internal carotid circulation occurred. The shunting of blood was partially reversed by removing the ligatures from the internal maxillary arteries, and this caused subsequent enhancement of external carotid blood flow.

Cannulation of blood vessels in the neck that has been subjected to prior neck dissection and/or irradiation increases the chance of wound infection or breakdown of the overlying skin. Patients with recurrent local-regional disease following neck dissection have considerable scarring in the neck as a result of previous surgery. This causes difficulties in identification and cannulation of the external carotid and thyrocervical trunk systems. In many cases several branches of the external carotid artery or the parent vessel itself have been ligated. We now routinely perform preoperative angiography of the external carotid and subclavian arteries on both sides of the neck in all patients who have had a previous neck dissection. In addition, a Doppler flow meter is utilized intraoperatively to aid in the identification of branches of the external carotid and thyrocervical trunk when dense scar tissue prevents easy identification. We have thus far explored the necks of three patients who had undergone previous neck surgery and have successfully implanted catheters in two.

Routinely, branches of the external carotid artery that are not supplying the tumor region, i.e., superior thyroid, lingual, and occipital arteries, are ligated at the time of catheter placement. Selective vessel ligation has the advantage of increasing the drug concentration in the tumor vasculature and limiting drug distribution to uninvolved normal tissues. In addition to the external carotid artery, the upper nasal passages and ethmoid sinuses receive blood supply from the internal carotid system through the anterior and posterior ethmoid arteries. We have treated two patients with ethmoid sinus cancer to date, and both patients have had ligation of the anterior and posterior ethmoid arteries.

Chemotherapeutic Regimens

Twenty evaluable patients have received 39 different treatment regimens using the implantable pump. Eighteen single-agent treatment regimens and 21 combination drug programs have been evaluated and are the source of a recent publication.[1] The versatility of the Infusaid System has allowed multiple therapeutic trials in individual patients. Five patients have received three separate treatment regimens, and eight have received two programs. Ten patients have responded to at least one regimen, and three additional patients have had minor response (25% to 50% tumor regression) of at least 5 months' duration. Seven of 14 patients who had the pump implanted over one year ago have received therapy for at least one year, and four patients have had functioning systems for over 2 years.

A total of fourteen objective responses were attained during these drug trials. The most efficacious regimen examined thus far has been the combination of cisplatin and FUdR (Table 3). The initial patients were treated with 50 mg/m² of cisplatin, and this was escalated to 100 mg/m² in later patients. The first patient treated received 0.1 mg/kg per day of FUdR and had disquamation over the infused side of the head. This dose rate was based on reported studies of intra-arterial FUdR. A dose-seeking study of FUdR was subsequently performed. The dose rates for FUdR delivered in combination, and the toxicity observed, were identical to the results obtained with single-agent FUdR. Cisplatin, therefore, appears to have little or no regional toxicity at this dose. FUdR was continuously administered for 14 days. Courses of therapy were repeated every 4 weeks.

Cisplatin was given with systemic hydration and mannitol. All patients experienced mild-to-moderate nausea and vomiting. Renal function was assessed by creatinine clearance prior to each dose of cisplatin. One patient had a fall in clearance to 40 to 45 ml/minute following the sixth course of therapy, and the drug was discontinued. All other patients maintained a clearance in excess of 50 ml/minute. No clinically evident hearing loss was noted in this population.

Objective partial responses were attained in eight of the ten patients. One of the nonresponders had received systemic cisplatin preoperatively 6 months prior to recurrence and pump implantation. The other nonresponder had received prior radiation therapy, but no previous chemotherapy. Two of the responders had previously received intra-arterial dichloromethotrexate. The median duration of response was 4 months with a range of 4 to 12 months.

DISCUSSION

Approximately 13,000 patients in the United States die yearly of squamous cell carcinoma of the head and neck.[2] Although the clinical incidence of distant me-

Table 3   Intra-arterial Cisplatin + FUdR

| | | | MTD | | Toxicity | | |
| | | | CP | FUdR (mg/kg/ | | | |
Pt.	Artery(s)	No. Course(s)	(mg/m²)	14 days)	Syst	Local	Resp.
1	ECA	1	50	0.1	N/V	SKIN	PR
2	ECA	4	50	0.015	N/V	MUC	PR
3	ECA	3	50	0.02	N/V	MUC	PR
4	ECA	2	50	0.025	N/V	MUC	
						SKIN	PR
5	ECA	4	50	> 0.03	N/V	NONE	PR
6	ECA	6	70	0.02	N/V	MUC	PR
7	ECA × 2	2	70	0.02	N/V	MUC	PR
8	ECA	4	100	0.02	N/V	MUC	PR
9	ECA	1	100	> 0.02	N/V	NONE	NR
10	ECA + TCT	2	100	0.01	N/V	MUC	NR

Abbreviations: MTD = maximum tolerated dose; CP = cisplatin; ECA = external carotid artery; TCT = thyrocervical trunk; N/V = nausea/vomiting; MUC = mucositis; PR = partial response; NR = no response.

tastases is increased in advanced disease, the majority of patients dying of their cancer die of local-regional disease.[3,4] It is this group of patients that will benefit from improved local control rates through new therapeutic approaches. Thus, head and neck cancer has an appropriate natural history for the application of a regional approach to therapy.

The rationale for regional therapy is based on the steep/dose/response curve exhibited by most antineoplastic agents.[5] Maximum cell kill occurs when the tumor exposure to drug concentration and/or exposure time is optimized. Since drug toxicity follows a similar steep curve, the value of chemotherapy delivered to any body region is proportional to the increase in tumor drug exposure with concomitant reduction in the exposure of normal tissues. The factors that favor a regional approach include (1) tumor natural history that demonstrates primarily loco-regional aggressiveness rather than early metastatic dissemination, (2) definable and accessible arterial supply that provides selected access to the tumor blood supply with inclusion of minimal normal tissue, (3) antineoplastic agent(s) with favorable pharmacokinetic properties (high total body clearance, rapid local tissue extraction), and (4) a reliable, predictable delivery system that minimizes patient inconvenience and permits long-term continuous infusion. We have demonstrated in previous communications that implantation of a catheter into the thyrocervical trunk can allow infusion of the cervical region, and can be used in conjunction with the standard craniofacial infusion through the external carotid artery.[6] The entire unilateral head and neck can theoretically be infused without cannulating the common carotid artery or the subclavian artery, thus maximizing drug delivery to the head and neck region and minimizing systemic distribution.

The infusion pump offers a convenient and versatile mode of access to veins, arteries, or body cavities. Drug dosage can be altered easily by emptying and refilling the pump with a different concentration of drug. Similarly, therapy can be intermittently discontinued by replacing the drug infusate with saline. Intra-arterial bolus chemotherapy can be accomplished through the auxiliary injection port of the pump.

A limiting factor in the use of this implantable pump is related to the infusion drug selected. The chemotherapeutic agents must not react with the titanium pump components, they must be of sufficiently low viscosity to permit infusion, and they must be chemically stable at physiologic temperatures over a period of 3 to 4 weeks. Therefore, drugs must be tested in vitro for stability and pump compatibility prior to clinical application.[7]

REFERENCES

1. Wheeler RH, Baker SR, Medvec B. Single-agent and combination drug regional chemotherapy for head and neck cancer using an implantable infusion pump. Cancer 1983, in press.
2. Silverberg E. Cancer Statistics, 1983. CA 1983; 33:9–25.
3. Probert JC, Thompson RW, Bagshaw MA. Patterns of spread of distant metastases in head and neck cancer. Cancer 1974; 33:127–133.
4. Million RR, Cassisi NJ, Wittes RE. Cancer in the head and neck. In: DeVita VT, Hellman S, Rosenberg SA, eds. Cancer Principles and Practices of Oncology. Philadelphia: JB Lippincott 1982:301.
5. Frei E III, Canellos GP. Dose: A critical factor in cancer chemotherapy. Am J Med 1980; 69:583–594.
6. Baker SR, Wheeler RH. Long-term intra-arterial chemotherapy infusion of ambulatory head and neck cancer patients. J Surg Oncol 1982; 21:125–131.
7. Keller JH, Ensminger WD. Stability of cancer chemotherapeutic agents in a totally implanted drug delivery system. Am J Hosp Pharm 1982; 39:1321–1323.

SECTION SEVEN / RECONSTRUCTION AND REHABILITATION

33. Microsurgical Reconstruction

INTRODUCTION

MAURICE J. JURKIEWICZ, M.D., F.A.C.S.

There is universal agreement that the advances made in reconstructive surgery in the past twenty years, and particularly in the past decade, have been truly remarkable. These advances are based on a solid understanding of the blood supply, not only to the integument, but also to muscle and bone. All the advances were made by clinical surgeons seeking reliable methods of immediate tissue transfer, particularly in head and neck cancer patients.

The concept of immediate reconstruction of head and neck cancer patients was articulated in 1953 by Edgerton[1]. That it was not universally embraced by head and neck surgeons is understandable. The methods available to accomplish that goal were based on an empiric understanding of flap physiology. Thus the methodology was uncertain and not altogether reliable.

In my view, the seminal paper that made the concept of immediate reconstruction a reality was published a decade later in 1963 by McGregor, entitled *The Temporal Flap in Intra-oral Cancer: Its Use in Repairing the Post-Excisional Defect*[2]. Here at once and at last was a reliable method of immediate closure of the defect left in the wake of an ablative cancer operation. The clinical experience on which the method was based was large and convincing, and the anatomic observations sound.

While at first the donor site defect was considered acceptable, the morbidity associated with it, particularly the appearance of the patient with a glabrous skin graft replacing his forehead, led surgeons to seek out additional ways to accomplish the objective of immediate reconstruction.

In 1965 Bakamjian introduced the deltopectoral flap based on perforating branches of the internal mammary artery[3]. Still a two-staged method, it did promote a further understanding of the blood supply of skin and represented a solid advance.

The groin flap, based on the superficial circumflex iliac artery, was described by McGregor and Jackson in 1970[4]. It was adapted to use in the head and neck cancer patient by utilizing an intermediate wrist carrier. The latter step was a necessary insertion because microvascular techniques awaited the necessary refinements of instrumentation then being worked on by Buncke in the United States and Acland in Glasgow, the latter stimulated by McGregor[5].

There followed then both refinements in microvascular technique and a better understanding of perioperative systemic and local factors in blood flow and thrombus formation; both are still evolving[6].

In the early 1970s came three events that changed the whole field of reconstructive surgery.

McGregor and Morgan published their anatomic observations on the blood supply to skin of the abdomen and generalized the following two important principles in flap physiology.

1. Flaps in general can be divided into two groups— axial pattern flaps with an in-built arteriovenous system and random pattern flaps lacking such a system.
2. The boundaries that exist between adjoining vascular territories do not have a basis in structure in the skin, but result from a dynamic pressure equilibrium in the blood vessels of each territory along the boundary line[7].

From 1970 to 1971 in the United States, McCraw and Furlow had worked out the anatomy of the dorsalis pedis flap. It was originally designed as an island transposition flap, but its adaptability to free flap transfer was obvious[8]. Again because of donor site problems and the occasional uncertainty of the anatomy, McCraw continued his search for a suitable free flap. Working in dogs he was able to consistently transfer a free flap of skin with the underlying rectus femoris muscle. He repeated the observations with gracilis and other muscles, and then worked out the myocutaneous flap principle[9].

Virtually at the very same time in 1973, Taylor and Daniel in Melbourne described the first successful free flap of skin in the human using microvascular techniques[10]. The defect was an avulsion injury in the foot, and the donor tissue was that of the groin and lower abdomen; the site originally investigated by McGregor.

The clinical and laboratory observations made in Glasgow, in Gainesville and Atlanta, and in Melbourne—taken together—have profoundly altered head and neck surgery as well as all of surgery. Ablation of disease, tumor or otherwise, can be undertaken with authority and boldness with the knowledge that certain means for wound closure and restoration of form and function are now readily at hand.

Although much has been learned, much is yet to be learned. The methods that have evolved in the past ten years remain imperfect and await all sorts of functional and aesthetic refinement. Nonetheless, the head and neck cancer patient can now be effectively rehabilitated and returned as a functioning member of society whether his wound was the result of operation, the radiation therapy, chemotherapy, or multimodality therapy.

Transfer of composite tissue by microvascular anastomosis is no longer experimental surgery. In the hands of the trained microvascular surgeon, the reliability of the transfer exceeds 90 percent and in elective circumstances now approaches 95 percent. Myocutaneous flap transfer is within the 95 percent confidence limit as well. Within the next decade, I am confident that we shall see remarkable progress in the surgical rehabilitation of the head and neck cancer patient.

REFERENCES

1. Edgerton MT. One-stage reconstruction of the cervical esophagus or trachea. Surgery 1952; 31:239.
2. McGregor IA. The temporal flap in intra-oral cancer: its use in repairing the post-excisional defect. Br J Plast Surg 1963; 16:381–385.
3. Bakamjian VY. A two-stage method for pharyngoesophageal reconstruction with a primary pectoral skin flap. Plast Reconstr Surg 1965; 36:173–184.
4. McGregor IA, Jackson IT. The groin flap. Br J Plast Surg 1972; 25:3–16.
5. Acland R. Signs of patency in small vessel anastomosis. Plast Reconstr Surg 1973; 52:325.
6. Acland R. Thrombus formation in microvascular surgery; experimental study of effects of surgical trauma. Plast Reconstr Surg 1973; 52:454.
7. McGregor IH, Morgan G. Axial and random pattern flaps. Br J Plast Surg 1973; 26:202–213.
8. McCraw JB, Fulow LT Jr. Dorsalis pedis arterialized flap. Plast Reconstr Surg 1975; 55:177.
9. McCraw JB, Dibbell DG. Experimental definition of independent myocutaneous vascular territories. Plast Reconstr Surg 1977; 60:212–220.
10. Taylor GI, Daniel RK. The free flap composite tissue transfer by vascular anastomosis. Aust NZ J Surg 1973; 43:1.

USEFUL ARTERIALIZED LOCAL FLAPS FOR HEAD AND NECK RECONSTRUCTIONS

JOHN BARRY McCRAW, M.D., F.A.C.S.

During the past ten years there have been explosive, parallel developments in both the "island" myocutaneous flap and microvascular "free" transfers. An apparent competition developed between these two schools of surgical methodology: one preferred "free" transfers to the exclusion of "island" muscle and myocutaneous flaps and the other preferred the latter local flaps to the virtual exclusion of "free" microvascular transfers. Today, these methods are known to be complementary, and the complete reconstructive surgeon should be conversant with both techniques in order to intelligently plan the best reconstruction for each patient.

It should be remembered that the "island" myocutaneous flap was developed for the *distinct purpose* of providing large vessels for free microvascular transfers.[1,2] In 1972, when this work was begun by McCraw and Vasconez, the microvascular instrumentation, microscopes, and sutures were in a rudimentary stage of development. A clinical "free" flap had not yet been performed, but it was the presumption that large vessels would facilitate such "free" transfers and also increase their reliability. The current trend to employ large vessels in "free" microvascular transfers has confirmed this earlier impression. From its halting start, microvascular transfers to the head and neck area were hampered because of the lack of suitable donor flaps. The initial flaps employed were the superficial groin flap and the dorsalis pedis flap. The disadvantages of bulk and small, short vessels for the groin flap and difficult technical manipulation of the dorsalis pedis flap with its associated skin-grafted donor site deformity were well known. This yielded the obvious criticism of lack of reliability and excessive operative time for "free" flaps. These drawbacks have been largely corrected by the many excellent microvascular donor sites that have been developed. Although these donor sites are too numerous to mention in this discussion, they have offered a level of reliability and operative time that is comparable to local head and neck arterialized flaps. Both groups of flaps should survive in an excess of 95 percent of their applications. The donor "free" flap can be elevated at the same time that the extirpative surgery is carried out, and both the performance of and the time consumed by the vascular anastomosis has become an inconsequential matter. "Free" flaps are still not "free," but they are, at least, our friends.

Today, there exists a pleasant dilemma of being able to choose between numerous, excellent well-vascularized local flaps and microvascular free flaps. It is therefore important to place each local flap into context with other local flaps so that comparisons can be made to the several "free" microvascular flaps available. This chapter presents the relative advantages and disadvantages of selected local arterialized flaps which are currently used in head and neck reconstructions so that such comparisons can be made.

REGIONAL FLAP CHOICES

Sternocleidomastoid Myocutaneous Flap

The sternocleidomastoid flap (SCM), one of the earliest arterialized flaps used for head and neck reconstructions, was first employed by Owens in 1949 and reported in 1955.[3] This reliable flap can be based either inferiorly or superiorly because of its tripartite vascular supply. When used with a superior base and pedicled on the occipital artery, it can be used for small defects of the palate, hypopharynx, and floor of the mouth. When based inferiorly on the thyrocervical trunk, it is also useful for covering defects of the larynx and trachea. It is often compared to the pectoralis minor muscle flap for these lower neck problems. However, the pectoralis minor is generally preferred for tracheal defects since it leaves a negligible donor site.

The SCM flap is no longer as popular, partly because the donor site defect may be cosmetically unacceptable. Removal of this muscle produces a deformity that is similar to that of a radical neck dissection. In addition, the wound requires vertical closure, which directly overlies the carotid vessels. Furthermore, several excellent alternatives are available. Recently, the temporalis muscle flap has been "resurrected" to directly compete with the superiorly based sternocleidomastoid flap for similar defects. The SCM flap is an extremely reliable flap, but its usefulness is limited by its donor site deformity.

Medially Based Deltopectoral Flap

In 1963, Bakamjian introduced the medially based deltopectoral flap.[5] Peerless at the time in its reliability, this flap was remarkable because it could be raised in a single stage to correct massive defects of the lower head and neck. It was originally compared to the Mutter flap, which is a random tranverse cervical flap first described in 1842,[6] and later modified by both Zovickian[7] and Chretien.[8] Unlike the Bakamjian flap, these random flaps required one or more "delaying" procedures and an obligatory orocutaneous fistula for intraoral use. The medially based deltopectoral flap has a reported 10 to 13 percent necrosis rate when used for intraoral purposes.[9] Since it was the only axial flap then available, it was used in some of the most difficult postradiation situations. This and operative inexperience probably artificially ele-

vated the expected rate of necrosis in this flap. Nevertheless, it is clearly less viable than the adjacent pectoralis myocutaneous flap when used for intraoral reconstruction. The donor site of the pectoralis myocutaneous flap can almost always be primarily closed, whereas the deltopectoral flap requires a skin graft for closure. For these reasons, the deltopectoral flap is now generally used for surface coverage of the neck rather than intraoral soft tissue replacement. However, as the first recognized "axial" flap, it remains a landmark contribution.

Pectoralis Major Myocutaneous Flap

The pectoralis major myocutaneous flap is based on the pectoral branch of the thoracoacromial artery trunk and is the "workhorse" of the head and neck area.[10-13] The entire skin overlying the pectoralis major muscle can be carried with this flap. However, the donor site defect would be similar to that of a Halsted mastectomy and would require a skin graft. Usually lesser skin requirements allow this flap to be employed with a primary closure that by design would not disturb the nipple or the breast conture.

The "skin paddle" modification is a way of describing a cutaneous segment that is partially attached to the muscle, but mainly supplied by the attached fascia of the anterior rectus abdominis and serratus anterior muscles. The paddle is usually designed overlying the inframammary fold and can be extended onto the margins of the chest wall and sternum. The flap, harvested with the patient in the supine position, has a long arc of rotation and can supply both external cover and internal lining at the recipient site. Although somewhat bulky when tubed, it can be used for circumferential pharyngeal defects as well. This excellent flap can provide a large amount of vascularized muscle and skin and is considered the "standard" for major flap reconstructions in the head and neck area.

Vertical Trapezius Myocutaneous Flap

The paraspinous skin overlying the trapezius muscle can be elevated and carried with this muscle, which is supplied by the thyrocervical trunk vessels. The vertical trapezius (VT) myocutaneous flap has the advantage of being a local flap to the posterior neck and occiput.[14-16] This region is not reached as well by any other major flap. Flap elevation prolongs a radical neck dissection by virtue of the necessity of preserving the transverse cervical artery. Therefore this flap is rarely used after a neck dissection because the supplying vessels may have been sacrificed. The VT myocutaneous flap is just as useful for intraoral problems as the pectoralis major myocutaneous flap, but it has been used less often because of poor accessibility on the back. If the width of the flap is less than 5 cm, the donor site is quite acceptable and can be primarily closed. The back requires a great deal of "stretchability"; a wide scar can be expected with a tight primary closure and a skin graft may be required.

Horizontal Trapezius Myocutaneous Flap

The horizontal or transverse trapezius myocutaneous flap is a modification of the random transverse cervical Mutter flap. McCraw and Magee first included the cervical (neck) portion of the trapezius muscle, based on the occipital artery, with the standard skin flap.[4] This increased its reliability in immediate elevation and enhanced its forward mobility. It was initially applied for intraoral reconstruction, but the necessary orocutaneous fistula required secondary closure and was an obvious disadvantage. This flap has an advantage over the deltopectoral flap in that the donor site is concealed on the back and not visible on the anterior chest. It is no longer used for intraoral problems, but is still useful for surface coverage on the neck with its excellent color match and very acceptable donor site defect.

Latissimus Myocutaneous Flap

The very large latissimus muscle has the advantage of its natural extension to the level of the iliac crest.[17-19] This muscle creates a flap that is based on the thoracodorsal artery and provides coverage to areas well above the level of the mandible and the mastoid process. The arch of rotation covers essentially the same areas as the pectoralis myocutaneous flap. However, it is less often used than the pectoralis "paddle" flap because of limited accessibility, which requires repositioning of the patient on the operating room table. Care must be taken to prevent a traction injury of the brachial plexus during arm manipulation. The greatest disadvantage of this flap concerns donor site complications, with a 50 percent seroma rate even with suction drainage. If more than 5 cm of skin is taken with the muscle, a widened scar may be expected; if more than 10 to 12 cm is required, there may be a need for skin grafting. The dissection for this flap is more tedious than for the pectoralis flap, but the latissimus is a very reliable flap. Because of its bulk, it has generally been used for large defects which encompass both the mouth and neck or massive defects of "core" resection, which require complete muscle coverage.

Platysma Myocutaneous Flap

The platymsa myocutaneous flap was originally described by Gersuny in 1887,[20] but more recently reintroduced by Futrell in 1983.[21] This compact flap, when based superiorly on its submental vascular pedicle, provides excellent surface cover for the chin and cheek. It has also been used for small intraoral defects, but it is then difficult to appropriately plan the neck flaps without harming their viability. If elevated to the level of the facial vessels, the platysma flap will reach the zygomatic and tonsillar areas. The donor site can often be closed primarily, but a skin graft in the lower neck is acceptable and sometimes required.

Temporalis Muscle

The temporalis muscle was originally utilized by Golovine in 1890 to reconstruct an orbital defect.[22] It has been commonly used in the past for obliteration of orbital exenteration defects and for problems of facial reanimation, but it can offer much wider applications. As a muscle flap it was nearly forgotten and only recently resurrected. The muscle has an arc of rotation of 8 to 10 cm in any direction from the coronoid process and can be used to replace the entire palate or floor of the mouth. The arc of rotation can be enhanced by separating the muscle from its insertion on the coronoid process. Access into the intraoral area is further improved by temporarily removing the zygomatic arch, which can be replaced after the flap is inset. The fact that it will re-epithelize without a skin graft is a major advantage for intraoral use, and the donor defect is quite acceptable.

Temporalis Muscle–Parietal Bone Flap

The temporalis muscle-parietal bone flap was first reported by Watson-Jones in 1933[23] and again suggested by Conley in 1972.[24] It has the advantage of providing abundant vascularized muscle bulk and cranial bone to facial defects and not requiring a second distant surgical site.

Provided the center of the axis of rotation is the coronoid process of the mandible, 12 to 15 cm of parietal bone length can be anticipated at the arc of the flap. With vascularized bone, there is less need to be concerned about infection, radiation to the field, or bone resorption.

The calvarium may be harvested as either full-thickness or partial-thickness bone. Temporary removal of the zygomatic arch may increase the arc of rotation of the flap and facilitate placement into its desired location.

Galeal Flaps

The galea is the deep fascia of the scalp and is supplied by four major vessels: the two occipital and two superficial temporal arteries. Unpublished data by Kaplan has demonstrated that injection of a single vessel with thin latex will fill all four vessels. The majority of the galea can therefore be raised on a single vessel providing a large surface area. Applications vary according to the artery used. Either pedicle allows coverage of the ear or the mastoid process. The flap, when supplied by the superficial temporal artery, easily resurfaces the ipsilateral forehead, orbit, and zygomatic areas. The only present disadvantage appears to be the need to do a "delayed" skin graft. The flap probably should be considered as a fascial layer containing large vessels, but devoid of the small vessels that facilitate skin graft survival. For this reason, it is preferable to perform a delayed skin graft. The full use of galeal flaps has not been completely delineated, but the thinness, malleability, and reliability of this flap will recommend it for many difficult problem areas in the future.

Tissue Expanders

Tissue expanders have offered a new dimension in "creating" cutaneous flaps. They have been used in the neck, forehead, and scalp to stretch skin and allow for primary closure after flap elevation. If the expansion is undertaken slowly, i.e., over a period of 6 to 8 weeks, very few problems will be encountered. If the expansion is too rapid, skin necrosis, exposure of the implant, hair loss, or late infection may result because of tissue ischemia. Early applications of skin expanders have provided some dramatic results, in spite of the associated complications.

SUMMARY

One should have good reasons to use either a local flap or a microvascular tissue transfer. Both have favorable features and their success rate has become comparable. It is necessary to closely consider the various local flap options offered in any small or large head and neck reconstruction because of certain salutary features offered by these flaps.

REFERENCES

1. McCraw JB, Dibbell DG. Experimental definition of independent myocutaneous vascular territories. Plast Reconstr Surg 1977; 60:212.
2. McCraw JB, Dibbell DG, Carraway JH. Clinical definition of independent myocutaneous vascular territories. Plast Reconstr Surg 1977; 60:341.
3. Owens N. A compound neck pedicle designed for massive facial defects. Plast Reconstr Surg 1955; 15:369.
4. McCraw JB, Magee WP, Kalwaic H. Uses of the trapezius and sternomastoid myocutaneous flaps in head and neck reconstruction. Plast Reconstr Surg 1979; 63:49.
5. Bakamjian VY. A two-stage method for pharyngoesophageal reconstruction with a primary pectoral skin flap. Plast Reconstr Surg 1965; 36:173.
6. Mutter TC. Cases of deformity from burns, relieved by operation. Am J Med Sci 1842; 4:66.
7. Zovickian A. Pharyngeal fistulas: Repair and prevention, using mastoid-occiput based shoulder flaps. Plast Reconstr Surg 1957; 19:355.
8. Chretien PB, et al. Extended shoulder flap and its use in reconstruction of defects of the head and neck. Am J Surg 1969; 118:752.
9. Mendleson BC, Masson JK. Treatment of chronic irradiation injury over the shoulder with a latissimus dorsimyocutaneous flap. Plast Reconstr Surg 1977; 60:681.
10. Magee WP, McGraw JB, Horton CE, McInnis D. Pectoralis "paddle" myocutaneous flaps: The workhorse of head and neck reconstruction. Am J Surg 1980; 140:507.
11. Ariyan S. One-stage repair of a cervical esophagotome with two myocutaneous flaps from the neck and shoulder. Plast Reconstr Surg 1979; 63:426.
12. Ariyan S. The pectoralis major for single-stage reconstruction of the difficult wounds of the orbit and pharyngoesophagus. Plast Reconstr Surg 1983; 72:468.
13. Theogaraj SD, Merritt WH, Acharya G, Cohen IK. The pectoralis major musculotaneous island flap in single-stage reconstruction of the pharyngoesophageal region. Plast Reconstr Surg 1980; 65:267.
14. Mathes SJ, Nahai F. Muscle flap transposition with functional preservation: technical and clinical considerations. Plast Reconstr Surg 1980; 66:242.
15. Demergasso F, Piazza M. Trapezius myocutaneous flap in reconstructive surgery of the head and neck: an original technique. Am J Surg 1979; 138:533.
16. Demergasso F. Colgajo cutaneos aislado a pediculo muscular. Nueva technica reconstructiva de cavidad oral en cancer de cabeza y cullo. Actas de la Sociedad de Cirugia de Rusario, 1976.
17. McCraw JB, Penix JO, Baker JW. Repair of major defects of the chest wall and spine with latissimus dorsi flaps. Plast Reconstr Surg 1978; 62:197.
18. Bostwick J, Nahai F, Wallace JG, Vasconez LD. Sixty latissimus dorsi flaps. Plast Recontr Surg 1979; 63:31.
19. Barton FE, Spicer TE, Byrd HS. Head and neck reconstruction with the latissimus dorsi myocutaneous flap: Anatomic observations and report of 60 cases. Plast Reconstr Surg 1983; 71:199.
20. Gersuny R. Plastischer Ersatz der Wagenscheimhaut. Zentralbl Chir 1887; 14:706.
21. Futrell JW. Platysma myocutaneous flap for intraoral reconstruction. Am J Surg 1978; 136:504.
22. Golovine SS. Procede de cloture plastique de l'orbite apres l'extenteration. Arch d'opht 1898; 18:679.
23. Watson-Jones R. The repair of skull defects by a new pedicle bone-graft operation. Br Med J 1933; 1:780.
24. Conley J. Use of composite flaps containing bone for major repairs in the head and neck. Plast Reconstr Surg 1972; 49:522.
25. Kaplan I. Personal communication 1984.

PRINCIPLES OF SUCCESSFUL FREE TISSUE TRANSFER IN THE HEAD AND NECK

ROBERT D. ACLAND, M.D.

Microvascular free tissue transfer offers the advantages of immediate reconstruction of the major head and neck defect at a single procedure, using an abundance of suitably thin and highly vascularized tissue, with no conspicuous donor site scarring, no bulky pedicles, and no deliberate fistulas.[1-6] Because its tissue is so much better vascularized than the tip of a pedicled flap, a free flap heals soundly, even under highly adverse conditions.

Certainly microvascular free tissue transfer is exacting work, and the margin for any error is very small indeed. The nature of the work is generally misunderstood by those not versed and trained in it. In particular, there is still a prevalent notion that the main business of the procedure is to put two pairs of vessel ends together. The difference between putting small vessels together and successfully carrying out a microvascular free tissue transfer procedure cannot be overstressed.

This chapter describes the factors which appear to be the main determinants of success in free tissue transfer. All these factors fall within a broad, rather than narrow, conception of "surgical technique". In the account which follows, the procedure described is an intraoral free skin flap transfer, though the essential features of the method would be the same for almost any other free tissue transfer procedure.

COMBINED TWO-TEAM APPROACH

A great amount of work and a number of different skills go into a combined procedure, which involves a major head and neck cancer excision followed by a free tissue transfer reconstruction. With two surgeons working together, one on the ablation and one on the reconstruction, the work goes quickly and every part of it is done well. I regard the single-team approach as dangerous, however skilled the surgeon, because of the increase in operating time and the likelihood of serious errors due to fatigue.

The two surgeons should work together regularly. They should see the patient in joint consultation and should jointly establish an agreed plan of operation. This works better for the patient than for one surgeon to be hauled in belatedly to "fill the other surgeon's hole".

Setting Up

Use a large operating room and a double nursing team. Put the patient's head on the foot end of the table so that the surgeon can be seated when doing the small vessel work. Have a two-man microscope so that the reconstructive surgeon and his assistant can work together from opposite sides when the time comes.

Physiology for Success

Warmth and hydration are better than all the vessel dilators in the pharmacopeia. Have the room warm (75°F) and warm the table, the IV fluids, and the inspired gases. Monitor the rectal temperature and make sure it stays above 98°F. Give the patient IV fluids from 12 hours prior to surgery and maintain good hydration throughout the procedure to give a urine output above 75 ml per hour. Monitor the patient's fluid status with a PA line in high-risk cases.

Raising a Good Flap

The difference between a well-raised and poorly raised flap is the difference between success and failure.

The details of free flap anatomy are best learned by repeated dissection in the fresh cadaver. There has been much recent progress in the development of better free flap donor sites. The earlier flaps all have quite severe disadvantages: the groin flap has small, short undependable vessels; the dorsalis pedis is hard to raise and has potentially severe donor site problems; and the latissimus skin muscle flap is unduly bulky. Three recently developed flaps are better suited for head and neck reconstruction: the scapular flap,[7] the radial forearm flap,[8] and the lateral upper arm flap.[9]

In raising a flap, use meticulous hemostatic technique throughout. Expose the vessels first before marking the full outline of the flap. To mark the outline, use a pattern carefully made of suitably flexible material and trimmed so that it fits the defect exactly. Raise the flap in such a way as to include all branches of its vascular tree. Dissect out a long enough vascular pedicle so that the intended vascular connections can be made without any tension.

Choosing the Recipient Vessels

The vessels to be used in the neck and the exact sites of anastomosis must fulfill several criteria:

1. Their preservation and use must not conflict with the performance of a conscientious ablative procedure.
2. They must be healthy, i.e., free from gross atheroma and away from any site of heavy irradiation.
3. They should be accessible without a struggle.
4. They must point in such a direction that with the anastomoses complete, the vessels of the flap will not be contorted.
5. They must be of appropriate diameter for either

471

end-to-end or end-to-side anastomosis. For end-to-end anastomosis, the recipient vessel should be the same size as the flap vessel or just a little larger. When the diameter ratio of the recipient and flap vessel is above 1.5:1, our preference for end-to-

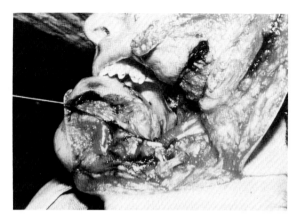

Figure 1 Excision of T3 N0M0 squamous cell cancer included partial hemimandibulectomy and resulted in a mucosal defect of 7 *mul* 5 cm, extending from the hard palate to the side of the tongue.

side anastomosis becomes strong; above 2:1, it becomes absolute.

Moving the Flap

On dividing the flap, rinse the vessel ends with heparinized Ringer's solution (20 units per ml). Under the microscope, dissect the artery and vein apart from one another so that each can go its own way without pulling on the other. Set the flap in place with a few temporary tacking sutures and carefully study the way the vessels will lie. Their comfort is most essential.

Vessel Comfort

The vessels must run from the anastomotic sites to their point of entry into the flap without compression, without tension, without kinking, and without twisting. These problems can only be foreseen and avoided by tacking the flap in its final position while the anastomoses are planned and the vessels trimmed and prepared. Once the vessel planning is complete, the tacking sutures can be undone and the flap laid

A

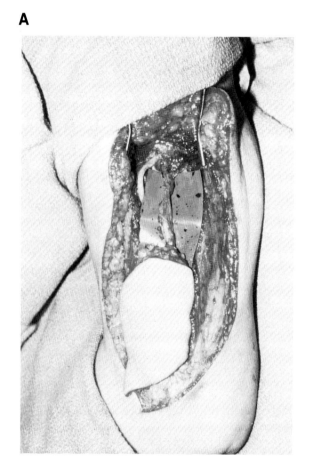

B

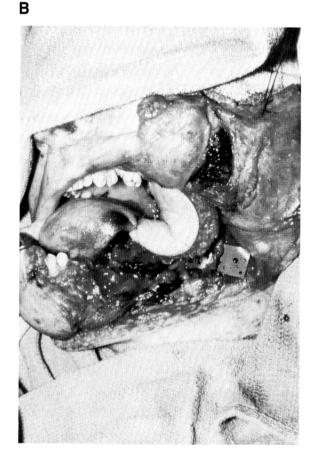

Figure 2 *A and B*, Reconstruction of defect shown in Figure 1 was done by means of a free lateral upper arm flap, tailored to the defect. The vessels were anastomosed to the superior thyroid artery and external jugular vein. (The mandible was not reconstructed). Duration of the two-team procedure was 7 hours. Postoperative hospitalization time was 11 days, with no complications.

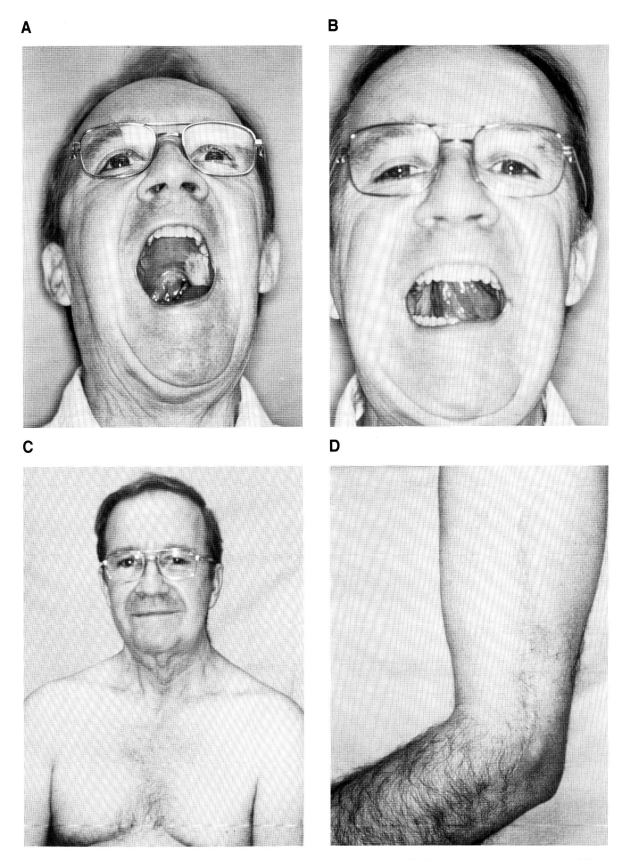

Figure 3 Postoperative result at $1^{1}/_{2}$ years (see Figs. 1 and 2). *A*, Upper one-third of the flap can be seen through patient's fully open mouth. *B*, Tongue movements are normal, and patient's speech and food handling are unimpaired. *C*, Face is almost completely symmetrical, and *D*, donor site scarring in upper arm is minimal.

loose if this will make the anastomoses themselves more convenient to perform.

Putting the Vessels Together

It is often said that microvascular anastomosis requires "good technique", but it is too seldom stressed that the "goodness" of the technique resides largely in the preparatory steps already described. The essentials of good small vessel anastomosis are precision, control, and economy of action.

Keep the operative field entirely free of blood with an indwelling sucker. Anastomose first whichever vessel lies deepest in the wound, keeping both vessels clamped until both vessels are anastomosed. Prepare each vessel well by mobilizing it, trimming the adventitia, and dilating it. For suturing, use 9-0 nylon with an effective cutting needle. In suturing, insist on seeing without question, the full thickness of each vessel wall with every stitch that is taken. Seeing clearly is the only way to make sure that the needle passes right through the full thickness of the vessel wall, including the intima, both going in and coming out. With each stitch, be sure to gain not only intimal apposition, but also a fair and equal coaptation of the circumferences of the two vessel ends.

Do not use any complex regimen of antithrombotic or anticoagulant medication. I generally use a single 300-mg rectal dose of aspirin given halfway through the procedure. I do not use heparin, dextran, or dipyridamole.

Once the clamps have been released and good perfusion of the flap is ascertained, suture the flap into place with a watertight double-layered suture closure. Make a final check on the state of flow in the flap vessels before closing the neck wound with appropriate drainage.

Postoperatively, monitor the condition of the flap by hourly checking of color and refill. Be prepared and equipped to reoperate if signs of vascular compromise develop. Monitoring techniques currently under development probably will lighten the task of postoperative monitoring in the future.

Figures 1 through 3 illustrate a typical example of a successful reconstruction by microvascular free tissue transfer.

At present, there is a widespread awareness of the potential of reconstructive microsurgery in the head and neck. Its more widespread use is still impeded in many centers by a stale "cookbook" attitude to reconstruction; by reluctance to implement a firm two-team operative approach; by reluctance to overcome time-honored interspecialty conflicts; and by failure at the institutional level to commit wholeheartedly the amounts of manpower, of operating time, and of training effort that are necessary for success.

REFERENCES

1. Acland RD. Microvascular surgery for reconstruction of the head and neck. In: Ariyan S, ed. Cancer of the head and neck. Baltimore; Williams & Wilkins, 1985.
2. Acland RD, Flynn MB. Immediate reconstruction of oral cavity defects using microvascular free flaps. Am J Surg 1978; 136:419–423.
3. MacLeod AM, Robinson DW. Reconstruction of defects involving the mandible and floor of mouth by free osteocutaneous flaps derived from the foot. Br J Plast Surg 1982; 35:239–246.
4. Reuther JF, Steinau HU, Wagner R. Reconstruction of large defects in the oropharynx with a revascularized intestinal graft: An experimental and clinical report. Plast Reconstr Surg 1984; 73:345–356.
5. Robinson DW, MacLeod A. Microvascular free jejunal transfer. Br J Plast Surg 1982; 35:258–267.
6. Zuker RM, Manktelow RT, Palmer JA, Rosen IB. Head and neck reconstruction following resection of carcinoma using microvascular free flaps. Surgery 1980; 88:461–466.
7. Barwick WJ, Goodkind DJ, Serafin D. The free scapular flap. Plast Reconstr Surg 1982; 68:779–785.
8. Soutar DS, Scheker LR, Tanner NSB, McGregor IA. The radial forearm flap: A versatile method for intraoral reconstruction. Br J Plast Surg 1983; 36:1–8.
9. Katsaros J, Schusterman M, Beppu M, Banis JC, Acland RD. The lateral upper arm flap—its anatomy and clinical applications. Ann Plast Surg 1984; 12:489–500.

FREE DEEP INFERIOR EPIGASTRIC ARTERY MUSCULOCUTANEOUS FLAP AND ITS APPLICATION TO HEAD AND NECK SURGERY

G. IAN TAYLOR, M.B., B.S.,
F.R.C.S.(Lond), F.R.A.C.S.

A plethora of local flaps is available for head and neck reconstruction following tumor resection, and these provide an adequate solution in the majority of cases. In the last decade, microsurgical techniques have introduced a one-stage method of repair with the donor scar hidden at a remote site.

Our approach has been a conservative one, and we have reserved such free transfers for situations in which (1) standard techniques have failed or (2) a superior result could be expected in a fit patient. A recent innovation, which followed extensive anatomic research in fresh cadavers, has been the free inferior rectus abdominis myocutaneous flap, designed on the deep inferior epigastric vessels.[1,3] This technique is rapid, safe, and reliable with the donor site at a distance, and may have considerable application to reconstruction of the head and neck.

Contrary to previous views, the major supply of the abdomen is from the deep inferior epigastric artery (DIEA).[1-3] This artery has an intimate relationship with the rectus abdominis muscle and, in the region of the umbilicus, provides major perforating vessels which pass directly through the muscle to reach the overlying skin. Below this level, the DIEA can be dissected from the muscle to provide a vascular pedicle 10 to 15 cm in length. The cutaneous perforators in the paraumbilical region radiate like "the spokes of a wheel" to communicate with other vessels supplying the abdominal skin. They connect with the superficial superior epigastric artery, the lateral intercostal perforators, the deep circumflex iliac artery (DCIA) perforators, the superficial circumflex iliac artery (SCIA), and the superficial inferior epigastric artery (SIEA). However, the predominant outflow is directed upward and laterally, parallel to the ribs.

A large skin flap can be designed on these perforating vessels, provided the segment of rectus muscle and its anterior sheath that contains these perforators is preserved. The pedicle can be dissected to its origin from the external iliac vessels. This flap may be raised in one stage from the groin to the anterior axillary fold. As an island it will reach the knee on the same side, the distal third of the opposite thigh, the buttocks, or the pelvic floor (Fig. 1).

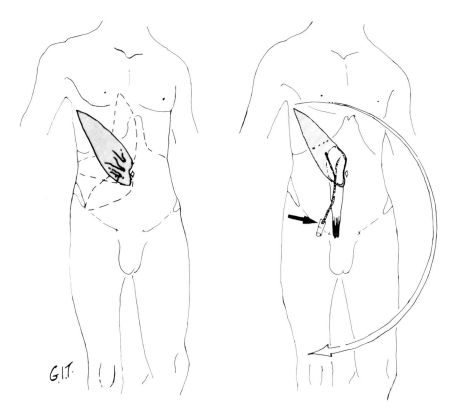

Figure 1 *Left*, The various flaps that can be based on the paraumbilical perforators of the DIEA, with the optimal flap radiating toward the inferior angle of the scapula, parallel to the ribs. *Right*, Arc of rotation of the inferior rectus abdominis thoracoumbilical flap (when dissected to the groin).

Alternatively, it may be used as a free flap, in which case it has many advantages (Fig. 2). It has a long pedicle with vessels of large diameter (the artery averages 3.4 mm, and there are always two venae comitantes which usually exceed 3 mm in diameter). Muscle may be taken alone and skin grafted at the recipient site. Alternatively the muscle can be combined with a large skin flap. Many designs are available (Fig. 3). The donor defect is minimal, and if care is taken when the graft is harvested, the anterior rectus sheath can be repaired directly in every case.

Although the superior epigastric artery (SEA) is currently in vogue for breast reconstruction, in fact the DIEA supplies a much larger vascular territory,[1,2] and this is reflected in the relative diameter of these two arteries (DIEA, 3.4 mm; SEA, 1.6 mm). The DIEA flap would appear to be the abdominal equivalent of the versatile latissimus dorsi flap.

DISSECTION OF THE GRAFT

The greatest number of major musculocutaneous perforators emerge from the rectus muscle in the paraumbilical region, especially from its middle and inner thirds.[1,2] These vessels are directed predominantly upward and laterally, and as they approach the costal margin, they connect with the lateral intercostal perforators. Because the paraumbilical perforators of the DIEA radiate like the spokes of a wheel, an axial skin flap can be designed in any direction with its base at the umbilicus. However, the longest flap is planned along a line between the umbilicus and the inferior angle of the scapula because this places the flap along the dominant vascular axis. The width of the flap is determined by the "pinch test," so that the wound can be closed directly.

The distal end of the flap is elevated first, and the areolar layer on the deep surface of the subcutaneous fat is included. This is an important anastomotic layer between the vascular territories incorporated in this flap. The flap is dissected medially until the lateral border of the rectus sheath is reached. Then it is carefully dissected from the outer third of the sheath to leave a sufficient fringe of this structure to facilitate direct repair of the donor defect. During this part of the dissection, fasciocutaneous perforators, which appear from the lateral border of the rectus muscle, are divided.

Next a disc of the rectus muscle and its sheath is isolated to preserve the cutaneous blood supply. The sheath and muscle at the upper border of the flap are divided, and the deep connections between the superior and inferior epigastric systems are ligated. The sheath is incised medially to leave a 5 to 10 mm fringe at the midline (again to aid the donor site repair). The tendinous intersection adjacent to the umbilicus is detached, and the muscle is separated easily from its posterior sheath. Next the lateral border of the rectus muscle is defined from its deep surface. The anterior sheath is divided in this region just lateral to the major skin perforators, leaving an outer fringe of rectus sheath 1 to 2 cm wide. Finally the lower part of the skin flap is divided, and the incision in the anterior rectus sheath is completed, taking care to incise the sheath above the level of the arcuate line.

This isolates the skin flap, which is now attached to the underlying muscle by a disc of the anterior sheath through which emerge the supplying perforators. This

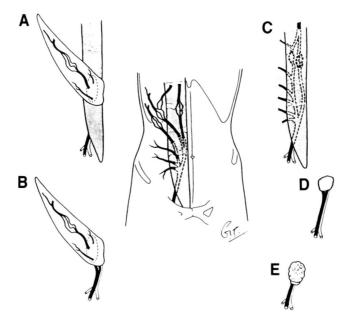

Figure 2 Diagram of several of the various combinations that we have used for free transfer, designed on the DIE system and its paraumbilical perforators. *A, B,* Myocutaneous flap with varying amounts of muscle. *C, D,* Versatile muscle flap with potential for segmental reinnervation. *E,* Myosubcutaneous flap.

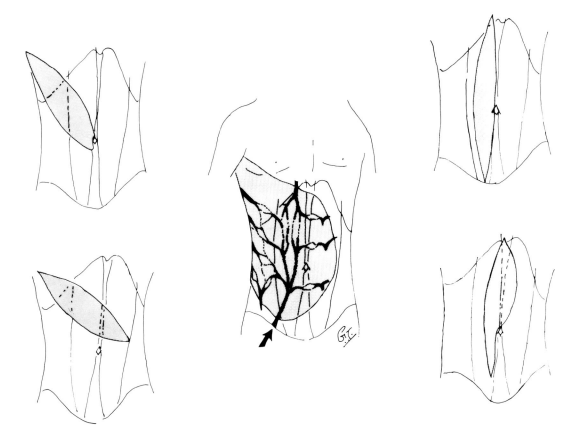

Figure 3 The clinical cutaneous vascular territory of the DIEA, (*center*) which extends via captured adjacent arterial territories to the midaxillary line laterally, superiorly to the axilla, and crosses the midline to the lateral border of the opposite rectus muscle. Several of the free skin flap designs that we have used successfully within this territory are illustrated, based on the perforators emerging through the anterior rectus sheath.

disc will be located over approximately the middle one-fifth of the length of the rectus muscle.

The pedicle is dissected last. This can be achieved through a paramedian incision, but we usually employ a transverse suprapubic (lipectomy) incision to isolate the pedicle. The anterior abdominal skin is then elevated from the muscle layers to join the upper dissection. A longitudinal incision is made in the anterior rectus sheath, and the muscle is dissected from its confines. The DIEA and its paired venae comitantes are found plastered to the undersurface of the muscle.

Near the pelvis, the DIE vessels diverge laterally toward the external iliac vessels. Most of the rectus muscle, except the disc through which the skin perforators course, can be discarded or left in situ. This requires a careful dissection of the pedicle with ligation of multiple branches. Nevertheless, it does provide a large skin flap with a small amount of muscle and a very long pedicle of 10 to 15 cm.

Alternatively, the muscle can be retained in the flap and simply filleted from its sheath. This latter method is a very quick and simple dissection.

Closure of the anterior rectus sheath above the arcuate line may be unnecessary. However, as an added precaution to prevent abdominal herniation, we have preserved a cuff of the anterior sheath, both medially and laterally, which has allowed us to restore its integrity in every case. As another precaution, we suture the anterior and posterior sheaths together at the arcuate line.

CONCLUSION

The rectus abdominis myocutaneous flap based on the deep inferior epigastric artery is an extremely versatile flap for use as either an island or a free flap. It is a speedy, simple, and safe procedure. There is a minimal donor site defect, especially if the anterior rectus sheath is repaired as described. This flap may be used to provide muscle only, as a myosubcutaneous flap, or as a large skin flap with a variable amount of muscle. The flap has a long pedicle with large vessels which are ideal for microvascular anastomosis.

In a series of over 40 patients, of whom 6 underwent this procedure on the face, the success rate has been 100 percent with an average operating time of $4^{1}/_{4}$ hours.

Disadvantages are those of a bulky graft in an obese patient and the possible onset of a late hernia. However, to date this latter problem has not occurred.

REFERENCES

1. Taylor, GI, Corlett RJ, Boyd JB. The extended deep inferior epigastric flap: a clinical technique. Plast Reconstr Surg 1983; 72:751.

2. Boyd JB, Taylor GI, Corlett RJ. The vascular territories of the superior epigastric and deep inferior epigastric systems. Plast Reconstr Surg 1984; 73:1.

3. Taylor GI, Corlett RJ, Boyd JB. The versatile deep inferior epigastric (inferior rectus abdominus) flap. Br J Plast Surg 1984; 37:330.

RADIAL FOREARM FLAP

IAN A. McGREGOR, Ch.M., F.R.C.S.

The radial forearm flap is a fasciocutaneous flap raised on the flexor aspect of the forearm which uses as its vascular basis the radial arteriovenous system, supplemented on occasion by a local superficial vein. The flap, used in intraoral reconstruction,[1] is transferred en bloc to the recipient site inside the mouth, and the vessels are anastomosed to suitable vessels in the vicinity. The secondary defect is split-thickness skin grafted. The flap is described as fasciocutaneous on the basis of the anatomic details of its blood supply.

ANATOMIC BASIS OF THE FLAP

The island that is transferred consists of skin, superficial fascia, and the investing layer of deep fascia (Fig. 1). It may be noted in passing that bone, a segment of radius, can be included in the transfer, but this extention of the method will not be considered in this paper. From the investing layer of the deep fascia, the radial artery and its venae comitantes are suspended by what is a virtual mesentery of deep fascia, which at the same time is acting as an intermuscular septum between brachioradialis and flexor carpi radialis. The muscles all around are supplied from a large number of small arteries and veins which are branching from the parent vessels. From these vessels many small arteries and veins also pass superficially to form a plexus on both the superficial and deep surfaces of the investing layer of fascia. It is from this plexus that the skin and superficial fascia are perfused. Venous drainage appears to be dual, both superficial veins and venae comitantes providing a pathway. An Allen test is invariably carried out to confirm the adequacy of the ulnar collateral supply.

When the flap, which has been raised under tourniquet, is ready for transfer, the radial artery and the veins can be divided according to the needs of the vascular anastomosis in the neck at any level from the brachial bifurcation to the wrist. In practice, the flap can be raised from any site on the forearm approximately overlying the vessels. In general, one avoids a hair-bearing site, although hair on the flap has not created a real problem, probably because it does not grow to a significant length.

CLINICAL USAGE AND RESULTS

It is used as a free flap transferred into the mouth, and since April 1982 we have used it in virtually all the intraoral sites (Fig. 2). Sixty patients have undergone reconstruction in this way, with a failure rate of 8 percent. At the same time, interspersed with our usage of the radial flap, we have used myocutaneous flaps when they were felt to be appropriate, mainly the pectoralis major flap. This has allowed us to make a comparative assessment between the two techniques, free flap and myocutaneous flap, using the radial forearm and the pectoralis major as representatives. We have also had sufficient experience with the main alternative free flaps, particularly dorsalis pedis and jejunal, in other roles, to make a valid comparison of the three free flaps. Clearly the two methods—free flap and myocutaneous flap—are not really in competition. Their roles in intraoral reconstruction are quite different.

It is not really feasible to use a pectoralis major flap unless a radical neck dissection has been carried out as part of the resection. A functional neck dissection which leaves sternocleidomastoid intact does not leave enough room for the muscle pedicle without compressing it in the neck. The skin paddle itself may be bulkier than is ideal in reconstructing certain defects, displacing the oral structures, tongue and fauces

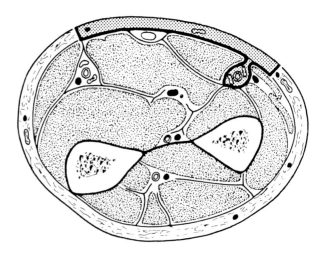

Figure 1 Transverve section of the forearm, showing the vascular basis of the radial forearm flap.

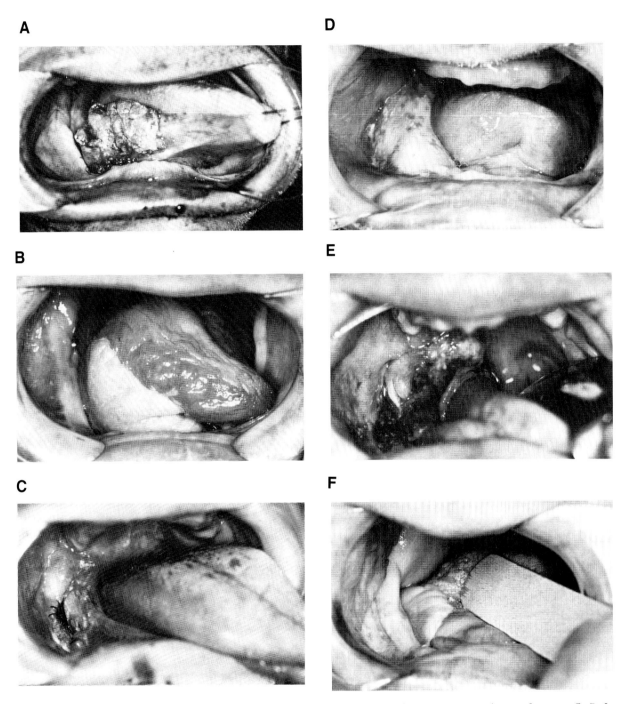

Figure 2 Examples of the use of the radial forearm flap in clinical practice. *A, B,* In a squamous carcinoma of tongue. *C, D,* In a squamous carinoma of retromolar trigone. *E, F,* In a squamous carcinoma of fauces extending medially onto the posterior third of the tongue and laterally onto the retromolar trigone.

for example, and producing dysphagia. Occasionally, however, the bulk of a myocutaneous flap is needed to fill a defect, and in such a situation it shows up particularly well. When mandible has been resected, the myocutaneous flap is excellent, but an intact mandible is less likely to leave a defect into which the flap can fit readily. It is then that the radial flap shows its virtues, with its thinness and its capacity to drape

itself over an irregular surface such as the tongue, floor of the mouth, lower alveolus, and fauces. It has been remarkable how well it sits into the defect, how quickly speech and swallowing have been restored, and how little there is in the way of flap contraction, early or late.

Viewed in relation to its free flap competitors, it has clear-cut advantages. Compared with the dorsalis pedis flap, the qualities of the tissue tranferred are approximately similar, but comparison of the donor sites shows up the deficiencies of the dorsalis pedis flap. It leaves a defect which prevents the patient from being mobilized early, quite apart from its other undesirable characteristics. The jejunal free flap involves an abdominal operation, and this must add markedly to the magnitude of the procedure, although the flap is otherwise a good one.

In contrast to both these flaps, the donor site of the radial forearm flap allows the patient to be mobilized quickly, and in the long term no disability has accrued to any of the patients from this aspect. In the short term, take of the graft has presented occasional problems, but in no patient has this resulted in a functional deficit.

It is routine for our patients to receive a full elective course of radiotherapy within 6 weeks of the resection-reconstruction, and the flap has tolerated this without ill effect. In sum we believe that it has significant advantages over the alternative free flaps, and that with proper patient selection it has a role which dovetails nicely with the myocutaneous flaps.

REFERENCES

1. Soutar DS, Scheker LR, Tanner NSB, McGregor IA. The radial forearm flap. Br J Plast Surg 1983; 36:1.

34. Reanimation of the Paralyzed Face

INTRODUCTION

IAN A. McGREGOR, Ch.M., F.R.C.S.

One fact that emerges from discussions of facial reanimation is that, judged by any objective standards, the results that are generally achieved remain considerably short of normality. Given the complexity of the problem, this is perhaps inevitable, but it does reflect the amount of knowledge still to be elucidated before we can improve these results.

In the face there is a mixture of movement patterns that are unique to that site. There is a pattern of voluntary movements, which generally involve one side of the face only, and a pattern of involuntary movements, which constantly reflect our emotional changes and are bilateral and symmetrical, the movements of one side a mirror image of the other. In their voluntary activity, the facial muscles and the nerve pathways that serve them are similar to the muscles and nerves elsewhere in the body. But in their emotional activity, the facial muscles are unique. No other muscle group has a comparable capacity. We assume that the peripheral nerve pathway is the facial nerve, since no alternative pathway appears to exist, but the central connections are certainly totally distinct since the distinction between the two forms of muscle function becomes so apparent when the muscles are reanimated after a facial palsy. Voluntary activity may be restored extremely effectively, but the emotional play of expression, normally bilateral and symmetrical, remains confined to the normal side. One must assume that the failure is central rather than peripheral, though the exact mechanism is totally unknown. Obviously it is not something that is amenable to re-education, though one wonders whether a child in the same clinical situation could be reeducated more effectively, given the known functional plasticity of the central nervous system in the young person.

In the adult, of course, a degree of reeducation does occur; witness the dissociation of tongue and facial movements that slowly develops after facial-hypoglossal anastomosis. However, this reeducation is confined to voluntary activity and falls short of achieving emotional movement patterns.

In facial palsy, the emphasis has passed from static fascial slings, with their limited objective of achieving resting symmetry, to efforts to achieve movement as well as symmetry, by restoring nerve continuity with suture or graft where possible, or by transfer of another nerve, usually the hypoglossal. Recourse has also been made to the transfer of muscles served by the trigeminal nerve, temporalis and masseter, but in the adult, adjustment involves a switch to a totally new and unnatural pattern of activity, and this limits the effectiveness of the methods in restoring normality. More recently, free muscle grafts have been tried, with a total lack of success, and the cross-facial nerve graft, which promised so much, has proved in most hands a virtually complete failure. At present, the way forward seems to be along the lines of transferring vascularized muscle, subsequently reinnervated to restore movement. The muscles used to date have not proved altogether satisfactory; failure to match the facial muscle patterns, even of voluntary movement, have resulted in mass movements rather than the refined patterns that characterize normality.

In sum, the current position remains a disappointing one. One hopes that refinements of technique, in muscle selection, and in adjusting nerve suture or graft to take better account of intraneural topography may yield better results one day. And beyond these lie the problem of restoring emotional muscle activity, a task that we have scarcely begun to tackle.

REANIMATION OF THE PARALYZED FACE: NERVE CROSSOVER, CROSS-FACE NERVE GRAFTING, AND MUSCLE TRANSFERS

DANIEL C. BAKER, M.D.

Patterns of facial paralysis vary in degree of involvement and duration, and no single surgical method can restore a complex combination of axonal and muscular degeneration. Careful preoperative selection of patients based on sound judgment of what can and cannot be achieved by the proposed surgical technique is paramount to a successful operation and a satisfied patient. A multiple or combined surgical approach often yields maximum results. The fact that the totally paralyzed face can never be made normal by any of the current methods of reconstruction does not detract from the measured and recognized success of these techniques.

NERVE GRAFTING

Nerve grafting is one of the most significant advances in the rehabilitation of the paralyzed face and in the treatment of malignant tumors of the parotid gland. It is applicable when there is a loss of the main trunk of the facial nerve or of the peripheral facial nerve system. It is obvious that if the ablation extends into the internal auditory meatus medially it is technically unrealistic to attempt to anastomose a nerve graft to the proximal stump as part of an extracranial technique without appropriate neurosurgical preparation. If the distal part of the facial nerve system and its muscle bed is ablated in a radical technique involving the mimetic muscles, then peripheral nerve anastomosis would be unrealistic and another concept of rehabilitation would have to be used. The majority of ablative procedures dealing with cancer of the parotid gland, and some traumatic and iatrogenic circumstances, lend themselves ideally to free autogenous nerve grafting. Again, the best time to carry out nerve anastomosis under these circumstances is at the time of the primary operation.

The usual donor areas are the sensory branches of the cervical plexus, with a segment of nerve containing four or five branches (Fig. 1). This graft is approximated to the proximal facial nerve stump with 8–0 to 10–0 atraumatic monofilament suture material. The peripheral branches are usually approximated with one suture. There is no question but that magnification with loupes or the dissecting microscope increases the precision of nerve approximation. Many of these grafts, however, have been placed without the aid of magnification with excellent return of function. The nerve graft is generous in length, thus eliminating any possibility of tension on the suture line. The suture line is encased in a soft nonconstrictive silicone tube, 1 cm long. All of these wounds must be drained.

When the foregoing criteria are applied, one can expect some degree of movement in the face in 95 percent of the cases. The first signs of return of movement appear in the cheek and about the commissure

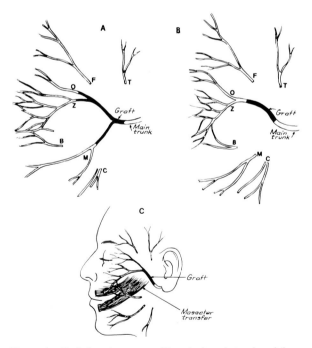

Figure 1 Variations in nerve grafting. *A*, A main trunk and three peripheral branches. *B*, A single graft is interposed between the main trunk and the dominant peripheral division (this can be confirmed by electrical testing on the operating table). Good return of movement could still be anticipated with this single graft because of numerous interconnections with other divisions of the facial nerve. *C*, If a single graft is used, we usually combine reconstruction with an immediate masseter muscle transposition. This immediately rehabilitates the lips and commissure and creates an ideal situation for myoneurotization.

of the mouth. The interval of time is from 6 to 12 months, depending upon the length of the graft, the accuracy of the anastomosis, and the volume of regenerating axons. The tone of the face during this interval is better than one would expect in a paralyzed face, and many individuals do not require an elective tarsorrhaphy. The movement spreads from the middle third of the face into the cheek and about the orbit. The forehead and platysma movement usually do not return. Improvement in tone, movement, and coordination continues for another 2 years. The movement is always weaker than that on the normal side. It is basically mass movement in character, and it exhibits varying degrees of dyskinesia. The natural response to emotional expression on the paralyzed side of the face is markedly limited, but can be improved by persistent training and awareness.

NERVE CROSSOVERS

Nerve crossovers employing the glossopharyngeal, accessory, and hypoglossal nerves, as well as the phrenic nerve, have been used for over 50 years. These techniques generally are used when direct suture or grafting is not feasible, as in the case of an obliterated central facial nerve segment with intact peripheral nerve segments and adequate mimetic muscles. They are particularly applicable to facial paralysis resulting from intracranial lesions or disorders of the temporal bone.

Nerve crossover techniques are advantageous in that they are simple, require only a single suture line, and serve as a powerful source of reinnervation. All of these techniques have been severely criticized because they result in associated and uncoordinated movements as well as in loss of function of the donor nerve. However, extensive clinical experience has demonstrated that many of these criticisms are overemphasized, particularly with regard to the hypoglossal-facial nerve crossover, which is the most popular crossover operation in use today.

Our experience with 137 cases of hypoglossal nerve crossover used for various causes of facial paralysis yielded the following results: 22 percent of patients had minimal atrophy of the tongue, 53 percent had moderate atrophy, and 25 percent had severe atrophy.[1] Patients who had hypoglossal nerve crossover performed immediately as part of the ablative procedure were much more satisfied than those who had delayed crossover. Perhaps because of their overriding concern about the success of their cancer program, patients in the "immediate" group complained very little about the interference with chewing, swallowing, and speaking. Only 3 percent complained about mastication; 2 percent, about swallowing; and 2 percent, about speech.

Ninety-five percent of all patients had some type and quality of movement, and 77 percent in the "immediate" group were classified as good, as opposed to 41 percent in the delayed group (Fig. 2). In patients with good return of movement, about 15 percent had hypertonia with overproduction of movement with eating, swallowing, and talking. Some patients were able to develop and refine this movement to obtain normal smiling and involuntary closing of the eye.

Hypoglossal nerve crossover is an extremely valuable technique, particularly when it is used as an integral part of the primary ablative operation for regional cancer. It provides excellent facial tone and normal appearance at rest, allows for protection of the eye, and permits intentional movement of the face controlled by movements of the tongue. Its disadvantages include minimal to moderate intraoral dysfunction, mass movement, and occasional hypertonia in the face (particularly in association with the act of chewing). The hypoglossal nerve crossover technique is not used to treat moderate general facial paresis, segmental paralysis, or regional paralysis.

CROSS-FACE NERVE GRAFTING

The newest crossover technique was introduced by Scaramella in 1970 at the Second International Symposium on Facial Nerve Surgery. Scaramella presented a case in which the intact buccal ramus on the nonparalyzed side had been sutured to the paralyzed stem of the facial nerve with a sural nerve graft. This technique has been further expanded and developed by Anderl,[2] Fisch,[3] Freilinger,[4] Samii,[5] and Smith.[6] The procedure is based on cross innervation from the nonparalyzed to the paralyzed side by means of sural nerve grafts that connect the reservoir of peripheral healthy facial nerve fascicles to the corresponding branches of specific muscle groups on the paralyzed side (Fig. 3). The Millesi technique of fascicular repair is used. The lengths of grafts vary from 6 to 18 cm. Anderl favors a two-staged procedure, allowing the nerve axons to grow to the opposite side and then resecting the neuroma to demonstrate success of axon growth before suturing the graft to the paralyzed side.[2] Smith and Samii, on the other hand, repair both junctures simultaneously, claiming good results.[5-6] There is also disagreement about whether reversal of the nerve graft will ensure that all axons entering tubules on the innervated side will present to the opposite end of the graft, or whether nonreversal permits axon outgrowth and neurotization through nerve branches along the way.

The concept of cross-face nerve grafting is ingenious, and its theoretical advantage is facial reanimation through specific nerve branches to specific mimetic muscle groups. The primary disadvantage, however, aside from the need for specialized techniques and long operating times, is the period required for return of function. The facial muscles undergo further atrophy during the time that is required for axonal growth through the long nerve grafts. Technical difficulties have been encountered in identifying the distal branches of the facial nerve because of the intimate plexus formation with the trigeminal

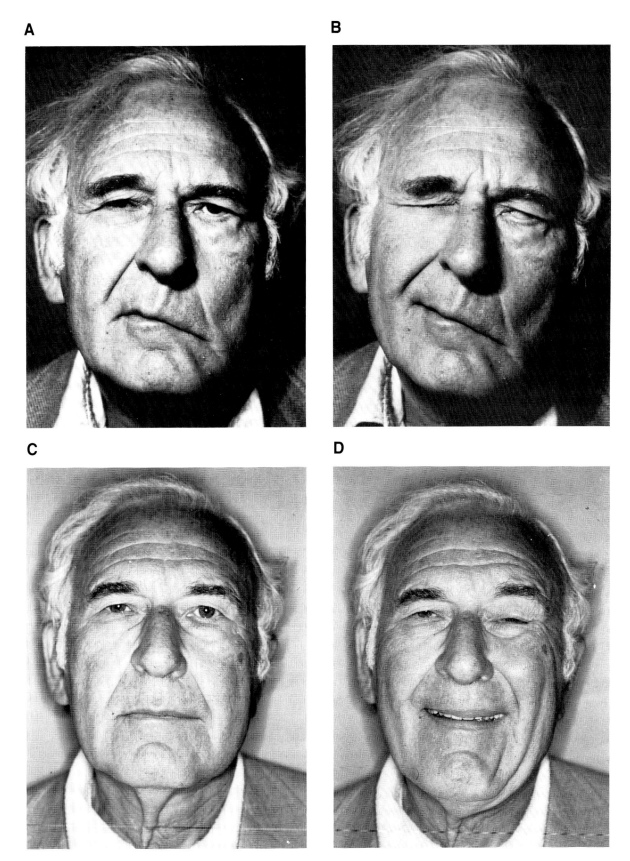

Figure 2   Complete paralysis one year after removal of an acoustic neuroma. The facial nerve did not respond to electrical testing. *A*, Preoperative view of the face in repose. *B*, Smiling and closing the eyes preoperatively. *C*, One year after a XII-VII nerve anastomosis, the face is normal in repose. *D*, Excellent movement mimicking a smile. Note the return of the frontal branch.

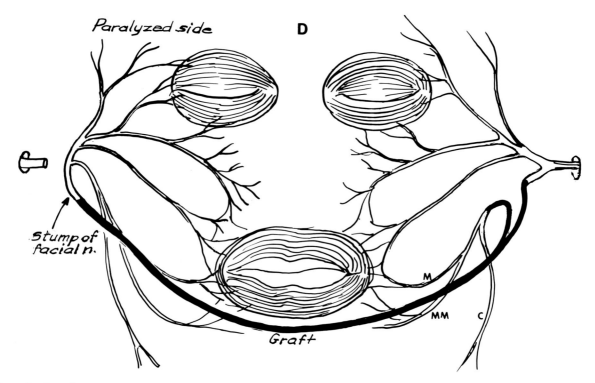

Paralyzed side   D

Stump of facial n.

Graft

M
MM   C

Figure 3   Cross-face nerve graft. My preferred technique is to anastomose the entire lower division of the normal side with the main trunk of the paralyzed side. Exposure is easily obtained with standard parotid incisions. The graft may be passed over the upper lip.

nerve, which varies considerably and cannot be standardized. Suturing of the sensory nerve branches of the infraoribital, buccal, zygomaticofacial, and mental nerves to branches of the facial nerve has been reported. Perhaps the greatest disadvantage of this technique, as noted by Samii[5] and Anderl,[2] is that only 50 percent of all nerve fibers of the facial nerve can be used from the normal side, and these are joined to about 50 percent on the paralyzed side, thereby limiting the amount of axonal input.

Samii reported on 10 such patients, five of whom showed symmetrical position of the face in repose, while one demonstrated good facial movement and the others showed some degree of movement.[5] One patient showed no evidence of reinnervation. Anderl reported on 15 patients, five of whom demonstrated good symmetry with some degree of movement.[2]

The present consensus is that the cross-face nerve graft is an alternative to accessory and hypoglossal nerve crossover and muscle interdigitation. In any case in which direct repair or grafting of the facial nerve is possible, there is no indication for this technique. The alternative of performing an immediate hypoglossal nerve crossover to restore tone and maintain muscular bulk and then to consider a cross-face nerve graft for more controlled facial movement is being studied. A further application consists of reinnervating a free muscle graft and combining a cross-face nerve graft with masseter and temporalis transposition.

MUSCLE TRANSFERS

Transfer of muscle to the paralyzed face is usually done under three circumstances: (1) in the absence of mimetic muscles following longstanding atrophy, (2) as an adjunct to the mimetic muscles to provide new muscle and myoneurotization, and (3) occasionally in combination with a nerve graft or crossover implanted in the transposed muscle. Although most of the available muscles about the head and neck have been transposed in whole or in part, by far the most popular muscle transposition techniques involve the masseter and temporalis.

The basic technique of masseter transfer was first delineated by Lexer in 1908 and is still used today. However, Lexer's original description of the procedure entailed rotating the anterior half of the muscle, a step that would introduce the possibility of transecting the nerve supply, as demonstrated by Correia and Zani. This muscle is ideally suited to give motion to the lower half of the face; commonly, three separate muscle slips are sutured to the dermis of the lower lip, oral commissure, and upper lip (Fig. 4). Overcorrection should be accomplished; if some mimetic muscles remain, the slips can be interdigitated with them. Postoperative immobilization and a liquid diet should be instituted for about 10 days to allow for healing. Chewing is then gradually begun, after which the patient is taught to practice control of facial move-

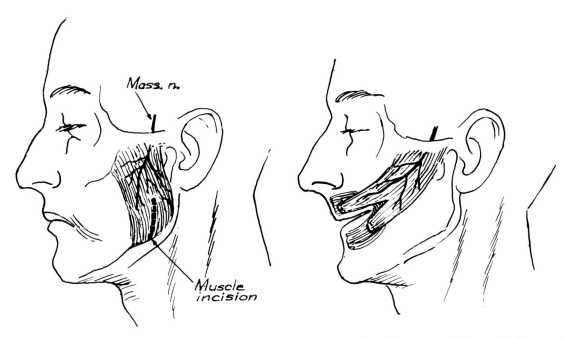

Figure 4 Transferring the entire masseter muscle. *Left*, Incision need only be several centimeters to avoid damage to the nerve. *Right*, Anterior portion of the muscle is sutured to the orbicularis oris and to the dermis anterior to the melolabial fold. The posterior portion of the muscle is sutured to the lower lip and commissure.

ments before a mirror. Masseter transfer has proved to be a valuable technique in certain cases of radical parotidectomy in which a nerve graft did not prove advantageous. Transposing the masseter with interdigitation into the freshly denervated mimetic muscles provides for maximum myoneurotization of all of the muscles in the middle third of the face (Fig. 5).

In facial rehabilitation, the temporalis muscle has enjoyed more popularity than has the masseter be-

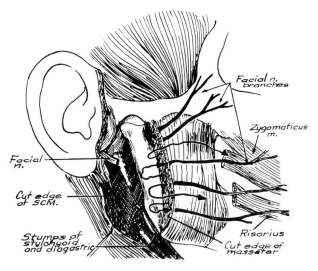

Figure 5 Representation of ideal circumstances for myoneurotization. Freshly denervated mimetic muscles (vascular supply intact) come in contact with transposed masseter muscle (neurovascular supply intact). Raw, living muscle is interdigitated with raw living muscle.

cause of its position, its facility for greater excursion of movement, and its adaptability to the orbit. Numerous ingenous techniques using various slings about the orbit and mouth have been described, as has been transposition of the muscle insertion with the coronoid process to the middle third of the face. The technique that is now most widely employed involves transfer and suturing of the muscle with its fascial extensions to the eyelids, the ala of the nose, the oral commissure, and the upper and lower lips (Fig. 6). The depression in the temporal area can be corrected by inserting a carved block of soft silicone. Although Rubin has indicated that the muscle is not long enough to go down to the face or reach the medial canthus without the fascial attachment,[7] the full muscle can be taken without difficulty to the canthi and commissure with a border of epicranium and suture slips.[8] This technique has several advantages, one of which is that the muscle provides bulk in the severely atrophic face. There is also direct muscular insertion on the structures to be moved. Finally, the possibility of myoneurotization is enhanced.

Because the impulse for muscle movement in temporalis and masseter transfers originates from the trigeminal nerve, facial movement is not physiologic. A facial nerve graft with nerve implantation into the transposed muscle to achieve specific innervation from the facial nerve can therefore be performed. Cross-face nerve grafts wiht muscle implantation have also been done, as have cross-face nerve grafts to the masseteric nerve at the foramen ovale. The results of these procedures have not yet been sufficiently evaluated to justify their routine use.

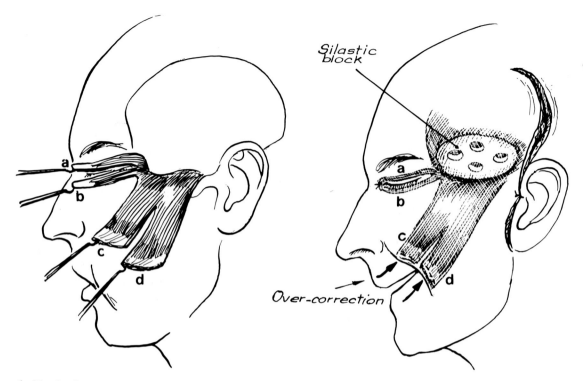

Figure 6 Muscle slips are transposed to upper and lower eyelids, upper lip and melolabial fold, lower lip and commissure. Over-correction is essential. The muscle should be sutured anterior to the melolabial fold and interdigitated with the orbicularis oris muscle in the upper lip.

In 1971, Thompson reported on the successful transplantation of free autogenous muscle grafts in humans, and in 1974 he established its clinical application in the treatment of unilateral facial paralysis.[9,10] Since then, other investigators have reported success with free muscle grafts. According to Thompson, the success of this procedure depends on three factors:[10] (1) the muscle belly selected for transplantation must be denervated 14 days prior to transplantation, (2) a full length of the muscle fiber must be preserved, and (3) the denervated muscle must be placed in direct contact with normal, fully innervated, and vascularized skeletal muscle at the recipient site before neurotization can occur. Thus a minimum of two operations is required, with an interval of 14 days between them. The technique consists of placing denervated muscle in contact with normal muscle on the nonparalyzed side of the face. The transplanted muscle tendon is then sutured to the appropriate area to obtain movement (e.g., the zygomatic arch for the oral sphincter and the lateral canthal tendon for the eye sphincter).

Thompson reports that of 54 patients treated for oral sphincter reconstruction, 90 percent had good results and 10 percent showed satisfactory improvement.[9,10] Seventeen percent of these 54 patients required another surgical procedure to tighten the tendon sling. In the reconstruction of paralyzed eyelids of 62 patients, 48 percent had good results and 45 percent had satisfactory results. Secondary operations to adjust tension or perform tenolysis were required in 22 percent of these 62 patients. The advantage of this technique is that movement is controlled by the normal side of the face.

In spite of the successful reports of Thompson[9,10] and Hakelius,[11] considerable skepticism exists about the reproducibility of free muscle grafting for reconstructive surgery. Watson's attempt to reproduce Thompson's experiments in dogs proved unsuccessful, and it is still uncertain which factors are responsible for the survival of free muscle grafts. In addition to this uncertainty, as well as reports that grafts have become fibrotic, other disadvantages include the multiple stages required, the high incidences of reoperation, and the intrusion on the nonparalyzed side of the face.

REFERENCES

1. Conley J, Baker DC. Hypoglossal-facial nerve anastomosis for reinnervation of the paralyzed face. Plast Reconstr Surg 1979; 63:63–72.
2. Anderl A (Moderator). Panel discussion No. 6: Rehabilitation of the face by VIIth nerve substitution. In: Fisch U, ed. Facial nerve surgery. Birmingham: Aesculapius Publishing Co, 1977:234.
3. Fisch U. Facial nerve grafting. Otolaryngol Clin North Am 1974; 7:517–529.
4. Freilinger G. A new technique to correct facial paralysis. Plast Reconstr Surg 1975; 56:44–48.
5. Samii M (Participant). Panel discussion No. 6: Rehabilitation of the face by VIIth nerve substitution. In: Fisch U, ed. Facial nerve surgery. Birmingham: Aesculapius Publishing Co, 1977:234.

6. Smith JW. A new technique for facial animation. In: Transactions of the Fifth International Congress of Plastic and Reconstructive Surgeons. Australia: Butterworths, 1971:125–138
7. Rubin L. The Moebius syndrome: Bilateral facial diplegia. Clin Plast Surg 1976; 3:625–636.
8. Baker DC, Conley J. Regional muscle transposition for rehabilitation of the paralyzed face. Clin Plast Surg 1979; 6:317–331.
9. Thompson N. Autogenous free grafts of skeletal muscle: A preliminary experimental and clinical study. Plast Reconstr Surg 1971; 48:11–27.
10. Thompson N. A review of autogenous skeletal muscle grafts and their clinical applications. Clin Plast Surg 1974; 1:349–403.
11. Hakelius L. Free muscle grafting. Clin Plast Surg 1979; 6:301–316.

OPTIMAL FACIAL REANIMATION SURGERY

ROGER L. CRUMLEY, M.D.

A myriad of surgical procedures has been introduced for rehabiliation of the paralyzed face. The objectives of all these procedures are quite similar, namely, restoration of meaningful facial movement with the establishment of symmetry during repose and all facial movements. However, once the facial nerve is transected, a symmetrical nonsynkinetic facial dynamism is not possible.

Consequently, the surgeon must be a knowledgeable neurophysiologist with respect to muscular paralysis and reinnervation phenomena so that he or she can best use the existing nerves and muscles in any given patient. Within this framework, I offer here a brief review of our facial reanimation protocol for consideration by the practicing head and neck surgeon.

Procedures which we feel have not found universal usage are not included in the protocol, but are mentioned for purposes of discussion. Patients are divided into three classes based on the presence of proximal and distal facial nerve segments (relative to the site of injury) and the presence or absence of muscles of facial expression.

CLASS I: Facial Muscles Present; Healthy Proximal Facial Nerve Present. In this group of patients, an attempt should be made to connect the viable proximal facial nerve with the facial muscles. Depending on the distal segment of the nerve, a variety of different methods may be used.

If a distal segment of facial nerve is present, a cable graft from a healthy section of proximal nerve, traversing the site of injury to connect with the healthy distal nerve, will provide a healthy milieu for regeneration into the distal stump and the facial muscles. If a patient is elderly, diabetic, suffering from malnutrition, or has been irradiated, the chances for success with this technique fall somewhat below that in the healthy subject.

When the distal facial nerve segment has been removed, as for parotid malignancy, it is often possible to route the distal end of the nerve graft directly to the most important facial muscles. In that regard the levator labii superioris, orbicularis oculi, zygomaticus major, and zygomaticus minor are thought to be the four most important facial muscles for purposes of reanimation. The distal end of the nerve graft can be implanted directly into these important midfacial muscles for neurotization.

Determination of facial muscle viability is most important. If less than 18 months has elapsed since injury, the facial muscles can be assumed to be viable (nondegenerated). If more time has elapsed, electromyography should be used to elucidate the viability of the muscles to be reinnervated, e.g., to prove that they have not undergone denervation atrophy.

CLASS II: Facial Muscles and Distal Facial Nerve Segment Intact; Proximal Facial Nerve Nonviable or Otherwise Unavailable for Grafting (e.g., Following Extensive Temporal Bone Surgery or Acoustic Neuroma). In this class the facial nerve will not regenerate satisfactorily to produce meaningful facial movement. As there is no innervation to the facial muscles from the ipsilateral facial nerve, a foreign nerve must be used if the muscles are to resume their contractile properties.

In this regard, it is my opinion that nerve transfer to reinnervate existing facial muscles is always preferred to muscle transfer, muscle grafting, or adynamic sling procedures. Only the existing muscles offer any chance for muscular movements to match to contralateral normal side. Accordingly, a temporalis muscle transfer and gracilis free flap muscle transfer, are *not* the operations of choice in this group of patients.

The procedure with the least donor dysfunction and the best postoperative results is that of hypoglossal-facial anastomosis. The large New York series of Conley and Baker has proved the relative insignificance of the donor defect produced by transection of one hypoglossal nerve.[1] A multitude of patients has confirmed that meaningful and strong facial movements are usually the result of this technique. Stennart's research has shown the similarity of some neural connections of the facial and the hypoglossal nerves to further confirm the physiologic basis for this operative procedure.[2] Experimental data from our institution have shown that most animals, including primates, are capable of central nervous system "plasticity" following nerve injury or transfer. This exciting principle may help us understand how patients can learn, at the involuntary level, how to integrate facial movements induced by nerve transfer, such as in hypoglossal-facial anastomosis. More importantly, it may ultimately elucidate techniques, exercises, or drugs that promote this neurologic neointegration.

When certain portions of the face remain innervated, it is possible to route all or a portion of the hypoglossal nerve to the denervated or paralyzed portions by means of hypoglossal-branch anastomosis or fascicular dissection within the pes anserinus. Combinations of hypoglossal facial anastomosis with facial nerve grafting and/or masseter transfer provide other possibilities for regional nonsynkinetic movement.

CLASS III: Muscles of Facial Expression Degenerated and/or Atrophic.

In this setting it matters not whether the proximal nerve is intact, as it has no distal end-organ to which it may be routed. No neural anastomosis or transfer of another nerve to the distal facial nerve will produce movement of the absent facial muscles. If tone at rest and elevation of an oral commissure is all that is desired, fascial suspension may effect the desired result. This approach might be used in the elderly patient or one with a short life expectancy.

However, in most instances it is possible and preferable to transfer muscle into the facial soft tissues to promote elevation of the oral commissure, movement in the cheek region stimulating smiling movements, and eye closure. A host of procedures have been proposed and discussed, but since the objective of this communication is a simplified protocol, the two most effective procedures in most surgeons' hands are described—masseter transfer and temporalis transfer.[3]

Determination of this class is based on the history and EMG findings. Generally, if the patient's facial muscles have been paralyzed longer than 2 years or if the electromyogram can find no voluntary, fibrillation, or other electrical myogenic potentials, the muscles can be assumed to be atrophic or otherwise absent. There is usually concomitant fat atrophy along with the muscular atrophy in such cases, and bidigital palpation reveals the buccal mucosa to be in close proximity to the overlying skin, with little interposed soft tissue.

In this situation the masseter muscle transfer provides expeditious and meaningful facial movement to the paralyzed oral sphincter and cheek region. The masseter operation can be done externally or intraorally. Although the latter approach avoids one of the external incisions, it is technically more difficult and less controllable. Consequently the external approach via a parotidectomy or rhytidoplasty incision is preferred. The muscle is detached at the undersurface of the mandible, being careful to transfer the mandibular periosteum with the muscle. The entire muscle belly is translocated anteriorly, avoiding the masseteric nerve supply coming from the sigmoid notch above. Overcorrection in pulling the oral commissure posteriorly is always necessary to achieve the desired end result

after 6 to 12 months. The masseter slips are sutured with 3–0 Mersiline or 4–0 Nylon interrupted sutures to the soft tissues of the oral commissural region.[4]

The masseter pull is largely posterior, and hence the oral commissure does not rotate superiorly. Thus in certain settings the temporalis procedure is preferred. It has been my experience, however, that of the two muscle transfers, the masseter approach is quicker and more dependable. The longer and thinner temporalis muscle has a tendency to stretch and to require more overcorrection, and also seems to have more undesirable effects such as bulging over the zygomatic arch and unnatural movements in the upper face.

One unmistakable advantage of the temporalis procedure, however, is its ability to rehabilitate the orbicularis oculi muscle in effecting eye closure.

When the temporalis is transposed, the entire muscle belly is turned downward, and the lateral temporalis fascia is sutured to the distal portion of the muscle. This fascia arises from the muscle's lateral (superficial) surface and superior border, which becomes inferior or distal to the muscle following transfer. While the assistant holds the oral commissure in a grossly overcorrected position, the surgeon ensures that the muscle slips and fascia are tightly approximated. The fascial strips are then sutured in and around the oral commissure with the same sutures described for the masseter procedure.

For the paralyzed orbicularis oculi, the strips are passed through subcutaneous tunnels in each eyelid and attached to the tendinous attachment of the medial canthal ligament. A lateral canthoplasty or tightening of the lateral canthal ligament sometimes improves eyelid closure when combined with this technique.[5,6]

CROSS-FACE NERVE GRAFT

Originally touted as the panacea for all facial paralysis, this operative approach has not withstood the test of time. Many authors have abandoned the approach (notably Conley) despite its ingenuity and theoretic potential for emotional rehabilitation.

Harii[7] and Alpert and Buncke[8] have described innervation of muscle transplanted via microvascular anastomosis (gracilis and serratus anterior) with more impressive movement than that which can be achieved by cross-face graft reinnervation of the existing facial muscles. However, the status of cross-face nerve grafting remains in limbo at this time.[9]

NEUROMUSCULAR PEDICLE

I have used this technique on a limited basis only, owing to questions raised regarding its mechanism of action. Its use in facial paralysis will be described by Tucker, whose results attest to some promise with the technique. (See chapter on The "Pyramid" Ap-

proach.) We have not used it in the context of the protocol described herein.

SUMMARY

I believe that facial reanimation is best accomplished by utilizing the patient's existing neuromuscular mechanism for facial expression. To this end, whenever facial muscles are intact and viable (as demonstrated by EMG), they should be reinnervated by the ipsilateral facial nerve stump, wherever it can be identified and attached to a nerve graft.

If the proximal facial nerve is unavailable, the hypoglossal nerve is the most effective reinnervation source for routing to the paralyzed facial muscles.

When the muscles are absent, masseter transfer is preferred for the oral commissure and cheek muscles, whereas temporalis muscle transfer offers some advantages in direction of pull and capability for rehabilitation of orbicularis oculi paralysis.

REFERENCES

1. Conley J, Baker D. Hypoglossal-facial nerve anastomosis for reinnervation of the paralyzed face. Plastic Reconstr Surg 1979; 63:63–72.
2. Stennart E, Chilla R. New aspects in facial nerve surgery. Clin Plast Surg 1979; 6:451–458.
3. Conley J, Baker DC. Regional muscle transposition for rehabilitation of the paralyzed face. Clin Plast Surg 1979; 6:317–331.
4. Conley J, Baker DC. The surgical treatment of extratemporal facial paralysis. Head Neck Surg 1978; 1:12.
5. Rubin LR. Entire temporalis muscle transposition. In: Rubin LR, ed. Reanimation of the paralyzed face: new approaches. St. Louis: C.V. Mosby Company, 1977:294.
6. May M. Muscle transposition for facial reanimation. Arch Otolaryngol 1984; 110:184–190.
7. Harri K. Microneurovascular free muscle transplantation for reanimation of facial paralysis. Clin Plast Surg 1979; 6:361–375.
8. Alpert B, Buncke H. Personal communication. San Francisco, 1983.
9. Conley J, Baker D. Myths and misconceptions in the rehabilitation of facial paralysis. Plast Reconstr Surg 1983; 71:538–539.

REANIMATION OF THE PARALYZED EYELID FOLLOWING CANCER SURGERY

MARK MAY, M.D., F.A.C.S.

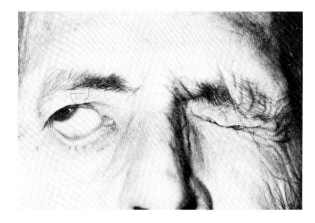

Figure 1 Ectropion, lagophthalmos, poor Bell's phenomenon, and corneal exposure resulting from facial paralysis.

Eyelid paralysis creates functional deficits that may lead to blindness (Fig. 1). Because such paralysis may occur when the facial nerve is sacrificed in resecting lesions of the temporal bone, parotid, and skull base, it is essential to include a plan to provide adequate corneal coverage in the management of patients undergoing resection of the facial nerve.

Tarsorrhaphy has been the classic method of providing such coverage. However, this procedure has many limitations. Because the procedure is static rather than dynamic, it produces a cosmetic blight (Fig. 2). With the tarsorrhaphy the patient looks through a small hole or slit, which limits vision on that side (Fig. 3). A lateral tarsorrhaphy limits vision in lateral gaze and a medial tarsorrhaphy limits vision in medial gaze, while both limit vision in upward gaze. On occasion the cornea breaks down and scars despite the procedure, causing permanent visual impairment. Even when facial function recovers enough to permit the tarsorrhaphy to be reversed, the eyelid margin may be notched, entropion may occur, the lashes may be di-

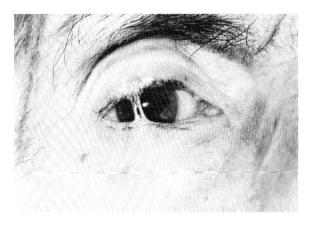

Figure 2 Ineffective tarsorrhaphy and cosmetic blight.

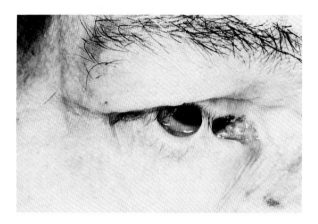

Figure 3 Tarsorrhaphy limits vision.

rected against the globe to produce irritation, and epithelial cysts may form.

This report details the advantages of implanting a gold weight or wire spring in the upper eyelid instead of performing a tarsorrhaphy, to reanimate the eyelid paralyzed by surgery or other causes.

METHODS AND MATERIALS

Patients

Between June 1978 and June 1984, the paralyzed eyelids of 77 patients were reanimated by insertion of a spring (45 patients) or gold weight (32 patients). Although in many patients paralysis was the result of surgery to resect a mass lesion, in some patients paralysis was due to trauma, Bell's palsy, herpes zoster cephalicus, inflammatory lesions, or congenital causes.

Techniques

Either a gold weight[1] or a wire spring[2] can be inserted in the upper eyelid by making an incision in the tarsal supratarsal fold.

Gold weights of 0.6 to 1.6 g have been used, but a 1-g weight seems to work best in most cases. The weight is placed on the upper border of the tarsus and is sutured in place with 8–0 Ethilon. The wound is closed with 6–0 mild chromic catgut.

A spring may be made with 0.01 orthodontic round wire and orthodontic pliers. It is inserted by passing a No. 19 spinal needle from the tarsus to the lateral orbital region, pushing the spring through the lumen of the needle, and then withdrawing the spinal needle. After the wire is in place, loops are made on the lower and upper limbs. The lower loop of the spring lies over the tarsus. The lower loop of the spring is then sutured into a Dacron envelope, which is closed with 8–0 Ethilon; this Dacron envelope has eliminated the problem of spring extrusion. The fulcrum of the spring is sutured with 5–0 Prolene to the lateral orbital periosteum just above the lateral canthal region, and the upper loop is sutured with 5–0 Prolene to the orbital periosteum beneath the lateral aspect of the eyebrow. Final adjustments in the tension of the wire are made by asking the patient to open and close the eyes. When the proper tension has been accomplished, the wound is closed with 6–0 mild chromic catgut.

RESULTS

In three of 32 patients in whom gold weights were implanted, a second procedure was required. In one patient the weight had rotated, creating an unsightly bulge in the lid; this was corrected by repositioning the weight and suturing it in place with 8–0 Ethilon to underlying tissues. The gold weight was replaced with a spring implant in the second patient and removed in the third because of dissatisfaction with eyelid droop created by the gold weight.

The initial results with the spring technique were discouraging because in three of the first ten patients the spring extruded and many adjustments were required. The Dacron envelope modification suggested by Levine[2] was then adopted, and in none of the last 30 patients has extrusion been a problem. However, a second procedure was performed in four of the last 30 patients: to improve spring function (2 patients); to replace the spring with a gold weight (1 patient); and to remove the spring entirely (1 patient) because the patient was unhappy with the eyelid droop that resulted with the spring in place.

DISCUSSION

When the facial nerve is resected in a procedure to remove cancer, paralysis of the eyelids must be a prime concern of the surgeon. The functional deficit that such paralysis produces leads to inadequate corneal coverage and ineffective distribution of the tear film. These in turn may lead to keratitis, corneal ulceration (Fig. 4), and even, should the ulcer heal, scarring (Fig. 5). An additional hazard of ulceration is eyelid perforation and permanent blindness. Although the cosmetic aspects of eyelid paralysis seem less important than preventing blindness, nevertheless the patient's self-image and presentation to others must not be neglected. Eye contact is an essential unavoidable concomitant of communication, and the nonblinking eyelid creates a major distraction for both observer and speaker.

Tarsorrhaphy has been the classic procedure of choice for protecting the eye when the eyelids have been paralyzed. However, 20 years ago two other procedures were introduced which restore dynamic eyelid function: spring implantation[3] and implantation of gold weights.[4]

Implantation of either a spring or a gold weight in a paralyzed eyelid is technically more difficult than performing a tarsorrhaphy; however, either of the former procedures offers better results in terms of improving function and appearance than does tarsorrha-

A

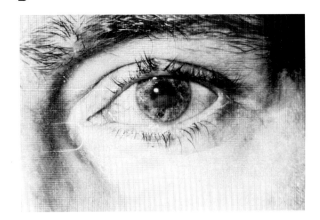

B

C

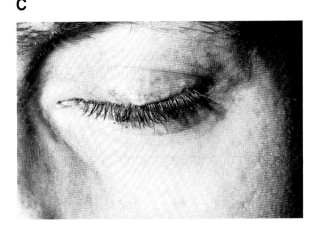

Figure 4 *A*, Keratitis and corneal ulceration due to paralyzed eyelids, and loss of tearing. *B*, Same patient; ulcer is healed, but there is residual scarring. *C*, In same patient, closure of the eye after implantation of an eyelid spring.

phy (see Figs. 4B and 4C). Either implantation procedure can be performed under local anesthesia on an outpatient basis: the gold weight technique requires approximately 20 minutes of operating time, whereas the spring requires about 1½ hours. Both techniques provide dynamic upper eyelid closure, separate eyelid closure from mouth movement, and are reversible without leaving any defects (see Fig. 5).

DIFFERENCES IN IMPLANTATION RESULTS

Eyelid closure is accomplished with the gold weight by the forces of gravity. For this reason this technique works best when the patient is upright, although eyelid closure is also improved when the patient is supine, as during sleep. This is becasue most patients sleep with the head slightly elevated on a pillow.

The spring, on the other hand, works by a different mechanism, unrelated to gravity. It allows for a faster blink and is preferred for patients with lid retraction or poor Bell's phenomenon, that is, where the cornea does not roll up under the protection of the upper lid with eyelid closure (See figure 1), and in whom the gold weight is ineffective. Most women prefer the cosmetic effect of spring implantation because the gold weight may leave a small bulge over the tarsal part of the lid. The reason for this can be better understood when one recognizes that in women the eyebrow sits just above the orbital rim and the supratarsal fold is not redundant. Therefore the fold does not hang over the tarsal part of the lid. In men, however, the brow is at the orbital rim level and the supratarsal fold is redundant covering most of the tarsal part of the lid. This characteristic in men camouflages the slight bulge created by the gold.

Gold weights do have the advantage over springs of being maintenance-free; springs may, on occasion, need adjustment. Both the gold weight and the spring may cause upper lid drooping, which may be camouflaged with tinted glasses if the patient is willing to wear them.

LOWER LID PROCEDURES

Although implanting a gold weight or a spring reanimates a paralyzed upper eyelid, it does not relieve lack of tone or the presence of ectropion of the lower lid. A lower lid-tightening technique may need to be combined with the gold weight or spring implantation procedure to restore maximal eyelid function.

A

B

C

D

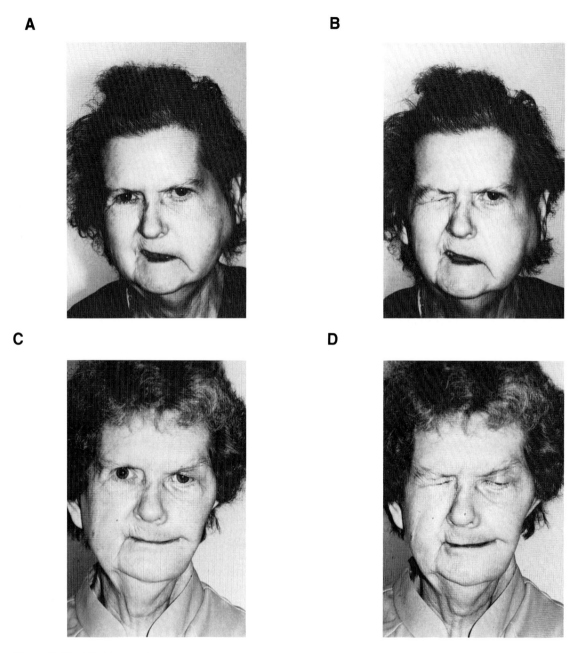

Figure 5 Total facial paralysis following excision of undifferentiated epidermoid carcinoma of the parotid. *A*, Attempting to smile. *B*, Closing eyes. *C and D*, Five weeks postoperative with eyelid spring implant and temporalis muscle transposition. *C*, In repose. *D*, Closing eyes.

CONCLUSIONS

I have found implantation of a gold weight or a spring in the upper eyelid to be the most successful way of restoring dynamic eyelid function when the eyelid has been paralyzed. Neither of these techniques is new, but they have not become popular, perhaps because of initially discouraging results. However, if meticulous attention is paid to using the proper implant material and surgical technique, the results will be gratifying to both surgeon and patient.

REFERENCES

1. Levine RE. Management of the eye after acoustic tumor surgery. In: House WF, Luetje CM, eds. Acoustic tumors. Vol. 2. Baltimore: University Park Press, 1979:105.
2. Jobe R. A technique for lid-loading in the management of lagophthalmos in facial palsy. Plast Reconstr Surg 1974; 53:29–31.
3. Morel-Fatio D, Lalardrie JT. Paliative surgical treatment of facial paralysis. The Palprebral spring. Plast Reconstr Surg 1964; 33:446.
4. Smellie GD. Restoration of the blinking reflex in facial palsy by a simple lid-load operation. Br J Plast Surg 1966; 19:279–283.

REANIMATION OF THE PARALYZED FACE: THE "PYRAMID" APPROACH

HARVEY M. TUCKER, M.D., F.A.C.S.

Facial nerve function may be lost due to trauma, disease, or congenital causes. The best recovery is generally achieved when continuity and eventual function of the ipsilateral facial nerve can be re-established. Unfortunately, in many cases of longstanding facial paralysis, this is not possible. Since no single means of reanimation now exists which satisfies all the criteria for an ideal repair (Table 1), the physician who endeavors to treat such patients must have at his disposal a number of procedures, all or any of which may be applied, depending on the peculiar needs of the case. Even more important, he must have a logical "game plan", which will permit selection of the proper timing and order in which each procedure will be utilized to achieve best results To this end, I have found what I call the "pyramid" approach most useful.

THE PYRAMID APPROACH

The first aim in rehabilitation of facial paralysis should be re-establishment of facial symmetry and tonus. Once this has been accomplished, attention can be turned to restoration of voluntary motion and, finally, to providing automatic and mimetic control of that motion. Each of these steps must be "built" upon the preceding one, much as the successive steps of a pyramid are built one upon the other (Table 2).

The procedure that comprises the base of the pyramid should be designed to arrest further degeneration of denervated facial muscles, to establish tonus and symmetry, and, if possible, to provide voluntary motion. In most hands today, this is attempted either by XII–VII crossover or, more recently, by masseter transposition. When successful, either of these approaches can achieve most of the aims listed for the "base" procedure. In my hands, however, the ansa hypoglossi nerve-muscle pedicle procedure, usually

combined with a temporalis muscle-fascia sling for rehabilitation of the eye as a single procedure (Fig. 1), has been successful and has certain advantages over the more widely employed techniques (Table 3).

In addition to the advantages listed, the nerve-muscle pedicle technique can be undertaken even when there remains some question whether or not the facial nerve may yet recover, since it does not require sectioning of the nerve for an anastomosis, as is required for XII–VII crossover, nor does it limit movement of the face, as may happen with onlay of masseter muscle transposition slips. Many of the patients I see have lost facial function because of intracranial procedures related to cerebellopontine angle tumors. In the majority of these cases, the surgeon has reported that cranial nerve VII was left mechanically intact. After several weeks or months with no evidence of return of function, one would like to begin efforts at rehabilitation, but may be reluctant to use a technique that might prevent spontaneous return of function until at least one year has gone by. Nerve-muscle pedicle technique can be employed as a first step in rehabilitation of such patients as soon after injury as circumstances permit, without interfering with spontaneous return of function.

Another important advantage of using nerve-muscle pedicle technique as a "base" procedure is that it does not occupy the neural tubules of the facial nerve in achieving restoration of tonus and some degree of voluntary motion. This becomes important in later stages of total rehabilitation, in which automatic and mimetic return of facial function is attempted. When fully successful, XII–VII crossover restores voluntary motion, but it is motion that must always be thought about separately from the spontaneous movement of the intact side. Even under the best of circumstances, patients can achieve a good, symmetrical smile, but betray themselves during ongoing animated conversation or sudden emotional expression. Only VII–VII crossover can provide any degree of spontaneous, mimetic function if the ipsilateral facial nerve is not available to re-establish function.

For this reason, I have employed limited VII–

TABLE 1 Criteria for Ideal Rehabilitation of Facial Nerve Paralysis

Single procedure
Rapid return of function
Restores symmetry at rest
Restores voluntary, symmetrical motion
No synkinesis
Motion is automatic and mimetic
Procedure does not incur other signficant functional or cosmetic deficits

TABLE 2 Pyramid Approach to Facial Reanimation

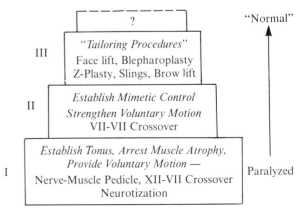

III	?
	"Tailoring Procedures" — Face lift, Blepharoplasty, Z-Plasty, Slings, Brow lift
II	Establish Mimetic Control, Strengthen Voluntary Motion — VII-VII Crossover
I	Establish Tonus, Arrest Muscle Atrophy, Provide Voluntary Motion — Nerve-Muscle Pedicle, XII-VII Crossover, Neurotization

"Normal" ↑ Paralyzed

493

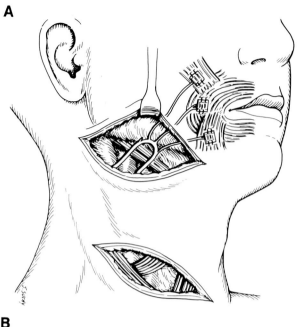

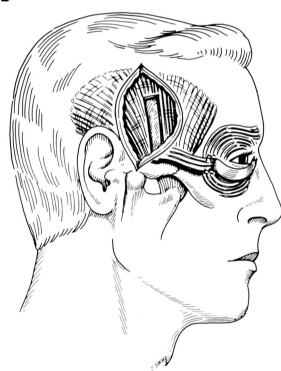

Figure 1 *A*, Nerve-muscle pedicle technique for selective reinneravation of muscles about the mouth. Branches of the ansa hypoglossi to various strap muscles in the neck are transposed as nerve-muscle pedicles to the levator anguli and orbicularis oris muscles. *B*, Temporalis muscle-fascia sling rehabilitation for the paralyzed eye. This procedure is simultaneously a static support and a potential animated rehabilitation for the eye, separate from the mouth. In this way synkinesis is avoided.

VII crossover as the second tier in the rehabiliation pyramid. The technique has been described elsewhere[2] (Fig. 2). It differs greatly from VII–VII crossover suggested as a means of total rehabilitation by Scar-

TABLE 3   Advantages of Nerve-Muscle Pedicle Technique for Facial Reanimation

Avoids synkinesis and inappropriate reinnervation
Does not paralyze other significant cranial nerves
Function returns within six months, if successful
Permits subsequent use of other techniques, whether successful (VII-VII crossover) or not (XII-VII crossover)
May be used even when some change of spontaneous recovery exists

amella,[3] Samii,[4] and others, in that it aims to *selectively* reinnervate the muscles about the upper lip only. Moreover, since the distance traversed is only from one buccal division to the other, a relatively short graft, which can be obtained from the greater auricular nerve, is usually sufficient. At the same time as this procedure is carried out, the surgeon may elect to perform certain adjunctive, or "tailoring", procedures. Both

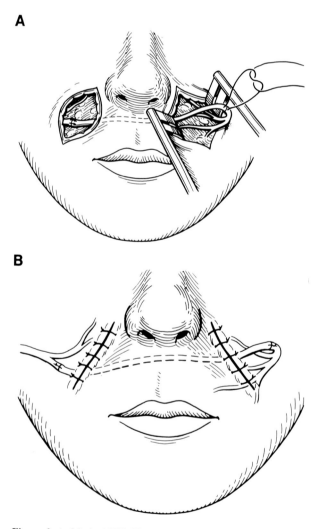

Figure 2 *A*, Limited VII–VII crossover graft for reanimation of muscles about the mouth. *B*, Completed procedure. When successful, this operation not only restores greater strength and mobility to the mouth (while slightly weakening the good side for better symmetry), but also restores mimetic facial expression to some degree.

facelift and nasolabial crease repositioning, for example, can be incorporated with limited VII–VII crossover to good advantage. Alternatively, such final adjustments may be carried out as separate "third tier" procedures.

DECISION MAKING AND PROCEDURE SELECTION

The decision as to what, if any further surgery for improvement of facial function should be performed, as well as when to do so, is an ongoing process. It must be the result of a continuous dialogue between the surgeon, the patient, and, if appropriate, the patient's family. At each point in the process, decisions must be made, based upon what has been achieved thus far, the patient's life status and needs, and any other factors that may pertain from time to time. The *least* important factor in this decision making process is the surgeon's satisfaction with the results achieved, whereas the *most* important is the patient's satisfaction. The process of rehabilitation of facial nerve function is completed when either the surgeon feels that the potential yield from further efforts does not justify the risks or expense, or when

the patient is either satisfied with the results or does not wish to proceed further.

CONCLUSIONS

A logical planned multi-tiered "pyramid" approach to facial nerve rehabilitation has served me well. Although certain preferred techniques are described in detail, this approach lends itself to optimal treatment planning and timing of operations, regardless of the actual procedures selected by the surgeon.

REFERENCES

1. Tucker HM. Restoration of function in long standing facial paralysis. Otolaryngol Clin N Am 1982; 15:69–76.
2. Tucker HM. Facial nerve crossover as an adjunct to nerve-muscle pedicle reinnervation in rehabilitation of the paralyzed face. In: Graham MD, House WF, eds. Disorders of the facial nerve. New York: Raven Press, 1982:523–531.
3. Scaramella LF. L'anastomosi Tra i due Nevi Facciali. Arch Ital Otol 1971; 82:209–215.
4. Samii M, Wallenborn R. Tierrexperimentelle Untersuchungen Uber Den Einfluss der Spannung auf den Regererationserfolg nach Nervennaht. Acta Neurochir (Wien) 1972; 27:87–110.

35. Reconstruction of the Mandible

INTRODUCTION

ROBERT W. CANTRELL, M.D.

The mandible is more than a bony structure of the face which projects the appearance of a person with strong resolve. It does contribute mightily to the appearance of the individual, but it does much more. The mandible, being the arch of the oral cavity, provides the foundation for the functions of articulation, deglutition, and mastication. Additionally, by serving as a support for the tongue, it permits respiration, which would otherwise be impossible if the tongue had no anterior attachment.

It is not known when man first attempted mandibular restoration, but in 1860, Ollier published a paper in the French journal of physiology detailing his experience with bone grafts and bone regeneration in lower animals and man.[1] Eighteen years later, the Scotsman Macewen removed from a 3-year-old lad a humeral shaft with osteomyelitis and restored the defect with wedges of tibia removed from donor patients.[2] Not much is said about who was willing to donate tibial wedges, but this was reported in 1881.

It represents perhaps the first reported case of homogenous bone grafting.

In 1891, the German surgeon Bardenheuer reported filling a bony and soft tissue defect of the lower jaw with a composite flap consisting of skin, periosteum, and bone from the forehead.[3] Skyoff, also of Germany, reported in 1900 the use of a free bone graft to restore a mandibular defect.[4]

Owing to the nature of trench warfare, World War I resulted in many casualties with facial trauma with which British, French, and German surgeons had to deal. Autogenous grafts of ilium, rib, or tibia were employed, and these materials continue to be used today. Excellent reviews of the history of mandibular restoration have been published by Ivy[5] and by Converse and Campbell.[6]

In 1951, Kreuz and co-workers at the National Naval Medical Center, Bethesda, Maryland prepared homografts for general use by freeze-drying them and thus permitted their preservation at room temperature indefinitely.[7] This technique utilized quick freezing at very low temperatures, followed by drying by sublimation in a high vacuum. Chalmers has shown that freeze-drying inactivates histocompatibility antigens.[8]

In 1954, Converse and Campbell reported their use of 42 autografts and 20 homografts to restore mandibular defects with only four failures.[6]

In 1967, DeFries and co-workers successfully used

a mandibular homograft packed with autogenous marrow and cancellous bone to restore a large, avulsive defect of the anterior mandible in a Marine who sustained this injury in Vietnam. This was reported in 1971.[9]

Boyne, in 1969, reported success in restoring mandibular defects by the use of a chrome-cobalt alloy cage cast in the shape of a mandible.[10] This was lined with a cellulose acetate microporous filter filled with autogenous marrow and cancellous bone.

Two theories of bone regeneration exist. One theory is that new bone formation results from functional activity of osteogenic cells present in periosteum, endosteum, and haversian canals.[11] This appears to be the major method by which fractures heal.

The other theory, based on observations of bone formation following transplants, is the "metaplasia theory". According to this concept, new bone formation is due to the transformation of surrounding connective tissue into bone. This transformation allegedly occurs because of presence of an osteogenetic substance called "osteogenin" by Lacroix,[12] which apparently diffuses from the transplant into the connective tissue.

It is doubtful that any osteoblasts in free bone grafts serve as the source of osteogenesis. Barth, in 1893, showed that *all* elements of transplanted bone die and are slowly replaced from adjacent living, bone-producing tissue by a process he called "creeping substitution".[13] According to this concept, the bone graft serves only as a scaffold for the invasion of bone cells from the host site.

Burwell has shown that homogenous bone washed free from marrow and then impregnated with fresh autogenous marrow forms a fresh composite homograft-autograft capable of forming new bone as readily as an autograft of fresh marrow-containing iliac bone.[14] Burwell believes that (1) the new bone formed by a fresh composite homograft-autograft is derived from its contained marrow, and (2) the initiation of osteogenesis in a proportion of such grafts is attributable to an interaction between bone and marrow.

In the chapters that follow, the current state of mandibular reconstruction is discussed. Ariyan discusses mandibular reconstruction by use of osteomusculocutaneous flaps. The chapter by Cummings is a discussion of the general aspects of mandibular reconstruction. DeFries presents a discussion of homograft reconstruction of the mandible. Finally, Taylor reports on his experience in reconstructing mandibles. (Attention is also called to the chapter on *Reconstruction: Yesterday, Today, and Tomorrow*, by Ian McGregor.)

REFERENCES

1. Ollier L. Recherches experimentales sur les greffes osseuses. J Physiol l'Homme Par 1860; 3:88–108.
2. Macewen W. The growth of bone. Glasgow: J. Mackhose, 1912.
3. Bardenheuer B. (A) Unter Kieferrection, (B) Oberkieferrection, Vorstellung zweier Patienten. Verh Dtsch Ges Chir Berl 1892; 21:68–69.
4. Skyoff W. Zur Frage der Knochen-plastik am Unterkiefer. Centralbl Chir 1900; 27:881–883.
5. Ivy RH. Collective review: Bone grafting for restoration of defects of the mandible. Int Abst Plast Reconstr Surg 1951; 7:33–341.
6. Converse JM, Campbell RM. Bone grafts in surgery of the face. Surg Clin North Am 1954; 34:375–401.
7. Kreuz FP, Hyatt GW, Turmer TC, Bassett AL. The preservation and clinical use of freeze-dried bone. J Bone Joint Surg 1951; 33A:863–872.
8. Chalmers J. Transplantation immunity in bone homografting. J Bone Joint Surg 1959; 41B:160–179.
9. DeFries HO, Marble HB, Sell KW. Reconstruction of the mandible: Use of homograft combined with autogenous bone and marrow. Arch Otolaryngol 1971; 93:426–432.
10. Boyne PJ. Restoration of osseous defects in maxillofacial casualties. J Am Dent Assoc 1969; 78:767–776.
11. DeBruyn PPH, Kabisch WT. Bone formation by fresh and frozen autogenous and homogenous transplants of bone, bone marrow, and periosteum. Am J Anat 1955; 96:375–417.
12. Lacroix P. L'Organisation des Os. Liege, Belgium: Desoer, 1949.
13. Barth A. Ueber Histologische Befunde nach Knochenimplantationen. Arch klin Chir 1893; 46:409–417.
14. Burwell RG. Studies in the transplantation of bone. VIII. Treated composite homograft-autografts of cancellous bone: an analysis of inductive mechanisms in bone transplantation. J Bone Joint Surg 1966; 48:532–565.

OSTEOMYOCUTANEOUS FLAPS FOR RECONSTRUCTION OF PARTIAL MANDIBULECTOMIES

STEPHAN ARIYAN, M.D.

One of the most difficult areas to reconstruct in the head and neck is the mandible. I do not believe there is really a good way to reconstruct a mandible. A number of people have devised various techniques to do this, some of which have been successful and some have not. I think that the best way to conceptualize what we should do with the mandible in cancer is to think of the very simple solution: that we should not resect the mandible unless we absolutely have to. All too often, the mandible has been resected because of the proximity of the cancer to this bone, rather than because the tumor has actually invaded the bone. However, in many instances the mandible needs to be partially removed for cancers of the floor of the mouth or along the lingual surface of the mandible, and a rim mandibulectomy is the best technique to use rather than taking out a segment or performing a hemimandibulectomy, which used to be fairly common a decade ago.

When the cancer has invaded the mandible, I believe the decision regarding the extent of the resection should be based on the horizontal dimensions rather than the vertical (depth). If cancer has invaded the mandible, the malignant cells invade the cancellous portion of this bone and spread in the horizontal direction. Thus curability is reduced because this is often associated with distant spread. Even with a segmental resection or a hemimandibulectomy, one cannot be assured that the microscopic limits of the tumor in the bone have been removed. I believe it is far better to resect the cancer and a very wide dimension of the mandible horizontally (that is, the alveolus and the cancellous portion of the bone) while preserving the inferior, thick cortical bone, which is rarely invaded by the cancer.

However, there are times when the mandible has to be resected or has been exposed and has resulted in osteoradionecrosis that needs to be reconstructed. Under those circumstances, we have to consider whether this area has been radiated , whether the area that is missing constitutes a segment or half the mandible, and whether the symphysis has been removed or a subtotal resection of the mandible has been performed. Once we have decided what is missing, we can think of several alternatives to reconstruct it.

The frequent failures of reconstructions of defects of the mandibular segment are often caused by poor vascularity in the recipient bed. This poor vascularity is usually a result of fibrosis or dermal scarring from previous injuries, surgical procedures, or radiation therapy. Consequently, successful reconstructions with bone grafts in these areas require the use of well-vascularized bone grafts or placement of bone grafts within tissue that has been transferred to the area to bring a blood supply.

In recent years, improved microvascular techniques have led to the use of free transfers of tissues to these compromised sites. The microvascular transfer of osteocutaneous flaps has been used for mandibular reconstruction to provide bone for the solid support of the jaw and soft tissue for either lining or contour, or both, in one stage. These microvascular transfers provide a permanent blood supply to ensure the viability of the bone graft even within the fibrotic bed.

Formerly, surgeons had stressed the need to use the segment of the posterior rib with the posterior intercostal artery for blood supply. This was based on the knowledge that the endosteal circulation to the rib is provided by the nutrient artery, a branch of the posterior intercostal, and the belief that this was the only satisfactory blood supply to the rib.[1-4] However, this approach was difficult and time-consuming, and required that the patient be kept in the prone position to harvest the rib; the patient is then turned supine after closure of the donor site to prepare the recipient site for the graft, resulting in a prolonged state of ischemia for the free flap. Furthermore, attempts at total mandibular reconstruction, using free osteocutaneous rib grafts with this posterior blood supply, had been unsuccessful because the circulation to the overlying skin was poor.[4,5] This then led some surgeons to advocate the use of the osteocutaneous groin flap to harvest the underlying attached iliac bone.[5,6]

In 1978, Ariyan and Finseth reported the first successful reconstruction of a chin and mandible with a free osteocutaneous rib transplant using the anterior intercostal vessels (Fig. 1).[7] This technique was based on the evidence that in the absence of the endosteal blood supply, the periosteal blood supply would take over. Additional cases of reconstruction using this technique confirmed the viability of the transplanted bone by observing the deposition of fluorochrome markers within the new osteoid laid down by the osteoblasts, as indicated by examination of thin sections of undecalcified bone.[8]

The confirmation of this concept of periosteal blood supply to the bone was concomitant with the development of the concept of musculocutaneous flaps for transporting paddles of skin of various size and shape, based on the musculocutaneous perforators from the muscle to the overlying skin. It became evident that any muscle that could be transported could also bring with it any overlying skin that was attached. It seemed reasonable, therefore, to expect that muscles would also transport the underlying attached bone by

A

B

C

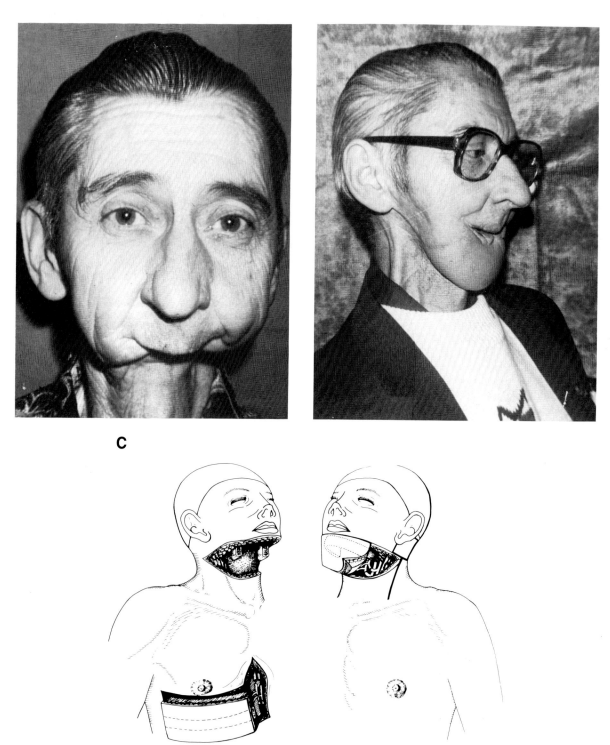

Figure 1 A total agnathia from resection of the jaw from angle to angle of the mandible was reconstructed in one stage using the anterior blood supply to the rib and overlying muscle and skin.

providing the circulation to the periosteum, which would then provide nourishment for the viable transfer of the bone. Using this principle, Cuono and Ariyan reconstructed a resected tongue, floor of mouth, two-thirds of a mandible, and overlying skin with a pectoralis major myocutaneous flap that incorporated a segment of the underlying fifth rib.[9] By means of fluorochrome markers, the viability of this rib was again

A

B

C

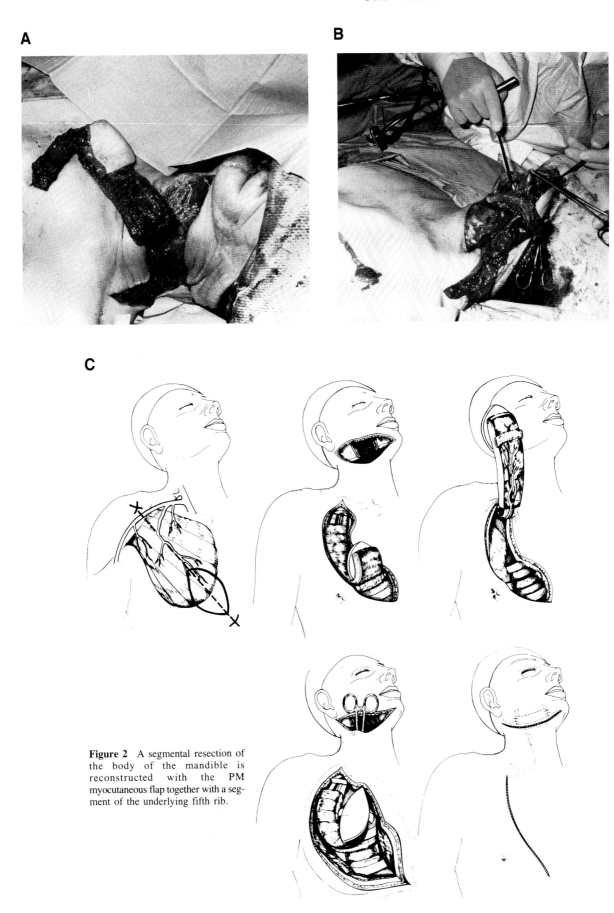

Figure 2 A segmental resection of the body of the mandible is reconstructed with the PM myocutaneous flap together with a segment of the underlying fifth rib.

confirmed postoperatively. This segment of rib is best suited for a segmental resection, although it has been used for subtotal resections of the mandible (Fig. 2). In young women with well-formed breasts, in order to avoid the deformity of taking the skin paddle and the rib from the midportion and medial aspect of the breast, the paddle of the skin can be outlined in the inframammary region.[10] In this way, the incision can be made in the inframammary fold and the breast completely elevated off the pectoralis major muscle. Then the skin paddle can be harvested below the inframammary fold with a portion of the pectoralis major muscle and a segment of the underlying attached fifth rib, and brought up into the neck through an infraclavicular incision for eventual reconstruction of the mandible (Fig. 3). The donor defect can then be closed by generous undermining and advancement to close the inframammary fold.

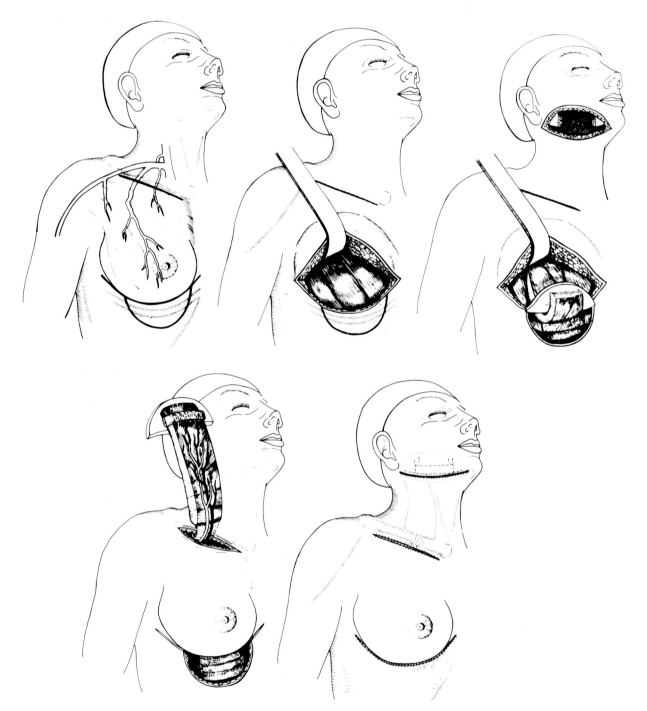

Figure 3 In female patients, the skin paddle may be outlined in the inframammary area. The breast is then dissected off the PM and the flap is transferred to the head and neck. The donor site is closed by advancement of chest skin.

For the major resections of the mandible, including the neck of the mandible and/or symphysis, reconstruction is better performed with iliac bone and the deep circumflex iliac artery,[11] or with the trapezius muscle and the attached acromion for the symphysis.

REFERENCES

1. Ostrup LT, Frederickson JM. Distant transfer of a free, living bone graft by microvascular anastomoses. Plast Reconstr Surg 1977; 59:737–738.
2. Ostrup LT, Frederickson JM. Reconstruction of mandibular defects after radiation, using free living bone graft transferred by microvascular anastomses. An experiment study. Plast Reconstr Surg 1975; 55:563–572.
3. Daniel RK. Free rib transfer by microvascular anastomses. Plast Reconstr Surg 1977; 59:737–738. (Letter to the Editor)
4. Serafin D, Villarreal-Rios A, Goergiade NG. A rib-containing free flap to reconstruct mandibular defects. Br J Plast Surg 1977; 30:263–266.
5. Daniel RK. Mandibular reconstruction with free tissue transfers. Ann Plast Surg 1978; 1:346–371.
6. Taylor GI, Miller GDH, Ham FJ. The free vascularized bone graft. A clinical extension of microvascular techniques. Plast Reconstr Surg 1975; 55:533–544.
7. Ariyan S, Finseth FJ. The anterior chest approach for obtaining free osteocutaneous rib grafts. Plast Reconstr Surg 1978; 62:676–685.
8. Ariyan S. The viability of rib grafts transplanted with the periosteal blood supply. Plast Reconstr Surg 1980; 65:140.
9. Cuono CB, Ariyan S. Immediate reconstruction of composite mandibular defect with a regional osteomyocutaneous flap. Plast Reconstr Surg 1980; 65:477.
10. Ariyan S, Cuono CB. Myocutaneous flaps for head and neck reconstruction. Head Neck Surg 1980; 2:321.
11. Taylor GI, Townsend P, Corlett R. Superiority of the deep circumflex iliac vessels as a supply for free groin flaps. Clinical work. Plast Reconstr Surg 1979; 64:745.

MANDIBULAR RECONSTRUCTION OTHER THAN OSTEOMYOCUTANEOUS HOMOGRAFTS

CHARLES W. CUMMINGS, M.D.
BRUCE LEIPZIG, M.D.

If a portion of the mandible is to be excised with the tumor, it must be established whether a need exists for mandibular replacement. It has been shown that replacement of the mandible is not a requisite if the posterior portion of the body and the ascending ramus represent all that needs to be excised. The cosmetic and functional deformity is measurable, but it is usually well tolerated by the patient. The urge to uniformly replace the mandible if it is removed may in fact be counter to the best interest of the patient's rehabilitative process. We must resist the surgical challenge if the benefits to the patient are not significant.

Another tenet with regard to mandibular surgery is that the indication for reconstruction increases as the defect projects further anteriorly, i.e., the severity of cosmetic and functional deformity increases as the defect moves forward. Unfortunately, the degree of difficulty with satisfactory reconstruction parallels the magnitude of the deformity. As we all know, reconstruction of the mandibular arch remains one of the great challenges in reconstructive head and neck surgery. Furthermore, there is no single method of mandibular reconstruction that clearly outshines alterna-

tive measures. In combination, the methods do not have a complementary effect.

There are certain baseline requisites which must be present to optimize the chances for success regardless of the technique involved. Most significant of these is the avoidance of salivary contamination after the graft has been introduced into the defect. Failure to provide an intact mucosal barrier to saliva will most assuredly result in devitalization, infection, and ultimately extrusion. If for some reason the mucosa breaks down at a later date prior to the completion of neo-osteogenesis, it will most assuredly have an adverse effect.

Immobilization of the graft segment is imperative to optimize the development of an intact graft and to avoid pseudarthrosis. The mandibular graft must intimately approximate the remaining mandibular segments. It has been shown that approximation of segments by compression plating is more effective than by simple approximation. The inward migration of periosteum and intermedullary osteoid material from the intact bone may be imparied by an interface of fibrous tissue, thus delaying reconstitution of a functional unit.

Another requisite for success is the reconstitution of proper intraoral configuration so that residual dentition abuts appropriately to promote normal mastication. If this can be achieved, the muscles of mastication are allowed to function properly, and referred pain associated with contralateral mandibular distortion assumes an insignificant role in the act of alimentation.

The primary requisite for success of mandibular reconstruction is that there be freedom from recurrent or persistent neoplasm. If such is not the case, concern over reconstruction and rehabilitation is spurious and inappropriate.

The methods available to reconstruct a mandibular defect are many. Almost every available biodegradable synthetic material has been tried at one time to span the defect created by a mandibular resection. Formed appliances, such as Vitallium, tantalum, titanium, or stainless steel prostheses, have their advocates.[1-5] However, these prostheses are not generally accepted as being sufficiently successful to use as a first-line method of repair. The same holds true for Silastic, Teflon, acrylic, and polyurethane materials if used alone. Ceramics and coralline hydroxyapatite are mentioned in the literature, but as yet have not replaced the more traditional methods of reconstruction.[6]

Biodegradable materials such as collagen have yet to be developed for clinical use, although the concept of a pre-shaped biodegradable scaffolding is attractive.

The standard workhorse for mandibular replacement is a combination of alloplast and autograft.[7-10] The alloplast may be in the form of a titanium or Vitallium metallic crib into which is placed a particulate marrow which is harvested from the iliac crest at the time of reconstruction. Recently the use of polyurethane crib has been introduced and has an advantage in that the crib may be shaped more easily than a metallic device. The technique for combined alloplast autograft will be described later in this chapter.

An alternative method to those previously mentioned is the use of autogenous bone (specifically from the patient's own mandible). This method cannot be used when there has been a traumatic avulsion of a mandibular segment, as from a gunshot wound, but is can be used satisfactorily in cases of tumor resection that involves removal of a mandibular segment or when the tumor involves the mandible. Cryogenic cytodestruction (to be described) is a method for rendering the mandible useful in the scaffolding procedure despite its previous involvement with tumor. Other methods of free grafts, such as iliac crest segments or isolated rib grafts, may be successful; however, these may fall short when compared to autograft mandible in terms of configuration and subsequent function.

Regardless of the method used to reconstruct the mandible, the timing of this event is of the utmost importance. Immediate reconstruction of the mandible at the time of extirpation has been shown to be successful less than 50 percent of the time.[1,10] Most failure eventuate because of postoperative wound infection or intraoral mucosal dehiscence with delayed exposure of the alloplast autograft. Delayed reconstruction, however, carries with it a high success rate because of the avoidance of salivary contamination. It therefore makes surgical sense to provide for stabilization of the remaining mandibular segments at the time of the initial resection, either by external devices, such as the biphase apparatus, or by an internal spanning device, such as K-wire or Champy plate. I prefer the external device because the internal spanning device has the increased potential for tenting up the mucosa, thus comprising mucosal vasculature and causing necrosis.

In the discussion of technique that follows, only the most significant defect, that of the mandibular arch, will be considered.

OPERATIVE TECHNIQUE: ALLOPLAST/AUTOGRAFT AND AUTOGRAFT

Tumor resection is performed with a mind set that has reconstruction as a secondary consideration. Complete circumferential expirpation obviously is the surgeon's primary goal. Regardless of the method of reconstruction and intraoral resurfacing, tracheostomy is an integral component of the surgical procedure to eliminate the potential for airway compromise and to rid the operative field of as many encumbrances as possible. A vascularized myocutaneous flap reconstruction is the most appealing because an independent blood supply may be thus delivered to an area compromised by surgery and perhaps radiation. This also allows for the insertion of a vascularized wall between the oral mucosal closure and the surgically created pocket which will house the replacement graft. It is important as well to apply the biphase apparatus so that the Vitallium screws are firmly inserted into the remaining mandibular segments. This is best done immediately subsequent to the resurfacing procedure. If one elects to use the cryogenically devitalized mandibular autograft, all of the soft tissue, periosteum, and gross tumor is removed from the mandibular arch by the rotating bur. This includes the medullary space of the mandibular segment. The graft is then submerged in liquid nitrogen for 10 minutes and warmed by immersion in Bacitracin solution at room temperature. Two complete cycles must be accomplished to ensure cytodestruction. Subsequently a horizontal incision is made in the left lower quadrant of the abdominal wall, and a space is developed immediately superficial to the external oblique fascia. The bony segment is then placed in this compartment for safeguarding while the intraoral reconstructive process heals. The wound is drained. If an alloplast autograft is to be employed, obviously this step in the process is omitted.

Subsequent to complete intraoral healing (usually 3 to 4 weeks), the patient is reanesthetized via the existing tracheostomy and a submental incision is made. A heated scalpel has been most helpful in controlling the bloody ooze that occurs in previously irradiated or surgically manipulated tissue. Dissection is carried out supralaterally to expose the anterior edges of the residual mandibular segments. Subsequently the dissection may be carried anteriorly to create a pocket that is large enough to receive the graft or alloplast. (A doubly gloved hand in the mouth at this time will enable the surgeon to avoid inadvertent entrance into the oral cavity, an absolute contraindication to continuance of the reconstructive process). Once the pocket has been created, the leading edge of the mandibular segment is freshened back to a bleeding bony edge. The recipient site is now ready for completion of the reconstructive process.

Siimultaneously, a second surgeon has harvested the mandibular segment from the left lower quadrant and denuded it of its fibrous capsule. It is then immersed in Bacitracin solution until ready for particulate marrow loading.

The particular marrow and osteoid material are harvested from the inner table of the iliac crest. A total of at least 10 cc of material is advised to maximize loading of the crib prosthesis, either alloplastic or allograft. This wound must be drained as well to eliminate the possibility of retroperitoneal hematoma.

The devitalized mandibular autograft is then shaped with a rotating bur so as to create a trough, preserving the inferior mandibular margin as well as the inferior one-third to one-half of the anterior and posterior cortices. A medium K-wire is then shaped to fit in the mandibular trough. A similarly sized drill hole is placed to a depth of 3 cm parallel to the inferior margin of the mandibular segments. Further, separate drill holes are placed in the mandibular segment and the autograft near the inferior margins to ensure fixation after proper seating of the autograft. The K-wires are then shortened to 2.5 cm, the autograft tray is filled with particulate marrow, and the graft is inserted into the surgical defect. No. 24 wire is then used for further stabilization after marrow loading of the graft-mandible interface.

The defect is drained inferiorly to prevent hematoma formation, which would impair viability of the particulate marrow. With this method of fixation, no external fixation is required subsequent to graft insertion and stabilization. A dental soft diet is introduced as soon as the cervical incision is healed.

This procedure is modified slightly when using the alloplast autograft method. The particulate marrow is harvested in a similar fashion. The alloplast (metal or polyurethane crib) is tailored to the defect.

Precautions here must include avoidance of tenting the intraoral lining superiorly, overcompensating for the mandibular defect. When properly sized, the crib is loaded with marrow and fixed to the mandibular segments using self-tapping screws. Again the wound is drained, and intravenous antibiotics are continued for the immediate postoperative period (72 hours or until the drain is removed).

Postoperative management involves documentation of proper placement by Panorex radiograph. Subsequently, technetium-99 MDP bone scans are obtained at 2 and 4 months to ascertain osteogenesis. The radiologic assessment at 6 months is routine and will show the presence of a calcified matrix.

Results

A moment must be taken to re-emphasize the now established fact that immediate replacement, whether alloplast autograft or autograft, yields an exceedingly high failure rate and thus is to be condemned. Patients with staged or delayed reconstruction tend to have a much higher rate of graft acceptance.

Both of us now utilize the delayed autograft reimplantation technique (Table 1). The experiences are somewhat different, perhaps because of modifications in the technique by each surgeon. In one series of four patients, one author (B.L.) performed reimplantation of an unmodified mandibular segment. These segments were large, ranging from 6 cm to 10 cm in length. Two patients were given postoperative radiation therapy. Three of these four mandibular reimplantations developed the complication of pressure necrosis of the overlying epithelium with subsequent exposure of the mandibular autograft. In all of these, there was isolated dry osteonecrosis; however, the autograft survived. The fourth patient died

TABLE 1 Results of Delayed Autograft Reimplantation Technique

Patient	Length of Resection	Interval in Storage	Intraoral Contamination	Post-op X-ray Therapy	Status	Fixation
J.H.	10 cm	4 mo	No	6,000 rads	Cutaneous fistula-bone viable, 5 mo	Biphase
E.C.	6 cm	4 mo	No	None	Died; distant metastasis; evidence of new bone growth	Biphase
D.G.	8 cm	8 mo	No	6,000 rads	Cutaneous fistula; bone intact, 13 mo	Biphase
D.S.	10 cm	3 mo	No	None	Cutaneous fistula 1 yr; Bone intact	Biphase
A.G.	7 cm	6 wk	Yes	None	Bone necrosis removal 7 mo; intraoral communication	Biphase
M.S.	7 cm	2 mo	No	None	Intact, normal appearance 5 yr	Biphase
P.W.	6 cm	10 mo	No	None	Intact, eating 9 mo	K-wire
E.W.	7 cm	4 mo	No	None	Intact, eating 10 mo	K-wire

of distant metastases 4 months after the implantation. There was evidence of viable osteoid material at the time of death.

The method currently used by C.W.C. involves reducing the vertical dimension of the mandibular autograft, forming a crib of the residual bone with a motorized burr, and subsequently fixing a preformed K-wire to the base of the autograft with a No. 24 stainless steel wire. After this is loaded with the particulate marrow, it is placed into the freshly created surgical envelope and fixed via the K-wire and a single No. 24 wire suture to the residual mandibular segments. No external biphase is used postoperatively. Two patients who underwent this particular procedure have fared well postoperatively. Two additional patients were treated in the same way except that external biphase apparatus was used in lieu of the internal fixation with the K-wire. One of these patients has normal configuration and function of the mandible 3³/₅ years after surgery. The second patient experienced a small intraoral communication with the surgical envelope at the time of mandibular reimplantation. As could be anticipated, a rather protracted process of graft necrosis and digestion ensued, eventuating in removal of the mandibular segment 7 months later. It is of interest that enough inflammatory reaction was created in that time span to hold the residual mandibular segments in approximately normal configuration.

From this small series some heartening information evolves. Trimming of the mandibular segment and using it as a biodegradable configuration-maintaining template warrants its continued use as one of the alternatives in mandibular replacement.

Conclusions

The autograft and alloplast autograft play a major role in the spectrum of successful mandibular reconstruction. Although there are exclusive indications for osteomyocutaneous flaps or free flaps, most of the needs may be serviced by the methods of reconstruction herein discussed.

Immediate reconstruction with this method is to be condemned. Delayed reconstruction employing interval biphasic fixation is the procedure of choice.

If available, one can achieve the optimum in configuration by using the autograft method of reconstruction.

Internal fixation as a delayed event shows promise to be effective and advantageous.

Because of the anatomic reality that neither the autograft nor the alloplast autograft carries its own blood supply, it is less apt to survive in a nonperfused recipient bed. Therefore, use of the vascularized muscular pedicle is to be encouraged with intraoral resurfacing.

REFERENCES

1. Lawson W, Biller HF. Mandibular reconstruction-bone graft techniques. Otolaryngol Head Neck Surg 1982; 90:589–594.
2. Maisel RH, Hilger PA, Adams GL, Giordano AM. Reconstruction of the mandible. Laryngoscope 1983; 93:1122–1126.
3. Schuller DE, Bardoch J, Monteith CG, Maves MD. Titanium tray mandibular reconstruction. Arch Otolaryngol 1982; 180:174–178.
4. Strelzaw UV. Mandibular reconstruction using implantable stabilization plates. Arch Otolaryngol 1983; 109:333–337.
5. Giordano A, Brady D, Foster C, Adams G. Particulate cancellous marrow crib graft reconstruction of mandibular defects. Laryngoscope 1980; 2027–2036.
6. Finn RA, Bell WH, Brammer JA. Interpositional "grafting" with autogenous bone and coralline hydroxyapatite. J Maxillofac Surg 1980; 8:217–227.
7. DeFries HO. Reconstruction of the mandible: Use of combined homologous mandible and autologous bone. Otolaryngol Head Neck Surg 1981; 694–697.
8. Kline SN, Rimer SR. Reconstruction of osseous defects with freeze-dried allogenic and autogenous bone. Am J Surg 1983; 146:471–473.
9. Hamaker RC. Irradiated autogenous mandibular grafts for primary reconstructions. Laryngoscope 1981; 91:1031–1050.
10. Leipzig B, Cummings CW. Immediate mandibular reconstruction: Human experience with autogenous frozen mandibular graft. Otolaryngol Head Neck Surg 1981; 89:879–881.

MANDIBULAR RECONSTRUCTION WITH HOMOLOGOUS AND AUTOLOGOUS BONE GRAFTS

HUGH O. deFRIES, M.D., D.D.S.

My experience in reconstructing the mandible has not been one of planned scientific study. Rather it has been a continuum, over a period of 15 years, of dealing with necessity, of drawing on the past experience of others, of formulating new concepts and observing the result in practice, of eventually drawing on my own experience, and finally developing further new concepts. The following summary of this experience is presented in the knowledge that it does not provide the final answer, but that it may provide some modest progress toward the solution to this difficult problem.

Much of what I initially learned about reconstructing the mandible was gained from the treatment of military patients who had lost portions of the mandible as a result of gunshot wounds. I subsequently learned that methods found to be successful in reconstructing the mandible in such patients frequently do not work in cancer patients. The obvious difference between these two groups of patients, both needing mandibular reconstruction, is their age and the fact that most cancer patients who have required mandibular resection have received, or will receive, significant doses of radiation to the prospective site of reconstruction. It is my belief that radiation therapy is the main cause of failure in such patients.

Prior to 1970, most attempts at mandibular reconstruction focused on the use of autologous iliac bone used in either single pieces or multiple pieces, cut, shaped, and wired together to achieve the desired bulk and form of the part to be replaced. Such grafts were found to be successful and useful in replacing simple segmental defects of the body of the mandible and small segmental defects of the symphysis. However, large segmental defects involving the symphysis were not easily replaced by such grafts because of the difficulty in reproducing the unique shape of the symphysis and in obtaining stability in a graft pieced together.

In 1970, some colleagues and I introduced the use of particulate bone grafts.[1,2] Such grafts consisted of particles of fresh autologous cancellous bone and bone marrow obtained from the ilium or ribs placed in either a metallic tray or in a tray of a preserved portion of human mandibular cortex. It was observed, in a large number of cases, that both such methods would restore bony continuity with a high degree of reliability, the principal difference between the two methods being that the metallic tray remained as a permanently implanted foreign body with all of the inherent well-known complications of extrusion, exposure, and infection. On the other hand, through animal experiments, human radiographic evidence, and histologic specimens obtained from patients, it was demonstrated that homologous bone trays were absorbed and replaced with living bone.[3] Thus it was clear that a successful composite graft of homologous cortical bone combined with autologous cancellous bone and bone marrow would provide the patient with a living bone graft in the shape of the part replaced and free of foreign material that could subsequently endanger the integrity of the graft through extrusion and infection.

The methods, criteria, and results of these clinical studies have been previously published.[4,5] A summary of the results is seen in Table 1.

On the basis of my experience since that study, I have concluded that there is no practical necessity for using either of these types of graft for segmental defects of the posterior mandible. Such defects, having largely linear and angular shape, may be replaced easily and successfully with solid autologous grafts from either the ilium or the ribs. However, both types of graft, the particulate and the solid, have been found to have marginal success in cancer patients who have previously received significant doses of radiation to the site of reconstruction, and recent publications supply ample evidence that postoperative radiation to the reconstruction site results in an unacceptable failure rate.[6] Table 2 clearly indicates the poor prognosis for reconstruction in an irradiated site with solid bone grafts.

TABLE 1 Combined Mandibular Homograft-Autograft

Type of Patient	No. of Patients	Success	Failure
Trauma	12	10	2
Cancer Resection			
without prior radiation	2	2	0
with prior radiation	12	2	10

TABLE 2 Mandibular Reconstruction: Solid Autologous Bone Grafts

Type of Patient	No. of Patients	Success	Failure
Trauma	7	6	1
Cancer Resection			
without prior radiation	2	2	0
with prior radiation	5	1	4

DISCUSSION

This experience, so far, has shown that with these two methods of reconstruction, cancer patients who have had significant doses of radiation therapy have a poor prognosis for successful reconstruction by conventional methods. Consequently, I have formulated the following strategy for reconstruction in such patients.

Preservation. If possible, mandible should be preserved, especially in the symphyseal area. Mandible that is preserved with its blood supply intact will survive radiation if adequately covered by connective tissue, skin, and mucosa.

Criteria to be used in determining whether the mandible can be preserved should be visual and radiographic (which are presumptive evidence) and confirmed by histologic examination. Although frozen sections of bone are not currently a practical reality, frozen sections of periosteum are easily obtained and can be used to determine whether there is a high probability of involvement of bone by an adjacent cancer. Bone seems to have a high degree of natural resistance to tumor invasion so that, if periosteum can be seen to be free of tumor and there is no clinical evidence of invasion of the cortex, the bone can be stripped of its periosteum and preserved with its internal blood supply intact on at least one side. Table 3 is a tabulation of the successful preservation of

TABLE 3 Preservation of Mandible (Clinical Carcinoma Involving Mucosa Or Gingiva Overlying Mandible; Periosteal Biopsy Negative; Postoperative Radiation)

Stage of Primary	No. Of Patients	Recurrence of Primary	No Recurrence of Primary
T2	3	1	3
T3	4	1	3
Adjacent fixed node	2	0	2
Total	9	2	7

mandible in patients who would normally, on clinical grounds, require mandibular resection.

Nonreplacement. Most mandibular resections posterior to the symphysis do not require replacement for functional reasons or even, in most cases, for cosmetic reasons. In fact, mandibular reconstruction in the posterior mandible following resection of large portions of the tongue, floor of mouth, or palate may create disorders of speech and swallowing that are worse than those in the majority of unreconstructed patients. Primary closure of the defect from composite resections results in a closure of the dead space that would be present were the original size of the oral cavity maintained. Since the mandible is a principal determinant of the size of the oral cavity, removal of a portion of the posterior mandible permits a reduction in the size of the oral cavity through primary closure of the cheek to the tongue. Thus the tongue, though reduced in size, still fills the oral cavity and oral pharynx and facilitates swallowing and speech.

Augmentation of Blood Supply. By growing a bone graft in an adjacent site with a good blood supply and subsequently transferring the graft as a part of a composite pedicle graft, bone can be successfully implanted in the desired previously irradiated site. Such a method has been tested by me in a small number of cases and has been found to be successful.

On the other hand, it is equally feasible to replace devitalized irradiated tissue with tissue having a good blood supply via a myocutaneous flap and to subsequently place a type of bone graft that has a high success rate in unirradiated patients. This method also has been used by me in a small number of cases with successful results. These two methods require delay of reconstruction in cases of postoperative radiation therapy. In cases in which these methods have been used, a delay of over one year has been observed.

Finally, the transfer of autologous bone through microvascular anastomosis has been shown to be successful and may well prove to be a consistently useful means of mandibular reconstruction.

CONCLUSIONS

Mandibular reconstruction is not difficult in the unirradiated patient. In the irradiated cancer patient, conventional grafts have a poor prognosis. A method of reconstruction that will provide consistently good results in such patients is still a subject for continued investigation.

REFERENCES

1. deFries HO, Marble HB, Sell KW. Reconstruction of the mandible. Arch Otolaryngol 1971; 93:426–432.
2. Boyne PJ. Restoration of osseous defects in maxillofacial casualties. J Am Dent Assoc 1969; 78:767–776.
3. Burwell RG. Studies in transplantation of bone. VIII. J Bone Facial Surg 1966; 48:532–563.
4. deFries HO. Reconstruction of the mandible: Use of combined homologous mandible and autologous bone. Otolaryngol Head Neck Surg 1981; 89:694–697.
5. Kreuz FP, Hyatt GW, Turner TC, et al. The preservation and clinical use of freeze-dried bone. J Bone Joint Surg 1951; 33:863–867.
6. Leipzig B, Cummings CW. Immediate mandibular reconstruction: human experience with autogenous frozen mandibular grafts. Otolaryngol Head Neck Surg 1981; 89:879–881.

MANDIBULAR RECONSTRUCTION WITH FREE ILIAC OSTEOCUTANEOUS FLAPS

G. IAN TAYLOR, M.B., B.S.,
F.R.C.S.(Lond.), F.R.A.C.S.

Major tumor resection or trauma to the head and neck frequently results in a defect of the mandible together with skin or intra-oral lining. In the early part of this century, either (1) such deficiencies were allowed to heal by contraction, and this produced the typical Andy Gump deformity, or (2) attempts were made to repair the defects with local flaps, and this commonly led to infection and fistula formation. Free bone grafts were particularly vulnerable when there was inadequate skin cover or lining.

The advent of the forehead flap, the deltopectoral flap, and more recently, the availability of new local flaps in this area (e.g., the trapezius and the pectoralis major myocutaneous flaps) have increased the surgeon's capabilities. These provide well vascularized soft tissue cover for free bone graffts and thus improve their chance of survival. To obtain one-stage reconstruction of these composite tissue defects, certain bones have been left attached to these local flaps in the expectation that they will retain some vascular supply. The clavicle has been transferred on the sternomastoid muscle, segments of the rib or sternum on the pectoralis major, and the acromiom on the trapezius muscle. There is evidence that the blood supply to these attached bones is at best tenuous, and this is reflected in their variable survival rate.[3-5] Our recent injection studies of the pectoralis major flap indicate that the supply to those ribs used most commonly (i.e., 6 and 7) is very poor or nonexistent. The major supply is to the third, fourth, and fifth ribs. Unfortunately, these ribs are more proximal to the base of the flap and thus their use is restricted in mandibular reconstruction.[6]

Manchester has shown excellent results for mandibular reconstruction by fashioning a corticocancellous replica of the lower jaw from the iliac crest and inserting it as a free graft into a healthy recipient bed.[2] Similar results have been achieved using split rib grafts placed in well-vascularized tissues. However, both of these techniques have limitations when there is a large soft tissue and bone gap. Previous radiotherapy compounds the problem. In this group of patients, a free vascularized flap of skin and bone provides the best solution. The skin is available for use as either external cover or internal lining, and the vascularized bone is more resistent to exposure and infection from the oral cavity.

A number of donor sites have been used for this purpose: (1) the rib and the overlying skin nourished by the intercostal vessels,[7] (2) the metatarsal and phalanges of the second ray, together with the skin on the dorsum of the foot based on the dorsalis pedis vessels,[1] (3) the iliac crest designed initially on the superficial circumflex iliac artery and more recently on the deep circumflex iliac artery (DCIA),[9,10] and (4) more recently, a segment of the radius combined with forearm skin and perfused by the radial vessels.[8]

I believe that the third alternative has a number of advantages, especially when the bone gap is considerable: (1) large amounts of both iliac bone and groin skin are available from an area that has a minimal donor site morbidity, both cosmetic and functional; (2) the vessels for anastomosis are large, 1.5 to 3.0 mm in diameter, permitting reliable anastomoses; (3) the pedicle is long, 5.0 to 8.0 cm; (4) the anatomy is familiar to most surgeons; (5) the iliac crest is the ideal shape for mandibular reconstruction, and sufficient bone is available in an adult to reconstruct an entire mandible with a vascularized graft from one hip; (6) the bone can be contoured, it can be split, or appropriate osteotomies can be performed to obtain an exact replica of the jaw; and (7) soft tissues other than skin may be included in the flap design to reconstruct muscle and ligamentous attachments to the lower jaw.

The main disadvantage of this graft is its bulk, especially in obese or very muscular patients. However, the skin and subcutaneous tissues can be omitted and the attached muscle sealed with a split skin graft. Alternatively, the skin flap may be thinned at a later stage.

DISSECTION OF THE FLAP

This dissection is conveniently divided into four steps: medial isolation of the pedicle, upper lateral division of the muscles of the anterior abdominal wall; lower lateral separation of the upper thigh muscles; and deep section of the ilium.

Medial Dissection

The skin is incised directly over the inguinal canal and the external ring located. The external oblique

aponeurosis is split parallel to and 1 cm above the free edge of the inguinal ligament. The external iliac artery is palpated through te posterior wall of the inguinal canal. The DCIA arises from its posterolateral side at the level of the inguinal ligament.[9]

The artery, together with its paired venae comitantes, courses upward and laterally in its own fascial sheath behind the inguinal ligament toward the anterior superior iliac spine (ASIS) (Fig. 1). The paired venae comitantes join to form a single vein 2 to 3 cm lateral to the external iliac artery. This vein then characteristically diverges upward from its artery to reach the external iliac vein. In so doing it crosses either in front of or behind the external iliac artery.

At this point of divergence, there is usually a communication with one of the venae comitantes of the superficial circumflex iliac artery. The pedicle is dissected laterally, dividing the arching fibers of the internal oblique and the transversus muscles from the inguinal ligament. A number of branches are distributed during this part of its course. Approximately 1 cm medial to the ASIS, a large ascending muscular branch is given off. This vessel pierces the transversus muscle and ascends the abdominal wall in the plane between this muscle and the internal oblique. It may be found reliably 1 cm above and lateral to the ASIS.

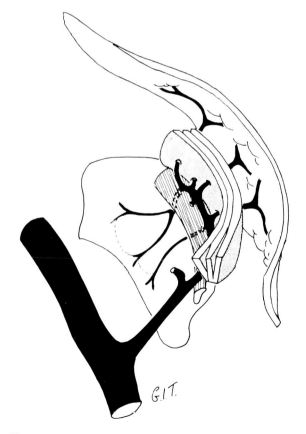

Figure 1 Diagram of the DCIA with its periosteal supply to the inner cortex of the ilium and the musculocutaneous perforators which pierce the three muscles of the abdominal wall at intervals to nourish the overlying skin. The iliacus muscle is cross-hatched.

It is often useful to look for this artery early in the dissection and trace it down to the main pedicle.

Rarely, the deep circumflex iliac vessels may lie in a more superficial plane, and when this occurs, the variation is usually associated with an abnormal obturator artery.

Upper Lateral Dissection

The key point in this part of the dissection is to include the musculocutaneous perforators to the skin. These vessels arise from the parent artery as it lies adjacent to the inner aspect of the ilium. They penetrate the muscles beyond the ASIS and emerge from the external oblique in a row approximately 1 cm above the iliac crest. The terminal part of the DCIA usually emerges as the largest perforator 8 to 10 cm from the ASIS.

To retain these perforators, a 1.5- to 2.0-cm wide strip of the three abdominal wall muscles is left attached to the bone, extending posteriorly for 8 to 10 cm. During the course of this dissection, the ascending branch of the DCIA is encountered (already discussed). This vessel is 1.0 to 1.5 mm in diameter and is usually suitable for anastomosis. It can be used to provide a distal runoff from the graft or to connect to another vessl (e.g., the superficial circumflex iliac artery) to augment the cutaneous circulation. After division of the three layers of the abdominal wall, the DCIA will be found situated in the fold between the overhanging transversus muscle and the iliacus. The iliacus muscle is divided 2 cm below and medial to this line, and the remaining muscle is swept from the surface of the iliac bone by blunt finger dissection. This preserves the periosteal supply.

Lower Lateral Dissection

Since the DCIA supplies the ilium from its medial side,[9] the muscles attached to its lateral aspect can be separated safely from the bone. However, it is useful in certain cases to retain some of the attachments to this side of the bone for use in mandibular reconstruction. A segment of the tensor fascia lata can be left on the outer lip of the iliac crest to reattach the masseter muscle. Similarly, the tendon of rectus femoris can be preserved at the anterior inferior iliac spine (AIIS) for reconstruction of the capsule of the temporomandibular (TM) joint.

The upper and lower lateral parts of this dissection are then joined beyond the tuberosity of the crest. The remaining muscle attachments are separated from the bone as far posteriorly as the posterior superior iliac spine (PSIS) if this length of bone graft is required. The terminal branch of the DCIA is thereby preserved in this part of the dissection. Finally, the inguinal ligament is detached from the ASIS, and the iliacus muscle is divided as it passes under the vascular pedicle. At this point the lateral cutaneous nerve of the thigh is encountered. In some cases its conti-

nuity can be retained: in others it may have to be divided and repaired.

Bone Section

Careful preoperative planning and the use of bone models provide an accurate assessment of the required length and shape of the bone graft.[9,10] The ilium is sectioned with an oscillating or reciprocating saw. The bone is eased medially to prevent tension on the vascular pedicle. Further contouring and osteotomies are performed *while the flap is in situ*. This shortens the ischemia time and permits circulatory readjustment in the flap before transfer.

Since the blood supply to the bone enters the medial cortex, it is possible to remove excess bone or indeed the entire outer cortex if desired. Osteotomies may be performed to adjust the curvature of the bone. In such circumstances, the integrity of the medial periosteum, together with the attachments of the transversus and iliacus muscle to the inner lip of the iliac crest, are preserved to ensure perfusion of the bone beyond the osteotomy.

Closure

Removal of the wing of the ilium creates a breach in the lateral abdominal wall which requires careful closure. It is essential to repair the transversus to the iliacus muscle or the remaining iliac bone. As the iliacus muscle is tenuous posteriorly, we have since found it useful to drill a number of holes in the cut edge of the ilium to reattach the transversus muscle. The remaining part of the closure involves suture of the glutei and the tensor fascia lata to the internal and external oblique muscles. A Tanner slide procedure may be useful if there is insufficient laxity in the external oblique.

In a series of over thirty patients, we have had only one minor area of herniation and this occurred in a man who gained 40 pounds in weight postoperatively. None of the patients have required a skin graft to the donor site as all have been closed directly.[11-13] The longest flap measured 33 cm and the widest 15 cm.

MANDIBULAR RECONSTRUCTION

The mandible may be designed from the iliac crest in one of three ways depending on the length of graft required and the position of the vascular pedicle (see Figs. 1 and 2).

1. The usual method utilizes the ipsilateral hip. The lower jaw is designed in such a way that the ASIS becomes the angle of the mandible, the AIIS becomes the head, and the iliac crest becomes the body of the mandible. The vascular pedicle will be situated behind the new angle of the jaw. Here it is readily accessible for anastomosis to one of

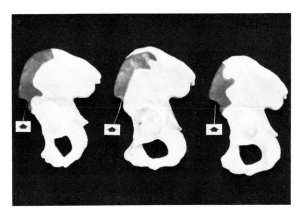

Figure 2 The three methods of designing the ramus and body of the mandible from the ilium. The first and third technique places the vascular pedicle (*arrow*) at the angle of the jaw. The second method sites the graft pedicle at the jaw midline where it will reach recipient vessels on either side of the neck.

the branches of the external carotid system (e.g., the facial artery). This design allows the greatest length of graft to be obtained for mandibular reconstruction. A wedge or step osteotomy is performed in the midline to adjust the curvature of the bone when the graft extends beyond the chin (Fig. 2, *left*).

2. Alternatively, the first pattern can be reversed so that the ramus is contoured from the posterior ilium and the body from the anterior part of the crest. This places the pedicle near the midline, and it will reach vessels on the opposite side of the neck. Because of the curvature of the crest, the graft must be designed from the opposite hip (Fig. 2, *center*).

3. Finally, for reconstruction of short mandibular segments, the bone graft may be designed so that the anterior iliac crest becomes the ramus of the jaw and the bone between the ASIS and the AIIS becomes the body (Fig. 2, *right*).

PREOPERATIVE PLANNING

Angiography

We perform angiography on the majority of patients. This is done under general anesthesia or regional anesthesia and provides valuable information regarding both the donor and the recipient vessels (Fig. 3). It outlines the effects of previous surgery, radiation, or tumor expansion on the vascular anatomy.

Our radiologists are experienced and have an extremely low morbidity rate associated with these procedures. The finding of an abnormal obturator artery in the groin is a preoperative warning that the course of the DCIA may be more superficial than normal, although we have yet to encounter this in a clinical case.[9]

The absence of suitable recipient vessels on one side of the neck following neck dissection or x-ray

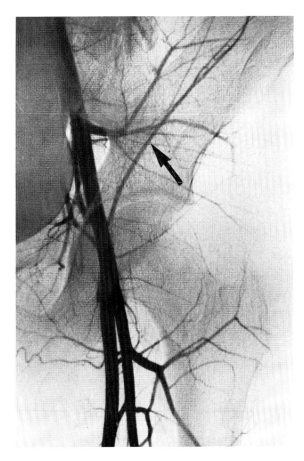

Figure 3 Angiogram showing the characteristic "paint brush stroke" of the DCIA passing upward and laterally at 45 degrees from the region of the hip joint.

therapy is identified, and this predicts the need for vein grafts or a modification of flap design.

Bone Models

An acrylic pelvis with detachable iliac crests is a useful aid when selecting the donor hip and for planning the correct orientation of the bone flap. A methyl methacrylate replica of the bone defect is made preoperatively and used both in the planning and as a preoperative check of the size and shape of the bone flap, both at the donor and at the recipient site (Fig. 4).

Cadaver Rehearsal

In spite of all the preoperative planning (already discussed), it may be difficult to anticipate some of the three-dimensional problems that are encountered during surgery. Rehearsal of the operation in a fresh cadaver has been invaluable in solving these problems before entering the operating room

Preoperative Marking

On the day prior to surgery, a plastic foam replica of the skin defect is shaped, and this pattern is

A

B

C

D

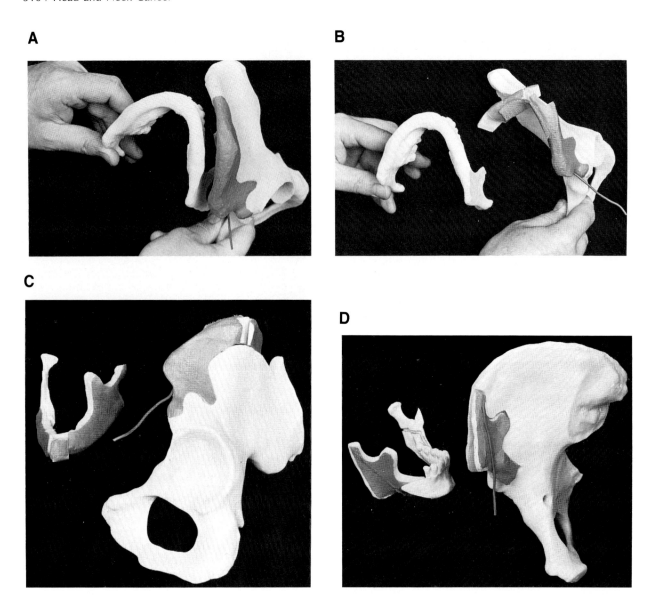

Figure 4 Bone models used in planning. *A*, The curve of the iliac crest matches the lower border of the body of the mandible to the chin and then veers away. *B*, Osteotomy, performed from the outer cortex to recreate the chin contour. This may be done as a step or a wedge osteotomy. *C*, Graft model. Note the keystone of bone at the chin point. *D*, Graft model. The graft was split from the inner aspect of the ilium in a child to leave the outer cortex and hemi-apophysis for normal hip contour and growth.

transferred to the hip, taking care to center it over the skin perforators. The skin flap is marked two-thirds above and one-third below the line of the anterior iliac crest (Fig. 5). This flap will survive as far medially as the femoral vessels, but it must incorporate the perforators which emerge above the iliac crest between 2 and 8 cm from the ASIS. The acrylic model is used to outline the bone flap.

Doppler studies can be used to locate the recipient vessels in the neck. The skin incisions are marked, and if vein grafts are required, these are also mapped out on a suitable arm.

OPERATIVE STRATEGY

Preferably, two or even three operating teams work simultaneously. One isolates that graft, another dis-

sects the recipient bed, and the third team harvests a vein graft if required.

The bone model facilitates the preparation of the recipient pocket in the face and the correct shape of the bone flap while it is still attached in the groin. We routinely leave the flap to perfuse for at least 20 minutes before transfer, and this provides a convenient coffee break.

After removing the flap, one team closes the donor site while another secures the bone flap and performs the anastomoses. If vein grafts are required, these may be attached to the flap on a side table under ideal conditions. A useful technique is to attach the vein graft as a loop between the flap artery and the vein, taking care to ensure that the valves are orientated correctly. After bone flap fixation, the loop can

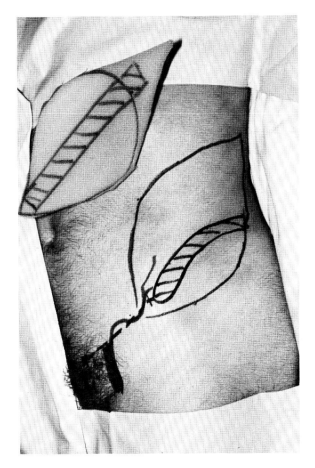

Figure 5 Pattern of the soft tissue and bone requirements transferred to the ipsilateral hip.

be cut at the required length and anastomosed in the neck (Fig. 6).[13]

RESULTS

At The Royal Melbourne Hospital, over a 16-year period, 110 patients have been treated for squamous cell carcinoma which involved the mandible. In 50 patients it was possible to perform a marginal resection, preserving the lower border of the jaw. Sixty patients required a full-thickness resection of the mandible, and of these patients, 20 underwent reconstruction of the jaw. The resections were performed by one surgeon.

In 14 patients a conventional nonvascularized bone graft was utilized; the rib was selected in 12 patients and the iliac crest in two. Three bone grafts were lost due to exposure and infection, thus providing a success rate of 80 percent.

In 6 patients in whom the defect was large, a free vascularized iliac osteocutaneous flap, designed on the deep circumflex iliac vessels, was used. In addition, a similar reconstruction was employed by me in a further eight patients, the majority of which followed tumor ablation. Of the 14 revascularized bone transfers, four bone flaps were used to reconstruct very large defects following extended hemimandibulectomy procedures, and in one of these patients, almost the entire mandible was repaired with bone from one hip. In eight cases, an osteotomy of the iliac bone was performed to recreate the chin contour, and six patients had received previous radiotherapy to the area. One case failed owing to complications with the vascular

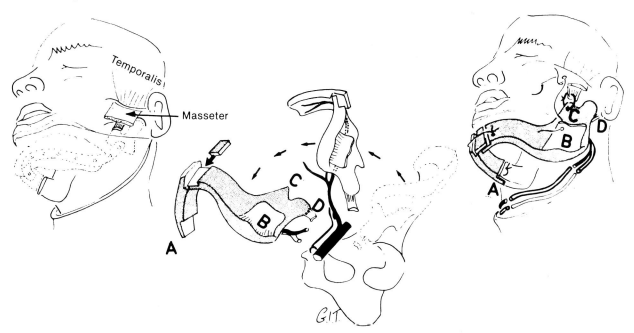

Figure 6 The procedure. *Left*, Resection of the entire mandible (except the right ramus) together with the tumor, the metal prosthesis, and the soft tissues from the lower lip to the level of the hyoid bone. *Center*, The graft designed from the ipsilateral hip. A segment of the rectus femoris tendon (*D*) provides capsular ligaments for the TM joint. A flap of fascia lata (*B*) allows reattachment of the masseter muscle. A coronoid process (*C*) is shaped from the blade of the ilium to secure the temporalis tendon. An osteotomy is made in the midline to recreate the chin and secured with a free bone keystone. The bone is step cut at *A* for fixation to the right ramus. *Right*, the graft in position with vein grafts needed to reach normal recipient vessels on the opposite side of the neck.

anastomosis, thus providing a success rate of 93 percent.

It is noteworthy that in three of the 13 successful cases, the bone flap was exposed in the floor of the mouth when the suture line broke down. In two of these patients, an osteotomy of the bone flap had been performed to recreate the chin contour, and it was the bone distal to the vascular pedicle which became exposed. In every case the defect healed spontaneously over 7 to 10 days by a process of granulation and epithelialization. This observation strongly supports the case for a free vascularized bone flap.

CONCLUSION

There have been many significant advances in the past twenty years for the reconstruction of major defects of the mandible and the associated soft tissues. Initially the forehead and the deltopectoral flap improved the soft tissue repair. They provided better cover for nonvascularized bone grafts taken usually from the iliac crest or the rib. Their reliability fell dramatically, however, when the area was heavily irradiated. The myocutaneous flap provides additional bulk as well as vascularized muscle to cover the carotid vessels. However, the supply to associated bone segments has not proved to be reliable.

The vascular territory of the DCIA encompasses a large amount of skin and bone. This can be used for one-stage transfer with reliability. The bone flap is well vascularized; it provides excellent contour for the mandible and a donor site that has minimal morbidity. In addition to skin, other soft tissue elements can be harvested with a common blood supply to provide a functional as well as an aesthetic result. The place of this composite graft is best suited for the difficult problems encountered in reconstruction of the head and neck especially where (1) the bone defect is large; (2) there is an associated soft-tissue defect of lining and/or cover; (3) the area has been or will be irradiated; and (4) the patient is fit enough to withstand a prolonged operation.

REFERENCES

1. Bell MSG. Personal Communication, 1979.
2. Manchester WM. Some technical improvements in the reconstruction of the mandible and temporomandibular joint. Plast Reconstr Surg 1972; 50:249.
3. Merritt WH, Acharya G, Johnson ML. Complications in forty-five island pectoralis major myocutaneous flaps for head and neck cancer reconstruction: A 13-month followup. Presented at the American Society of Plastic and Reconstructive Surgeons, New York, New York, October 23, 1981.
4. Baek S, Lawson W, Biller HF. An analysis of 133 pectoralis major myocutaneous flaps. Plast Reconstr Surg 1982; 69:460–467.
5. Mehrhof A, Rosenstock A, Niefeld J, Merritt WH, Theogaraj SD, Cohen IK. The pectoralis major myocutaneous flap in head and neck reconstruction: an analysis of complications. Am J Surg. In Press.
6. Reid C, Taylor GI. The vascular territory of the acromiothoracic axis. Br J Plast Surg April 1984; 37:194.
7. Rosen IB, Bell MSG, Barron PT, Zuker RM, Manktelow RT. Use of microvascular flaps including free osteocutaneous flaps in reconstruction after composite resection for radiation–recurrent oral cancer. Am J Surg 1979; 138:544.
8. Serrafin D, Bunke HJ, eds. Vascularized rib periosteal transplantation. In: Microsurgical composite tissue transplantation. St. Louis: Mosby, 1979.
9. Soutar DS, Scheker LR, Tanner NSB, McGregor IA. The radial forearm flap: a versatile method for intra oral reconstruction. Br J Plast Surg 1983; 36:1–8.
10. Taylor GI, Townsend P, Corlett RJ. Superiority of the deep circumflex iliac vessels as the supply for free groin flaps; Experimental work. Plast Reconstr Surg 1979; 64:595.
11. Taylor GI, Townsend P, Corlett RJ. Superiority of the deep circumflex iliac vessels as the supply for free groin flaps; Clinical work. Plast Reconstr Surg 1979; 64:745.
12. Taylor GI. Reconstruction of the mandible with free composite iliac bone grafts. Ann Plast Surg 1982; 9:361.
13. Taylor GI. Aesthetic aspects of microsurgery: composite tissue transfer to the face. Clin Plast Surg 1981; 8:333.
14. Taylor GI. The current status of free vascularized bone grafts. Clin Plast Surg 1983; 10:185.

36. Vocal Rehabilitation after Laryngectomy

INTRODUCTION

JEROME C. GOLDSTEIN, M.D., F.A.C.S.

The larynx is a marvelous organ. Not only does it function as the organ of voice, but more importantly, it is the guardian of the airway. It is responsible for the prevention of aspiration.

The oncologic surgeon is concerned not only with curing the patient of his disease, but also with the restoration of form and function following our ablative surgery. This concept is not new. Gussenbauer created an external shunt for Billroth's first laryngectomy patient in 1873. This was followed by a century more of different attempts, some with devices, many with innovative surgical efforts. It must not be forgotten that the purpose of surgery is to cure the patient of his disease. Some innovative surgical improvisations necessitated the preservation of mucosa (as, for example, in the Staffieri method), which occasionally was related to higher than acceptable recurrence rates.

The reintroduction and improvement of the puncture technique by Singer and Blom was a most important step in this evolution. Resse Gutman's original observations of his butcher patient in the late 1920s and his attempt to reproduce this in the early 1930s were fortunately resurrected by these authors. Their introduction of the small Silastic "duckbill" valve constituted the missing link for the success of this procedure.

The question now is "What is the proper application of this procedure?" Is the following statement true or false? "The acquisition of good esophageal speech is the best means of vocal rehabilitation following a laryngectomy." What in fact is the best rehabilitation today? Where are we now in this regard in 1984? These challenges are discussed in the chapters that follow. Gates has organized one of the few prospective studies of esophageal speech acquisition. He stresses the functions of the voice in emotional expression (laugh, whistle) and its role in total rehabilitation, as well as the goals and choices of rehabilitative efforts. Weinberg, who has been involved with many of the basic pressure studies done on these prostheses, discussed various perspectives involved in speech rehabilitation following total laryngectomy. He

emphasizes that cancer treatment is a unified process of which rehabilitation is an integral part. He tells us that voice production is but one part of the total speech process and the restoration of speech involves more than just "restoring the voice". He reviews the airway resistance of the currently available prostheses. Panje further modified the puncture technique so that it can be performed on an outpatient basis under local anesthesia. He is now performing the procedure primarily at the time of laryngectomy and will introduce us to his "scoop instrument", which he utilizes in the performance of this procedure. He has ten specific indications for the performance of his surgical technique and will review these for us.

In their chapter, Singer and Bloom present their present criteria, modifications, and results for this procedure.

The reader should be aware of the areas of disagreement as well as agreement among the authors. For example, Panje believes that parasurgical irradiation may be an indication to delay performance of TE puncture, whereas Singer does not. The relative importance of the airway resistance of the prosthesis is another area of vigorous discussion. All of this makes this surgical frontier exciting for the experienced surgeon as well as a fruitful research area for the young residents and fellows.

CURRENT STATUS OF LARYNGECTOMEE REHABILITATION

GEORGE A. GATES, M.D.

REHABILITATION CONSEQUENCES OF TOTAL LARYNGECTOMY

Physiologic Effects

Loss of voice is the most important rehabilitation consequence of laryngectomy. Although some focus upon this mutilative aspect of the surgery, it is important to remember that it is the cancer that destroys the voice, not the operation. Today it is unusual to find a patient with an early lesion in whom voice preservation is not possible. Thus, total loss of voice can be avoided if patient awareness is high and prompt diagnosis is rendered.

Because voice is the primary modality of human communication, it serves as the carrier for language in which are embedded the entire range of human emotions, feelings, and thoughts. Nonetheless, alternative methods of oral and nonoral communication exist

and may be utilized in rehabilitation. It is also important to remember that postlaryngectomy rehabilitation involves more than voice restoration. Substantial adjustments need to take place postoperatively in many other areas of function as well.

Loss of the emotional expression and of the other contributions of the larynx to normal function of the upper air passages is an important aspect of postlaryngectomy rehabilitation. Laryngectomees are well aware, by their absence, of the importance of chuckles, guffaws, and good old-fashioned belly laughs and indicate considerable regret at being unable to express themselves through laughter. Less noticeable, perhaps, but of importance, especially to women laryngectomees, is loss of the ability to express sorrow physically through sobbing, sighing, and crying.

Related airway functions such as nasal clearance (sneeze, sniff, blow), the sense of smell, and the ability to whistle are also lost after laryngectomy. Many larynx-related functions are taken for granted, especially the ability to clear the nasal passages through sneezing, sniffing, and blowing. Loss of smell results principally from the inability to pass ordorant-containing air over the olfactory epithelium, located high in the nose, where the sensation of smell is initiated. Also a factor is loss of olfactory sensors located in the supraglottic larynx. Other airway actions lost following laryngectomy are the ability to whistle or blow out a candle. These are examples of medically minor but personally important consequences of laryngectomy.

Psychosocial Effects

Psychosocial effects are profound. Self-image and self-esteem are reduced substantially, in part, because organ removal generally is a psychologic equivalent of castration, and because, in many cases, the patient is well aware that the cancer is self-induced (secondary to smoking), and the operation is viewed as punishment. While we may view these as strange perceptions, considering the life-saving value of the procedure, it is nonetheless the patients' perceptions which greatly influence their behavior. Few patients fail to describe an alteration of their self-image when given appropriate psychologic tests. The extent to which this impairs subsequent adjustment is variable and may, in some cases, adversely influence rehabilitation.

All patients pass through an episode of substantial depression in the immediate postoperative period when the impact of what has transpired becomes a reality. This is usually transient, provided there is substantial support from family and friends and the problem has been addressed preoperatively. In some cases the depression may persist indefinitely and strongly impair recovery. Some who are alcoholics preoperatively seemingly intensify their withdrawal after surgery.

Interpersonal relationships are usually affected. Some withdraw from relationships for the aforementioned reasons. Most find that stable relationships readjust satisfactorily after the surgery; indeed, some note increased closeness because of the enhanced bonding that occurs through the stress of the illness. All spouses must pass through an adjustment period, a fact that is often overlooked in rehabilitation programs.

Socioeconomic Consequences

Occupational considerations are important for those with laryngeal cancer because absence of a normal voice can be disqualifying for many jobs. Most employers are able to take advantage of the person's skills and experience and relocate or reassign the employee satisfactorily, but sometimes with a demotion in status or pay.

Because the average age of a laryngectomee is 55 and job relocation may not be acceptable, many who are near retirement age opt for early retirement or retirement because of medical disability. This aspect of rehabilitation deserves study and attention toward optimal use of employee skills and experience.

For laryngectomees with communication handicaps (i.e., esophageal speech that cannot be heard in a noisy factory), alternative methods for communication may need to be developed. There are many choices for successful restoration of job-related communication ability. Unfortunately, cancer patients are often excluded from government sponsored rehabilitation programs, and the patient must turn to the private sector for assistance.

REHABILITATIVE CHOICES

Avoid Total Laryngectomy

Today there are more alternatives to total laryngectomy than ever before. For small lesions, radiation therapy should be considered. For large lesions strategically placed, subtotal laryngectomy via the classic hemilaryngectomy or the supraglottic subtotal laryngectomy are useful alternatives. Pearsons' near-total operation with a speaking shunt offers voice retention, but with a permanent tracheostomy.

Mutism

Some patients are quite content to remain mute and noncommunicative. Attempts to teach esophageal speech to such patients will obviously fail. It is important for the surgeon and speech instructor to ascertain preoperatively the goals and needs of the patient in this regard.

Communication Devices

The classic Western Electric artifical larynx, the Cooper Rand device, and a variety of other models and types of communication devices are available and should be employed extensively in the early postoperative and posthospitalization periods to facilitate communication until a permanent method is achieved. Some patients find these devices to be satisfactory long-term methods.

Esophageal Speech

Long the mainstay of postlaryngectomee rehabilitation, esophageal speech has declined in the minds of many as the ideal method because (1) only one-third of today's laryngectomees are able to acquire esophageal speech,[1] (2) because of low volume and flexibility, many are turning to a speech fistula technique, and (3) as experience and satisfaction grow with the newer techniques, there will be less incentive for patients and teachers alike to struggle with learning esophageal speech. Better predictors of the ability to acquire esophageal speech as well as techniques for integrating esophageal voice with other methods are needed.

Surgical Speech Fistula

Passing through a long line of methods, most of us have settled on the surgically created midline tracheoesophageal fistula, which is kept open (and impervious to aspiration) by a plastic tube with a one-way valve, such as Blom-Singer's or Panje's devices. These permit rapid acquisition of an "esophageal" voice that is much louder and more versatile than the classic esophageal speech. Either an external valve or the patient's finger must be used to occlude the tracheostoma in order for air flow and voicing to occur.

FACTORS LIMITING ACQUISITION OF ESOPHAGEAL SPEECH

From 1975 to 1976, my associates and I evaluated 103 patients with suspected (or proven) laryngeal cancer prior to definitive therapy. This cohort was accrued from all the hospitals within San Antonio at the time and represented an unselected nearly total sample of all available cases. Of these, 53 underwent total laryngectomy and 47 were evaluated 6 months after completion of cancer therapy.[1] The characteristics of those who acquired and used esophageal speech and those who did not are displayed in Tables 1 and 2. The most important factors that affect the acquisition of esophageal speech are to be discussed.

Extent of Cancer Therapy

Radiation therapy impedes the acquisition and use of esophageal speech in two ways: (1) the fibrosis

stiffens tissues and limits flexibility, and (2) the intense mucositis of the pharynx that occurs during radiotherapy is usually given postoperatively and precludes practicing esophageal speech.

Extended operations which remove large parts of the pharynx, base of tongue, or soft palate usually preclude acquisition of esophageal speech. In such instances, good planning should include alternative methods for speech production.

Vigor (Performance Status)

Advanced age or its sequelae often diminish physical energy to the point that learning an effortful new skill such as esophageal speech may not be possible. Age, per se, is not a factor. Hearing loss that accompanies old age does interfere with the learning of esophageal speech.

Lowered performance status is not an unusual result of multimodality therapy used in the treatment of head and neck cancer. For advanced lesions, chemotherapy, surgery, and radiation therapy may all be used, and each takes away from patients' physical reserves.

Stricture and Dysphagia

The development of a pharyngeal/esophageal stricture virtually precludes acquisition of esophageal

TABLE 1 Personal Characteristics of Esophageal Speakers (ES) and Nonesophageal Speakers (ES) Groups

	ES (N=12)	ES (N=35)	Significance of Difference
	(Mean and standard error of the mean)		
Age (years)	61 ± 2.5 years	60 ± 1.3	P 0.701*
Income ($)	$5,084 ± 1,155	$7,043 ± 1013	P 0.305*
No. homemates	1.8 ± .5	1.3 ± 1.2	P 0.260*
Phonation time (sec)	13.8 ± 2.2	8.8 ± 1.2	P 0.032*
Sex (M:F)	9 M; 3 F	26 M; 9 F	P 0.961†
Education (8: 9 yrs)	6 eighth grade or less; 6 ninth grade or more	8 eighth grade or less; 27 ninth grade or more	P 0.076†

*(Student's t-test of independent means)
†(Chi-square test)
Reprinted with permission from Gates GA, Ryan W, Cooper JC Jr, et al. Current status of laryngectomee rehabilitation. Part II, Causes of failure. Am J Otolaryngol 1982;3:8–14.

TABLE 2 Treatment and Six-month Outcomes of Esophageal Speakers (ES) and Nonesophageal Speakers (ES)

	ES (N=12)		ES (N=35)		
	No	Yes	No	Yes	Significance of Difference
Radical neck dissection	4	8	5	30	P 0.148*
Postoperative radiotherapy	8	4	12	23	P 0.06*
Postoperative fistula	8	4	25	9	P 0.650*
Difficulty swallowing	11	1	17	17	P 0.011*
Recurrent cancer	8	4	25	10	P 0.756*
Physical scale (x ± SEM)	3.25 ± 0.3		2.3 ± 0.2		P 0.021†

*(Chi-square)
†(Student's t-test of independent means)
Reprinted with permission from Gates GA, Ryan W, Cooper JC Jr, et al. Current status of laryngectomee rehabilitation. Part II, Causes of failure. Am J Otolaryngol 1982;3:8–14.

speech. Dysphagia from any cause increases the likelihood of failure.

Motivation

To learn and use esophageal speech well requires great desire on the part of the patient. No amount of cajoling from family or therapist can replace intrinsic motivation. Certainly, without motivation esophageal speech cannot be acquired. It is often the case that patients who are strongly motivated learn esophageal speech. The converse implication, i.e., that those who fail do not really try, does not have validity in my opinion and may result in an undeserved sense of failure, as described earlier.

RECOMMENDATIONS

Team Approach

The ideal rehabilitative environment requires, in my opinion, a functional relationship between the surgeon, speech teacher, and other support personnel (cancer nurse, psychologist, social worker). It is important, for planning, that evaluations regarding rehabilitation be done preoperatively and that the patient meet and identify with the speech teacher before the surgery so that goals can be established early on.

Flexibility

It is clear that no one method is best and that, given today's variety of rehabilitative options, due consideration should be given to individualization of technique to meet each patient's specific needs.

REFERENCES

1. Gates GA, Ryan W, Cooper JC Jr, et al. Current status of laryngectomee rehabilitation. Part II, Causes of failure. Am J Otolaryngol 1982; 3:8–14.

SPEECH REHABILITATION FOLLOWING TOTAL LARYNGECTOMY: SOME PERSPECTIVES

BERND WEINBERG, Ph.D.

In this presentation, I would like to share some views about treatment and research in speech rehabilitation of laryngectomized patients from my perspective as a speech pathologist. These should reveal something about the current status of treatment and research and identify some goals or philosophies that might guide future research and treatment.

ONCOLOGY, REHABILITATION, AND SPEECH

Initially, I would like to explore briefly two general perspectives. The first is that the various facets of cancer treatment (.e.g., total laryngectomy surgery, speech rehabilitation following larynx removal), are highly integrated or related parts of what should be a unified clinical process. This perspective is not an original one, but an important perspective that should guide both current and future treatment and research. Stated differently, rehabilitation (e.g., speech, psychosocial) should not be regarded as independent, postsurgical activities, but should form integral parts of treatment protocols developed during the intial visit(s) by patients to physicians' offices.

In actual practice, cancer treatment in the form of total laryngectomy and postsurgical speech rehabilitation are often carried out as two relatively independent activities. The rationale on which surgeons rely for removing the larynx and reconstructing the patient is largely influenced by oncologic principles and considerations. The consequences of these actions on the restoration of speech are enormous. Total laryngectomy occasions radical alteration in body systems used to produce speech. These changes have far-reaching consequences on speech reacquisition which require laryngectomized patients to produce speech using nonconventional air stream, phonatory, articulatory, and timing mechanisms.[1,2]

It is clear that total laryngectomy always results in a sacrifice of tissue essential to normal vocal function. For example, both esophageal speech and tracheoesophageal speech depend on the use of surgically reconstructed tissue for voice production. Speech pathologists are therefore called on to develop speech in individuals who rely on surgical residue for voice-producing sources.[1] Variations in reconstructive technique would be expected to influence function of the voicing sources used by many laryngectomees. The point is simply that surgical treatment and rehabilitation are related parts of a single process. It should be high research priority to identify and gain control over the determinants for successful alaryngeal voice/speech reacquisition. Efforts must be undertaken to define and develop rationales for reconstruction which are based on rehabilitative considerations. Reconstruction should be undertaken to facilitate or optimize reacquisition of speech/voice and to optimize tumor control.

Improvements in both current practice and future treatment protocols would be expected through aggressive integration of oncology treatment and post-surgical rehabilitation. Significant advances in communication rehabilitation can be expected only after the realities of the integrated nature of cancer treatment and rehabilitation are incorporated into clinical practice and research.

These realities suggest a need for broad, preferably shared, educational and clinical experiences between head and neck surgeons and speech specialists. Surgeons need to understand how speech is produced and relate this understanding to the problem of acquiring speech after larynx removal. Speech pathologists need to understand what cancer is, how it is treated, and how to relate this understanding to the management of head and neck cancer from both oncology and rehabilitation perspectives. At a minimum, shared educational and clinical experiences between surgeons and speech specialists would be expected to heighten awareness of the relation that exists between oncology treatment and speech rehabilitation, to foster improvements in total care and management, and to enhance the depth and breadth of knowledge shared by practitioners and scholars in both professions.

The title of this part, *Vocal Rehabilitation after Laryngectomy*, serves as an effective platform for introducing the second perspective. There should be universal agreement that a fundamental rehabilitation aim following total laryngectomy is the restoration of oral communication or speech.[1,2] It is apparent that many clinicians and investigators in our mutual fields do not clearly distinguish between, and perhaps fail to comprehend what is meant by, the terms voice and speech. For example, a review of recent papers published about the tracheoesophageal puncture method reveals that all but a few paper titles and contents focus on the voice restoration aspects of this approach.[3-21] Human voice production does represent an essential part of the speech act. However, voice production is but one part of the speech production process and an even larger communication process. This issue is raised because it has enormous treatment and research implications and because it represents more than a mere semantic error. Focus on voice restoration serves to oversimplify the rehabilitative aim sought for all laryngectomized patients—restoration of oral communication. Speech rehabilitation for laryngectomized patients involves far more than voice restoration or vocal rehabilitation.

There is ample evidence to support the view that the process of speech production is more generally and profoundly altered following larynx removal.[1,2] Restoration of speech involves much more than merely getting the voice back! Speech rehabilitation for laryngectomized patients should involve routine management of speech rate, phrasing and temporal difficulties, alteration of articulatory and intelligibility errors, elimination of extraneous behaviors and noises,

development of prosody (stress, intonation, and juncture), in addition to a concern for voice return in a generic sense.[1,2] Speech pathologists and surgeons who fail to address speech rehabilitation broadly may fail to fully comprehend the communication–speech process and may seriously underestimate the contributions therapy can provide. Treatment that merely deals with the fitting of prostheses, teaching patients to use these devices, and/or early voice return seriously undercuts the ultimate levels of speech proficiency patients might reasonably be expected to achieve. From a communication perspective, the ultimate rehabilitative outcomes achieved by patients undergoing puncture type methods of treatment are not solely dependent on surgery or surgical-prosthetic factors. Our second perspective is a simple one. Although voice restoration is an important part of speech rehabilitation, voice restoration and speech rehabilitation are not necessarily synonomous treatment endeavors.

SPEECH ALTERNATIVES

A fundamental rehabilitation aim following total laryngectomy is the restoration of oral communication. There are three major contemporary approaches used to achieve this goal: teaching laryngectomized patients to speak with various types of artificial larynges, to develop esophageal speech, and to develop speech with some form of surgical–prosthetic assistance. These approaches provide speech specialists, physicians, and patients with a reasonably large set of rehabilitative alternatives. The current state-of-the-art is such that it would be appropriate to conclude that no patient undergoing uncomplicated, total laryngectomy should be without some method of functionally serviceable speech. This conclusion is made in full recognition that all contemporary approaches to communication restoration are characterized by a set of clearly identifiable assets as well as liabilities. All approaches are not universally applicable to all laryngectomized patients. Large numbers of laryngectomized patients have been successfully rehabilitated using each of these three primary methods of speech restoration, whereas a significant number of patients have not been or cannot be successfully rehabilitated by means of each of these methods. Stated simply, there are successes and failures in all approaches, and there is no univerally applicable rehabilitative solution.

Given these realities, some discussion about future goals and directions appears fruitful. A significant number of laryngectomized patients rely on artificial larynges to produce speech. Unfortunately, major advances or improvements have not been made in the design of artificial larynges. The speech of users of these devices is characterized by a non-normal electronic or mechanical quality and linguistically limiting variation in fundamental frequency (pitch) and intensity (loudness). Given the current state of knowledge, technology, models, and theory, efforts should be undertaken to design efficient, linguistically acceptable, more esthetically pleasing and human sounding artificial voicing sources.

In this context, we should acknowledge that contemporary knowledge and understanding of important aspects of alaryngeal speech production are not based on strong theoretical formulations or models. As suggested earlier, human voice production is an important component of human speech production. Contemporary knowledge, treatment, and research on phonation with a larynx are supported by a rich array of theoretic formulations and a variety of models. This framework provides a powerful investigative platform from which advances in treatment, understanding, and inquiry can emerge.

In both esophageal and tracheoesophageal phonation, surgically reconstructed tissue is used as a voicing source. In the former, air insufflated into the esophagus is used to power the voicing source; in the latter, pulmonary air is used. In either case, a theory or model of phonation does not exist. The absence of a strong theoretic or model base seriously impairs the quality of investigation and diminishes the prospect for attaining significant advances.

Significant future advances in communication rehabilitation of laryngectomized patients require accelerated investigation of both a basic and an applied type. As indicated, both esophageal and tracheoesophageal speech rely on surgically reconstructed tissue as voicing sources. In both cases, phonation is accomplished with air in the esophagus and with esophageal distention. There is a clear need to enlarge current understanding of both normal and surgically altered/reconstructed esophageal anatomy and function. Basic studies of the innervation and physiological mechanisms underlying function of the esophagus, particularly under conditions of insufflation and distention, are needed. Studies of this type are essential because differences in structure and function of the esophagus, particularly in the region of the upper esophageal inlet or sphincter, would be expected to influence directly the acquisition and quality of (tracheo)esophageal speech. Esophageal air insufflation and distention are reported to mediate reflex responses (airtight closure, spasm, peristalsis) in the upper esophageal inlet and body.[17,18,22] Carefully controlled investigation of these responses in both normal and laryngectomized patients is limited. More research is needed to resolve a number of important rehabilitative questions. For example, does normal function of the esophagus represent an influence that is detrimental (negative) to the acquisition of functionally serviceable (tracheo)esophageal voice?[22] Would the production and acquisition of functionally serviceable (tracheo)esophageal speech be facilitated by deliberately compromising the function of the esophageal body and its upper inlet?[22] Do laryngectomized patients who exhibit airtight closure of the upper esophageal inlet in response to or in association with esophageal air insufflation and distention exhibit an abnormal response?[17,18,22] Can patients learn to inhibit this response? What factors mediate this response?[17,18,22] What is the rationale for performing selective myotomy on patients who exhibit airtight closure?[18,22,23] Is selective myotomy being performed to minimize or eradicate an "abnormal response"[17,18] or is it being completed to deliberately compromise function and alter a "normal response" in order to optimize rehabilitation.[22] Finally, it would be highly valuable to define, on an a priori basis, both the necessary and sufficient physiologic properties of the (tracheo)esophageal voicing source essential to optimization of air insufflation and voicing. Efforts must be undertaken to begin to design reconstructive phases of surgical treatment in such a manner as to be able to create this physiologically optimizing situation on a reliable basis.

In concluding this phase of this presentation, the highly significant investigative opportunities tracheoesophageal puncture methods have provided should be highlighted. These methods provide scientists and clinicians with an opportunity for direct, relatively noninvasive monitoring of respiratory input (e.g., volumes, pressures, flows), chest wall kinematics, and changes in the response state of the voicing source. This opportunity represents a powerful new experimental advantage which should enable investigators to make significant future advances in treatment and research.

TRACHEOESOPHAGEAL PUNCTURE: SOME PERSPECTIVES

In recent years, we have all witnessed a dramatic resurgence of interest and activity related to surgical–prosthetic methods of speech rehabilitation, and many of us have taken active and significant roles in this treatment development. I would like to raise a few perspectives about this treatment approach from my orientation as a speech pathologist. Initially, I would emphasize again that contemporary surgical–prosthetic approaches represent speech (communication) restoration methods.[2] They are not merely voice restoration techniques, and the ultimate outcomes of these approaches are not solely mediated by surgical–prosthetic factors. Second, as a consequence of recent papers[7] and advertisements (ASHA, May, June, 1984), there is a need to express concern about efforts to popularize the notion that prostheses used in conjuction with tracheoesophageal puncture are prosthetic larynges. For example, the title of a recent paper by Henley-Cohn and his associates, *Artifical Larynx Prostheses: Comparative Clinical Evaluation*[7], and the prominent use of the text, *A Prosthetic Larynx—an Alternative to the Electrolarynx or Esophageal Speech*, in a recent advertisement by American V. Mueller represent two vivid examples of this form of unnecessary popularization. Two types of prosthesis are used in conjunction with tracheoesophageal puncture methods: tracheoesophageal puncture prosthesis and tracheostomal breathing valves. Neither of these devices constitutes prosthetic larynges. Rather, the prostheses referred to by Henley-Cohn and American V. Mueller and Singer-Blom are tracheoesophageal puncture prostheses. Tracheoesophageal puncture prostheses are one-way air shunts.[3-31] Hence, the implication that a larynx has been developed is both misleading and unnecessary, particularly in publications and advertisements directed toward informed, professionally educated readers and consumers.

A few words about these prostheses. At this time, several one-way valved tracheoesophageal puncture prostheses have been developed to the point that they are being manufactured and distributed on a commercial basis. All tracheoesophageal puncture prostheses serve three primary functions: (1) they are used to maintain patency of the puncture tract; (2) they permit air to be shunted from the trachea to the esophagus; and (3) they prevent blackflow of contents of the esophagus (e.g., air, liquids) into the airway. The design objectives and performance characteristics of such devices can be carefully specified on an a priori basis.[25,31] In addition, all of these devices are relatively simple mechanical systems which respond or behave in ways that can be modeled and investigated in terms of known theory (e.g., spring constants, fluid dynamics).[25] In view of these realities, it would not be unreasonable to expect developers of such devices to at least specify design objectives and determine performance characteristics prior to commercialization and wide clinical use by human subjects.

With respect to the primary functions identified, all puncture prostheses properly sized for patients appear to function adequately as stents. These devices also appear to function competently as one-way valves, although this function has not been investigated thoroughly in a controlled experimental fashion. With respect to the air-shunting function, tracheoesophageal puncture prostheses exhibit substantial differences.

We are interested in quantifying the functional attributes of these devices.[24-26,28-31] In particular, we have characterized the efficiency with which these devices permit air to be shunted from the trachea to the esophagus. To accomplish this goal, the degree of opposition such devices offer to airflow through them has been calculated.[24-26,28-31] This opposition is called airway resistance, a quantity calculated from the ratio between the magnitude of pressure occasioned by the presence of these devices and the volume flow rate through them. We are interested in specifying device resistance or opposition for at least three major reasons. First, quantification of the magnitude of airway resistance or opposition to airflow provides a useful index of prosthesis efficiency. Second, reduction in airway resistance properties of these devices would be expected to enhance the efficiency of voice and speech production. This is true simply because less work would be required to overcome reduced opposition to airflow through these prostheses. These prostheses form an integral part of the speech mechanism, and their airway resistance contributes significantly to the magnitude of work required of the patient during speech/voice production. In other words, higher airway resistance of tracheoesophageal puncture prostheses results in higher magnitudes of work and decreased efficiency of voice/speech production. Third, reduction in airway resistance would be expected to facilitate retention and optimize use of tracheoesophageal breathing valves. Significant reduction in airway resistance leads to an appreciable reduction in tracheal pressure. For example, halving airway resistance results in a halving of the pressure build-up behind a device at a given flow rate. Since a major problem underlying the retention of breathing valve housing on the neck relates to the persistent presence of elevated tracheal pressures, reduction in airway resistance of these devices would be expected to facilitate retention.

Airway resistance properties of four puncture prostheses available on a commercial basis are illustrated in Figure 1. Substantial differences in airway resistance properties exist among devices.[31] Panje Voice

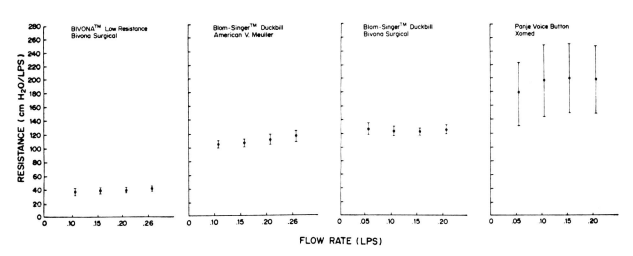

Figure 1 Airway resistance of four tracheoesophageal puncture prostheses.

Buttons exhibit the highest opposition to flow (means range from 180 to 200 cm H_2O/LPS) and the largest variability in performance. The original Blom-Singer duckbill devices manufactured by Bivona Surgical Instruments Inc. and duckbill devices Blom-Singer now marketed through American V. Mueller exhibit the second highest opposition to flow, with average resistance in the range of 110 to 125 cm H_2O/LPS. The Bivona Low Resistance devices exhibit the lowest opposition, with airway resistance of about 40 cm H_2O/LPS. Parenthetically, average airway resistance offered by the human larynx during the production of vowels falls in the range of 30 to 45 cm H_2O/LPS. These differences in device performance are substantial and can be attributed to differences in the design features among these prostheses.[25,31] The results of our independent investigations suggest that among major devices available commercially, Bivona Low Resistance tracheoesophageal puncture prostheses maximize the efficiency of speech/voice production and increase the likelihood of optimizing the use of tracheostomal breathing valves. Panje Voice Buttons contribute substantial magnitudes of opposition, are the least efficient shunts, and would be expected to contribute substantially to tracheostomal breathing valve retention problems.

I recognize that the results of in vitro testing of prostheses performance has been undertaken and described. However, it is essential to define how prosthetic devices function on an in vitro basis prior to defining their in vivo performance. In vitro experimentation enables estimation of performance under optimal, controlled conditions, a form of evaluation that should be undertaken prior to implementation of large-scale clinical trials or widespread patient use. In vivo studies of device performance and patients' response to these devices are important. Hence, there is a need for independent, appropriately ordered, comparative in vitro and in vivo investigation.

In conclusion, I would like to share some final perspectives about speech rehabilitation in abbreviated form. Recently developed surgical–prosthetic methods of speech restoration represent significant milestones for the disciplines of surgery and speech pathology. At present, carefully controlled studies have not been completed which enable workers in our fields to definitively determine treatment outcomes on a comparative or method-by-method basis. The problems associated with evaluation of treatment outcomes are numerous and certainly not unique to this field.[30] One problem associated with treatment outcomes research relates to a view that outcomes expressed in terms of speech cannot be measured objectively or are ''hard to quantify''.[7] This simply is not the case. Stated concisely, outcomes expressed in terms of speech results are not hard to quantify. Objective, controlled, comparative studies using dependent speech measures can be completed. Methods are available which permit specification of valid and reliable speech and vocal outcomes.

In this context, there is a need to specify and distinguish influences of surgical–prosthetic intervention from those occasioned by nonsurgical-prosthetic factors. As indicated, rehabilitative outcomes achieved by patients undergoing puncture-type methods of rehabilitation are not solely dependent on surgery or on surgical–prosthetic factors. Rather, outcomes are mediated by complex interactions among surgical, prosthetic, behavioral, psychosocial, patient, physician, and therapist influences. The interactions among these influences merit more careful study, and the methods for studying these interactions are available.

Although evaluation of treatment outcomes has been discussed in terms of speech and communication indices, outcomes must also be evaluated in nonspeech terms. Here, too, methods are available. Finally, it is important to note that patient selection can significantly bias outcome. Patients considered for tracheoesophageal puncture are evaluated and selected (or rejected) on the basis of explicit or implicit criteria. These criteria exert a significant bias on outcome and need to be considered in comparative work of this type.

REFERENCES

1. Weinberg B. Readings in speech following total laryngectomy. Baltimore: University Park Press, 1980.
2. Weinberg B. Speech and voice restoration following total laryngectomy. In: Perkins W, ed. Current therapy in communication disorders-voice disorders. New York: Thieme-Stratton, 1983, Chapter 13.
3. Blom ED, Singer MI, Hamaker RC. Tracheostoma valve for postlaryngectomy voice rehabilitation. Ann Otol Rhinol Laryngol 1982; 91:576–578.
4. Bors EFM, De Boer GHA, Schutte HK. Speech training for esophageal voice by using a button. Logopedic en Foniatric 1983; 55:356–359.
5. Donegan JO, Gluckman JL, Singh J. Limitations of the Blom-Singer technique for voice restoration. Ann Otol Rhinol Laryngol 1981; 90:495–497.
6. Henley-Cohn J. New technique for insertion of laryngeal prostheses. Laryngoscope 1981; 91:1957–1959.
7. Henley-Cohn J, Hausfeld JN, Jakubczak G. Artificial larynx prostheses: comparative clinical evaluation. Laryngoscope 1984; 94:43–45.
8. Johns ME, Cantrell RW. Voice restoration of the total laryngectomy patient. The Singer-Blom technique. Otolaryngol Head Neck Surg 1981; 89:82–86.
9. Knapp BA, Panje WR. A voice button for laryngectomees. Assoc Operating Nurses J 1982; 36:183–192.
10. Nijdam HF, Annyas AA, Schutte HK, Leever H. A new prosthesis for voice rehabilitation after laryngectomy. Arch Oto Rhino Laryngol 1982; 237:27–33.
11. Panje WR. Prosthetic vocal rehabilitation following laryngectomy. Ann Otol Rhinol Laryngol 1981; 90:116–120.
12. Panje WR, VanDemark D, McCabe BF. Voice button prosthesis rehabilitation of the laryngectomee: additional notes. Ann Otol Rhinol Laryngol 1981; 90:503–505.
13. Pearson BW. Subtotal laryngectomy. Laryngoscope 1981; 11:1904–1911.
14. Pearson BW, Woods RD, Hartman DE. Extended hemilaryngectomy for T3 carcinoma with preservation of speech and swallowing. Laryngoscope 1980; 12:1950–1961.
15. Shapiro MJ, Ramanathan V. Tracheo stoma vent voice prosthesis. Laryngoscope 1982; 92:1126–1129.

16. Singer MI, Blom ED. An endoscopic technique for restoration of voice after laryngectomy. Ann Otol Rhinol Laryngol 1980; 89:529–533.

17. Singer MI, Blom ED, Haymaker RC. Further experience with voice restoration after total laryngectomy. Ann Otol Rhinol Laryngol 1981; 90:498–502.

18. Singer MI, Blom ED. Selective myotomy for voice restoration after total laryngectomy. Arch Otolaryngol 1981; 107:670–673.

19. Wetmore SJ, Johns ME, Baker SH. The Singer-Blom voice restoration procedure. Arch Otolaryngol 1981; 107:674–676.

20. Wetmore SJ, Krueger K, Wesson K. The Singer-Blom speech rehabilitation procedure. Laryngoscope 1981; 1109–1116.

21. Wood BG, Rusnov MG, Tucker HM, Levine HL. Tracheoesophageal puncture for alaryngeal voice restoration. Ann Otol Rhinol Laryngol 1981; 90:492–494.

22. McGarvey S, Weinberg B. Esophageal insufflation testing in normal adults. J Speech Hearing Dis August, 1984; 49:272–297.

23. Chodosh P, Giancarlo H, Goldstein J. Pharyngeal myotomy for vocal rehabilitation postlaryngectomy. Laryngoscope 1984; 94:52–57.

24. Moon J, Weinberg B. Airway resistance of Blom-Singer tracheoesophageal puncture prostheses. J Speech Hearing Dis 1982; 47:441–442.

25. Moon J, Weinberg B, Sullivan J. Evaluation of Blom-Singer tracheoesophageal puncture prostheses. 1983; 26:459–463.

26. Moon J, Weinberg B. Airway resistance characteristics of voice button tracheoesophageal prostheses. J Speech Hearing Dis August, 1984; 49:326–328.

27. Shedd DP, Weinberg B. Surgical-prosthetic approaches to speech rehabilitation. Boston: GK Hall, 1980.

28. Weinberg B. Airway resistance of the voice button. Arch Otolaryngol 1982; 108:498–500.

29. Weinberg B, Horii Y, Blom E, Singer M. Airway resistance during esophageal phonation. J Speech Hearing Dis 1982; 47:194–199.

30. Weinberg B. Speech assessment and treatment of the laryngectomized patient. In: Costello J, ed. Recent advances in speech, hearing and language. San Diego: College Hill Press, in press (1985).

31. Weinberg B, Moon J. Aerodynamic properties of four tracheoesophageal puncture prostheses. Arch Otolaryngol 1984; 110:673–675.

PANJE PROCEDURE AND PROSTHETIC RESTORATION OF SPEECH AFTER LARYNGECTOMY

WILLIAM R. PANJE, M.D., F.A.C.S.

The Panje Voice Prosthesis, used in conjunction with appropriate speech therapy, provides an effective primary means of voice rehabilitation for the total laryngectomy patient. The Panje prosthesis, or "voice button", is a miniature, bi-flanged, one-way silicone valve that was developed and first used by me in 1979. It makes possible tracheoesophageal speech in the laryngectomee, while successfully preventing excessive aspiration of food and liquid in the trachea.

Tracheoesophageal fistula speech is essentially esophageal speech created by driving tracheal air through a fistula created between the trachea and esophagus. This eliminates the necessity of gulping and belching air to produce the pharyngoesophageal vibrations that create new speech sound. A number of devices have been developed that are used in conjunction with a permanent tracheoesophageal fistula to produce tracheoesophageal fistula speech.[1,2] Many of these devices are expensive, bulky, and difficult to clean. With some of these, aspiration and stenosis have been serious problems. The voice button procedure and device enable the laryngectomee to achieve tracheoesophageal fistula speech with the following advantages: (1) the fistula is created by an outpatient procedure than can be done in 15 to 30 minutes, re-

quiring no special instrumentation; (2) the fistula can be created at the time of laryngectomy, which avoids nasogastric feeding tube and allows early speech rehabilitation; (3) the prosthesis is self-contained within the tracheostoma; (4) usually, there is no specific size requirement with the prosthesis; and (5) if it becomes necessary to discontinue use of the prosthesis for any reason, the fistula site will, in nearly all cases, heal spontaneously.

For successful results with the voice button, it is important that the otolaryngologist and speech pathologist work together as a team. This optimizes the chances for complete vocal rehabilitation of the laryngectomy patient. In the laryngectomee's attempt to regain speech with the Panje prosthesis, it is important for the patient to obtain some measure of successful voice production as soon as possible after creation of the fistula. This helps the patient to believe that he or she can return to a productive life as an individual who can successfully communicate and provides motivation to continue the rehabilitation process. Patients who have had the guidance and counsel of the speech pathologist during the initial tracheoesophageal fistula speech production are more successful in their early speech efforts and are less likely to become discouraged with the process of voice rehabilitation.

PATIENT SELECTION

Patients to be considered for the Panje Voice Prosthesis should be evaluated in terms of the following requirements. The patient selected should:

1. Have total laryngectomy (simultaneous or delayed).

2. Have no evidence of locally persistent or recurrent

cancer (metastatic cancer is not a contraindication to the procedure).

3. Have a tracheostoma area 1.5 cm square (for example, 1.5×1 cm or 3×0.5 cm, and so forth). The stoma must be of adequate size so that the voice button can be inserted, yet small enough so that the patient can occlude the stoma.

4. Have good manual dexterity in occluding the trachestoma with a finger or thumb (this would exclude patients with severe arthritis or tremulous conditions).

5. Have good pulmonary status (this excludes patients with severe chronic pulmonary disease, asthma, and recurrent pneumonia).

6. Have not had radiation therapy for 3 to 6 months, and/or are not undergoing concomitant radiation or chemotherapy at the time of the tracheoesophageal fistula formation.

7. Be in positive nitrogen balance because negative nitrogen balance increases the danger of wound infection and widening of tracheoesophageal puncture site.

8. Have communication skills that are not satisfactory to him or her, have little success with esophageal speech, or desire better speech in order to communicate more readily. Be cautious of performing tracheoesophageal fistula in long-term esophageal speakers who will need extensive retraining for voice button speech.

9. Have good attidude and personal hygiene.

In addition, excessively tense patients or patients with psychologic problems should be considered with caution.Each patient who has had a laryngectomy and is considered as a potential candidate for the Panje prosthesis should be evaluated by both the speech pathologist and the otolaryngology–head and neck surgeon. The speech pathologist assesses the patient in terms of adequacy of current speech, ability to close the stoma, air supply, general tension, and hygiene. The otolaryngology–head and neck surgeon evaluates the patient in regard to stoma size, evidence of further disease, and appropriateness of surgical site.The criteria presented herein can assist in the selection of patients who would be most suitable to receive the Panje Voice Prosthesis. However, predicting which of the selected patients would achieve good tracheoesophageal fistula speech with the voice button appears to be just as difficult as attempting to predict which patients will succeed with esophageal speech. The factors that influence the development of esophageal speech will also influence the development of tracheoesophageal fistula speech. These factors include patient age, stage of disease, extent of radical neck dissection, extent of radiation therapy, upper esophageal sphincter function, hearing capacity, patient motivation, degree of personal stress, and quality of verbal training.[3]

SURGICAL PROCEDURE FOR THE ESTABLISHED LARYNGECTOMEE

The procedure that creates the tracheoesophageal fistula, making possible the placement of the voice button, is a simple outpatient tracheoesophageal stab operative technique.[4,5] Surgical instrumentation includes a headlight, suction equipment, and soft tissue surgical instruments.

Thirty minutes before beginning the procedure, the patient is given by mouth 30 mg of codeine to decrease the cough reflex and 5 mg of Valium to reduce anxiety. The upper aerodigestive system is anesthesized by having the patient swallow 15 cc of 2% viscous lidocaine with 0.5% Dyclone gargle. The trachea, oral cavity, and pharynx are sprayed copiously with 5% cocaine solution.

Once the patient is under local anesthesia, he or she swallows an appropriately sized Hurst or Maloney dilator that has been previously emptied of mercury (Fig. 1). The size of the dilator can range from 34 for a small person to 46 for a large individual. If the patient cannot swallow a 34 dilator, the surgeon should consider trying to actively dilate the esophagus up to the size of a 34 dilator before attempting the fistula

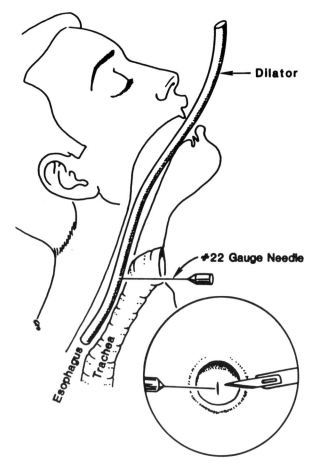

Figure 1 Making T-E fistula.

operation. Thus, the patient may have to wait until the esophagus has been dilated to an appropriate size before undergoing the operation.

With the patient supine, his or her face should be pointed straight ahead, not to one side or the other. Wearing a headlight and looking into the tracheostoma, the surgeon notes that as the esophageal tube passes the tracheostoma, a bulge develops at the posterosuperior verge of the stoma and proceeds inferiorly as the dilator is advanced. It is crucial to determine the point of maximum bulge of the posterior tracheal wall because this represents the anterior midpoint (maximum lumen diameter) of the esophagus.

The midpoint of the esophagus is injected through the membranous tracheal wall with 0.5 cc of 1% lidocaine with epinephrine. A 22-gauge spinal needle is then inserted through the intended fistula site into the rubber esophageal tube (it is critical that the dilator should not contain mercury when the spinal needle is inserted). The spinal needle should be inserted into the rubber dilator approximately 1.5 to 2 cm below the superior verge of the tracheostoma. The fistula is usually then located just above the level of the lower verge of the stoma. With a No. 15 Bard-Parker blade, a midpoint incision is made vertically along the spinal needle down to the esophageal dilator. The incision is approximately 7 to 10 mm in length.

When the fistula has been established, a 14F Foley catheter is passed through the fistula site and inserted 6 to 8 cm toward the stomach (Fig. 2). Simultaneously, the esophageal dilator is removed. The balloon of the catheter is filled with 1.5 cc of fluid, preventing inadvertent extrusion of the catheter during the healing period.

The catheter is tied to the patient's neck in the same manner as a tracheostomy tube. It is important to occlude the catheter by tying the string (No. 4 silk) tightly to avoid regurgitation of fluids and to prevent the escape of water from the balloon through the catheter. The upper part of the Foley catheter is then cut away.

The cut edges of the fistula do not need to be sutured together unless there is excessive bleeding. The tracheal and esophageal mucosa will heal together over the catheter in 10 to 14 days.

POSTOPERATIVE CARE AND PATIENT TEACHING

At the completion of the procedure, the patient is given a few sips of water. If the patient, on swallowing, demonstrates excessive leakage around the 14F Foley catheter through the fistula, a larger catheter is inserted after removal of the original catheter. The patient is instructed to return in 2 or 3 days. During that visit, the catheter is removed and the surgical site is cleaned. The next size smaller catheter is inserted (e.g., 18F to 16F, or 16F to 14F). This reduction in the size of the catheter should be made every 3 days until a 14F Foley catheter can be inserted. It is rec-

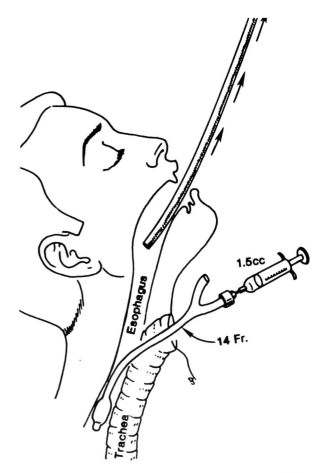

Figure 2 Stenting of T-E fistula with 14F Foley catheter. Note only 1.5 cc of fluid used to partially fill Foley balloon.

ommended that the patient refrain from speaking during this period.

Since the upper aerodigestive tract has been surgically violated, the patient is placed on a 5- to 7-day course of prophylactic antibiotics.

The patient is instructed not to remove the catheter. The patient is told that if the catheter does inadvertently become dislodged, it should be immediately reinserted. The catheter should not come out unless the balloon bursts or the catheter is intentionally cut. The patient is warned that during the first 24 postoperative hours, the liquids that he drinks leak around the catheter, but this leakage can be reduced if he or she eats solid food at the same time liquids are taken. Therefore, during the first 2 or 3 days after the procedure, fluids should be taken only with meals. It is emphasized that food should be well chewed while the patient is wearing the partially filled Foley catheter.

In approximately 10 to 14 days following formation of the fistula, the patient returns and the final catheter is removed. At that time, if the fistula is healed, the patient can be introduced to tracheoesophageal speech.

SURGICAL PROCEDURE AT TIME OF LARYNGECTOMY

Excellent-to-good tracheoesophageal speech results have been achieved in the established laryngectomee. Recently, some initial reports have suggested that even better success can be achieved when the tracheoesophageal fistula is performed at the time of laryngectomy. I have also found this latter statement to be true in the properly prepared patients (Fig. 3).

I essentially perform a tracheoesophagostomy in nearly all of my patients at the time of laryngectomy. A simple instrument made from modifying a ring forceps allows the surgeon to make the tracheoesophagostomy (Fig. 4) 1.5 to 2 cm inferior to the superior

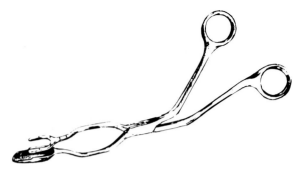

Figure 4   Panje-Shagets tracheoesophageal forceps.

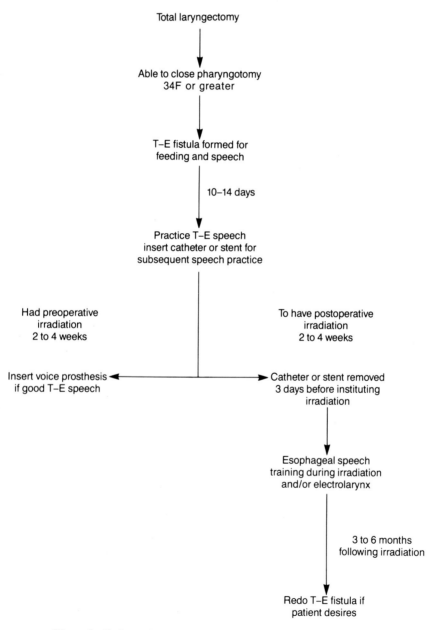

Figure 3   Patient selection for T–E fistula at time of laryngectomy.

cut edge of the trachea (Fig. 5).[6] The cup part of the forceps is introduced into the esophagus through the resultant pharyngotomy following removal of the larynx; the other arm of the forceps (the U-shaped part of the clamp) is inserted into the trachea, and with gentle approximation of the clamp, the tracheoesophageal tissues become aligned for creation of the fistula. A No. 15 or No. 11 knife blade is used to make a 1-cm vertical incision in the midpart of the U-shaped clamp. The cup arm of the forceps prevents inadvertant cutting of the posterior esophageal wall and allows for proper insertion of a 14- to 16-F feeding tube into the stomach. The feeding tube is sutured or tied to the neck with string in such a manner as not to cross over the tracheostoma (Fig. 6). If the feeding tube traverses the stoma, an inordinate amount of crusting can develop in the postoperative period. At 7 to 10 days postoperatively, the feeding catheter is removed and a 14- to 16-F Coudé catheter or Panje Fistula Stent (Xomed, Inc.) is then inserted through the fistula. Tracheoesophageal fistula speech can usually be introduced to the patient at this time if the wound has healed well. The catheter or stent is removed from the fistula only during those times in which the patient is practicing tracheoesophageal fistula speech, as outlined in the following section on initial voice production. Again, I am not anxious to place the voice prosthesis until the patient has achieved good tracheoesophageal fistula speech and can comfortably manage obturating the fistula with the catheter.

I have been able to establish 23 fistulas at the time of laryngectomy. Of the 23, if the pharynx and cervical esophagus could be closed over a 34F or 36F Hurst dilator (16 patients), all were able to achieve tracheoesophageal fistula speech. Although too early to prove, we do think that this selected population of

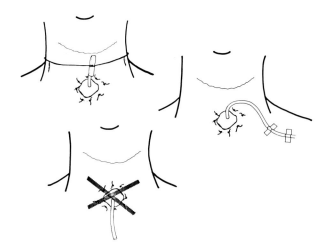

Figure 6 Illustration demonstrating appropriate placement of stent or feeding table after T-E puncture. The tube should not cross stoma entrance.

laryngectomees (immediate tracheoesophageal fistula and closure of viscus over a 34 Hurst dilator) will have better long-term success with the voice prosthesis as well as subsequent or concommitant development of esophageal speech.

INITIAL VOICE PRODUCTION

The speech pathologist plays an important role in helping the patient to achieve initial tracheoesophageal fistula speech. The approach used by the speech pathologist to first introduce the patient to tracheoesophageal fistula speech is an important factor in the overall success of the voice rehabilitation process (Table 1).

INSERTING THE PROSTHESIS

First, the appropriate length prosthesis is chosen. The Panje Voice Prosthesis is made in three lengths based on interflange distance (short = 7 mm; medium = 9 mm; long = 12 mm). Most patients require the medium or long prosthesis. If the patient is not retaining the prosthesis, the next longer prosthesis should be tried.

The most common difficulty encountered in in-

TABLE 1 Initiation of Tracheoesophageal Speech

1. Remove catheter or stent.
2. Patient takes small breath.
3. Speech pathologist or surgeon occludes tracheostoma with minimal digital pressure.
4. Patient attempts to say "ahh."
5. Patient instructed in stomal occlusion.
6. Patient attempts to say "ahh," a, e, i, o, and sing short verses of well-known songs.
7. Short sentences are produced.
8. Patient practices speech four to six times per day for 15 to 30 minutes each time at home or at work.
9. Catheter or stent replaced after practice session.

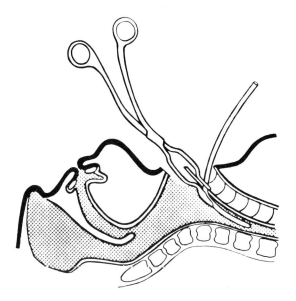

Figure 5 Panje-Shagets tracheoesophageal forceps inserted through pharyngotomy at time of laryngectomy. A 14F feeding tube is being inserted through fistula site.

serting the prosthesis is failure to insert it far enough into the fistula. In some cases, difficulty with insertion can be caused by less than optimal placement of the fistula site.

After insertion of the voice button, most patients find that voice production requires a bit more effort than with the "naked" fistula. It is for this reason that the patient should feel confident in voice production before the prosthesis is inserted.

Once the Panje Voice Prosthesis is inserted into the tracheoesophageal fistula the patient may experience the need for an inordinate amount of pulmonary force to achieve sound. In fact, some patients may not be able to make any sound after insertion of the voice button, whereas without the prosthesis they have acceptable speech. Some investigators believe that the reason for failure to achieve tracheoesophageal fistula speech in patients wearing the voice button is that the prosthesis produces excessive resistance to pulmonary air flow into the esophagus. I (as well as a number of other investigators) have not found this to be a major reason for failure to achieve speech with the voice prosthesis. My results, as well as comparative studies between the voice prosthesis and the Blom-Singer "duckbill" prosthesis, have demonstrated essentially no difference in the ability to achieve or sustain speech as well as intelligibility. I must conclude that if the surgeon or speech pathologist encounters a tracheoesophageal fistula patient with inordinate difficulty in achieving speech after voice prosthesis placement, other reasons than that of prosthesis airway resistance should be explored.

RESULTS AND DISCUSSION

The Panje Voice Prosthesis procedure provides a highly successful, reproducible, reversible, and inexpensive method of voice rehabilitation for the laryngectomee. Our success rate for establishing the fistula in 120 cases has been 100 percent (Table 2). A success rate of 85 percent can be expected for initial sound production (having the patient phonate against the occluded tracheostoma without the voice button in place). Of the patients who achieve success with initial sound production, only 5 to 10 percent will be unable to wear the voice button due to a thick tracheoesophageal wall, or an inability to insert the prosthesis, or incorrect stoma size. The success rate for short-term use of the voice button (using effective tra-

TABLE 2 Results of Panje Procedure

No. of Patients	Result
97/97	Established T–E fistula as an outpatient.
23/23	Established T–E fistula at time of laryngectomy.
102/102	Produced T–E sound.
8/120	Unable to wear Panje voice prosthesis.
94/120	Intelligible T–E — prosthesis speech.
62/120	Intelligible T–E — prosthesis speech 6 months or longer.

cheoesophageal fistula speech for less than 6 months) approaches 78 percent. The rate for long-term success with the prosthesis (using effective tracheoesophageal speech for more than 6 months) is 52 percent. Reasons for failure with the voice button include: inability to retain the prosthesis; poor phonatory qualities; inability to attain good stomal occlusion; and the patient's decision not to use the voice button (more comfortable with original communication, i.e., electrolarynx, esophageal speech; did not like volume or pitch of speech; or salivary soiling of occluding digit was repulsive), even though they successfully attained effective speech with the prosthesis.

I believe that greater success with the Panje Voice Prosthesis can be attained by a coordinated effort of the speech pathologist, or knowledgeable nurse, and the otolaryngologist–head and neck surgeon. Such an approach can help the laryngectomee to maintain the confidence and motivation necessary to achieve voice rehabilitation at the highest level of success, and in the shortest possible time.

REFERENCES

1. Dworkin JP, Sparker A. Surgical vocal rehabilitation following laryngectomy; a state-of-the-art report. Clin Otolaryngol 1980; 5:339–350.
2. Shedd D, Weinberg B, eds. Surgical and prosthetic approaches to speech rehabilitation. Boston: GK Hall, 1980.
3. Gates GA, Ryan W, et al. Current status of laryngectomee rehabilitation. I. Causes of failure. Otolaryngol 1982; 3:8–14.
4. Panje WR. Prosthetic vocal rehabilitation following laryngectomy; the voice button. Ann Otol Rhinol Laryngol 1981; 90:116–120.
5. Panje WR, VanDemark D, McCabe BF. Voice button prosthesis rehabilitation of the laryngectomee; additional notes. Ann Otol Rhinol Laryngol 1981; 90:503–505.
6. Shagets F, Panje WR. Primary tracheoesophageal fistula formation for feeding and voice rehabilitation. Accepted for publication, Laryngoscope, 1984.

VOCAL REHABILITATION AFTER TOTAL LARYNGECTOMY: CURRENT STATUS AND FUTURE DIRECTIONS

MARK I. SINGER, M.D., F.A.C.S.
ERIC D. BLOM, Ph.D.
RONALD C. HAMAKER, M.D., F.A.C.S.

Laryngeal carcinoma is a disease that annually threatens life and its dignity for nearly 11,000 Americans. Inadequate treatment leads to inevitable demise and functional incapacitation of communication, deglutition, and respiration. Many patients fear the loss of speech more than the loss of life itself. Efforts to preserve the human capability for verbal communication have included subtotal laryngectomy and differing methods of therapeutic radiation for voice preservation. The total laryngectomy is often a salvage treatment, relegating the patient to an uncertain fate with esophageal speech, artificial laryngeal communication, or silence.

A debate continues among advocates of conservation treatment methods, subtotal laryngectomies, and radical total laryngeal extirpation. Although alaryngeal speech rehabilitation by shunt was known as early as 1873, the success of esophageal speech in the twentieth century made shunt speech an inconvenient method for rehabilitation. Contemporary treatment of laryngeal carcinoma ranges from extensions of conservative surgical techniques to innovative radiation schemes and reconstructions employing cartilage remnants or tracheal shunts.

In 1978, two of us (MIS and EDB) proposed, after the unsatisfactory preliminary experience with "neoglottic reconstructions," a simple endoscopic puncture technique to establish a short horizontal tracheoesophageal fistula.[1] This was obturated to maintain its patency with a cylindrical valve incorporating a "slit" for unilateral airflow from the trachea. The puncture behaved differently from a fistula in that there was lack of dilatation and there was comfortable maintenance of the valve. Specialized instrumentation or training has not been required for patient or clinician.

In a series of over 300 patients dissatisfied with current alaryngeal speech rehabilitation, 93 percent were capable of comfortable, intelligible speech production with the valve prosthesis after a minimum time expenditure. Long-term follow-up over a 5-year period demonstrates continued use of tracheoesophageal phonation/prosthetic speech in nearly 80 percent, the decrease being explained by intercurrent and/or recurrent disease or mechanical failures of the valve (e.g., stoma size or retention). Nevertheless, this success rate exceeds the accepted rates of reported acquisition of esophageal speech. Furthermore, intelligibility studies and acoustic analysis of tracheoesophageal phonation point out clear advantages over conventional esophageal speech.

The ease of the endoscopic voice restoration permitted rapid accumulation of a series. The simplicity of tracheoesophageal airflows allowed for early identification of a subpopulation of alaryngeal speech failures who displayed pharyngoesophageal spasm during insufflation of the esophagus.[2] It was reasoned that this behavior represented unexpected activity of the cricopharyngeus and pharyngeal constrictor muscles after partial denervation and mechanical alteration after separation of their insertions from the laryngo-hyoid complex. Confirmation of this theory of constrictor opposition was made by videofluoroscopic study during esophageal insufflation with and without pharyngeal plexus anesthetic blockade. Additional confirmation was achieved by selective myotomy of the constrictor muscle mass, permitting satisfactory airflows for tracheoesophageal phonation. Alterations of the cricopharyngeus muscle or pharyngoesophageal segment to enhance alaryngeal speech acquisition is contrary to the previous experience with esophageal speech. The tracheoesophageal puncture permitted a useful vantage point to better evaluate the esophageal speech mechanism by direct assessment rather than by static x-ray studies or manometric probes with their necessary introduction of significant artifacts. The tonicity of the pharyngoesophagus during esophageal air charge is important for fluent speech production, but of equivalent importance is the ability of the constrictor mass to relax for trans-segment airflows during speech. From our series, nearly 40 percent of patients have failure of consistent airflow because of sustained pharyngoesophageal sphincter resistance, and benefit from myotomy procedures. This spastic behavior of the laryngectomized pharynx has no analogue in normal patients and cannot be deconditioned or pharmacologically released. It is unique to the altered state of the laryngectomy, and recognition of its considerable role will eventually reduce the number of unsuccessful esophageal speakers and improve the quality of resultant speech.

The simplicity of tracheoesophageal puncture and the techniques of shunt formation compel us to investigate this method as a primary speech rehabilitation applied at the laryngectomy procedure. The additional steps include a short tracheoesophageal puncture made via the pharyngotomy, a meticulous posterior midline constrictor myotomy, and a dynamic tracheostomal construction to enlist the forces of scar contracture to maintain patency and to prevent stenosis.

A series of 50 consecutive laryngectomies underwent the additional phonatory reconstructive method and experienced 86 percent successful speech rehabilitation for 6 months or more.[3] The success rate was improved by a better silicone valve prosthesis (American V. Mueller Blom-Singer Voice Prosthesis), a durable stoma, and a better understanding of tracheoesophageal airflows with reference to pharyngoesophageal resistance.

This speech rehabilitative method was safely applied because of its elimination of tracheal aspiration, a considerable problem plaguing earlier shunt techniques and neoglottic reconstructions. Even greater significance must be attached to the avoidance of compromise of treatment of malignant disease. The accepted total laryngectomy is not altered regarding margins, and T3 lesions receive radiation therapy without delayed observation for disease or shielding the trachea. The introduction of these simple methods at laryngectomy presents an important rehabilitative potential for patients facing total laryngectomy and the uncertainty of prolonged rehabilitation.

In 1980, we stated that surgical-prosthetic speech rehabilitation for the laryngectomized patient required the team effort of the surgeon and speech pathologist as an interdisciplinary approach to the communication-impaired patient.[4] The role of the speech clinician is altered by tracheoesophageal phonation and must be expanded to provide a better understanding of the mechanics of the prostheses and the physiology of the laryngectomized pharynx. Tradiational speech therapy with respect to articulation training, breath control, and phrasing are reduced to a minor role in this patient population, and to demand such peripheral activities diminishes the efficiency of this rehabilitation and actually impedes the patient's progress. The necessary prerequisite is involved clinicians to provide the environment for rapid independent recovery from laryngectomy.

In 1974, the Centennial Conference on Laryngeal Cancer convened in Toronto, Canada, to commemorate the 100 years' progress since Billroth's historic first laryngectomy. As Bryce stated, "The Centennial Conference, because of the stature of its faculty, had a great challenge to be a source of information and to develop an unequaled bank of information which can be widely disseminated across the world."[5] It was the hope that out of the Conference would come a "great leap forward" to stimulate new efforts in the treatment of cancer of the larynx.

Ten years have passed since the Toronto meeting, and a perspective has developed on the variety of techniques for speech preservation after laryngectomy. It is important to understand earlier efforts in order to learn about problems and unfulfilled promises. Intellectual honesty is critical to progress, free of unsubstantiated claims, competitiveness, and commercialism. As we learn from past experience, we also learn from each other, and in this way the laryngeal cancer patient is the beneficiary. Surgical rehabilitation of these patients is fraught with exaggerated claims,

emotionalism, and great public interest. It is the obligation of the investigators to adhere to disciplined reporting and to prevent unrealistic expectations among patients.

The second ten years after the Centennial demands careful criteria for successful methods and their evaluation. It is not adequate to say "good speech" or "results equivalent to good esophageal speech." Furthermore, it is incorrect to eliminate an entire treatment modality, for example, radiation therapy, in the interests of preservation of a tenuous shunt reconstruction. Careful analysis of other oncology disciplines will avoid misquotation and misinterpretation. Accurate evaluation of the laryngeal cancer patient demands careful treatment planning to prevent both overtreatment and inadequate treatment.

It is understood that alaryngeal patients may acquire voice by the vibration of pharyngoesophageal mucous membranes through skilled air trapping or various tracheal shunts. The valved silicone devices placed in a controlled tracheoesophageal puncture permit voice production generated by exhaled air and provide needed airway protection for physiologic deglutition. The laryngectomized pharynx, free of cricoid and hyoid remnants, and relaxed by myotomy, can be effectively enlisted for patient rehabilitation with no compromise of the accepted principles of surgical oncology. Combinations of modern silicone valve technology, a simple horizontal tracheoesophageal shunt, and skilled patient instruction will permit natural vocal rehabilitation for most laryngectomized patients. Although the laryngeal cancer patient is threatened by voicelessness, it is accepted that a dignified and good-quality life may resume. The eventual direction for laryngectomy procedures in rehabilitative cancer surgery must be to the end of restoration of the upper airway. This will permit oro-nasal respiration with the restoration of olfaction and gustation. The tracheobronchial tree will be rehabilitated by the more physiologic air conditioning of the pharyngeal and oral nasal environments. This must be accomplished without risking tracheal aspiration during deglutition and without gambling with the patient's survival with narrow margins in the presence of malignant disease.

This reconstruction must demand airway patency and protection with the reliability expected of a cardiac replacement valve. The challenge is complicated by the contaminated environment of the pharynx and the adjunctive treatment method of radiation therapy. The possibility of implantation of an artificial device in this milieu is unlikely. The total laryngeal extirpation leaves scant tissue for tubulation or transposition for a neolarynx. Nevertheless, innovations in muscle and cartilage transposition with improved understanding of the complex neuroanatomy of the laryngopharynx may open the way for reconstruction that stimulates the physiologic elegance of the larynx.

Restoration of the voice has been and remains as important as the effective treatment of laryngeal carcinoma. The historical record reveals generations of efforts refining earlier ideas and methods with a continued improvement in the understanding of the mechanisms of voice production. Future reports will appear with improvements based on a critical understanding of earlier methods, with the eventual aim of a better cancer treatment and preservation of the continuity of the aerodigestive system.

REFERENCES

1. Singer MI, Blom ED. Preliminary results with tracheoesophageal fistula technique of Amatsu. In: Shedd DP, Weinberg B, ed. Surgical Prosthetic approaches to speech rehabilitation. Boston: GK Hall, 1980:3.
2. Singer MI, Blom ED. A selective myotomy for voice restoration after total laryngectomy. Arch Otolaryngol 1981; 107:670–673.
3. Hamaker RC, Singer MI, Blom ED, Daniels H. Primary voice restoration after total laryngectomy. Presented at Annual Meeting of the American Society of Facial Plastic and Reconstructive Surgery, May 1984.
4. Singer MI, Blom ED. An endoscopic technique for restoration of voice after laryngectomy. Ann Otol Rhinol Laryngol 1980; 89:529–533.
5. Bryce DP. The Conacher Memorial Lecture: One Hundred Years of Effort. Laryngoscope 1975; 85:241.

37. Nonsurgical Rehabilitation

INTRODUCTION

EUGENE N. MYERS, M.D., F.A.C.S.

The topic of nonsurgical rehabilitation of the patient following head and neck cancer concerns issues having to do with quality of life. However, the issue of rehabilitation cannot be separated from treatment. Generally, the more extensive the ablative procedure, the greater the disability inflicted upon the patient. In recent years, there have been numerous creative attempts to surgically reconstruct the region. In some cases, however, this is not possible or feasible. Therefore, nonsurgical means of rehabilitation are often employed.

Nowhere in medicine does the team approach to the patient play a more prominent role than in the management of head and neck cancer. The surgeon, radiation therapist, and medical oncologist are certainly responsible for the patient's treatment program. However, all of these professionals must be aware of the need for rehabilitation. Playing a prominent role in the rehabilitation phase are maxillofacial prosthodontists, specialized nurses, speech pathologists, nutritionists, and physical medicine and rehabilitation personnel. There must always be a leader of a team, and I believe that this should be the surgeon.

In his chapter, Wenger presents a general overview of the rehabilitation issues and some of the unique ways in which the Milton Dance Center, part of the Greater Baltimore Medical Center, has made an effort to solve these problems. Wenger's group places great emphasis on rehabilitation of the patient and quite correctly evaluates the patient in the pretreatment, particularly presurgical, phase with a view toward rehabiliation. Playing prominent and important roles on this team are maxillofacial prosthodontists, speech pathologists, nurses, and social workers. The weekly staff conferences discuss all of the issues involved in the patient's care. The group quite correctly places great emphasis on intensive counseling of the patients and their families. The importance of follow-through during the convalescent phase and subsequent discharge planning is also emphasized.

Weaver's contribution addresses the rehabilitation of swallowing. He too emphasizes the team approach and introduces the concept of the "dysphagia therapist". Weaver states that the primary dysphagia therapist remains to be identified in many institutions. However, it appears to me that nationally the speech pathologists who have a special interest in that area are probably the best motivated and best qualified to fill this role. Weaver makes the important point that even in our high technology world the best way of evaluating the degree of impairment of nutritional status is the patient's estimation of his weight loss and a description of the patient's diet and general appearance.

In his chapter, Schweiger provides us with excellent insights into preoperative planning in the case of the patient undergoing partial mandibulectomy. His technique of extracting a tooth and placing the bone cut in the extraction socket is an excellent way of preserving adjacent teeth. His technical point on removing the ramus of the mandible in segmental mandibulectomy is also most important in preventing superior and medial displacement of the fragment, which later interferes with swallowing and rehabilitation. Schweiger also presents us with important insights into postoperative considerations such as intermaxillary fixation, jaw exercises, the use of mandibular glide plane appliances, and the use of the incline occlusal plane.

Saunders has worked for many years in concert with the Physical Medicine Rehabilitation Department at Ohio State. His chapter brings to us long years of experience in the prevention of diability of the shoulder following radical neck dissection. Certainly the guidelines and techniques are within our province, and yet the responsibility for the rehabilitation of the shoulder and prevention of pain is clearly a reflection of the motivation of the patient.

Research efforts in the field of nonsurgical rehabilitation have lagged behind efforts in development of treatment protocols. Perhaps the difficulties encountered in defining objectives and effectively measuring outcome militate against such studies. The payoff for such studies is potentially great for these patients. Workers in this field should be encouraged to design research protocols, and funding agencies should be encouraged to provide not only financial resources but leadership in this most important health care area.

NONSURGICAL REHABILITATION

ALVIN P. WENGER, M.D.

In 1977, through the generosity of Mr. and Mrs. Milton J. Dance, Jr., funds were provided to establish a nonsurgical rehabilitation center for head and neck cancer patients at the Greater Baltimore Medical Center. Before construction of the center was undertaken, 2 years were devoted to planning and visiting leading oncology centers in the country to study the physical design and the clinical arrangements, and to discuss with the directors the problems that were faced in the administration of such centers. Visits and planning were carried out by a team consisting of Dr. Robert Chambers, other members of the Department of Otolaryngology, Head and Neck Surgery, and me. I would like to express our gratitude to the centers visited and for the help that they gave us. We are especially grateful to Roswell Park and Dr. Shedd for their warm reception and detailed discussions and advice which proved so helpful in our planning.

THE STAFF

The administrative head of the center is the medical director. The staff itself is divided into a full-time (or core) staff and a part-time staff, which includes other members of the general hospital staff. The core staff consists of the center director, a charge nurse, a social service worker, a speech therapist, and a secretary. The part-time staff includes the operating surgeons, an internist, a prosthodontist, a psychiatrist, and a physical therapist.

The physical planning of the center consists of an examining area provided with fiberoptic equipment for the examination of nose, throat, larynx, and upper trachea, and for making video tapes of the areas examined. There are also devices to make simultaneous recordings of the voice. A speech therapy area is provided and consultation rooms are available; these areas also used by members of the part-time staff for examinations of the patients. The director's office, secretarial space, and waiting area complete the physical plan.

PROGRAM FOR THE FULL-TIME STAFF

One morning each month is devoted to continuing education, which includes lectures from the otolaryngology and head and neck staff to familiarize the core staff with terminology, with the process of tumor staging, and with local anatomy, and to demonstrate flaps and other ongoing surgical procedures. A second morning each month is devoted to establishing policies, procedures, and fees. Decisions concerning these are placed in a manual, and any alterations or approved ideas are periodically entered.

One morning each week the full-time and the part-time staff meet to exchange information on new and old patients. This is the most important and most critical meeting held in the center. Here information is exchanged concerning the progress of old patients and presentation of new patients. Plans for the care of new patients are made during these discussions. Review of the old patients includes discussion concerning alteration of the treatment protocol to include any approved new therapies. This meeting serves to promote optimal patient care on an interdisciplinary basis and acts as a learning experience for the resident trainees, the nurses, and other professional personnel. All rehabilitation plans must be made with the responsible surgeon and approved by him and the patient's attending physician. These meetings are conducted by the medical director, with the responsible surgeon playing a major role.

Once a month the center devotes an evening to a social gathering for the patients and their families. This provides an opportunity for them to exchange experiences and discuss their individual rehabilitation programs and problems. This evening has been a very successful addition to our program.

Grand rounds for the entire department are conducted at 7:30 AM once a week, during which interesting cases are presented. Much of the material is now presented on video tape, and this practice reduces the incidence of patient examination during the rounds. The presentation of new patients includes the following: (1) history and physical findings, presented by the responsible surgeon, (2) laboratory reports, available photographs, and tapes, (3) discussion of the treatment plan, including contemplated surgery and preoperative consultations with, for example, an internist, psychiatrist, and prosthodontist, and (4) plans for indoctrinating the patient concerning his planned course in the hospital and his later rehabilitation.

Following new patient presentations, the progress of old patients is discussed, their hospital course, their condition on discharge, and arrangements for family care and for local transportation. Decisions are made concerning home nursing requirements and arrangements made for the installation of any special equipment in the home. The protocol adopted for the care of each new patient is discussed in the sections that follow.

PREOPERATIVE REHABILITATION ASSESSMENT OF THE PATIENT

The majority of the patients come to the center preoperatively as outpatients, at which time they undergo (1) video-laryngeal photography and voice recordings, and (2) the beginning of their education and that of their family. This education is of paramount importance. In the past it was believed that the head and neck surgeons were not informing and instructing the patient in all the aspects of the proposed surgery, but subsequently it has been found that this is incorrect. These patients do not accept what is being told them, or they actually do not listen or understand what is said, and there can be total rejection of everything that is presented to them. In many patients, the psychological impact of hearing the word cancer is far greater than has previously been realized. Their psychologic state at this time is such that they do not want to hear or accept what is being told. We have found that education of the family plays a most important role in solving this problem. Rejection by the family is not unusual when faced with the problem of cancer surgery. The spouse and the family must understand the procedures that the patient must face and the subsequent problems that must be solved for the rehabilitation of the patient, such as psychologic support. They must also understand the problems of transportation, home care, and the like. To aid in this educational process, pamphlets have been prepared describing the care of the stoma, the use of the suction apparatus, and some instructions for esophageal speech. This is done to help the patient and the family in the future home care routine. The introduction of the patient to the facilities of the hospital is the next step. He is shown an operating room suite, the recovery room, and the intensive care ward. In addition, whenever possible, the incoming patient has the opportunity to see and talk with an individual who has had the same operation that is being planned for him. Our center is fortunate in having a group of volunteers who give freely of their time and are very conscientious in cooperating with new patients. The patients that do not live in the Baltimore area are admitted to the hospital 3 days before surgery and undergo the preparation just described. Counseling is needed for the problems with which the patient and the family members must cope. Such counseling is provided by the social service worker and the charge nurse. (The aforementioned evening meetings for groups of families to get together prove to be an effective means of helping individuals deal with their problems by sharing experiences and feelings with postoperative patients. The focus of such a group must be supportive and educational. The content of each session varies considerably, depending on the need of the families present.)

The charge nurse and the social service worker spend a great deal of time counseling patients under the guidance of the operating surgeon and the center director. Alcohol and smoking problems are among the most frequent and difficult to address, and counseling must include the documentation of their association with malignant tumors of the head and neck. In spite of all of our efforts to counsel such patients, the center has had its share of failures in this area.

The speech therapist is responsible for the teaching of esophageal voice. She also demonstrates the various speech prostheses that are available for the postoperative patient and helps to individually select devices most helpful for the patient's specific disability. Deglutition is often a problem to be solved following head and neck surgery, and the center has developed a fiberoptic recording of barium swallows which has proved most helpful. The dietitian plays an important role in the establishment of the nutritional requirements of each patient, laying specific emphasis on caloric intake, supplementary feeding, and the counseling of the family on the necessary diet. She also shows them feeding techniques that may have to be used. Other staff members—such as the prosthodontist, the psychiatrist, the physiotherapist, and the medical illustrator—all play a role in each of the multidisciplinary conferences concerning the patient. It is the responsibility of the dental personnel to see that prostheses are available at the time of surgery, and that every precaution for the prevention of dental caries is exercised in patients who are about to receive radiation therapy. The role of the radiation therapist and that of the chemotherapist are discussed in these conferences, and plans for their services are made at that time. The center also employs a moulage expert to provide artificial ears, eyes, nose, and other structures.

The basic decisions concerning the long-term requirements of the patient are formulated during these discussions. The leader of such discussions invariably is the operating surgeon. This is as it should be because he has the responsibility for the patient.

Preparatory to the patient's discharge, a pre-discharge conference is held with the patient and the patient's family with the core faculty in attendance. This conference provides an opportunity for the patient and the family to ask questions, and for the staff to reinforce recommendations, identify gaps in understanding, and clarify misconceptions. Following this conference, plans are made for the discharge, and these include any arrangements that may be necessary for placing the patient in a nursing home, arrangements for continued care by visiting nurses, the provision of supplies, drugs, and equipment, and transportation for follow-up visits to the center. When financial need exists, referrals to economic resources are supplied. Arrangements are made for any subsequent special services, such as radiation therapy and outpatient follow-up. Plans are made for further education of the family regarding the patient's care at home. Any special instructions, e.g., with regard to wound redressing or special dietary problems, are discussed at this meeting.

OUTPATIENT CARE

Outpatient care in the rehabilitation center is important as it serves to review the patient's progress and identify new special rehabilitation and medical problems. Many of these topics may have been covered in previous group meetings with the families. Many patients need help on an outpatient basis to deal with psychosocial issues that confront them after discharge from the hospital and when they are attempting to resume their place in the community. Contin-

ued counseling is needed for patients who have alcohol and tobacco problems because frequently these abuses are used as an outlet for their emotional instability.

LESSONS LEARNED

The staff must consist of individuals drawn from the medical and paramedical disciplines working together, making decisions together, and planning long-term rehabilitation programs together. Essential to the success of the program is early indoctrination of the patient to his rehabilitation plan before surgery, explaining to him that rehabilitation may continue for months after hospital discharge.

The center must provide emotional support for the patient and his family and must instruct the patient and his family in their respective roles at home. It must give support to the family in arranging bedside nursing care, special equipment, and transportation for outpatient visits. It must also give the patient time for continued training in speech and help in the problems of deglutition and postoperative care.

A center for rehabilitation and a hospital head and neck surgical program are greatly strengthened by a good residency training program. Conversely, such a center and program greatly strengthen the residency training in that hospital.

It is important to have a sufficient number of patients participating in a rehabilitation program. Without a full supply of patients, it is difficult to (1) do clinical research on rehabilitation programs, and (2) recruit and satisfy a core faculty. Furthermore, we believe that patients help patients, particularly those with similar disabilities.

SWALLOWING REHABILITATION

ARTHUR WEAVER, M.D.
SUSAN FLEMING, Ph.D.

Head and neck cancer frequently disables the vital functions by which we eat, speak, and swallow. The swallowing function begins in utero and continues throughout life to provide not only essential nutrition for the body, but significant pleasure as well. The ability to chew, savor, and swallow food requires complex neuromuscular coordination and reflexes of voluntary and autonomic origin. Maintenance of appropriate nutrition is dependent on the metabolism, appetite, psyche, cultural background, and food preferences of the patient. Successful ingestion and deglutition of food in the normal adult is dependent on

appropriate function of the entire upper aerodigestive tract. Detailed descriptions of the anatomic structures and physiologic function of deglutition are available, and representative resources are included in the references for this chapter.[1-4] A fundamental understanding of these functions is essential for persons treating head and neck cancer.

Normal swallowing is usually described as being involved with three phases: (1) oral, (2) pharyngeal, (3) esophageal. Deglutition is a rapid synchronous process that is dependent on a complex system of reflexes. Once the food is placed in the mouth it is necessary to be able to close the lips in order to prevent drooling. Combined function of the jaws, teeth, tongue, cheek, and mastication muscles are then integrated to masticate, mix, and move the food to the dorsum of the posterior tongue, where the bolus may be voluntarily thrust into the pharynx. This initiates the pharyngeal stage of deglutition. At this juncture, the soft palate rises to close the nasopharynx, and the food bolus is divided into two lateral streams while the larynx rises and is moved anteriorly, opening the piriform sinuses to accept the food bolus on either side. The tongue rises against the elevated palate to close off possible regress into the mouth while the cricopharyngeus relaxes, and the pharyngeal constrictors propel the food into the upper esophagus. This entire pharyngeal phase of swallowing is accomplished in less than a second. The food is then carried downward through the esophagus by peristaltic action of the striated and smooth involuntary muscles.

Facilitating the swallowing mechanism is a rapid outpouring of salivary juices and mucous lubricants which "grease the skids" and allow the smooth transit of the food bolus. This whole process is made pleasurable through appropriate functions of taste and smell as well as the many psychosocial associations frequently experienced with the eating ritual.

DYSPHAGIA ON THE HEAD AND NECK SERVICE

The dysphagia associated with head and neck cancer may be either tumorigenic or iatrogenic. Cancer involvement of any the vital structures associated with the swallowing process can produce significant dysphagia. The patient, when confronted with possible surgical loss of these important functions, sometimes resists the idea of operative ablation of the cancer. The patient who refuses appropriate cancer therapy, however, usually finds that the cancer will as effectively destroy the swallowing function as will the surgeon, but without any associated chance for survival. Unfortunately, postoperative and postradiotherapy patients are often left with significant swallowing defects. In all too many instances, the patient is left to struggle alone with his dysphagia without an integrated support team to aid and encourage him toward rehabilitation of these lost functions.

PREOPERATIVE EVALUATION AND NUTRITION INTERVENTION

Recently, there has been a flurry of interest by surgical oncologists in the role of nutrition in cancer therapy. Particular emphasis has been placed on pretreatment evaluation of cancer patients. Many studies have been done in an attempt to select patients who require nutritional intervention prior to therapy. Numerous formal evaluations have been suggested. We now have methods for determining lean body mass, fat stores, visceral functions, hepatic protein synthesis, immunologic functions, cellular defense mechanisms, nonspecific humoral defense mechanisms, and somatic protein synthesis.[5-7] For each of these areas, numerous tests have been designed, including weight loss, weight-height ratio, creatinine-height ratio, triceps skin-fold thickness, midarm and midthigh muscle circumference, plasma albumin concentration, plasma transferin concentration, concentrations and turnover of proteins (i.e., thyroxine-binding prealbumin, retinol-binding protein), lymphocyte count, T rosette formation, delayed hypersensitivity skin tests, neutrophil migration index, opsonic index, IgG, IgM,

C3, and many others.[8-10] On the head and neck service, perhaps the majority of the patients would present abnormalities in a significant number of these tests. In fact, Mullen and co-workers, in applying a number of these risk factors to patients in the Veterans Administration Hospital, found that according to their standard criteria, only 3 percent of the hospital population was considered normal.[11] Bassett and Dobie applied a battery of nutritional assessment tests consisting of anthropometric measurements, skin tests, laboratory assessment of visceral somatic proteins, and a patient questionnaire to characterize the nutritional status of 50 consecutive new head and neck tumor patients. They concluded that the best predictor of impaired nutritional status was the patient's description of his recent diet. A normal diet predicted a very good score and a soft or liquid diet predicted a fair or poor nutritional score with an overall accuracy of 72 percent.[12]

At present, it appears that adequate information regarding the patient's current nutritional status can best be obtained by a simple history of weight loss and current dietary intake. If the patient has lost 10 percent or more of his normal body weight and is currently receiving inadequate caloric intake, that patient should have immediate nutritional intervention concomitantly with his tumor work-up.

We have discovered that many patients frequently inflate their report of current food intake. A calorie count by the dietitian on the ward may give an objective evaluation quite different from the patient's assessment. In many instances, adequate nutritional intake can be ensured by simply paying attention to patient's food preferences and supplying needed blenderized or mechanically softened foods.

Some patients benefit greatly when their diets are supplemented with one of the many available commercial liquid nutritional supplements. When oral intake proves inadequate, a small nasogastric tube may be used for preoperative nutritional enhancement. Great caution should be used, however, in patients who are markedly nutritionally depleted and have severely diminished oral intake. Fatal aspiration may occur from overloading the stomach via nasogastric tube. These patients often have edematous stomachs from protein depletion. The gastric musculature has also been weakened by lack of use, producing a marked delay in gastric emptying. Such stomachs overload easily. Food may then be regurgitated into the pharynx, and because the patient is unable to swallow, aspiration and death may occur.

Patients in a cachectic state should initially be given small feedings with a larger nasogastric tube. The stomach should be emptied prior to the start of each new feeding until such time as no significant residual is found in the stomach. If it is determined that sufficient calories are not permissible by enteral alimentation, intravenous hyperalimentation may be instituted concomitantly or independently of small nasogastric feedings.

ESTIMATING POSTTREATMENT SWALLOWING DEFECTS

The complexity and variability of surgical and radiotherapeutic treatment regimens and patient variability are such that absolutes are impossible in the prediction of swallowing defects.

The patient is best served, however, when the nature and likelihood of posttreatment swallowing is anticipated in the pretherapy work-up. It is generally possible to anticipate and prepare for such problems. The entire deglutition therapy team should be involved in pretreatment evaluation and counseling.

PROSTHETIC PLANNING

An experienced prosthodontist is a valuable adjunct to any head and neck cancer service. In many instances a properly fabricated prosthesis is the simplest method for handling surgical defects. This is particularly true for defects involving the hard palate or maxilla. Defects of the soft palate, tongue volume deficiency, and mandibular loss can also frequently be benefited by appropriate prosthesis. The prosthodontist can best make needed dental impressions prior to surgery or radiotherapy. Often a prosthesis may be premanufactured and modified as necessary in the operating room to permit immediate placement. Artificial feeding mechanisms in the postoperative period can thus be avoided.

DETERMINING THE NEED FOR AIRWAY DIVERSION

Careful evaluation of a patient's anticipated therapy should, in most instances, allow for pretreatment determination of need for airway diversion. In some instances it may be best to permit an interval of trial feedings before permanently committing the patient to alaryngeal speech. Occasionally the patient may be allowed to choose between rather normal eating and normal speech mechanisms. In our experience, most patients, when given this choice, would prefer to eat rather normally and use an alternative communication method. Fortunately we now have a number of methods available for speech rehabilitation. We strongly believe that patients might better be counseled to accept airway diversion as a primary procedure than be forced into a prolonged period of trial feedings without a significant chance of success. A prolonged interval of unsatisfactory feeding with ultimate realization of failure is disheartning to both patient and therapist.

RADIOTHERAPY

The contribution of radiotherapy to the dysphagia of head and neck cancer patients is frequently underestimated. All swallowing problems resulting from surgical resection are aggravated acutely and chronically by radiotherapy. We have seen several patients who had large pharyngeal masses that were controlled by radiotherapy alone, but who were never able to swallow effectively following this therapy. Radiotherapy acutely affects swallowing by causing edema and inflammation of the mucosa and musculature in the treatment field. On a chronic basis, the effect is one of edema, fibrosis, and atrophy of the musculature and prolonged mucosal edema. The loss of lubrication of the mucosal surfaces from saliva and mucus can be a particular problem for many patients. Any deficit in the swallowing mechanism expected from surgery is usually significantly upgraded in the patient who will have either pre- or postoperative radiotherapy.

GLOSSECTOMY

Patients tolerate removal of as much as 50 percent of their lateral tongue without significant swallowing defect. An occasional patient with as little as one-third of the posterior tongue remaining does learn to swallow successfully without airway diversion. A myocutaneous flap to add bulk for replacement of the removed segment of tongue appears to be beneficial. Resection of the anterior tongue produces greater speech disability, whereas resection of the base of the tongue has a more profound effect on the swallowing mechanism. Some surgeons report that total glossectomy may be done with a reasonable expectation of swallowing without airway diversion. This has not been our experience. Although an occasional patient may successfully accomplish this feat, we believe that the percentage of individuals who can do so is so small that airway diversion is indicated for patients with total glossectomy.

HYOMANDIBULAR COMPLEX

Resection of large, floor-of-the-mouth lesions may be deceptively destructive of the swallowing mechanism. The hyomandibular complex is vital to the whole swallowing process and is responsible for lifting the larynx anterosuperiorly, thus closing the larynx against the base of the tongue and epiglottis and opening the piriform sinuses and pharynx. Large floor of the mouth lesions may involve most of these laryngeal lifters. This is particularly true when resection of the anterior arch of the mandible is required. Large lesions in this area may also encroach on the hypoglossal nerves. When the anterior mandible has been removed along with the laryngeal lifters, suspension of the larynx is lost. It is our general policy to replace the mandibular arch either with autogenous bone or with mandibular prosthesis, which may help to support the larynx postoperatively. Resection of both hypoglossal nerves makes successful swallowing postoperatively highly unlikely.

PHARYNGEAL RESECTION

It is probable that as much as one-third of the pharynx may be successfully removed and primarily closed. In most instances, if there is no other significant surgical defect, a patient can expect reasonable postoperative swallowing function. A large adynamic skin or myocutaneous flap for hypopharyngeal reconstruction, however, is incompatable with successful swallowing without airway diversion. Small flaps high in the nasopharynx and upper pharynx are better tolerated.

NEURAL DEFECTS

One hypoglossal nerve can be sacrificed without significant problems in deglutition, unless other major surgical defects coexist. Resection of the vagus nerve high in the neck is sometimes necessary with vagal tumors or carotid resection. This creates a significant problem in deglutition. Even as an isolated procedure, resection of the vagus nerve mandates a temporary tracheostomy. Most patients can overcome the flaccid pharynx associated with this nerve loss. A period of re-education is necessary, and a tracheostomy helps prevent serious pulmonary complications during this time of learning. Bilateral vagal nerve loss is incompatable with a combined food track and airway.

PARTIAL LARYNGECTOMY

In general, patients with vertical or hemilaryngectomy have minimal swallowing problems in the postoperative period. Patients with supraglottic laryngectomy can generally anticipate a significant immediate dysphagia postoperatively. Patients whose supraglottic resection includes the epiglottis and one aryepiglottic fold, false cord, and one superior laryngeal nerve have a satisfactory outcome. Patients who have lost both their aryepiglottic folds and epiglottis with preservation of one superior laryngeal nerve can learn to swallow, particularly if radiation is not included. Patients who lose both superior laryngeal nerves and aryepiglottic folds, false cords, and epiglottis are most unlikely to develop successful airway coping mechanisms. Radiation in addition to the supraglottic laryngectomy can be expected to worsen any anticipated swallowing defect.

SURGICAL PLANNING TO MINIMIZE DYSPHAGIA

The oncologic surgeon must be careful to see that his goals in rehabilitation do not lead him into compromising his surgical therapy. It is certain that many patients have lost their lives owing to misguided attempts at preserving vital function. The surgeon, however, should be fully aware of the implications of any surgical ablation, and needless destruction of even "minor anatomic parts" should be avoided. Many patients, for example, have needless destruction of the nerve to the mylohyoid. The submaxillary triangle is seldom involved with lesions of the larynx and hypophyarynx, and in most instances the nerve to the mylohyoid can and should be preserved when these

lesions are being treated. The mylohyoid muscle, which is one of the lifters of the tongue, allows the food to be squirted into the back of the mouth and pharynx. The mylohyoid nerve also supplies the anterior belly of the digastricus, which aids in elevation and anterior displacement of the larynx during swallowing. Preservation of this nerve, for example, might allow a patient who has undergone supraglottic laryngectomy to swallow, who might otherwise not do so. Another nerve that is frequently treated with indifference during neck dissection is the ansa hypoglossi. In many operations, the descending branch of the hypoglossal nerve which contributes innervation to the strap muscles, can be easily preserved without compromising nodal dissection of the neck. In some instances, the cervical component to the ansa passes posteriorly to the jugular vein and can also be preserved. The strap muscles are ancillary muscles of deglutition, and again these nerves should not be sacrificed without thought. We have seen patiaents with previous supraglottic laryngectomy and one dissected neck who were able to swallow prior to, but not after, a second neck dissection.

The piriform sinus is frequently overlooked as an important necessity for normal swallowing. Patients having a supraglottic laryngectomy in which both piriform sinuses are partially obliterated may indeed expect significant difficulty in swallowing or experience total dysphagia. A number of patients in whom we have evaluated dysphagia following supraglottic laryngecotomy have been rehabilitated by reconstruction of the piriform sinus. This reconstruction allows the food to spill lateral to, rather than over, the top of the larynx.

DYSPHAGIS THERAPY

Team Concepts

Responsibility for therapy in many of the disabilities encountered in the hospital population have been clearly identified. Physiotherapists, for example, are employed with good advantage in the rehabilitation of the muscular skeletal system. Speech pathologists have aided greatly in the recovery of communication skills. Responsiblity for aiding patients with dysphagia, however, remains largely unstructured in most institutions. We believe that the dysphagic patient's best interests are served by a team of cooperative, coordinated, and communicating individuals with definite responsibilities.

Physician's Role

The physician who is managing the care of the patient with dysphagia should head the rehabilitation team. In cooperation with other members of the team, he should set the rehabilitation goals and time the various interventions. Most patients who undergo major resections for cancer of the head and neck area return from the operating room with some type of nasogastric feeding tube and tracheostomy tube in place. In some patients the respiratory status may be critical, and premature feeding with aspiration could be disastrous. Medical clearance is therefore essential before oral feeding can be instituted. The physician should be aware of any possible anatomic distortions produced by surgery and anticipate complications that might result from radiotherapy or chemotherapy.

SUPPORT TEAM

Nurses play an integral part in the nutrition therapy, both in the tube feeding phase and in beginning oral alimentation. They should be aware of and quickly note and report any suggestion of feeding tube misplacement; they can effectively use the tracheostomy vent for tracheal toilet in case of food aspiration.

The dietitian on the team ideally is concerned with the patient's caloric intake, nitrogen balance, and weight progress. The dietitian also provides a liaison with the hospital kitchen for the preparation of foods of appropriate consistency.

The primary dysphagia therapist, however, still remains to be identified in most institutions. On a national basis, no professional group has claimed responsibility for this neglected and somewhat difficult role. The physician and nurse are generally too busy with other responsibilities. The occupational and physiotherapists are generally not well trained in the anatomy and physiology of the aerodigestive tract. The respiratory therapists seem content to limit their interest to pulmonary function, and speech pathologists, until recently, have limited themselves to rehabilitation of communicative disorders. We believe that the speech pathologist who has additional training in dysphagia therapy is probably best suited to this role. There is an intimate relationship between the anatomic and physiologic functions of the speech and swallowing processes, and many patients with head and neck cancer suffer from disability in both these areas. A speech pathologist properly trained in dysphagia therapy can be of tremendous service as a member of the dysphagia therapy team. Currently, there is an active interest by some speech pathlogists in exploring the role of their specialty in this area.

POSTOPERATIVE EVALUATION AND THERAPY FOR DYSPHAGIA

Before oral feedings are begun, a careful evaluation of the patient's status from all aspects is mandatory. An immediate assessment on entering the patient's room can give a good indication of whether the patient is ready for oral feedings to begin. Several observations should be made automatically. What is the patient's respiratory status? If a tracheostomy tube is present, is the cuff inflated or deflated? Is the patient alert and is he relating to the environment about him? Does he appear able to hear and answer questions and follow directions? More importantly, how is the patient handling his own secretions? Perhaps one of the more vital indications of when to begin oral feedings is the absence of the bag of used facial tissues at the patient's bedside. There is little use in starting oral feedings in someone who is unable to swallow hiw own saliva. Observation of the patient can also indicate whether he has mouth control, whether his lips are competent, and what his general motivation appears to be.

TRACHEOSTOMY TUBES

Tracheostomy tubes, so essential in the head and neck cancer patient to prevent possible respiratory obstruction and to provide tracheal toilet for any aspirated secretions, are a mixed blessing in dysphagia therapy. The tracheostomy tube helpfully provides a good toilet for aspirated oral intake; however, it also serves to interfere with the swallowing mechanism. Following the normal human swallow, an individual always exhales to clear the laryngeal aditus. In the patient with a tracheostomy, this air is shunted through the tracheostomy tube and does not clear the larynx. In addition, the tracheostomy tube tends to fix the trachea and larynx to the skin, thus making the elevation of the larynx more difficult.[11] As a basic rule, the tracheostomy tube should not be removed until there is a likelihood of good swallowing without significant aspiration. It should be removed, however, at the earliest date consistent with the patient's progress. Many patients have cuffed tracheostomy tubes in place following surgery. The cuff should be deflated early in the patient's postoperative care, and the patient should be encouraged, when feasible, to speak around the tracheostomy tube. This encourages use of the tongue and accessory muscles of speech and, we believe, facilitates swallowing. If the tracheal toilet is adequate, it is well to reduce progressively the size of the tracheostomy tube. In many instances, the tracheostomy tube can be plugged as a test of the patient's ability to handle his secretions before starting oral feedings. It is also helpful on test feedings to have the tracheostomy tube plugged. This allows for expulsion of air through the larynx to clear the laryngeal aditus. Once swallowing progress without significant aspiration is ensured, the tracheostomy should be removed promptly if there is no evidence of respiratory obstruction.

Feeding tubes as well as tracheostomy tubes should be removed as soon as consistent with maintaining the patient's nutrition by oral means. The feeding tube itself interereres with the swallowing process and frequently keeps the throat slightly sore. It also promotes reflux of gastric content into the pharynx with possible aspiration. Large feeding tubes should be avoided except for initial feedings in the emaciated patient. We have found a 10 Fr feeding tube to be about the ideal size. This size is easily kept open by irrigation and yet is small enough to be no more than a minimal annoyance to the patient.

BEGINNING ORAL FEEDING

When it is apparent that the patient is now becoming successful in handling his secretions, and if there are no complicating medical respiratory problems, oral feedings may begin. The deglutition therapist or nurse should always be present with the patient during these initial feedings. The tracheostomy tube is best plugged before trial feeding. Suction apparatus and saline irrigation should be available for tracheal toilet if this proves to be needed. For most patients with surgical defects of the head and neck area, semisolid lubricating-type foods are best tolerated. Custards and thin purees are ideally suited for initiating the swallowing process. Patients with dysphagia from radiotherapy swallow liquids well. The dysphagia therapist should be well aware of any anatomic defect and be prepared to handle any emergency that might arise during the feeding. The process of eating should be explained thoroughly to the patient, and he should be given opportunity to explain his problems as he sees them. The patient should be seated upright with the head up and the chin extended, or he may lie in a semireclined position if drooling is a problem. If defects exist in the lips, anterior tongue, or mouth, it may be necessary to use some type of feeding device to place the food in the posterior aspect of the oral cavity. A feeding syringe with an attached plastic or rubber tube or a glossectomy-type feeding spoon may be a valuable adjunct for these patients. The food bolus should be adequately prepared. The patient should be instructed to inhale, hold his breath, give a good strong swallow, and then exhale. Initially, consecutive boluses of food should be avoided. Any evidence of aspiration should be noted, and success in swallowing also should be observed, documented, and encouraged. A number of techniques are available to the educated therapist which involve manipulation of the swallowing reflexes, permit desensitization of the gag reflexes, and prevent nasogastric regurgitation. When difficulty in swallowing is encountered, a careful observation should be made as to the nature of this difficulty and the types of food that may be involved. A cooperative examination of the patient's swallowing by the physician and deglutition therapist should permit identification of the cause of the specific swallowing problem. Often, surgically correctable defects may be identified. Videofluoroscopy may be of significant benefit to the clinician in making this determination. Problems encountered during the pharyngeal phase of swallowing are often best delineated by radiographic assessment.

Although surgical rehabilitation of the swallowing mechanism is outside the scope of this chapter, we would emphasize that in many instances, surgical rehabilitative procedures may salvage what appears to be a hopeless swallowing situation.

REFERENCES

1. Bosma J. Deglutition: Pharyngeal stage. Physiol Rev 1957; 37:275–300.
2. Doty RW. Neural organization of deglutition. Handbook Physiol 1968; 4:1861–1902.
3. Ekberg O, Nylander G. Cineradiography of the pharyngeal stage in 150 individuals without dysphagia. Br J Radiol 1982; 55:253–257.
4. Miller A. Deglutition. Physiol Rev 1982; 62:129–184.
5. Blackburn GL. Manual for the nutritional metabolic assessment of the hospitalized patient. Presented at the 62nd Annual Clinical Congress of the American College of Surgeons, Chicago, Oct. 11–15, 1976.
6. Shils ME. Principles of nutritional therapy. Cancer 1979; 43:2093.
7. Harvey KB, Bothe A, Blackburn GL. Nutritional assessment and patient outcome during oncological therapy. Cancer 1979; 43(2065).
8. Chencharick JD, Mossman KL. Nutritional consequences of the radiotherapy of head and neck cancer. Cancer 1983; 51:811–815.
9. Blackburn GL, Maini BS, Bistrian BR, McPermott WV Jr. The effect of cancer on nitrogen, electrolyte and mineral metabolism. Cancer Res 1977; 37:2348–2353.
10. Harvey KB, Bothe A, Blackburn GL. Nutritional assessment and patient outcome during oncological therapy. Cancer 1979; 43:2065–2069.
11. Mullen JL, Buzby GP, Walman MT, Gertner MH, Hobbs CL, Rosato EF. Prediction of operative morbidity and morality by preoperative nutritonal assessment. Surg Form 1979; 30:80–82.
12. Bassett MR, Dobie RA. Patterns of nutritional deficiency in head and neck cancer. Otolaryngol Head Neck Surg 1983; 91:119–125.
13. Bonanno P. Swallowing dysfunction after tracheostomy. Am Surg 1971; 174:21–33.

PROSTHETIC REHABILITATION OF THE MANDIBULECTOMY PATIENT

JAMES W. SCHWEIGER, D.D.S., M.S.

One of the most complex challenges facing the prosthodontist today is the management of the mandibulectomy patient. These patients, because of the nature and extensiveness of their operative procedures, frequently are subject to major postoperative problems that affect deglutition, speech, mastication, and appearance. This paper will address these major problems, the appropriate treatment regimens, the major prosthodontic rehabilitation techniques, and preventive measures.

PROBLEMS IN DEGLUTITION

The first major problem patients have is with swallowing because they cannot elevate the tongue in a coordinated reflex to push the bolus of food posteriorly into the oral pharynx. The status of the remaining tongue is an important diagnostic indicator for successful use of dentures. If the motor and sensory control of the tongue has been significantly compromised by the resection, the prognosis is not good. The position of the tongue is also an important factor. If the base of the tongue has been removed, the tongue is located in a more posterior position, which prevents proper seal of the lower denture; therefore, adequate retention cannot be gained.

IMPAIRED SPEECH

Impaired speech occurs when part of the tongue has been resected in order to remove the tumor. In addition, if during a resection, nerve innervation to the tongue has been injured or interrupted, the movement of the tongue is affected, and adequate elevation of the tongue during speech cannot be achieved.

A further complication that will impair speech occurs when a portion of the tongue is removed and the patient receives radiation therapy. Patients who receive radiation therapy experience changes in the volume and consistency of their saliva. The combined lack of tongue tissue and changes in volume and consistency of saliva result in difficulty in prolonged speaking.

Patients who have had part of their tongue resected usually need speech therapy in order to improve articulation. Scott (1970)[1] investigated the potential benefit of speech therapy for mandibulectomy patients.[2] The number of patients in the study group was small. A total of 20 patients participated, and these were subdivided into four groups. There were two groups of five patients each with a prosthesis and two groups of five patients each without a prosthesis. Two of the four groups, one with the prosthesis and the other without a prosthesis, were selected to receive 6 weeks of intensive speech therapy. Although the sample selection was small, Scott arrived at two decisive conclusions after the data were collected and analysed. First, he determined that placement of a prosthesis, although it improves the quality of speech sound, does not improve discourse. Second, it was determined that intensive speech therapy improves speech significantly for patients both with and without a prosthesis.

MASTICATION

Mandibular deviation and character of mandibular movements are important factors to consider in mastication. Patients with severe deviation of the mandible and angular paths of closure have difficulty in wearing dentures because of instability, and they can only apply masticatory force on the nonresected side. If the mandible is viewed in the frontal plane, a rotation of the mandible away from the occlusal contact on the resected side is noted (Fig. 1). This is caused by the contraction of the masseter and internal pterygoids on the nonresected side, which results in a rotation around the occlusal table on the nonresected side (Fig. 2). In patients who have a considerable amount of floor of mouth and tongue resected, there is also an imbalance in the closing and opening musculature of the mandible. The lateral pterygoid muscle is a major contributor to this deviation. The mylohyoid and digastric muscles on the nonresected side do not have antagonists, and this contributes to the deviation (Fig. 3). If a considerable amount of soft tissue is removed, as with a radical neck dissection, this adds to the deviation. On closing, the mandible takes a diagonal path. When the internal pterygoid muscle and the masseter contract, the diagonal path of clo-

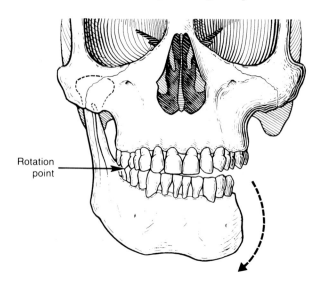

Figure 1 Rotation of mandible away from the occlusal contact.

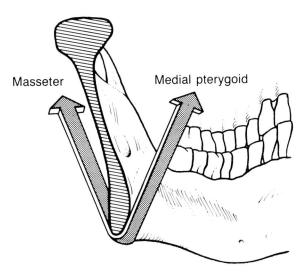

Figure 2 View of the mandible from psoterior to anterior on the nonresected side. It shows the contraction of the internal pterygoids and masseter muscles on the nonresected side. The direction of pull is emphasized.

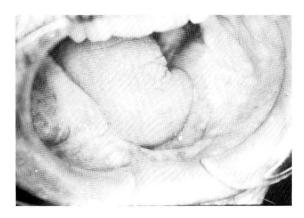

Figure 4 View of an anterior inner-table resection. Shows lack of attached mucosa and obliteration of the vestibule.

sure is greater, resulting in instability of the lower denture. This also affects the patient's ability to masticate.[2,6]

Defects with Mandibular Continuity. These types of defects can occur either in the anterior segment or the posterior segment of the mandible. The case demonstrated shows an anterior inner table resection (Fig. 4). The lack of attached mucosa and the obliteration of the vestibule could require a vestibuloplasty and skin graft.[4] Frequently, bands of scar tissue cross the residual anterior ridge. These must be removed if a satisfactory prosthesis is to be constructed. The prosthesis for these patients provides support for the lower lip and cheek, improving speech and aesthetics.

Lateral Discontinuity Defects. Edentulous patients with lateral discontinuity defects of the mandible never achieve preoperative masticatory efficiency. The extent of the bony and soft tissue resection determines the success of the prosthesis. If the resection involves considerable soft tissue, loss such

as a resection of a portion of the tongue, floor of mouth, or buccal mucosa, the prosthetic results will not be as good as for a patient who has only the mandible removed. A patient with large amounts of soft tissue removed has increased mandibular deviation and trismus as well as tongue and lip disability. The location of the bony resection is a good indicator of the prosthetic success.[3–5]

If the resection is posterior to the canine or anterior curvature of the mandible, the prognosis is more favorable than if the resection is to the midline (Fig. 5). The status of the remaining tongue is also an im-

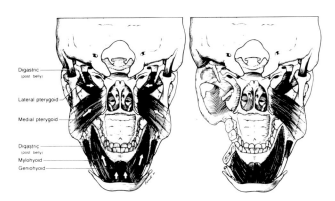

Figure 3 Shows the muscles that are responsible for the directional pull of the deviation.

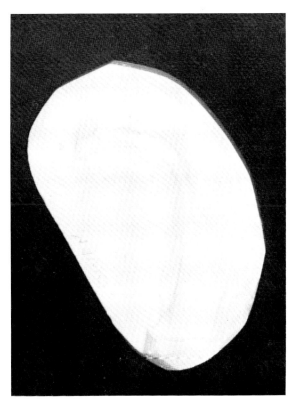

Figure 5 A model of a lateral discontinuity defect in which the anterior curvature of the mandible is maintained.

portant prognostic indicator. If motor and sensory control of the tongue have been significantly compromised by the resection, the prognosis is not good.

Anterior Discontinuity Defects. Patients with anterior discontinuity defects have a poor prognosis for prosthetic reconstruction without initial surgical reconstruction. Even though the patient has teeth, because of the disharmony in movement of the two mandibular segments, it is difficult and almost impossible to make a successful removable mandibular prosthesis. If the patient is edentulous and rehabilitation is desired, surgical mandibular reconstruction must be considered before prosthetic replacements can be made.

Patients with lateral discontinuity defects of the mandible never achieve presurgical maxillary efficiency. Complete dentures are mainly for aesthetics, and in some patients they may improve articulation in speech. According to Beumer,[6] a number of factors affect the patient's ability to function: (1) stability, support, and retention of mandibular denture is compromised; (2) oral mucosa is fragile and easily irritated because of radiation therapy; (3) reduction of salivary output affects retention of denture and compromises lubrication of the denture-mucosal interface; (4) angular path of closure induces lateral stresses that unseat the denture; (5) deviation of mandible creates a poor jaw relationship so that teeth cannot be placed over the ridge; and (6) impairment of motor and sensory control of tongue, lip, and cheek prevents the patient from controlling the prosthesis.

COSMETIC CONSIDERATIONS

A major facial disfigurement that occurs after surgery of a lateral discontinuity defect is the deviation of the mandible to the resected side (Figs. 6 and 7). If an adequate prosthesis can be constructed, this brings the mandible into proper alignment with the maxilla in the frontal aspect (Figs. 8 and 9). If there is an anterior discontinuity defect, there is the possibility of constant drooling from the mouth, which can be overcome by surgical reconstruction.

PROSTHETIC REHABILITATION CONSIDERATIONS

The several major issues to be considered in prosthetic rehabilitation are (1) whether the patient is dentulous or edentulous; whether the patient is receiving radiation therapy; whether the patient is going to receive radiation therapy; the extent of tongue mobility; the extent of the resection and the degree of soft tissue contracture; and the extent of mandibular range of motion.

In treating denulous patients following lateral mandibulectomy it is current practice to place Ivy loops or arch bars prior to surgery and then place the patient into intermaxillary fixation following surgery (Fig. 10). This procedure is followed by removing the intermaxillary fixation and placing the patient on oral ex-

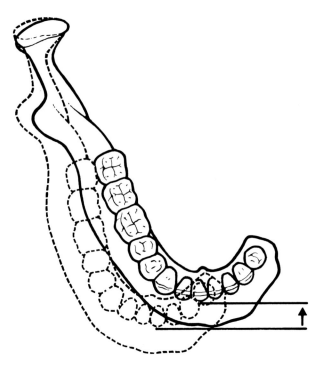

Figure 6 Drawing of lateral posterior deviation of mandible following resection.

ercises. These are demonstrated to the patient, who continues to be monitored closely. After these exercises, if the dentulous patient still has problems achieving a proper mandibular relation, a guidance prosthesis is used on an interim basis. At this time, if the patient is to be rehabilitated with a removable partial prosthesis, some type of inclined occlusal plane is constructed to bring the mandible over into proper centric position.

For the patient who is edentulous, it is current practice to place the patient on a jaw exercise program after surgery. This too is monitored closely, to ensure that the patient can bring the mandible over to the midline. After healing has taken place, in approximately 4 to 6 weeks, maxillary and mandibular

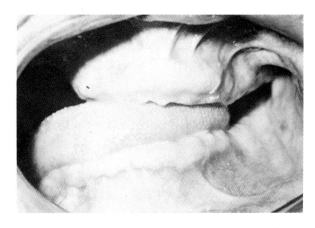

Figure 7 Rotation of the mandible after resection.

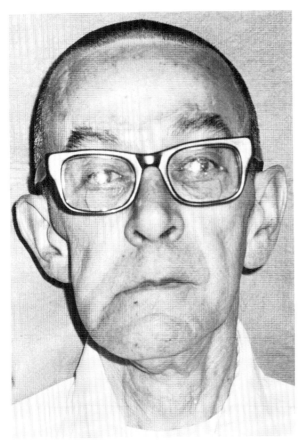

Figure 8 Frontal view of patient shows deviation without prosthesis in place.

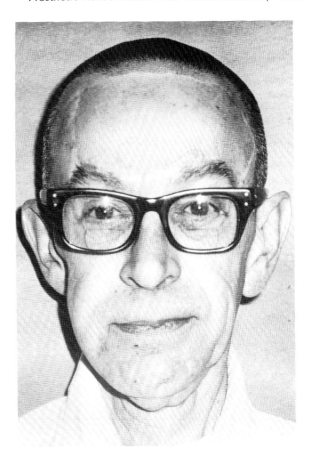

Figure 9 Frontal view of patient with prosthesis in place.

prostheses are constructed with occlusal incline ramps to bring the mandible into proper inner occlusal relationship. A guidance prosthesis is not used on an edentulous patient because it makes the maxillary and mandibular prostheses unstable.

A dentulous or edentulous patient who is to receive radiation therapy is monitored closely during the course of radiation therapy and afterward to prevent

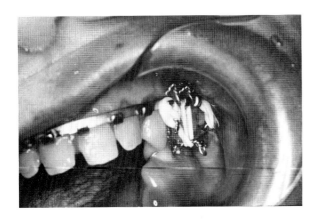

Figure 10 Placement of intermaxillary fixation with use of arch bars.

scar tissue from forming, as this can bring the mandible over into an abnormal occlusal relationship. Considerable time is spent with the patients, instructing them in the proper jaw exercises and informing them of complications that can result if the program outlined is not followed.

When a patient is to receive an anterior mandibulectomy and has teeth, it is advisable to place this patient into intermaxillary fixation during the healing phase after operation. This prevents the mandibular segments from rotating medially and upward and thereby causing soreness of the roof of the mouth. It also aids in proper alignment of the posterior segment if reconstruction is contemplated.

If the patient is edentulous and rehabilitation is desired, the posterior fragments should be held at the proper alignment. This can be achieved with either an intraoral rigging appliance which is placed at the time of surgery, or an external fixation appliance, which should be placed prior to the mandibular resection. At present, reconstruction of these anterior defects is being achieved with an iliac crest placement.

If the patient is going to have a lateral discontinuity defect reconstructed surgically, it is imperative that the mandibular segment be in proper alignment before the surgical procedure. The case illustrated in

Figures 11 through 13 is that of a mandible that was removed for an ameloblastoma, after which a microvascular free bone graft taken from the iliac crest was inserted. At the time of placement of the bone graft there was intermaxillary fixation. This was maintained until healing had taken place, approximately 10 weeks after graft placement.

Our experience with these grafts has been limited; however, the surgical results so far have been reasonable. At present, we are constructing a mandibular prosthesis for this type of mandibular reconstruction.

PREVENTIVE MEASURES

Preoperative Evaluation. All patients who are considered for mandibulectomy should be evaluated preoperatively to determine the condition of the oral cavity. Radiographs must be taken of the remaining teeth to evaluate them for possible disease at the apices of the teeth. A periodontal evaluation must also be included to ascertain the amount of bony support around the teeth. Diagnostic models provide a valuable guide in assessing the occlusion of the patient. The past dental history must be evaluated to determine whether the patient has been interested in, and has maintained, good dental health.

Surgical Considerations. If a lateral mandibulectomy is to be performed, the ramus of the mandible should be removed so that it will not interfere with later placement of a prosthesis. If the ramus is not removed, it will be displaced superiorly and medially and impinge on the tuberosity of the resected side, thereby causing a problem in prosthetic reconstruction (Fig. 14). During mandibulectomy in the dentulous patient, the bone should be cut through the socket of the tooth and not between the teeth. Extracting a tooth and cutting through its socket provides maximal height

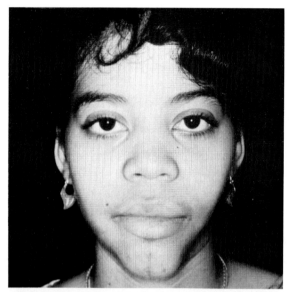

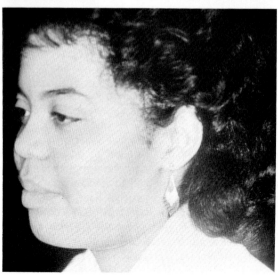

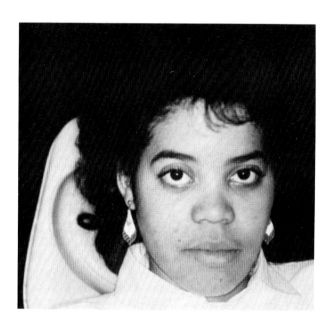

Figure 11   Frontal view of patient after mandibulectomy.

Figure 12   Frontal view of patient after surgical reconstruction.

Figure 13   Side view after reconstruction.

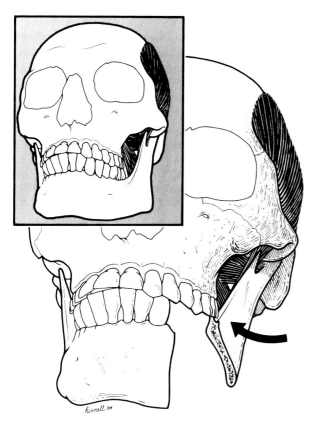

Figure 14 Illustration of results if ramus is not removed at the time of surgery. Ramus is displaced superiorly and medially.

for bone supporting the posterior aspect of the last remaining tooth (Fig. 15).

Postoperative Considerations. For the dentulous patient undergoing either an anterior mandibulectomy or a lateral mandibulectomy, either Ivy loops or maxillary mandibular arch bars should be placed to immobilize the mandible after surgery. These procedures prevent the initial deviation of the mandible to the resected side. The immobilization should remain intact for approximately the first 10 days to 2 weeks following surgery. After that period, the Ivy loops or arch bars are removed, and jaw exercises are initiated. The patient is taught how to forcibly move the mandible over to the nondefective side. This will

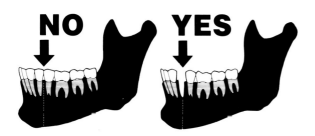

Figure 15 Illustration demonstrates proper bone cut to allow for maximal height of bone on terminal tooth.

help in the final cosmetic disfigurement, and the patient's teeth will line up and intercusp properly. After these two procedures have been accomplished, if the patient is still having problems with proper occlusion, a guidance restoration can be used to guide the mandible into proper occlusion (Figs. 16 and 17). If a guidance appliance is used, it is only used on an interim basis until a proper occlusal relationship and proper proprioception are re-established. Once this has been accomplished, the guidance appliance can be discarded, or it can be used occasionally to reinforce the appropriate proprioceptive mechanisms. Some patients feel more comfortable wearing a guidance appliance while sleeping as it prevents the mandible from drifting to the resected side.

Lateral mandibulectomy generally requires an inclined occlusal table because the path of closure of the mandible is from the resected to the nonresected side (Figs. 18 and 19). The size and inclination of the inclined occlusal table depend on the angle of closure. These tables bring the mandible into proper intercuspation during mandibular function.

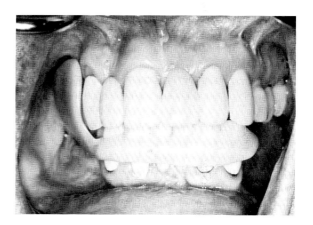

Figure 16 Acrylic guidance appliance. Used to prevent deviation of the mandible.

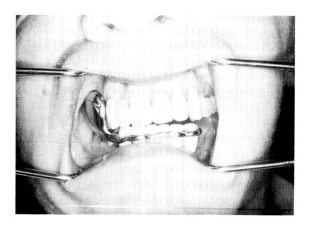

Figure 17 Permanent guidance appliance. Used to prevent deviation of the mandible.

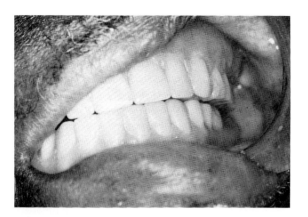

Figure 19 Illustrates function of the occlusal table with the prosthesis in place.

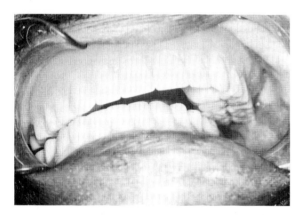

Figure 18 Inclined occlusal table as it appears in a denture prosthesis.

SUMMARY

The prosthetic management of patients with resection of part of the mandible, tongue, floor of mouth, and regional lymph nodes is challenging. These patients present extensive rehabilitation problems. Restoration of defects of the mandible can be accomplished with a properly constructed prosthesis. Early intervention of prosthodontic procedures enhances the success of rehabilitation efforts.

REFERENCES

1. Scott L. Speech rehabilitation for oral cancer patients, a pilot investigation, Master of Arts thesis, University of California, Santa Barbara, 1970.
2. Aramany M, Meyers E. Dental occlusion and arch relationship in segmental resection of the mandible. In: Sessions GA, Tardy ME (eds). Plastic and Reconstructive Surgery of the Face and Neck. Proceedings of the Second International Symposium. New York: Grune and Stratton, 1977.
3. Cantor R, Curtis TA. Prosthetic management of edentulous mandibulectomy patients. Part I. Anatomic and physiologic considerations. J Pros Dent 1971; 446–451.
4. Cantor R, Curtis TA. Prosthetic management of edentulous mandibulectomy patients. Part II. Clinical considerations. J Pros Dent 1971; 546–555.
5. Cantor R, Curtis TA. Prosthetic management of edentulous mandibulectomy patients. Part III. Clinical considerations. J Pros Dent 1971; 670–678.
6. Beumer J III, Curtis TA, Fertell DN. Acquired defects of the mandible etiology, treatment, and rehabilitation. In: Maxillofacial Rehabilitation: Prosthodontic and surgical considerations. St. Louis: CV Mosby, 1979; 90–188.
7. Loré JM. An Atlas of Head and Neck Surgery. Vol I 2nd Ed, Philadelphia: WB Saunders, 1973; 454–483.

SHOULDER REHABILITATION

WILLIAM H. SAUNDERS, M.D.

After division of the spinal accessory nerve supplying the trapezius muscle, there is weakness and deformity and often pain in the shoulder. A number of surgeons performing a neck dissection prefer the classic or complete radical operation to the various modified or conservative procedures designed to preserve the nerve because they believe that the radical operation removes metastatic disease more effectively. They are willing to accept the resulting functional deformity if they gain better control of the malignant process.

Other surgeons, however, have questioned the additional effectiveness of the classic radical neck dissection as compared with modified neck dissections, especially when there is no palpable lymphadenopathy in the neck. Bocca, in particular, saves the internal jugular vein, the sternocleidomastoid muscle, and all major nerves and blood vessels. His procedure removes the facial compartments around the muscles, vessels, and nerves. Still other surgeons remove the internal jugular vein and the sternocleidomastoid muscle, but spare the spinal accessory nerve to save the function of the shoulder. Finally, it has been demonstrated that grafting between the cut ends of the spinal accessory nerve, using the greater auricular nerve, affords adequate neural supply to the trapezius muscle.

THE TRAPEZIUS

The trapezius has three parts: upper, middle, and lower. It resembles a fan and is attached medially to the vertebrae and at the other end to the spine of the scapula. It functions to rotate the scapula upward and downward and to retract it. Muscles that compensate for loss of the trapezius are the levator scapulae and the rhomboids.

My test for function of the trapezius is to have the patient hold both arms in full abduction and then to pull down on each arm against resistance. On the weakened side, the patient cannot maintain his arm in the elevated position, whereas on the normal side,

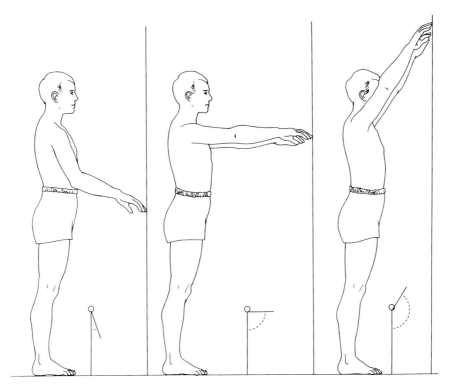

Figure 1 Scapulohumeral ROM.

he readily can. Another test for the middle and lower segments of the trapezius may be done by having the patient lie prone with arms outstretched and then having him raise his arms upward. This maneuver brings the middle and lower segments of the trapezius muscle into prominence.

In paralysis the vertebral border of the scapula is flared, and this is accentuated if the arm is abducted from the side against resistance. Patients with marked loss of shoulder abduction, 70° or less, characteristically try to compensate for contralateral flexion of the trunk. Even though the spinal accessory nerve has been cut and the trapezius is paralyzed, the patient may be able to elevate the arm in a forward position by using the serratus anterior to stabilize the scapula.

Thus, in evaluating shoulder function, one must be careful to note that the patient with paralysis of the trapezius cannot abduct the arm laterally to raise it overhead, but that he can raise it anteriorly using flexors.

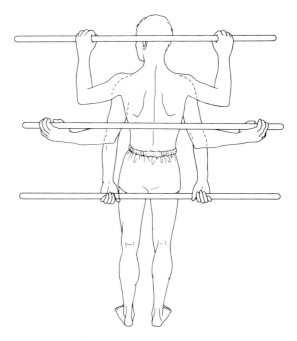

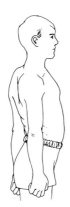

Figure 2 Stretch protractors.

Figure 3 Stretch protractors.

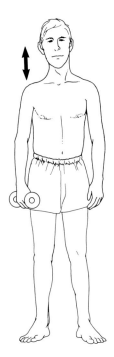

Figure 4 Strengthen elevators and retractors.

OTHER PROBLEMS

In some cases the scapulohumeral joint tends to lose motion and may develop a *periarthritis* or adhesive capsulitis. This tends additionally to limit motion, especially in the early postoperative weeks in response to pain associated with surgery, and discourages use of the shoulder joint.

Pain may be caused by stretching of compensating muscles, particularly the rhomboids and the elvator scapulae. These muscles are stretched by the unbalanced pull of the serratus anterior. Pain also may be produced by periarthritis of the scapulohumeral joint and, less frequently, by osteoarthritis of the sternoclavicular joint on the side of the paralysis, which occurs as a result of longstanding stress imposed by the unbalanced scapulohumeral complex.

TREATMENT

THe exercises demonstrated in Figures 1 through 4 are beneficial in that they increase shoulder motion and relieve pain. The patient should be instructed by a physical therapist for two or three sessions and then checked every several weeks to ensure progress. The usual result of treatment is relief of pain, then an improvement in posture, and finally functional improvement of the arm as shoulder motion increases. Also helpful is exposure to an infrared luminous 250-watt lamp and massage.

As one might expect, the results are directly proportional to the persistence and effort made by the patient, and these in turn are dependent on the encouragement of his physician and physical therapist. Many patients believe that the effort is too great and shortly discontinue the program.

SECTION EIGHT / NEW TREATMENT MODALITIES

38. New Treatment Modalities

INTRODUCTION

DANIEL MILLER, M.D., F.A.C.S.

Therapeutically, the goal of the oncologic surgeon, the medical oncologist, and the radiation therapist is to destroy the cancer cell in any way possible and at the same time to avoid as much as possible the destruction or injury of the normal cell.

The advent of newer techniques revolves around such a philosophy. The fine line that separates the ability of an injured cell to repair itself, whether normal or abnormal, is the gray area that concerns the therapist no matter what the modality of therapy employed. In reality we are searching for the best destructive tool for that particular cancer, whether this tool be used locally or in conjunction with systemic therapy.

The chapters of this book reveal a profound historical experience in the use of time-honored modalities such as radiation therapy, scalpel surgery, and, of recent vintage, chemotherapy—singly or in combinations, and in varying methods of application. This wealth of information has given us increasing hope for greater survival associated with a reasonable quality of life.

From time to time thinking oncologists report preliminary studies in the area of newer modalities to eradicate cancer. In essence, the question arises as to what is the best destructive tool we have available to accomplish our goal of help for the particular patient afflicted with a particular cancer and its local geography and topography. The chapters in this part report on the use of three modalities that have gained ground and, of greater importance, are still gaining the respect of the oncologic therapists who have been exposed to and gained experience in their proper utilization.

Strong, who is one of the world's greatest contributors in the development of and utilization of laser surgery, reports on his experience using the CO_2 laser, the argon laser, and now the neodynium-YAG laser. He brings into proper perspective the present and future value of this modality in the management of cancer of the head and neck, with a goal of palliation and/or cure.

DeSanto, who has made many contributions to the understanding and application of cryosurgery, writes about this modality. This destructive tool, like the laser, has many applications in the management of cancer of the head and neck. The author's experiences and recommendations as to the proper place of this modality in our therapeutic regimen, although perhaps controversial, are of considerable interest and importance.

Dougherty, in his chapter, reports on another modality, photoradiation, which is not well known but rapidly gaining ground. Photoradiation for the treatment of malignant disease is based on the concentration of the photosensitizing agent hematoporphyrin derivative (HPD) in tumor cells with resultant necrosis of these cells when light of the appropriate wave length is applied.

As one of the pioneers in the field, Dougherty has demonstrated that a red light with wave length of 630 nm that is used to illuminate a cancer containing HPD will cause selective necrosis. He discusses here the possible therapeutic potential of this process, the method of utilization of HPD in patients, the possible phototoxicity associated with this modality, and the management program of the patient so treated. He prefers to call the modality "photodynamic therapy" to avoid its being equated with ionizing radiation.

ROLE OF LASERS IN HEAD AND NECK CANCER

M. STUART STRONG, M.D.

The physical attributes and the soft tissue effects of CO_2, neodymium-YAG (Nd-YAG), and argon lasers make them all worthy of consideration for possible use in the management of head and neck cancer. Although the effects vary between one laser and another, they all have some features in common that require amplification.

The effect of laser radiation on soft tissues is entirely thermal; the degree of thermal injury depends on the selective absorption of the electromagnetic energy by the target tissue. The absorption of the laser energy results in photocoagulation of the tissues and hemostasis in small blood vessels.

If the absorption of energy is high, the tissue destruction may go on to carbonization and even vaporization. The degree of tissue destruction is dose-dependent and is therefore under good to excellent control; with clinical experience it can be predetermined how much tissue destruction will be produced by a given amount of laser irradiation, taking into account the power density of the focused beam (watts per square centimeter), the duration of the exposure (in seconds), the power setting (in watts) of the instrument, and the absorption characteristics of the target tissue. Shock-impact is not a problem with continuous wave lasers, such as the CO_2, Nd-YAG, and argon. The first laser to be used in experimental tumors was a *pulsed* neodymium laser;[1] this resulted in widespread scattering of viable tumor cells by the shock-impact effect. This phenomenon does not occur with continuous-wave lasers.

POTENTIAL ADVANTAGES OF LASER USAGE

Laser application is a *non-touch technique*, so that incision or vaporization of a tissue can be carried out without introducing an instrument into the field and obscuring the view of the target area; the lack of contact eliminates manipulation of vascular lesions prior to coagulation.

The hemostatic effect of lasers is a great advantage in that it allows good visibility and precise control over tissue destruction.

Since lasers can be applied whenever the target tissue can be viewed, lasers allow tissue destruction to be carried out readily in inaccessible areas.

SELECTION OF LASER WAVELENGTH

The selection of a particular laser depends on the nature of the clinical problem as well as the treatment plan; the different effects of each laser usually indicate which instrument should be selected.

The CO_2 laser (wavelength 10.6μ) is absorbed by all biologic tissues so that it is ideal for carrying out controlled tissue destruction or excisional biopsy of all lesions, except those that are conspicuously vascular. The amount of scar formation following healing of a CO_2 laser-induced wound is so minimal that excellent mobility of the tongue, palate, and vocal cord are frequently preserved after laser dissection. The finding that there is little pain in the immediate postoperative period allows early feeding of the patient (on the same day) and early discharge from the hospital (most often the next day); the modality is therefore cost-effective.

The neodymium-YAG laser (wavelength 1.06μ) has the capacity to penetrate deep into the tissues and produce deep coagulation at a distance of 1 to 1.5 cm from the surface; this attribute, of course, makes it ideal for the management of very vascular tumors, such as carcinoids or paragangliomas. The degree of coagulation that follows neodymium-YAG usage makes it unsuitable for excisional biosy when histologic detail must be preserved.

The argon laser (wavelength 0.488μ) has the characteristic of being absorbed by black and red targets, which suggests its value in the treatment of pigmented melanomas. Unfortunately, the lack of adequate power makes the achievement of adequate power densities impossible, except with the use of a very small spot size; this renders the use of the instrument impractical in the management of established macroscopic tumors.

The purpose of this presentation is to review the clinical experience in the use of lasers in the management of head and neck cancers and to place lasers in the context of other treatment modalities.

CLINICAL APPLICATIONS

CO_2 Laser

This laser is ideal for carrying out excisional biopsy of all small, superficial, potentially dysplastic lesions of the oral cavity, oropharynx, and larynx, which on histologic examination may prove to be keratosis, atypia, or carcinoma in situ. The removal of all of the lesions unequivocally establishes the diagnosis and may provide cure.

Excisional biopsy of all micro (less than 2 mm) and mini (2 to 5 mm) cancers of the glottis is ideally carried out with the CO_2 laser; the diagnosis is established unequivocally, and if the margins are histologically free, no further treatment is needed. After healing has been completed, an acceptable quality of voice is preserved; this may be better than that present preoperatively. Ninety percent 3-year tumor-free survival has been achieved with these patients. Patients whose tumor margins are not free should be treated by radiotherapy for cure; these patients have been found

548

to have a 90 percent 3-year tumor-free survival as well. Large verrucous carcinomas and spindle-cell carcinomas have been consistently excised successfully in this manner.[2]

Exploration with a view to doing an excisional biopsy of T1 glottic cancer radiotherapy failures is ideally carried out with the CO_2 laser. Because tumors treated by radiotherapy do not necessarily shrink concentrically, it is more difficult to be certain of the surgical margins than in an untreated case. If histologically free margins cannot be obtained, it is usually because of subglottic spread dictating the need for total laryngectomy. Tumor-free margins have been achieved in this way and have resulted in 40 percent 3-year tumor-free survival.[2]

In the presence of bulky tumors, intratracheal intubation can often be achieved, but after completion of the examination of the larynx, there may be concern about the wisdom of extubating the patient without performing a tracheostomy; it is usually not difficult to excise the redundant, obstructing portions of the tumor with the CO_2 laser, thus restoring the airway so that extubation can be completed safely and comfortably. Tumor reduction in this way has been most satisfactory, allowing definitive surgery such as laryngectomy to be carried out at a later date in the absence of a contaminated tracheostomy stoma.

Palliation of obstructive endotracheal and endobronchial tumors can often be achieved with the CO_2 laser via a rigid bronchoscope; in the presence of slow-growing tumors, such as adenoid-cystic carcinoma, palliation often lasts for a year or more before the treatment needs to be repeated. It is usually not worthwhile opening up the orifice of secondary bronchi because recurrence takes place so quickly—in a week or two.[3]

The limitations of the use of the CO_2 laser are that (1) good visibility is needed at all times, (2) the field must be dry, and (3) vessels larger than 0.5 mm will not be coagulated by the CO_2 beam. Foreknowledge of these prerequisites makes it easy to avoid the use of the laser in unsuitable situations.

Neodymium-YAG Laser

This laser is of limited value in head and neck cancer management, but it has been found to be effective in the palliation of obstructive lesions of the esophagus; the laser is applied via the flexible esophagoscope.[4]

At present, its use in the palliation of lesions of the tracheobronchial tree is experimental and is being explored under the auspices of the Food and Drug Administration.[5]

The limitations of the neodymium-YAG laser are due to limited absorption of the energy and transmission deep into the tissue for distances of 1 to 1.5 cm; the thermal injury is therefore delayed in onset, and its full effect (necrosis) is not evident for several days. It is possible to achieve some tumor vaporization with the neodymium-YAG after some charring has taken place, but this is much less predictable that with the CO_2 laser.

Argon Laser

The absorption of the energy, by other than red or black targets, is so low that it is difficult to produce tissue destruction. At high-energy densities, using a very small spot size of around 200 microns, some vaporization can be achieved, but under these conditions the hemostatic effect is partially lost.

The argon laser is not a practical instrument for achieving tumor destruction in the head and neck.

SUMMARY

Excisional biopsy with the CO_2 laser is the preferred method of management of premalignant and early malignant disease of the upper air and food passages. It has proved consistently reliable in the excision of verrucous carcinoma and spindle-cell carcinoma of the head and neck.

The CO_2 laser is valuable in (1) the exploration of T1 glottic cancers that have failed radiation to determine the extent of additional needed surgery if tumor-free margins cannot be obtained; (2) relieving airway obstruction in the presence of larger laryngeal tumors and thus avoiding tracheotomy in the prelaryngectomy state; and (3) the palliation of obstructing tumors of the tracheobronchial tree.

The neodymium-YAG laser has a limited role in head and neck cancer, but it is useful in palliation of cancer of the esophagus and perhaps of the tracheobronchial tree.

The argon laser has no part to play in head and neck cancer management.

REFERENCES

1. Ketcham AS, Hoyes RC, Riggle GC. A surgeon's appraisal of the laser. Surg Clin North Am 1967; 47:1249–1263.
2. Blakeslee D, Vaughan CW, Shapshay SM, Simpson GT, Strong MS. Excisional biopsy in the selective management of T1 glottic cancer: A three-year follow-up study. Laryngoscope 1984; 94:488–494.
3. Shapshay SM, Davis RK, Vaughan CW, Norton ML, Strong MS, Simpson GT. Palliation of airway obstruction from tracheobronchial malignancy: Use of the CO_2 laser bronchoscope. Otolaryngol Head Neck Surg 1983; 91:615–619.
4. Fleischer De, Sivah MV Jr. Endoscopic laser therapy as palliation for esophagastric cancer: Parameters effecting initial outcome. Gastroenterology 1984; 86:1078.
5. Dumon JF, Reboud E, Garbe L, et al. Treatment of tracheobronchial lesions by laser photoresection. Chest 1982; 81:278–284.

CURATIVE, PALLIATIVE, AND ADJUNCTIVE USES OF CRYOSURGERY IN THE HEAD AND NECK

LAWRENCE W. DeSANTO, M.D.

The usual experiences with cryogenic surgery of head and neck tumors have been directed to palliation of accessible growths after maximal conventional treatment has failed.[1-3] This random and uncontrolled use of cryosurgery in a previously operated and often heavily irradiated anatomic region has given disappointing results. Usually, the destructive capability of profound cold is exploited. The hemostatic, adhesive, and immunogenic properties are less well understood and appreciated. In a sense, we are exploring the clinical potential of a powerful therapeutic agent while developing the basic knowledge necessary for optimal therapeutic effectiveness. A few experiments have only been suggestive of the tissue variations in the susceptibility to cryonecrosis, the relationship of blood supply to cryonecrosis, the potential of vascular exclusion to augment destruction of tissues, and the possibility of in situ cryonecrosis as a stimulant to tumor-specific immunity.[4] This deficiency in fundamental data hinders clinical effectiveness.

BACKGROUND

Freezing for organ and cell preservation, as in blood and spermatozoa banks and food preservation, is common. However, tumor necrosis requires more than just lowering the tissue temperature. The variables that determine success or failure in cryosurgery are (1) rate of freeze, (2) depth of homogeneous freeze, (3) use of repetitive freezing after spontaneous thaw, (4) effect of ischemia, and (5) adequate treatment of the entire tumor.

Rate of Freeze.   The rate of freeze depends on the size of the probe tip, the cryogenic agent, and the vascularity of the tissue. Using liquid nitrogen (boiling point, $-196°C$), Neel et al showed that cure rates in syngeneic mouse tumor-host systems increased significantly as the rate of freeze increased if temperatures were lowered below $-30°C$.[5] There are no specific guidelines to determine the optimal rate of cooling in order to obtain maximal necrosis, but the usual rule is to cool as rapidly as possible, according to tumor accessibility. How rapidly a tissue cools varies with the organ, its vascularity, and the position of the organ in relationship to large blood vessels. At the cellular level, the difference in the mechanism of producing cell death between slow and rapid freezing is

specific. During slow cooling (temperature changes of 1 to 10°C per minute), extracellular ice crystals form at or below the eutectic freezing point of the extracellular fluid. Water is then extracted from within cells through intact cell membranes and joins the growing ice crystals. Intracellular electrolytes concentrate to toxic levels, and cells collapse from dehydration and die. In contrast, during rapid cooling (temperature changes of 10 to 100°C per minute), both extracellular and intracellular ice crystallization form. A cell with ice in it becomes severely damaged and usually dies.[6]

In clinical cryosurgery for cancer, the rate of freeze depends on the size of the probe and the size of the tumor. The larger the surface area of the cryoprobe, the more rapid will be the rate of freeze. Open-spray and open-chamber probes are very effective because liquid nitrogen at $-196°C$ comes into direct contact with the tumor surface. There is rapid extraction of heat with temperature changes of 10 to 100°C per minute. Intracellular crystallization, which presumably is essential for predictable cell death, is ensured. The limitations of open-spray or open-chamber use are apparent. They can be safely applied only to very accessible surface lesions and anterior oral growths. With growths in these areas, adjacent normal tissue can be protected better from the splatter of free liquid nitrogen.

Lowest Temperature of Freeze.   The proportion of cells that die is the greatest when temperatures are reduced below $-30°C$.[5] Extending temperatures to below $-50°C$ does not increase the lethality of cold if the rate of temperature change is relatively constant. The number of minutes that a tissue must remain in the superfrozen state to ensure death is not known. If rapidly cooled to below a critical temperature, a cell probably will die, regardless of how long it remains at that temperature. The rate of freeze and rate of thaw to a low temperature is more important than the length of time a single cell remains at its lowest temperature. Our experience with clinical cryosurgery for tumor necrosis confirms that holding the periphery of a tumor mass at temperatures below -20 or $-30°C$ for 2 to 3 minutes usually ensures homogeneous cell death if the other requirements are met.

Spontaneous Thaw and Refreeze.   With unassisted spontaneous thaw, intracellular ice crystal formation continues as temperatures increase from -10 to 0°C. The enlarging crystal of ice further damages cells and may kill the cells that survived the rapid freeze. In contrast, an assisted rapid thaw causes the ice crystals to melt rather than enlarge, and the probability of cell survival increases; this decreases the chance that the entire cell population will die.[4] To ensure the death of every cell, a second and third refreeze with a spontaneous thaw between is recommended. Neel et al have demonstrated that the cure rate in experimental tumors progressively increases with the second and third applications of the probe.[5] The likelihood of success increases for several reasons: (1) repeated freezing increases the change that an individual cell is exposed to lethal intracellular ice formation; (2) each preceding freeze potentiates the effectiveness of later treatment because of associated impairment of circulation; with this compromise to the vascular supply, heat transfer is diminished and cold conductivity is increased, and a larger ice ball with lower tissue temperatures can be obtained by subsequent freezes; and (3) the tissue ischemia created by cryogenic intravascular coagulation and direct injury to the vessel wall further limits the microcirculation of the tumor and can itself produce the cell death of viable survivors after a freeze-thaw-refreeze tissue insult.

Organ Ischemia. Transient organ ischemia can potentiate effectiveness of freezing and ensure more certain cell death. Inflow vascular occlusion has quadrupled the volume of cryonecrosis in the experimental situation.[7] Vascular occlusion increases the effectiveness of treatment by lessening the rate of heat delivery and increasing the rate and volume of cooling. Vascular compromise is a practical adjunct to cryosurgery in certain head and neck neoplasms and requires clinical trial.

Pitfalls to Successful Cryonecrosis. Successful cryosurgery to control cancer obviously requires adequate treatment of the entire tumor cell population. To accomplish this, a rather precise estimate of tumor borders is necessary. In the oral cavity, this is not difficult. The surgical estimate acquired by observation and palpation can be reasonably accurate. Estimating the boundaries of tumor infiltration caudal to the area of the tonsillar fossa at the base of the tongue and in the hypopharynx is more hazardous. As in excisional surgery, in which a margin of normal tissue is usually removed, in tumor cryosurgery, the ball of frozen tissue must extend beyond the specific tumor into adjacent normal tissue. Thermocouple monitors placed 1 to 1.5 cm beyond the estimated boundaries in every dimension will ensure adequate treatment of all the tumor if the thermocouple temperatures can be reduced rapidly to below -20 or $-30°C$. Theoretically, if the rate of freeze of the boundary tissue is too slow, tumor cells could be forced peripherally through tissue planes into normal tissue by a slowly advancing cold front and be implanted beyond the area of lethal freezes. Tumor implantation is less likely with a rapidly advancing front. Mobile cells are more likely to be trapped within a freezing mass than to be pushed beyond the area of lethal temperatures. The less accessible a tumor is, the more likely it is that treatment will fail, because all requirements are not met. The paramount requirement for success in clinical cryosurgery is accessibility.

To summarize, every cell of a tumor must be properly treated to ensure tumor control. The requisites of cell death are well known from experimental models: a lethal subzero temperature of about $-30°C$, a rapid rate of freeze to this critical temperature, and a slow spontaneous thaw, with repetition of this sequence. Normal tissue beyond the tumor margins similarly must be included in a treated tissue mass to ensure that cells forced by advancing ice mass are rendered nonviable.

Three groups of patients who have been treated with cryosurgery were (1) patients with malignant tumors of the upper aerodigestive system who were treated for cure, (2) patients with malignant tumors who were treated for palliation, and (3) patients with nonmalignant tumors who were treated primarily with conventional surgery, but in whom cold was used to facilitate excisional surgery by limiting loss of blood.

Each patient was treated in the operating room with the use of sterile equipment and techniques. A self-pressurized cryosurgery unit (Brymill model SP5) and a laryngoscopic unit were used. Most patients were treated while under general endotracheal anesthesia. A few patients who had surface and accessible anterior oral cancers or recurrent cancers within maxillectomy cavities were treated with the use of the anesthetic properties of cold supplemented by the intravenous analgesic agents diazepam and ketamine.

The choice of cryoprobe depends on the site of the tumor and its accessibility. The open-spray or the open-chamber probes are preferred for surface growths, those within the maxillectomy defect, and some tumors of the anterior oral cavity and tongue. These open probes allow maximal rate and area of freeze. The oral tumors that are posterior to the mobile portion of the tongue, such as on the base of the tongue and hypopharymx, are treated with closed probes of either the surface type or the insertable prong-tipped type. When the prolonged probe is used, it is inserted into the tumor mass. This probe is preferred for the more posterior oral and pharyngeal growths because with it a larger tumor area can be treated effectively. Tissue temperatures are monitored by needle thermocouples placed at the periphery of the growth when a tumor was treated for cryonecrosis. Tumors are repeatedly frozen at least three times and allowed to thaw spontaneously between freezes. To treat an entire tumor mass, five or six freeze-thaw cycles are sometimes necessary. Each freeze cycle continues for 3 minutes after tissue temperatures of $-20°C$ are established at the thermocouple. Treatment is continued until every area of tumor is frozen to temperatures of $-20°C$ or lower.

Rubber mouth gags and wooden tongue blades are used to expose tumors of the oral cavity, whereas the suspension laryngoscope is used to expose tumors of the tongue base and hypopharynx. Adjacent normal tissue is protected with Styrofoam insulating material and packing impregnated with petroleum jelly.

DISCUSSION

Curative Cryosurgery. Because of the serious responsibility of substituting a new therapeutic method for an established mode of therapy, cryosurgery for cure is offered only in carefully selected situations.

Each growth treated for cure was considered ideally accessible for cryosurgery. In addition, every patient who was treated with cryosurgery was considered unsuitable for conventional excision because of age or existing blood dyscrasias or because the patient refused mutilating surgery.

Of an earlier series of eight patients who underwent cryosurgery with the objective of cure, three were cured of their cancer. Three other patients died of second primary cancers; one patient (an 82-year-old man) died of natural causes 14 months after treatment; and one patient died from cryosurgically induced hemorrhage one month after ligation of the common carotid artery.

This experience represents the early steps in the evaluation of a new tool for the control of cancer and has been helpful in establishing criteria for patient selection. Since the initial trials, cyrosurgery use has been to carefully selected cases.

Deeply infiltrative tumors with poorly defined margins are seldom suitable for cryosurgery. Particularly unsuitable are those infiltrative growths caudal to the tonsillar fossa at the base of the tongue and the hypopharynx. In these tumors, the depth of the growth is difficult to determine accurately, the exposure is limited, and several weeks must pass before the necrotic slough clears and the depth of the wound can be evaluated.

In contrast, superficially infiltrative exophytic or verrucose cancers that are anterior to the tonsillar pillars are particularly suitable to primary cryosurgery. Specifically suitable are tumors of the buccal mucosa, retromolar triangle, floor of the mouth and tongue, and the palate. Bony cellular elements and tumor infiltration into bone can be destroyed with proper cryogenic techniques. Bone repair can be anticipated. Cryosurgery is an attractive alternative to excisional surgery when conventional ablation necessitates the loss of portions of the upper or lower jaw.

Naturally, cryosurgery can be directed only to the primary growth. Nodal deposits require separate treatment, usually neck dissection.

The morbidity of cryosurgery deserves mention. Every patient in our experience either had or required tracheotomy, except one patient with nasal cancer, one with a small cancer on the floor of the mouth, and one with cancer of the anterior buccal mucosa and alveoli. Two patients experienced major hemorrhage after cryosurgery. Both had hypopharyngeal squamous tumors; each had received extensive radiation therapy to the primary site months or years before cryogenic therapy; and each had previous excisional surgery in the anastomosis region. One of the patients who hemorrhaged required common carotid artery ligation to control the bleeding and eventually died after the ligation. One patient experienced severe trismus after cryosurgery on a retromolar squamous cancer and required months of effort with the use of the mouth stretcher for rehabilitation. Because the patient was 82 years old, the trismus was a major compli-

cation and may have hastened his death. One patient required a feeding esophagostomy for 8 weeks. This 62-year-old man had undergone cryosurgery rather than excision after external radiation had failed to control a squamous cancer in the base of the tongue. Cryosurgery was selected because the patient had a serious bleeding disorder. Although free of disease for 18 months after treatment, he ultimately died from a solitary pulmonary cancer that was either a second primary lesion or a massive solitary metastatic lesion.

Whether the rates for control and survival after cryosurgery will justify its broader use in head and neck cancer remains to be determined. Our early experience indicates that profound cold is a potent destructive agent. It can be effectively used to destroy totally accessible head and neck malignant tumors. The morbidity in cryosurgery occurs not only because of the profound tissue destructiveness of cold, but also because the cold is delivered to a tissue substrate that has been altered by previous external irradiation. Our experience encourages us to continue this work and to judiciously substitute primary cryosurgical therapy for external fractionated radiation or excisional surgery in selected patients with accessible head and neck malignant tumors.

Palliative Cryosurgery. The primary malignant tumors of 27 patients were treated palliatively when there was disseminated disease. The therapeutic goals were relief of pain (through destruction of sensory nerves), reduction of bulky tumor masses, and elimination of bleeding. In every instance, these goals were accomplished, but whether palliation was worthwhile when morbidity was considered is a value judgement. Three patients in this group had serious hemorrhages within weeks after cryosurgery, but no patient died as a direct result of bleeding. Hemorrhage in experimental cryosurgery is unusual. In the unusual clinical setting, however, it is not surprising that vascular necrosis occurs, resulting in serious bleeding. Each patient in the palliative group already had received high doses of external radiation therapy. Cryonecrosis of a tissue depleted of its reparative potential by previous irradiation results in an occasional major vessel blowout. Another serious complication of palliative cryosurgery is oral cutaneous fistula. Such a fistula occurred in one patient who had previously received high doses of external radiation after cryosurgery to the tongue and floor of the mouth.

Results of cryosurgical palliation have been disappointing in our experience. Cryosurgery that was used because "nothing else was available" only converted large problems into enormous ones; nevertheless, when a specific palliative objective can be accomplished with cryosurgery, such treatment may be justified. Examples of circumstances in which cryosurgery should be used in the absence of a realistic chance for cure are limited. In our palliative group, three patients with local maxillectomy cavity recurrences were helped in that they were able to wear maxillary prostheses until their death. Another patient with a huge disseminated parotid mucoepidermoid cancer was relieved of a bleeding bulky mass that could not be easily concealed, but this benefit was sustained for only 2 months. Another patient with a huge ulcerating basal cell cancer at the root of the nose retained the sight of his only useful eye for 3 extra months. Beyond these modest accomplishments, palliative cryosurgery was of no value.

Adjunctive Cryotherapy. Cryosurgery as a supplement to excisional surgery has been proposed as particularly suitable during surgery on vascular neoplasms. In this situation, the hemostatic and sometimes the adhesive properties of cold are exploited. The tumors are frozen into an ice ball (to limit loss of blood) and are excised. Three patients were so treated: two had juvenile nasopharyngeal angiofibromas and one had a nasal hemangiopericytoma. The adjunctive use of cryosurgery for this type of tumor is not very helpful and for larger tumors impractical.

REFERENCES

1. Shibata HR, Tabah EJ. The use of cryosurgery in the control of locally recurrent tumors. Can Med Assoc J 1970; 103:134–139.
2. Miller D. Three years experience with cryosurgery in head and neck tumors. Ann Otol Rhinol Laryngol 1969; 78:786–791.
3. Goldstein JC. Cryotherapy in head and neck cancer. Laryngoscope 1970; 80:1046–1052.
4. Shulman S. Cryo-immunology: The production of antibody by the freezing of tissue. In: Rand RW, Rinfret AP, von Leden H, eds. Cryosurgery. Springfield, IL: Charles C Thomas 1968; pp 78–91.
5. Neel HB III, Ketchman AS, Hammond WG. Requisites for successful cryogenic surgery of cancer. Arch Surg 1971; 102:45–48.
6. Mazur P. Physical-chemical factors underlying cell injury in cryosurgical freezing. In: Rand RW, Rinfret AP, von Leden H, eds. Cryosurgery. Springfield, IL: Charles C Thomas, 1968; pp 32–51.
7. Neel HB III, Ketcham AS, Hammond WG. Ischemia potentiating cryosurgery of primate liver. Ann Surg 1971; 174:309–318.

PHOTODYNAMIC THERAPY OF SOLID TUMORS

THOMAS J. DOUGHERTY, Ph.D.

Photodynamic therapy (PDT) utilizes a photosensitizing drug (hematoporphyrin derivative–Hpd) or its purified form, dihematoporphyrin ether (DHE), and activating visible light (usually red, near 630 nm) to treat a variety of localized solid tumors in man and animals. The therapy is based on a combination of properties of the photosensitizer; it is relatively nontoxic (except for a temporary, generalized photosensitivity), is photochemically active, can be activated in situ by relatively penetrating visible light (i.e., red), and perhaps most unique of all, it is retained in nearly all malignant and some premalignant lesions to a higher degree and longer than in many of the surrounding normal tissues (exceptions are liver, kidney, spleen).

Results of the first clinical trials were reported by Dougherty and colleagues in 1978[1] and 1979.[2] Since that time PDT has been applied in a wide range of tumors including those of the lung,[3–5] esophagus,[6] head and neck,[7] bladder,[8] skin,[9] eye,[10] and brain.[11] Duration of response has exceeded 4 years to date in some patients. Areas demonstrating special efficacy are in the treatment of lung cancer (both carcinoma in situ and frank carcinoma), metastatic breast cancer (soft tissue), and bladder cancer. PDT probably will have its major import in treating primary and early-stage cancers, although debulking of even rather large tumors has been accomplished by this method when other

treatments have failed. The primary limitations are depth of effect, 5 to 15 mm unless repeated interstitial techniques are used, and the temporary induced porphyria resulting from retention of the current drugs in the skin. This requires patients to remain out of bright light (especially sunlight) for 20 to 30 days. In a few cases patients have reported remaining photosensitive for up to 80 days.

Since the attractiveness of PDT is the ability to selectively destroy tumors with little deleterious effects on normal tissues, many investigators have attempted to demonstrate selective uptake or retention of Hpd or DHE in malignant cells in culture. Most studies have been negative in this regard, i.e., in most cases the nonmalignant control cells (more or less normal in culture) have taken up and retained the drug in the same manner as the malignant cells.[12] However, there are a few reports indicating selectivity for transformed cells in culture, e.g., a thyroid cell line and its transformed counterpart,[13] but it is more likely that the selectivity in vivo is based on tissue properties of tumor rather than the cells per se. Animal studies indicate uptake and retention in reticuloendothelial cells in general including macrophages, mast cells, and live Kupfer cells.[14] Therefore, tissues such as liver, kidney, and spleen, which contain a high proportion of such cells, retain large amounts of the drug (although at nontoxic levels). Retention in the skin is probably also due to the large number of macrophages present in skin. In experimental tumors, the Hpd and DHE are found to be concentrated in the vascular stroma and probably in macrophages and mast cells. However, a measurable level of the drug is also found in and around the tumor cells themselves long after normal tissue cells and serum have cleared the drug.[14] For example, it has been reported that 60 hours after administration of Hpd to rabbits with induced transitional cell carcinoma of the bladder, the relative fluorescence is >15:1 in tumor versus normal urothelium.[15] In patients with bladder tumors or dysplastic tissue of the bladder, a similar high selectivity has been found by Benson.[8] It is likely that at least a contributing factor to tumor retention is the leaky neovasculature of tumors and carcinomas in situ, which allows influx of large molecules (i.e., serum proteins) that have difficulty in leaving because of a nonexistent or nonfunctioning lymphatic system. The active component of Hpd appears to be an ether formed by combining two molecules of hematoporphyrin. This material has a very strong tendency to self-associate or polymerize to large molecules which remain associated even in serum. Thus it is possible that these aggregates or polymers leak into the tumor interstitial fluid along with the other serum components and become trapped there for long periods of time. It is known that these aggregates bind strongly to cell surfaces, undergoing slow disaggregation and binding to cellular components, primarily membrane components, the exact nature of which is unknown. This disaggregation and cellular binding are probably necessary prerequisites for the light-induced tumor destruction. Other porphyrins, equally effective photochemically in vitro, which circulate as small molecules bound to serum proteins, are ineffective for PDT since they do not remain localized in the tumor after serum clearance, a necessary requirement for selective treatment.

An early effect of photoactivating the drug in situ is apparent in the vasculature of the tumors; red cells coagulate, blood flow ceases, and ultimately the vessels rupture. In experimental systems it has been observed that within a few hours the tumor cells themselves die with complete eradication of the tumor in many cases. This can be done without excessive damage to normal tissue exposed to the same light dose. The exact mechanism whereby the tumor vasculature is so completely destroyed is not known, but it may be that the tumor endothelium itself retains the porphyrin at relatively high levels for an extended time after serum clearance with consequent destruction by the light.

In the early clinical trials, all patients were considered to be failures on all conventional therapies, i.e., surgery, chemotherapy, and radiation therapy. Most of these patients had cutaneous and subcutaneous tumors, usually metastatic breast cancer. Also in the early stages of development, broad-spectrum light sources were used, whereas currently most investigators use an argon pumped dye laser producing 630 nm light, the optimun wavelength for in vivo activation of Hpd and DHE. Nonetheless, the early results were sufficiently positive to continue and expand the study. Follow-up in this group is up to 4 years without recurrence. In some cases, recurrence and/or new disease following PDT has been treated a second and third time by PDT over a period of 1 to 2 years. The majority of these patients had received tolerance doses of ionizing radiation in addition to other therapies. It has been found that PDT can be effectively applied over a radiation field without causing additional normal tissue damage; however, if the skin is severely compromised from past treatment and/or disease, skin breakdown may occur. In spite of this, healing generally occurs normally although frequently very slowly. In order to cause minimal damage to normal skin, the proper selection of drug dose and light dose are important as well as the time interval between injection and light treatment.

Patients who have large ulcerating lesions over a wide area rarely benefit from PDT because the trauma and pain of causing necrosis of a large amount of tumor in a short period is excessive. Provided these larger lesions are confined to a small area, they also can be treated by interstitial methods. For patients to receive maximum benefit from PDT they should be treated at an early stage of occurrence or recurrence before the disease has gotten out of control. Furthermore, since PDT does not compromise subsequent chemotherapy or radiation therapy, it can be used earlier in the overall management of the patient's disease when maximum benefit is to be expected.

Hayata and colleagues at the Tokyo Medical College were the first to apply PDT for treatment of lung tumors.[3] Using the 630 nm light directed through the bronchoscope by means of the quartz fibers already described, they have treated carcinoma-in-situ, early-stage lung tumors, and more advanced, recurrent cases. Their first patient remained alive, free of disease, more than 3 years post-treatment. This patient had an early-stage squamous cell carcinoma of the bronchus and refused surgery. Currently, several centers are treating lung cancer by PDT. To date more than 200 patients in a variety of stages of lung cancer have been treated. Most cases have been recurrent advanced-stage cancers of the bronchus and trachea. Cortese at the Mayo Clinic is currently confining this method to treatment of early-stage and CIS tumors,[4] whereas the other groups treat cases even when complete obstruction has occurred. In this latter group, it is important to select patients carefully. Those with severely impaired respiratory function can be put at considerable risk following PDT owing to the resulting edema and heavy secretions that may occur. However, most investigators suggest a "clean-up" bronchoscopy 1 to 4 days after PDT to remove secretions and necrotic tumor debris (necrosis of tumors occurs almost immediately). Balchum and Doiron at USC have treated the largest number of lung cancer patients in the United States by PDT and have devised criteria for patient selection and treatment that are producing excellent results.[5] They are careful to select patients whose main current problem is the endobronchial tumor. They use light delivery fibers with specially designed diffusers to provide peripheral illumination over 5 to 15 mm, delivering approximately 400 mW for each 10-mm length of fiber. Treatment time is 8 to 10 minutes. If at all possible, the fiber is placed directly into the tumor. In a group of 35 patients treated this way, 33 have had complete opening of the airways for follow-up ranging to more than one year. Fifteen of the patients were able to resume a normal work schedule. None of these patients experienced the severe edema and exudate problems seen in the earlier cases, which were treated more aggressively and tended to be in respiratory difficulty prior to PDT.

One of the most promising applications of PDT is in the treatment of localized and diffuse bladder cancer. This type of cancer tends to involve wide areas of the bladder while remaining superficial or simply in the dysplastic stage. Thus patients who present initially with a solitary bladder tumor are likely to develop disease involving the entire bladder, frequently necessitating a radical cystectomy. Other methods for controlling this tumor include instillation of drugs and radiation therapy, which have limited success. Benson at the Mayo Clinic has demonstrated highly selective uptake of Hpd in carcinoma-in-situ and dysplastic tissue of the bladder.[8] This has been confirmed by groups in Japan and Germany as well. This has been followed by PDT treatments for both CIS and transitional cell carcinoma. Although the groups at the Mayo Clinic (Benson[8]) and in Japan (Hisazumi,[16] Ohi[17]) have treated local tumors in the bladder, the patients in other studies were treated by whole-bladder illumination for widespread tumor, CIS, and dysplasia. These patients were treated by using a light-delivering fiber with a bulb-type arrangement to provide isotropic illumination to the whole bladder through the cystoscope. Patients frequently experience some pain, hematuria, and difficulty in urination as well as discharge of necrotic debris within a few days of treatment. These symptoms subside over a few days. With complete responses ranging up to 2 years for the Japanese group treated for transitional cell carcinoma and the early but encouraging results for CIS lesions, PDT may become the treatment of choice for certain bladder cancer patients and may prevent or at least delay the trauma of a cystectomy.

Other cancers, most less advanced than those already cited, for which PDT is being tested clinically are esophageal cancers (several instances of relief of obstruction with palliation have been reported), gynecologic tumors, tumors of the eye (choroidal melanoma, retinoblastoma), and head and neck tumors. PDT has also been used as an adjuvant to surgery for recurrent tumors or those likely to recur locally (e.g., retroperitoneal sarcomas, glioblastomas). The application of PDT to early esophageal cancer is being carried out in China. Reviews of these studies and other aspects of PDT are available.[18-21]

CONCLUSION

PDT is found to be especially useful in the treatment of early stage disease because of its relative selectivity, its localized effect, and its compatability with most other forms of cancer therapy. It has also been found to be useful as palliative therapy in certain advanced cancers of the bronchus, esophagus, and skin metastasis. Most types of tumor respond to PDT, the overall response rate being over 70 percent. Among early-stage cancers, the response rate is over 80 percent. Tumors that do not respond are generally those that are poorly vascularized and very slow-growing (e.g., certain liposarcomas and chondrosarcomas). Since most tumors take up the photosensitizing drug, most will respond to treatment provided a sufficient light dose is delivered. The ease of doing so depends on size, site, and, to some extent, geometry. With fiberoptic endoscopes and special ends on the light delivery fibers, these limitations are rapidly being overcome. Because of the early stage of development, it is difficult to make a direct comparison with other therapies except to point out the high degree of response to most malignant tumors. PDT undoubtedly will be used where appropriate in the overall management of the patient's disease since it is compatible with the other modalities. For patients who have run out of viable options, PDT may offer the possibility of treatment with palliation. For other patients for whom current treatments are inadequate, PDT may be the treatment of choice, as in widespread CIS of the bladder or early-stage, nonoperable lung cancer.

REFERENCES

1. Dougherty TJ, Kaufman JE, Goldfarb A et al. Photoradiation therapy for the treatment of malignant tumors. Can Res. 1978; 38:2628–2635.
2. Dougherty TJ, Lawrence G, Kaufman J et al. Photoradiation in the treatment of recurrent breast carcinoma. J Natl Cancer Inst 1979; 62:231–237.
3. Hayata Y, Kato H, Konaka C et al. Hematoporphyrin derivative and laser photoradiation in the treatment of lung cancer. Chest 1982; 81:269–277.
4. Cortese DA, Kinsey JH. Hematoporphyrin derivative phototherapy in the treatment of bronchogenic carcinoma. Chest 1984; 86:8–13.
5. Balchum OJ, Doiron DR, Huth GC. Photoradiation therapy of endobronchial lung cancers employing the photodynamic action of hematoporphyrin derivative. Lasers Surg Med 1984; 4:13–20.
6. Aida M, Hirashima T. Cancer of the esophagus. In: Hayata Y, Dougherty TJ, eds. Lasers and Hematoporphyrin Derivative in Cancer. Tokyo and New York: Igaku-Shoin, 1983:57.
7. Wile AG, Coffey J, Nahabedian MY et al. Laser photoradiation of cancer: An update of the experience at the University of California, Irvine. Lasers Surg Med 1984; 4:5–12.
8. Benson RC Jr, Kinsey JH, Cortese DA et al. Treatment of transitional cell carcinoma of the bladder with hematoporphyrin derivative phototherapy. J Urol 1984; 130:1090–1095.
9. Dougherty TJ. Photoradiation therapy for cutaneous and subcutaneous malignancies. J Invest Derm 1981; 77:122–124.
10. Bruce RA Jr. Photoradiation for choroidal malignant melanoma. In: Andreoni A, Cubeddu R, eds. Porphyrins in Tumor Phototherapy. New York: Plenum, 1984:455.
11. Laws ER, Cortese DA, Kinsey JH et al. Photoradiation therapy in the treatment of malignant brain tumors. A phase I (feasibility) study. Neurosurgery 1981; 9:672–678.
12. Henderson BW, Dougherty TJ. Studies on the mechanism of tumor destruction by photoradiation therapy (PRT). In: Doiron DR, Gomer CJ, eds. Porphyrin Localization and Treatment of Tumors. New York: AR Liss, 1984: in press.
13. Andreoni A, Cubeddu R, De Silvestri S et al. Effects of laser

irradiation on hematoporphyrin-treated normal and transformed thyroid cells in culture. Can Res 1983; 43:2076–2080.

14. Bugelski PJ, Porter CW, Dougherty TJ. Autoradiographic distribution of hematoporphyrin derivative in normal and tumor tissue of the mouse. Can Res 1981; 41:4606–4612.

15. Jocham D, Staehler G, Chaussy CH et al. Laserbehandlung von blasentumoren nach photosensibilisierung mit hematoporphyrin-derivat. Urolge A 1981; 20:340.

16. Hisazumi H, Misaki T, Miyoshi N. Photodynamic therapy of bladder tumors. In: Hayata Y, Dougherty TJ, eds. Lasers and Hematoporphyrin Derivative in Cancer. Tokyo and New York: Igaku-Shoin, 1983:85.

17. Ohi T, Tsuchiya A. Superficial bladder tumors. In: Hayata Y, Dougherty TJ, eds. Lasers and Hematoporphyrin Derivative in Cancer. Tokyo and New York: Igaku-Shoin, 1983:79.

18. Dougherty TJ, Weishaupt KR, Boyle DG. Photodynamic therapy and cancer. In: DeVita VT et al, eds. Principles and Practice of Oncology. (2nd ed), Philadelphia: JB Lippincott, 1985: in press.

19. Hayata Y, Dougherty TJ, eds. Lasers and Hematoporphyrin Derivative in Cancer. Tokyo and New York: Igaku-Shoin, 1983.

20. Doiron DR, Gomer CJ, eds. Porphyrin localization and treatment of tumors. New York: AR Liss, 1984: in press.

21. Andreoni A, Cubeddu R, eds. Porphyrins in Tumor Phototherapy. New York: Plenum, 1984.

SECTION NINE / IMMUNOLOGY AND IMMUNOTHERAPY

39. Immunology and Immunotherapy

INTRODUCTION

PAUL B. CHRETIEN, M.D.

Thus far, there have been a number of attempts to control head and neck squamous carcinomas (HNSCa) by manipulation of immunologic responses.[1-15] All of these trials were pilot studies, since they consisted of small populations with great heterogeneity in tumor sites, stages, and treatments. Almost all utilized agents that subsequently have been found to have negligible clinical activity in trials with other malignant tumors, and although there was evidence for tumor control in several groups of patients, none of the trials yielded results that were sufficiently promising to provoke additional similar investigations.

Despite these discouraging initial results with immunotherapy of HNSCa, the rationale for such trials is relatively ideal, in that patients with HNSCa display far greater frequencies of abnormal levels of serum and cellular factors that influence systemic immune responses than do patients with other histologic types of malignant diseases.[16,17] Most of these abnormalities appear to be due to the effects of factors associated with the development of HNSCa, i.e., consumption of tobacco (see chapter by Weiss) and exposure to the herpes simplex virus (HSV).[18-22] These abnormalities are invaluable for their usefulness in providing rationale for development of new approaches to the control of HNSCa. For example:

1. Serial monitoring of the quantitative levels of the abnormalities may provide a means of assessing the early effect of immune therapy regimens, especially if the immediate goal of the therapy is correction of immune deficits. In view of the correlations between the levels of immune reactivities and clinical course in head and neck cancer,[16,17] monitoring of the levels may give insight into the effectiveness of the primary therapies and provide a basis for the early institution of adjunctive immunotherapies.

2. The immune abnormalities support the investigation of the effects of immune modulating or restorative agents that recently have been shown to increase tumor control in other solid malignant tumors.

It is relevant that sufficient documentation has now accumulated concerning the immune deficits associated with HNSCa, as well as the deficits that result from the primary therapies, to allow the design of regimens that maximize the potential gain from the newer immunotherapy agents.

3. In view of the high incidences of second primary cancers in patients previously treated for HNSCa, —up to 30 percent in several surveys,[23-26] the potential for lowering these incidences by long-term administration of immune restorative agents should be investigated. In these studies, correlations would be sought between the freedom from new primary cancers and the quantitative restoration of immune responses achieved by the immunotherapy.

4. The cross-reactivity, and possible similarity in identity, between the tumor-associated antigens (TAA) of HNSCa and HSV-induced antigens[18-22], raises the speculation that these TAA could be generated in large quantities from HSV infected cultures, as compared with the current technique of isolation of the small quantities of TAA available from individual tumors obtained by surgical excision. Since the TAA of HSV origin potentially offer a means of specific immunotherapy for HNSCa, investigations are needed now to confirm and further define the relationships between these antigens. Production of HSV culture-generated TAA would allow extension of the current intensive investigations of local delivery in high concentrations of cytotoxic drugs to the malignant cells by coupling of the drugs to anti-TAA antibodies.

5. The unique abnormal responses to HSV in smokers and in patients with HNSCa provide rationale for vaccination against HSV not only for prevention of the acute infectious disease but also against HNSCa and other tumors potentially induced by HSV, e.g., squamous carcinoma of the cervix (SCaCx).

6. The immune abnormalities induced by chronic tobacco consumption which precede the primary HNSCa could be used to reduce the incidence of HNSCa, since these abnormalities offer a mechanism for the precipitation of HNSCa by tobacco products and provide a scientific rationale for the cessation of tobacco consumption—both in smokers and in patients previously treated for HNSCa—and for interdiction of sales promotion of tobacco and government subsidies for producers of tobacco. The data on the immune abnormalities induced by tobacco also may further serve as a guide for the investigation of the

mechanisms of carcinogenesis by other suspect environmental agents.

Currently, several pilot vaccination trials against primary HSV infection in young subjects are in progress. If successful, the incidence of HNSCa in the vaccinated subjects during the adult decades of high risk will provide the conclusive evidence of the etiologic role of HSV in the genesis of HNSCa and offer the ideal approach for the elimination of the malignant tumor.

In the following chapters, the authors present the results of recent studies of immunologic responses that could give rise to these new clinical approaches to the control of HNSCa. Weiss surveys the immune abnormalities precipitated by cigarette smoking, with emphasis on increases in immune depressive humoral factors that may predispose to neoplastic transformation by HSV. Veltri presents the recently detected increases in circulating immune complexes containing immunoglobulin A (IgA) in patients with HNSCa. These findings give importance to the elevations of anti-HSV-specific IgA previously detected in these patients[27,28] and give importance also to the determination of the specificity for HSV of the IgA in the complexes. Ibrahim demonstrates cross-reactive TAA in the sera and tumors of patients with HNSCa and with SCaCx. The data parallel earlier reports of HSV-induced nonvirion antigens that reacted similarly with antibodies in the sera of the patients with HNSCa and ScaCx.[18-11]. Ibrahim's data thus are important extensions of this evidence for a common origin of squamous carcinomas of the head and neck and cervix, which is further supported by the reports of increased incidences of SCaCx in women who consume tobacco. The mechanism whereby tobacco products may exert effects localized to the cervix is provided by the recent demonstration of nicotine in the cervical mucus of cigarette smokers that appears to be secreted in high concentrations by the cervical mucus glands.[29] Aurelian provides important clinical applications for the immunologic properties of HSV origin that are shared by HNSCa and SCaCx. Serum levels of antibodies to transformation-related HSV proteins isolated by the author correlated with extent of tumor in patients with cervical neoplasia, suggesting the potential of antibodies to HSV transforming sequence in HNSCa as adjuncts in monitoring course of disease and as carriers of chemotherapeutic agents. Pearson supports the optimism expressed for HSV vaccinations against HNSCa with his description of the prevention of infections by the Epstein-Barr virus (EBV) in nonhuman primates by vaccination with EBV antigens. The effectiveness of vaccination against EBV in preventing infections in humans is currently under investigation.

These comments on the following chapters illustrate that each author presents unique data on immunologic abnormalities in HNSCa that are critically important for the development of new approaches to control of the malignant tumors. Unfortunately, only a few similar investigations have been conducted by others. The dirth of activity in this area of clinical research is a significant impediment since a major commitment of resources, both manpower and money, will be needed to initiate and continue the trials needed to develop these new approaches. It is hoped that the advanced research achieved by the authors of the following chapters, combined with their descriptions of the potential clinical relevance of their data, will stimulate others to initiate or contribute to the implementation of their findings in appropriate clinical investigations.

REFERENCES

1. Cunningham TJ, Antemann R, Paonessa D, Sponzo RW, Steiner D. Adjuvant immuno and/or chemotherapy with neuraminidase-treated autogenous tumor vaccine and bacillus Calmette-Guerin for head and neck cancers. Ann NY Acad Sci 1976; 277:339.
2. Richman SP, Livingston RB, Gutterman JU, Suen JY, Hersh EM. Chemotherapy versus chemo-immunotherapy of head and neck cancer: Report of a randomized study. Cancer Treat Rep 1976; 60:535.
3. Olkowski Z, McLaren J, Skeen M. Effects of combined immunotherapy with levamisole and bacillus Calmette-Guerin on immunocompetence of patients with squamous cell carcinoma of the cervix, head and neck and lung undergoing radiation therapy. Cancer Treat Rep 1978; 62:1651.
4. Amiel JL, Sancho-Garnier H, Vandenbrouck C, Eschwege F, Droz JP, Schwaab G, Wibault P, Stromboni M, Rey A. First results of a randomized trial on immunotherapy of head and neck tumors. Recent Results Cancer Res 1979; 68:318.
5. Beuchler M, Mukherji B, Chasin W, Nathanson L. High dose methotrexate with and without BCG therapy in advanced head and neck malignancy. Cancer 1979; 43:1095.
6. Papac R, Minor DR, Rudnick S, Solomon LR, Capizzi RL. Controlled trial of methotrexate and bacillus Calmette-Guerin therapy for advanced head and neck cancer. Cancer Res 1978; 38:3150.
7. Olivari AJ, Glait HM, Guardo A, Califano L, Pradier R. Levamisole in squamous cell carcinoma of the head and neck. Cancer Treat Rep 1979; 63:983.
8. Wanebo HJ, Hilal EY, Strong EW, Pinsky CM, Mike V, Oettgen HF. Adjuvant trial of levamisole in patients with squamous cancer of the head and neck: A preliminary report. Recent Results Cancer Res 1979; 68:324.
9. Szpirglas H, Chastang C, Bertrand JC. Adjuvant treatment of tongue and floor of the mouth cancers. Recent Results Cancer Res 1979; 68:309.
10. Bier J, Rapp HJ, Borsos T, Zbar B, Kleinschuster S, Wanger H, Rollinghoff M. Randomized clinical study on intratumoral BCG-cell wall preparation (CWP) therapy in patients with squamous cell carcinoma in the head and neck region. Cancer Immunol Immunother 1981; 12:71.
11. Cheng VS, Suit HD, Wang CC, Raker J, Kaufman S, Rothman K, Walker A, McNulty P. Clinical trial of Corynebacterium parvum (intra-lymph node and intravenous) and radiation therapy in the treatment of head and neck carcinoma. Cancer 1982; 49:239.
12. Vogl SE, Schoenfeld DA, Kaplan BH, Lerner HJ, Horton J, Creech RH, Barnes LE. Methotrexate alone or with regional subcutaneous Corynebacterium parvum in the treatment of recurrent and metastatic squamous cancer of the head and neck. Cancer 1982; 50:2295.
13. Hirsch B, Johnson JT, Rabin BS, Thearle PB. Immunostimulation of patients with head and neck cancer. In vitro and preliminary clinical experiences. Arch Otolaryngol 1983; 109:298.
14. Taylor SG, Sisson GA, Bytell DE, Raynor WJ Jr. A randomized trial of adjuvant BCG immunotherapy in head and neck cancer. Arch Otolaryngol 1983; 109:544.

15. Wara WM, Neely MH, Ammann AJ, Wara DW. Biologic modification of immunologic parameters in head and neck cancer patients with thymosin fraction V. Goldstein AL, Chirigos MA, eds. In: Progress in Cancer Research and Therapy, Vol 20: Lymphokines and Thymic Hormones. New York: Raven Press, 1981:257.

16. Browder JP, Chretien PB. Immune reactivity in head and neck squamous carcinoma and relevance to the design of immunotherapy trials. Semin Oncol 1977; 4:431.

17. Johns ME. Immunological considerations in head and neck cancer. Batsakis JG, ed. In: Tumors of the Head and Neck. Baltimore: Williams and Wilkins, 1979:501.

18. Hollinshead AC, Lee O, Chretien PB, Tarpley JL, Rawls WE, Adam E. Antibodies to herpesvirus nonvirion antigens in squamous carcinomas. Science 1973; 182:713.

19. Silverman NA, Alexander JC Jr, Hollinshead AC, Chretien PB. Correlation of tumor burden with in vitro lymphocyte reactivity and antibodies to herpesvirus tumor-associated antigens in head and neck squamous carcinoma. Cancer 1976; 37:135.

20. Hollinshead AC, Chretien PB, Lee OB, Tarpley JL, Kerney SE, Silverman NA, Alexander JC Jr. In vivo and in vitro measurements of the relationship of human squamous carcinomas to herpes simplex virus tumor-associated antigens. Cancer Res 1976; 36:821.

21. Notter MF, Docherty JJ. Reaction of antigens isolated from herpes simples virus-transformed cells with sera of squamous cell carcinoma patients. Cancer 1976; 36:4394.

22. Notter MF, Docherty JJ. Comparative diagnostic aspects of herpes simplex tumor-associated antigens. J Natl Cancer Inst 1976; 57:483.

23. Wagenfeld DJH, Harwood AR, Bryce DP, et al. Second primary respiratory tract malignancies in glottic carcinoma. Cancer 1980; 46:1883.

24. Wagenfeld DJH, Harwood AR, Bryce DP, et al. Second primary respiratory tract malignant neoplasms in supraglottic carcinoma. Arch Otolaryngol 1981; 107:135.

25. Silverman S, Giorsky M, Greenspan D. Tobacco usage in patients with head and neck carcinomas: A follow up study on habit changes and second primary oral/oropharyngeal cancers. JAMA 1983; 106:33.

26. Aygun C, Salazar OM, Castro-Vita H, et al. Secondary tumors in head and neck cancer patients. Proceedings of the International Conference on Head and Neck Cancer, Baltimore, July, 1984.

27. Smith HG, Horowitz N, Silverman NA, Henson DE, Chretien PB. Humoral immunity to herpes simplex viral-induced antigens in smokers. Cancer 1976; 38:1155.

28. Smith HG, Chretien PB, Henson DE, Silverman NA, Alexander JC Jr. Viral-specific humoral immunity to herpes simplex-induced antigens in patients with squamous carcinoma of the head and neck. Am J Surg 1976; 132:541.

29. Sasson IM, Haley NJ, Hoffmann D, Wynder EL, Hellberg D, Nilsson S. Cigarette smoking and neoplasia of the uterine cervix: Smoke constituents in cervical mucus. N Engl J Med 1985; 312:315.

INTERRELATIONSHIP OF IMMUNE RESPONSE, CIRCULATING PROTEINS, AND ETIOLOGIC FACTORS FOR HEAD AND NECK CANCER

JOSEPH F. WEISS, Ph.D.
PAUL B. CHRETIEN, M.D.

Tobacco usage is a clear risk factor for head and neck squamous tumors, although it does not appear to be a major etiologic factor for nasopharyngeal cancer (NPC).[1] Apart from the potential direct effects on initiation or promotion of cancer by substances in tobacco, there is the possibility that tobacco smoke or extracts have immunologic effects that may contribute to the development of head and neck cancer.[2] A number of studies have clearly shown immunologic abnormalities in patients with head and neck tumors, which often persist even after apparent cure, and there may be further derangements due to treatment such as radiation therapy.[3] Immunologic responses and interrelationships may play a somewhat different role in the etiology of head and neck cancer compared with tumors at other sites because of, for example, the role of viruses (the association of Epstein-Barr virus (EBV) with NPC and herpes virus type 1 with head and neck squamous tumors) and the importance of the mucosal immune system. Immune responses may also be affected by risk factors other than tobacco products: increased alcohol consumption with the consequent relative nutritional deficiencies, age, occupation, and genetic factors.[1] This review will concentrate on the immunologic effects of cigarette smoking. Data from our laboratory will emphasize changes in smokers of circulating proteins other than immunoglobulins. The importance of the evaluation of systemic immunity, compared to cellular immune parameters only, is based on increasing evidence that systemic immunity is the result of the interaction of circulating immune-reactive white blood cells and multiple serum factors.[4]

IMMUNOLOGIC RESPONSES IN SMOKERS

Some reported alterations in immunologic factors or responses that contribute to systemic immunity in smokers are shown in Table 1. Because of space limitations, these are not individually referenced, but the majority of the reported alterations are discussed in References 2 and 5 through 8. There have been conflicting reports on some of these observations, and they and the speculations made in this paper are open to debate and continued investigation. Alterations have been reported in humoral immune responses in patients with head and neck cancer and in smokers. One of the most interesting observations was an elevation of serum IgA specific for herpes virus among smokers as well as in patients with head and neck squamous tumor.[6] A potential role in the development of head and neck squamous tumor could be proposed in that serum anti-herpes IgA antibodies that were found to be elevated in cigarette smokers could function as

TABLE 1 Reported Alterations in Systemic Immunity in Smokers Compared to Nonsmokers

Humoral Immunity
  ↓ Antibody formation but ↑ antibodies to cigarette smoke components; ↑ autoantibodies
  ↓ IgG, IgM; ↑ IgD, IgE (? ↓ in heavy smokers)
  ↑ Serum IgA specific to herpes virus type 1

Cell-Medicated Immunity
  ↓ Delayed-type hypersensitivity
  ↑ Leukocytes, lymphocytes, pulmonary alveolar macrophages (but ↓ some functional abilities)
  ↑ T-cells and lymphocyte reactivity to PHA in younger smokers, but ↓ lymphocyte reactivity in older smokers
  ↓ NK cell activity
  ↑ Helper/suppressor ratio (but may be ↓ in heavy smokers)

Systemic Factors
  ↑ Carcinoembryonic antigen (or related antigen)
  ↑ C-reactive protein, fibrinogen, haptoglobin; ? ↓ α_2HS-glycoprotein
  ↑ α_1-Antitrypsin and ceruloplasmin, but ↓ functional capacity
  ↑ Arachidonic acid metabolites from platelets

blocking antibodies, preventing detection of single transformed cells that would lead to proliferation of these cells and gross carcinoma. An immunosuppressed state could also result owing to immune complex formation from antibodies to smoke products.

Among the circulating noncellular factors altered are the acute-phase proteins (to be discussed). Prostaglandins and other arachidonic acid metabolites are known to have immunomodulatory properties. Head and neck tumors are among the tumors producing increased quantities of prostaglandins. Increased production of these substances in smokers could be due, in part, to increased platelet stimulation. Carcinoembryonic antigen (or related antigens) is increased in smokers and suggests that antigenic derepression may be occurring. Carcinoembryonic antigen (CEA) is also believed to be an immunosuppressive factor. The elevation in CEA in smokers and in the aged is only one of a number of changes observed in immune responses in humans and experimental animals exposed for long periods to polluted atmospheres, which in many respects resemble changes seen with aging, and may therefore represent an acceleration of what is essentially a ''normal'' process.[2]

The chronic overstimulation due to smoking may result in accelerated aging of the thymus-dependent immune processes. From consideration of animal data and limited human studies, continued exposure to cigarette smoke would appear to produce a biphasic pattern of change in T-cell-dependent immunologic functions, with moderate exposure enhancing, and prolonged exposure ultimately depressing reactivity.[2] One aspect of this appears to be increased lymphocyte reactivity to phytohemagglutinin (PHA) in young smokers, but a depressed reactivity in older smokers, suggesting that chronic stimulation by tobacco products leads to eventual exhaustion of immunologic reactivity.[9] In such a setting, agents that induce head and neck cancer, which normally would be controlled, would then be more effective in inducing cellular transformation and neoplasia. The role of suppressor cells in these processes needs to be clarified.

Besides extent of smoking, the reversal of changes in immune function associated with smoking is an important aspect to be considered. Lymphocyte counts decreased, natural killer cell activity increased, and serum IgG and IgM levels increased in subjects who ceased smoking.[7] In another study, T-cell subsets were reversed after cessation of smoking.[8] Future studies should carefully consider all the immunologic changes shown in relation to age, extent of smoking, immediate effects of smoking, and changes due to cessation of smoking.

IMMUNE-REACTIVE PROTEINS IN CANCER PATIENTS

Levels of certain naturally occurring serum proteins, other than immunoglobulins, are altered in cancer patients with solid malignant tumors, in relation to tumor burden or stage.[4] In general, the serum proteins increased to the greatest extent are the major acute-phase proteins: α_1-acid glycoprotein (AGP), α_1-antitrypsin or α_1-protease inhibitor (ATr), haptoglobin (Hp), and ceruloplasmin (Cer). Other proteins sometimes referred to as negative acute-phase proteins are often depressed in cancer patients: α_2HS-glycoprotein (HS), albumin (Alb), and prealbumin (PA). Levels of some of these proteins also related to immune status in cancer patients.[4] In patients with impaired delayed-type hypersensitivity (DTH) to dinitrochlorobenzene, Hp and AGP were higher and HS and PA were lower than in cancer patients with normal DTH. Levels of Hp and AGP correlated inversely with lymphocyte reactivity, and levels of HS correlated directly with lymphocyte reactivity. The immunologic importance of these proteins suggested by these correlations is supported by other studies showing an immunoregulatory role for serum glycoproteins. In general, the positive acute-phase proteins can be thought of as immunosuppressive[4,10,11] (to be discussed). The negative acute-phase proteins, PA and HS, have immunorestorative properties.[4] These immune-reactive proteins may relate to tumor histology, but definite changes are usually seen in patients with tumors in which

TABLE 2 Median Serum Protein Levels in Normal Subjects and in Patients with Head and Neck Squamous Carcinoma

	Nonsmokers (n = 140)	Smokers (n = 132)	Patients NED ≥ 5 years (n = 51)	Nontreated Patients (n = 90)	Patients with Recurrent Tumors (n = 11)
α_1–Acid glycoprotein (mg/dl)	74	74	88	114	142
α_1–Antitrypsin (mg/dl)	249	292	252	285	353
Haptoglobin (mg/dl)	165	182	218	327	378
α_2HS–glycoprotein (mg/dl)	68	67	66	60	57
Prealbumin (mg/dl)	29	30	31	22	26
Albumin (g/dl)	4.8	4.8	4.5	4.4	4.0

smoking is an etiologic factor. Table 2 compares the median serum protein levels in patients with head and neck squamous tumors and in smoking and nonsmoking controls.[5,12] The data indicate that in the total group of nontreated patients, ATr did not differ from the level in smokers, which was significantly higher than that in nonsmokers. When patients were divided according to tumor stage (I through IV, AJC-1977), however, serum levels of ATr and AGP increased progressively with increasing tumor stage, and serum HS decreased progressively.[12] Studies of proteins during therapy suggested that HS levels may be as useful as T-cells for monitoring immune reactivity. In patients with NPC,[13] elevated antibody titers to EBV-associated antigens were related to tumor presence, but not significantly to clinical tumor stage. Serum levels of immune-reactive proteins, particularly Hp, were directly related to clinical tumor stage. Furthermore, serum Hp levels correlated directly with anti-Epstein-Barr nuclear antigen antibody titers and serum levels of IgA.

IMMUNE-REACTIVE PROTEINS IN SMOKERS

Because serum protein patterns appeared to be of value in assessing cancer patient status and as indicators of host systemic immunity, a more detailed analysis of the effects of smoking and age on levels of serum proteins altered in patients with head and neck cancer was necessary.[5] Serum protein levels in nonsmokers and smokers shown in Table 2 were further analyzed according to age and extent of smoking. Table 3 summarizes the correlations and levels of significance among age, pack-years, and serum proteins. Because of the correlation of serum proteins with age and, to a lesser extent, with sex, a final comparison was made of the protein levels in smokers and nonsmokers after matching the persons in both groups by sex and age (±2 yrs). The number of individuals in each group was reduced to 101 owing to elimination of cases that could not be matched. Figure 1 shows the regression of positive acute-phase protein levels on age in the matched groups. There is a unique association of ATr levels with smoking habit, independent of age or smoking extent, although there is a suggestion of greater ATr levels in smokers less than 40 years of age in our study and in another study[14] of more than 1000 male subjects. In the latter study, it was found that ATr levels returned rapidly to normal among subjects who stopped smoking. We found a direct correlation of Hp levels with age and pack-years in smokers. Since Hp did not increase with age in nonsmokers, as does AGP, Hp levels are probably increased due to smoking extent.

Evidence that the positive acute-phase proteins (increased due to smoking and/or aging) have im-

TABLE 3 Correlations Among Serum Protein Levels, Age, and Pack-Years

	Nonsmokers (N = 140)								Smokers (N = 132)							
	Age	AGp	Hp	ATr	HS	PA	Alb		Age	AGp	Hp	ATr	HS	PA	Alb	Pack Years
Age		*					*(−)	Age		*	**				**(−)	**
AGp			**	**	●			AGp			**					●
Hp				●				Hp								●
ATr							●(−)	ATr					*			
HS								HS						**		
PA							●	PA								
Alb								Alb								**(−)

● 0.05 < p ≤ 0.10
* 0.01 < p ≤ 0.05
**p < 0.01
Based on Spearman correlation coefficients.
AGp, α_1-acid glycoprotein; HS α_2HS-glycoprotein; Hp; haptoglobin; PA, prealbumin; ATr, α_1-antitrypsin; Alb, albumin.

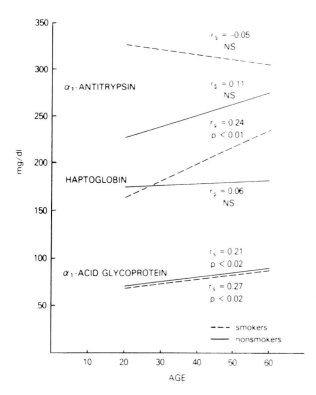

Figure 1 Regression of α_1-antitrypsin, haptoglobin, and α_1-acid glycoprotein levels on age in groups of nonsmokers (n=101) and smokers (n=101) matched for age and sex.

munoregulatory functions is included in studies that show modulation of lymphocyte reactivity in vitro by ATr, AGP, Hp, fibrinogen, Cer, and C-reactive protein.[4,10] Hp, fibrinogen, and AGP inhibited the chemotactic response of monocytes.[10] Combinations of Cer, ATr, and AGP had a much greater inhibitory effect on lymphocyte proliferation than the single proteins alone.[10] This suggests that sera from cancer patients or smokers, and especially patients with head and neck squamous tumor who continue to smoke, may have a pronounced immunosuppressive effect on immune function. Suppression of effector cell function may involve binding of these proteins to surface receptors of lymphocytes and monocytes. As "nonspecific blocking factors", the acute-phase proteins could be involved in the protection of tumors against the host's immunologic attack.[11]

The unique early increase in ATr levels in smokers requires a more detailed discussion of its potential role as an immunosuppressive substance. Although there are a number of antiproteases of importance in serum, ATr is quantitatively the most important. It occurs in large quantities in lung and has been identified in various immune cells: neutrophils, monocytes, alveolar macrophages, and mast cells. ATr has a wide range of activities and acts against a number of enzymes involved in the regulation of cell function and various immunologic and inflammatory responses (leukocyte proteases, elastase, collagenase, trypsin, thrombin, kallikrein).[15] For example, trypsin is able

to directly activate lymphocytes, suggesting that there is an enzyme cleavage step involved in lymphocyte transformation. ATr is localized on the surface of mitogen-transformed T-cells and is not detectable on nonstimulated cells, whereas the addition of ATr to lymphocyte cultures suppresses blastogenesis. Patients with severe ATr deficiency have significantly enhanced lymphocyte responses to PHA.[15] Other clinical studies of patients with mildly deficient phenotypes of ATr indicate that they are likely to have exaggerated immunologic and inflammatory responses due to lymphocyte responses, complement activation, and leukocyte migration.[15]

Smoking results in an inactivation of the antielastase activity of ATr as well as its antitrypsin activity.[16] The decrease in activity of both of these activities is about 20 percent in serum, but it is probably greater in cells and tissues where there is direct contact with cigarette smoke. The inactivation of elastase activity is due to oxidation of the methionyl residue, but inactivation of the antitrypsin activity may occur by a different mechanism. Events leading to increased production of oxygen free radicals by phagocytic cells could also result in ATr inactivation. The liver produces much of the ATr transported to other tissues, and increased synthesis of ATr might occur in response to the local functional deficiency caused by smoking. We propose that immunosuppressive effects could result from the increased levels of total, but functionally altered, ATr in the form of nonspecific effects of ATr at cell surfaces or due to an imbalance of proteolytic enzyme activity /ATr, in immune-reactive cells (Fig. 2). Ceruloplasmin (Cer), the antioxidant acute-phase protein, may provide some extracellular protection from oxidative damage to ATr.[17] Because of the importance of oxidative processes in macrophage and PMN function, Cer has been proposed to have a role in immunomodulation. The effects of smoking on Cer are apparently analogous to the effects on ATr: Cer levels are increased, but its antioxidant capacity appears to be decreased.[17] Since oxidative processes appear to be involved in the deleterious effects of smoking on immune-reactive pro-

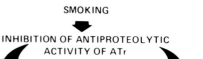

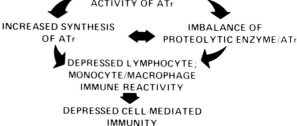

Figure 2 α_1-Antitrypsin (ATr) and immunosuppression.

teins, and probably on some immune cell populations, it is possible that antioxidant vitamins, such as vitamins A and C, can provide some protection against these effects. The modulation of smoking effects by nutritional factors could play a role in the etiology of head and neck cancer.

With respect to treatment of head and neck cancer, the changes in proteins due to smoking and age, already described, should be considered when using protein levels as monitors of treatment efficacy or immune reactivity. The further effects of immunosuppressive treatment regimens, as well as immunotherapeutic measures, on levels of immune-reactive proteins should be evaluated.

SUMMARY

A number of alterations in immunologic factors and responses have been reported to occur as a result of cigarette smoking. These changes include both cell-mediated and humoral immune responses, as well as circulating factors, such as acute-phase proteins, that contribute to host systemic immunity. A number of hypotheses can be offered, based on these alterations, that should stimulate future studies on the interrelationship of the factors constituting the immune status of smokers and provide definitive information on the role of immune factors in the etiology and treatment of head and neck cancer. These include immunosuppression due to increased immune complex formation, depressed cell-mediated responses due to chronic stimulation by tobacco products leading to eventual exhaustion of immunologic reactivity, and immunosuppression due to increased levels of acute-phase proteins. These latter effects of "immune-reactive proteins" shown to be increased due to smoking and aging (haptoglobin, α_1-acid glycoprotein, α_1-antitrypsin, ceruloplasmin) have been emphasized in this review. The deleterious effects of smoking are exemplified by inactivation of α_1-antitrypsin and its increased synthesis, which, it is proposed, results in nonspecific immunosuppressive effects and/or an imbalance of antitrypsin/proteolytic enzyme activity in immune cells.

REFERENCES

1. Decker J, Goldstein JC. Risk factors in head and neck cancer. N Engl J Med 1982; 306:1151–1155.
2. Holt PG, Keast D. Environmentally induced changes in immunological function: Acute and chronic effects of inhalation of tobacco smoke and other atmospheric contaminants in man and experimental animals. Bacter Rev 1977; 41:205–216.
3. Scully C. The immunology of cancer of the head and neck with particular reference to oral cancer. Oral Surg 1982; 53:157–169.
4. Chretien PB, Weiss JF. Clinical applications of acute phase proteins. In: Hadden JW, Chedid L, Dukor P, Spreafico F, Willoughby D (eds). Advances in Immunopharmacology 2. Oxford: Pergamon, 1983: 517–524.
5. Weiss JF, Wolf GT, Edwards BK, Chretien PB. Effects of smoking and age on serum levels of immune-reactive proteins altered in cancer patients. Cancer Detec Preven 1981; 4:211–217.
6. Chretien PB. The effects of smoking on immunocompetence. Laryngoscope 1978; 88:11–13.
7. Hersey P, Prendergast D, Edwards A. Effects of cigarette smoking on the immune system. Follow-up studies in normal subjects after cessation of smoking. Med J Aust 1983; 2:425–429.
8. Miller LG, Goldstein G, Murphy M, Ginns LC. Reversible alterations in immunoregulatory T cells in smoking. Analysis by monoclonal antibodies and flow cytometry. Chest 1982; 5:526–529.
9. Silverman WA, Potvin C, Alexander JC, Chretien PB. In vitro lymphocyte reactivity and T-cell levels in chronic cigarette smokers. Clin Exp Immunol 1975; 22:285–292.
10. Samak R, Edelstein R, Israel L. Immunosuppressive effect of acute-phase reactive proteins in vitro and its relevance to cancer. Cancer Immunol Immunother 1982; 13:38–43.
11. Apffel CA, Peters JH. Tumors and serum glycoproteins. The 'symbodies'. Prog Exp Tumor Res 1969; 12:1–54.
12. Wolf GT, Chretien PB, Elias EG, Makuch RW, Baskies AM, Spiegel HE, Weiss JF. Serum glycoproteins in head and neck squamous carcinoma. Correlations with tumor extent, and T-cell levels during chemotherapy. Am J Surg 1979; 138:489–500.
13. Baskies AM, Chretien PB, Yang CS, Wolf GT, Makuch RW, Tu SM, Hsu MM, Lynn TC, Yang HM, Weiss JF, Spiegel HE. Serum glycoproteins and immunoglobulins in nasopharyngeal carcinoma. Correlations with Epstein-Barr virus associated antibodies and clinical tumor stage. Am J Surg 1979; 138:478–488.
14. Lellouch J, Claude JR, Thevenin M. α_1-Antitrypsine et tabac, une etude de 1296 hommes sains. Clin Chim Acta 1979; 95:337–345.
15. Breit SN, Penny R. The role of α_1 protease inhibitor (α_1 antitrypsin) in the regulation of immunologic and inflammatory reactions. Aust NZ J Med 1980; 10:449–453.
16. Janoff A. Proteases and lung injury. A state-of-the-art mini-review. Chest 1983; 5:54S–58S.
17. Gladston M, Leytska V, Schwartz MS, Magnusson B. Ceruloplasmin. Increased serum concentration and impaired antioxidant activity in cigarette smokers, and ability to prevent suppression of elastase inhibitory capacity of alpha$_1$-proteinase inhibitor. Am Rev Respir Dis 1984; 129:258–263.

IMMUNE REGULATION IN CARCINOMA OF THE HEAD AND NECK

ROBERT W. VELTRI, Ph.D.

A major contribution to our improved knowledge of immunity in cancer and its application to the management of this disease by the clinicians has been derived in part from the passage of the National Cancer Act in 1971. A decade of contract-funded research was committed to seeking improved methods to treat the disease. This program supported research and development of new biochemical and immunologic markers for all types of cancer as well as new sophisticated instrumentation for the diagnosis and treatment of cancer. Some of these developments are presented in two recently published monographs.[1,2]

The leading etiologic factors consistently implicated in head and neck cancer are tobacco and alcohol consumption.[3,4] The products of pyrolysis produced during the burning of tobacco yield numerous chemical irritants and carcinogens. Such substances, when combined with the effects of radiant and thermal heat, serve to initiate as well as promote the process of carcinogenesis. The alcohol consumption factor provides additional promoter activity in this complicated process. Ancillary consideration must be given to the possible cofactorial and/or etiologic role of viruses in the cause of head and neck cancer. A number of studies have linked Epstein-Barr virus (EBV) to nasopharyngeal carcinoma[5,6] and implicated herpes simplex virus (HSV) in the etiology of other types of head and neck cancer.[7,8] A high degree of variability with respect to the incidence and demographic distribution of the various types of head and neck cancer may be attributable in part to nutritional status of the host,[9] the immunologic status of the host, and/or the biologic diversity of the tumor itself in terms of its invasive properties and factors elaborated from the tumor cells which could affect the latter property. We now realize that tumors exhibit numerous properties that exemplify their biologic heterogeneity. Some examples of this diversity include variability with respect to pigment production and metastatic potential as in the B-16 melanoma,[10] in vitro production of carcinoembryonic antigen (CEA) by colon carcinoma cell lines,[11] and in vivo and in vitro expression of ectopically produced hormones and other proteins by lung tumor cells.[12]

This review will direct its attention to immunity in head and neck cancer and factors that contribute to maintenance of the persistent immunodepressed status of both cured and uncured patients.

HUMORAL FACTORS IN HEAD AND NECK CANCER

In an analysis of the humoral immune limb and factors produced during the development of head and neck cancer, it is appropriate to assess both the local and the systemic compartments. Several early reports on the salivary IgA response locally to infectious agents, such as viruses, provided a basis for investigations of the specific IgA local immune response to EBV-coded antigens in patients with nasopharyngeal carcinoma.[13] The results were most encouraging in this patient sample and produced other studies on the local IgA response which proved relevant to head and neck cancer.

A direct relationship to head and neck cancer is provided in a study by Brown et al,[14] demonstrating an association between both salivary and serum IgA levels and status of 102 patients with squamous cell carcinoma of the head and neck. These authors found the highest levels of salivary IgA in patients with advanced or recurrent disease, but even if the patients were cured, the IgA levels were well above the control. In the event that new head and neck TAA were eventually identified, the local IgA immune response to such antigens will have to be assessed.

The serum immunoglobulin response in head and neck cancer was thoroughly assessed in patients with squamous cell carcinoma by Katz et al.[15] This prospective analysis demonstrated a significant elevation of serum IgA levels both before and after therapy. Many investigators have used changes in host immunoglobulin levels to monitor a patient's response to therapy. Katz observed that major differences in circulating serum immunoglobulin levels reside with the IgA and IgE classes. An evaluation of 245 patients with carcinomas of the head and neck and 111 controls showed no significant difference between the two groups when IgG, IgM, or IgD levels were compared. With IgE, however, 26.2 percent of the patients had values in excess of 200 IU/ml, whereas only 7.2 percent of the controls had similar levels. With IgA, 41.6 percent of the head and neck patients had IgA levels greater than 325 mg/dl, but only 14.1 percent of the controls were elevated above this level. Both of these values were significant at $p < 0.0001$ by the Chi square test.

Katz also compared the foregoing immunoglobulin data with the success or failure of treatment in these patients (personal communication). He found that the treatment failure rate was inversely proportional to the serum IgE level and directly proportional to the serum IgA level. Of the 13 patients in this study with IgE values greater than 1000 IU/ml, only two were treatment failures. Seven patients presented with IgE levels lower than 100 IU/ml, but IgA levels greater than 600 mg/dl. Six of these were treatment failures. In patients whose IgE was under 1000 IU/ml, a more favorable prognosis was associated with a higher IgE value. However, the IgA level had impact on the rate of treatment failures in that the number of failures increased as the IgA level increased. A serum immunoglobulin prognostic index (SIPI), using multiple immunoglobulin markers, was formulated based on the patient's IgE, IgA, and IgD levels. A positive SIPI indicated a relative excess of IgA over IgE and IgD and was associated with increased failure rates. When this formula was applied to the test groups, it was found to be accurate in predicting treatment failures and successes when the SIPI score was either highly positive or negative. However, the overall accuracy of the SIPI was 60.5 percent. The accuracy of these markers was increased when combined with patients' clinical information such as stage, age, and lymphocyte count.

Our laboratories at West Virginia University conducted similar prospective immunoglobulin studies of head and neck cancer patients which have been presented elsewhere.

A brief summary of immunoglobulin levels of our patient sample is provided in Table 1, and the IgA levels were persistently elevated throughout the course of our study. A more recent analysis by Ockhuizen et al,[16] utilizing part of our West Virginia University serum panel, confirmed the elevated IgA levels and, in addition, demonstrated for the first time a significantly increased incidence of the Km(1) IgA phenotype marker (p <0.001). Additional data on elevated IgA levels have been reported for nasopharyngeal cancer (NPC) in both the American and the Chinese populations.[17] However, the majority of these studies were correlated with specific antibody responses to the EBV-coded antigens, which is a unique opportunity since this virus is very closely related to the cause of this type of cancer. These types of data would indicate the possible existence of head and neck cancer tumor-associated antigens (TAA), and the approach may have a broader application to understanding head and neck cancer etiology if applied to both virion and non-virion antigens of herpes simplex virus.[7] In this case it will be necessary to determine whether the relationship is a primary or cofactorial one or whether the virus is serving as a passenger virus or has been reactivated from a latent state.

Additional support for an immune response to TAA in head and neck cancer is derived from observations of immunoglobulin-secreting plasma cells either in or bordering the tumor. In a study of 202 patients by Loning and Burkhardt,[18] high numbers of both IgA- and IgG-secreting plasma cells were observed in cases of leukoplakia with dysplasia, and much fewer such cells were seen in well-differentiated tumors. The relationship of elevated serum and salivary immunoglobulins, specific antiviral antibodies, local antibody-producing cell infiltrates into the tumor site, and related studies (to be discussed) focus our attention on the possible existence of specific tumor antigens and immune responses to them in head and neck cancer.

The foregoing analysis of immunoglobulins and specific antibodies in head and neck cancer also sets the stage for presenting new and interesting studies of soluble circulating immune complexes (CIC) in cancer of the head and neck. Our laboratory reported the existence of such CIC in a high percentage of these patients, at least 75 percent, using the Raji cell assay.[19] Another collaborative effort with Baskies et al in patients with nasopharyngeal cancer also showed a similar universal elevation of CIC.

Table 2 summarizes data on these patient samples using the polyethyleneglycol (PEG) method of Digeon[21] combined with the measurement of total precipitable protein by the Lowery method. Statistically significant increases in PEG-CIC levels were demonstrable both before and after therapy. As a follow-up to the historical data gathered on head and neck

TABLE 1   Immunoglobulin Levels Before and After Therapy in Head and Neck Cancer Sera

Immunoglobulin	Cancer Patients (mg %)			Normal Donors (mg %)			
	Visit	Mean	CI_{95}	Visit	Mean	CI_{95}	Alpha*
IgG	1†	1107	(955–1258)	1	1022	(880–1163)	n.s.
	3‡	1078	(1064–1091)	3	975	(834–1115)	0.01
	5§	0899	(729–1066)	5	981	(871–1090)	n.s.
IgA	1	319	(266–371)	1	0214	(168–259)	0.001
	3	325	(263–386)	3	0223	(159–286)	0.01
	5	296	(234–357)	5	0215	(172–257)	0.01
IgM	1	286	(234–336)	1	0253	(202–301)	n.s.
	3	294	(238–348)	3	0200	(155–244)	n.s.
	5	253	(194–310)	5	0225	(173–274)	n.s.
IgD	1	4.07	(2.50–5.63)	1	2.83	(1.14–4.51)	n.s.
	3	2.99	(1.80–4.12)	3	2.00	(1.23–2.76)	n.s.
	5	2.90	(1.65–4.14)	5	2.08	(0.825–3.33)	n.s.

*Student's t-test for independent samples.
†Pre-therapy sample.
‡3–5 months after therapy.
§5–7 months after therapy.

TABLE 2   Immune Complex in Head and Neck Cancer

	Cancer Patients (g/ml PEG–Protein)			Normal Donors (g/ml PEG–Protein)			
Visit	Mean	CI_{95}	Visit	Mean	CI_{95}	Alpha*
1†	1107	(387–729)	1	223	(152–293)	.001
3‡	1078	(295–478)	3	226	(147–302)	.01
5§	0899	(296–482)	5	182	(126–236)	.001

*Student's t-test for independent samples.
†Pre-therapy sample.
‡3–5 months after therapy.
§5–7 months after therapy.

cancer which demonstrated elevations in serum IgA and CIC, working in our laboratories at Cooper-Biomedical, Inc., Dr. Michael Baseler developed an IgA-specific immune complex enzyme immunoassay (IgA-IC).

The data summarized in Table 3 illustrates the significant increases in this unique category of CIC, and a complete manuscript on this subject is now in preparation. Recent evidence in support of the importance of IgA-CIC to the pathogenesis of head and neck cancer comes from an investigation which has revealed an IgA-like substance in cancer sera capable of abrogating the in vitro lymphocyte mitogenic response to EBV.[22] At this time we have the knowledge and technology to more completely assess the role of such CIC in immunoregulation as well as to delineate the types of cancer-associated antigens contained in these unique IgA-CIC substances.

CELL-MEDIATED IMMUNITY IN HEAD AND NECK CANCER

The analysis of cell-mediated immunity (CMI) in carcinoma of the head and neck has been much more extensive, and at least one review of the subject which covers methodology and the authors' original results has been published.[23] In general, during the last ten years authors have assessed one or more of the following in vivo and in vitro CMI correlates in head and neck cancer patients:

1. In vivo dinitrochlorobenzene (DNCB) sensitization, afferent and efferent limb
2. In vivo specific recall antigen testing of efferent limb

TABLE 3   Serum — IGA Immune Complex Levels in Head and Neck Cancer

	Sample Size	Serum IgA–IC* (g/ml)	Alpha*
Normals	57	5.12 ± 4.07	—
Head & neck cancer (WVU Study)	42	11.38 ± 12.54	.0025
Nasopharyngeal cancer (NCI Study)	37	13.36 ± 17.56	.0025

*IgA-IC specific ELISA developed by Dr. Michael Baseler.

3. Total small lymphocyte count
4. Surface lymphocyte marker analysis for lymphocyes T and B
5. In vitro CMI correlates: Polyclonal mitogenesis; Specific recall antigen mitogenesis; Leukocyte adherence inhibition; Leukocyte migration inhibition

The most consistent and reproducible results have been produced by means of the in vivo DNCB sensitization protocol. The earliest report was by Maisel and Ogura,[24] who tested 55 patients with head and neck cancer and found 88 percent of the positive reactors to be alive and tumor-free one year after diagnosis and successful treatment. Of interest, however, was the 53 percent of nonresponders who also were disease-free and hence provide the first evidence that CMI defects can persist in successfully treated head and neck cancer. Twomey et al[25] and Eilber et al,[26] in 1974, extended and verified these observations in a similar patient sample. In 1976, Maisel and Ogura published a follow-up of their previous patient sample as well as some new patients.[27] The results extended the positive correlation of the value of DNCB sensitization to assess both the afferent and efferent limbs of the CMI system and also showed that 85 percent of the recurrent tumors fell into the nonresponder group of patients. Other clinical investigators attempted to use DNCB to determine patient prognosis and found its value to be limited to early stage I and II carcinoma of the head and neck. In advanced head and neck cancer (stage III and IV), in addition to depressed delayed cutaneous hypersensitivity responsiveness to DNCB in sensitized head and neck cancer patients, other investigators used in vitro CMI correlates to substantiate a persistent state of immunodepression.[23] These studies employed one or more of the following assays: total small lymphocyte count, polyclonal mitogenesis, T-lymphocyte count, and, more recently, suppressor T-lymphocyte subset counts determined with monoclonal OKT8+.

An apparent relationship between circulating humoral factors and depressed CMI surfaced during studies of circulating immune complexes and cell-mediated immunity in head and neck cancer patients.[27] The results indicated a consistent relationship between elevated CIC and depressed CMI functions when analyzed by in vitro CMI methods. Alternatively, extensive prospective longitudinal studies by Wolf et al have demonstrated that selected serum glycoproteins elevated during head and neck carcinogenesis correlate to the depressed immune state of these patients.[28] Also, as mentioned previously, an IgA-like CMI blocking factor has been demonstrated in NPC patients' sera.[22] It therefore becomes apparent that circulating humoral as well as cellular factors may combine to collectively exert a negative control over the immune response in head and neck cancer.

The only additional data to support the existence of immunity to head and neck cancer-associated antigens has resulted from the application of some rather controversial, yet acceptable in vitro assays. Using the leukocyte adherence-inhibition (LAI) method, several authors have reported positive reactions to crude head and neck cancer antigen preparations.[29] The very best results were obtained using a homogeneous laryngeal carcinoma patient sample and the homologous extract, whereby the results were 86 percent positive for the test population.[30] Laryngeal cancer-associated antigens are suggested by data obtained using the leukocyte inhibition factor (LIF) release assay with 3M KCL extracts of homologous tumors in the presence and absence of adherent cells.[31] Finally, the results of Hollinshead bear repeating in this section since she obtained her best results for HSV nonvirion antigens in laryngeal cancer patients.[7]

New methodology in cellular immunology, immunochemistry, and monoclonal technology should provide ample opportunities to conduct new and innovative research regarding the etiology and pathogenesis of head and neck cancer.

REFERENCES

1. Sell S. Cancer Markers: Diagnostic and Developmental Significance. The Humana Press; 1980.
2. Rosenberg SA. Serologic Analysis of Human Cancer Antigen. New York: Academic Press; 1980.
3. Fraumeni JF. Respiratory carcinogenesis: An epidemiological appraisal. J Natl Cancer Inst 1975; 55:1039–1046.
4. Decker J, Golstein JC. Risk factors in head and neck cancer. N Engl J Med 1982; 306:1151–1155.
5. Binnie WH, Rankin KV, Machenzie IC. Etiology of squamous cell carcinoma. J Oral Pathol 1983; 12:11–29.
6. Ho HC, Ng MH, Kwan HC, Chau JCW. Epstein-Barr virus specific IgA and IgG specific antibodies in nasopharyngeal carcinoma. Br J Cancer 1976; 34:656–659.
7. Hollinshead A. DHR-ST, LMIT and CF tests to identify herpes simplex tumor-associated antigens and antibody. In: Heberman RB (ed). Compendium of Assays for Immunodiagnosis of Human Cancer. New York/Amsterdam/Oxford: Elsevier-North Holland, 1979: 489–497.
8. Shillitoe EJ, Greenspan D, Greenspan JS, Silverman S. Immunoglobulin class of antibody to HSV in patients with oral cancer. Cancer 1983; 51:65–71.
9. Cunningham-Rundles S. Effects of nutritional status on immunological function. Am J Clin Nutrition 1982; 35:1202–1210.
10. Fidler IJ, Hart IR. Biological diversity in metastatic neoplasms. Origins and implications. Science 1982; 217:998–1003.
11. Shi ZR, Tsao D, Kim YS. Subcellular distribution synthesis and release of carcinoembryonic antigen in cultured human colon adenocarcinoma cell lines. Cancer Res 1983; 4045–4049.
12. Primack A. The production of markers by bronchogenic car-

cinoma. A review. Semin Oncol 1974; 1:235–244.
13. Order SE, Klein JL, Leichner PK. Antiferritin IgG antibody for isotopic cancer chemotherapy. Oncology 1981; 38:154–160.
14. Brown AM, Lally ET, Frankel A, Harwick R, Davis LW, Rominger CJ. The association of IgA levels of serum and whole saliva with the progression of oral cancer. Cancer 1975; 35:1154–1162.
15. Katz AE, Yoo TJ, Nysather JO, Harker LA, Krause CJ. Serum immunoglobulin concentrations in carcinoma of the head and neck. In: Neiburgs HE (ed). Prevention and Detection of Cancer. New York: Marcel Dekker, 1980: 1335–1349.
16. Ockhuizen T, Pandey JP, Veltri RW, Arlen M, Fundenberg HH. Immunoglobulin allotypes in patients with squamous cell carcinoma of the head and neck. Cancer 1982; 49:2021–2024.
17. Baskies AM, Chretien PB, Yang CS, Wolf G, Makuch RW, TU SM, Hsu MM, Lynn TC, Yang HM, Weiss JF, Spiegel HE. Serum glycoproteins and immunoglobulins in nasopharyngeal carcinoma. Correlations with Epstein-Barr virus-associated antibodies and clinical tumor stage. Am J Surg 1979; 138:478–488.
18. Loning T, Burkhardt A. Plasma cells and immunoglobulin synthesis in oral pre-cancer and cancer. Virchows Arch Pathol Anat Histol 1979; 384:109–120.
19. Veltri RW, Sprinkle PM, Maxim PE, Theophilopoulos AN, Rodman SM, Kinney CL. Immune monitoring protocol for patients with carcinoma of the head and neck. Preliminary report. Ann Otol Rhinol Laryngol 1978; 87:692–701.
20. Baskies AM, Chretien PB, Maxim PE, Veltri RW, Wolf GT. Circulating immune complexes correlate with levels of serum immune reactive proteins and clinical tumor stage in head and neck squamous carcinoma. Surg Forum 1980; 31:526–527.
21. Digeon M, Laver M, Riza J, Bach JF. Detection of circulating immune complexes by siplified assays with polyethylene glycol. J Immunol Methods 1977; 16:165–183.
22. Sundar SK, Ablashi DV, Kamraju L, Levine PH, Faggione A, Armstrong GR, Pearson GR, Krueger GRF, Hewetson JF, Betram G, Sesterhenn K, Menexes J. Sera from patients with specific Epstein-Barr virus antigen-included lyphocyte response. Int J Cancer 1982; 29:407–412.
23. Wanebo H. Immunobiology of head and neck cancer. Basic Concepts. Head Neck Surg 1979; 2:42–55.
24. Maisel RH, Ogura JH. Abnormal dinitrochlorobenzene skin sensitization as a prognostic sign of survival in head and neck squamous cell carcinoma. Laryngoscope 1973; 83:2012–2019.
25. Twomey PL, Catalona WJ, Chretien PB. Cellular immunity in cured cancer patients. Cancer 1974; 33:435–440.
26. Eilber FR, Morten DL, Ketcham AS. Immunologic abnormalities in head and neck cancer. Am J Surg 1974; 128:534–538.
27. Maisel RH, Ogura JH. Dinitrochlorobenzene sensitization and peripheral lymphocyte count. Predictors of survival in head and neck cancer. Ann Otol Rhinol Laryngol 1976; 84:517–522.
28. Wolf G, Chretien PB, Elias EG, Makuch RW, Baskies AM, Spiegel HE, Weirs JF. Serum glycoproteins in head and neck squamous carcinoma. Correlations with tumor extent, clinical tumor stage, and T-cell levels during chemotherapy. Am J Surg 1979; 128:489–500.
29. Vetto RM, Burger DR, Vandenbark AA, Jenke PE. Changes in tumor immunity during therapy determined by leukocyte adherence-inhibition and dermal testing. Cancer 1978; 41:1034–1039.
30. Yetto RJ, Sako K, Dasmahapatra K, Raina S, Rajack S, Holojoke ED, Golrosen MH. Detection of tumor immunity by the computerized tube leukocyte adherence-inhibition assay in patients with squamous cell carcinoma of the head and neck. Tumor Diagnostik 1981, 2.74–78.
31. Cortesina G, Bussi M, Morra B, Cavallo GP, Beatrice F, Fortunato V Di, Poggio E, Orecchia R, Gabriele P, Rendine S, Sartoris A. Specific LIF production in laryngeal cancer patients. Evidence of suppressor activity exerted by adherent cells. IARC Med Sci 1982; 10:243–244.

TUMOR-ASSOCIATED ANTIGENS IN HEAD AND NECK CANCER TISSUES AND IN SERA OF TUMOR-BEARING PATIENTS

ADLY N. IBRAHIM, D.V.M., Sc.D.
RUTH ANN TUCKER, M.S.
LEE MARR, M.S.
AHMED ABDELAL, Ph.D.

We have previously demonstrated tumor-associated antigens (TAA) in herpes simplex virus type 2 (HSV-2)-associated hamster sarcomas and in sera of tumor-bearing animals.[1] In addition, we have determined antigenic relationships between HSV-2, the hamster sarcomas, and human cervical cancer.[2] Therefore, we explored the possibility of detecting TAA in cervical cancer tissues (CaCx) and circulating TAA (C-TAA) in sera of cervical cancer patients (CaCxS).

Using precipitin-in-gel methods, anti-CaCx sera, adsorbed with pooled normal cervical tissue antigen preparations (NCx) and with pooled normal human serum (NHS), demonstrated TAA in CaCx and circulating TAA (C-TAA) in sera of patients with cervical cancer and those with head and neck cancers. Statistical analysis of data obtained by testing 96 coded sera from National Cancer Institute-Mayo Clinic Serum Bank showed that the results were significant and that specificity was high, but sensitivity was relatively low. Further analysis of the data based on the time the serum was drawn from the patient showed that the C-TAA is more frequently detected in sera obtained before or shortly after operation than in those obtained years after surgery.[3]

In addition, other investigators reported that antibodies against HSV-related antigens were frequently detected in sera of patients with these malignant tumors.[4-7] Therefore, it was of interest and importance to determine (1) the antigenic relationship between CaCx TAAs and cancer of larynx (CaLa) TAAs, (2) the antigenic relationship between CaLa and certain human proteins, (3) the potential use of enzyme immunoassay for immunodiagnosis of head and neck cancer by demonstration of C-TAA in sera of tumor-bearing patients, and (4) methods of purification of anti-CaLa sera.

METHODS

Tissues

Invasive squamous cell CaCx and CaLa as well as NCx and NLa were obtained at time of surgery.

The specimens were kept in sterile saline containing penicillin (100 U/ml) and streptomycin (100 μg/ml) and stored at $-20°C$ until used.

Tissue Antigen Preparations

Antigens were prepared from pooled CaCx, from CaLa, and from normal tissue (NT) specimens.[8] The crude antigens were partially purified.

Purification of Antisera

Attempts were made to purify anti-CaCx and anti-CaLa by elimination of antibodies to normal tissue and serum components. Two methods were used for this purpose: the first has been described previously in the literature[1] and the second method consisted of subjecting each antiserum to ion-exchange followed by affinity chromatography. Briefly the immunoglobulins were separated from other serum proteins by application to DEAE-sephadex. Isolation and purification of antibodies against TAAs were achieved by subjecting the immunoglobulins to affinity chromatography using immobilized NT and NHS.

Test Sera

Test specimens included sera from patients with cancer of the larynx and patients with cancer of the cervix. Sera from normal individuals (NHS) were used as controls. In addition, coded sera were obtained from NCI-Mayo Clinic Serum Bank.

Serologic Methods

The following serologic methods were used: (I) The immunodiffusion methods[8] to determine the antigenic relationship between CaCx and CaLa. Anti-CaCx serum, adsorbed with NT and NHS, was placed in the central well of the left side of the ID slide (Fig. 1). The central well of the pattern on the right side was filled with adsorbed anti-CaLa serum. The peripheral wells of both left and right sides were filled with: (1) CaCx, (2) CaLa, (3) CaLaS, (4) CaCxS, (5) NHS, and (6) NT. (II) Cross-adsorption tests: To determine whether CaLa and CaCx are antigenically identical, the cross-adsorption immunodiffusion test was carried out. Anti-CaCx serum was successively adsorbed with CaLa and NHS in the central well of an ID slide as shown on the left in Figure 2. Anti-CaLa serum was adsorbed with CaCx and NHS in the central well of the slide (right side pattern). The peripheral wells of both left and right patterns were filled with (1) CaCx, (2) CaLa, (3) CaLaS, (4) CaCxS, (5) NHS, (6) NT. (III) Enzyme immunoassay (EIA): The indirect method of EIA was employed. Briefly, the flat-bottom microtiter EIA plates were employed. The wells were sensitized with the test sera (cancer patients' or normal control sera). They were then reacted in succession with: (1) purified anti-CaLa serum,

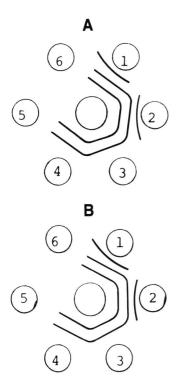

Figure 1 Immunodiffusion reaction patterns, *A*, central well: rabbit anti-CaCx serum adsorbed with normal tissues and normal sera. Peripheral wells: (1) CaCx, (2) CaLa, (3) CaLaS, (4) CaCxs, (5) NHS, (6) NT. *B*, Same as *A* except that the central well contains anti-CaLa serum.

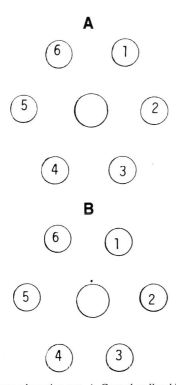

Figure 2 Cross adsorption test. *A*, Central well: rabbit anti-CaCx serum adsorbed with CaLa and NHS. *B*, Central well: rabbit anti-CaLa serum adsorbed with CaCx and NHS. *A and B*, Peripheral wells: (1) CaCx, (2) CaLa, (3) CaLaS, (4) CaCxS, (5) NHS, (6) NT.

(2) peroxidase-labeled goat anti-rabbit immunoglobulins, (3) O-phenylenediamine as the enzyme substrate. The change of color of the substrate resulting from its degradation was read spectrophotometrically. Saline containing 0.05 percent Tween 20 was employed for washing after each step except after adding the substrate.

Antigenic Relationship Between CaLa TAAs and Certain Human Proteins

CaLa antigen was placed in the central well of an ID slide. The peripheral wells were filled with the following reagents: (1) anti-CaLa serum adsorbed with NT and NHS, (2) NHS to serve as a control for adequate adsorption of the antiserum which was placed in well No. 1, (3) unadsorbed anti-ferritin serum, (4) adsorbed anti-CaLa serum (exactly as in well No. 1), (5) as in well No. 3, (6) NT antigen to serve as another control for adequate adsorption of anti-CaLa serum of well No. 1 (Fig. 3).

A similar ID slide has been used for each of the following antisera: anti-lactoferrin, anti-fibrinogen, anti-α_2 macroglobulin, anti-α_2 HS glycoprotein, anti-α_2 ZN glycoprotein, anti-α_2 AP glycoprotein, anti-alpha fetal protein (AFP) anti-ceruloplasmin, and anti-chorionic Gonadotropin (HCG).

Immunologic Approach

The following six figures serve to illustrate schematically and explain the immunologic approach used to demonstrate the TAAs in cancer tissues and C-TAA in sera of cancer patients. Figure 4 shows that when a normal cell is transformed into a cancer cell it acquires newly synthesized tumor-associated antigens (TAA) on the cell membrane and inside the cell. For the sake of simplicity, the TAA is schematically presented as a triangle and the normal tissue antigen as a circle. The TAA is thought to be shed into circulation where it is called C-TAA. For the immunologic detection of TAA and C-TAA, antisera are prepared against cancer tissues in animals such as rabbits. The antiserum contains antibodies to normal tissue components as well as antibodies against TAAs (Fig. 5). When such an antiserum is reacted with normal or

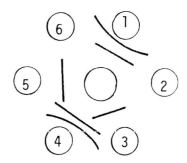

Figure 3 Central well: CaLa. Peripheral wells: (1 and 4) anti-CaLa serum adsorbed with NHS and NT, (2) NHS, (3 and 5) anti-human ferritin serum, (6) NT.

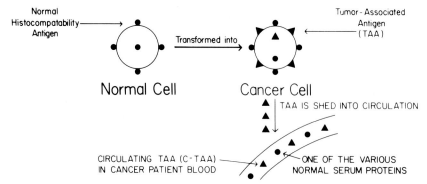

- ● Representative of one of the various normal-tissue histocompatibility antigen (NTA) or normal serum proteins
- ▲ Representative of one of the tumor-associated antigen (TAA)

Figure 4 Schematic presentation of TAA and C-TAA.

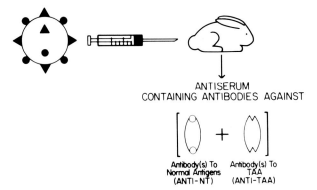

Figure 5 Schematic presentation of preparation of antisera against crude cancer tissue antigens.

cancer tissues, it reacts positively with either antigen preparation (Fig. 6). Figure 4 shows that in order to eliminate antibodies against normal tissue antigens, one has to resort to one of 3 approaches (a) isolate and purify TAAs and prepare antiserum against the purified TAAs, (b) purify and isolate anti-TAA sera, or (c) prepare monoclonal antibodies against TAAs (not shown in Fig. 7). Figure 8 shows that purified anti-TAA serum would react only with cancer antigen preparation (demonstrating TAA) or with cancer patients' serum (demonstrating C-TAA). A typical immundiffusion reaction of a purified antiserum with normal and cancer tissue antigens and sera is shown in Figure 9.

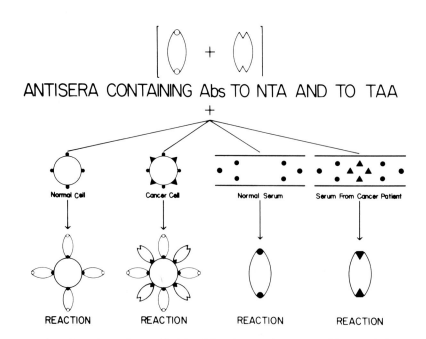

Figure 6 Schematic presentation of reactions of unpurified (crude) anticancer tissue sera with normal tissue, cancer tissue, normal serum, and serum from cancer patients.

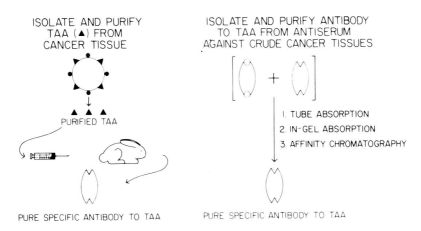

Figure 7 Methods for obtaining purified anti-TAA sera.

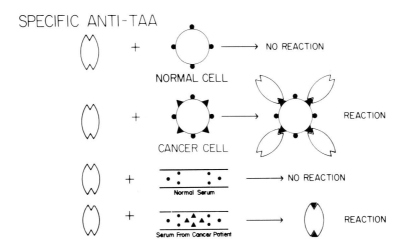

Figure 8 Schematic presentation of reactions of purified anti-TAA with normal tissue, cancer tissue, normal serum, and serum from cancer patient.

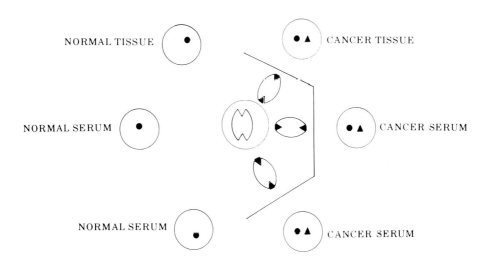

Figure 9 Schematic presentation of ID reaction using purified anti-TAA serum (central well) with the following antigens in peripheral wells. Clockwise, starting at one o'clock: cancer tissue antigen, serum from cancer patient, another serum from cancer patient, normal serum, another normal serum, and normal tissue.

RESULTS

Antigenic Relationship Between CaLa and CaCx

Each of anti-CaCx and anti-CaLa sera, adsorbed with pooled NT and NHS (see Fig. 2), was tested against the homologous and heterologous antigen preparations (wells 1 and 2). Each showed three precipitin lines representing TAA-1 (close to central well), TAA-2 (middle), and TAA-3 (close to peripheral well). Two lines of identity appeared with CaLaS and CaCxS (wells 3 and 4). No reaction appeared with the NHS or NT controls (wells 5 and 6), indicating that the adsorption-in-gel of the antiserum was adequate for elimination of antibodies to normal tissue and serum components. When each of CaLa and CaCx antigen preparations were titrated, the titers of TAA-1, TAA-2, and TAA-3 were 1:32, 1:8, and 1:2 respectively. The patterns of reaction shown in Figure 2 suggested antigenic identity of CaLa and CaCx. However, to confirm the identity of the two antigen preparations, the cross-adsorption test was performed (see Fig. 2). Anti-CaCx serum was adsorbed with the heterologous CaLa and with NHS. Similarly, anti-CaLa serum was adsorbed with the heterologous CaCx and with NHS. No reaction appeared with the homologous or heterologous antigens or sera from cancer patients.

Antigenic Relationship Between CaLa and Certain Human Proteins

Figure 3 shows that the adsorption-in-gel of anti-CaLa serum (well 1 and 4) with NT and NHS was adequate since no reaction appeared with the adjacent wells containing NHS (well 2) or with NT (well 6). The adsorbed anti-CaLa sera (wells 1 and 4) showed two precipitin lines with the homologous CaLa (central well). The unadsorbed anti-human ferritin serum gave one line with CaLa. This line did not meet with any of the two lines formed with the adsorbed anti-CaLa serum. Essentially the same results were obtained when a similar ID slide was used for each of the following antisera against fibrinogen: α_2-macroglobulin, α_2 HS glycoprotein, and α_2 ZN glycoprotein. However, the following antisera did not react with CaLa: lactoferrin, ceruloplasmin, α_2 AP glycoprotein, α-fetoprotein (AFP), and human chorionic gonadotropin (HCG).

Purification of Antisera

Both methods used—(1)adsorption-in-gel and (2) ion-exchange followed by affinity chromatography—were successful in eliminating antibodies to normal tissue and serum components. However, the chromatographic method seemed to be superior.

Evaluation of EIA for the Detection of C-TAA In Sera of Patients with Head and Neck Cancer

Ten out of 20 sera from head and neck cancer patients which were obtained earlier from NCI-Mayo

Clinic Serum Bank were used to evaluate EIA in detection of C-TAA. Forty-five percent were reported positive using ID test.[3] Table 1 shows that 80 percent of these sera were positive employing the purified antiserum in EIA.

DISCUSSION

In a previous publication,[3] we reported that rabbit anti-CaCx sera detected C-TAA in sera of patients with cervical cancer and those with head and neck cancer. In addition, other investigators reported that antibodies against herpes simplex virus-related antigens were frequently detected in sera of patients with these neoplasias.[4-7] Therefore, it was of interest and importance to determine the antigenic relationship between CaCx TAAs and CaLa TAAs. Adsorbed anti-CaLa or anti-CaCx gave identical precipitin-gel reactions with CaLa, CaCx, CaLaS, and CaCxS. Three lines appeared with each cancer tissue antigen preparation, suggesting that each consists of at least three antigens (1) TAA-1, highest in titer and probably lowest in molecular weight since it is curved toward the antiserum well, (2) TAA-2, intermediate in titer with approximately the same molecular weight as TAA-1, and (3) TAA-3, lowest in titer and highest in molecular weight since it is curved toward the antigen well. Patterns of identity prevailed between CaLa and CaCx antigens as well as between CaLaS and CaCxS. Circulating TAAs are most likely related to tissue TAAs since patterns of identity are observed with the lines formed with patients' sera and cancer tissue antigens. The results of cross-adsorption tests suggest strongly the antigenic identity of CaLa TAAs and CaCx TAAs.

The presence of common antigens among CaLa and CaCx as well as shared C-TAA in sera of patients with both types of malignant tumor suggest a possible virus etiology. Our previous studies, as well as those of others,[4-7] have demonstrated common antigens between herpes simplex virus type 2 (HSV-2) and cervical cancer. However, whether HSV-2 is etiologically related to CaCx and head and neck cancer is still

TABLE 1 Evaluation of Enzyme Immunoassay for the Detection of Circulating Tumor-Associated Antigen in Sera of Patients with Head and Neck Cancer obtained from NCI-Mayo Clinic Serum Bank

	Code No.	Diagnosis	EIA
1	1452	Tongue, SCC, St III	+
2	1483	Soft palate, SCC	+
3	1730	Nasopharynx, lymphoepithelioma	+
4	1745	Oropharynx, SCC	+
5	8255	Larynx, Gr 3 SCC	0
6	11967	Neck, palate, Gr2 SCC	0
7	390–228	Neck and mouth, SCC	+
8	390–369	Larynx, SCC	+
9	390–424	Larynx, SCC	+
10	391–135	Head, neck, back of tongue, SCC	+
			8/10 (80%)

unresolved and needs further investigation. The precipitin reaction patterns of anti-human ferritin serum with CaCx suggest a partial antigenic relationship between CaCx and human ferritin. The same finding was observed with fibrinogen, α_2-macroglobulin, α_2 HS glycoprotein, and α_2 ZN glycoprotein. Other markers, which have been observed in association with other types of malignant tumors, appeared unrelated to CaLa or CaCx. These markers were: lactoferrin, ceruloplasmin, α_2 AP glycoprotein, AFP, and HCG. Ion exchange followed by affinity chromatography was successful in eliminating antibodies to normal tissue and serum components from antisera against partially purified cancer tissue antigens. The chromatographic methods appeared to be superior to the purification in-gel previously used.[1] The use of purified antiserum EIA for the detection of C-TAA in sera of patients with CaLa was promising for immunodiagnosis of head and neck cancer. Eighty percent of cancer patients' sera were positive.

These results suggest the antigenic identity of CaLa TAAs and CaCx TAAs. They further indicate a potential use for purified anti-CaCx or anti-CaLa serum in EIA as an immunodiagnostic procedure.

Further improvement is needed in the specificity and sensitivity of the procedure by using highly purified antisera, such as monoclonal antibodies, for quantitative measurement of C-TAA.

REFERENCES

1. Ibrahim AN, Ray M, Nahmias A. Tumor antigens in hamster with sarcomas associated with herpes virus type 2. Proc Soc Exp Biol Med 1975; 148:1025–1028.
2. Ibrahim AN, Ray M, Megaw J, et al. Antigenic interrelationships between herpes simplex virus 2 hamster-associated tumors and cervical cancer. Proc Soc Exp Biol Med 1976; 152:343–347.
3. Ibrahim AN, Robinson RA, Marr L, et al. Tumor-associated antigens in cervical cancer tissues and in sera from patients with cervical cancer or with head and neck cancer. J Natl Cancer Inst 1979; 63:319–323.
4. Hollinshead AC, Lee O, Chretien PB, et al. Antibodies to herpes virus nonvirion antigens in squamous carcinoma. Science 1973; 182:713–715.
5. Hollinshead AC, Chretien PB, O'Bong L, et al. In vivo and in vitro measurements of herpes simplex virus tumor-associated antigens. Cancer Res 1976; 36:821–828.
6. Notter MF, Docherty JJ. Reaction of antigens isolated from herpes simplex virus-transformed cells with sera of squamous cell carcinoma patients. Cancer 1976; 36:4394–4401.
7. Notter MF, Docherty JJ. Comparative diagnostic aspects of herpes simplex tumor-associated antigens. J Natl Cancer Inst 1976; 57:483–488.
8. Ibrahim AN, Rawlins D, Abdelal A, et al. Tumor-associated antigens in lung cancer tissues and in sera of tumor-bearing patients. Cell Mol Biol 1980; 26:327–333.

HSV ANTIGENS AS DIAGNOSTIC AND/OR THERAPEUTIC MARKERS IN SQUAMOUS CANCER OF THE CERVIX AND HEAD AND NECK

LAURE AURELIAN, Ph.D.

At least two problems must be addressed when considering the role of the immune system in neoplastic disease. The first relates to the biology of the neoplastic process. It argues that novel protein(s)/antigen(s) are synthesized during carcinogenesis, thereby becoming unique tumor markers that can be used in cancer detection and/or immunotherapy. The second question that must be considered within the context of the role played by the immune system in neoplastic disease relates to non-tumor-specific immunostimulation (or immunodepression) and its effect on tumor growth.

Over the past 25 years, major efforts have been made to identify new antigens that are specifically related to human malignant tumors. In the case of virus-associated human neoplasms, this effort has focused on viral antigens, as experimental data indicate that such antigens are unique to the tumor cells with which they are associated in a biologically meaningful fashion. The major human cancers that have been studied in this context, and in which a virus etiology has become a generally accepted concept, are African Burkitt's lymphoma and certain histopathologic types of nasopharyngeal carcinoma in which EBV has been implicated as a causative factor, and squamous carcinoma of the cervix in which herpes simplex virus type 2 (HSV-2) has been implicated as a causative factor. (In his chapter, Pearson describes his exciting findings pertaining to the diagnosis and prevention of EBV-associated malignant disease). I will discuss cervical cancer, and the possible significance of the findings, with respect to squamous cell malignant tumors of the head and neck.

HSV-2 AND CERVICAL CANCER

There is a paucity of information pertaining to the role of nonspecific immunity in cervical cancer. However, novel viral antigens have been described, and their properties and potential role in the carcinogenic process have been analyzed. Specifically, the following questions have been addressed:

Is HSV Oncogenic, and if so, Are Viral Protein(s) Related to the Oncogenic Process?

In principle, cancer could be viewed as a population of cells that has escaped regulatory controls, thereby achieving immortality. Accordingly, several laboratories have focused on the mechanism of HSV-2-induced neoplastic transformation as a means of providing a better understanding of the role played by HSV-2 in cervical cancer. Inactivated HSV-2 and HSV-1, the HSV associated with facial lesions, transform rodent cells from a normal to a neoplastic phenotype.[1] Recent studies indicate that the transformed cells must retain and express viral DNA sequences in order to maintain a neoplastic phenotype. The acquisition of phenotypic changes characteristic of transformation strongly correlates with the maintenance of viral DNA, and all independently established lines express a viral protein designated ICP-10. Some but not all lines also express another protein, designated ICP-12.[1,2]

Based on these findings, two approaches were taken by our laboratory in order to identify a specific viral protein responsible for transformation. The first sought to define viral proteins that are associated with the ability of a focus of morphologically transformed cells to survive subculture and grow into anchorage-independent, tumorigenic lines. Cells from three of 11 independently isolated foci stained with monospecific antiserum to ICP-10, and two of these three foci survived subculture and grew into anchorage-independent and tumorigenic lines. All the other foci, including two that stained with anti-ICP-12 serum, senesced within two to five further subculture passages.[2] The second approach taken in order to define viral protein(s) necessary for transformation used two temperature-sensitive mutants of HSV-2 (tsA8 and tsH9). Both mutants have been mapped in the region of the HSV-2 genome that lies within or near the coding sequences for the 130K major DNA-binding protein, but they fail to complement each other; tsA8 has a secondary mutation in the ICP-10 region. Diploid cells were transformed at the permissive temperature (34°C) and assayed for anchorage-independent growth (in 0.3% agarose) at the permissive and nonpermissive (39°C) temperatures. At postinfection passages (pips) 14–40, both tsA8-established lines, but neither one of the two lines established with tsH9 or with the wild type virus evidenced a significantly reduced cloning efficiency in 0.3% agarose at 39°C. Beyond this passage level, all lines cloned equally well at 34°C and 39°C.[2] These findings suggest that ICP-10 is required for the acquisition of the transformed phenotype, but only before pip 33-39. Possibly, the maintenance of a carcinogenic potential is due to the rearrangement of integrated viral DNA sequences, giving rise to lines that are no longer dependent on ICP-10. Alternatively, viral DNA sequences, although retained and expressed, are no longer required for the maintenance of a transformed phenotype.

To identify the viral genes that are responsible for transformation, cells were transformed by defined viral DNA fragments. These studies indicated that when established cell lines, rendered heteroploid by factors other than HSV (viz., NIH 3T3), are exposed to the Bgl II N fragment of HSV-2 DNA (0.58 to 0.63, map units), they become morphologically altered and evidence a reduced serum requirement for growth. The transforming region is located in a 2.1 kb fragment within Bgl II N bounded on the left by a BamHI site. Originally, it was shown that cells transformed by Bgl II N do not retain the 2.1 kb sequences, but instead retain sequences from the right-hand end of the Bgl II N fragment.[3] However, recent evidence suggests that a 227 base pair fragment from within the 2.1 kb transforming sequences is maintained in the transformed cells.[4] Not one of the proteins encoded by Bgl II N is fully encoded within the 2.1 kb transforming sequences, and viral proteins are not expressed in the cells transformed by Bgl II N.[3]

On the other hand, the transformation of normal diploid cells is mediated by the Bgl II C fragment of HSV-2 DNA that is positioned between 0.419 and 0.582 map units. Transformation appears to involve at least two stages. Thus cells transfected with sequences spanning the left 64 percent end of the Bgl II C fragment (0.419 to 0.525 map units) escape senescence and grow into immortal lines. However, these lines remain nontumorigenic as late as posttransfection passage (ptp) 60 (immortalizing sequences). The right-hand 35 percent of the Bgl II C fragment, extending from 0.525 to 0.582 map units, is required for the conversion of the preneoplastic immortal lines to a tumorigenic state ("presumptive neoplastic" sequences).[5]

Significantly, a tumor line derived from Bgl II C transformed cells retains a 7.8 kb DNA fragment that is homologous to the "presumptive neoplastic" sequences within Bgl II C. This 7.8 kb band is not observed in normal hamster or human cell DNA.[2] Cell-free translation of mRNA selected from HSV-2-infected cells by the cloned HSV-2 DNA fragment that encompasses the "presumptive neoplastic" sequences encodes two proteins, a 52K and a 144K that are structurally and antigenically identical to ICP-10.[2]

In their totality these findings indicate that HSV-2 genes can transform normal diploid cells by themselves (Bgl II C fragment) or in concert with other factors that modify the cells by immortalizing them (Bgl II N fragment). If viral proteins mediate the acquisition of tumorigenic potential by immortalized cells, the 144 K (ICP-10) and 52K proteins are the only possible candidates. Based on our data with inactivated virus, ICP-10 is a particularly attractive candidate. However, since the mRNA that specifies ICP-10 is encoded by sequences that overlap with Bgl II N,[6,9] and the latter does not transform diploid cells,[5] the data are amenable to three interpretations. First, the entire reading frame for ICP-10 may be located within the Bgl II C fragment. Alternatively, a truncated ICP-10 protein may be involved in the establishment and/or maintenance of anchorage-independent lines, or ICP-10 may not be involved in transformation by viral DNA fragments, although it is related to transformation by the virus itself. Although further studies are required in order to differentiate between these interpretations, it must be stressed that viral proteins appear to be involved in the carcinogenic process, since (1) prolonged exposure of the mouse cervix to inactivated HSV-2 results in dysplasia (65.8% of infected animals), microinvasion (13.4% of infected animals), and invasive cancer (10.5% of infected animals), and (2) immunization against HSV-2 prevents the oncogenic response of the mouse cervix to inactivated HSV-2.[7]

What is the Function, if any, of the Transformation-Related Viral Proteins (viz., ICP-10 and ICP-12)?

Recent studies indicate that a virus-encoded enzyme, the ribonucleotide reductase, is encoded by DNA sequences that map at the same site on the HSV genome as the DNA sequences that encode ICP-10,[8] and immunoprecipitation competition analyses indicate that ICP-10 is at least one of the enzyme components.[9] What does this mean with respect to carcinogenesis? The answer to this question is not clear. However, the following speculations seem appropriate. Ribonucleotide reductase catalyzes the first unique step in DNA synthesis by direct reduction of all four ribonucleotides to the corresponding deoxyribonucleotides. Enzymatic activity is enhanced in rapidly proliferating tissues, an increase that parallels tumor growth rates.[10] Several determinants of DNA replicative fidelity, such as base addition or substitution, altered proofreading (if it exists), or error-prone nonscheduled repairs could be affected by alterations in the dNTP pools. Derangements in the dNTP pools have been shown to increase the rate of spontaneous mutation,[11] and increases in these pools have been linked to transformation and progression.[12] Indeed, ribonucleotide reductases altered in their regulatory control have been shown to confer a mutator phenotype.[11] However, it has been suggested that some specific function other than the production of deoxynucleotides (such as direct participation in the replicative complex[13]) may be involved in tumor progression. In this context it may be particularly significant that ICP-12, the other viral protein that is expressed in some of the transformed cells, is the major viral DNA-binding protein.[14]

Are the transformation-related viral protein(s) (viz., ICP-10 and ICP-12) expressed in human squamous cervical cancer tissue?

ICP-10 is expressed in cervical tumor (but not normal) tissue,[15] and it induces specific antibody in patients with cervical cancer and those with precancerous lesions (e.g., dysplasia, carcinoma in situ). Normal control subjects and individuals with cancer at other sites do not have antibody to ICP-10.[16-18] An-

tibody to ICP-10 is IgM.[16,17] Seroconversion occurs during primary infection with HSV-2, but it is transient. Antibody is no longer detectable around 20 to 40 days post-primary infection, in direct contradistinction from neutralizing antibody to HSV-2, which is primarily IgG, and persists for the life-time of the infected host. Therefore, most (86%) normal subjects without cancer are ICP-10 seronegative even if they have a history of recurrent HSV-2 disease, and are positive for neutralizing antibody to the virus.[16-18] The presence of ICP-10 in the cervical tumor cells causes the reappearance of the specific antibody, thereby rendering the patients with cervical cancer (or precancerous lesions) ICP-10 seropositive (Fig. 1). These findings were reproduced using a panel of sera supplied by the NCI,[18] and they were confirmed in other laboratories in the United States and abroad as well as in a large-scale epidemiologic analysis of 1325 patients.[16]

Another viral protein expressed in cervical tumor cells is ICP-12 (or AG-e). This protein is the homologue of ICSP-11/12, the major viral DNA binding protein[14] independently described in cervical cancer cells.[19] However, direct comparison indicates that ICP-12 is expressed only in a fraction of the ICP-10-positive cervical tumor cells,[15] a finding that is similar to that obtained with virus-transformed cells. ICP-12 induces a specific antigen-driven immune response in patients with cervical cancer and precancerous lesions. Thus, lymphocytes from 75 percent of patients with cervical dysplasia, CIS, or invasive cancer respond to this antigen in leukocyte migration inhibition assay. This compares with 13 percent of the matched control women without cancer and 16 percent of patients with other cancers.[20] These findings are summarized in Table 1.

Can ICP-10 and/or ICP-12 be used in cancer screening and/or immunotherapy?

Our data indicate that ICP-10 seropositivity is highly correlated with the extent of disease (from dysplasia to invasive cancer). Furthermore, successfully treated patients are virtually all ICP-10 seronegative (8.1% positivity), whereas most of those with recurrent disease (96%) are ICP-10 seropositive. ICP-10 antibody is lost in patients with a successfully removed tumor mass, but reappears in patients with cancer recurrence.

From a clinical standpoint, the finding that ICP-10 seropositivity reflects the growth of the cervical tumor is particularly significant. Thus, although it is generally agreed that cervical neoplasia runs the gamut from dysplasia/CIS to invasive cancer, a measure of uncertainty remains. In fact, only 5 to 20 percent of mild dysplasias and 40 percent of the severe ones progress to cancer. The questions remain: What proportion of CIS lesions eventually become invasive? At what rate do cervical dysplasias progress to cancer or even CIS? Is there any way of distinguishing be-

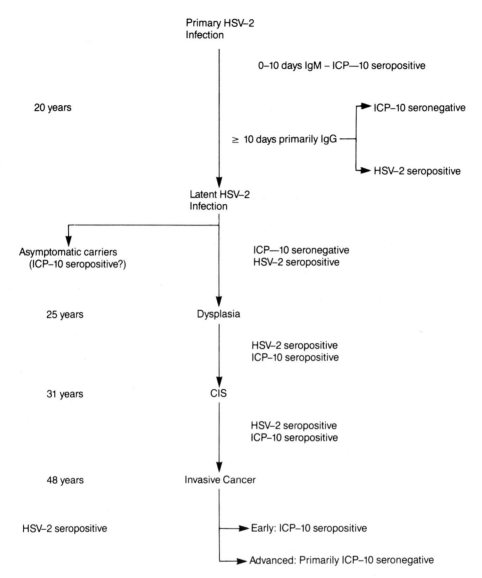

Figure 1 Schematic representation of the natural history of carcinoma of the cervix based on mean age at diagnosis incorporates the concepts of (1) the progression from precursor lesions to invasive disease and (2) the temporal relationship to HSV-2. The development of humoral immune response against viral antigen ICP-10 and the virion (HSV-2) is described.

TABLE 1 Transformation-Related Viral Antigens and Antibody in Patients with Cervical Cancer

Patient*	ICP-10 (AG-4)	ICP-12/ICP-14 (AG-e)	VP-143‡
Atypical cells	+	+	TC§
Antibody (serum)	+ (IgM)	+ (IgG)	+ (IgG)
CMI (lymphoid cells)	−	+ (LIF)†	U#

*Patient with cervical dysplasia, CIS, cancer.
†Leukocyte migration inhibition factor assay.
‡VP143 and ICP-12/14 are different nomenclatures for the major DNA binding protein.
§Tissue-cultured cells from invasive cancer.
#Uknown.

tween premalignant lesions that are destined to advance (high-risk patient) and those that are not?

Answers to these questions are not readily available. The diagnosis of dysplasia or other presumed precursor lesions requires surgical excision that in turn may cure, partly miss, or otherwise modify its biological behavior. However, it seems reasonable to conclude that if a certain precursor lesion is indeed destined to undergo malignant transformation, whereas others are not, the two types may be biochemically, immunologically, or otherwise distinguishable. In theory, the existence of a test capable of differentiating between those cervical precursor lesions with neoplastic or invasive potential and those without such a potential could, when combined with exfoliative cytology, have a major impact on the efficacy and yield of cancer screening programs as well as on the precision and validity of clinical diagnosis. For example, if a patient's initial smear is classified as inconclusive, atypical, or suggestive of neoplasia, the physician may not be certain about his course of action. The physician may wish to observe the patient for a period of time, obtain repeat ctyologic smears, and reexamine her later. However, should the woman be unreliable, mobile, or potentially noncompliant, the physician may feel constrained to take a biopsy or perform conization earlier than is his usual practice. Improvement in the diagnostic precision of the initial cytologic smear could, when applied to precancerous lesions, prevent unnecessary procedures and lead to a more rational clinical management. These issues become particularly relevant in our present-day cost-efficient and consumer-oriented society, in which the cost of the cytologic procedure vs. its effectiveness (cost/benefit ratio) and the possible increase in morbidity associated with mass screening are loudly voiced criticisms.

The potential use of ICP-10 serology as an adjunct to exfoliative cytology was examined for patients for whom the ctyologic reports were inconsistent. In all but one case, ICP-10 serology correlated well with the results of the subsequent hysterectomy reports. Furthermore, ICP-10 seropositivity proved to be an early warning of malignant disease in patients diagnosed as normal or benign (squamous metaplasia) disease.[16] As ICP-10 serology proves to be a diagnostic adjunct to exfoliative cytology, a rational triage of patients could be affected. Women showing suggestive exfoliative findings without ICP-10 antibodies could be reassured and seen less frequently. The physician could thus direct more time and attention specifically to those patients who are at a considerably greater manifest risk of developing cervical cancer. The obvious advantage of such an approach, both in lowering the cost while still retaining all the benefits of the screening program and in reducing unnecessary morbidity associated with screening, has been independently discussed.

ICP-10 testing has another clinical potential. It appears to serve as a simple method for monitoring the completeness of the therapeutic procedure at least for patients with dysplasia, CIS, and early invasive cancer. This conclusion is exemplified by the data summarized in Table 2 for a number of patients followed prospectively. Thus, patient 215 was considered clinically negative for 12 months while ICP-10

TABLE 2   Correlation between AG–4 Seropositivity and Clinical Status after Treatment for Cervical Anaplasia

		Inital Diagnosis*	AG–4†	Subsequent Diagnosis‡
Patient 194 (post rad.)		Dysplasia (mild)	16	Metastatic Ca.
Patient 221 (post cone)		Inconclusive	2	Mod. atypia
Patient 350 (post cone)	5/76	Dysplasia (mild)	4	CIS
	6/76	Negative	4	
	10/77	Inconclusive	4	
		3/78 Recurrent (?)	8	Dysplasia (mild)
Patient 215 (post rad.)	5/76	Negative	4	
	7/76	Negative	4	
		1/77 Dead		Metastatic disease
Patient 340 (post rad.)	5/76	Negative	0	
	9/76	Negative	2	
		5/77 Recurrent (?)	2	Vulvar CIS
Patient 490 (post TVH)	8/76	Negative	4	
	9/76	Negative	8	
	4/77	Negative	4	
		3/78 Recurrent (?)	4	Dysplasia
Patient 449 (post rad.)	7/76	Negative	4	
		7/76 Recurrent (?)	8	
		9/76 Recurrent	16	Liver metastases
		12/76 Dead		
Patient 219 (post rad.)	7/76	Negative	0	
	2/77	Negative	2	
	1/78	Negative	4	
	9/79	Negative	16	
		2/80	ND	Recurrent disease

*Clinical, cytology, and/or histology.
†Titer expressed as reciprocal of highest serum dilution that fixes ≥ 10% complement.
‡Clinical, histology, exploratory.
post rad. = 1–5 years after treatment by radiation for invasive carcinoma; post cone = 1 year after treatment by conization; post TVH = 1 year after treatment by total vaginal hysterectomy; ND = not done.

seropositive. She died with metastatic cancer. Patient 340 was considered negative for 8 months while ICP-10 seropositive. When the possibility was finally considered that she might have recurrent disease, a vulvar CIS lesion was found. Patient 449 was first considered negative and then a possible recurrence case within the same month. She was consistently ICP-10 seropositive and died with disseminated metastatic disease. Since patients with recurrent cervical anaplasia appear to become ICP-10 seropositive before the development of a relatively large tumor mass, periodic serologic testing of cervical cancer patients could provide their physicians with an early warning system vis-a-vis clinical recurrence or metastases and could lead to more effective control and increased survival. However, it should be pointed out that there is also a small proportion (9.6%) of patients for whom we still do not have any correlation between ICP-10 seropositivity and clinical status. This may represent a false-positive response, since the level of ICP-10 seropositivity in the control groups ranges between 7.7 percent (cancers at other sites) and 11.7 percent (normal controls).[16–18]

HSV-1 AND SQUAMOUS CANCER OF THE HEAD AND NECK

How do these findings relate to squamous cancer of the head and neck? A number of extrapolations seem reasonable. First, available data establish the oncogenic potential of both HSV-1 and HSV-2. They indicate that this transforming potential resides within the viral genetic information and that at least one viral protein, ICP-10, is involved in the HSV-2-induced carcinogenesis. Specific HSV-2 DNA sequences that impart neoplastic potential upon normal diploid cells were identified (Bgl II C). Other viral DNA sequences were shown to require previous cellular immortalization by other co-factors, as indicated by the Bgl II N-mediated transformation of the immortalized NIH 3T3 cells.

HSV-1 DNA sequences capable of transforming immortalized NIH 3T3 cells have also been identified. They do not overlap with the HSV-2 transforming sequences, but rather reside at 0.30 to 0.45 map units on the HSV-1 genome,[21] the region that encodes for the 130K major DNA-binding protein designated ICP-8 for HSV-1 and ICP-12[1,15] or ICSP-11/12 for HSV-2.[1];4

Squamous cancer of the head and neck has been associated with HSV-1 in epidemiologic and serologic studies. Carcinoma of the lip has occurred more frequently at sites of recurrent HSV-1 infection than at other sites of the lip.[22] Antibodies to a nonvirion antigen induced in human tissue culture cells by HSV were elevated in patients with head and neck cancer as compared with patients with nonsquamous malignant lesions and normal adults.[23] A protein antigenically indistinguishable from this antigen has been isolated from an extract of lip cancer and is considered

to be a tumor-associated antigen induced by HSV (HSV-TAA).[24] Patients (90%) with squamous carcinoma were shown to have antibody to HSV-TAA in contrast to patients with nonsquamous cancer (11%) or normal individuals (4%). Recent studies by Tarro's laboratory indicate that the antigenic reactivity resides in a 70,000 daltons glycoprotein that appears to be host encoded and virus induced.[25] To increase the sensitivity and specificity of the antibody detection procedures, these investigators have developed an enzyme-linked immunoabsorbent assay (ELISA). The results obtained with this assay are similar to the original data, with 74 percent seropositivity in the head and neck cancer sera as compared to 8 percent in sera from normal controls and 6 percent in patients with other malignancies.[25]

Transforming DNA sequences that can impart a neoplastic phenotype on normal diploid cells have not been described for HSV-1. Therefore, any co-factors that may induce cellular immortalization could be visualized as acting in concert with HSV-1 to cause neoplastic transformation. In this context, it is particularly significant that tobacco has been clearly shown to be a significant risk factor for head and neck cancer. However, HSV-1 also appears to be involved, since a greater percentage of sera from patients with squamous cancer of the head and neck (61%) was shown to have IgA anti-HSV-1 antibodies than heavy smokers without cancer (57%), normal nonsmokers (8%), or patients with nonsquamous malignant tumors (11%). The titers of the IgA antibodies to HSV-1 were also higher in the patients with head and neck cancer than in the normal heavy smokers, and the percentage of positive sera was significantly lower (44%) in patients who were tumor-free for 3 years.[26]

It would be of utmost interest to study the head and neck cancers along the lines described for cervical cancer. Possibly HSV-1 has a transforming DNA sequence that overlaps with HSV-2 Bgl II C fragment that has not yet been identified. Transformation studies using the continuous passage assay of normal diploid cells transfected with various HSV-1 DNA fragments should help resolve this question. Although the cervical cancer studies have shown that only HSV-2 specific domains on the ICP-10 protein are recognized by the immune system in cancer patients,[17,27] the protein itself has both type-common (i.e., shared by HSV-2 and HSV-1) and type-specific determinants. The type-common determinants are shared with a HSV-1 protein designated ICP-6,[9,28] which is well characterized and should be relatively easy to study within the context of head and neck cancer. Even if, by analogy to ICP-10, the type-specific determinants on the HSV-1 ICP-6 protein are the only ones that are expressed in the head and neck cancer patients, monoclonal antibodies that recognize unique as well as shared epitopes on ICP-6 have been developed,[28] and they could be used to study these malignancies.

If a transforming DNA sequence that overlaps the HSV-2 Bgl II C fragment is not identified, monoclonal antibodies to proteins that are encoded within the presently established HSV-1 transforming region are presently available, and they could be used to identify viral proteins in head and neck cancer tissues. One such protein is the 130K major binding protein (designated ICP-8 for HSV-1 and ICP-12 for HSV-2) that has already been identified in cervical cancer, and has been shown to induce a specific antigen-driven cell-mediated immune response in patients with invasive and precancerous cervical lesions.

Monoclonal antibodies against HSV-TAA have also been recently developed, and they should be evaluated for direct analysis of antigen presence and location (viz., cytoplasm or membrane) within the tumor cells. In this context it is of particular significance to notice that recent studies by Tarro and his colleagues suggest that HSV-TAA antibody is no longer detectable in patients with long-term clinical histories, many undergoing chemotherapy, whereas 78 percent of the patients with progressive tumors are HSV-TAA-positive.[25] These findings suggest that HSV-TAA may be clinically helpful as a marker for monitoring the completeness of therapy, as discussed earlier for ICP-10 in cervical cancer.

Finally, it should be pointed out that in both head and neck and cervical cancers, novel unique antigens may prove to be an ideal immunotherapeutic tool. Monoclonal antibodies directed against these antigens can be used to target delivery of appropriate drugs and/or radioactive compounds, thereby achieving the required high doses in the tumor cells while maintaining the high tissue selectivity that is desirable when using toxic compounds.

In contrast to the foregoing, there is significantly more information on the nonspecific immune status of the head and neck cancer patients. Indeed, as discussed throughout this book, head and neck cancer has been associated with persistent immune depression. Low levels of T cells, specific increases in suppressor T cells, decreased NK and lymphokine activities, soluble suppressor factors of tumor or immune origin, and soluble immune complexes (primarily of the IgA type) have been related to this state of immune depression. Immunotherapy designed to achieve nonspecific immune stimulation, such as treatment with BCG, levamisole, or thymosin, has been attempted, but so far it has not resulted in a significant difference in survival.

An exciting, though at present entirely speculative, scenario argues that HSV-1 is involved in this nonspecific immune depression. Previous data,[29] as well as recent findings from our laboratory (Wachsman and Aurelian, in preparation), indicate that latently infected patients often show HSV-1 antigen in their oral secretions in the absence of herpetic lesions. Not only can this antigen lead to the generation of immune complexes, but we have also found that such virus reactivation induces a transient state of immunosuppression, characterized by an increased proportion of suppressor T cells, the generation of soluble suppressor factors (apparently mediated by monocyte-produced PGE_2), and the inhibition of lymphokine activity.[30] If, as suggested by this interpretation, HSV-1 plays a role in the immune depression that is characteristic of head and neck cancer, immunotherapeutic approaches specifically directed toward the regulation of the HSV-induced lymphoid cell modulation should be significantly more effective than the nonspecific immunostimulatory approaches used in the past.

REFERENCES

1. Aurelian L, Manak MM, McKinlay M, Smith CC, Klacsmann KT, Gupta PK. The herpesvirus hypothesis; are Koch's postulates satisfied? Gynecol Oncol 1981; 12:S56–S87.
2. Aurelian L, Manak MM, Ts'o, POP. HSV-2 and cervical cancer: the transformation lesson. In: Giraldo G, Beth E, eds. The Role of Viruses in Human Cancer. Vol. II New York: Elsevier North Holland 1984:73.
3. Galloway DA, McDougall JK. The oncogenic potential of herpes simplex virus: evidence for a hit and run mechanism. Nature 1983; 302:21–24.
4. Galloway DA, Weinheimer SP, Swain MA, McDougall JK. A molecular basis for HSV-2 mediated "hit and run" transformation. Proc. Int. Herpes Virus Workshop, Oxford, 1983; p 70.
5. Jariwalla RJ, Aurelian L, Ts'o POP. Immortalization and neoplastic transformation of normal diploid cells by defined cloned DNA fragments of herpes simplex virus type 2. Proc Natl Acad Sci 1983; 80:5902–5906.
6. Galloway DA, Goldstein LC, Lewis JB. Identification of proteins encoded by a fragment of herpes simplex virus type 2, DNA that has transforming activity. J Virol 1982; 42:530–537.
7. Wentz WB, Heggie AD, Anthony DD, Reagan JW. Effect of prior immunization on induction of cervical cancer in mice by herpes simplex virus type 2. Science 1983; 222:1128–1129.
8. Dutia BM. Ribonucleotide reductase induced by herpes simplex virus has a virus-specified constituent. J Gen Virol 1983; 64:513–521.
9. Iwasaka T, Smith CC, Aurelian L, Ts'o POP. Proteins encoded by the transforming Bgl II C fragment of herpes simplex virus type 2 include ICP-10. Submitted for publication.
10. Elford HL, Freeze M, Passamani E, Morris HP. Ribonucleotide reductase and cell proliferation. I. Variation of ribonucleotide reductase activity with tumor growth rate in a series of rat hepatomas. J Biol Chem 1970; 245:5228–5233.
11. Weinberg G, Ullman B, Martin DW Jr. Mutator phenotype in mammalian cell mutants with distinct biochemical defects and abnormal deoxyribonucleoside triphosphate pools. Proc Natl Acad Sci 1981; 78:2447–2451.
12. Weber G. Biochemical strategy of cancer cells and the design of chemotherapy. Cancer Res. 1983; 43:3466–3492.
13. Prem Veer Reddy G, Pardee AB. Multienzyme complex for metabolic channeling in mammalian DNA replication. Proc Natl Acad Sci 1980; 77:3312–3316.
14. Powell K, Sittler E, Purifoy D. Nonstructural proteins of herpes simplex virus. II. Major virus specific DNA binding protein. J Virol 1981; 39:894–902.
15. Aurelian L, Smith CC, Klacsmann KT, Gupta PK, Frost JK. Expression and cellular compartmentalization of a herpes simplex virus type 2 protein (ICP-10) in productively infected and cervical tumor cells. Cancer Invest 1983; 4:301–313.
16. Aurelian L, Kessler II, Rosenshein NB, Barbour G. Viruses and gynecologic cancers. Herpesvirus protein (ICP-10/AG-4) a cervical tumor antigen that fulfills the criteria for a marker of carcinogenicity. Cancer 1981; 48:455–471.
17. Arsenakis M, May JT. Complement fixing antibody to the AG-4 antigen in herpes simplex virus type 2 infected patients.

Infect Immun 1981; 33:22–28.

18. Aurelian L. Coitus and cancer. Bull NY Acad Med 1976; 52:910–934.

19. Dreesman GR, Burek J, Adam E, Kaufman RH, Melnick JL, Powell KL, Purifoy DJ. Expression of herpesvirus induced antigen in human cervical cancer. Nature (Lond) 1980; 285:591–593.

20. Bell R, Aurelian L, Cohen G. Proteins of herpes virus type 2. IV Leukocyte inhibition responses to type common antigen(s) in cervix cancer and recurrent herpetic infections. Cell Immunol 1978; 41:86–102.

21. Camacho A, Spear PG. Transformation of hamster embryo fibroblasts by a specific fragment of the herpes simplex virus genome. Cell 1978; 15:993–1002.

22. Kvasnich A. Relationship between herpes simplex and lip carcinoma. IV. Selected cases. Neoplasma 1965; 12:61–70.

23. Hollinshead AC, Lee O, Chretien PB, Tarpley JL, Rawls WE, Adam E. Antibodies to herpes virus non-virion antigens in squamous carcinomas. Science 1973; 182:713–715.

24. Hollinshead AC, Tarro G. Soluble membrane antigens of lip and cervical carcinomas: reactivity with antibody for herpes virus non-virion antigens. Science 1973; 139:698–700.

25. Tarro G, Flaminio G, Cocchiara R, DiAlessandro G, Mascolo

A, Popa G, DiGioia M, Geraci D. Herpes simplex virus tumor associated antigen (HSV-TAA) detected by the enzyme-linked immunosorbent assay (ELISA). In: Giraldo G, Beth E, eds. The role of viruses in human cancer. Vol. I. New York: Elsevier/North-Holland, 1980:109.

26. Smith HG, Chretien PB, Henson DE, Silverman NA, Alexander JC Jr. Viral specific humoral immunity to herpes simplex induced antigens in patients with squamous carcinoma of the head and neck. Am J Surg 1976; 132:541–548.

27. Kawana T, Cornish JD, Smith MF, Aurelian L. Frequency of antibody to a virus-induced tumor-associated antigen (AG-4) in Japanese sera from patients with cervical cancer and controls. Cancer Res 1976; 36:810–820.

28. Showalter SD, Zweig M, Hampar B. Monoclonal antibodies to herpes simplex virus type 1 proteins including the immediate early protein ICP-4 Infect Immun 1981; 34:684–692.

29. Douglas GR, Couch RB. A prospective study of chronic herpes simplex virus infection and recurrent labialis in humans. J Immunol 1970; 104:289–295.

30. Sheridan JF, Donnenberg AD, Aurelian L. Immunity to herpes simplex virus type 2. IV. Impaired lymphokine production correlates with a perturbation in the balance of T lymphocyte subsets. J Immunol 1982; 129:326–331.

ADVANCES TOWARD DIAGNOSIS AND PREVENTION OF EPSTEIN-BARR VIRUS (EBV)-ASSOCIATED MALIGNANT DISEASE

GARY R. PEARSON, Ph.D.

Major efforts have been continuing over the past 30 years to identify new antigens associated with animal and human malignant tumors. Such antigens could serve as targets for immunotherapeutic approaches for the treatment of cancer. In addition, antibodies produced against such tumor-associated antigens could be of potential importance to the clinician for the diagnosis and clinical management of patients with specific types of cancers. In general, studies directed at identifying tumor-associated antigens have met with variable success. However, in animal systems, virus-induced tumors consistently express new antigens with defined specificities. Such tumors expressing new antigens have in fact been treated successfully by both specific and nonspecific approaches to immunotherapy.

Because of the success in identifying new tumor-associated antigens in virus-associated animal cancers, numerous investigators have attempted to identify similar antigens in human cancer with apostulated

virus etiology. The major human cancers that have been under study are those in which the Epstein-Barr virus (EBV) and herpes simplex virus type 2 (HSV-2) have been implicated as possible etiologic agents. EBV has been implicated as a major factor in the etiology of African Burkitt's lymphoma, B-cell lymphomas in immunocompromised individuals, and certain histopathologic types of nasopharyngeal carcinoma (NCP).[1] HSV-2 has been implicated as the causative factor of cervical cancer.[2] With these different diseases, antibodies produced against viral antigens associated with these cancers have been evaluated extensively as possible new diagnostic and prognostic markers. In addition, there have been major advances in the development of vaccines against these viruses which might have potential importance to the prevention of these specific cancers. In the chapter on HSV antigens as markers, Aurelian discusses some of the newer information concerning the diagnosis, treatment, and prevention of HSV-2-associated cancers. My discussion will concentrate on EBV, particularly in relation to NPC.

IMMUNOLOGIC APPROACHES TOWARD THE IDENTIFICATION OF VIRUS-INDUCED TUMOR-ASSOCIATED ANTIGENS

A number of different humoral and cell-mediated immunity assays have been employed to identify new antigens in animal and human cancers. Some of the major assays are listed in Table 1. Humoral antibody assays include complement fixation, immunofluorescence, various radioimmune assays with increased sensitivity, and antibody-dependent cellular cytotoxicity (ADCC). This last assay has proved to be of particular clinical importance in regard to NPC (to be discussed), possibly because it measures a functional

TABLE 1 In Vitro Tests used to Study Tumor Immunology

Humoral antibody assays
  Immunofluorescence
  Cytotoxicity
  Complement fixation
  Radioimmune assays
  ADCC
  ELISA
Cell-mediated assays
  Colony inhibition
  Microcytotoxicity
  Lymphocyte transformation
  Lymphokine production

quality of the antibody molecule.[3] Most studies using these immunologic assays have been directed at defining membrane-associated antigens in tumor cells which could serve as the targets for immunotherapy. In addition to the humoral assays, cell-mediated immunity methods have also been employed for purposes of identifying tumor antigens in virus-associated cancers. These assays include cytotoxicity methods such as colony inhibition and microcytotoxicity as well as assays based on the production of specific lymphokines as a measure of a specific cell-mediated immune response. In general, such assays have been successfully used in animal systems to identify new surface antigens in virus-induced tumors which serve as targets for the cellular immune responses. Similar antigens have been identified in EBV-associated cancers including NPC.

CLINICAL VALUE OF ANTIBODIES TO EBV ANTIGENS FOR THE DIAGNOSIS OF NASOPHARYNGEAL CARCINOMA

Early studies on EBV concentrated on the use of sero-epidemiologic approaches to identify specific disease states associated with infection by EBV. These studies were instrumental in establishing leads which pointed to an etiologic association between this virus and certain human cancers.[4] However, these studies also identified antibody responses to certain EBV-associated antigens which followed a disease-related pattern and were therefore of potential clinical value to the diagnosis of EBV-associated cancers. This was particularly true for NPC. Based on results originally reported by the Henles,[5] a number of laboratories have now reported findings that demonstrate that certain antiviral antibodies are of importance to the diagnosis of certain histopathologic types of NPC. Of particular importance to this disease is the presence of IgA antibodies to EBV antigens. Such antibodies are present at a high frequency in the sera of patients with NPC as opposed to a much lower frequency in the sera of various control populations, including patients with other head and neck cancers. Further studies established that the specificity of this antibody response was related to tumor histopathology according to the

WHO classification scheme.[6] This is illustrated in Table 2 for North American patients with this disease. As shown in this Table, greater than 80 percent of the sera from individuals with the less well-differentiated forms of NPC were positive for IgA antibodies to VCA as opposed to 5 to 15 percent of the sera from different control groups. The frequency of positivity for patients with the well-differentiated WHO 1 histopathologic types was similar to that for the control populations. This specificity could be improved by examining sera for both IgA anti-VCA antibodies and IgG antibodies to the early antigen (EA) complex. Previous studies established that both of these antibodies were present in sera at an increased frequency compared to controls.[4] When the sera of North American NPC patients were analyzed in this manner, the specificity was improved (Table 3). Approximately 76 percent of the patients with WHO 2 and WHO 3 carcinomas were positive for both of these antibodies at diagnosis as opposed to 3 to 11 percent of the control sera. Because of this specificity, these assays have now proved useful for the diagnosis of the occult form of this disease and for screening tests for identifying individuals at risk for developing NPC.[7]

TABLE 2 Frequency of IgA–Positive Sera in Different Disease Categories

Disease	No. Sera Positive/ No. Tested	% Positive
NPC		
WHO 1	5/51	10
WHO 2 and 3	206/249	83
Other head and neck cancers	51/324	15
Benign head and neck diseases	57/428	13
Other malignant tumors including lymphomas	7/73	10
Normals	18/405	5

TABLE 3 Frequency of Sera Positive for Both IgA Anti-VCA and IgG Anti-EA Antibodies in Different Disease Categories

Disease	No. Sera Positive/ No. Tested	% Positive
NPC		
WHO 1	4/51	8
WHO 2 and 3	189/249	76
Other head and neck cancers	35/324	11
Benign head and neck diseases	34/428	8
Other malignant tumors including lymphomas	5/73	7
Normals	8/405	2

PROGNOSTIC VALUE OF EBV SEROLOGY IN PATIENTS WITH NPC

Results from retrospective studies indicated that increases in antibody titers to certain EBV antigens following treatment of patients with NPC reflected the development of recurrent or metastatic disease.[4] These increases were frequently noted even before there was clinical evidence of recurrent disease. In contrast, stable or decreasing titers tended to reflect a good prognosis. These conclusions have now been supported by findings from a number of prospective studies on patients with NPC in different geographic locations throughout the world. Based on the results of these studies, therefore, it is now possible to monitor the course of NPC following treatment by periodically measuring antibodies to specific EBV proteins. The utilization of such viral markers should be helpful in the future in aiding the clinician in the management of patients with this disease.

A second assay that appears promising in relation to prognosis is the ADCC assay, which measures a cytotoxic antibody against an EBV protein expressed in the membrane of EBV-infected or transformed cells.[3] A recently completed prospective study on North American patients with NPC established the clinical value of this assay.[8] In general, disease progression ultimately resulting in death, in this patient population, occurred mainly in individuals who presented with low ADCC titers at diagnosis. Patients with high titers in general survived disease-free for significant periods of time following treatment. Approximately 75 percent of the patients with high titers at diagnosis have remained disease-free for 3 years or longer as opposed to approximately 30 percent of the individuals in the low-titered group. The results from this prospective study have been quite striking and suggest that this assay is of potential importance for predicting disease course following treatment. The results suggest further that this antibody might be active in immunity in vivo, possibly through an ADCC mechanism. Approaches to enhance this antibody level through an appropriate vaccine or by passive transfer of high-titered serum could therefore be of therapeutic importance for patients with this EBV-associated malignant tumor.

PROSPECTS FOR PREVENTION OF EBV-ASSOCIATED CANCERS

With the accumulation of data concerning the association of EBV to NPC and other human cancers, efforts have been initiated to prevent or treat such diseases with an appropriate vaccine. Such a vaccine has to be free of EBV DNA since the genome of this virus contains a gene capable of changing a normal cell into a cell with neoplastic properties. Therefore, research directed at preparing a vaccine against EBV has concentrated on the development of a component or subviral vaccine free of viral DNA. The relevant antigens

TABLE 4   Conclusions on the Clinical Application of EBV Immunology

The most specific antibody response for the diagnosis of the less-differentiated histopathologic types of NPC is the presence of serum IgA anti-EBV antibodies. Detection of this antibody has proved useful to the clinician for the diagnosis of NPC including the occult form.

Antibody titers to EBV antigens detected by immunofluorescence generally increase in parallel with the development of metastatic disease. Decreasing or stable titers tend to reflect a good prognosis.

Low antibody titers at diagnosis as determined with the antibody-dependent cellular cytotoxicity assay in patients with NPC in general reflect a poor prognosis.

Serum with high ADCC titers or an appropriate vaccine for inducing the formation of such antibodies might prove to be useful adjuncts to conventional therapy for the treatment of NPC.

are those expressed in the membranes of infected cells and also in the envelopes of mature virions. These are the proteins responsible for the induction of neutralizing antibodies to the virus and cytotoxic antibodies to the infected cell. The relevant proteins have now been isolated and purified by a number of different laboratories. Such purified antigens induce neutralizing and cytotoxic antibodies.[9] Preliminary findings suggest that nonhuman primates immunized with such antigens are protected from infection by EBV. Further studies are needed, however, to establish the applicability of this vaccine to human populations either as a preventive measure or a form of immunotherapy. In addition, efforts are ongoing to produce this subviral vaccine through gene cloning techniques. Success with this approach should enhance the possibility of producing a relatively inexpensive vaccine in large quantities for administering to human populations.

CONCLUSIONS

The studies on EBV over the past twenty years have established that this virus is a factor in the etiology of some forms of human cancers. The experimental studies have also resulted in the identification of certain immune parameters of importance to the clinician for the diagnosis and management of patients with EBV-associated cancers. Some conclusions concerning the application of EBV immunology to NPC are listed in Table 4. Utilization of these tests in the clinical laboratory should lead to earlier detection of primary or recurrent disease, which should enhance the effectiveness of treatment of these cancers. In addition, advances have been made which could eventually lead to the eradication of EBV-associated cancers.

REFERENCES

1. De The G. Role of Epstein-Barr virus in human disease: infectious mononucleosis, Burkitt's lymphoma and nasopharyngeal carcinoma. In: Klein G, ed. Viral oncology. New York: Raven Press, 1980:769.
2. Pearson GR, Aurelian L. Immunology of herpesvirus-associ-

ated cancers. In: Nahmias AJ, ed. The human herpesviruses. New York: Elsevier Press, 1981:297.

3. Pearson GR. In vitro and in vivo investigations on antibody-dependent cellular cytotoxicity. Curr Top Microbiol Immunol 1978; 80:65–96.

4. Pearson GR. Epstein-Barr virus: immunology. In: Klein G, ed. Viral oncology. New York: Raven Press, 1980:739.

5. Henle G, Henle W. Epstein-Barr virus-specific IgA serum antibodies as an outstanding feature of nasopharyngeal carcinoma. Int J Cancer 1976; 17:1–7.

6. Pearson GR, Weiland LH, Neel HB III, Taylor W, Earle J, Mulroney SE, Goepfert H, Lanier A, Talvot ML, Pilch B, Goodman M, Huang A, Levine PH, Hyams V, Moran E, Henle G, Henle W. Application of Epstein-Barr virus (EBV) serology to the diagnosis of North American nasopharyngeal carcinoma. Cancer 1983; 51:260–268.

7. Neel HB III, Pearson GR, Weiland LH, Taylor WF, Goepfert HH. Immunologic detection of occult primary cancer of the head and neck. Otolaryngol Head Neck Surg 1981; 89:230–234.

8. Pearson GR, Neel HB III, Weiland LH, Mulroney SE, Taylor W, Goepfert H, Huang A, Levine P, Lanier A, Pilch B, Goodman M. Antibody-dependent cellular cytotoxicity and disease course in North American patients with nasopharyngeal carcinoma: a prospective study. Int J Cancer 1984; 33:777–782.

9. Qualtiere LF, Chase R, Pearson GR. Purification and characterization of a major Epstein-Barr virus-induced membrane glycoprotein. J Immunol 1983; 129:814–819.

SECTION TEN / INTERVENTION APPROACHES TO PREVENTION

40. Interventional Approaches to Prevention

INTRODUCTION

WILLIAM D. DeWYS, M.D.

The topic addressed in the chapters that follow is the question whether human cancer can be prevented. In the past, physicians tended to take a fatalistic position and answer this question in the negative. Today we can respond to this question with a qualified "yes" or "yes, sometimes". Authors of the following chapters review the basis for this optimism and highlight the need for further research in this area.

We base our enthusiasm for the prospect of cancer prevention on leads from the laboratory, leads from epidemiologic studies, and very preliminary leads from clinical trials (Fig. 1).

Laboratory research relevant to cancer prevention can be broadly divided into basic research and applied research. Basic research elucidates the principles of carcinogenesis. These principles provide the conceptual framework on which to build hypotheses for applied research. Leads for applied research come from basic research or from epidemiologic research. Laboratory research in turn provides leads to epidemiologic research, resulting in an enriching interaction between laboratory research and epidemiologic research (see Fig. 1).

When results from laboratory research or from epidemiologic research support the possibility of cancer prevention, these leads should be subjected to further study in clinical trials. If clinical trials give positive results, the emphasis should then shift to wide application of these results to the relevant segments of the general population (see Fig. 1).

Why do we need clinical trials in cancer prevention?

1. Epidemiologic studies may lack specificity. By specificity we mean the ability to reach conclusions that apply to one and only one specific factor. This would mean that in an epidemiologic study the population under scrutiny differs in only one factor when compared to a control population. This is rarely the case in epidemiologic studies. For ex-

ample, if we observe that a population of cancer patients has a lower dietary intake of vitamin A than a control group, we must remember that a diet which is low in vitamin A is also likely to be low in vitamin C and folic acid, and thus we cannot specifically attribute the protection of vitamin A.

2. There is a need to determine the relevance or predictive value of animal models and other laboratory research to interpretation in humans. For example, is an animal model in which a single large dose of carcinogen is painted on the skin relevant to the human situation in which exposure to low doses of carcinogens may occur over long periods of time? Also, is the metabolism of carcinogens or of preventive agents similar in the animal model and in humans?

3. We need to evaluate participant acceptance of the intervention. Acceptance might be low either because of poor motivation within the target population or because of unpleasant side effects of the intervention.

4. Clinical trials will address issues of risk/benefit ratio and cost/benefit ratio. Few, if any, interventions which might be considered are free of risk. The question is, do the benefits outweigh the risks? Similarly, we need to assess all of the costs of the intervention to be sure that the intervention represents a wise use of the resources of society.

Carcinogenesis may be viewed as a two-step process, namely, initiation followed by promotion (Fig.

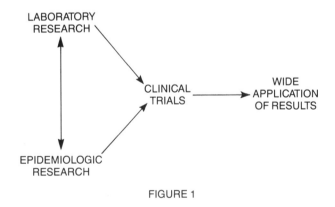

FIGURE 1

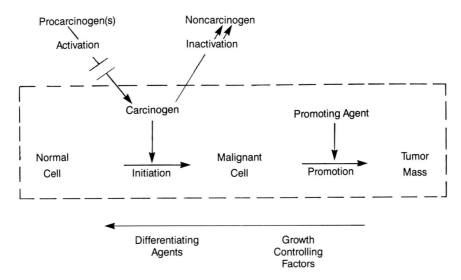

Figure 2 Theoretical model of carcinogenesis (inside dashed line) and cancer prevention (outside of dashed line).

2). Initiation may be prevented by avoidance of exposure to carcinogens, interference with activation of precursors of carcinogens, or enhanced deactivation of carcinogens. Theoretically, initiation could also be reversed by application of a differentiating agent. Promotion may be prevented by avoidance of exposure to promoting agents, use of antipromoters, or use of growth controlling factors.

Initiation is often viewed as an instantaneous event, whereas promotion extends over a long period of time. Interference with initiation in general must be applied prior to or during the initiating event: interference with promotion can occur long after initiation.

In the following chapters, Thomas reviews epidemiologic studies relevant to prevention of cancer of the head and neck region. I review examples of laboratory research that may be relevant to prevention of human cancer. Stitch and Rosin report on pilot clinical trials. I concluded the presentations with a brief discussion of factors which should be considered in the design and conduct of a prevention clinical trial.

SINONASAL, NASOPHARYNGEAL, ORAL, PHARYNGEAL, LARYNGEAL, AND ESOPHAGEAL CANCERS: EPIDEMIOLOGY AND OPPORTUNITIES FOR PRIMARY PREVENTION

DAVID B. THOMAS, M.D., Dr. P.H.

In this chapter, the epidemiologic features and known and suspected causes of carcinomas of the upper respiratory and digestive systems will be summarized, and opportunities for their primary prevention will be reviewed. Carcinomas of five distinct sites will be considered. In order of their numeric impor-

tance in the United States, they are neoplasms of the buccal cavity and pharynx, larynx, esophagus, nasal cavity and paranasal sinuses, and nasopharynx. In the aggregate, these neoplasms constitute about 6 percent of all cancers in the United States (exclusive of nonmelanotic skin cancers), including over 8 percent of all cancers in men and 2 percent in women. Their average annual incidence rates in the United States, and the proportion of all cancers that each constitutes, are shown in Table 1.

CARCINOMAS OF THE NASAL CAVITY AND PARANASAL SINUSES

Approximately one-half of all sinonasal tumors arise from the nasal cavity, about a third originate in the maxillary sinuses, and most of the remainder occur in the ethmoid sinuses.[6] Data from the Third National Cancer Survey showed that about two-thirds of all sinonasal carcinomas in men and about half in women were squamous cell, 9 percent in men and 14 percent in women were adenocarcinoma, 15 percent in men and 5 percent in women were not classified

TABLE 1 Incidence Rates of Cancer of the Upper Respiratory and Digestive Systems in the United States

Site	Incidence rates*			% of all cancers		
	Total	Male	Female	Total	Male	Female
Nasal cavity and paranasal sinuses	0.6	0.8	0.5	0.2	0.2	0.2
Nasopharynx	0.6	0.9	0.3	0.2	0.2	0.1
Buccal cavity and pharynx†	10.6	16.5	5.9	3.2	4.3	1.9
Esophagus	3.6	5.9	1.9	1.1	1.6	0.6
Larynx	4.6	8.5	1.3	1.4	2.2	0.4
All sites	331.5	379.3	304.1	100.0	100.0	100.0

*Average annual age-adjusted (1970 standard) incidence rates per 100,000 population for all races, SEER program, 1973–1977.
†Excluding nasopharynx.

as to histologic type, and rare histologic entities constituted the remainder.

These tumors rarely occur before age 30, and thereafter their incidence rates increase steadily with age. They occur about twice as frequently in men as in women in most countries. The variation in incidence rates among countries and ethnic groups is not as great as for most other cancers. Higher than average incidence rates have been noted in Japan, in some parts of Africa, in native Hawaiians, and in American Indians. Incidence rates for American whites and blacks are similar, although mortality rates in blacks are about 50 percent higher, probably due to delayed diagnosis. In the United States the incidence of these tumors has changed little with time, at least since 1969.

Nearly all known causes of sinonasal carcinomas are chemicals and dusts to which individuals have been occupationally exposed. These substances (and the occupational site of exposure) include: nickel and nickel compounds (nickel refining), isopropyl oil (isopropyl alcohol manufacturing), chromates (chrome-based paint manufacturing), and β-dichlorethyl sulfide (mustard gas manufacturing). Other high-risk occupations, in which the specific carcinogen has not been identified, include: woodworkers, boot and shoe makers and repairmen, textile and clothing manufacturers, and possibly workers in the chemical, petroleum, and coal gas industries. In addition, individuals who inhale snuff have been reported to develop carcinomas of the nasal cavity.

Ionizing radiation can also cause sinonasal carcinomas. The radium dial painters, who usually developed osteosarcomas, also occasionally developed carcinomas of the nasal cavity and sinuses; and the contrast material thorium dioxide undoubtedly caused carcinomas of the sinuses after intrasinus injection.

Primary prevention of sinonasal cancer can obviously be accomplished by reducing exposures in those industries where workers are not adequately protected from the established and suspected causes. However, the proportion of all sinonasal cancers that can be explained by these causes is unknown.

These diseases are of sufficient rarity that their occurrence should stimulate the alert clinician to inquire about prior chronic exposure to dusts and chemicals. This could lead to the identification of additional causes of these neoplasms and new opportunities for primary prevention.

NASOPHARYNGEAL CARCINOMAS

Nasopharyngeal carcinomas arise from the epithelium of the nasopharynx. Squamous cell, nonkeratinizing, and undifferentiated histologic types are recognized, but there is little evidence that they are of different etiologies, and they will be considered together in this discussion.

The striking feature of nasopharyngeal carcinoma is the marked variation in incidence rates among ethnic groups. The highest rates in the world have been recorded in the Chinese populations of California, Singapore, and Hawaii. Individuals in and from southern China are at particularly high risk. Other groups with unusually high rates include the Eskimos, Malays, native Hawaiians, and some populations in North Africa. Chinese in San Francisco and Eskimos in Alaska, respectively, have rates over 20 and over 12 times higher than rates of San Francisco whites.

In the Chinese, the incidence increases with age from about 15 until 50 years of age, and then declines. The decline after age 50 is not evident in low-risk countries such as Sweden, and in North Africa a bimodal distribution with an initial peak in early adulthood has been reported. In most areas, rates in males are about twice those in females.

The incidence rates in Chinese born in the United States are about half as great as the rates in the Chinese who immigrated, suggesting that environmental factors are at least partly responsible for the high rates in Chinese. Rates have remained stable over time in Chinese populations in Asia, which implies that these factors are deeply ingrained in Chinese culture.

The Epstein-Barr virus (EBV) has been implicated strongly as a cause of nasopharyngeal cancer. Antibodies against a variety of EBV antigens have been detected in serum from nearly 100 percent of cases tested, and also in nasopharyngeal washings. Serum antibody titers are elevated in approximately 85 percent of cases, and the levels increase with the extent and size of the tumor, and decline following treatment. Viral DNA has been demonstrated in the epithelial cells of tumors from many geographic areas. However, the distribution of EBV in human population does not correspond to the occurrence of nasopharyngeal carcinoma, and only a small proportion of infected individuals ultimately develop the tumor. Other environmental or genetic factors must also play an important etiologic role.

Of the many other environmental factors that have been studied, evidence is strongest for salted fish eaten by certain Chinese ethnic groups. Nitrosamines have been identified in samples of salted fish, and rats fed these fish have developed nasal and paranasal malignant disease. Case-control studies in Hong Kong and Malaysia have shown risk to be highest in individuals fed salted fish when weaned, and inversely related to the age at which a person first began eating these fish.

One small study in Kenya purported to show low levels of β-carotene in serum from cases of nasopharyngeal carcinoma, but this has not been confirmed elsewhere.

Some studies have found individuals who lived in poorly ventilated smoky rooms, or who were occupationally exposed to fumes, smoke, or chemicals, to be at increased risk, but the evidence for these associations is either meager or inconsistent among studies. Other studies have found more cases than controls with a prior history of previous nasal infections.

Genetic susceptibility to the carcinogenetic effect of the environmental factors is likely to play an important etiologic role. Studies of HLA antigens have shown nasopharyngeal carcinoma to be associated with an increased frequency of first locus antigen (HLA-2), and with a decreased frequency of the second locus antigen (SIN-2).

In summary, it appears reasonable to hypothesize that EBV may lead to nasopharyngeal infection in genetically susceptible individuals who have also been exposed at an early age to dietary carcinogens, perhaps nitrosamines in salted fish. The roles of inhaled carcinogens later in life and vitamin A deficiency are unclear.

Primary prevention should be directed toward high risk ethnic groups. Reduction of salted fish consumption, particularly by children, should be encouraged, as this is the only preventive measure currently available. A vaccine against EBV may provide the means to protect against this tumor in the future. If additional studies show beta carotene or retinol to be protective, dietary modification or supplementation with vitamin A-like substances may also be of value.

CARCINOMAS OF THE ORAL CAVITY AND PHARYNX

Carcinomas of the oral cavity and pharynx include those arising from the mucosa of the lips, tongue, mouth, oropharynx, and hypopharynx. They are predominately squamous cell, although adenocarcinomas and other rarer histologic types do occur. The occurrence of these tumors is largely dependent on the frequency of use of alcohol and tobacco products.

Estimates of the risk of oral and pharyngeal carcinomas in smokers compared to nonsmokers vary from close to one to over 10, and average about three. The relative risks are about the same for smokers of cigars, pipes, and cigarettes, except that the increase in risk of lip cancer is restricted largely to pipe smokers. In areas of the world where the lighted end of the cigarette is inserted into the mouth, oral cancers tend to develop on the hard palate.

A large number of studies of various designs have clearly shown rates of oral and pharyngeal cancers to be increased in those who drink alcoholic beverages, and risk tends to increase with the amount consumed. Distilled spirits, wine, and beer have all been implicated. It is not known whether alcohol acts independently to alter the risk of these neoplasms or only as a cofactor in the presence of other carcinogens. Some studies have shown smoking and alcohol to influence the risk of oral cancer independently, but others have found alcohol to either increase risk only in smokers or increase the risk to a greter extent in smokers than in nonsmokers, suggesting a synergistic effect of alcohol and tobacco smoke.

Use of snuff and chewing tobacco have both been implicated as causes of oral and pharyngeal cancers in the United States. Snuff is finely ground or powdered tobacco that is not chewed, but retained between the cheek or lip and lower gum. Snuff dipping, as this practice is called, is common among women in the southern United States, and studies of such women have clearly shown risks of oral and pharyngeal cancer to be increased in snuff dippers. The risk increases with the duration of use, and the cancers tend to occur where the snuff is habitually kept. In one study the risk of carcinomas of the buccal mucosa and gum was 50 times greater in snuff dippers than in nondippers.

Chewing tobacco is sold as solid plugs and in a more loosely packed form, both of which are both chewed and retained in the mouth. In the United States, chewing tobacco is used almost exclusively by men. Most men who chew also smoke, and it has therefore been difficult to study the separate effect of chewing tobacco on risk. Some studies show an independent effect of chewing tobacco, but others do not; and synergism between smoking and chewing tobacco has been reported.

In parts of Asia, oral cancers have been strongly linked to chewing pan (betel nut, slaked lime, tobacco, and other ingredients wrapped in a betel leaf) and nass (a mixture of tobacco, lime, ashes, oil, and other substances). It is likely that the tobacco in these substances is at least partly responsible for their carcinogenic effects, but the influence of other ingredients cannot be ruled out. Synergism between smoking and pan chewing has been reported.

Unlike tobacco smoke, which contains a large number of carcinogens, nitrosamines are the only carcinogenic substances that have been identified in unsmoked tobacco, and it is likely that these substances play a role in the genesis of oral and pharyngeal cancers.

Ill-fitting dentures and poor dentition have been related to oral cancers. Poor oral hygiene could therefore be of etiologic importance. Studies of the influence of oral bacteria on nitrosamine production in the mouth would be of interest. Mouth wash has been implicated as a cause of oral cancers in nonsmokers and nondrinkers. Either some mouth washes contain carcinogenic substances or frequent use of mouth wash is an indicator of poor oral hygiene.

Consumption of smoked meats and home-cured ham has been related to risk of oral and pharyngeal cancers in one study.[7] Such products could contain carcinogens from the smoke or potential precursors of nitrosamines such as amines and nitrites.

Two studies in India and Pakistan showed lower serum levels of vitamin A (retinol) and beta carotene in oral and pharyngeal cancer cases than in controls. Two dietary studies in the United States have shown risk of these cancers to be inversely related to consumption of foods rich in vitamin C and beta carotene (fresh fruits and vegetables). One also related risk to low intake of retinoids, whereas the other did not. Vitamin C can inhibit the formation of nitrosamines from amines and nitrites, beta carotene can quench singlet oxygen, and retinol can reverse oral leukoplakia and reduce tumor production in animal models. There is thus ample reason to suspect that dietary factors can alter the risk of oral and pharyngeal carcinomas.

It has been estimated that approximately 75 percent of all cancers of the mouth and pharynx in American men are due to use of tobacco and alcohol. The proportion for women may be smaller, although in areas where snuff dipping is practiced, most of the tumors in women are probably due to this practice. Cessation of use of tobacco in all of its forms and reduction in use of alcohol, especially in those who use tobacco, are obvious preventive measures that would have a large impact on risk of these neoplasms.

CARCINOMAS OF THE ESOPHAGUS

Over 95 percent of all carcinomas that arise from the esophageal epthelium are squamous cell. A striking feature of esophageal carcinomas is the marked geographic and ethnic variation in incidence rates. High-risk groups and areas include blacks in southern and eastern Africa and the United States, Indians in Bombay, some Latin American countries, and a large portion of Asia extending from Turkey in the east, across northern Iran and Afghanistan and the Asian Soviet Republics, to Mongolia, parts of China, and parts of Japan. Even within relatively small areas, such

as the Transkei in southern Africa, the Caspian Littoral in Iran, and Brittany in France, large differences in incidence exist. In the United States, the ratio of black to white rates is approximately four for males and three for females.

Rates are usually higher in men than in women. In the United States the sex ratio is about 3. The sex ratio tends to be lower in high-risk areas. The incidence rates increase markedly with age in all areas. In the United States, rates in blacks have increased in succeeding birth cohorts.

In the United States and other Western countries, use of tobacco and alcohol is a strong determinant of risk. Many studies clearly show risk to increase with the number of cigarettes and the grams of alcohol consumed per day. Other forms of smoked tobacco also increase risk. One study showed risk in nonsmokers to be related to alcohol consumption, and risk in nondrinkers to be related to amount smoked.[9] Alcohol thus exerts an influence on risk in the absence of smoking, and vice versa. The effect of these two factors has been shown to be multiplicative in some studies, with risks in heavy smokers and drinkers over 100 times greater than in persons who consume little or no alcohol or tobacco. Experimental studies have shown alcohol to enhance the penetration of the esophageal mucosa of the rat by benz(a)pyrene. The amount of penetration increased with the concentration of alcohol used. Alcohol could similarly enhance absorption of carcinogens in tobacco smoke in humans. Distilled spirits have been more strongly related to risk of esophageal cancer than beer or wine, but most studies show all forms of alcohol to exert some influence on risk. In some parts of the world, esophageal carcinomas may be caused by contamination, by nitrosamines or other carcinogens, of home-brewed drinks such as maize beer in parts of Africa and rum in Puerto Rico, but evidence for this is weak. Pan chewing, with or without tobacco, may enhance risk in India, and chewing the residue in pipes used for smoking tobacco in Transkei and opium in Iran have been causally implicated. These residues contain mutagenic substances.

Estimates of the proportion of esophageal cancers attributable to alcohol and tobacco in North America and Western Europe range to over 90 percent. However, in some high-risk parts of the world, such as northern Iran where alcohol consumption is proscribed by Muslim law and cigarette smoking is rare, nearly all of the esophageal carcinomas must be due to other factors.

Hot tea and tea gruel have been related to risk of esophageal cancer and, like alcohol, could act as solvents for carcinogens. Alcohol and hot beverages could also act as chronic irritants to the esophageal mucosa.

A number of dietary deficiencies have been related to risk of esophageal cancer. Sideropenic dysphagia (Plummer-Vinson or Paterson-Kelly syndrome) was formerly common in parts of Europe, particularly in women, and was associated with subsequent development of esophageal carcinomas. This syndrome, although related to iron deficiency, probably is a result of other deficiencies as well, including vitamin C and riboflavin.

Dietary studies in Puerto Rico and several countries of Asia have shown individuals in high-risk areas to consume diets poor in riboflavin and in vitamins A and C. Five case-control studies in the United States[8] and studies of similar design in France, Japan, and Iran have also consistently shown risk to be related to low intake of fresh fruits and vegetables (sources of beta carotene and vitamin C). Some of these studies have also found inverse relationships between risk and intake of dairy products and fresh meat (sources of retinol), thiamin, and riboflavin. One study in China found lower levels of zinc in hair and blood specimens from cases than from controls. Levels of many of these dietary substances are highly correlated in normal diets, and it is not currently possible to determine exactly which deficiency or combination of deficiencies predisposes to esophageal cancer. Reasonable biologic explanations for all appear in the literature.

It has been hypothesized that these dietary deficiencies lead to atrophic changes in the esophageal mucosa, that hot drinks and strong alcoholic beverages further insult the tissues and serve as solvents for carcinogens, and that the carcinogens from tobacco, opium residue, or other unknown sources then can penetrate to the basal epithelial cells from which the carcinomas arise. Considerable additional research needs to be conducted to test and clarify elements of this hypothesis.

In the United States, the primary prevention of most esophageal carcinomas could be effected by cessation of smoking, reduction of alcohol consumption, especially of distilled beverages, and maintenance of a diet adequate in fresh fruits and vegetables, and possibly meats and dairy products.

LARYNGEAL CARCINOMAS

Nearly all carcinomas of the larynx are squamous cell. Approximately 40 percent arise from the supraglottic portion of the larynx, i.e., superior to the true vocal cords. Nearly all of the rest are glottic and arise from the true vocal cords. Only about 1 percent are subglottic in origin. Rates in the United States are 6.5 times higher in men than in women, and increse markedly with age in both sexes.

Smoking and alcohol consumption are the major factors that determine the pattern of occurrence of laryngeal cancer.[10] Risk in cigarette smokers relative to nonsmokers (uncorrected for alcohol consumption) varied from 6.1 to 13.6 in eight large prospective studies, and risk has consistently been shown to increase with the number of cigarettes smoked. Smokers of pipes and cigars are also at increased risk; and relative risks for smokers of these forms of smoked tobacco are nearly as great as those for cigarette smokers. A study in India found risk of laryngeal cancer to be increased in men who chewed tobacco (RR = 4.6) as well as in those who smoked cigarettes (RR = 7.7); in men who habitually did both, the relative risk was over 20.

Most studies show an increase in risk of laryngeal cancer with the amount of alcohol consumed per day; and at least four case-control studies have shown a synergistic effect of alcohol and smoking on risk. Alcohol definitely increases the risk in smokers. There is limited evidence that it does not do so in nonsmokers, but additional research is needed to clarify this point. One study found that tumors in heavy drinkers more frequently developed in the supraglottic region of the larynx, which is the portion that comes in direct contact with imbibed alcohol. Unfortunately, few other investigations have reported findings separately for supraglottic and glottic tumors.

In areas where cigarette smoking is common and rates of lung cancer are high, the ratio of lung to laryngeal cancer rates is relatively high. Conversely, in areas where unsmoked tobacco is commonly used and oral cancer rates are high, the ratio of lung to laryngeal cancer rates is lower. Since lung cancer is related to smoking, but not to alcohol, these observations also suggest that a portion of laryngeal cancer is due to alcohol or to other factors that influence the risk of oral, but not lung, cancers. Additional evidence that the laryngeal cancers with an etiology similar to that of oral cancer tend to be supraglottic is provided by the observation that second primary cancer of the mouth and pharynx, and also esophagus, occur much more frequently in laryngeal cancer cases with supraglottic lesions than in those with glottic lesions.

It thus seems reasonable to conclude that carcinomas of the supraglottic region are etiologically similar to oral and pharyngeal cancers, whereas carcinomas of the glottic region are etiologically more like lung cancer. Additional investigations are needed to further clarify the epidemiologic and etiologic features of tumors arising from these two regions of the larynx.

In most western countries, lung cancer rates have increased markedly during this century as consumption of tobacco has increased, but laryngeal cancer rates have tended to change little until recent years. Time trends in rates of laryngeal cancer in England, Australia, and France have been shown to correspond to changing patterns of alcohol consumption and (in England and Australia) use of chewing tobacco. A decline in use of chewing tobacco and distilled spirits, until relatively recently, probably countered the effect of the increasing use of cigarettes.

The only other known or suspected causes of laryngeal cancer are occupational exposures. Increased risk has been documented in mustard gas manufacturers, individuals exposed to isopropyl oil used in the production of propanol, and persons exposed to diethyl sulfate used in making ethanol. Asbestos workers may also be at increased risk, but this association has

TABLE 2 Summary of Opportunities for Primary Prevention of Cancers of the Upper Respiratory and Digestive Systems in the United States

Site	% in US due to tobacco and alcohol	Evidence for effect of vitamin deficiency*	Dietary excess implicated	Occupational exposures implicated
Nasal cavity and paranasal sinuses	< 1%	non-existent	none	yes
Nasopharynx	0%	weak for beta carotene	salted fish	no (?)
Buccal cavity and pharynx	75%	moderate	? smoked and cured meats	no
Esophagus	85%	strong	hot tea and tea gruel	no
Larynx	75%	moderate	none	yes

*Including fresh fruits and vegetables, vitamin A, beta carotene, victamin C, and riboflavin.

not been observed consistently in all studies of asbestos workers. It is likely that occupational exposures account for only a very small proportion of all laryngeal carcinomas.

One case-control study has found risk of laryngeal cancer to be related to a low consumption of fresh vegetables rich in vitamin C and beta carotene. The protective effect of these micronutrients in individuals exposed to tobacco and alcohol should be evaluated further.

Although firm estimates of the proportion of all laryngeal cancers in the United States that are due to alcohol and tobacco are not available, 75 percent is probably a conservative figure. Discontinuance of tobacco use and reduction of alcohol consumption (especially in smokers) would thus prevent most laryngeal cancers. A diet rich in fresh fruits and vegetables might be of additional benefit.

SUMMARY AND OPPORTUNITIES FOR PRIMARY PREVENTION

Current opportunities for primary prevention include reduction of use of tobacco and alcohol, dietary modification, and control of occupational exposures. As summarized in Table 2, probably three-quarters of all carcinomas of the buccal cavity, pharynx, and larynx, and an even higher proportion of esophageal cancer in the United States are due to use of tobacco and alcohol.[2] Since the effect of alcohol on risk of these cancers is probably small in the absence of tobacco, but the effect of tobacco is large even without alcohol, by far the most important preventive measure to be taken is cessation of use of all forms of tobacco. Use of alcohol only in moderation, or not at all, would also be of some additional benefit, particularly in those who continue to smoke.

All of the cancers considered except those of the nasal cavity and paranasal sinuses have been related either to low intake of fresh fruits and vegetables, or low serum or consumption levels of one or more of the following: beta carotene, vitamin A, vitamin C, or riboflavin. Amounts of these substances and other micronutrients are often highly correlated in American diets, and it is not currently possible to determine which specific deficiencies or combinations of deficiencies, if any, predispose to any neoplasm. However, the bulk of the evidence currently available suggests that it would be beneficial to encourage more consumption of fresh fruits and vegetables. This would certainly do no harm. There is not sufficient evidence to warrant taking commercial vitamin preparations to prevent cancer, and use of these products for this purpose should be restricted to controlled clinical trials until results of such experiments are available.

The remaining possibilities for primary prevention are not likely to have a large impact on the occurrence in the United States of any of the cancers under consideration, although selected measures directed toward high-risk populations may be beneficial in some situations. These include reduction of salted fish consumption in Chinese immigrants and their descendents, perhaps reduction in use of smoked and home-cured meats in rural areas of the South, and reduction of implicated exposures in selected industries.

It must be emphasized, however, that in the United States, over two-thirds of all of the tumors of the head and neck of the type that have been considered in this presentation would not occur if tobacco products were no longer used. Therefore, the bulk of our efforts to prevent these cancers should be directed against the use of tobacco in all of its forms.

REFERENCES

1. Schoffenfeld D, Fraumeni JF Jr, eds. Cancer epidemiology and prevention. Philadelphia: WB Saunders, 1982, Chapters 7, 8, 15, 16, 20, 23, 29, 30, 31, 33, and 34.
2. Rothman KJ. The proportion of cancer attributable to alcohol consumption. Prev Med 1980; 9:174–179.
3. Willett WC, MacMahon B. Diet and cancer—an overview (First of two parts). N Engl J Med 1984; 310:633–638.
4. Willett WC, MacMahon B. Diet and cancer—an overview (Second of two parts). N Engl J Med 1984; 310:697–701.
5. Graham S. Results of case-control studies of diet and cancer in Buffalo, NY. Cancer Res 1983; 43(Suppl):2409s–2413s.
6. Roush GC. Epidemiology of cancer of the nose and paranasal sinuses: current concepts. Head Neck Surg 1979; 2:3–11.

7. Winn DM, Ziegler RG, Pickle LW, Gridley G, Blot WJ, Hoover RN. Diet in the etiology of oral and pharyngeal cancer among women from the southern United States. Cancer Res 1984; 44:1216–1222.

8. Ziegler RG, Morris LE, Blot WJ, Pottern LM, Hoover RN, Fraumeni JF Jr. Esophageal cancer among black men in Washington, D.C. II. Role of nutrition. JNCI 1981; 67:1199–1206.

9. Tuyns AJ. Oesophageal cancer in non-smoking drinkers and in non-drinking smokers. Int J Canc 1983; 32:443–444.

10. Rothman KJ, Cann CI, Flanders D, et al. Epidemiology of laryngeal cancer. Epidemiol Rev 1980; 2:195–209.

PREVENTION OF HEAD AND NECK CANCER: LEADS FROM LABORATORY RESEARCH

WILLIAM D. DeWYS, M.D.

Numerous studies in animal models support the hypothesis that the development of cancers of epidermoid tissues can be modulated or prevented under the influence of certain specific chemicals. Relevant studies include those showing an increased incidence of cancer in the presence of a nutrient deficiency, a decreased incidence of cancers in the presence of an excess of a specific nutrient, and a decreased incidence of cancers in the presence of synthetic analogs which may or may not retain the normal physiologic effects of the parent compound.

ILLUSTRATIVE EXAMPLES OF CHEMOPREVENTION

A representative example of a study showing an increased incidence of cancer in the oral cavity in the presence of a nutrient deficiency was reported by Rowe and Gorlin.[1] In their study, oraal cancers were induced in golden hamsters by the carcinogen 7, 12-dimenthyl-1,2-benzanthracene dissolved in liquid solution and applied with a cotton swab to the left cheek pouch. In hamsters receiving a nutritionally adequate diet, 33 percent (9/27) developed oral cancers. In contrast, in a group of hamsters receiving a diet that was deficient in vitamin A, 59 percent (16/27) developed oral cancer. Because the group receiving the vitamin A-deficient diet lost weight, a pair-fed group was included in this study to monitor the effect of weight loss per se on the incidence of cancer. Weight loss tends to reduce the incidence of cancer (25% incidence in the pair-fed, vitamin A-adequate group), thus making the increased incidence in the vitamin A-deficient group even more significant.

A representative example of studies of the effect of vitamin A supplementation on carcinogenesis of an epithelial surface is a study reported by Saffiotti et al.[2] These investigatorsused a tracheal instillation of benzo(a) pyrene to induce lung cancers. In a group receiving an adequate diet, lung tumors developed in 32 percent (17/53) of the Syrian golden hamsters. In a group receiving supplemental amounts of vitamin A, the incidence of lung tumors was reduced to 11 percent (5/46). The contrast between the two groups was even more striking when the effect on squamous cell cancers was evaluated. In the adequate diet group, 21 percent (11/53) developed squamous cell cancers compared to a 2 percent (1/46) incidence of squamous cell cancers in the vitamin A supplemented group.

A similar pattern in humans for vitamin A having a protective effect, especially for the development of squamous cell cancers, has recently been reported.[3] In this epidemiologic study, a group of humans with a high vitamin A intake had about one-fourth as many squamous cell lung cancers as did a group having a low intake of vitamin A. A weaker protective effect was seen for small cell lung cancer, and there was no protective effect for other cell types.

The effects of vitamin A and analogs of vitamin A on carcinogenesis in animal models has recently been reviewed by Hill and Grubbs.[4] They catalogued cancer-preventive effects for a spectrum of anatomic sites. Their review may be summarized by noting the number of studies showing positive results (preventive effects) compared to the total number of studies reported as follows: skin 10/11, bladder 8/10, breast 7/9, lung 5/10, esophagus 1/1, cervix 1/1, colon 1/3, and salivary glands 1/1. These protective or preventive effects were seen with native vitamin A as well as with synthetic analogs of vitamin A having less toxicity than native vitamin A.[4]

PRINCIPLES OF CHEMOPREVENTION

Experiments in animals collectively establish a series of principles that should be considered in human application of these results (Table 1). The route of administration may not be important. Protective effects have been seen with administration in the drinking water, administration in food or with topical ap-

TABLE 1 General Principles Derived from Studies of Chemopreventive Effects of Retinoids in Experimental Animals

Route of administration is not important
Retinoids must be given after carcinogen
Continued treatment is necessary
A spectrum af analogs may be effective
The effect is dose-dependent
The preventive effect may be overwhelmed by large doses of carcinogens

plication (skin cancer prevention). The timing is important in that the retinoid must be given after the administration of the carcinogen in order to demonstrate maximum effectiveness. This suggests that vitamin A and its analogs have their predominant effect on the promotional phase of carcinogenesis rather than on the initiation phase (see my introduction to this group of chapters).

Another principle is that continued treatment is necessary for optimal preventive effects. Short-term treatments may delay the appearance of cancer, but long-term continuous treatment is needed to maximally reduce the incidence of cancer. The preventive effect is dependent on the dose of vitamin A administered up to and including toxic doses of vitamin A. Because vitamin A is toxic in high doses, an important research area has been the synthesis of vitamin A analogs having the cancer preventive effects of vitamin A but a reduced incidence of toxicity. This research has generated a spectrum of analogs some of which have greater protective effects than native vitamin A while having a reduced potential for toxicity. Some of these analogs may have their greatest effect on one anatomic site; others may have a greater effect on other sites. In part, these differences in therapeutic index and site of effect may be attributable to differences in tissue distribution of the analogs. An analog that concentrates in body fat may be protecive against mammary carcinogenesis, whereas a water-soluble analog may protect against bladder carcinogenesis.

Finally, the preventive effect may be influenced by the dose of the carcinogen. The preventive effect may be most striking against low or moderate doses of carcinogen, but large doses of a carcinogen may overwhelm the preventive effect of the retinoid. This observation may be relevant to human studies. For example, if we were to study the ability of a retinoid to prevent cancer in smokers, we should not limit our study to the heaviest smokers who have smoked for a very long time. Their heavy dose of carcinogen might overwhelm any protective effect. We should also include in such a study persons who were moderately heavy smokers for shorter periods of time so as to provide a fair test of the potential preventive agent.

POSSIBLE MECHANISMS OF EFFECT IN CANCER PREVENTION

Laboratory research has contributed significantly to our understanding of the process of carcinogenesis and to our understanding of possible mechanisms of cancer prevention (Table 2). Carcinogenesis is considered to have at least two distinct stages—initiation and promotion. Recently, several investigators have subdivided the promotion stage into two substages— early promotion and late promotion.

Cancer preventive agents may have effects that counter initiation, for example, the effects of beta carotene, the provitamin form of vitamin A. Beta carotene has the ability to quench singlet oxygen. For-

TABLE 2 Possible Mechanisms of Effect in Cancer Prevention

Anti-initiation
Antipromotion
   Ornithine decarboxylase inhibition
   Direct antipromoter effects
   Growth factor inhibition
Immunologic alterations
Cell membrane effects (contact inhibition)
Effects on cellular differentiation (steroid hormone-like effects)

mation of singlet oxygen may be an important step leading to damaged DNA in chemical or radiation carcinogenesis. Beta carotene, by scavenging this singlet oxygen, may prevent DNA damage and thus prevent initiation of carcinogenesis.

There are several proposed mechanisms by which preventive agents may counter the promotion phase of carcinogenesis. Chemicals may have direct antagonistic effects against promoting chemicals, for example, by competitively binding to the cellular binding site for the promoting agent. A second possible antipromotion mechanism may be antagonism of ornithine decarboxylase. This enzyme increases dramatically in cells during the promotion phase of carcinogenesis. Chemicals that inhibit this enzyme have antipromotion effects. A third possible antipromotion mechanism is inhibition of growth-stimulating factors. During promotion, cells elaborate factors that stimulate growth of cells. These growth factors may be autocrine (i.e., a cell stimulates itself to grow) or paracrine (i.e., a cell stimulates cells surrounding it to grow). Receptors exist on cell surfaces for binding of these growth factors. An antipromoting chemical may counter these growth factors either by inhibiting their formation or by binding to their receptors to inhibit their action.

Another possible cancer preventive mechanism is the immune system. Cancers often elicit a weak reaction of the immune system. Theoretically, if this immune reaction could be strengthened while the tumor is still microscopic in size, the development of a clinically detectable cancer could be prevented.

Still another possible mechanism of cancer prevention is via effects on cell membranes. When normal cells are grown in tissue culture, their growth stops when the glass surface in the tissue culture vessel is fully covered. This process is called contact inhibition. The in vivo correlate of this is the orderly arrangement of normal cells along epithelial surfaces. In contrast, the growth of malignant cells is not controlled by contact inhibition. In tissue culture they continue to grow, forming a population several layers thick along a glass surface. The in vivo correlate is the disorderly piling up of malignant cells on epithelial surfaces. If a chemical could restore the property of contact inhibition to malignant cells, disorderly growth could be made orderly and the cells would appear to be normal cells.

A chemical may directly affect cellular differentiation via a steroid hormone-like effect. This involves binding to a specific receptor on the cell surface followed by transport to the cell nucleus. There, specific biochemical effects occur which may result in alterations in protein synthesis and change of the cell to a differentiated phenotype.

In conclusion, much has been learned in laboratory research which can now be applied in efforts to prevent human cancer. Laboratory research has confirmed information from epidemiologic studies regarding possible risk factors and possible preventive factors in carcinogenesis. Laboratory research has elucidated a series of principles which must guide the formulation of human prevention research. Laboratory research has also elucidated possible mechanisms for cancer prevention which will assist us in monitoring and interpreting prevention studies in humans.

REFERENCES

1. Rowe NH, Gorlin RJ. The effect of vitamin A deficiency upon experimental oral carcinogenesis. J Dent Res 1959; 38:72–83.
2. Saffiotti U, Montesano R, Sellakumar AR, Borg SA. Experimental cancer of the lung: inhibition by vitamin A of the induction of tracheobronchial squamous metaplasis and squamous cell tumors. Cancer 1967; 20:857–864.
3. Kvale G, Bjelke E, Gart J. Dietary habits and lung cancer risk. Int J Cancer 1983; 31:397–405.
4. Hill DL, Grubbs CJ. Retinoids as chemopreventive and anticancer agents in intact animals. Anticancer Res 1982; 2:111–124. (Review)

USE OF THE MICRONUCLEUS TEST TO TRACE THE PROGRESS OF INTERVENTION STUDIES WITH CAROTENOIDS ON POPULATION GROUPS AT HIGH RISK FOR ORAL CANCER

HANS F. STICH, Ph.D.
MIRIAM P. ROSIN, Ph.D.

The removal of carcinogens from man's environment would appear to be the simplest and most direct way to reduce hazardous exposure. However, this approach is unrealistic if the carcinogenic mixture is part of a regular diet, provides pleasure, or has a ritualistic significance. In such cases, chemoprevention should be applied with the aim of either trapping the carcinogens before they can induce cellular changes or inhibiting the formation of preneoplastic colonies from which neoplastically transformed cells could arise.

SELECTION OF END POINTS

To avoid confusion, intervention programs should be placed into three categories which apply different methodology and seek different responses. (1) Chemopreventive agents are applied to cancer patients who have had a primary cancer removed. The recurrence of carcinomas in such patients would be used as an end point to reveal the success of the treatment. (2) Chemopreventive agents are applied to patients with well-defined preneoplastic lesions to suppress a progression toward benign or malignant tumors. For example, changes in leukoplakias within the oral cavity,[1,2] bronchial metaplasia in smokers,[3] and esophageal dysplasias[4] have been successfully used as end points. (3) Chemopreventive agents are applied to population groups which are exposed to chemical or physical carcinogens, but which do not show any detectable clinical signs of preneoplastic or neoplastic lesions. In the first and second cases, tissues may already contain transformed cells or cells irreversibly programmed for transformation. Thus a chemopreventive regimen would aim to alter the behavior of an already committed cell. The third approach aims to trap or inactivate carcinogens before they can either enter the target cells or react with target molecules. In this case, chemopreventive agents must be applied to large numbers of people at elevated risk for cancer over periods of extensive exposure to carcinogenic agents.

If the aim of a chemopreventive regimen is to prevent cells from becoming committed to neoplastic transformation, the treatment must be done in the early stages of carcinogenesis at the time of exposure to carcinogens. Reliable markers which can quantitate exposure of a tissue to carcinogens or promoters had to be found to estimate the efficacy of a chemopreventive regimen. The use of exfoliated cells would have many advantages. Since these cells can be readily obtained by noninvasive procedures, large population groups can be screened and placed on intervention trials.[5] As markers suitable to quantitate exposure patterns, one could consider the frequency of micronuclei,[5,6] immunofluorescent localization of DNA adducts,[7] and the ^{32}P postlabeling technique for known as well as unknown DNA adducts.[8]

These studies were supported by the National Cancer Institute of Canada. Dr. H.F. Stich is a Research Associate of the National Cancer Institute of Canada. Dr. M.P. Rosin is a staff member of the British Columbia Cancer Foundation of Vancouver, B.C.

SELECTION OF POPULATION GROUPS AT ELEVATED CANCER RISK

An easy identification of the population group at elevated risk for cancer appears to be a prerequisite for any intervention program. Such groups can frequently be recognized by their particular habits (e.g., chewing tobacco), physical changes (e.g., red mouth of betel quid chewers), or clinical symptoms (e.g., blood in the urine of *Schistosoma haematobium* infected individuals). In many instances, the cancer sites can be correlated to particular customs. Khaini chewers place the carcinogenic tobacco/lime mixture within the lower gingival groove, some betel quid chewers prefer to keep the pan at the right or left side of the oral cavity, users of nass keep the tobacco/lime/cotton oil mixture under the tongue, snuff dippers may place the tobacco in the oral vestibule between the gum and cheek, and inverted smokers (chutta smokers in India, the Philippines, or several regions of Africa) keep the burning end of their cigars close to the palate and upper surface of the tongue. In each of these cases, carcinomas develop preferentially at the site that is in closest contact with the carcinogenic mixtures. Obviously, any cell marker that is to be used to measure the progress of an intervention trial must be applicable to the site of the oral cavity from which carcinomas are most likely to develop.[6]

SELECTION OF A CHEMOPREVENTIVE PROTOCOL

There are several ways to reach a decision with regard to the most promising chemopreventive protocol. One could rely on animal models. However, the metabolism and vitamin requirements of animals differ greatly from those of man. Epidemiologic evidence from human population groups points to the consumption of fruits or green/yellow vegetables as being inversely related to the incidence of cancer at several sites.[9] Unfortunately, the resolution of most epidemiologic studies is not fine enough to uncover the chemicals involved in the inhibition of carcinogenesis. One can base the choice of anticarcinogenic agents on the type of vitamin or trace element deficiencies that occur in a population group. This approach is based on the assumption that a particular deficiency is actually associated with the development of a cancer. Finally, one could simulate in vitro the conditions prevailing in vivo and use in vitro systems in the search for the most active chemopreventive agents.

The most troublesome feature of chemoprevention is a shocking lack of knowledge about the initiators of carcinogenesis and the nature of promoters involved in the etiology of human cancers. Since one does not know the solubility characteristics of the carcinogens and promoters, it becomes difficult to decide between polar and nonpolar scavengers. Also unresolved is the issue whether efforts should be directed to trap the carcinogen and scavenge the free radicals *before* they can interact with cellular target molecules, or whether one should concentrate on agents that may protect by, for example, affecting repair mechanisms or controlling gene regulation, *after* a carcinogen-DNA bond (or methylation) has been established.

CHEMOPREVENTIVE APPLICATION OF A VITAMIN REGIMEN TO BETEL QUID CHEWERS

To learn about the usefulness of the micronucleus test as a tool to follow the progress of an intervention program, several pilot trials were conducted. Betel quid chewers were selected since they met several prerequisites. Epidemiologic evidence points to a quantitative relationship between the incidence of oral carcinomas and the extent of chewing betel quid.[10] The examined betel quid chewers in India[11] and the Philippines[5] had elevated frequencies of micronucleated buccal mucosa cells. Increases as high as 15-fold over those found in the nonchewing population were observed. Exfoliated cells can be readily obtained from the sites at which betel quid is in close contact with the oral epithelium. The formation of micronucleated buccal mucosa cells is probably due to the strong clastogenicity of the saliva of betel quid chewers.[12] The chemistry of the clastogenic agents and their synergistic effects are known, at least in part. Thus the frequencies of micronuclei in exfoliated cells from various sites of the buccal mucosa are a good indicator of exposure to the carcinogenic betel quid, and should also respond to the application of successful chemopreventive agents.

Vitamin A and beta-carotene appear to be the most promising chemopreventive agents in protecting the mucosa of the oral cavity and esophagus. The use of beta-carotene would be particularly attractive since it is virtually nontoxic and obtainable from several dietary sources.[13] Interest in vitamin A as a chemopreventive agent is based on the observations that the vitamin preserves the integrity of epithelial tissues, that vitamin A-deficient rodents show an increased susceptibility to the induction of cancer,[14] and that the administration of vitamin A and retinoic acid analogs has been found to reduce the incidence of chemically induced rodent and human cancers.[15,16] Additional support comes from epidemiologic studies, which point to a relationship between a deficient intake of vegetable-derived carotenoids and elevated risks for carcinomas of the bladder,[17] lung,[18] stomach,[9] and larynx.[19] In connection with our objectives, the link between low plasma carotene levels and increased incidence of oral cancers is of particular interest.[20]

The volunteers who belonged to the hill tribe, Ifugaos (Philippines), were daily chewers of betel quid which, as a rule, consisted of one-quarter of a fresh areca nut (*Areca catechu*), part of a betel leaf (*Piper betle*), lime, and dried tobacco leaves. The number of quids chewed per day varied from 4 to 15. One capsule of vitamin A (50,000 units) and three capsules of beta-carotene (total, 150,000 units) were administered twice weekly. Exfoliated oral mucosal cells were sampled prior to the onset of the vitamin regimen, once a month throughout the trial and once a month after cessation of the vitamin treatment (for more detailed information, see Stich et al[5]). The results are shown in Figures 1 and 2. Following the twice-weekly administration of vitamin A and beta-carotene over a 3-month period, the frequencies of micronucleated

mucosa cells were greatly reduced in both buccal sides of 30 individuals (Fig. 1A) and in only one buccal side of three persons (Fig. 1B). Three chewers did not respond to the intervention regimen within the 3-month period. The protective effect seems to be maintained for at least 3 months after cessation of the vitamin regimen.

The administration of a vitamin cocktail can create a dilemma. On the one hand, the chance of obtaining a positive response is obviously higher with a mixture of several chemopreventive agents than that obtained following administration of a single compound. On the other hand, the cocktail approach has two serious drawbacks. First, it does not reveal the compound with the most effective chemopreventive effect. Second, an ethics issue could be raised if a successful application of a mixture is followed by trials using individual chemicals whose efficiency is unknown. In our pilot study, we compared the response of the oral mucosa of betel quid chewers (Philippines) to the vitamin A/beta-carotene mixture, beta-carotene which changes into vitamin A, and canthaxanthin (4,4'-diketo-beta-carotene), which shows a good protective effect against photosensitization[21] and against UV- (or DMBA + UV) induced tumors in mice,[22] but which cannot be converted to vitamin A. The results clearly show that vitamin A and beta-carotene reduce the frequencies of micronucleated buccal mucosa cells among betel quid chewers, whereas canthaxanthin has no detectable effect at the dose used (Fig. 2).

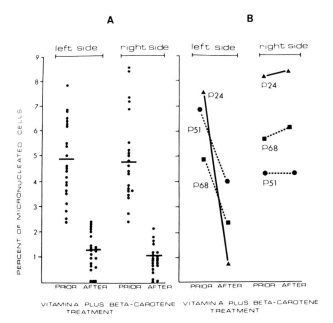

Figure 1 *A,* Reduced frequencies of micronucleated buccal mucosa cells of the left and right side of 30 betel nut/tobacco chewers prior to and after administration of vitamin A/beta-carotene. Bars show averages. For both the left and right buccal mucosa, the mean frequency of micronucleated cells after the 3-month treatment period was significantly different from the mean frequency prior to treatment (P<0.001). *B,* The different responses between the left and right sides of the buccal mucosa of 3 treated individuals.

OUTLOOK

Undoubtedly, the application of chemopreventive agents that are naturally occurring or have already been approved as food additives by regulatory agencies to groups at elevated risk for cancer of the oral cavity is a highly promising approach. However, some issues remain unresolved and others require improvement. For example, the precise relationship between the frequency of micronucleated mucosa cells and the incidence of oral leukoplakias or carcinomas is still unknown. One could argue that the formation of abnormal chromosome complements which prevail in oral and esophageal carcinomas requires years of random chromatid breakages and the reshuffling of chromatid segments. If these chromatid translocations result in a transposition of oncogenes followed by their activation,[23] one could conceivably see a causal relationship between the frequency of micronuclei, which are a by-product of this reshuffling process, and the risk of developing a neoplastically transformed cell.

The scoring procedures require improvement and adaptation to examine the large numbers of subjects that are desirable in any intervention trial. The current practice of screening hundreds of slides of exfoliated cells for micronuclei is time-consuming. Similarly, the quantitation of immunofluorescence in individual nuclei or cells stained with immunofluorescent antibodies against DNA adducts requires time and man-

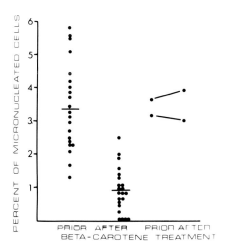

Figure 2 Reduced frequencies of micronucleated buccal mucosa cells of the right cheek of 22 betel nut/tobacco chewers prior to and after administration of beta-carotene (150,000 IU) twice weekly for 9 weeks. Two individuals did not respond to the treatment.

TABLE 1 Analysis of Micronucleated Cells in a Pooled Sample of Exfoliated Cells from the Palate of 20 Betel Nut/Tobacco Chewers

	% Frequency of Micronucleated Cells	
Type of Analysis	Individual Cases	Average
Each smear was examined	3.7, 5.4, 3.2, 2.0, 3.6, 3.3, 4.2, 3.3, 3.0, 6.3, 5.1, 3.6, 6.4, 6.2, 4.4, 5.5, 3.7, 7.2, 4.9	4.5
Cells of all cases were pooled and one smear analyzed	—	4.7

power. This technical difficulty could be overcome by pooling cell samples taken from individuals. From the pooled sample, cells can be withdrawn, smeared on one slide, stained, and screened for micronuclei or fluorescence-labeled nuclei. The prerequisites are that the numbers of cells taken for pooling from different samples are comparable and that a thorough mixing of the pooled cells occurs. The validity of the pooling procedure can be seen in Table 1, which compares the arithmetic average of scores on buccal smears of 20 chewers with the results obtained from one slide after the exfoliated cells from the same 20 individuals have been pooled.

In summary, one can state that the application of the micronucleus test to exfoliated cells will provide information on the genotoxic damage induced by carcinogens and carcinogenic mixtures in the tissue from which carcinomas arise, and can be used to estimate the response of carcinogen-exposed tissues to chemopreventive agents.

REFERENCES

1. Ryssel HJ, Brunner KW, Bollag W. Die perorale Anwendung von Vitamin-A-Säure bei Leukoplakien, Hyperkeratosen und Blattenepithelkarzinomen: Ergebnisse und Verträglichkeit. Schweiz Med Wschr 1971; 101:1027–1030.
2. Koch HF. Biochemical treatment of precancerous oral lesions: the effectiveness of various analogues of retinoic acid. J Maxillofac Surg 1978; 6:59–63.
3. Gouveia J, Hercend T, Lemaigre G, Mathé G, Gros F, Santelli G, Homasson JP, Angebault M, Lededente A, Parrot R, Gaillard JP, Bonniot JP, Marsac J, Pretet S. Degree of bronchial metaplasia in heavy smokers and its regression after treatment with a retinoid. Lancet 1982; 1:710–712.
4. Munoz N. IARC Annual Report, International Agency for Research on Cancer, Lyon, France, 1982.
5. Stich HF, Rosin MP, Vallejera MO. Reduction with vitamin A and beta-carotene administration of proportion of micronucleated buccal mucosal cells in Asian betel nut and tobacco chewers. Lancet 1984, 1:1204–1206.
6. Stich HF, Rosin MP. Micronuclei in exfoliated human cells as an internal dosimeter for exposures to carcinogens. In: Stich HF, ed. Carcinogens and mutagens in the environment. Vol. II. Naturally occurring compounds: Endogenous formation and modulation. Boca Raton: CRC Press, 1983; 17.
7. Poirier MC, Santella R, Weinstein IB, Grunberger D, Yuspa SH. Quantitation of benzo(a)pyrene-deoxyguanosine adducts by radioimmunoassay. Cancer Res 1980, 40:412–416.
8. Gupta RC, Reddy MV, Randerath K. ^{32}P-Postlabelling analysis of nonradioactive aromatic carcinogen-DNA adducts. Carcinogenesis 1982; 3:1081–1092.
9. Hirayama T. Epidemiology of human carcinogenesis: a review of food-related diseases. In: Stich HF, ed. Carcinogens and mutagens in the environment. Vol. I. Food products. Boca Raton: CRC Press, 1982; 13.
10. Hirayama T. An epidemiological study of oral and pharyngeal cancer in Central and Southeast Asia. Bull WHO 1966; 34:41–69.
11. Stich HF, Stich W, Parida BB. Elevated frequency of micronucleated cells in the buccal mucosa of individuals at high risk for oral cancer: betel quid chewers. Cancer Lett 1982; 17:125–134.
12. Stich HF, Stich W. Chromosome-damaging activity of saliva of betel nut and tobacco chewers. Cancer Lett 1982; 15:193–202.
13. Peto R, Doll R, Buckley JD, Sporn MB. Can dietary beta-carotene materially reduce human cancer rates? Nature (Lond.) 1981; 290:201–208.
14. Nettesheim P, Snyder C, Kim JCS. Vitamin A and the susceptibility of respiratory tract tissues to carcinogenic insult. Environ Health Perspect 1979; 29:89–93.
15. Sporn M, Roberts AB. Role of retinoids in differentiation and carcinogenesis. Cancer Res 1983; 43:3034–3040.
16. De Luca LM. Essential function deficiency as the result of tumor promotion and the establishment of biological autarchy. J Natl Cancer Inst 1983; 70:405–407.
17. Mettlin C, Graham S. Dietary risk factors in human bladder cancer. Am J Epidemiol 1979; 110:255–263.
18. Bjelke E. Dietary vitamin A and human lung cancer. Int J Cancer 1975; 15:561–565.
19. Graham S, Mettlin C, Marshall J, Priore R, Rzepka T, Shedd D. Dietary factors in the epidemiology of cancer of the larynx. Am J Epidemiol 1981; 113:675–680.
20. Ibrahim K, Jafarey NA, Zuberi SJ. Plasma vitamin 'A' and carotene levels in squamous cell carcinoma of oral cavity and oro-pharynx. Clin Oncol 1977; 3:203–207.
21. Anderson SM, Krinsky NI. Protection action of carotenoid pigments against photodynamic damage to liposomes. Photochem Photobiol 1973; 18:403–408.
22. Mathews-Roth MM. Antitumor activity of β-carotene, canthaxanthin and phytoene. Oncology 1982; 39:33–37.
23. Rowley JD. Human oncogene locations and chromosome aberrations. Nature (Lond.) 1983; 301:290–291.

GUIDELINES FOR PREVENTION: CLINICAL TRIALS

WILLIAM D. DeWYS, M.D.

In the previous chapter by Stick and Rosin, several illustrative examples of human studies of potential cancer preventive agents are presented. The end point in these studies was the micronucleus assay which was presumed to be a proxy for a cancer end point. In this chapter I will proceed from these specific examples to a discussion of general principles for cancer prevention clinical trials.

OBJECTIVES OF A TRIAL

An important initial step in formulating a clinical trial is the selection of the objective(s) of the trial:

1. Prevent precursor lesions
2. Reverse precursor lesions
3. Prevent progression of precursor to malignancy
4. Reduce incidence of malignancy
5. Reduce mortality due to malignancy
6. Reduce total mortality

The presence of precursor lesions or precancerous lesions may be used to select a study population at high risk for developing cancer. In such a population one may have as the study end point the reversal of precursor lesions or the prevention of progression from a precursor state to overt malignant disease. In some clinical settings, a precursor lesion may not exist, or the relationship between a precursor lesion and the development of a malignant tumor may be unpredictable. Then the only meaningful end point may be a reduction in the incidence of malignant disease. The study should be designed to include follow-up of all incident cases so that an impact on cancer mortality may also be monitored. Finally, one would like to know whether the intervention reduces total mortality or only affects cancer mortality. An example would be cessation of smoking which would be expected to reduce both cancer and heart disease. Thus its impact on overall mortality might be greater than its effect on cancer mortality.

SELECTION OF STUDY PARTICIPANTS

After deciding the objectives of a prevention trial one must consider the selection of the study participants appropriate to address the study objective(s) (Table 1). Generally, prevention trials concentrate on populations who are at increased risk for developing malignancy. Risk factors have often first been identified by astute clinicians and then evaluated in quantitative terms by epidemiologists. Undoubtedly other risk factors remain to be identified. Some of the more prominent risk factors are outlined in Table 1 and are discussed in detail by Thomas in his chapter on epidemiology (q.v.).

Another approach to selection of study participants who are at increased risk for malignancy is selection based on presence of precursor or preneoplastic lesions.[1] A significant proportion of persons so identified will be expected to develop cancer. Another group at high risk are persons with a previous cancer of the head and neck or lung. The high risk for developing cancer probably reflects the combined effects of exposure to risk factors listed in Table 1 and poorly understood individual susceptibility factors.

An important additional selection criteria for prevention trials is an estimate of the individual's ability to comply with the requirements of the study and to return for follow-up on a long-term basis.

SELECTION OF THE INTERVENTION

Many different types of preventive interventions may be considered, including risk avoidance, use of protective devices in an occupational setting, change in diet, or use of a chemopreventive agent. I will focus this discussion on chemoprevention, but many of the points raised apply also to other types of interventions. The selection of intervention agent is based on leads from epidemiologic research, laboratory research, or previous clinical trials (discussed in other chapters in this Part of the book). The guidelines for selection of the intervention agent are as follows:[1]

1. Based on leads from epidemiology, laboratory, and clinical research.
2. If analogs available, consider relative effectiveness, relative toxicity, and tissue distribution.
3. Unless dose-response curve has a plateau, use maximum tolerated dose.
4. Schedule based on pharmacokinetics, mechanism of action, and compliance considerations.

In chemoprevention research, one thrust is the development of synthetic analogs which may have less

TABLE 1 Selection of Participants for a Cancer Prevention Clinical Trial

At risk based on epidemiologic and clinical observations
  Life style factors: smoking, alcohol, snuff and chewing tobacco, betel quid
  Occupational factors
  Diet
  Viruses
  Genetic factors
Presence of precursor lesions
Previous cancer of head and neck or lung
Potential for compliance and long-term follow-up

risk of toxicity, greater effectiveness, or both. The pattern of toxicity or effectiveness may in part be determined by patterns of tissue distribution.

The selection of the dose of the intervention agent is based on the nature of the dose-response relationship both for efficacy and for toxicity. If the dose-effectiveness relationship does not show a plateau, one should use the largest tolerable dose so as to maximize the chance of observing a preventive effect. This dose must be chosen with great care and usually on the basis of pilot studies. If too high a dose is chosen and toxicity leads to noncompliance, the result may also be negative.

The scheduling of the drug should take into account knowledge about the pharmacology of the agent, its mechanism of action, and compliance considerations. A drug with a rapid metabolism and clearance from the body may need to be taken frequently in order to have an effect. A drug that acts to block formation of a chemical in ingested food would need to be given with each meal. For example, carcinogenic nitrosamines may be formed by the reaction of nitrite in saliva and amines within the food. This reaction may be blocked by vitamin C, and maximal effects would then require taking vitamin C with each meal. Factors favoring frequent administration must be balanced against the truism that compliance varies inversely with the daily frequency of administration. Thus, in selection of an agent, one requiring once-daily administration would be favored over more frequent administration if all other factors were equal.

INTERVENTION PLAN FOR A CANCER PREVENTION TRIAL

The many details which must be considered in a prevention trial are beyond the scope of this brief chapter, but a few key details will be discussed:

1. Randomized study
2. Doubled-blinded study
3. Monitoring for compliance
4. Monitoring for toxicity
5. Dose modifications

Generally, trials require a control group with randomized assignment to intervention and control groups. Even in high risk populations, the incidence of disease or the risk of progression from a precursor to malignant tumor is sufficiently unpredictable so that there can be no substitute for a concurrent control group. The assignment to the control and intervention groups must be randomized to avoid bias in the assignment.

The assignment to control and intervention groups should be double-blinded, that is, neither the participant nor the researcher should know the treatment assignment. If the participant were to learn that he or she were in the control group, he or she might obtain the active agent through sources outside the study, and thus eliminate the difference between the two groups. If the researcher were to learn the assignment, he or she might be biased in his or her examination of study participants, and this could bias observations, such as time of appearance of disease.

Study participants must be monitored regularly for detection of study end points (see Table 1), for assessment of compliance, and for assessment of toxicity. Assessment of compliance might include use of a questionnaire, counting of remaining tablets, or measurement on a blood sample. The measurement on the blood sample might measure the active agent in the intervention group (e.g., beta carotene ingestion elevates the blood level) or measure some other tracer in the placebo tablets (e.g., a subtherapeutic amount of phenobarbital might result in detectable blood levels). Assessment of toxicity might utilize a questionnaire, physical examination, or blood tests, depending on the anticipated toxicity.

The study protocol must include a plan for modification of drug dose if evidence of toxicity develops. This may raise a concern about revealing the assignment of the study participant (often called breaking the blind). If the toxicity is life-threatening, it may be necessary to break the blind, thus removing the participant from the trial. If the toxicity is not life-threatening, the toxicity may be handled by omitting the study agent until the toxicity clears and then reinstituting reduced doses. If the pattern of toxicity is such that it is not specifically and distinctly characteristic of the intervention agent, its occurrence will not reveal the treatment assignment. For example, dry lips may be a side effect of vitamin A ingestion, but may also be seen in the placebo group due to exposure to the elements.

STATISTICAL CONSIDERATIONS

The development of a prevention trial generally should involve collaboration with a statistician familiar with design of clinical trials. The size of the population to be studied depends on the frequency of the end point and the magnitude of the difference expected to develop between the control and the intervention groups. For a cancer end point, even in high-risk groups, the end point occurs infrequently and a very large population needs to be studied. In animal studies, the difference between the control and intervention groups is often a greater than 50 percent reduction in cancer incidence. However, in human studies, we have less certainty that all conditions are optimized, and therefore a 25 to 35 percent reduction in cancer incidence would seem more realistic.

The sample size must also be adjusted for an anticipated rate of noncompliance or "drop-outs" since these would detract from the anticipated difference between the study group and the control group. If the intervention being studied is commercially available, some persons in the control group may begin taking the agent being studied, a so-called drop-in. This also will detract from the difference between the control and study groups and must be adjusted for.

Also to be considered is the possibility of a pre-existent cancer, one that is present at the time the study is started. This cancer could be so small as to be below the level of detection, but it could be beyond the scope of the effect of the preventive agent. This problem is usually handled by deciding that the cancers appearing within a certain time interval of the start of the study will not be included in the analyses.

Consideration of the foregoing factors leads to an estimate of a large sample size requirement for cancer prevention studies. For example, several of our current studies are enrolling 20–30,000 participants. Others, which focus on special very high-risk groups, may have several thousand participants. Reaching these sample sizes often requires collaboration between multiple institutions.

I believe the time is ripe for trials of prevention of head and neck cancer. Epidemiologic studies can guide the selection of high-risk subjects. Laboratory studies suggest agents which may be effective. Preliminary clinical studies indicate that a cancer-related end point can be reversed by a chemopreventive agent. The challenge, then, is for a group of investigators to organize such a trial and obtain funding for the study. NCI is interested in supporting prevention trials in head and neck cancer.

REFERENCE

1. DeCosse J. Precancer—an overview. Cancer Surveys 1983; 2:347–355.

INDEX

Page numbers in *italics* refer to figures; page numbers followed by t refer to tables.